Clinical
Men's Health

Clinical
Men's Health
EVIDENCE IN PRACTICE

Joel J. Heidelbaugh, MD
Clinical Assistant Professor, Department of Family Medicine,
University of Michigan Medical School, Ann Arbor, Michigan
Medical Director, Ypsilanti Health Center,
Ypsilanti, Michigan

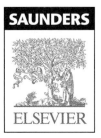

SAUNDERS

ELSEVIER

SAUNDERS
ELSEVIER

1600 John F. Kennedy Boulevard,
Suite 1800
Philadelphia, PA 19103-2899

CLINICAL MEN'S HEALTH: EVIDENCE IN PRACTICE ISBN: 978-1-4160-3000-3
Copyright © 2008, Elsevier Inc. All rights reserved.

Notice

Knowledge and best practice in this field are constantly changing. As new research and experience broaden our knowledge, changes in practice, treatment and drug therapy may become necessary or appropriate. Readers are advised to check the most current information provided (i) on procedures featured or (ii) by the manufacturer of each product to be administered, to verify the recommended dose or formula, the method and duration of administration, and contraindications. It is the responsibility of the practitioner, relying on their own experience and knowledge of the patient, to make diagnoses, to determine dosages and the best treatment for each individual patient, and to take all appropriate safety precautions. To the fullest extent of the law, neither the Publisher nor the Editors assumes any liability for any injury and/or damage to persons or property arising out or related to any use of the material contained in this book.

The Publisher

Library of Congress Cataloging-in-Publication Data

Clinical men's health: evidence in practice / edited by Joel J. Heidelbaugh, Eric R.M. Jauniaux (international editor), Mark B. Landon. – 1st ed.
    p. ; cm.
  Includes bibliographical references and index.
  ISBN 978-1-4160-3000-3
    1. Men–Health and hygiene. 2. Men–Diseases. 3. Andrology. I. Heidelbaugh, Joel J.
II. Jauniaux, E. III. Landon, Mark B.
    [DNLM: 1. Health Status. 2. Men. 3. Clinical Medicine–methods. 4. Health. 5. Sex Factors. WA 300 C641 2007]

  RC48.5.C55 2007
  613'.04234–dc22   2007026211

Acquisitions Editor: Rolla Couchman
Developmental Editor: John Ingram
Senior Production Manager: David Saltzberg
Design Direction: Steve Stave

Working together to grow
libraries in developing countries
www.elsevier.com | www.bookaid.org | www.sabre.org

ELSEVIER   BOOK AID International   Sabre Foundation

Printed in the United States of America.
Last digit is the print number: 9 8 7 6 5 4 3 2 1

For my family, my mentors, and my colleagues
For the advancement of men's health worldwide

Contributors

Alon Avidan, MD, MPH
Associate Professor
Director, UCLA Neurology Clinic
Associate Director, UCLA Sleep Disorders Clinic
Department of Neurology
University of Califoria, Los Angeles
Los Angeles, California
Neurology

R. Scott Chavez, PhD, MPA, PA
Vice President
National Commission on Correctional Health
  Care
Chicago, Illinois
The Incarcerated Male

Sandro Cinti, MD
Assistant Professor
Department of Internal Medicine
Division of Infectious Diseases
University of Michigan
Ann Arbor VA Medical Center
Ann Arbor, Michigan
Infectious Diseases

A. Evan Eyler, MD, MPH
Associate Professor
Departments of Family Medicine and
  Psychiatry
University of Vermont College of Medicine
Attending Physician
Psychiatric Consultation Service and Family
  Medicine Service
Associate Director
Family Medicine Residency Program
Fletcher Allen Health Care,
Burlington, Vermont
*Diagnostic Bias in Men's Healthcare; The
  Transsexual Male*

Gary J. Faerber, MD
Associate Professor
Department of Urology
University of Michigan
Ann Arbor, Michigan
Urology

Jamie Feldman, MD, PhD
Assistant Professor
Department of Family Medicine and Community
  Health
University of Minnesota
Minneapolis, Minnesota
The Transsexual Male

Sheila Gahagan, MD, MPH
Clinical Professor
Department of Pediatrics and Communicable
  Diseases
Assistant Research Scientist
Center for Human Growth & Development
University of Michigan
Ann Arbor, Michigan
The School-Aged Male Child

Naila Goldenberg, MD
Clinical Lecturer
Division of Metabolism, Endocrinology, and
  Diabetes
Department of Internal Medicine
University of Michigan
Ann Arbor, Michigan
Endocrinology

Grant Greenberg, MD, MA
Assistant Professor
Department of Family Medicine
University of Michigan Medical School
Ann Arbor, Michigan
Medical Director
Chelsea Health Center
University of Michigan
Chelsea, Michigan
The Newborn/Infant Male

Keyvan Hariri, MD
Attending Physician
Family Medicine and Urgent Care
Care Station Manhattan Beach
Manhattan Beach, California
Stress and the Modern Male

Masahito Jimbo, MD, PhD, MPH
Assistant Professor
Department of Family Medicine
University of Michigan
Ann Arbor, Michigan
Organizing Preventive Healthcare in Men; Nephrology

Michael T. Kernan, MD
Associate Professor
Department of Family Medicine
SUNY Upstate Medical University
Vice Chairman and Associate Residency Director
Department of Family Practice
St. Joseph's Hospital Health Center
Syracuse, New York
Medical Director
Department of Family Medicine
Heritage Family Medicine
Fayetteville, New York
The Collegiate/Professional Male Athlete

Sean Kesterson, MD
Assistant Professor
Departments of Internal Medicine and General
    Medicine
University of Michigan
Ann Arbor, Michigan
Medical Director
Brighton Health Center
Brighton, Michigan
The Executive Male

Robert Kiningham, MD
Associate Professor
Director Sports Medicine Fellowship
Department of Family Medicine
University of Michgan
Ann Arbor, Michigan
Exercise and Fitness

Daniel A. Knight, MD
Associate Professor, Program Director, and
    Acting Chairman
Department of Family and Preventive Medicine
University of Arkansas for Medical Sciences
Little Rock, Arkansas
The Homosexual Male

Arno K. Kumagai, MD
Associate Professor
Division of Metabolism, Endocrinology, and
    Diabetes
Department of Internal Medicine
Director
Intensive Insulin Therapy Clinic
University of Michigan
Ann Arbor, Michigan
Endocrinology; Exercise and Fitness

William M. Kuzon, Jr., MD, PhD
Reed O. Dingman Professor of Surgery
Section Head, Section of Plastic Surgery
Department of Surgery
University of Michigan
Staff Surgeon
Department of Surgery
Ann Arbor VA Medical Center
Ann Arbor, Michigan
Cosmetic Plastic Surgery

Jerilyn M. Latini, MD
Assistant Professor
Department of Urology
University of Michigan
Ann Arbor, Michigan
Urology

Anurag Malani, MD
Clinical Lecturer
Department of Internal Medicine
Division of Infectious Diseases
University of Michigan
Ann Arbor, Michigan
Infectious Diseases

Raman Malhotra, MD
Clinical Lecturer
Director, Sleep Disorders Clinic
Department of Neurology
University of Michigan
Ann Arbor, Michigan
Neurology

Arik V. Marcell, MD, MPH
Assistant Professor
Department of Population, Family and
    Reproductive Health
Bloomberg School of Public Health
Department of Pediatrics
The Johns Hopkins University School of
    Medicine
Baltimore, Maryland
The Adolescent Male

Tarannum Master-Hunter, MD, CAQ
Clinical Instructor
Department of Family Medicine
University of Michigan
Ann Arbor, Michigan
Exercise and Fitness

Jason Michael Matuszak, MD
Chief Resident
Department of Family Medicine
St. Joseph's Hospital
Syracuse, New York
The Collegiate/Professional Male Athlete

Bob Maurer, PhD
Associate Clinical Professor
Department of Family Medicine
University of California, Los Angeles
Los Angeles, California
Stress and the Modern Male

Mark H. Mirabelli, MD
Senior Instructor
Department of Family Medicine
Department of Orthopaedics and
  Rehabilitation
University of Rochester
Attending Physician
Department of Family Medicine
Highland Hospital
Attending Physician
Department of Orthopaedics and
  Rehabilitation
Strong Memorial Hospital
Rochester, New York
Nutrition

M. Haskell Newman, MD
Professor
Section of Plastic Surgery
Department of Surgery
University of Michigan
Ann Arbor, Michigan
Cosmetic Plastic Surgery

Bhuvana Raja, MD
Resident Physician
Department of Family Practice
St. Joseph's Hospital
Syracuse, New York
The Collegiate/Professional Male Athlete

David P. Rakel, MD
Assistant Professor and Director of University of
  Wisconsin Integrative Medicine
Department of Family Medicine
University of Wisconsin School of Medicine and
  Public Health
Madison, Wisconsin
Integerative Medicine

James Riddell IV, MD
Assistant Professor
Department of Internal Medicine
Division of Infectious Diseases
University of Michigan
Ann Arbor, Michigan
Infectious Diseases

William W. Roberts, MD
Assistant Professor
Department of Urology
University of Michigan
Ann Arbor, Michigan
Urology

Douglas Michael Sammer, MD
House Officer
Section of Plastic Surgery
Department of Surgery
University of Michigan
Ann Arbor, Michigan
Cosmetic Plastic Surgery

Timothy G. Schuster, MD
Assistant Professor
Department of Urology
University of Michigan
Ann Arbor, Michigan
Urology

David Charles Serlin, MD
Clinical Instructor
Family Medicine Newborn Service Chief
Department of Family Medicine
University of Michigan
Ann Arbor, Michigan
The Newborn/Infant Male

Lisa Seyfried, MD
Clinical Lecturer
Department of Psychiatry
University of Michigan Medical School
Ann Arbor, Michigan
Suicide

Ramsey Shehab, MD
Primary Care Sports Medicine Fellow
Department of Family Medicine
Wake Forrest University
Winston-Salem, North Carolina
Nutrition

Jennifer N. Stojan, MD
Resident
Department of Internal Medicine and Pediatrics
University of Michigan
Ann Arbor, Michigan
The School-Aged Male Child

Contributors

Denise K.C. Sur, MD
Associate Clinical Professor
Department of Family Medicine
University of California, Los Angeles
Attending Physician and Officer of Executive
    Medical Board
Department of Family Medicine
Santa Monica-UCLA Medical Center
Santa Monica, California
Stress and the Modern Male

L. Susan Taichman, RDH, MPH, PhD
Adjunct Clinical Assistant Professor
Department of Periodontics and Oral Medicine
University of Michigan School of Dentistry
Ann Arbor, Michigan
Oral Health

Lourdes Velez, MD
Assistant Professor
Department of Family Medicine
University of Michigan
Ann Arbor, Michigan
The Aging Male/End of Life Issues

Alan Keith White, PhD, MSc, BSc(Hons) RN
Professor
Centre for Men's Health
Leeds Metropolitan University
Leeds, England
*Men and the Problem of Help Seeking; Global
    Disparities in Men's Health*

Gary Yen, MD
Clinical Lecturer
Department of Family Medicine
University of Michigan Medical School
Ann Arbor, Michigan
Lifestyle Risks

Brian D. Zamboni, PhD
Clinical Psychologist
Assistant Professor
AASECT Certified Sex Therapist
Department of Family Medicine and Community
    Health
Program in Human Sexuality
University of Minnesota Medical School
Minneapolis, Minnesota
Sexual Health

Samuel Zwetchkenbaum, DDS, MPH
Clinical Assistant Professor
Department of Oral and Maxillofacial Surgery/
    Hospital Dentistry
University of Michigan School of
    Dentistry
Section Chief, Hospital Dentistry
Department of Maxillofacial Surgery/Hospital
    Dentistry
University of Michigan Health System
Ann Arbor, Michigan
Oral Health

Preface

What is men's health? "Guy problems. You know, prostate and genital problems. They die of heart attacks and strokes mostly. Working out at the gym. Oh yeah, some cancers too. And stupid, risky behaviors. Guys like to take chances, and don't always think about what might happen to them. We should know better. Yeah, that should just about cover it..."[1]

While the above answer is obviously superficial in its scope, it is widely known that men worldwide share a common factor in that they are at a higher risk of premature death from the majority of adverse health conditions that one would expect to affect men and women in equal incidence. According to the National Center for Health Statistics, of the top 15 causes of mortality in the US in 2003, men had higher death rates than women for 12 of these causes, and approximately equal death rates to women for only 2 causes.[2] Interestingly, population data have demonstrated via numerous surveys that an average of one in four men did not see a physician within the past year, nearly one-third of men admit to not having a definable "regular doctor," and just less than one-half of men deny receiving any preventive healthcare services within the past year. Statistically, men have a shorter average life expectancy than women worldwide, and perennially they have higher rates of injury; suicide; homicide; and tobacco, alcohol, and illicit substance abuse when compared with aged-matched women.

Ultimately, men's health as a subgenre of medicine needs to progress beyond a discussion simply reflecting morbidity and mortality statistics, and focus on the circumstances that influence men to either seek or not seek routine medical care. In the past decade, the field of men's health has begun to evolve, not simply as an answer to "women's health," but more formally to recognize, research, and address medical and social issues predicated upon inherent disparities affecting male gender.

An outstanding review by Salzman and Wender[3] in 2006 highlights the following key points regarding disparities in men's health and gender:

- Male gender is a major determinant of public health in the US and worldwide
- Although major health disparities exist between men and women, few health initiatives have either acknowledged or addressed them in an adequate fashion
- Discrepancies in health issues between men and women cannot be explained solely by biologic differences, although these differences do play a critical role
- A deeper understanding of the many factors that influence the health decisions and behaviors of men must be investigated, and the global healthcare community must be willing to impact the culture of men

In reviewing numerous primary care and specialty-oriented men's health-affiliated journals and textbooks, I saw a growing need for primary care clinicians to have a current and evidence-based reference guide to the diseases and disorders that affect male patients of all ages, with a comparative epidemiologic focus. Although the majority of references for this target audience on general pediatric and adult medical problems are considered to be comprehensive and up-to-date, few are specifically targeted at those diseases and disorders that unequally affect male patients.

While it is a formidable challenge to provide a complete and exhaustive primary care–based document that encompasses every potential aspect of men's health, I have opted to focus on several main tenets for this textbook:

- A general overview of the construct of men's health, with special attention given to an in-depth evaluation of organizing preventive healthcare in men, diagnostic bias in men's healthcare, gender disparities on a global level, and the problem of help-seeking in men
- A focus on pertinent medical and biopsychosocial issues in the developing male from infancy through school-age to adolescence
- A comprehensive review of common system-based disease conditions that unequally impact adult men

- An overview of special concerns and unique populations of today's adolescent and adult males

The scope of the chapters includes specific epidemiology centered on men; the etiology and pathophysiology of various disorders; and diagnosis and treatment guidelines based upon randomized controlled trials, meta-analyses, and Cochrane reviews when available. Otherwise, best evidence practices and recommendations are presented in the context of the various topics covered in each section.

The collection of authors assembled for this textbook represents a cohort of nationally and internationally recognized scholars, clinicians, and researchers, many of whom are leading experts on their respective topics. They have provided current evidence-based reviews and practice recommendations on common clinical concerns and disorders in men's health, in accordance with the Strength of Recommendation Taxonomy (SORT) ratings used by the *American Family Physician* journal.[4] Several chapters highlight guidelines and evidence-based recommendations from additional sources, including the United States Preventive Services Task Force, and are specifically noted within the text.

I would like to sincerely thank all of the authors who donated their extremely valuable time and energy to believe and participate in this textbook project. A very special thanks is given to Dr. Lee Green, Professor of Family Medicine at the University of Michigan Medical School, for his assistance in preparing the SORT ratings for many chapters. I also thank Mr. Rolla Couchman, Mr. John Ingram, and their kind staff at Elsevier for their assistance in the production and timely publication of this textbook.

It is my hope that this textbook spawns a devout interest in recognizing and addressing disparities in men's health and provides a practical reference for clinicians who care for common disorders in male patients across the globe.

Joel J. Heidelbaugh, MD

References:

1. *Random male patient interview conducted by editor, when soliciting advice on what to include in a textbook on men's health* Ypsilanti Health Center: Ypsilanti, Michigan, June 11, 2004.
2. Hoyert DL, Heron M, Murphy SL, et al Deaths: Final Data for 2003. National Center for Health Statistics, *Natl Vital Stat Rep* 54(13):1–120, 2006.
3. Salzman BE, Wender RC Male sex: a major health disparity. In Haines CA, Wender RC (eds): *Primary Care: Clinics in Office Practice, Men's Health*, Vol. 33, No. 1. Philadelphia, 2006, Saunders.
4. Ebell MH, Siwek J, Weiss BD, et al: Strength of Recommendation Taxonomy (SORT): A Patient-Centered Approach to Grading Evidence in the Medical Literature, *Am Fam Phys* 69(3):548–556

Additional publications and websites dedicated to men's health:

Davidson N, Lloyd T (eds): *Promoting Men's Health: A Guide for Practitioners*. Edinburgh, 2001, Bailliere-Tindall/Royal College of Nursing.

Haines CA, Wender RC (eds): *Primary Care: Clinics in Office Practice, Men's Health*, Vol. 33, No. 1. Philadelphia, 2006, Saunders.

The Journal of Men's Health and Gender. Editor-in-Chief: Dr. Siegfried Meryn.

Kirby RS, Carson CC, Kirby MG, Farah RN (eds): *Men's Health*, ed 2. London and New York, 2004, Taylor & Francis.

The Men's Health Forum, available at: http://www.menshealthforum.org.uk/.

The Men's Health Network, available at: http://www.menshealthnetwork.org/.

Simon HB: *Harvard Medical School Guide to Men's Health: Lessons from the Harvard Men's Health Studies*. New York, 2002, The Free Press.

Contents

Contents

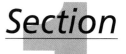

Overview of Men's Health

Organizing Preventive Healthcare in Men

Masahito Jimbo, MD, PhD, MPH

Key Points

- Patient and physician reminders are effective tools in providing preventive healthcare (strength of recommendation: B).
- Interventions geared toward organizational change are effective (strength of recommendation: B).
- Physicians should proactively schedule dedicated health maintenance visits (strength of recommendation: C).
- Physicians should have a contingency plan for implementing preventive care services at the time of acute office visits (strength of recommendation: C).
- Follow-up plans should be incorporated to ensure that the preventive services are maximally effective (strength of recommendation: C).

Introduction

When organizing preventive healthcare for men, primary care physicians face several challenges. First, many preventive care services are both time and labor intensive, adding stress and strain to the already sparse resources of physicians and their staff. Second, patients often bring multiple, competing agendas to the visit, adding even more time pressure to the provision of preventive services; it is during these visits that acute care often takes precedence over preventive care.[1] Third, most primary care practices do not possess an adequate system to ensure timely provision of preventive healthcare services and adequate follow-up for abnormal or unexpected results to their patients. Last, general biopsychosocial characteristics of male patients may place them at a unique disadvantage compared with women, and these need to be considered.

This chapter seeks to address these various challenges in more detail. The current age- and risk factor–appropriate guidelines for routine health maintenance examinations, screening tests, immunizations, chemoprophylaxis, and counseling will be outlined according to the most current evidence-based recommendations. Subsequently, a discussion will follow regarding steps that may be taken in the ambulatory care setting to ensure that patients are receiving the appropriate preventive care at the right intervals and that abnormal findings are followed up or referred expeditiously. Finally, methods in which practices may address the unique facilitators and barriers that male patients bring to their own healthcare will be proposed.

In this chapter, the term *men* is defined as adult males aged 18 years or older. The discussion of organizing preventive healthcare in men will be limited to the ambulatory care setting, including private physician offices and academic and community health centers. Community-targeted interventions requiring the participation of larger organizations, including health insurance plans and state and federal agencies, will be outside the scope of this chapter.

Challenges to Implementing Appropriate Preventive Healthcare for Men

Substantial time and effort are required to provide adequate and appropriate preventive healthcare services. In 1996, the second edition of the US Preventive Services Task Force (USPSTF) found that approximately 50 different preventive services are effective.[2] A recent study estimated that 7.4 hours per workday would be required for physicians to implement all of the preventive services recommended by the USPSTF for their patients.[3] Obviously, this is a time allotment that primary care physicians simply do not have, especially with their responsibility to provide acute and chronic illness care, in addition to preventive care that includes counseling.[1]

Most primary care offices lack systems to ensure timely implementation and follow-up of preventive healthcare for all patients. This is not surprising, since adequate provisions of preventive healthcare require multiple steps that include the following:

- Identifying specific preventive care measures recommended at the appropriate interval
- Notifying the patient of the recommended preventive care
- Scheduling the patient for the appropriate preventive care services, which may or may not require an office visit
- Ensuring that the patient followed up with the preventive care
- Obtaining the results from screening tests and determining their significance
- Notifying the patient of the results in a timely fashion
  - If normal, scheduling the patient for recommended preventive care at the next appropriate interval
  - If abnormal, arranging for appropriate follow-up treatment and/or referral
- Ensuring that the patient followed through with the follow-up and/or referral
- Obtaining the results of the follow-up and/or referral
- Referring the patient for further testing and management if indicated

This complex series of steps is further complicated by several factors including the following:

- Various recommended time intervals for different modalities of preventive care (e.g., blood pressure monitoring every 1–2 years vs. fasting lipid profile every 5 years)
- A varying time schedule for the same test depending on a patient's risk (e.g., fasting lipid profile every 5 years for a patient with no risk of heart disease vs. annually for a diabetic patient)
- The multiple choice of tests with different time schedules and risk/benefit ratios for the same screening objective (e.g., annual fecal occult blood testing versus colonoscopy every 10 years for colorectal cancer screening)
- Discussion of preventive healthcare services in a dedicated, scheduled health maintenance visit or opportunistically during an acute visit (e.g., offering tetanus prophylaxis to an overdue patient who came in for treatment of an ankle sprain)[4]
- The dilemma of whether certain preventive healthcare options should be offered at all (e.g., annual digital rectal examination and prostate-specific antigen test for prostate cancer screening)

Unfortunately, considerable evidence from surveys of both patients and physicians demonstrates that physicians fall short of providing all of the necessary preventive care for their patients. In a population-based telephone survey of 13,275 adult patients and physicians in 12 metropolitan areas in the United States, only 54.9% and 52.2% reported receiving preventive healthcare and screening, respectively, determined by the RAND Corporation's Quality Assessment Tools system.[5] In a self-report survey of 3881 primary care physicians randomly sampled from the professional associations representing family medicine, internal medicine, pediatrics, and obstetrics/gynecology, the percentage of physicians who provided adequate clinical preventive service (defined as providing the service to more than 80% of their patients who were indicated to receive them) varied from 60.2% to 87.2% for screening, from 26.6% to 44.7% for immunizations, and 21.3% to 47.7% for counseling.[6] Even when the initial preventive service is implemented appropriately, one study found that fewer than 75% of patients receive adequate follow-up care.[7] From the findings of these and other related studies, deficiencies in the provision of preventive care are classified predominantly as underutilization, although inappropriate utilization (e.g., performing a digital rectal examination to assess for fecal occult blood in lieu of three take-home fecal occult blood test cards[8]) could also occur.

The various reasons why clinical preventive services are not implemented as well as they should be are numerous and complex. Physicians may not adhere to recommended clinical practice guidelines due to lack of awareness, lack of familiarity, disagreement with the recommendation, lack of self-efficacy (i.e., belief that they could effectively perform the recommended service), lack of outcome expectancy (i.e., belief that the performance of the recommended service will lead to the desired outcome), inertia of previous practice, and external barriers including lack of adequate time, resources, and reimbursement.[9] External barriers arising from the complexity of the healthcare delivery system, such as lack of continuity of care and breakdown in communication, may be bigger factors than the individual physician attributes.[10] The vagaries of each practice may be a particularly relevant issue in the United States, where preventive service delivery is dependent on individual patient and physician interactions and is not delivered through centrally organized programs as seen in Europe and Japan, which increase the potential for variability in implementation and follow-up.[11]

Common issues regarding preventive healthcare have been shown to be both unique to male patients as well as more amplified. A survey by Sandman et al. determined the following[12]:

- One of four men (24%) did not see a physician within the past year, three times the rate found in women (8%).
- Thirty-three percent of men do not have a definable "regular doctor," compared with 19% of women.
- Forty-one percent of men did not receive preventive services in the past year, compared with 16% of women.

Various adverse health outcomes that are more prevalent in men include the following[13,14]:

- Higher mortality from heart disease
- Higher mortality from cancer
- Shorter than average life expectancy
- Higher rates of injury and death from accidents, including industrial and motor vehicle injury
- Higher suicide rates
- Higher homicide rates
- Higher rates of smoking
- Higher rates of alcohol abuse
- Higher rates of substance abuse

The gender gap illustrated above is even greater among men younger than 30 years old, men in minority groups, and men in lower socioeconomic class. Successful interventions to have men actually present for preventive care visits have neither been implemented nor evaluated in detail and compose an area for further research.

Fortunately, this gender gap virtually disappears once men are aged 65 years or older.

It is important to note that not all gender differences are statistically disadvantageous to men. For example, more men have been found to exercise 3 or more days per week than women (51% and 39%, respectively).[14] Provision of counseling on smoking cessation (30% men vs. 31% women), diet (44% vs. 49%), exercise (46% vs. 52%), alcohol and drug abuse (22% vs. 24%), safety (6% vs. 9%), and sexually transmitted diseases (14% vs. 17%) is unacceptably low for both men and women.[14]

Several conclusions may be drawn from the above data trends. Many, if not most, primary care physicians' offices fall short of providing appropriate preventive care to all of their patients. Second, the data support the difficulty of organizing appropriate preventive care for all patients in primary care physicians' offices; the barriers include lack of adequate time during an office visit, complexity of the recommendations, complexity of the healthcare delivery system, and physician beliefs and behaviors. Third, men have health behavior characteristics that place them at an increased risk for morbidity and mortality from a variety of conditions, their greater lack of adequate preventive care compounds the situation. Last, organizing preventive care for men in a physician's practice will entail organizing the care for all patients in the practice.

Current Age- and Risk Factor–Appropriate Guidelines for Routine Examinations, Screening Tests, Immunizations/Prophylaxis, and Counseling in Men

Recent evidence from the literature supports a set of preventive services tailored to an individual's age, gender, and risk factors, rather than a one-size-fits-all battery of examinations and screening tests.[2,15] With this in mind, one of the challenges involved in implementing appropriate preventive care is the seemingly constant changes in guidelines. Fortunately, the USPSTF, considered by many healthcare professionals to be the most authoritative of the guidelines for preventive services, has a Web site that is frequently updated with the most current evidence-based recommendations.[16] Other organizations that have Web sites that are regularly updated for provision of preventive services include the

American Academy of Family Physicians (AAFP)[17] and the National Guideline Clearinghouse (NGC).[18] A particularly useful Web site for vaccination recommendation updates is that of the Centers for Disease Control and Prevention (CDC). For example, timely information is available on the recent recommendation by the Advisory Committee on Immunization Practices (ACIP) regarding the routine use of combined tetanus, diphtheria, and acellular pertussis (Tdap) vaccinations in adolescents aged 11–18 years in place of the previously recommended tetanus and diphtheria toxoid (Td) vaccinations. The routine use of a single dose of Tdap for adults 19–64 years of age, as well as for adults who have close contact with infants younger than 12 months of age, is now to replace the subsequent booster dose of Td vaccine.[19]

The age-appropriate guidelines that will be highlighted here are based predominantly on the recommendations for preventive healthcare screening published by the USPSTF. These guidelines cover the areas of the routine clinical examination, screening tests, immunizations, chemoprophylaxis, and counseling. The USPSTF incorporates an evidence rating system as highlighted in Tables 1-1 and 1-2. By definition, "A" and "B" level recommendations as determined by the USPSTF correspond to "A" and "B" recommendations by the Strength of Recommendation Taxonomy system[20]; this system is used to provide a framework for the "Key Points" section listed at the beginning of every chapter in this text. To be consistent with the USPSTF recommendations, the ratings based on this system are used in the recommendations that follow. Only those guidelines with "A" or "B" level recommendations have been included. The exception to this schematic is the prostate cancer screening guideline, which was included despite the "I" recommendation, on account of its widespread use and ongoing debate. In addition, some

Table 1-1. The US Preventive Services Task Force Strength of Recommendations

Strength of Recommendations	Explanation
A	The USPSTF strongly recommends that clinicians provide the service to eligible patients. (Good evidence that the service improves important health outcomes; benefits substantially outweigh harms)
B	The USPSTF recommends that clinicians provide the service to eligible patients. (At least fair evidence that the service improves important health outcomes; benefits outweigh harms)
C	The USPSTF makes no recommendation for or against routine provision of the service. (At least fair evidence that the service can improve health outcomes; the balance of benefits and harms is too close to justify a general recommendation)
D	The USPSTF recommends against routinely providing the service to asymptomatic patients. (At least fair evidence that the service is ineffective or that harms outweigh benefits)
I	The USPSTF concludes that the evidence is insufficient to recommend for or against routinely providing the service. (Evidence that the service is effective is lacking, of poor quality, or conflicting; the balance of benefits and harms cannot be determined)

Adapted from: US Preventive Services Task Force: *Guide to Clinical Preventive Services,* ed 2. Baltimore, Md, 1996, Williams & Wilkins.

Table 1-2. The US Preventive Services Task Force Level of Evidence

Level of Evidence	Explanation
Good	Consistent results from well-designed, well-conducted studies in representative populations that directly assess effects on health outcomes
Fair	Sufficient to determine effects on health outcomes, but the strength of the evidence is limited by the number, quality, or consistency of the individual studies, generalizability to routine practice, or indirect nature of the evidence on health outcomes
Poor	Insufficient to assess the effects on health outcomes because of limited number or power of studies, important flaws in their design or conduct, gaps in the chain of evidence, or lack of information on important health outcomes

Adapted from: US Preventive Services Task Force: *Guide to Clinical Preventive Services,* ed 2. Baltimore, Md, 1996, Williams & Wilkins.

recommendations, such as subjective screening for hearing loss in patients aged 65 years or older, were recommended prior to the advent of the current USPSTF evidence rating system, and this fact is noted where appropriate. Immunizations are not included in the USPSTF recommendations; therefore, the ACIP guidelines from the CDC Web site were used[21] and the USPSTF ratings were not. When additional resources including the American Cancer Society (ACS) or ACIP were used elsewhere, a notation is made next to the individual recommendation. Recommended intervals are noted next to each item if they have been included in the USPSTF or other comparable guidelines; if the recommended screening interval is not present, then the guidelines and recommendations are left to the physician's discretion. Although these compilations are not meant to be exhaustive, the reader is referred to the USPSTF and other related Web sites for further details and guidance.

Routine Examinations and Screening Tests

Men 18–39 Years Old

- Blood pressure measurement every 1–2 years (strength of recommendation: A)
- Height and weight measurement to calculate body mass index (BMI), defined as weight (kg) divided by height (cm) squared (strength of recommendation: B)
- Screening for depression (strength of recommendation: B)
- Fasting lipid profile after the age of 35 years* (strength of recommendation: A), or from age 20 years if coronary risk factors are present (strength of recommendation: B), including the following:
  - Diabetes mellitus
  - Family history of cardiovascular disease before the age of 50 years in male relatives or 60 years in female relatives
  - Family history suggestive of familial hyperlipidemia

---

*Of note, the National Cholesterol Education Program of the National Heart, Lung, and Blood Institute recommends in its Third Report of the Expert Panel on Detection, Evaluation, and Treatment of High Cholesterol in Adults that all adults aged 20 years and older should be offered a fasting lipid profile every 5 years. Physicians who wish to take a more aggressive approach than those recommended by the USPSTF may consider this approach.[22]

- Multiple coronary heart disease risk factors as listed above, including tobacco abuse and hypertension
- Fasting plasma glucose, if hypertension or hyperlipidemia are present, every 3 years (strength of recommendation: B)
- Screening for human immunodeficiency virus (HIV) if increased risk of infection is present, based on individual risk or care received in a high-prevalence or high-risk clinical setting (strength of recommendation: A), including the following:
  - Men who have had sex with men after 1975
  - Unprotected sex with multiple partners
  - Past or present injection drug use
  - Exchange of sex for money or drugs, or having sex partners who do
  - Past or present sex partners who were/are HIV infected, bisexual, or injection drug users
  - Treatment received for sexually transmitted diseases (STDs)
  - History of blood transfusion between 1978 and 1985
  - Request for HIV test
  - STD clinics
  - Time spent living in a homeless shelter
  - Time spent in a correctional facility
  - Time spent in a tuberculosis clinic
  - History of time in a clinic serving men who have sex with men
- Consider colorectal cancer (CRC) screening for those at increased risk (e.g., those with a first-degree relative who received a diagnosis with colorectal cancer before 60 years of age) or high risk (e.g., those with inflammatory bowel disease) [USPSTF mentions that initiating screening at an earlier age is reasonable but does not assign strength of recommendations. For detailed recommendations, refer to the ACS Web site[23]; further information can be found in Chapter 24, Cancer Incidence, Screening, and Prevention.]

Men 40–49 Years Old

- Blood pressure measurement every 1–2 years (strength of recommendation: A)
- Height and weight measurement to calculate BMI (strength of recommendation: B)
- Screening for depression (strength of recommendation: B)
- Fasting lipid profile every 5 years (strength of recommendation: A)

- Fasting plasma glucose, if hypertension or hyperlipidemia are present, every 3 years (strength of recommendation: B)
- Screening for HIV if increased risk of infection is present, based on individual risk or care received in a high-prevalence or high-risk clinical setting (strength of recommendation: A)
- Consider CRC screening for those at increased risk or high risk. [USPSTF mentions that initiating screening at an earlier age is reasonable but does not assign strength of recommendations. For detailed recommendations, refer to the ACS Web site[23]; further information can be found in Chapter 24, Cancer Incidence, Screening, and Prevention.]
- Consider screening men aged 40 years and older for prostate cancer if risk factor(s) present (strength of recommendation: I), including the following:
  - African American ethnicity
  - First-degree relatives with prostate cancer

Men 50–64 Years Old

- Blood pressure measurement every 1–2 years (strength of recommendation: A)
- Height and weight measurement to calculate BMI (strength of recommendation: B)
- Screening for depression (strength of recommendation: B)
- Fasting lipid profile every 5 years (strength of recommendation: A)
- Fasting plasma glucose, if hypertension or hyperlipidemia is present, every 3 years (strength of recommendation: B)
- Screening for HIV if increased risk of infection is present, based on individual risk or care received in a high-prevalence or high-risk clinical setting (strength of recommendation: A)
- Screening for CRC (strength of recommendation: A); although the USPSTF does not recommend specific intervals for each screening modality, the ACS recommends the following[23]:
  - Fecal occult blood test every year
  - Flexible sigmoidoscopy every 5 years
  - Double-contrast barium enema every 5 years
  - Colonoscopy every 10 years
- Consider screening for prostate cancer (strength of recommendation: I)

Men 65 Years and Older

- Blood pressure measurement every 1–2 years (strength of recommendation: A)
- Height and weight measurement to calculate BMI (strength of recommendation: B)
- Screening for depression (strength of recommendation: B)
- Subjective screening for hearing loss (recommendation made before the USPSTF started its strength of recommendation rating system)
- Fasting lipid profile every 5 years (strength of recommendation: A)
- Fasting plasma glucose, if hypertension or hyperlipidemia present, every 3 years (strength of recommendation: B)
- Screening for HIV if increased risk of infection is present, based on individual risk or care received in a high-prevalence or high-risk clinical setting (strength of recommendation: A)
- Screening for CRC (strength of recommendation: A)
- Screening for abdominal aortic aneurysm once via ultrasound for men aged 65–75 years who have ever smoked (strength of recommendation: B)

Immunizations

- Tetanus booster every 10 years (For men aged 18–64 years or who have close contact with infants younger than 12 months of age, consider the routine use of a single dose of Tdap.)
- Varicella vaccination, two doses 4 weeks apart, if not immune
- Measles, mumps, and rubella vaccination once, if born after 1956 and not immune
- Influenza vaccination annually, if aged 50 years or older or if in a risk group, including the following:
  - Chronic disorders of the cardiovascular or pulmonary systems, including asthma
  - Chronic metabolic diseases, including diabetes mellitus, renal dysfunction, hemoglobinopathies, or immunosuppression (including immunosuppression caused by medications or HIV)
  - Any condition that compromises respiratory function or the handling of respiratory secretions or that can increase the risk for aspiration (e.g., cognitive dysfunction, spinal cord injury, seizure disorder, or other neuromuscular disorder)
  - Asplenia

- Time spent as a healthcare worker or employee of long-term care or assisted-living facility
- Residence in a nursing home or other long-term care or assisted-living facility
- Likelihood of transmission of influenza to persons at high risk (e.g., in-home household contacts and caregivers of children aged 0–23 months, or persons of all ages with high-risk conditions)
- Wish to be vaccinated
- Pneumococcal vaccination at the age of 65 years or younger if risk factors are present, including the following:
  - Chronic disorders of the pulmonary system (excluding asthma)
  - Cardiovascular diseases
  - Diabetes mellitus
  - Chronic liver diseases, including liver disease as a result of alcohol abuse (e.g., cirrhosis)
  - Chronic renal failure or nephrotic syndrome
  - Functional or anatomic asplenia (e.g., sickle cell disease or splenectomy)
  - Immunosuppressive conditions (e.g., congenital immunodeficiency, HIV infection, leukemia, lymphoma, multiple myeloma, Hodgkin's disease, generalized malignancy, or organ or bone marrow transplantation)
  - Chemotherapy with alkylating agents, antimetabolites, or long-term systemic corticosteroids
  - Cochlear implants
  - Alaska Native and certain American Indian ethnicities
  - Residence in a nursing homes or other long-term care facility
- Hepatitis A (HAV) vaccination if in a high-risk group, including the following:
  - Persons with clotting-factor disorders
  - Persons with chronic liver disease
  - Men who have sex with men
  - Users of illegal drugs
  - Persons working with HAV-infected primates or with HAV in a research-laboratory setting
- Hepatitis B (HBV) vaccination if in a high-risk group, including the following:
  - Patients receiving hemodialysis
  - Patients who receive clotting-factor concentrates
  - Healthcare workers and public safety workers who have exposure to blood in the workplace
  - Persons in training in schools of medicine, dentistry, nursing, laboratory technology, and other allied health–related professions
  - Injection drug users
  - Persons with more than one sex partner during the previous 6 months
  - Persons with a recently acquired STD
  - Men who have sex with men
  - Household contacts and sex partners of persons with chronic HBV infection
  - Clients and staff members of institutions for developmentally disabled persons
  - All clients of STD clinics
  - Inmates of correctional facilities

Chemoprophylaxis

- Aspirin prophylaxis for men older than 40 years and those aged 40 years and younger with coronary risk factors (strength of recommendation: A), including the following:
  - Diabetes
  - Hypertension
  - Smoking

Counseling

- Tobacco use screening and counseling (strength of recommendation: A)
- Alcohol abuse screening and counseling (strength of recommendation: B)
- Diet counseling for men with cardiovascular risk factors (strength of recommendation: B), including the following:
  - Hyperlipidemia
  - Hypertension
  - Family history of heart disease
  - Overweight/obesity
  - Smoker
  - Sedentary lifestyle
- Injury prevention (recommendation was made prior to the USPSTF strength of recommendation rating system), including the following:
  - Using lap and shoulder belts while driving
  - Using motorcycle and bicycle helmets
  - Avoiding driving under the influence of alcohol
  - Household and recreational safety precautions regarding the following:
    - poisoning
    - fire
    - proper hot water temperature (< 125 °F)

- o drowning
- o firearms
- o cardiopulmonary resuscitation training
- Fall prevention (age 65 years and older)
- STD risk reduction (recommendation was made prior to the USPSTF strength of recommendation rating system)

It should be emphasized that the above lists are suggested guidelines for age-appropriate preventive services to be implemented in the physician's office. Because the USPSTF uses a very rigorous evaluation methodology, many preventive services, such as drug abuse screening and counseling, were concluded to have insufficient evidence to recommend for or against implementation. In addition, some screening tests including screening for visual impairment in men aged 65 years and older have not been recently addressed by the task force. Therefore, the above lists should be used as a framework from which physicians may consider modifications (in terms of intervals) and additions or deletions where applicable (in terms of services). Other useful references include the Web sites of the AAFP[17] and the NGC.[18]

In deciding which preventive services to prioritize, useful information can be obtained from a study by Coffield et al. that assessed the relative value of each preventive service.[24] Value scores were defined as the combined score of clinical preventable burden and cost-effectiveness being 7 or greater on a scale of 2–10. Of the preventive services concluded to be of high value by the study authors, the following are applicable to men, in the order of descending priority (the combined scores are listed in parentheses):

- Tobacco use screening and counseling[9]
- Screening for vision impairment among men aged 65 years and older[9]
- CRC screening for men aged 50 years and older[8]
- Blood pressure measurement to screen for hypertension[8]
- Influenza vaccination for men aged 65 years and older[8]
- Pneumococcal vaccination for men aged 65 years and older[7]
- Fasting lipid profile for men aged between 35 and 65 years[7]
- Alcohol abuse screening and counseling[7]

Implementing Preventive Healthcare Services for Men in the Office

Many studies have been performed with the outcome goal of finding ways to improve the rate of providing preventive healthcare in the ambulatory care setting. Extrapolation of data from these study findings to design an effective strategy for other physician practices has been difficult to interpret. One reason is that the complexity of each practice creates unique barriers that defy straightforward implementation of tools, even if they showed efficacy in other settings.[25,26] Another reason is that many successful studies rely on external assistance through funding during the course of the research project, and once the study ends and the funded external assistance is removed, the implemented systems tend to disappear.[27]

Nevertheless, several excellent reviews have arrived at similar conclusions in terms of effective interventions in the delivery of preventive healthcare services.[28–31] Patient and physician reminders have been shown to be effective tools. Although these reminders do not need to be electronic, computer-generated prompting and reminding has the advantage of both efficiency and responsiveness.[32] The availability of a complete electronic medical record system would also have the additional benefit of a lower incidence of missing clinical information relevant to patient care.[33]

In addition, interventions geared toward organizational change have been shown to be effective. These include the use of separate clinics devoted solely to prevention, the use of a planned care visit for prevention (e.g., delivering the services during health maintenance/periodic health examinations rather than opportunistically during acute or chronic visits), and the designation of non-physician staff to conduct specific prevention activities. The importance of being cognizant of the organizational characteristics of the physician practice when effecting a change cannot be overestimated, and the evaluation of the organizational structure and culture is now recognized to be the key step warranted before implementing any such intervention.[34] A large practice network–based study that assessed the effect of interventions to improve preventive care concluded that the *organizational composition* of the practice, defined as teamwork and tenacity, was more important than the actual tools being used to effect change.[35]

Based on a systematic review of the literature, several steps can be envisioned in organizing preventive healthcare in men. The steps are consistent with the quality improvement models using the Plan-Do-Study-Act cycle[36] and are necessarily abstract to accommodate the uniqueness of each practice:

- Set a clear goal among the healthcare team, composed of physicians, midlevel providers, and support staff, in which organizing and improving preventive healthcare among the practice patients is of paramount importance.
- Take an inventory of the current workflow and preventive service implementation in the practice and determine the areas for improvement. The series of steps reviewed in the early section of this chapter, as well as the list of recommended services and priorities, may serve as a useful guide.
- Specify the roles that each team member will play in organizing the preventive healthcare service.
- Consider allocating dedicated health maintenance visits for each patient. This is particularly important for men who underutilize healthcare services.
- Have a contingency plan for those men who come in only for acute visits to also implement preventive care at the time of the visit.
- Create or use the reminder tools available through professional organizations such as the AAFP. These can be either electronic, such as via personal digital assistants,[37] or manual flow sheets.[38]
- Ensure that an appropriate follow-up process is in place.
- After a trial period, reassess how well the process has been implemented and adjust accordingly.

Conclusion

In organizing preventive healthcare for men, the key is to implement a system for the entire practice encompassing all patients, not just men. Emphasis should be placed on organizational change and reminders. For men, enticing them to actually come in for healthcare visits is crucial. Proactively scheduling health maintenance examinations and having a contingency plan for implementing preventive care at the time of the acute visits are also possible solutions. A follow-up plan should be incorporated into practices to ensure that the preventive services are maximally effective.

References

1. Jaen CR, Stange KC, Nutting PA: The competing demands of primary care: a model for the delivery of clinical preventive services, *J Fam Pract* 38:166–171, 1994.

2. US Preventive Services Task Force: *Guide to clinical preventive services*, ed 2, Baltimore, Md, 1996, Williams & Wilkins.

3. Yarnall KSH, Pollack KI, Ostbye T, et al: Primary care: is there enough time for prevention? *Am J Public Health* 93(4):635–641, 2003.

4. Flocke SA, Stange KC, Goodwin MA: Patient and visit characteristics associated with opportunistic preventive services delivery, *J Fam Pract* 47: 202–208, 1998.

5. McGlynn EA, Asch SM, Adams J, et al: The quality of health care delivered to adults in the United States, *N Engl J Med* 348(26):2635–2645, 2003.

6. Ewing GB, Selassie AW, Lopez CH, et al: Self-report of delivery of clinical preventive services by U.S. physicians, *Am J Prev Med* 17(1):62–72, 1999.

7. Bastani R, Yabroff KR, Myers RE, et al: Interventions to improve follow-up of abnormal findings in cancer screening, *Cancer* 101(5 Suppl): 1188–1200, 2004.

8. Nadel MR, Shapiro JA, Klabunde CN, et al: A national survey of primary care physicians' methods for screening for fecal occult blood, *Ann Intern Med* 142(2):86–94, 2005.

9. Cabana MD, Rand CS, Powe NR, et al: Why don't physicians follow clinical practice guidelines? *JAMA* 282(15):1458–1465, 1999.

10. Crabtree BF: Individual attitudes are no match for complex systems, *J Fam Pract* 44(5):447–448, 1997.

11. Miles A, Cockburn J, Smith RA, et al: A perspective from countries using organized screening programs, *Cancer* 101(5 Suppl):1201–1213, 2004.

12. Sandman D, Simantov E, An C: Out of touch: American men and the health care system, Commonwealth Fund Men's and Women's Health Survey Findings March 2000. Available at: http://www.cmwf.org/usr_doc/sandman_outoftouch_374.pdf.

13. Schofield T, Connell RW, Walker L, et al: Understanding men's health and illness: a gender-relations approach to policy, research, and practice, *J Am Coll Health* 48:247–256, 2000.

14. Williams DR: The health of men: structured inequalities and opportunities, *Am J Public Health* 93(5):724–731, 2003.

15. Han PKJ: Historical changes in the objectives of the periodic health examination, *Ann Intern Med* 127 (19):910–917, 1997.

16. US Preventive Services Task Force: *Guide to clinical preventive services*, ed 3. Available at: http://www.ahrq.gov/clinic/cps3dix.htm.

17. American Academy of Family Physicians: Summary of recommendations for clinical preventive services. Revision 6.3, March 2007. Available at: http://www.aafp.org/online/en/home/clinical/exam.html.

18. Institute for Clinical Systems Improvement: Preventive services for adults. June 1995 (revised October 2005). National Guideline Clearinghouse. Available at: http://www.guidelines.gov/summary/summary.aspx?doc_id=10040&nbr=005340.

19. Centers for Disease Control and Prevention: National Immunization Program (NIP): Tdap

vaccine: combined tetanus, diphtheria, and pertussis (Tdap) vaccines. Available at: http://www.cdc.gov/nip/vaccine/tdap/default.htm.

20. Ebell MH, Siwek J, Weiss BD, et al: Strength of Recommendation Taxonomy (SORT): a patient-centered approach to grading evidence in the medical literature, *Am Fam Phys* 69(3):548–556, 2004.

21. Centers for Disease Control and Prevention: Recommended adult immunization schedule—United States, October 2005–September 2006, *MMWR* 54:Q1–Q4, 2005. Available at: http://www.cdc.gov/mmwr/PDF/wk/mm5440-Immunization.pdf.

22. National Cholesterol Education Program: *Third report of the National Cholesterol Education Program (NCEP) Expert Panel on the Detection, Evaluation, and Treatment of High Blood Cholesterol in Adults (Adult Treatment Panel III), executive summary*, NIH Publication no. NIH 01–3670. Bethesda, Md, 2001, National Cholesterol Education Program, National Institutes of Health, National Heart, Lung, and Blood Institute.

23. American Cancer Society: Detailed guide: colon and rectum cancer. Can colorectal polyps and cancer be found early? Colorectal cancer screening. Available at: http://www.cancer.org/docroot/CRI/content/CRI_2_4_3X_Can_colon_and_rectum_cancer_be_found_early.asp?sitearea=.

24. Coffield AB, Maciosek MV, McGinnis M, et al: Priorities among recommended clinical preventive services, *Am J Prev Med* 21(1):1–9, 2001.

25. Stange KC: One size doesn't fit all: multimethod research yields new insights into interventions to increase prevention in family practice [editorial], *J Fam Pract* 43:358–360, 1996.

26. McVea K, Crabtree BC, Medder JD, et al: An ounce of prevention? Evaluation of the "Put Prevention into Practice" program, *J Fam Pract* 43:361–369, 1996.

27. Solberg LI, Kottke TE, Brekke ML: Will primary care clinics organize themselves to improve the delivery of preventive services? A randomized controlled trial, *Prev Med* 27:623–631, 1998.

28. Stone EG, Morton SC, Hulscher ME, et al: Interventions that increase use of adult immunization and cancer screening services: a meta-analysis, *Ann Intern Med* 136:641–651, 2002.

29. Smith WR: Evidence for the effectiveness of techniques to change physician behavior, *Chest* 118: 8S–17S, 2000.

30. Grimshaw JM, Shirran L, Thomas R, et al: Changing provider behavior: an overview of systematic reviews of interventions, *Med Care* 39:II-2–II-45, 2001.

31. Garg AX, Adhikari NKJ, McDonald H, et al: Effects of computerized clinical decision support systems on practitioner performance and patient outcomes: a systematic review, *JAMA* 293:1223–1238, 2005.

32. Nease DE Jr, Green LA: ClinfoTracker: a generalizable prompting tool for primary care, *J Am Board Fam Pract* 16(2):115–123, 2003.

33. Smith PC, Araya-Guerra R, Bublitz C, et al: Missing clinical information during primary care visits, *JAMA* 293(5):565–571, 2005.

34. Wears RL, Berg M: Computer technology and clinical work: still waiting for Godot [editorial], *JAMA* 293(10): 1261–1263, 2005.

35. Carpiano RM, Flocke SA, Frank SH, et al: Tools, teamwork, and tenacity: an examination of family practice office system influences on preventive service delivery, *Prev Med* 36:131–140, 2003.

36. Coleman MT, Endsley S: Quality improvement: first steps, *Fam Pract Manage* 6(3):23–27, 1999. Available at: http://www.aafp.org/fpm/990300fm/23.html.

37. Lewis M: Using your Palm-Top's date book as a reminder system, *Fam Pract Manage* 8(5):50–51, 2001. Available at: http://www.aafp.org/fpm/20010500/50usin.html.

38. Moser SE, Goering TL: Implementing preventive care flow sheets, *Fam Pract Manage* 8(2):51–56, 2001. Available at: http://www.aafp.org/fpm/20010200/51impl.html.

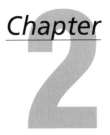

Diagnostic Bias in Men's Healthcare

A. Evan Eyler, MD

Key Points

- The cognitive processing of large amounts of information requires the use of unconscious mental mapping, that is, generalizations and assumptions. This is particularly true in situations that require the rapid assimilation and evaluation of a large amount of information for a particular purpose, such as the practice of medicine (strength of recommendation: C).
- The use of gender-based assumptions and stereotyping in the practice of medicine is usually a function of unconscious cognitive processes, reflecting the beliefs of the larger culture. Its consequences can be damaging to both women and men. For example, the characterization of coronary artery disease as primarily a disease of men of European ancestry has been detrimental to women and minority-identified men who suffer cardiac events (strength of recommendation: B).
- Medical conditions that occur (or are diagnosed) more commonly among women than men, such as osteoporosis and some psychiatric illnesses, sometimes become regarded as "women's health problems." Men who experience them may experience misdiagnosis or diagnostic delay (strength of recommendation: B).
- Very few illnesses are truly the province of only one gender. Clinical research should include members of all population groups that experience the illness or condition under investigation. Study of clinically relevant differences based on factors such as

gender, race, age, and sexual orientation can be used to improve medical care (strength of recommendation: C).
- Clinical stereotypes and invalid assumptions can best be countered by making *covert* bias *overt* and therefore open to scrutiny by physicians and their patients. Unconscious assumptions and prejudices remain inaccessible, but those that are brought into conscious awareness can be questioned and positively countered with more accurate information (strength of recommendation: C).

Introduction

Stereotyping and gender-based assumptions are ubiquitous in medical practice, as in society at large. Treating each patient as a unique individual, and scrutinizing assumptions regarding potential physical and mental illnesses, remain challenging aspects of clinical practice for physicians and other healthcare personnel. This chapter discusses gender-based generalization as a complicating factor in the diagnosis and treatment of male patients.

Clinical Assumptions and Diagnostic Bias

The Merriam-Webster Dictionary[1] defines *assumption* as synonymous with *supposition*, with its root referring to something that is "mistakenly believed." A *stereotype* is defined as "something agreeing with a pattern: especially an idea that many people have about a thing or a group and that may often be untrue or only partly true." The term *bias* has a more negative connotation and is synonymous with *prejudice*: "to judge before full hearing or examination...an opinion made without adequate basis," as well as the damage that can result from its exercise. A *stigma* refers to a stereotype that is fundamentally damaging in nature: "a mark of disgrace or discredit."

Social scientists note that cognitive processing of the large amount of information that confronts human beings on a daily basis requires the use of unconscious mental mapping. This process relies on inferences from the general to the specific: "Generalization devoid of judgment is generally adaptive and helps everyone understand the world."[2] This is particularly true in situations that require the rapid assimilation and evaluation of a large amount of information for a particular purpose, such as the practice of medicine. Although this is a morally neutral phenomenon, its unconscious exercise can be harmful, both to particular individuals who do not fit the expected clinical pattern, and to entire population groups, particularly those who are in some way stigmatized, such as racial minorities and residents of economically depressed communities. Because this process rarely comes to conscious awareness, it can be particularly difficult to avoid or remedy. Perrin notes the following:

> Social stereotyping is so powerful that it transcends individual recognition. Stigmatization is fundamentally reflective of an unequal distribution of power with regard to a particular characteristic; those who are unaffected generally do not even notice its effects...No one *intended* to create inequities in healthcare between Caucasian patients and people of color, and yet such social disparities are documented repeatedly. When a highly qualified candidate is passed over for a job, her obesity is not consciously seen as an explanation.[2]

Similarly, when inappropriate assumptions or bias enter the particular clinical encounter, this is usually a reflection of the social generalizations held by the physician, patient, or both, rather than the result of ill will or lack of competence.

Consequences

Although the use of assumptions and stereotyping in the clinical setting is usually without malignant intent, its consequences can be quite serious. The evaluation and management of cardiovascular disease provides an example of the differential treatment of population groups (in this case, both by gender and by race) through prevalent patterns of clinical decision making, rather than by policy or intent.

Differences in the evaluation of chest pain and treatment of coronary artery disease by race[3–5] and gender[6–8] have been reported for decades. Despite some inconsistency in these findings[9,10] and proposed explanations for these differences in clinical care,[11] unconscious bias on the part of physicians and other healthcare providers has been difficult to exclude.

Schulman and colleagues[12] investigated physician recommendations for managing chest pain using videotaped standardized patient presentations and a computerized survey instrument. The effects of gender and race on physician recommendations were evaluated while controlling for the effects of age, type of chest pain, and other clinical factors. In discussion of their finding that women and African Americans were less likely to be referred for cardiac catheterization than were men and patients of European ancestry, respectively, the authors noted:

> Our finding that the race and sex of the patient influence the recommendations of physicians independently of other factors may suggest bias on the part of the physicians. However, our study could not assess the form of bias. Bias may represent overt prejudice on the part of physicians or, more likely, could be the result of *subconscious perceptions rather than deliberate actions or thoughts*. Subconscious bias occurs when a patient's membership in a target group automatically activates a cultural stereotype in the physician's memory regardless of the level of prejudice the physician has.[12] [emphasis added]

The work of Schulman and colleagues[11] has been criticized on the grounds that cardiac catheterization carries the risk of complications, including death, and that the possibility of overtreatment was not well addressed in this study. However, other research has found gender differences in rates of utilization of noninvasive and low-risk treatments, including intensive care unit admission for evaluation of chest pain,[6] noninvasive testing and pharmacotherapy,[7] and cardiac rehabilitation,[8] in addition to cardiac catheterization and revascularization procedures. Differences in cardiac care by gender have been reported by European investigators[7,8] as well as in the United States, suggesting that Schulman et al.'s results are consistent with widespread, likely inadvertent, clinical gender stereotyping, rather than representing an artifact or methodologic flaw in any single study.

Educational messages aimed at both physicians and patients are attempting to improve the cardiac care of women and minority-identified men by bringing these unconscious assumptions into conscious scrutiny and countering them with evidence-based medical recommendations. For example, in the "Pearls and Pitfalls" section of their recent review regarding the diagnosis and management of ST-segment elevation myocardial infarction, Hahn and Chandler[13] state:

> Certain groups of patients are less likely to be offered reperfusion therapy, including women, ethnic minorities, and the elderly, despite demonstrated benefit from intervention. *Be particularly vigilant when evaluating these groups for possible ACS.* [emphasis added]

Similarly, the American Heart Association Web site contains public information that specifically addresses clinical stereotyping as part of an effort to improve cardiovascular health among women and minority-identified men:

> What comes to mind when you think of heart disease? A middle-aged white man dying suddenly from a heart attack? Well, think again. Cardiovascular disease, including stroke, is the leading cause of death for African-American men and women...[14]

Practicing physicians also report success in improving patient care and outcomes by purposefully addressing diagnostic bias in cardiac care. Desantis[15] reports telling a woman patient with coronary artery disease that he would like to treat her, medically, as "one of the guys," that is, as a patient for whom intensive, comprehensive treatment is indicated. He made this statement after learning that her four sisters had all died of complications of coronary artery disease, while her five brothers had received more aggressive treatment of the same condition and were all still living.

These examples demonstrate efforts to evaluate the validity of clinical stereotypes, and then to counteract invalid assumptions (in this case, that coronary artery disease is primarily a disease of men of European ancestry) by making *covert* bias *overt*, and therefore open to scrutiny by physicians and their patients. Unconscious assumptions and prejudices remain inaccessible, but those that are brought into conscious awareness can be questioned and positively countered with more accurate information.

Clinical Bias and Men's Health

Clinical bias that negatively affects women's healthcare is sometimes the residual of previous medical policy. For example, until the mid 1990s, most clinical research regarding conditions that were common to both women and men was conducted using exclusively male volunteers, often only men of European ancestry. The US Food and Drug Administration (FDA) Web site[16] understatedly reports that:

> Historically, investigators have been reluctant to include female subjects in clinical trials due, in part, to concerns with potential birth defects. In addition, the 1977 FDA guideline entitled *General Considerations for the Clinical Evaluation of Drugs* excluded women of childbearing potential from early drug development studies. This may have further contributed to a general lack of females participating in drug development studies and thus, to a paucity of information about drug and biologic product effects in females... In order to reverse this real or perceived regulatory barrier to the participation of women of childbearing potential in clinical trials the agency has taken a number of initiatives... The 1988 document entitled *Guideline for the Format and Content of the Clinical and Statistical Sections of New Drug Applications* emphasized the importance of including analyses of demographic data in [new drug] applications.... The 1993 *Guideline for the Study and Evaluation of Gender Differences in Clinical Evaluation of Drugs* provides guidance regarding inclusion of both genders in drug development, analysis of clinical data by gender, and assessment of potential pharmaco-kinetic differences between genders.

Nonetheless, the legacy of previous policy continues to affect the clinical care of women and racial minority–identified men. Pharmacologic and biologic treatments produced after 1992 are more likely to have been clinically tested in racially diverse sample populations that include both genders. However, many products and procedures developed prior to that time have not been reevaluated according to current guidelines. In addition, clinical research that excludes particular population groups may inadvertently communicate to the medical community that the condition under study is primarily a concern of the chosen study population—as has likely been the case regarding coronary artery disease and men of European ancestry.

Faulty clinical assumptions and bias that negatively affect the health and medical care of men have often been more subtle. Rather than being based on specific policies or exclusionary research, it has usually reflected the statistical probabilities associated with particular clinical conditions, sometimes influenced by prevailing gender stereotypes and unconscious diagnostic bias. Unfortunately, medical conditions that occur (or are diagnosed) more commonly among women than men sometimes become regarded as "women's health problems"; men who experience them may then undergo misdiagnosis or diagnostic delay. Men who experience illnesses for which women are more likely to seek care may also experience negative emotional responses to being treated for a condition that is not "masculine." In addition, clinical stereotypes regarding illness and gender can persist after the disease prevalence has been altered by changes in population health behaviors or demographic shifts, such as widespread reduction in levels of physical activity and the increasing life expectancy of men. In some cases, prevalent stereotyping of an illness—as both "feminine" and socially stigmatizing—may make clinicians reluctant to appropriately assign the diagnosis when the patient is male.

Despite physician efforts to maintain clinical objectivity, the practice of medicine contains a significant subjective element, as befits a *biopsychosocial* field. In addition, healthcare exists within the context of the larger culture and is influenced by societal trends, including economic forces. For example, Metzl[17] notes that advertisements for psychotropic medications during the last several decades have disproportionately used visual images of women, "giving the impression that many more women visit psychiatrists and other health professionals than actually do. Clinicians and health-policy experts have... connected such ads to the prescribing patterns of physicians, suggesting that the overrepresentation of women in them *may work to expand epidemiological norms*" [emphasis added]. In other words, patterns of clinical diagnosis and treatment recommendation are influenced by unconscious assumptions and stereotyping, which then become reinforced and self-perpetuating. This may work either to the benefit of male patients (as with the diagnosis and management of coronary artery disease) or to their detriment (as in some psychiatric conditions).

Detecting and correcting gender bias in medical care can be extremely problematic due to the ambiguous nature of many clinical presentations.[18] Applicable research is often extremely scant. The multiple lines of investigation regarding gender and racial stereotyping bias in the evaluation and treatment of coronary artery disease have gradually illuminated a persistent pattern in need of change. However, many aspects of gendered healthcare remain to be adequately investigated. The implications of these difficulties are discussed below through several illustrative cases.

Case Discussions from a Men's Health Perspective

Case 1: An Elderly Man with Osteoporosis

Highlights: Clinical stereotyping, diagnostic delay, and lack of clinical research

WR is a 76-year-old semi-retired physician with back pain, which was diagnosed as musculoligamentous in etiology and treated conservatively. He subsequently experiences a T9 vertebral compression fracture while lifting a 10-lb computer monitor. More detailed evaluation follows, during which it is noted that he has lost more than 2 inches in height. Dual-energy x-ray absorptiometry reveals severe osteoporosis. WR's only risk factors for this illness are European ancestry and advanced age.

Osteoporosis is a clinical condition defined by the loss of bone mineralization to the level at which skeletal integrity can no longer be maintained, resulting in pathologic fractures. Compression or "crush" vertebral fractures and fractures of the femoral neck are the sequelae that produce the greatest burden of morbidity and mortality among older adults. In the United States, 18% of women and 6% of men experience at least one hip fracture due to osteoporosis; 16% of women and 5% of men have vertebral fractures. Genetic factors influence the likelihood of bone demineralization, and significant differences in prevalence exist among adults of different racial ancestries. However, at least 13% of American men older than 50 years will experience at least one fracture due to skeletal calcium depletion.[19] Overall, nearly one third of osteoporotic fractures occur in men.[20] Osteoporosis risk is also significantly higher among older men. Cancurtaran and colleagues[21] evaluated 464 male patients admitted to an inpatient geriatric unit in Turkey; 45.9% were found to be osteoporotic and 36.6% osteopenic.

Osteoporosis prevalence is lower among men than women due to several factors. On average, men enter adulthood with a greater skeletal mass than their female peers and experience a more gradual decline in the production of sex steroids. Estrogens, rather than androgens, maintain the skeletal mineralization; in males, this is achieved through the peripheral conversion of testosterone to estradiol.[22,23] Women who do not take supplemental estrogen or use other protective measures experience a rapid loss of bone integrity in the early menopausal years. Andropause is a more gradual phenomenon, with serum testosterone levels declining from an average of 600 ng/dl (20.8 nmol/l) at the age of 30 years to approximately 400 ng/dl (13.9 nmol/l) by age 80.[24] In addition, the average life expectancy of women is greater than that of their male peers, so that loss of skeletal mass proceeds over a longer period of time and becomes gradually more severe. Nonetheless, osteoporosis will afflict a significant minority of the men who survive into the older adult years. The effects of increasing life expectancy in many parts of the world and the concurrent decrease in physical activity among both boys and girls may serve to further increase the prevalence of this serious illness among both women and men.

Until very recently, osteoporosis was considered a disease of older women. Few texts and articles discussed osteoporosis in men except as a consequence of concurrent pathology, such as the nonjudicious use of corticosteroids (results of National Library of Medicine search, 1956–2006). WR's physician did not consider osteoporosis in the differential diagnosis of his back pain because he did not think of it. Unconscious gender-based assumptions prevented him from perceiving a likely clinical reality, much as gender stereotyping regarding cardiovascular disease can interfere with clinical reasoning when the patient is female or African American. In the work of Wright and colleagues,[25] 27% of men with distal forearm fractures were found to have osteoporosis on subsequent evaluation; only 10% of the osteoporotic patients had been given information about this illness at the time of the fracture.

Although further research regarding osteoporosis among both men and women is clearly needed, current knowledge raises some significant concerns for older male patients. Morbidity and mortality after osteoporotic fracture may be higher among men than among their female peers.[19,26] Some evidence suggests that the onset of pathologic fractures occurs at higher average levels of bone mineral density among men than women.[27] Colles' fractures are more likely to be followed by vertebral or hip fracture when the patient is male.[28] Prostate cancer is commonly treated by androgen deprivation, which increases the likelihood of bone demineralization among older men,[29] many of whom are already osteopenic prior to the onset of treatment.[30]

Optimum detection and treatment of osteoporosis requires further investigation, particularly among men. The fundamental aspects of prevention are the same for women and men: participation in weight-bearing physical activity throughout life, maintaining adequate nutrition, and limiting use of alcohol and tobacco. Treatment with bisphosphonates is effective in men[31,32] and additional agents, such as selective androgen receptor modulators, are in development. However, many areas of ambiguity remain. Diagnostic measures such as bone area and width, bone mineral density, etc. have different means among women and men,[33] and testing for osteopenia is being reevaluated in this light. Secondary causes of osteoporosis are detected more commonly among male patients with this condition.[26] Excess alcohol consumption is one of the most common of these, suggesting the need for additional preventive messages directed at men in this regard.

Conclusion: Osteoporosis should no longer be solely regarded as a women's illness.

Case 2: A Middle-Aged Man with Lupus

Highlights: Clinical stereotyping and misperceptions regarding diagnosis and treatment

RE is a 48-year-old office manager who presents with a history of profound fatigue of approximately 6 months' duration and some mild joint aching. Initial laboratory studies reveal mild neutropenia but are otherwise unremarkable. Clinical investigation by his internist includes screening for alcoholism and discussion of life stress; cardiac risk factors are also evaluated.

A diagnosis of systemic lupus erythematosus is made 18 months after initial presentation. RE wonders why his diagnosis remained elusive for such a lengthy period, particularly as he had been having difficulty remaining productive at work due to the fatigue and psychological malaise. He begins reading about lupus; the first text that he consults states that this condition "occurs mainly in young women." His physician tells RE that his is "a rare case" and that "the few men who develop lupus" are often not correctly diagnosed for extended periods of time. RE's subsequent self-education causes him to cast doubt on this assessment as well.

RE's case illustrates the confusion that can occur when clinical thinking is strongly influenced by gender stereotypes applied to particular symptoms and medical conditions. Lupus is a common autoimmune illness whose prevalence varies greatly in different population groups and is affected by age, gender, and racial ancestry. Many continuing medical education reviews and general medical texts emphasize the effect of race, and particularly gender, on disease prevalence, with descriptions such as "Essentials of Diagnosis: occurs mainly in young women..."[34] However, despite the marked female predominance (8–9:1) of this illness during the mid-second through fifth decades, men of RE's age are approximately as likely to develop lupus as are their female peers.

RE's experience with regard to the length of time between symptom onset and correct diagnosis is also rather typical for this disease. Lupus has been called "the disease with a thousand faces" because its presentations are variable and often initially subtle. Intervals of 2–3 years between onset and diagnosis are not uncommon.[35,36] In two series,[37,38] men with lupus were diagnosed *more rapidly*, on average, than were women. In a sample of African American men, this finding persisted even when cases presenting with nephritis were excluded.[37] RE would likely have been correctly diagnosed more swiftly had his signs and symptoms been more severe—though he is fortunate that they were not. In many,[37–40] but not all,[41,42] clinical series, manifestations of illness have been more dramatic (e.g., fever) or severe (e.g., nephritis, pericarditis) at the time of presentation among men with lupus than among their female peers.

Patients who are newly diagnosed with a chronic illness often feel anxious, vulnerable, and suddenly separated from the "normal" world. Information can help to restore feelings of self-efficacy and control. The choice of information and the manner in which it is presented can foster inclusiveness or can maintain a more narrow focus. For example, the Lupus Canada Web site public information section includes the frequently asked question, "Who gets lupus... Anyone can: women, men, children. Between the ages 15 and 45, eight times more women than men get lupus. In those under 15 and over 45, both sexes are affected equally."[43] RE's physician might have been more helpful in fostering adjustment to living with this chronic illness had he been more knowledgeable regarding its epidemiology and less reliant on gender-based stereotypes.

Conclusion: Illnesses such as lupus that occur more commonly among women than men should remain in the differential diagnosis when the patient is male.

Case 3: A Young Man with Depression, Social Anxiety, and Adjustment

Highlights: The "masculine" or "feminine" qualities of illness—gender stereotyping in mental health

MH is a 20-year-old university student with social anxiety and depression. He has responded well to treatment with a serotonin-specific reuptake inhibitor (SSRI) prescribed by his family physician and has recently begun psychotherapy to address his difficulties in social situations and concerns related to his coming out as a gay man. On a follow-up visit, MH informs his physician that he has been reading about depression. He asks, "Isn't this something mainly for women?"

Case 4: A Middle-Aged Man with Alcohol Dependence and Borderline Personality Disorder

Highlights: Gender stereotyping, stigma, and incomplete treatment

BN is a 48-year-old carpenter with a long history of alcohol dependence. He is admitted to the internal medicine inpatient service for inpatient alcohol detoxification and management of withdrawal, due to his history of seizures during withdrawal in the outpatient setting. BN is transferred to the inpatient psychiatry service after a suicide "gesture" (attempting to stab himself with a plastic knife) while on the medicine service.

Review of BN's hospital record reveals numerous visits to the emergency department for treatment of orthopedic injuries and lacerations and several previous admissions to inpatient psychiatry due to suicidal ideation or threats following romantic breakups. On further discussion, BN admits that most of the injuries were self-inflicted: He has thrown himself down stairs and burned himself during periods of emotional upset. Although full examination reveals that he clearly meets the diagnostic criteria for borderline personality disorder (BPD), this diagnosis is not recorded in his medical record. When he again leaves the hospital against medical advice, he is given information regarding resources for treatment of alcohol dependence, but none pertaining to treatment of the emotional dysregulation associated with BPD.

A thorough discussion of gender bias and stereotyping in psychiatric diagnosis and treatment is well beyond the scope of this chapter. Some psychiatric disorders vary in prevalence by gender. In addition, diagnosis and treatment recommendations are influenced by sometimes unconscious gender stereotyping and bias. Some conditions become more closely associated with women, or with men. The consequences of this process can be either favorable to male patients (e.g., historically greater availability of substance dependence treatment for men in many areas) or unfavorable, as is the case when diagnoses are overlooked and remain untreated.

Unipolar depressive illnesses, such as major depressive disorder and dysthymia, and most anxiety disorders, are more common among women than men. However, due to the substantial lifetime prevalence of these conditions (24% for anxiety, at least 6% for major depressive disorder) large numbers of men experience these illnesses. Some convergence occurs over time: Men and women older than 50 years are equally likely to suffer from depression. Compared with the epidemiologic data, women are over-represented relative to men in media images of anxiety and depression sufferers, including pharmaceutical advertising.[17] Men who would benefit from treatment of anxiety or depression may be reluctant to seek care, at least in part due to gender stereotypes regarding "masculine" and "feminine" illnesses. Panic disorder is especially unappealingly named, perhaps particularly from a masculine perspective. The effect of gender stereotyping on physicians and other mental health clinicians remains to be adequately addressed, although some research has proven illuminating, as described below.

BPD is a psychiatric illness characterized by an impaired capacity to form stable interpersonal relationships, identity disturbance (usually manifested as chronic feelings of emptiness or boredom), affective instability ("mood swings"), use of primitive defenses such as splitting and sometimes brief reactive psychotic states, and recurrent suicidal or parasuicidal behaviors, such as self-mutilation.[44] Etiologies are both neurobiologic and experiential. Paris and colleagues found that major loss and trauma, particularly sexual trauma, as well as relationship problems with fathers, were important risk factors for the

development of BPD in men.[45] Streeter and colleagues found a much higher prevalence (42% versus 4%) of prior head injury among male veterans diagnosed with BPD than among matched control subjects with other psychiatric diagnoses.[46] Genetic factors have also been implicated. BPD shares some characteristics with many other psychiatric illnesses, including post-traumatic stress disorder (PTSD), bipolar disorder, intermittent explosive disorder, and some other personality disorders. Persons diagnosed with BPD are more likely to be female, and those diagnosed with antisocial personality disorder (ASPD) are more likely to be male, though with regard to the former, Skodol and Bender note that, "True prevalence by gender is unknown."[47]

Becker and Lamb[48] investigated gender bias in the diagnosis of BPD and PTSD among mental health professionals. Study participants, including psychiatrists, psychologists, and clinical social workers (n = 311), reviewed standardized case vignettes in which criteria for diagnosis of BPD and PTSD were present in equal measure, such that diagnostic ambiguity was substantial. Some participants received a version in which the subject was identified as male, others as female. Among other differences, respondents were more likely to recommend a diagnosis of BPD if the client was female and were more likely to recommend a diagnosis of ASPD if the client was male. Becker and Lamb note the following:

> The finding that clinicians rated female clients higher for applicability of the BPD diagnosis than they rated male clients suggests that sex bias may be influencing the application of this diagnosis. Some argue that when the base rates for a given disorder are higher for women than for men, as is the case with BPD, clinicians who diagnose in accordance with the base rates when judging an ambiguous case are not necessarily showing bias in clinical judgment...
>
> However, *few cases with which therapists are actually presented are unambiguous*; furthermore, some researchers suggest that the base rates for a given disorder are themselves the result of clinician diagnoses and that those base rates may be used by therapists to rationalize bias in decision making...[48] [emphasis added]

Eubanks-Carter and Goldfried[49] conducted a similar study in which clinical psychologists (n = 141) evaluated a hypothetical client who exhibited behaviors consistent with either a sexual identity crisis or BPD (e.g., unstable and intense interpersonal relationships, unstable self-image, impulsivity) but who lacked the symptom chronicity and severity needed to diagnose BPD. Study participants were substantially more likely (61% vs. 36%) to assign a diagnosis of BPD if the hypothetical male client was perceived as having a strong likelihood of being gay or bisexual than if he was perceived as likely to be heterosexual. Participants were more likely to evaluate the client as having a positive prognosis, and to express confidence in working with the client, if the vignette presented the individual as female rather than male.[49]

Widiger[50] describes a number of ways in which differential prevalence rates for certain personality disorders, by gender, may reflect gender bias. These include "biased diagnostic constructs, biased thresholds for diagnosis, biased population sampling, biased application of diagnostic criteria, biased instruments of assessment, and biased diagnostic criteria."[50] Self-report inventories can also contain gender biases.[51]

Making the correct diagnosis of personality disorders can be clinically challenging yet crucially important. Approximately 30–40% of suicides are committed by persons with personality disorders[52]; a majority of persons who commit suicide is male. Lesage and colleagues[53] evaluated case histories of 75 young men in cities in Ontario, whose lives ended by suicide, compared with 75 living matched control subjects, and found that BPD was identified in 28% of the men who committed suicide, compared with 4% of controls.[53] Many persons with BPD can learn to modulate affect and reduce self-harming behaviors with treatment. At present, the majority of research regarding treatment of BPD has been conducted among women.

Men with BPD often suffer from other psychiatric comorbidities. Darke and colleagues[54] found a high co-occurrence of BPD and ASPD among 615 Australian heroin users: 46% met criteria for BPD, 71% for ASPD, and 38% for both. Paris[55] questions whether ASPD and BPD may in fact represent two aspects of the same pathology. Compared with women with this illness, men with BPD are more likely to also meet diagnostic criteria for substance use disorders, ASPD, and intermittent explosive disorder, though less likely to suffer from eating disorders.[56] Nonetheless, level of overall impairment among men and women is not different.[56]

Treatment of personality disorders is more complex and less pharmacologically based than treatment of mood and psychotic disorders. In addition, BPD remains a highly stigmatized diagnosis, with many clinicians regarding patients with this condition as unpleasant, manipulative, and refractory to treatment. As Nehls[57] notes,

In North America, there may be no other psychiatric diagnosis more laden with stereotypes and stigma than borderline personality disorder... [There are] stigmatizing practices and limited services for seriously ill persons with borderline personality disorder diagnoses.

Some clinicians do not record a suspected diagnosis of BPD, particularly if the patient is male. Nonetheless, being diagnosed with ASPD can also be damaging, particularly if the diagnosis is incorrect. Smallwood notes,[43]

...this disorder is difficult, if not impossible, to treat...the most effective form of treatment appears to be in confined settings, such as prisons, where external constraints can substitute for their moral deficits...behavioral therapy with a strong emphasis on legal sanctions is the most effective method of treatment.

In other words, both BPD and ASPD are highly stigmatized, but one is regarded as potentially treatable and the other as primarily requiring containment and supervision. Women with PTSD who are misdiagnosed as having BPD and men with BPD who are misdiagnosed as antisocial will both likely be stigmatized and mistreated or undertreated, though in different ways and with different consequences to themselves and their families.

Bias in psychiatric diagnosis and treatment, including stereotyping based on gender or sexual orientation, merits additional research, discussion, and scrutiny. Anxiety, depression, and BPD occur commonly among both women and men. Men with these or other psychiatric disorders should be encouraged to seek effective treatment.

Conclusion

The use of gender-based assumptions and stereotyping in the practice of medicine is usually a function of unconscious cognitive processes, reflecting the beliefs of the larger culture. Although it may be without ill intent, the inherent consequences can be damaging to both women and men. Research regarding bias in diagnosis and treatment, as has been conducted regarding coronary artery disease, can help to illuminate these errors. Once brought into conscious scrutiny, biases can be reassessed and rectified.

Medical conditions that occur (or are diagnosed) more commonly among women than men sometimes become regarded as "women's health problems," yet very few illnesses not directly connected with reproductive anatomy and physiology are truly the province of either gender. Clinical research should include members of all population groups that experience the illness or condition under investigation. Study of clinically relevant differences based on factors such as gender, race, age, and sexual orientation can be used to improve medical care.

In medical practice, each patient remains a unique individual, rather than simply a member of a group. Medicine is based on the importance of the individual and recognition of common humanity.

Before I built a wall I'd ask to know

What I was walling in or walling out,

And to whom I was like to give offense.

Something there is that doesn't love a wall,

That wants it down.

"Mending Wall," by Robert Frost

References

1. Mish FC, editor-in-chief: *The Merriam-Webster Dictionary*, Springfield, MA, 1997, Merriam-Webster.
2. Perrin EC: *Sexual Orientation in Child and Adolescent Health Care*, New York, 2002, Kluwer Academic/Plenum, pp 5, 7.
3. Ford E, Cooper R, Castaner A, et al: Coronary arteriography and coronary bypass survey among whites and other racial groups relative to hospital-based incidence rates for coronary artery disease: findings from NHDS, *Am J Public Health* 79 (4):437–440, 1989.
4. Ferguson JA, Tierney WM, Westmoreland GR, et al: Examination of racial differences in management of cardiovascular disease, *J Am Coll Cardiol* 30 (7):1707–1713, 1997.
5. Ibrahim SA, Whittle J, Bean-Mayberry B, et al: Racial/ethnic variations in physician recommendations for cardiac revascularization, *Am J Public Health* 93(10):1689–1693, 2003.
6. Green LA, Ruffin MT, 4th: Differences in management of suspected myocardial infarction in men and women, *J Fam Pract* 36(4):389–393, 1993.
7. Daly C, Clemens F, Lopez JL Sendon, et al: Gender differences in the management and clinical outcome of stable angina, *Circulation* 113(4):490–498, 2006.
8. Cottin Y, Cambou JP, Casillas JM, et al: Specific profile and referral bias of rehabilitated patients after an acute coronary syndrome, *J Cardiopulm Rehabil* 24(1):38–44, 2004.
9. Taylor AJ, Meyer GS, Morse RW, et al: Can characteristics of a health care system mitigate ethnic bias in access to cardiovascular procedures? Experiences from the Military Health Services System, *J Am Coll Cardiol* 30(4):901–907, 1997.
10. Ben-Ami T, Gilutz H, Porath A, et al: No gender difference in the clinical management and outcome of unstable angina, *Isr Med Assoc J* 7(4):228–232, 2005.
11. Schwartz LM, Woloshin S, Welch HG, et al: Misunderstanding about the effects of race and sex on physicians' referrals for cardiac catheterization, *N Engl J Med* 341:279–283, 1999.
12. Schulman KA, Berlin JA, Harless W, et al: The effect of race and sex on physicians' recommendations for cardiac catheterization, *N Engl J Med* 340: 618–626, 1999.
13. Hahn S, Chandler C: Diagnosis and management of ST elevation myocardial infarction: a review of the recent literature and practice guidelines, *Mount Sinai J Med* 73(1):469–480, 2006.
14. 2005–2006 African American Heart Health Kit. Available at: http://www.americanheart.org. Accessed on September 3, 2006.
15. Desantis. New York State Academy of Family Physicians Winter Weekend and Scientific Assembly at the Lake Placid Hilton. January 2006.
16. 1993 guideline for the study and evaluation of gender differences in clinical evaluation of drugs. Available at: http://www.fda.gov. Accessed on September 3, 2006.
17. Metzl JM: *Prozac on the Couch: Prescribing Gender in the Era of Wonder Drugs*, Durham, NC, 2003, Duke University Press.
18. Becker D, Lamb S: Sex bias in the diagnosis of borderline personality disorder and posttraumatic stress disorder, *Prof Psychol Res Pract* 25(1):55–61, 1994.
19. Amin S: Male osteoporosis: epidemiology and pathophysiology, *Curr Osteoporos Rep* 1(2):71–77, 2003.
20. Blain H: Osteoporosis in men: epidemiology, pathophysiology, diagnosis, prevention and treatment, *Rev Med Interne* 25(Suppl 5):S552–S559, 2004.
21. Cancurtaran M, Yavuz BB, Halil M, et al: General characteristics, clinical features and related factors of osteoporosis in a group of elderly Turkish men, *Aging Clin Exp Res* 17(2):108–115, 2005.
22. Gooren LJ, Toorians AW: Significance of oestrogens in male (patho)physiology, *Ann Endocrinol (Paris)* 64 (2):126–135, 2003.
23. Alexandre C: Androgens and bone metabolism, *Joint Bone Spine* 72(3):202–206, 2005.
24. Snyder PJ: Hypogonadism in elderly men—what to do until the evidence comes, *N Engl J Med* 350 (5):440–443, 2004.
25. Wright S, Beringer T, Taggart H, et al: A study of male patients with forearm fractures in Northern Ireland, *Clin Rheumatol* 26(2):191–195, 2007.
26. Kamel HK: Male osteoporosis: new trends in diagnosis and therapy, *Drugs Aging* 22(9):741–748, 2005.
27. Sone T: Diagnosis of male osteoporosis [Japanese], *Clin Calcium* 13(8):1047–1050, 2003(abstract).
28. Haentjens P, Johnell O, Kanis JA, et al: Evidence from data searches and life-table analyses for gender-related differences in absolute risk of hip fracture after Colles' or spine fracture: Colles' fracture as an early and sensitive marker of skeletal fragility

in white men, *J Bone Miner Res* 19(12):1933–1944, 2004.

29. Gilbert SM, McKiernan JM: Epidemiology of male osteoporosis and prostate cancer, *Curr Opin Urol* 15(1):23–27, 2005.

30. Conde FA, Aronson WJ: Risk factors for male osteoporosis, *Urol Oncol* 21(5):380–383, 2003.

31. Drake WM, Kendler DL, Rosen CJ, et al: An investigation of the predictors of bone mineral density and response to therapy with alendronate in osteoporotic men, *J Clin Endocrinol Metab* 88(12): 5759–5765, 2003.

32. Gonnelli S, Cepollaro C, Montagnani A, et al: Alendronate treatment in men with primary osteoporosis: a three-year longitudinal study, *Calcif Tissue Int* 73(2):133–139, 2003.

33. Fukunaga M, Sone T: Guideline for diagnosis and therapy of osteoporosis from a point of view of sex difference [Japanese], *Clin Calcium* 13(11): 1399–1404, 2003(abstract).

34. Hellmann DB, Stone JH: Arthritis and musculoskeletal disorders, In Tierney LM Jr, McPhee SJ, Papadakis MA (eds): *Current Medical Diagnosis and Treatment 2005*, New York, 2005, Lange Medical Books/McGraw-Hill, pp 781–836.

35. Bujan S, Ordi-Ros J, Paredes M, et al: Contribution of the initial features of systemic lupus erythematosus to the clinical evolution and survival of a cohort of Mediterranean patients, *Ann Rheum Dis* 62:859–865, 2003. Available at: http://ard.bmjjournals.com/cgi/content/full/62/9/859.

36. Ozbek S, Sert M, Paydas S, et al: Delay in the diagnosis of SLE: the importance of arthritis/arthralgia as the initial symptom, *Acta Med Okayama* 57 (4):187–190, 2003.

37. Arbuckle MR, James JA, Dennis GJ, et al: Rapid clinical progression to diagnosis among African-American men with systemic lupus erythematosus, *Lupus* 12(2):99–106, 2003.

38. Garcia MA, Marcos JC, Marcos AI, et al: Male systemic lupus erythematosus in a Latin-American inception cohort of 1214 patients, *Lupus* 14:938–946, 2005. Available at: http://www.lupus-journal.com.

39. Molina JF, Drenkard C, Molina J, et al: Systemic lupus erythematosus in males: a study of 107 Latin American patients, *Medicine (Baltimore)* 75(3): 124–130, 1996.

40. Mayor AM, Vila LM: Gender differences in a cohort of Puerto Ricans with systemic lupus erythematosus, *Cell Mol Biol (Noisy-le-grand)* 49(8): 1339–1344, 2003.

41. Mok CC, Lau CS, Chan TM, et al: Clinical characteristics and outcome of southern Chinese males with systemic lupus erythematosus, *Lupus* 8(3):188–196, 1999.

42. Voulgari PV, Katsimbri P, Alamanos Y, et al: Gender and age differences in systemic lupus erythematosus: a study of 489 Greek patients with a review of the literature, *Lupus* 11(11):722–729, 2002.

43. Smallwood P: Personality disorders. In Stern TA, Herman JB, editors: *Psychiatry Update and Board Preparation*, New York, 2003, McGraw-Hill, p 193.

44. Paris J, Zweig-Frank H, Guzder J: Risk factors for borderline personality disorder in male outpatients, *J Nerv Ment Dis* 182(7):375–380, 1994.

45. Paris J, et al: Available at: http://www.lupuscanada.org. Accessed on September 3, 2006.

46. Streeter CC, Van Reekum R, Shorr RI, et al: Prior head injury in male veterans with borderline personality disorder, *J Nerv Ment Dis* 183(9):577–581, 1995.

47. Skodol AE, Bender DS: Why are women diagnosed borderline more than men? *Psychiatric Q* 74 (4):349–360, 2003.

48. Becker D, Lamb S: Sex bias in the diagnosis of borderline personality disorder and posttraumatic stress disorder, *Prof Psychol: Res Pract* 25(1):55–61, 1994.

49. Eubanks-Carter C, Goldfried MR: The impact of client sexual orientation and gender on clinical judgments and diagnosis of borderline personality disorder, *J Clin Psychol* 2006. Available at: http://www.interscience.wiley.com. DOI: 1.1002/jclp.20265.

50. Widiger TA: Invited essay: sex biases in the diagnosis of personality disorders, *J Personal Discord* 12 (2):95–118, 1998.

51. Lindsay KA, Sankis LM, Widiger TA: Gender bias in self-report personality disorder inventories, *J Personal Discord* 14(3):218–232, 2000.

52. Duberstein PR: Personality disorders and completed suicide: a methodological and conceptual review, *Clin Psychol: Sci Pract* 4(4):359–376, 1997.

53. Lesage AD, Boyer R, Grunberg F, et al: Suicide and mental disorders: a case control study of young men, *Am J Psychiatry* 151(7):1063–1068, 1994.

54. Darke S, Williamson A, Ross J, et al: Borderline personality disorder, antisocial personality disorder and risk-taking among heroin users: findings from the Australian Treatment Outcome Study (ATOS), *Drug Alcohol Dep* 9(74):77–83, 2004.

55. Paris J: Antisocial and borderline personality disorders: two separate diagnoses or two aspects of the same pathology? *Compr Psychiatry* 38(4):237–242, 1997.

56. Zlotnik C, Rothschild L, Zimmerman M: The role of gender in the clinical presentation of patients with borderline personality disorder, *J Personal Discord* 16(3):277–282, 2002.

57. Nehls N: Borderline personality disorder: gender stereotypes, stigma, and limited system of care, *Issues Ment Health Nurs* 19(2):97–112, 1998.

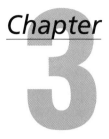

Global Disparities in Men's Health

Robert Winn, MD

Key Points

- Men have a higher disease burden and a lower life expectancy than women (strength of recommendation: A).
- Globally, HIV/AIDS is the fourth leading cause of death (strength of recommendation: A).
- Reducing the common attributable risk factors for the leading causes of death will significantly reduce global disease burden and increase life expectancy in all countries, developed or developing (strength of recommendation: B).

Introduction

Men are disproportionately affected by multiple chronic disease states in the United States and around the world. Within the United States, different subpopulations of men, particularly among racial minorities, show disparate rates of the leading causes of mortality. The global burden of disease differs both by region and gender. Although cardiovascular disease, cancer, and stroke predominate perennially as the top killers of men worldwide, the devastating effects of human immunodeficiency virus (HIV)/acquired immunodeficiency syndrome (AIDS) and violence are large among certain groups. Understanding the risk factors associated with these disease states helps to define public health efforts aimed at reducing disease, resource, and financial burden.

Over the past century, the differences in health between men and women have been the focus of much debate and research in the United States and around the world. Scientists have moved away from the notion that all humans are equal with regard to health status or health outcomes and that a single intervention strategy can address the health of all. Nowhere is this more apparent than in the biopsychosocial differences in health between men and women. Studies repeatedly demonstrate that being male is a health disparity in and of itself.[1] Until recently, however, the issues surrounding specific issues of men's health had not been specifically and adequately addressed. These issues include increased risk for heart disease, cancer, stroke, HIV/AIDS, and interpersonal violence. This chapter provides an overview of some of the most important issues affecting men's health from a global perspective.

Epidemiology

The women's health movement was critical in advancing the health of women and persuading researchers (and supporters of that research) to focus on the specific medical needs of women.[2] What was created was a concentration on female health leading to an increased understanding of gender differences. Although one compelling reason for this change was that most previous research was completed with men as subjects and then extrapolated to women, this perspective excluded issues specific to men. It has become

Table 3-1. Age-adjusted Death Rates by Race and Sex, United States, 2003 (per 100,000 Persons)

	White Men	White Women	Black Men	Black Women	Hispanic Men	Hispanic Women
Hypertension	6.1	6.5	18.6	16.6	7.1	7.5
Heart disease	282.9	185.4	364.3	253.8	286.6	190.3
Cerebrovascular disease	51.7	50.5	79.5	69.8	54.1	52.3
Diabetes mellitus	27.0	19.9	50.7	47.5	28.9	22.5
HIV/AIDS	4.2	0.9	31.3	12.8	7.1	2.4
Prostate cancer	24.4	—	57.4	—	26.5	—
Lung cancer	71.1	42.3	92.4	40.2	71.7	41.3
Colon cancer	22.4	15.7	31.9	22.8	22.9	16.2

Adapted from: Hoyert DL, Heron MP, Murphy SL, Kung HC: Deaths: final data for 2003, *National Vital Statistics Reports* 54:1–120, 2006.

clear that *gender and health* is not only a term to be used to describe women's health, but one that needs to examine the disparities in the health of both sexes equally.

The average life expectancy for men and women in the United States in 2003 was 74.8 and 80.1 years, respectively.[3] This trend of women living longer than men was seen for each decade of life from age zero to 100. Many explanations of this finding have been postulated and researched, and much effort has been placed on discovering the factors related to the morbidity and mortality disparities in men. Although there are undoubtedly significant genetic and biologic causes of the differential health outcomes and disease burden between the sexes, they do not explain the majority of the disparities seen in the statistics.

In the United States, the leading causes of age-adjusted death rates among men and women have been established (Table 3-1). Cardiovascular disease, cancer, and cerebrovascular disease are the top three causes of death for both men and women year after year. However, men consistently have 1.5 times the mortality rate for heart disease and cancer compared with women[4]; these diseases have remained the leading causes of mortality in the United States for decades. Many of the public health efforts focused on cancer, heart disease, and stroke have led to decreases in all forms of these health disparities over time. Still, men are more likely to die in each category. Men are less likely to visit clinicians in times of poor health and to seek preventive care.[5] In terms of health risks, men have historically been more likely to smoke tobacco, a factor which contributes to all three major causes of death.[4] In fact, a large portion of the decrease in the gap between life expectancy between men and women is attributable to the increase in smoking among women. Even still, the exact mechanisms attributable for the poorer health seen in men are not well understood.

In an effort to address the health of the population, the US government has developed an extensive public health plan. *Healthy People 2010*, published in 2000, is a US-based plan developed by the Department of Health and Human Services to promote health.[6] There are 10 leading health indicators are outlined in this plan, and for each indicator a comprehensive plan was developed and measurable goals defined with the objective of achieving these goals by 2010 (Table 3-2). The major outcome measures in this plan relate to the reduction in morbidity and mortality from the leading causes of death in

Table 3-2. Healthy People 2010 Leading Health Indicators for the United States

Leading Health Indicators
Physical activity
Overweight and obesity
Tobacco use
Substance abuse
Responsible sexual behavior
Mental health
Injury and violence
Environmental quality
Immunization
Access to health care

Adapted from: US Department of Health and Human Services: *Healthy People 2010: Understanding and Improving Health*, 2000, US Department of Health and Human Services, Washington, DC.

the United States, namely heart disease, cancer, and stroke. Underlying health risk behavior such as tobacco use, inactivity, poor diet, and unsafe sexual practices play a significant role in relation to these disease states and are addressed below. Although aimed at reducing the leading causes of mortality, this plan does not specifically address the differential impact on the health of men and women.

Race

While overall health disparities between men and women are striking, the differences become even more compelling when subdivided by racial group. The clearest differences exist among African American, Hispanic, and white populations. In the United States, African Americans and Hispanics are more likely to live in poverty and to suffer discrimination including having poor access to regular healthcare.[7] In addition, there are some cultural and social differences among these groups that may account for some of the disparity. For example, African American men are socially conditioned to be "strong" and to not seek help,[8] have an historical mistrust of the healthcare system,[9] and often lack the financial resources to seek care.[10] For Hispanic men, these same issues play a role in their lack of connection with a healthcare provider.[11]

African Americans composed 12.3% of the US population in the 2000 census.[12] This is a substantial minority population, yet the disease burden in this group is significantly higher. African American men rank highest in almost every category of diseases causing death burden in the United States (see Table 3-1). African Americans and non-Hispanic whites share the top three causes of death (i.e., heart disease, cancer, and stroke), yet in each category, African Americans have a much higher mortality rate. Of the top 10 causes of death in whites, African Americans share seven; however, HIV and homicide are among the top causes of mortality among African American men.[13] Many explanations for these differences include socioeconomic status, lifestyle behaviors, social environment, and access to care, all of which have been found to play a large role in this disparity.[7]

Hispanic/Latino populations mimic white populations in terms of disease burden, with a few key exceptions. According to 2000 census data, Hispanics compose 13.3% of the US population and are the fasting growing minority group.[12] Again, the top three causes of death for Hispanic men are heart disease, cancer, and stroke. Unlike African American men, however, mortality rates are much closer to the rates for white men (see Table 3-1). Like African American men, HIV and violence are also leading causes of death. Research aimed at understanding this observed disparity is needed to make valiant attempts at improving this trend.

The health status of men in the United States is determined by multiple factors. Using the leading causes of death as a guide to public health policy is one way to approach changing the disparities seen. However, taking into account that the US population is ever diversifying and that different populations have different risks and outcomes will ultimately lead to better health and a decrease in observed health disparities. Specifically, addressing the underlying causes of increased violent deaths and infection with HIV among African Americans and Hispanics has the potential to favorably affect these minority groups.

Global Health

Measuring the health of any population, even within one country, is difficult to accomplish. Within the United States, for example, governmental agencies like the Centers for Disease Control and Prevention are tasked with the duty of outlining the status of the public's health. Collection of data varies by region of the country and by decade of collection. Consequently, defining trends in health is problematic as the data are not always measuring the exact same end point or collected on the same sample of the population. Determining consistent and comparable data sets among the nations of the world presents an even more difficult task. Each country has a different approach to its measure of public health and collects different kinds of data. In addition, many of the poorer nations do not have the infrastructure or capacity to create the kinds of databases that exist in the developed world. Consequently, public health researchers have been working on methods to overcome these barriers. Over the past few decades, the World Health Organization has defined global expectations of public health measurements and helped the many countries that are members of the organization to build standard databases and collection instruments. Therefore, most recent world health data are thought to have a higher degree of reliability and accuracy.

There are many ways to measure global health disparities. The most simplistic way to accomplish this is to simply compare causes of death among countries; another way is to compare measures of burden of disease. Given this challenge, one must take into account some determination of life expectancy to better understand why differences among nations occur. Three of the most commonly used measures of life expectancy widely seen in the literature include the following: (1) the disability-adjusted life-year (DALY), (2) the healthy life expectancy (HALE), and (3) the disability-adjusted life expectancy (DALE).[14] The DALY is used to describe life-years lost to a certain condition or risk factor, whereas the latter two terms are measures of years of life expected to be lived in full health (HALE) and in total (DALE).[14-16] The DALY is used most often to describe the impact of a certain condition on life expectancy. The HALE and DALE measures are used to compare the life expectancy of different large populations. For example, it is often used to define *health status* among the various nations of the world.

Life expectancy in the world as a whole has increased over the past century. Many factors have contributed to this increase, including advances in medicine and pharmaceuticals, improvement in environmental conditions, and health education around the world. The overall global life expectancy at birth in 1999 was 64.5 years.[15] This is an increase of almost 6 years since the same measure in 1979. Taken alone, this might appear to be a good outcome measure for global health. However, when examined by region, the health disparities that exist are extreme (Table 3-3). Public health researchers have investigated these differences and have developed strategies to eliminate the disparities by defining the risk factors and predicting the level of influence these factors have on disease state.

Global health life expectancy in 1999 was 57.8 years for women and 55.8 years for men.[14] Differences in life expectancy among regions in the world vary tremendously. Japan had the highest statistic in the world at 77.2 years for women and 71.9 years for men. In the same year, the United States was 24th with a measure of 70.0 years for men and 72.6 years for women.[17] Across the globe men have a shorter HALE than women, with a few exceptions: the largest gap between men and women was found in Russia with women at 66.4 years and men at 56.1 years of healthy life expectancy. This gap is thought to be due to a high incidence of male alcohol abuse leading to accidents, violence, and early cardiovascular disease.[14]

The 10 countries with the lowest HALE scores were all in sub-Saharan Africa, as the HIV/AIDS epidemic is most prevalent in these countries. It is estimated that life expectancy has been reduced by 15–20 years as a direct result of HIV infection, yet a few regions do not show this trend. In Northern Africa and the Middle East, men and women have very similar life expectancies. For example, Saudi Arabian men (65.1 years) and women (64.0 years) and Qatar men (64.2 years) and women (62.8 years) do not demonstrate the common global pattern of women living longer than men. This is an unusual finding; however, these countries have a higher female infant and child mortality rate and higher rates of maternal mortality compared with Europe and the Americas, both of which are thought to contribute to this finding.[14]

Defining reliable and comparable risk assessments and their effects on morbidity and mortality is a difficult task within a community, much less from a global perspective. In 2002, Ezzati

Table 3-3. Percentage of 2001 Deaths by Cause and Global Region

	High Mortality, Africa	Very Low Mortality, Americas	Very Low Mortality, Europe	High Mortality, Europe
HIV/AIDS	28.4	0.5	0.1	0.5
Colon cancer	0.2	2.7	3.5	1.7
Lung cancer	0.2	6.4	5.1	2.8
Prostate cancer	0.3	1.5	1.7	0.4
Ischemic heart disease	2.6	22.6	18.1	32.4
Hypertension	0.5	1.8	1.7	1.1
Violence	1.1	0.7	0.01	1.6
Diabetes mellitus	0.6	2.8	2.2	0.6

Adapted from: World Health Organization: *World Health Report 2002: Reducing Risks, Promoting Healthy Life,* Geneva, 2002, World Health Organization.

Table 3-4. Ten Leading Risk Factors for Global Disease Burden

Rank	Risk Factor
1	Underweight
2	Unsafe sex
3	High blood pressure
4	Tobacco
5	Alcohol
6	Unsafe water, sanitation, and hygiene
7	Cholesterol
8	Indoor smoke from solid fuels
9	Iron deficiency
10	Overweight

Adapted from: World Health Organization: *World Health Report 2002: Reducing Risks, Promoting Healthy Life,* Geneva, 2002, World Health Organization.

and colleagues attempted to outline estimates of the contributions of selected major risk factors on global disease burden.[18] This analysis was based on data from the World Health Report 2002.[15] Table 3-4 outlines the 10 leading risk factors associated with global deaths. Although the risks of hypertension, tobacco use, and high cholesterol were the primary sources of significant worldwide mortality, unsafe sex and underweight status disproportionately affected health in high-mortality developing regions. In terms of morbidity, the DALY lost attributed to unsafe sex and underweight status became the two leading causes of lost healthy life-years. Table 3-5 outlines the ranking of DALY lost by global region.

The burden of disease is also varied across countries. These differences can be attributed to a collection of common risk factors, some of which are modifiable. Blood pressure, serum cholesterol levels, overweight status, and lack of physical activity are among the leading factors that contribute to the leading causes of morbidity and mortality. In addition, the risks of unsafe sex and violence predominate the attributable risk profiles of developing regions.

Unsafe Sexual Practices

Although HIV/AIDS is not one of the top 10 causes of death in the United States, it is the fourth leading cause of death in the world. The World Health Report 2004 dedicated its entire document to define the scope of this global pandemic and offered a roadmap to changing the approach to this devastating disease.[19] Seventy percent of the 40 million people afflicted with HIV live in Africa, but the rates are rising rapidly in Eastern Europe and Asia.[20] The impact of HIV/AIDS is seen most dramatically in Africa. Specifically, life expectancy in sub-Saharan Africa, which is currently 47 years, would be an estimated 62 years without the existence of AIDS. This disease is devastating communities in this region, killing people at an early age and leaving multitudes of orphaned children in an already impoverished region on the world. Unsafe sexual practice is the primary route of transmission for HIV and accounts for 2.9 million global deaths (5.2% total deaths). The global problem of HIV/AIDS is compounded by the high cost of

Table 3-5. Rank of Burden of Disease by Risk Factor on Attributable DALY

Rank	High-mortality Developing Regions	Lower-mortality Developing Regions	Developed Regions
1	Underweight	Alcohol	Tobacco
2	Unsafe sex	High blood pressure	High blood pressure
3	Unsafe water	Tobacco	Alcohol
4	Solid fuels	Underweight	High cholesterol
5	Zinc deficiency	High BMI	High BMI
6	Iron deficiency	High cholesterol	Low fruit/vegetable intake
7	Vitamin A deficiency	Low fruit/vegetable intake	Physical inactivity
8	High blood pressure	Solid fuels	Illicit drugs
9	Tobacco	Iron deficiency	Unsafe sex
10	High cholesterol	Unsafe water	Iron deficiency

DALY, Disability-adjusted life-year; BMI, body mass index.
Adapted from: Ezzati M, Lopez AD, Rodgers A, et al, and the Comparative Risk Assessment Collaborating Group: Selected major risk factors and global and regional burden of disease, *Lancet* 360:1347–1360, 2002.

treatment for the disease, a cost many of these countries simply cannot afford.

In developed nations, HIV/AIDS is often viewed as a problem of homosexual men and intravenous drug abusers. However, in the rest of the world where the disease is one of the leading causes of death, heterosexual unprotected sexual encounters are the predominant mode of transmission. Much advocacy around homosexual men's health has produced a significant decline in the rates of these men infected with HIV. In the United States, the fastest growing populations of HIV infection are among people of color, particularly in urban underserved areas.[21] Although men who have sex with men account for 44% of new infections, African Americans and Hispanics together account for 69% of all reported HIV/AIDS cases from 2001 to 2004. This is particularly true in urban centers in the United States.[22]

This pattern mimics the epidemiology of HIV/AIDS in developing countries. Although access to highly active antiretroviral therapy to treat HIV is much more readily available in the United States, only recently have public health campaigns begun to tackle reducing the risks of transmission of HIV. Globally, controversy has existed with regard to the moralistic overtones placed on sexual health promotion and education. To combat this growing problem, public health efforts must promote safer sexual practices and encourage HIV testing among populations at risk.

Violence

Interpersonal violence is a global phenomenon that is a significant cause of morbidity and mortality for many populations. In the United States, minority populations are far more likely to experience intentional violence than their white counterparts.[15] Homicide rates also differ by region of the world, as death rates per 100,000 people in 2000 were the following: 22.2 in Africa, 19.2 in the Americas, 8.4 in Europe, and 5.8 in Southeast Asia. Although this problem was most significant in Africa, the homicide rate in the Americas was much greater than that of the rest of the world. Interestingly, this factor does not rank in the top 10 overall causes of death in the United States; yet, when examined by racial group, violence does appear as a major health concern.

Collective violence consists of war, conflict, and acts of genocide. This type of violence is difficult to measure, but in 2000 an estimated 310,000 people died as a result of collective violence, mostly in Africa and Southeast Asia.[15] As the world attempts to deal with growing terrorism and conflict in the Middle East, increased casualties as a result of war are being seen, the vast majority of which are men. The lives lost are increasing among military combatants and from the collateral damage among civilians living in the regions at war. It is expected that future World Health Reports will document a rise over the past decade in deaths due to this kind of violence.

Diet, Hypertension, Hyperlipidemia, and Obesity

Worldwide, malnutrition is one of the leading causes of death, particularly in underdeveloped and developing nations.[15] Although this is a major public health concern, it is not the primary cause for most developed nations and is therefore not the focus of many of the efforts in the United States or Europe. Dietary modification in developed countries, however, is a major concern for preventing premature death and is a major modifiable risk factor in the development of hypertension, diabetes mellitus, and obesity.

Hypertension is a major health issue in all countries affecting millions of people. The major modifiable risk factors contributing to hypertension are diet, exercise, and excessive alcohol intake. In addition to being a health issue alone, hypertension is a risk factor for many of the leading causes of death. Globally, 62% of stroke and 49% of ischemic heart disease can be attributed to elevated blood pressure.[15] Hypertension is estimated to cause 7.1 million deaths per year, representing 13% of total deaths worldwide.[15] A major focus of the Healthy People 2010 initiative is on lowering blood pressure with both lifestyle changes and increased medical treatment.

Lipid disorders are due to both environmental and genetic factors. Treatment of hypercholesterolemia is a primary health topic in the developed world and is the focus of multiple pharmaceutical industry competitive product production. This condition has a substantial impact on both heart disease and stroke risk. Elevated cholesterol levels are estimated to cause 18% of strokes and 56% of ischemic heart disease, accounting for 4.4 million or 7.9% of total deaths worldwide.[15] Although dietary changes can have a substantial impact on lowering serum cholesterol levels, medication is often required to adequately control lipid disorders and minimize cardiovascular risk.

Significant focus in recent years has been placed on the large increase in the percent of the US population that is obese. Each decade the problem expands, and recent figures suggest that this problem is in epidemic proportions in the developed world, particularly in the United States.[23] Being overweight contributes to approximately 58% of diabetes mellitus and 21% of ischemic heart disease.[15] The impact globally varies depending on the region. In Europe and the United States, this risk factor contributes to 8–15% of DALY lost, whereas it only contributes 3% in developing nations[15]; these developing regions are more likely to experience malnutrition and underweight conditions among its populations.

Even when food is not scarce, the kinds of food that people eat can contribute to poor health. Low fruit and vegetable intake has been linked to multiple disease states. Although in the developed world the lack of fresh food intake is often by choice, for many developing countries it is simply unaffordable or not available. Low intake of fresh fruits and vegetables has been linked to the development of cancers of the digestive system as well as other health conditions.[24] Nineteen percent of gastrointestinal cancers, 31% of cases of ischemic heart disease, and 11% of incidence of stroke have been attributed to poor intake of these foods. This risk accounts for 2.7 million deaths (4.9%) worldwide.[15]

The Impact of Reducing Risks

Based on the data from the World Health Report 2002, Ezzati and colleagues determined the 20 leading risk factors that contribute to the global burden of disease and leading causes of death.[25] From this data, they developed a model demonstrating the effects of elimination of these risk factors. Collectively, these risks account for 72% of lung cancers, 83–89% of ischemic heart disease, and 70–90% of strokes. This amounts to 47% of mortality and 39% of disease burden in the world. Complete removal of these risks would have a dramatic impact on global health. It is predicted that HALE would increase from 56.2 to 65.5 years if these risks were completely addressed. The impact would be large in each region of the world, although more dramatic increases in HALE would be seen in the developing countries including those in America and Europe, as they would an average of a 36% increase in HALE. By contrast, there would be a 57% increase in developing counties in Africa and a 49% increase in developing countries in Europe. Although the authors did not define the differential impact of risk reduction on men

versus women, it would be expected to have a greater impact on men. As outlined in this chapter, men have a higher incidence of and death rate from the leading causes of death in the world. Risk reduction targeted toward men, taking into account the impact of regional and cultural health concerns, should lead to overall improvement in men's health and a reduction in the gender disparities seen for men.

Conclusion

Men and women share risk factors for disease and die from the same causes. However, men tend to experience morbidity earlier in life and die younger than women from the same diseases. Within the United States, these rates vary not only between men and women, but also among cultures, geographic regions, and among racial groups. The underlying factors contributing to these disparities are many, but they have to do with barriers to access, cultural differences in health approach, and lifestyle risks. In a similar way, the worldwide burden of disease varies according to many factors; most strongly related is economic development, with developing nations having the worst outcomes in terms of healthy life expectancy. The same 20 modifiable risk factors, if eliminated, would substantially increase health in all regions of the world, even more dramatically in underdeveloped countries. Public health promotion programs should therefore be directed at regional and cultural differences in health outcomes and health behavior to focus on the biggest issues facing the population at hand.

References

1. Grumbach M: To an understanding of the biology of sex and gender differences: "an idea whose time has come," *J Men's Health Gender* 1:12–19, 2004.
2. Courtenay WH: Constructions of masculinity and their influence on men's well-being: a theory of gender and health, *Social Sci Med* 50: 1385–1401, 2000.
3. Arias E: United States life tables, 2003, *National Vital Statistics Rep* 54:1–40, 2006.
4. Hoyert DL, Heron MP, Murphy SL, Kung HC: Deaths: final data for 2003, *National Vital Statistics Rep* 54:1–120, 2006.
5. Doyal L: Sex, gender and health: the need for a new approach, *Br Med J* 323:1061–1063, 2001.
6. US Department of Health and Human Services: *Healthy people 2010: Understanding and Improving Health*, 2000, US Department of Health and Human Services, Washington, DC.

7. Williams DR, Neighbors HW, Jackson JS: Racial/ethnic discrimination and health: findings from community studies, *Am J Public Health* 93: 200–208, 2003.

8. McCord CFH: Excess mortality in Harlem, *N Engl J Med* 322:173–177, 1990.

9. Gamble V: Under the shadow of Tuskegee: African Americans and health care, *Am J Public Health* 87:1773–1778, 1997.

10. Sandman D, Simantov E: *Out of Touch: American Men and the Health Care System,* New York, 2000, The Commonwealth Fund.

11. Diaz V: Cultural factors in preventive care: Latinos, *Prim Care* 29:503–517, 2002.

12. *Profile of General Demographic Characteristics: 2000 Census of Population and Housing,* 2001, US Census Bureau. Available at http://www.census.gov/Press-Release/www/2001/tables/dp_us_2000.pdf.

13. Centers for Disease Control and Prevention: Health disparities experienced by black or African Americans—United States, *MMWR* 54:1–3, 2005.

14. Mathers CD, Sadana R, Salomon JA, Murray CJ, Lopez AD: Healthy life expectancy in 191 countries, 1999, *Lancet* 357:1685–1691, 2001.

15. World Health Organization: *World Health Report 2002: Reducing Risks, Promoting Healthy Life,* Geneva, 2002, World Health Organization.

16. Mathers CD, Iburg KM, Salomon JA, et al: Global patterns of healthy life expectancy in the year 2002, *BMC Public Health* 4:24, 2004.

17. World Health Organization: *World Health Report. Health Systems: Improving Performance,* Geneva, 2000, World Health Organization.

18. Ezzati M, Lopez AD, Rodgers A, Vander Hoorn S, Murray CJ, Comparative Risk Assessment Collaborating Group: Selected major risk factors and global and regional burden of disease, *Lancet* 360: 1347–1360, 2002.

19. World Health Organization: *World Health Report: Changing History 2004,* Geneva, 2004, World Health Organization.

20. *Report on the Global HIV/AIDS Epidemic,* Geneva, 2002, Joint United Nations Programme on HIV/AIDS.

21. Centers for Disease Control and Prevention: Racial/ethnic disparities in diagnoses of HIV/AIDS—33 states, 2001–2004, *MMWR* 55:121–125, 2006.

22. Centers for Disease Control and Prevention: The global HIV/AIDS pandemic, 2006, *MMWR* 55: 841–844, 2006.

23. Wyatt SB, Winters KP, Dubbert PM: Overweight and obesity: prevalence, consequences, and causes of a growing public health problem, *Am J Med Sci* 331:166–174, 2006.

24. World Cancer Research Fund and American Institute for Cancer Research: *Food, Nutrition and the Prevention of Cancer: a Global Perspective,* Washington, DC, 1997, American Institute for Cancer Research.

25. Ezzati M, Hoorn SV, Rodgers A, et al: Estimates of global and regional potential health gains from reducing multiple major risk factors, *Lancet* 362:271–280, 2003.

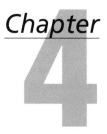

Chapter

4

Men and the Problem of Help Seeking

Alan Keith White, PhD, MSc, BSc(Hons), RN

Key Points

- Men are at an age-adjusted greater risk of premature death than women for causes that should affect men and women equally (strength of recommendation: B).
- An understanding of masculinity and the implications of male socialization helps to explain why men have a different relationship with their health and help-seeking behavior (strength of recommendation: C).
- Targeting young men to empower them to have a better understanding of their healthcare needs and how to use existing services should be considered (strength of recommendation: C).
- Perceived challenges in access to healthcare and an unwillingness to undergo what many men construe as an ordeal are significant barriers to men seeking appropriate help and proper healthcare (strength of recommendation: C).

Introduction

According to *Health, United States, 2005*, an annual publication from the National Center for Health Statistics, over 400 million visits were made to physician offices in the ambulatory care setting by men, as healthcare expenditures resulted in one of the largest proportions of the US gross national product compared with that of other nations.[1] Despite this trend, American men—as well as many men worldwide—share a common factor in that they are at a higher risk of premature death from the majority of conditions that should affect men and women equally. These data suggest that the examination of men's health as a sub-genre of medicine and separate category all its own needs to move beyond a discussion simply reflecting the numbers of men who access services; it must also consider the circumstances that influence men to seek medical care as well as what occurs when men are evaluated by medical professionals. The impetus for a broader perspective of men's healthcare stems from an increasingly recognized notion that there are many issues in the way men use healthcare services that can have profound effects not only on the health of the individual, but also on an entire nation.[2] This chapter examines these important issues and describes links to masculinity and factors inherent in men, regarding help-seeking behavior as it pertains to their pursuit of appropriate healthcare.

Epidemiology

The disparities in men's health are increasingly recognized as being problematic, with headline figures demonstrating that biologic differences between men and women should be considered, as well as variations among men from differing socioeconomic and racial backgrounds that are a cause for concern.[1] An epidemiologic study by White and Cash[3,4] examined the extent of premature death in European men and highlighted that a shorter life expectancy in males was not only limited to accidents and coronary heart disease, but also that men were dying sooner from

Table 4-1. Comparison of the Ratio of Total Deaths of Men to Women Across Major Disease Classification Groups at Ages 1–24 Years, 25–74 Years, and 75+ Years

	1–24 Years	25–74 Years	75+ Years
Mental and behavioral disorders	4.2	2.8	0.4
External causes of injury and poisoning	3.4	3.1	0.7
Symptoms, signs, abnormal findings, ill-defined causes	2.7	2.5	0.4
Total of all causes of death	2.4	1.8	0.7
Diseases of the genitourinary system	2.1	1.4	0.8
Diseases of the nervous system and the sense organs	1.7	1.3	0.6
Diseases of the digestive system	1.6	2.0	0.6
Diseases of the blood-forming organs, immunologic disorders	1.6	1.8	0.6
Diseases of the circulatory system	1.6	2.1	0.6
Infectious and parasitic diseases	1.5	2.0	0.6
Diseases of the respiratory system	1.4	2.0	0.9
Neoplasms	1.4	1.6	1.0
Congenital malformations and chromosomal abnormalities	1.3	1.1	0.7
Endocrine, nutritional, and metabolic diseases	1.2	1.3	0.5
Diseases of the musculoskeletal system/connective tissue	0.7	0.7	0.3
Diseases of the skin and subcutaneous tissue	0.0	0.9	0.4

Adapted from: White A, Cash K: *The state of men's health in 17 European countries,* Brussels, 2003, European Men's Health Forum.

the majority of conditions that should have affected men and women equally at the same age (Table 4-1).

A more recent epidemiologic study[5] explored mortality patterns across 44 countries for both men and women aged 15–44 years. Within this study, which used data from the World Health Organization Mortality Database,[6] six main causes of death were highlighted within the analysis:

- Accidents and adverse effects
- Suicide and self-inflicted injury
- Diseases of the cardiovascular system
- Malignant neoplasms
- Chronic liver disease and cirrhosis
- Homicide and injury purposely inflicted by other persons

Among persons in the age ranges of 15–24 and 25–34 years across the majority of countries, the highest rates of mortality were as a result of non-disease causes, including accidents, adverse effects, and suicide, with a rapid increase observed in the 35–44-year age group in disease-related deaths.[5]

When data specific for US males were examined for persons in the 15–24 and 25–34-year age groups, a similar trend was observed in that non-disease processes predominate; the highest mortality rates were as a result of accidents and adverse effects, suicide, and homicide (Figure 4-1). In the 35–44-year age group, there was a rapid increase in the number of deaths as a result of cardiovascular disease, neoplasms, and chronic liver disease and cirrhosis.[4] In comparison with women, a similar pattern was observed in that there is an increase in the mortality as a result of disease processes in the 35–44-year age groups, specifically that of malignant neoplasms (Figure 4-2). The mortality rate in men in the 35–44-year age groups as a result of malignant cancer was 32.9 per 100,000, whereas the mortality rate for women including gender-specific cancers was 40.9 per 100,000.[5] If the gender-specific cancers were excluded from these figures, there is almost no observable change for men due to the very low level of male-specific cancers prevalent at these age groups, yet there was a significant decrease to 24.3 cases per 100,000 for women. These data suggest that men are succumbing to a greater number of non–gender-specific cancers that should affect both men and women equally in these age groups.* These data also suggest that there may be significant health problems developing in these earlier age groups in men that attribute to increased

---

* This represents additional analysis of the data from the Patterns of Mortality study.

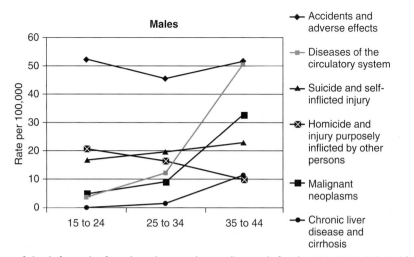

Figure 4-1. Rates of death for males for selected causes, by age (in years), for the USA, 2000. (Adapted from: White A, Holmes M: Patterns of mortality across 44 countries among men and women aged 15–44, *J Men's Health Gender* 3[2]:139–141, 2006.)

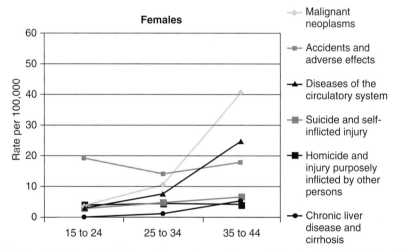

Figure 4-2. Rates of death for females for selected causes, by age (in years), for the USA, 2000. (Adapted from: White A, Holmes M: Patterns of mortality across 44 countries among men and women aged 15–44, *J Men's Health Gender* 3[2]:139–141, 2006.)

mortality rates, and although the etiology of these problems may be related to lifestyle factors (e.g., cigarette smoking and other risk-taking behaviors), the lack of use of healthcare services may play a role leading to this disparity in premature mortality rates in men.

Years of Life Lost

The impact of premature mortality in males is best illustrated when one considers the number of years of life lost for each individual male as a result of premature deaths compared with the total number of deaths. Years of life lost are calculated by determining the difference between the age of death and a set time period. For example, if a boy dies at age of 15 years as a result of suicide and the current average life expectancy is 75 years of age, then he has lost 60 years of life prematurely. Data from the National Center for Health Statistics from 2003 reveal that when examining years of life lost for various causes in men compared with women up to the age of 75 years, men have a significantly higher

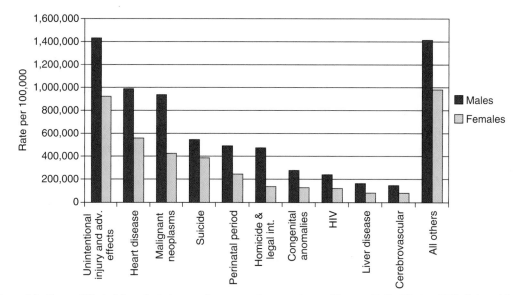

Figure 4-3. Years of life lost for selected causes for men and women to age 75 years, United States, 2003. (Adapted from: National Center for Health Statistics: *Health, United States, 2005: With Chartbook on Trends in the Health of Americans,* Hyattsville, Md, 2005, National Center for Health Statistics. Available at: http://www.cdc.gov/nchs/hus.htm.)

number of years of life lost for every category (Figure 4-3).[1]

Men's Use of Healthcare Services

When data pertaining to men's current use of health services are closely examined, it is evident that there are still many questions that need to be answered regarding how and when men use available healthcare provisions. However, exploration of current statistics does provide some interesting insight. Across the lifespan, there is little difference between men and women with regard to the distribution of ambulatory visits by primary diagnosis (Table 4-2). With the exception of the approximately 5.5% of female visits attributed to normal pregnancy and routine gynecologic examinations, the majority of diagnostic conditions fall within a 1–2-percentage-point range of similarity in total visits between the sexes. However, these age-standardized data mask variations that occur across the lifespan, as the analysis undertaken by White and Cash[3,4] suggests that the problem of the increased premature mortality rate in men is a feature of men's seemingly increased susceptibility to problems across the disease spectrum at an earlier age (see Table 4-1).

Men's use of healthcare services varies considerably with age, as boys younger than 18 years have similar if not greater access to services than girls, yet once they move beyond this age, the data reflect service use that is significantly lower than that for women until the age of 75 years (Figure 4-4). It was once thought that women overuse healthcare services and that similar use by men was an appropriate amount, but now it seems reasonable to conclude that it is men who underuse available healthcare resources.[7]

The increase in use of healthcare provisions for women in the 18–44-year age group has been attributed to their peak years of reproductive health, yet it is also notable that women have a higher consumption of prescription medications (Figures 4-5 and 4-6). When specific data on prescription trends are explored comparing men and women aged 18–44 years, women have been found to have a higher rate of prescription use for every category of medication surveyed, despite a proven higher incidence of premature mortality in men (Figure 4-7). Examination of prescription trends in the 45–64-year age group again reveals a higher use rate for women than for men for the majority of medication classifications (Figure 4-8). Exceptions to this trend in the older age group include anti-hyperlipidemic agents, angiotensin-converting enzyme inhibitors, and non-narcotic analgesics.

Table 4-2. Percent Distribution of Office Visits, by Selected Primary Diagnosis Groups, According to Patient Sex, United States, 2002

	Male[*]	Female[†]
Essential hypertension	5.4%	5.4%
Routine infant or child health check	5.2%	3.2%
Acute upper respiratory infections, excluding pharyngitis	3.7%	3.1%
Diabetes mellitus	3.5%	2.3%
Arthropathies and related disorders	2.4%	2.8%
General medical examination	2.6%	2.5%
Spinal disorders	2.3%	2.3%
Rheumatism, excluding back	2.1%	1.9%
Normal pregnancy	N/A	3.3%
Otitis media and eustachian tube disorders	2.2%	1.6%
Malignant neoplasms	2.1%	1.5%
Chronic sinusitis	1.6%	1.6%
Allergic rhinitis	1.4%	1.7%
Asthma	1.3%	1.5%
Gynecologic examination	N/A	2.2%
Disorder of lipoid metabolism	1.6%	1.1%
Heart disease, excluding ischemic	1.5%	1.2%
Ischemic heart disease	1.9%	0.8%
Acute pharyngitis	1.2%	1.1%
Follow-up examination	1.2%	1.0%
All other diagnoses	56.5%	57.7%

NOTE: Numbers may not add to 100% due to rounding.
*Based on 360,905,000 visits made by males.
†Based on 529,075,000 visits made by females.
N/A, Not applicable.
Adapted from: Woodwell DA, Cherry DK: National Ambulatory Medical Care Survey (NAMCS): 2002 summary. National Center for Health Statistics. Available at: http://www.cdc.gov/nchs/about/major/ahcd/ahcd1.htm.

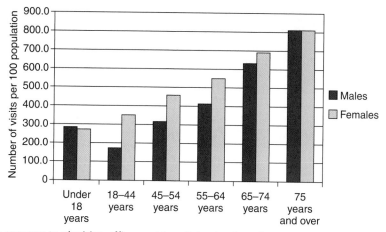

Figure 4-4. Visits per year to physician offices and hospital outpatient departments by sex and age, United States, 2003. (Adapted from: National Center for Health Statistics: *Health, United States, 2005: With Chartbook on Trends in the Health of Americans,* Hyattsville, Md, 2005, National Center for Health Statistics. Available at: http://www.cdc.gov/nchs/hus.htm.)

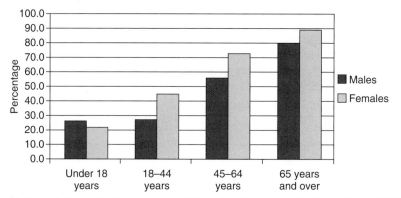

Figure 4-5. Percent of population with at least one prescription drug in past month, United States, 2003. (Adapted from: National Center for Health Statistics: *Health, United States, 2005: With Chartbook on Trends in the Health of Americans,* Hyattsville, Md, 2005, National Center for Health Statistics. Available at: http://www.cdc.gov/nchs/hus.htm.)

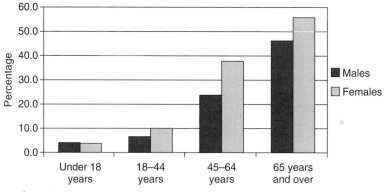

Figure 4-6. Percent of population with three or more prescription drugs in past month, United States, 2003. (Adapted from: National Center for Health Statistics: *Health, United States, 2005: With Chartbook on Trends in the Health of Americans,* Hyattsville, Md, 2005, National Center for Health Statistics. Available at: http://www.cdc.gov/nchs/hus.htm.)

Women are more likely to receive preventive healthcare services from primary care specialists than age-matched control subjects in men older than 15 years of age (Figure 4-9). These data include multiple visits for antenatal care in the peak years of female fertility between 15 and 44 years, but even after these data are subtracted, the rate of visits for preventive healthcare remains much higher for women than for men (54.8 visits per 100 females per year compared with 34.6 visits per 100 males per year).[8] This trend is compounded by the fact that there is a much larger percentage of men who have admitted to having no regular and definable access to healthcare (21.8 % of men compared with 11.6% of women).[1] Thus, it is not surprising that when men are admitted to hospitals they are more likely to require a longer length of stay compared with women, although these data suggest that this

trend is largely attributable to recovery from serious accidents and human immunodeficiency virus (HIV) infection and its resultant complications (Figure 4-10). It has also been assumed that if men are not using their primary care physicians for their routine healthcare needs, then they will generally access healthcare via the emergency department. This belief has also been proved to be incorrect, in that 21.8% of women compared with 18.2% of men visited the emergency department one or more times over the course of 2003 and 8.4% women compared with 5.6% of men for two or more visits over the same time period.[1]

Links to Masculinity

Men's apparent underuse of healthcare services can be attributed to many suggested causes, but there is still a dearth of research that has

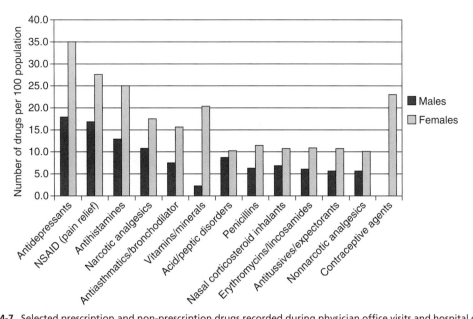

Figure 4-7. Selected prescription and non-prescription drugs recorded during physician office visits and hospital outpatient department visits, for men and women aged 18–44 years, United States, 2002–2003. NSAID, Nonsteroidal anti-inflammatory drug. (Adapted from: National Center for Health Statistics: *Health, United States, 2005: With Chartbook on Trends in the Health of Americans,* Hyattsville, Md, 2005, National Center for Health Statistics. Available at: http://www.cdc.gov/nchs/hus.htm.)

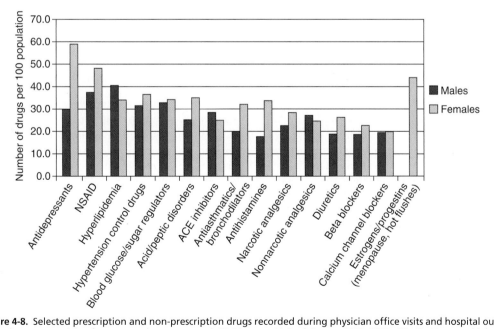

Figure 4-8. Selected prescription and non-prescription drugs recorded during physician office visits and hospital outpatient department visits, for men and women aged 45–64 years, United States, 2002–2003. NSAID, Nonsteroidal anti-inflammatory drug; ACE, angiotensin-converting enzyme. (Adapted from: National Center for Health Statistics: *Health, United States, 2005: With Chartbook on Trends in the Health of Americans,* Hyattsville, Md, 2005, National Center for Health Statistics. Available at: http://www.cdc.gov/nchs/hus.htm.)

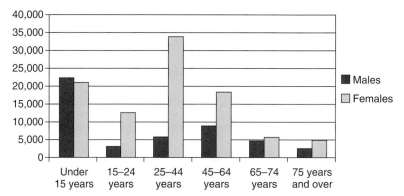

Figure 4-9. Number of preventive care office visits, United States, 2002. (Adapted from: Woodwell DA, Cherry DK: National Ambulatory Medical Care Survey [NAMCS]: 2002 summary. National Center for Health Statistics. Available at: http://www.cdc.gov/nchs/about/major/ahcd/ahcd1.htm.)

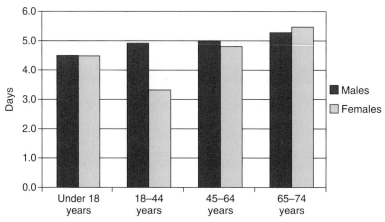

Figure 4-10. Average length of stay in non-federal short-stay hospitals, according to sex, United States, 2003. (Adapted from: National Center for Health Statistics: *Health, United States, 2005: With Chartbook on Trends in the Health of Americans,* Hyattsville, Md, 2005, National Center for Health Statistics. Available at: http://www.cdc.gov/nchs/hus.htm.)

adequately explored this issue. It is possible, however, to see explanations in both the way men are socialized into managing their healthcare as well as structural issues in relation to the availability of the services to men that make the physical act of seeking healthcare problematic.

The personal issues men face with regard to the social expectations relating to their health and healthcare they seek and receive can be more easily labeled as the impact of their masculinity. Although the term *masculinity* has now been recognized as being more of a composite of many different forms of roles and expectations placed on men today and is now commonly referred to as *masculinities*,[9] it is still a useful starting point when examining men and help-seeking behavior. From birth, it is often seen that the social pressures placed on boys are different from those placed on girls, with a differing tolerance being given to the manner in which boys and girls respond to various physical and emotional challenges. The old adage "big boys don't cry" is a typical and almost universal signifier of how we expect boys to meet the challenges they face and to react in a stereotypical fashion of not engaging help.

Although there has been a significant devotion to the research of masculinity, it is only within the last 10 years that research has started to focus on the health consequences of men's expected roles within our society.[10] The completed work to date suggests that the differing use of healthcare services between men and women is not surprising; however, this is not an excuse for accepting it as inevitable. Research has shown that men have been found to admit to caring about their health, yet it is the specific management of routine healthcare and disease that makes this problematic, and that when services are made more "male friendly" then the response rate is more favorable. It is wrong for healthcare providers to assume that all men are poor at obtaining and using healthcare services; this is patently untrue, and the timely and appropriate use of services is certainly encountered for many men. Men have the capacity to adapt their help-seeking behavior in response to changing circumstances, yet it is also apparent that many men do not use available healthcare services in an appropriate or timely fashion. It is this particular issue on which those clinicians interested in men's healthcare and its inherent disparities should focus their attention. Current research on men and help-seeking behavior has taken a number of different forms, as addressed below.

Men and Help Seeking

Current research and literature reviews pertaining to men and help-seeking behavior suggest that this is a key area of concern pertaining to men and their overall health.[11–15] Male socialization, which militates against showing vulnerability and an inability to cope, coupled with problems in accessing healthcare services, creates significant problems for men in knowing when and how to access appropriate assistance. In 2001, White[16] conducted a scoping study on men's health for the past Public Health Minister for the United Kingdom. This review was conducted over an intensive 4-week period involving all of the key national stakeholders who were deemed to have an opinion on men's health, with the chief goal of exploring the "scope" of the problem of men and their health. Four key areas emerged as being central to the discussion on the factors influencing men and their health:

- Access to health services
- Lack of awareness of their health needs
- Inability to express their emotions
- Lack of social networks

Although all of these factors are interlinked, the issue of men accessing healthcare services has been seen as a principal cause for concern in this study, with the survey respondents noting the following as key factors in men's unwillingness to attend to their healthcare:

- A lack of understanding of the processes of making appointments and negotiating with female receptionists

- Inappropriate office-opening times, which tend to coincide and conflict with work commitments
- An unwillingness to wait for appointments
- A feeling that the service is primarily for women and children, and that sitting in the waiting room is uncomfortable for them
- The name "health centre" identified as problematic
- The negative response many men feel they get when presenting with difficulties that are not quickly dealt with
- A lack of trust in the healthcare system, mainly around the issue of confidentiality, especially within the gay community and regarding disclosure of HIV status
- Great fears relating to shame if their concerns are judged to be of little consequence, or having to admit to another person that they may have a problem, namely one that they cannot solve themselves
- Lacking the vocabulary they feel necessary to discuss issues of a sensitive nature, with the result that it is easier to go to the doctor with a non-embarrassing physical illness than when depressed or faced with the symptoms of, for example, colorectal cancer or erectile dysfunction

As a result, it seems that there are two main barriers regarding men and help seeking—that of perceived challenges in access to healthcare and that of an unwillingness to undergo what many men construe as an ordeal. The latter issue relates to the threat of a man submitting to either a personal failing and loss of control over a situation or the fear of what may be discovered in a medical setting related to his health.[17]

Courtenay's[7] observations on what it means to be a "proper man" provide an insight into the pressures that men fall under when they consider the impact posed by a threat to their health or independence:

> In exhibiting or enacting hegemonic ideals with health behaviors, men reinforce strongly held cultural beliefs that men are more powerful and less vulnerable than women; that men's bodies are structurally more efficient than and superior to women's bodies; that asking for help and caring for one's health are feminine; and that the most powerful men among men are those for whom health and safety are irrelevant.

Although this quotation may be seen as an extreme version of manhood, there is an apparent social pressure on men to be reluctant to seek help of any kind and in any situation, to be in control, and to not to take time off from work such that the "Patriarchal Dividend" can be seen to be a burden as well as an advantage to men.[18]

Nevertheless, although the majority of research suggests that men delay seeking help from healthcare services, there are some studies that seem to refute the idea that men and women differ in their access to necessary healthcare. Macintyre and colleagues,[19] in a review of the West of Scotland Twenty - 07 Study, found no concrete evidence that men were less willing to report health-related symptoms or to seek healthcare, and that there was no difference in the degree of suffering that men in comparison to women experienced before seeking help. Reviewing the same data set, Wyke and colleagues[20] presented the respondents with a check list of 33 symptoms of minor illness and asked whether they had at any time over the previous month experienced any of the inherent symptoms and whether they had consulted a general practitioner. The researchers found that although women were more likely to have consulted a general practitioner for at least one of the symptoms, there was no difference in consultation rates when only those who had reported symptoms within the last month were included in the analysis, suggesting that men and women seem to respond in a similar fashion to the experience of symptoms. Similarly, Adamson and colleagues[21] found no significant difference between men and women in the likelihood of either group seeking healthcare advice, based on socioeconomic and ethnic background.

Another key factor in men and help seeking is in relation to the structural constraints under which men find themselves.[22] An analysis of current healthcare provisions in many countries reveals that the majority are female and child oriented, with services predominantly provided during the daytime, when it is acknowledged that a higher proportion of men work full-time, have less opportunity for flexible schedules, and are often in precarious employment where taking time off for healthcare visits may be perceived as a sign of vulnerability, not only by the men themselves but also by their peers and/or employers.[16] Another structural issue with a significant impact on men's use of healthcare services relates to the overall cost of healthcare, a well-recognized barrier within predominantly insurance-based healthcare systems. Royster and colleagues[23] conducted an epidemiologic study that detailed the experiences of African American men, suggesting that they felt excluded from mainstream healthcare services as a result of their race and economic status, highlighting the concern that different cross-sections of society may not able to derive similar benefits from the same healthcare system. Certain men have precarious personal circumstances and may be homeless,[24] asylum seekers,[25] or illegal immigrants,[26] and these persons carry an additional burden of increased health risk as well as an unfortunately minimized opportunity to gain medical assistance unless specific provisions are provided for them.

A further angle to the challenges of men and help seeking that should also be explored is the male patient-physician relationship during a consultation. Studies that have explored this area have suggested a profound difference between the conversations male and female physicians have with their male patients and in regard to the type of conversations men initiate compared with female patients,[27] with the suggestion being that practitioners should be aware of their own communication skills in managing the care of male patients. This may simply require the clinician to recognize that the path men have chosen to seek help may have been more tortuous compared with that of female patients, and that men may not be as articulate in either recognizing or describing what is ailing them. As will be discussed, this can be a significant barrier with regard to problems with men's mental health.

Men and Help Seeking With Physical Illness

From adolescence through early adulthood, many women obtain healthcare services for contraception and antenatal- or child-related reasons, and as such have an early introduction to the healthcare service model as a place of "health delivery" and "health promotion" as well as ill-health treatment. Women are also invited to see healthcare practitioners earlier in their lives on a more regular basis as a result of formal cervical and breast cancer screening programs, yet there are few formal reasons for men to attend in the same way.

The impressions of an unchanging nature of men's bodies throughout their early years of adulthood further influence their relationship with healthcare services. With neither monthly hormonal changes nor childbearing function, the male body can often remain in relative biophysical homeostasis for decades after adolescence, with a large majority of health problems being acquired as a result of external factors, including preventable habits such as cigarette smoking, alcohol consumption and illicit drug use, sedentary lifestyle, and poor diet leading to weight gain and decreased metabolism, accidents, and infection.

Research examining male views on accessing healthcare services suggests that there is a reluctance to "bother the doctor" with problems that may be identified as trivial. Men also report that their doctor is a person whom one visits when one is feeling physically unwell. This belief, therefore, requires a man to be able to discern whether his signs or symptoms are in fact as a result of a disease process.[2,28] Even when a man's healthcare problems are thought to be extreme, it is not necessarily in a straightforward fashion that men will seek healthcare. White and Johnson[17] examined male responses to chest pain: within this cohort, there were a number of men who were able to attribute their pain to other non-cardiac causes, even when they were experiencing what they described as the worst pain they had ever felt. The fact that more women than men report skin cancer yet more men die from this condition strongly suggests that women are reporting the disease in its earlier stages and therefore have a greater chance of a full recovery.[29]

With regard to sexual health, there is an obvious need for men to access healthcare services for screening, as the number of men who develop sexually transmitted diseases is increasing. Forrest[30] and Marcell and colleagues[31] both found men to be very reluctant users of sexual healthcare services, in part as a result of men's general avoidance of health-seeking behavior, but also as a direct result of fear of what might be found and the potential for negative judgments or lack of confidentiality. With regard to testicular cancer, the incidence is rising, yet the total number of deaths is miniscule in proportion to other etiologies of male mortality. The advances in curative therapies may suggest that those men who do die probably do so as a result of delay in seeking help.

Many men, despite the wide increase in publicity over the last 5–10 years regarding prostate cancer, still have little understanding of the prostate gland and what symptoms herald problems either as a result of benign enlargement or cancer. Practitioners still encounter men dismissing potential serious and life-threatening problems to advancing age rather than seeking a definitive diagnosis, which leaves them more vulnerable to advanced disease, a delay in diagnosis, and opportunities to undergo various potential treatment options.[32]

Men and Help Seeking With Emotional Issues

The early research of Padesky and Hammen[33] identified that men were less likely to seek professional help to address and discuss their depressive symptoms than women. More recently, Möller-Leimkühler[34] identified this problem as being a discrepancy of need, both in recognizing men's symptoms as requiring health advice and also in terms of the possible consequences of seeking help with the fear of loss of status, loss of control and autonomy, incompetence, dependence, and potential damage of identity. These are important points to make clear because the minority of men who actually enter psychotherapy are often very willing to engage with the process. Therefore, it cannot be appropriately stated that men are unable to benefit from therapy; rather, it is more a problem of getting them integrated into the services in the first place.[35]

The issue of men being less likely to seek help regarding psychosocial problems is compounded by the possibility that, for many men, the way in which their mental health difficulties emerge are different from those experienced by women. Brownhill and colleagues[36] suggest that the current diagnosis of depression is based on the female presentation of signs and symptoms and that for men the presentation is more covert, with men overcompensating for their loss of control leading to overworking or violence or maladjusted behavior either toward themselves or others. The reason this phenomenon occurs requires an exploration of how men are socialized as children and ultimately trained to deal with their mental well-being.

Studies on young men at school[37,38] highlight that discussing their emotions, feelings, and relationship issues are frowned upon by boys and construed as being a female-orientated occupation. Being viewed as overly concerned with emotional issues results in sanctions from others from the peer group, resulting in bullying, name calling, chastising, and physical abuse, all used to make the boy recognize his "wayward" activity. This negative social pressure is also seen to act against boys and men who wish to lead any form of alternative lifestyle to the mainstream, with young gay men especially often experiencing anxiety and depression. Missing out on this formative time for developing a vocabulary and introspection about their feelings (an emotional literacy) may explain why men are thought to be at a higher risk of emotional difficulties in their adolescence and adult life, adding to their reluctance to seek healthcare support.[39] The most tragic consequence of this could be directly related to high rates of suicide in men, with similar patterns of mortality seen across many nations.[5]

This lack of early socializing in men is compounded by the perceived social stigma of being identified as having a "mental health" illness and for some a distrust of the healthcare services themselves.[40,41] The very term *counseling* can have negative implications for men with a fear of having to acknowledge vulnerability creating a significant barrier to accepting many forms of psychotherapy.[42] It is interesting to note, however, that as men become more aware of their health this reluctance may be reducing[43]; despite this notion, the majority of men have to be persuaded to seek help with their emotional problems.[44]

When men often present with emotional health problems, it is in the form of a physical symptom. For example, if a man's partner leaves him, he may develop financial problems, he may become angry and frustrated and develop clear problems with anxiety management, but only when he develops either headaches or stomach problems does he present to the doctor. This somatization of emotional health problems can then result in medical treatment of a symptom rather than dealing with the root cause of the problem, as pertinent information regarding the actual stressor may be withheld from the inquiring physician.[40]

Conclusion

Throughout the panoply of illnesses that can affect men, there are examples of delay that can only be minimized to an inability, for various reasons, to poorly use available healthcare services. What we do know from current research is that the vast majority of men do care about their health, and it is therefore imperative, if there are barriers in place as a result of male socialization or due to structural constraints that prevent men from accessing healthcare in an appropriate and timely manner, that they be appropriately minimized.

When we search for solutions on how to improve men's response time to problems and to achieve a better use of healthcare services, we have to tackle some fundamental issues. Parents, schools, and others responsible for the early social development of boys must have a greater awareness of the impact of negative messages relating to physical and emotional well-being. Healthcare providers at all levels must look to their own provision and identify how welcoming and supportive they can be toward their male patients in an effort to eliminate any potential barriers and allow men to access and achieve their desired and deserved healthcare benefits.

References

1. National Center for Health Statistics: *Health, United States, 2005: With Chartbook on Trends in the Health of Americans,* Hyattsville, Md, 2005, National Center for Health Statistics. Available at: http://www.cdc.gov/nchs/hus.htm. Accessed June 6, 2006.
2. Bonhomme J: Cultural and attitudinal barriers to men's participation in the health care system. Presented at the 2nd World Congress on Men's Health, University of Vienna, October 27–29, 2002.
3. White AK, Cash K: *The State of Men's Health Across 17 European Countries,* Brussels, 2003, The European Men's Health Forum.
4. White AK, Cash K: The state of men's health in Western Europe, *J Men Health Gender* 1(1):60–66, 2004.
5. White AK, Holmes M: Patterns of mortality across 44 countries among men and women aged 15–44, *J Men Health Gender* 3(2):139–141, 2006.
6. The World Health Organization: The World Health Organization Statistical Information Service Mortality Database. 2005. Available at: http://www3.who.int/whosis/menu.cfm?path=whosis&language=english.
7. Courtenay WH: Constructions of masculinity and their influence on men's well-being: a theory of gender and health, *Soc Sci Med* 50(10):1385–1401, 2000.
8. Woodwell DA, Cherry DK: National Ambulatory Medical Care Survey (NAMCS): 2002 National Center for Health Statistics. Available at: http://www.cdc.gov/nchs/about/major/ahcd/ahcd1.htm.
9. Connell RW: *Masculinities,* Oxford, 1995, Polity Press.
10. White AK: Men's health in the 21st century, *Int J Men's Health* 5(1):1–17, 2006.
11. Addis M, Mahalik JR: Men, masculinity, and the contexts of help seeking, *Am Psychol* 58(1):5–14, 2003.
12. Davies J, McCrae BP, Frank J, et al: Identifying male college students' perceived health needs, barriers to seeking help, and recommendations to help men adopt healthier lifestyles, *J Am Coll Health* 48:259–267, 2000.
13. Mansfield AK, Addis ME, Mahalik JR: "Why won't he go to the doctor?": the psychology of men's help seeking, *Int J Men's Health* 2(2):93–109, 2003.
14. O'Brien RK, Hunt K, Hart G: "It's caveman stuff, but that is to a certain extent how guys still operate": men's accounts of masculinity and help seeking, *Soc Sci Med* 61:503–516, 2005.
15. Galdas P, Cheater MF, Marshall P: Men and health help-seeking behaviour: literature review, *J Adv Nurs* 49(6):616–623, 2005.
16. White AK: *Report on the Scoping Study on Men's Health,* London, 2001, The Department of Health.
17. White AK, Johnson M: Men making sense of their chest pain—niggles, doubts and denials, *J Clin Nurs* 9(4):534–541, 2000.

18. White AK, Fawkner H, Holmes M: The health of men and women: a case for differential treatment? (Health Policy – Viewpoint), *Med J Aust* 185(8): 454–455, 2006.
19. Macintyre S, Ford G, Hunt K: Do women 'over-report' morbidity? Men's and women's responses to structured prompting on a standard question on long standing illness, *Soc Sci Med* 48:89–98, 1999.
20. Wyke SK, Hunt K, Ford G: Gender differences in consulting a general practitioner for common symptoms of minor illness, *Soc Sci Med* 46(7): 901–906, 1998.
21. Adamson J, Ben-Shlomo Y, Chaturvedi N, et al: Ethnicity, socio-economic position and gender—do they affect reported health-care seeking behaviour? *Soc Sci Med* 57:895–904, 2003.
22. Banks I: No man's land: men, illness and the NHS, *Br Med J* 323(7320):1056–1060, 2001.
23. Royster M, Richmond A, Eng E, et al: Hey brother, how's your health? A focus group analysis of the health and health-related concerns of African American men in a southern city in the United States, *Men Masculinities* 8(4):389–390, 2006.
24. Brush BL, Powers EM: Health and service utilization patterns among homeless men in transition: exploring the need for on-site, shelter based nursing care, *Schol Inq Nurs Pract* 15(2):143–154, 2001.
25. Harris MF, Telfer BL: The health needs of asylum seekers living in the community, *Med J Aust* 175:589–592, 2001.
26. Torresa A, Sanz B: Health care provision for illegal immigrants: should public health be concerned? *J Epidemiol Commun Health* 54:478–479, 2000.
27. Kiss AJ: Does gender have an influence on the patient-physician communication? *J Mens Health Gender* 1(1):77–82, 2004.
28. Richardson C, Rabiee F: A question of access: an exploration of the factors that influence the health of young males aged 15–19 living in Corby and their use of the health service, *Health Educ J* 60(1): 3–16, 2001.
29. White A, Banks I: Help-seeking in men and the problems of late diagnosis, In Kirby R, et al., editors: *Men's Health*, London, 2004, Martin Dunitz & Parthenon Publishing, pp 1–7.
30. Forrest K: Men's reproductive and sexual health, *J Am Coll Health* 49(6):253–266, 2001.
31. Marcell A, Raine T, Eyre S: Where does reproductive health fit into the lives of adolescent males? *Perspect Sex Reprod Health* 35(4):180–186, 2003.
32. Kelsey S, White A, Julie O: The experience of radiotherapy for localised prostate cancer: the men's perspective, *Eur J Cancer Care* 13:272–278, 2004.
33. Padesky C, Hammen C: Sex differences in depressive symptom expression and help-seeking among college students, *Sex Roles* 7(3):309–319, 1981.
34. Möller-Leimkühler AM: Barriers to help seeking by men: a review of sociocultural and clinical literature with particular reference to depression, *J Affect Dis* 71:1–9, 2002.
35. Emslie C, Ridge D, Ziebland S, et al: Men's accounts of depression: reconstructing or resisting hegemonic masculinity? *Soc Sci Med* 62:2246–2257, 2006.
36. Brownhill S, Wilhelm K, Barclay L, et al: "Big build": hidden depression in men, *Aust N Z J Psychiatry* 39:921–931, 2005.
37. Frosh S, Phoenix A, Pattman R: *Young Masculinities: Understanding Boys in Contemporary Society*, Houndmills, Basingstock, UK, 2002, Palgrave.
38. Mac an Ghaill M: *The Making of Men: Masculinities, Sexualities and Schooling*, Buckingham, UK, 1994, Open University Press.
39. White AK: Men and mental wellbeing: encouraging gender sensitivity. Personal perspective, *Ment Heath Rev J* 11(4):3–6, 2006.
40. Whaley A: Ethnicity/race, paranoia, and hospitalization for mental health problems among men, *Am J Public Health* 95:78–81, 2004.
41. Miller A: Men's experience of considering counselling: "entering the unknown." *Couns Psychother Res* 3(1):16–24, 2003.
42. Lee C, Owens RG. *The Psychology of Men's Health*. Buckingham, 2002, Open University Press.
43. McCarthy J, Holliday E: Help-seeking and counselling within a traditional male gender role: an examination from a multicultural perspective, *J Counsel Dev* 82:25–30, 2004.
44. Cusack J, Deane FP, Wilson CJ, et al: Who influence men to go to therapy? Reports from men attending psychological services, *Int J Adv Counsel* 26 (3):271–283, 2004.

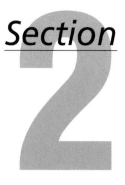

Section

2

The Developing Male

The Newborn/Infant Male

Grant Greenberg, MD, MA, David Serlin, MD

Key Points

- There is no significant difference in efficacy between surgical and hormonal treatments for cryptorchidism (strength of recommendation: B).
- Neonatal circumcision reduces the risk for urinary tract infections (strength of recommendation: A), sexually transmitted disease transmission (strength of recommendation: B), and HIV transmission (strength of recommendation: C).
- Analgesia for circumcision is safe, effective, and beneficial to the infant (strength of recommendation: A).

Introduction

The medical care of a newborn male infant poses several unique care considerations. Although the number of conditions of concern in the neonatal period are limited, early recognition and treatment are essential to improve long-term outcomes. Specific considerations include inherited conditions that may manifest in the neonatal period, anatomic abnormalities, and elective neonatal circumcision.

Behavioral Considerations

The newborn period is one of great adjustment for parents, family members, and the infant himself. One of the challenges is an expectation of behavioral differences between male and female infants. This is driven by cultural factors that likely influence the perception of a difference in gender. There have been attempts to demonstrate innate behavioral and physiologic differences between male and female infants, but these have yielded inconsistent and inconclusive findings. For example, a common perception is that male infants have greater motor activity than females. This is perception stems from casual observation that male infants have more vigorous motor activity; however, there is no clear evidence of a quantitative difference.[1] As an example from a physiologic perspective, no difference has been discovered between male and female infants in response to external stimuli such as music.[2] Despite studies such as these, there is a persistent belief in physiologic and behavioral differences that, even if present, are not likely to be of any clinical significance such as differences in metabolism, sleep patterns, and perceived constitution.

Inherited Metabolic Disorders with Expression in the Neonatal Period

There are numerous rare inherited, X-linked genetic disorders that can affect the male infant (Table 5-1). Many of these disorders have either subtle or delayed expression and do not typically affect care during the immediate neonatal period. The conditions of greatest immediate physiologic concern include hemophilia, Fabry's disease (i.e., alpha-galactosidase A deficiency resulting in impaired lipid metabolism), glucose-6-phosphate dehydrogenase deficiency, and those with obvious anatomic manifestations such as fragile X syndrome (i.e., mutation in the *FMR1* gene on the X chromosome), Wiskott-Aldrich syndrome

Table 5-1. X-Linked Inherited Disorders

Disorder	Incidence in Males
Autosomal Dominant	
Coffin-Lowry syndrome	<1:200,000
Familial rickets	0.2/1000
Hereditary nephritis	>1:1000
Incontinentia pigmenti	<1:200,000
Autosomal Recessive	
Androgen insensitivity syndrome	<1:200,000
Becker muscular dystrophy	3–6:100,000
Deuteranopia	1% in Caucasians
Duchenne's muscular dystrophy	1:6000
Fabry's disease	1:50,000
Fragile X syndrome	1:2,000
Glucose-6-phosphate dehydrogenase (G6PD) deficiency	2–28% Africans
	11% African Americans
	2–6% Asians
	4–19% Indians
	2–35% Greeks/ Sardinians
Hemophilia	1:5,000
Menkes disease (kinky hair disease)	4.9:1,000,000
Progressive spinobulbar muscular atrophy	0.19:100,000
Protanopia	1.5%
Red-green color blindness	5–8%
Wiskott-Aldrich syndrome	<1:200,000
X-linked agammaglobulinemia	1:10,000

Incidence data adapted from: Medline Plus. Available at: http://www.nlm.nih.gov/medlineplus/encyclopedia.html.

(i.e., immunodeficiency disorder with insufficient immunoglobulin M production and often thrombocytopenia), and Coffin-Lowry syndrome (i.e., craniofacial and skeletal abnormalities, mental retardation, short stature, and hypotonia). Those disorders with delayed detection include androgen insensitivity syndrome (genetic male [XY] but phenotypic female), which may not be determined until the early teenage years with the occurrence of primary amenorrhea; Duchenne's muscular dystrophy, which may not manifest until 1–2 years of age with the onset of proximal muscle weakness or observation of delay in reaching motor developmental milestones; and Becker's muscular dystrophy, which may not manifest until early adulthood.

There are a variety of color-blindness conditions that are of little significance in the newborn period. These include deuteranopia (i.e., difficulty distinguishing between blue/green and red/green due to a lack of the receptors for long wavelengths of light), protanopia (i.e., difficulty distinguishing between red/purple and green/purple due to a lack of the receptors for medium wavelengths of light), and tritanopia (i.e., difficulty distinguishing between yellow/green and blue/green due to lack of receptors for short wavelengths of light).

As a result of neonatal circumcision, the inherited disorders of most immediate concern in the newborn period are hemophilia A (factor VIII deficiency) and hemophilia B (factor IX deficiency). Hemophilia occurs in approximately 1 in 5000 male births and occurs worldwide in all racial groups. A diagnosis can be made prenatally through chorionic villous sampling, amniocentesis, cordocentesis, or DNA analysis of fetal cells in the maternal circulation. Postnatally, testing infants with a known familial history can be performed through a venous cord blood sample for either factor VIII or factor IX because these do not cross the placenta. Despite these testing options, most infants with hemophilia are diagnosed after a bleeding episode.[3] In addition to circumcision, common causes of these bleeding episodes include intracranial hemorrhage, subdural hemorrhage, and punctures for diagnostic testing via venipuncture, the newborn screen, and capillary blood samples.[4]

Despite the potential for a bleeding complication, circumcision can still be performed when there is a family history of a bleeding disorder (Table 5-2). Bleeding risk can be reduced, even in the absence of an inherited bleeding disorder, by administering 1 mg of vitamin K intramuscularly as a prophylactic measure, which has been shown to reduce complications from hemolytic disease of the newborn based on data from two randomized controlled trials in a Cochrane review.[5]

Anatomic Considerations
Congenital Hernia and Hydrocele

Congential inguinal hernia occurs most frequently in male infants. During normal fetal development, the testes pass through the inguinal canal to the scrotum through the processus vaginalis (Figures 5-1, *A* and 5-2, *A*). Normally, the processus vaginalis closes at approximately 32 weeks of gestation. However, if it persists or is still present at birth, as could be the case in a preterm

Table 5-2. Laboratory Tests to Determine Circumcision Safety with Bleeding Disorders

Hemophilia
If PTT < 36 seconds and factor VIII level is within normal range, then proceed with circumcision.
Von Willebrand's Disease (VWD)
Type I, IIa, III: If PTT < 36 seconds, then proceed with circumcision.
Type IIb: If PTT < 36 seconds and platelets >100,000, then proceed with circumcision.
Maternal Thrombocytopenia (ITP, HELLP, Type IIb VWD)
If platelets >100,000, then proceed with circumcision.
Familial Anemia
No contraindication to circumcision is present.
Platelet Function Disorder
Defer circumcision.

PTT, Partial thromboplastin time; ITP, idiopathic thrombocytopenic purpura; HELLP, hemolysis, elevated liver enzymes, low platelet count.

delivery, a variety of anatomic consequences can occur that are then diagnosed at birth. If the opening is present but narrow, only peritoneal fluid can pass through, and the resulting consequence is called a *hydrocele* (Figures 5-1, *B* and *C*). If the opening is large enough such that intestinal contents can pass through the inguinal ring, it is termed a *hernia,* and generally a bulge can be visualized or palpated in the groin area (Figure 5-2, *B*). This bulge may be more noticeable when the infant strains or cries. Often, both conditions will occur concurrently. To clinically differentiate between a hydrocele and hernia, the clinician can attempt transillumination of the scrotum. Visible shadowing of the testis is indicative of hydrocele only. However, this technique is imperfect, and when clinical concern is present, use of adjunctive technology such as ultrasonography is recommended. Management of an inguinal hernia is surgical, whereas hydroceles may be observed over time and often resolve without surgical intervention. Delaying surgical intervention in the treatment of inguinal hernias carries a risk of incarceration; in one study,[6] more than half of infants with an incarcerated hernia before the age of 1 year had known inguinal hernias. If there is a persistence of a hydrocele, surgery may delayed until 2–3 years of age but timing of surgery may vary.

Cryptorchidism

Much less common but still an important diagnosis to make in the neonatal period is the presence of cryptorchidism. This condition occurs 10 times more frequently in preterm infants and in up to 5.9% of term newborns.[7] Diagnosis is generally accomplished by physical examination, where the lack of a palpable testis may indicate cryptorchidism but may be easily confused with a retractile testis. Treatment generally does not occur in the immediate neonatal period. Options for treatment may include hormonal treatment, but an

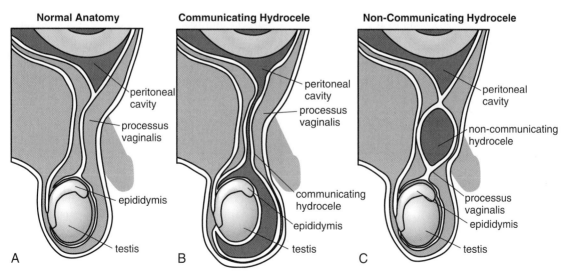

Figure 5-1. A, Normal male anatomy. **B,** Communicating hydrocele. **C,** Non-communicating hydrocele. (Adapted from: Hydrocele treatment for children. Cleveland, Ohio, 2005, The Cleveland Clinic. Available at: http://www.clevelandclinic.org/health/health-info/docs/0200/0227.asp?index=4312.)

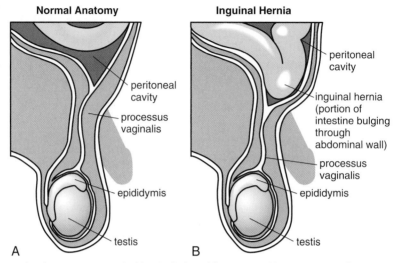

Normal Anatomy　　　　　　　**Inguinal Hernia**

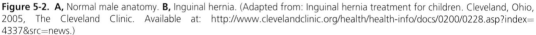

peritoneal cavity

processus vaginalis

epididymis

testis

A

peritoneal cavity

inguinal hernia (portion of intestine bulging through abdominal wall)

processus vaginalis

epididymis

testis

B

Figure 5-2. A, Normal male anatomy. **B,** Inguinal hernia. (Adapted from: Inguinal hernia treatment for children. Cleveland, Ohio, 2005, The Cleveland Clinic. Available at: http://www.clevelandclinic.org/health/health-info/docs/0200/0228.asp?index= 4337&src=news.)

evidence-based review found no clear benefit over surgical management.[8] Treatment at an earlier age may be beneficial to the patient from a psychosocial perspective in later life. Patients with larger testicular size as adults who had cryptorchidism treated at ages ranging from 10 months up to 13 years had a positive correlation with increased sexual activity as an adult.[9] However, age at surgery, termed *orchiopexy*, does not seem to affect the potential for future paternity.[10] Although surgery may be delayed until the child is close to 12 months in age, referral as early as 6 months of age may be warranted if there is persistent cryptorchidism on examination to ease parental concerns and to allow for earlier discussion of timing of surgical intervention.

Hypospadias

Hypospadias (Figure 5-3) classically presents as a combination of a malpositioned urethral meatus, ventral penile curvature (also known as a *chordee*), and foreskin that can have a "hooded" appearance.[11] However, more subtle cases are often not detected until later in the boy's childhood when the foreskin begins to retract or during the process of reducing foreskin adhesions during the circumcision procedure. When hypospadias is diagnosed, circumcision should be deferred to facilitate subsequent surgical reconstruction of the urethral meatus. Surgically correctable features include restoring meatal position, glans shape, scars, scrotum, and overall general appearance. Penile size, thickness, and

volume of the glans are generally not correctable.[12] Surgery timing is variable, but most sources agree that earlier repair (age younger than 1 year) reduces any potential for long-term psychosocial impact stemming from genital abnormalities.[12] Referral to a pediatric urologist at the time of diagnosis is helpful to facilitate evaluation, to provide optimal reassurance and information to parents, and to facilitate timing of surgical repair if deemed necessary.

Circumcision

Circumcision is the world's oldest documented surgery and today is becoming one of the more controversial. It also happens to be the most common procedure performed over the last century, with roughly one sixth of the world male population having undergone circumcision.[13] There has been a significant increase in US circumcision rates from 1988 to 2000, rising from 48.3% to 61.1%.[14] Many factors influence the rate of circumcision, and there is regional variation due to demographic, cultural, and insurance reimbursement differences. Proponents of the procedure include those believing in circumcision for religious or cultural reasons as well as those citing the various medical benefits. Opponents focus on the costs of an elective procedure as well as pain and suffering of the male infant.

Culture and tradition play a major role in the decision whether to have a male infant circumcised. Traditional Jewish and Muslim cultures demand circumcision. Although not mentioned

Hypospadias

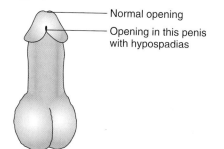

— Normal opening
— Opening in this penis
with hypospadias

Figure 5-3. Hypospadias. Opening in hypospadias can be anywhere along the underside of the penis. (Adapted from: Department of Health and Human Services, Centers for Disease Control and Prevention: Birth defects: frequently asked questions. Available at: http://www.cdc.gov/ncbddd/bd/faq1.htm.)

directly in the Koran, circumcision is mentioned in the Old Testament of the Bible (Genesis 17), where instructions are to fulfill the covenant between God and Abraham by performing the procedure on the eighth day of life. To this day, many Jews abide by this, having a *mohel,* a special religious figure, perform the ceremony. A graphic description of the *bris milah,* or Jewish ritual circumcision, is described in ancient handbooks known as Sifrei-Ha Mohelim, the equivalent of a modern textbook.[15]

Proponents of circumcision promote the procedure based on a variety of potential medical benefits. The evidence ranges from quite strong and incontrovertible to weak associations. Active research is currently focused on a number of promising areas examining this relationship. Evidence demonstrating protective effects of circumcision against the development of penile cancer has been known since the early 1900s. However, although the incidence of penile cancers is quite low in the United States at approximately 1 in 100,000, it is approximately three-fold higher in uncircumcised men.[16] Given the low incidence in the United States, recommending universal circumcision for penile cancer prevention is difficult to justify.[17]

Treatment and prevention of *phimosis,* the inability to fully retract the foreskin, has traditionally been one of the most common indications for circumcision. However, treatment with potent topical steroids such as betamethasone over the course of up to 2 months has been shown to be effective in resolving phimosis up to 75% of the time in a case-controlled study.[18]

Many studies have found that newborn circumcision markedly reduces the risk of urinary tract infections (UTIs), especially in the first year of the male infant's life. Schoen and colleagues[19] demonstrated a 9.1-fold reduction in UTI rates with a 10-fold decrease in cost to manage these infections in one small study, although cost savings was not significant when the cost of the circumcision procedure was factored in. This reduction in morbidity may make the recommendation of routine neonatal circumcision a reasonable choice.

Newer evidence includes emerging data suggesting that circumcision significantly reduces the transmission of human immunodeficiency virus (HIV). Although the exact mechanisms have not been proven in vivo, it has been shown in vitro that viruses and bacteria are less able to adhere and propagate in the keratinized epithelium in the circumcised penis compared with the uncircumcised prepuce. It is theorized that the more fragile epithelial cells in the uncircumcised prepuce are at a higher risk for microtrauma and thus easier transmission of HIV. Similar recent studies have now demonstrated a significant risk reduction for ulcerative sexually transmitted infections including syphilis, chancroid, and herpes simplex.[20] Circumcision also appears to reduce the risk of transmission of *Chlamydia trachomatis* infection from men to their female partners both in monogamous and nonmonogamous relationships by up to 82%.[21]

Both meta-analyses and a Cochrane review have examined the relationship between male circumcision and HIV transmission. These reviews document a significant correlation between circumcision and decreased risk of both acquiring and transmitting HIV, which is even greater when examining high-risk populations in sub-Saharan Africa. However, the reviewers note that there are significant limitations to these studies, none of which are randomized controlled trials. Several trials are currently underway that will hopefully further elucidate the connection between circumcision and disease risk reduction. Therefore, recommending circumcision as a means to reduce HIV transmission is somewhat premature but does appear promising, especially in high-risk populations.[22]

Human papilloma virus (HPV) represents the final infective agent thought to be influenced by circumcision. Castellsague and colleagues[23] found that male circumcision is associated with a reduced risk of penile HPV infection. Additionally, in a high-risk population, defined as males with a history of multiple sexual partners (defined as more than 6 partners), this study found a reduced risk of cervical cancer (odds ratio, 0.42) in their current female partners.

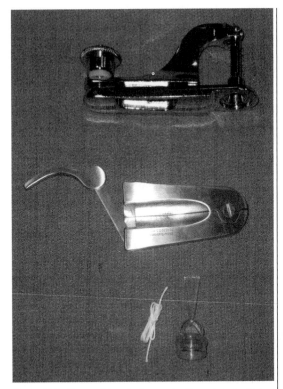

Figure 5-4. Circumcision instruments. From top to bottom: Gomco clamp, Mogen clamp, Plastibell. (Photos courtesy of Dr. David Serlin, Clinical Instructor, Department of Family Medicine, University of Michigan Medical School.)

Although the circumcision procedure itself is beyond the scope of this chapter, there are three main modalities used in current practice. The Gomco and Mogen clamps and the Plastibell (Figure 5-4) are currently the most common instruments used to perform circumcisions. There are advantages and disadvantages to each modality. The Mogen clamp allows for the fastest procedure but removes the least amount of foreskin. It also generally causes less pain response in infants, but this may also be related to the speed at which the procedure can be performed with this device.[24] Patients undergoing circumcision with Mogen or Gomco clamps go home with the procedure completed, whereas those with the Plastibell leave with the equipment still attached to the foreskin until it falls off 4–7 days later.

Adequate analgesia is an important aspect of any surgical procedure. In the past, it was thought that infants did not experience pain in the same way as adults, and thus circumcisions were performed without anesthesia. Research over the past decades has proved this to be a misconception. Brady-Fryer and colleagues performed a sys-

tematic Cochrane review[25] addressing this issue. Modalities reviewed included the dorsal penile nerve block (DPNB), application of a eutectic mixture of local anesthetics (EMLA) cream to the foreskin, oral sucrose, and oral analgesics (e.g., acetaminophen suspension) against placebo. The meta-analysis concluded that DPNB was superior to EMLA, and that both modalities were superior to oral agents and placebo. The oral analgesic and oral sucrose trials were inconclusive compared with placebo, although limited data demonstrated that oral sucrose decreased heart rate and crying time. The authors noted that no modality studied completely eliminated pain response during circumcision.[25]

Despite these findings, the use of anesthesia during circumcision may indeed have longer-term benefit to the infant. Taddio and colleagues[26] demonstrated that circumcised male infants who did not have analgesia had a stronger pain response to routine immunizations than both uncircumcised infants and those who received analgesia for the procedure. Our recommended best practice at the University of Michigan uses a combination of DPNB or ring block (i.e., circumferential infusion of subcutaneous lidocaine at the base of the penile shaft) with concentrated oral sucrose solution administered on a pacifier during the procedure, as supported by a recent clinical trial.[27] Acetaminophen administered before circumcision did not have any significant effect on pain scores; however, given postoperatively, acetaminophen did reduce pain response within the first 24 hours.[28]

Those arguing against circumcision point to the elective nature of the procedure, including the costs and the complications that can ensue, yet complication rates are low and mostly minor in nature. One study estimated the rate of complication at 0.2%, with most representing minor bleeding that can be controlled with direct pressure to the glans and no resulting long-term morbidity. This is followed distantly by local infection, again with little evidence of long-term morbidity.[29]

Lastly, opponents criticize circumcision as causing sexual dysfunction. A variety of studies[30,31] found no difference in tactile stimulation, and one large study[32] demonstrated a higher incidence of sexual difficulties in uncircumcised men but no significant difference in the likelihood of contracting sexually transmitted diseases. Another recent study[33] showed no difference between circumcised and uncircumcised men with regard to ejaculation, erection, sexual drive, and overall sexual satisfaction.

In conclusion, circumcision is a controversial procedure in the United States and worldwide. Cultural or aesthetic reasons are the main reasons to support elective neonatal circumcision; however, emerging evidence does indicate that the procedure is protective against a number of medical problems and infections, especially in high-risk populations. Whether the procedure is cost-effective remains an elusive target to study accurately. Therefore, parents should be given all the current medical data available, including the risks and benefits of the procedure, to allow them to make the most informed choice for their newborn sons. If they choose to proceed, adequate anesthesia using a penile nerve block, concentrated sucrose on a pacifier, and postoperative acetaminophen at a dose of 15 mg/kg every 4–6 hours should be used, along with one of the three devices, preferably the Mogen or Gomco clamp.

Care of the Uncircumcised Penis

No current data support that any special intervention is required to care for a patient with an uncircumcised penis during the neonatal period. It is not necessary to manually retract the foreskin for hygienic purposes.

References

1. Parmelee AH, Stern E: Development of states of infants. In Clemente CD, Purpura DP, Meyer FE, editors, *Sleep and the Maturing Nervous System*, New York, 1972, Academic Press.
2. Dureau SJ: The effect of gender on one-day-old infants' behavior and heart rate responses to music decibel level, *J Music Ther* 42(3):168–184, 2005.
3. Kulkarni R, Lusher JM: Perinatal management of newborns with haemophilia, *Br J Haematol* 112:264–274, 2001.
4. Kulkarni R, Lusher JM: Intracranial and extracranial hemorrhages in newborns with hemophilia: a review of the literature, *J Pediatr Hematol/Oncol* 21 (4):289–295, 1999.
5. Puckett RM, Offringa M: Prophylactic vitamin K for vitamin K deficiency bleeding in neonates, *Cochrane Database Syst Rev* 4:CD002776, 2005.
6. Niedzielski J, Kr IR, Gawlowska A: Could incarceration of inguinal hernia in children be prevented? *Med Sci Monit* 9(1):CR16–18, 2003.
7. Pillai SB, Besner GE: Pediatric testicular problems, *Pediatr Clin North Am* 45:813–830, 1998.
8. Bertelloni S, Baroncelli GI, Ghirri P, et al: Hormonal treatment for unilateral inguinal testis: comparison of four different treatments, *Hormone Res* 55(5): 236–239, 2001.
9. Takinen S, Hovatta O, Wikstrom S: Sexual development in patients treated for cryptorchidism, *Scand J Urol Nephrol* 31(4):361–364, 1997.
10. Lee PA, O'Leary LA, Songer NJ, et al: Paternity after cryptorchidism: lack of correlation with age at orchidopexy, *Br J Urol* 75(6):704–707, 1995.
11. Mouriquand P, Persad R, Sharma I: Hypospadias repair: current principles and procedures, *Br J Urol* 76(Suppl 3):9–22, 1995.
12. Woodhouse CR, Christie D: Nonsurgical factors in the success of hypospadias repair, *Br J Urol Int* 96:22–27, 2005.
13. Dunsmuir WD, Gordon EM: The history of circumcision, *Br J Urol Int* 83(Suppl 1):1–12, 1999.
14. Nelson CP, Dunn R, Wan J, Wei JT: The increasing incidence of newborn circumcision: data from the nationwide inpatient sample, *J Urol* 173(3):978–981, 2005.
15. Zwi Werblowsky RJ, Wigoder G, editors: Circumcision. In *The Oxford Dictionary of the Jewish Religion*, New York, 1997, Oxford University Press, p 161.
16. Maden C, Sherman KJ, Beckmann AM, et al: History of circumcision, medical conditions, and sexual activity and risk of penile cancer, *J Natl Cancer Inst* 85:19–24, 1993.
17. Schoen EJ, Oehrli M, Colby CJ, Machin G: The highly protective effect of newborn circumcision against invasive penile cancer, *Pediatrics* 105(3):e36, 2000.
18. Elmore JM, Baker LA, Snodgrass WT: Topical steroid therapy as an alternative to circumcision for phimosis in boys younger than 3 years, *J Urol* 4:1746S–1747S, 2002.
19. Schoen EJ, Colby CJ, Ray GT: Newborn circumcision decreases incidence and costs of urinary tract infections during the first year of life, *Pediatrics* 105:789–793, 2000.
20. Weiss HA, Thomas SL, Munabi SK, Hayes RJ: Male circumcision and risk of syphilis, chancroid, and genital herpes: a systematic review and meta-analysis, *Sex Trans Infect* 82:101–110, 2006.
21. Castellsague X, Peeling RW, Franceschi S: *Chlamydia trachomatis* infection in female partners of circumcised and uncircumcised adult men, *Am J Epidemiol* 162(9):907–916, 2005.
22. Siegfried N, Muller M, Volmink J, et al: Male circumcision for prevention of heterosexual acquisition of HIV in men, *Cochrane Database Syst Rev* 3: CD003362, 2006.
23. Castellsague X, Bosch FX, Munoz N, et al: Male circumcision, penile human papillomavirus infection, and cervical cancer in female partners, *N Engl J Med* 346:1105–1112, 2002.
24. Kurtis PS, DeSilva HN, Bernstein BA, et al: A comparison of the Mogen and Gomco clamps in combination with dorsal penile nerve block in minimizing the pain of neonatal circumcision, *Pediatrics* 103(2): E23, 1999.
25. Brady-Fryer B, Wiebe N, Lander JA: Pain relief for neonatal circumcision, *Cochrane Database Syst Rev* 4:CD004217, 2004.

26. Taddio A, Katz J, Ilersich Al, Koren G: Effect of neonatal circumcision on pain response during subsequent routine vaccination, *Lancet* 349 (9052):599–603, 1997.

27. Razmus IS, Dalton ME, Wilson D: Pain management for newborn circumcision, *Pediatric Nurs* 30 (5):414–417, 427, 2004.

28. Howard CR, Howard FM, Weitzman ML: Acetaminophen analgesia in neonatal circumcision: the effect on pain, *Pediatrics* 93:641–646, 1994.

29. Wiswell TE, Geschke DW: Risks from circumcision during the first month of life compared with those of uncircumcised boys, *Pediatrics* 83:1011–1015, 1989.

30. Masood S, Patel HRH, Himpson RC, et al: Penile sensitivity and sexual satisfaction after circumcision: are we informing men correctly? *Urol Int* 75 (1):62–66, 2005.

31. Bleustein CB, Fogarty JD, Eckholdt H, et al: Effect of neonatal circumcision on penile neurologic sensation, *Urology* 65(4):773–777, 2005.

32. Laumann EO, Masi CM, Zuckerman EW: Circumcision in the United States: prevalence, prophylactic effects, and sexual practice, *JAMA* 277 (13):1052–1057, 1997.

33. Collins S, Upshaw J, Rutchik S, et al: Effects of circumcision on male sexual function: debunking a myth? *J Urol* 167:2111–2112, 2002.

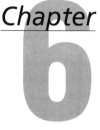

The School-Aged Male Child

Jennifer Stojan, MD, Sheila Gahagan, MD, MPH

Key Points

- The diagnosis of ADHD requires the use of standardized reports of symptoms by parents and teachers (strength of recommendation: B).
- The most effective treatment for ADHD is a combination of pharmacologic and behavioral interventions (strength of recommendation: B).
- The combination of behavioral and medication management has the highest rate of favorable outcomes for childhood functional constipation and soiling (strength of recommendation: A).
- Bullying may coexist with ADHD, oppositional defiant disorder, depression, or anxiety (strength of recommendation: C).
- Childhood body mass index greater than or equal to the 95th percentile increases the risk for adult obesity (strength of recommendation: B).
- Screening for type 2 diabetes mellitus and hyperlipidemia is recommended for overweight children (strength of recommendation: C).
- Family-centered counseling to make nutritional and physical activity changes in a stepwise fashion to control a child's weight gain is recommended (strength of recommendation: C).

Introduction

For male children, life between the ages of 6 and 12 years is perhaps the healthiest period of all.

The health risks of infancy are past, and the risks of accident, injury, and the mental health problems of adolescence are barely emerging. This chapter on the health of preadolescent boys focuses on four potentially chronic conditions with a male predominance that have lifelong consequences. These conditions, which include attention-deficit/hyperactivity disorder (ADHD), bullying, encopresis, and obesity, are common and their identification is often delayed or neglected.

Bullying is not classically considered to be a health problem per se, yet its role in the development of lifelong mental health disorders elevates its importance. Bullying is different from most medical conditions because it involves at least two people, the victim and the perpetrator; we consider the consequences for both in our discussion. Bullying is believed to affect at least 10% of older school-aged children; boys are at three times the risk for bullying compared to girls.[1] Encopresis, or chronic constipation with soiling, is reported in up to 2% of 6 year olds, yet it is a diagnosis which is commonly missed.[2] Its prevalence in boys is three times that of girls.[3,4] Obesity is important as an emerging public health problem that is frequently considered only in adults. It has become a steadily rising predicament that has the potential for ominous future outcomes as well as enormous financial consequences. All four of these conditions require the special attention of primary care physicians aimed at prevention, early identification and intervention. Innovative thinking and research are needed to limit the financial, physical, and emotional costs of these four conditions.

Attention-Deficit/ Hyperactivity Disorder

Definitions

Attention-deficit/hyperactivity disorder is the most common childhood mental health condition in the United States. This neurobehavioral disorder typically manifests in early childhood, presenting with symptoms of inattention, hyperactivity, and impulsivity as described by the *Diagnostic and Statistical Manual of Mental Health Disorders*, fourth edition (DSM-IV) (Table 6-1).[5] ADHD is often responsible for poor school performance and social problems that can have ramifications throughout life. These problems, in turn, can cause difficulties in peer and family interactions and result in lower self-esteem.

Primary care physicians provide the vast majority of ADHD evaluation and treatment in the United States because there are few child psychiatrists. ADHD care includes evaluation using standardized questionnaires, advice about behavioral plans, communication with schools, prescription medications, monitoring and referral for counseling, and other mental health interventions.

To accurately diagnose ADHD, DSM-IV criteria require that symptoms be present in more than one setting and for at least 6 months.[5] Additionally, the definition requires that symptoms are developmentally inappropriate beginning before the age of 7 years. Furthermore, diagnostic criteria are met only if the symptoms disrupt social, occupational, or academic functioning. ADHD can be divided into three subtypes based on the predominant symptom: (1) inattentive, (2) hyperactive-impulsive, and (3) combined. Children with *inattentive* ADHD typically fail to pay close attention to detail and have difficulty sustaining attention. They may not listen, even when spoken to directly. Organizing tasks is difficult, and they may avoid work or play requiring sustained mental effort. Forgetfulness in daily activities due to distractibility is not uncommon. The child with *hyperactive-impulsive* ADHD is described as always "on the go": fidgeting, squirming, running, climbing, talking excessively, blurting out answers, and interrupting. Remaining seated is often difficult for these children. The *combined* subtype includes symptoms of both inattentive and hyperactive-impulsive ADHD.

Epidemiology

ADHD is one of the most common childhood disorders in the United States and has a notable male predominance.[6] ADHD affects approximately 9% of school-aged boys.[7] In the United States, boys are at least three times as likely to be diagnosed with ADHD as girls.[8] Furthermore, boys with ADHD are twice as likely to have the hyperactive-impulsive type as girls with ADHD.[9]

Differential Diagnosis

The differential diagnosis for the predominant symptoms of ADHD—inattention, impulsivity, and hyperactivity—is nonspecific and may mimic other disorders. For example, childhood chronic illness may interfere with attention and impair a child's school performance. Attention is also affected by multiple factors including sleep, pain, and emotional distress. Medical conditions including seizure disorders, hypothyroidism, lead poisoning, and iron deficiency can present with inattention. Hearing, visual, and cognitive impairments can be mistaken for ADHD. Mentally handicapped children may appear impulsive and more hyperactive than "normal" children of the same age. Fetal alcohol syndrome, autism, and hyperthyroidism also commonly present with hyperactivity.

Similarly, learning disabilities can be misinterpreted as ADHD. Major life stressors such as violence in the home, death, and divorce can cause inattention, distractibility, and impulsivity. Chronic symptoms including pain and constipation similarly cause preoccupation with bodily function, which is distracting. Psychiatric conditions including depression, anxiety disorder, and posttraumatic stress disorder may present with symptoms of inability to concentrate, restlessness, and inattention. Therefore, careful attention must be taken when diagnosing a school-aged child with ADHD because there may be many possible explanations for their symptoms of inattention, impulsivity, and hyperactivity. The diagnosing physician is advised to carefully consider the differential diagnosis for each child during the evaluation process.

Clinical Approach

Medial History

The diagnosis of ADHD is made on clinical grounds based on reports from parental and child interviews with input from teachers and other caregivers. Guidelines from the American Academy of Pediatrics (AAP) for the diagnosis and treatment of ADHD recommend evaluation for children between 6 and 12 years of age who present with inattention, hyperactivity, impulsivity, academic underachievement, or

Table 6-1. DSM-IV Diagnostic Criteria for Attention-Deficit/Hyperactivity Disorder

A. Either 1 or 2
1. Six (or more) of the following symptoms of inattention have persisted for at least 6 months to a degree that is maladaptive and inconsistent with development level:
Inattention
a. Often fails to give close attention to details or makes careless mistakes in school work, work, or other activities
b. Often has difficulty sustaining attention in tasks or play activities
c. Often does not seem to listen when spoken to directly
d. Often does not follow through on instructions and fails to finish schoolwork, chores, or duties in the workplace (not due to oppositional behavior or failure to understand instructions)
e. Often has difficulty organizing tasks and activities
f. Often avoids, dislikes, or is reluctant to engage in tasks that require sustained mental effort (such as schoolwork or homework)
g. Often loses things necessary for tasks or activities (e.g., toys, school assignments, pencils, books, or tools)
h. Is often easily distracted by extraneous stimuli
i. Is often forgetful in daily activities
2. Six (or more) of the following symptoms of hyperactivity-impulsivity have persisted for at least 6 months to a degree that is maladaptive and inconsistent with developmental level:
Hyperactivity
a. Often fidgets with hands or feet or squirms in seat
b. Often leaves seat in classroom or in other situations in which remaining seated is expected
c. Often runs about or climbs excessively in situations in which it is inappropriate (in adolescents or adults, may be limited to subjective feelings of restlessness)
d. Often has difficulty playing or engaging in leisure activities quietly
e. Is often "on the go" or often acts as if "driven by a motor"
f. Often talks excessively
Impulsivity
g. Often blurts out answers before questions have been completed
h. Often has difficulty awaiting turn
i. Often interrupts or intrudes on others (e.g., butts into conversations or games)
B. Some hyperactive-impulsive or inattentive symptoms that caused impairment were present before 7 years of age.
C. Some impairment from the symptoms is present in two or more settings (e.g., at school [or work] or at home).
D. There must be clear evidence of clinically significant impairment in social, academic, or occupational functioning.
E. The symptoms do not occur exclusively during the course of a pervasive developmental disorder, schizophrenia, or other psychotic disorder and are not better accounted for by another mental disorder (e.g., mood disorder, anxiety disorder, dissociative disorder, or personality disorder).

Code based on type:

   314.01 Attention-Deficit/Hyperactivity Disorder, Combined Type: if both criteria A1 and A2 are met for the past 6 months.

   314.00 Attention-Deficit/Hyperactivity Disorder, Predominantly Inattentive type: if criterion A1 is met but criterion A2 is not met for the past 6 months.

   314.01 Attention-Deficit/Hyperactivity Disorder, Predominantly Hyperactive-Impulsive Type: if criterion A2 is met but criterion A1 is not met for the past 6 months.

   Reprinted with permission from the *Diagnostic and Statistical Manual of Mental Disorders,* Fourth Edition, Text Revision, (Copyright 2000). American Psychiatric Association.

behavioral problems.[6,10] The diagnostic interview is based on the DSM-IV criteria mentioned above. Medial history focuses on age of onset, duration of symptoms, degree of impairment, and where the symptoms occur. Classroom teachers should report on core symptoms and timing of problems, behavioral disturbances, and degree of impairment. Direct observations during school and after-school activities are valuable. School-based multidisciplinary reports are an additional source of information. Rating scales completed by parents and teachers provide a method of comparative standardization and validation of reported symptoms. ADHD-specific rating scales can effectively distinguish between children with and without ADHD, with a sensitivity and specificity of at least 94%.[11] Commonly used behavioral rating scales include the Conner Rating Scale[12] and the Vanderbilt Assessment Scale.[13] The Vanderbilt Assessment Scale is part of the AAP and National Initiative for Children's Healthcare Quality ADHD toolkit and can be accessed at http://www.aap.org/healthtopics/adhd.cfm.

A comprehensive medical and developmental history including information about the perinatal period, in utero exposure to drugs or alcohol, brain trauma, and current medications allows idiopathic ADHD to be differentiated from ADHD associated with an underlying disorder. Sleep deprivation can lead to attention difficulties, as can inadequate nutrition. For certain conditions, including hyperthyroidism and lead poisoning, treatment of the underlying disorder may eliminate ADHD symptoms. Family medical history often reveals additional family members with ADHD, which suggests a genetic or gene-environment component to etiology. Because hyperactivity and inattention are nonspecific symptoms, psychological events or life stressors may induce these symptoms. Therefore, strict attention to both family psychiatric and social history is important.

Physical Examination

The physical examination allows the physician to investigate other potential diagnoses contributing to learning difficulties and behavioral problems including chronic illness, sensory impairment, and potential genetic defects or birth defects that were previously undiagnosed. Fetal alcohol syndrome[14,15] and fragile X syndrome both have clinical symptoms that overlap with ADHD.[16] An observational examination of the child's behavior can reveal whether the child can attend to tasks in the doctor's office. This environment is usually quiet and nonstimulating, albeit often associated with discomfort and anxiety. Children with ADHD may not manifest symptoms of hyperactivity or inattention in a structured clinical atmosphere that provides little distraction or stimulation.

Diagnostic Tests

Diagnostic tests are not routinely recommended for the establishment of a diagnosis of ADHD. Laboratory and radiographic studies may be performed to rule out an alternative etiology of

inattentive or hyperactive behavior such as lead poisoning, iron deficiency anemia, or hyperthyroidism. Evaluation of comorbid conditions such as encopresis may require some laboratory or radiographic testing.

Comorbidities

Children with ADHD are at an increased risk for several medical and psychiatric conditions. Encopresis is associated with ADHD, as are sleep disorders. More than one third of children with ADHD have a second mental health disorder including oppositional defiant disorder, conduct disorder, anxiety disorder, or depression.[11] ADHD is also associated with injuries because children with ADHD are more likely to be injured as pedestrians or bicyclists and to incur self-inflicted injuries compared with children without ADHD. These children experience an increased risk of multiple injuries over simple injuries and head injuries over bodily injuries compared with children who do not have ADHD.[17,18] Suicide and injury resulting from assault are also associated with a diagnosis of ADHD.[19,20] In males 6–24 years old with ADHD, the estimated relative risk for suicide is 2.9 of that for age-matched males without ADHD.[17,18] It is likely that this association is due the higher prevalence of both conduct disorder and depression in those with ADHD.

Treatment

Treatment for ADHD begins with education, demystification, and removing blame from the child because it is a chronic disease that will require ongoing management. The primary care physician is in an important position to educate the patient and family members on the need for ongoing treatment strategies. Encouraging the family to set short-term behavioral and educational goals for the child lays the foundation for a combined pharmacologic and behavioral intervention. The child's family can begin by providing structure and routines that promote the child's ability to organize and attend. Although most children with ADHD do not need psychotherapy, they do need special assistance in learning how to focus, family support for organization, and often special accommodations in school. They also benefit from social skills training as well as feedback about the consequences of impulsivity. Although behavioral therapy is essential, data suggest that multimodal therapy is superior to behavioral therapy alone.[21]

Pharmacologic treatment includes psychostimulant medication, antidepressants, and alpha-2 adrenergic agonists (Table 6-2). Methylphenidate and dextroamphetamine are the most commonly prescribed stimulants used in the treatment of ADHD. Although there are individual differences in response to different stimulants and formulations, no clear difference in efficacy among different stimulants has been found.[10] Stimulant medications are effective in managing inattention, hyperactivity, and distractibility but have common adverse effects including appetite suppression, decreased weight gain, and sleep disturbances. Neuromotor tics can be unmasked by stimulant medication, presenting earlier than they would have if the child had not received medication. In the United States, the Food and Drug Administration has placed a black box warning on stimulant medications to warn physicians of the rare but serious risk of sudden cardiac death associated with stimulant use. Before prescribing stimulant medications, physicians are advised to evaluate the patient for any risk of underlying cardiac disease. Prescribing stimulant medications at the lowest effective dose is prudent. Furthermore, informing families of potential risk is essential. Second-line treatment including antidepressants or an alpha-2 agonist (e.g., clonidine [Catapres] or guanfacine [Tenex]) is considered when two or more stimulant drugs have been ineffective in controlled behavior or have produced intolerable adverse effects.

Successful treatment of ADHD includes long-term monitoring of the patient's degree of symptomatic relief, medication compliance, and the presence of adverse effects. Families often have worries regarding medications that can decrease adherence to treatment; for example, parents are often concerned that the use of medications to treat ADHD may increase their child's risk of developing substance abuse problems later in life. Families can be reassured that research suggests that the risk of developing a substance abuse disorder is almost two times less in children with ADHD treated with stimulants compared with those who were not treated.[22]

Table 6-2. Medications Used in the Treatment of Attention-Deficit/Hyperactivity Disorder

Generic Class (Brand Name)	Daily Dosage Schedule	Duration	Prescribing Schedule
Stimulants (First-Line Treatment)			
Methylphenidate			
Short-acting (Ritalin, Metadate, Methylin)	BID to TID	3–5 hr	5–20 mg BID to TID
Intermediate-acting (Ritalin SR, Metadate ER, Methylin ER)	QD to BID	3–8 hr	20–40 mg QD or 40 mg in the morning and 20 mg early afternoon
Long-acting (Concerta, Metadate CD, Ritalin LA*)	QD	8–12 hr	18–72 mg QD
Amphetamine			
Short-acting (Dexedrine, Dextrostat)	BID to TID	4–6 hr	5–15 mg BID or 5–10 mg TID
Intermediate-acting (Adderall, Dexedrine spansule)	QD to BID	6–8 hr	5–30 mg QD or 5–15 mg BID
Long-acting (Adderall-XR*)	QD		10–30 mg QD
Antidepressants (Second-Line Treatment)			
Tricyclic antidepressants (Imipramine, Desipramine)	BID to TID		2–5 mg/kg/day†
Bupropion			
(Wellbutrin)	QD to TID		50–100 mg TID
(Wellbutrin SR)	BID		100–150 mg BID

BID, Twice a day; TID, three times a day; QD, once a day.
*Not FDA approved at time of publication.
†Prescribing and monitoring information in *Physicians' Desk Reference*.
From American Academy of Pediatrics, Subcommittee on Attention-Deficit/Hyperactivity Disorder and Committee on Quality Improvement: Clinical practice guideline: treatment of the school-aged child with attention-deficit/hyperactivity disorder, *Pediatrics*; 108 (4):1033–1044, 2001.

Gender Differences

Several key differences exist across gender in the school-aged child pertaining to ADHD:

- Boys with ADHD engage in more rule-breaking and externalizing behaviors than girls with ADHD.[23]
- Boys with ADHD have higher scores on the Conner scale for hyperactivity, inattention, impulsivity, and externalizing problems compared with girls.[24]
- Boys with ADHD are more likely to have learning disability, behavior problems, comorbid major depression, conduct disorder, and oppositional defiant disorder than girls with ADHD.[25]
- Boys with ADHD are rated as more annoying to their teachers than girls.[25]
- Boys with hyperactive-impulsive type ADHD have symptoms that interfered more with peer activities when compared with girls with ADHD.[26]
- Boys with ADHD have poorer grades in school than girls with ADHD.[13]

Prognosis

Childhood ADHD has the potential to have a dramatic impact on later life. Adults who have had ADHD as children have documented lower social and academic outcomes compared with age-matched control subjects.[27] During adolescence, those who had ADHD were found to have lower grades on standardized tests, to fail more classes, and to have fewer friends than control subjects.[28] By young adulthood, this group had completed less schooling and had lower-ranking employment, poorer self-esteem, and worse social skills compared with controls. Antisocial disorders are also more common in this group.[29] Treatment using behavioral therapy, school accommodations, and when indicated, psychopharmacologic therapy promotes scholastic and social success.[30] ADHD usually persists into adolescence. However, some symptoms lessen during this period, particularly hyperactivity. In longitudinal studies of persons who had ADHD as children, approximately one half continue to demonstrate symptoms during adulthood.[31]

Bullying

Bullying, defined as the repeated assertion of power through aggression with the deliberate intent to harm or disturb a victim through social, emotional, or physical means, occurs in the context of either real or perceived imbalance of power.[1,32–35] *Direct bullying*, more commonly seen in boys, is overt and encompasses such activities as hitting, kicking, shoving, slapping, stealing, threatening with a weapon, name calling, public humiliation, racial slurs, sexual harassment, threatening or obscene gestures, or intimidation. *Indirect bullying*, more commonly seen in girls, is covert and typically manifests as rumor spreading, social rejection, exclusion from peer groups, and ignoring. Three types of individuals are described within the bullying paradigm: bullies, victims, and bully/victims. *Bully/victims* are defined as those children who have been bullied and who also engage in bullying behavior.

Since there are often severe consequences for both bullies and their victims, early identification and intervention is paramount. The National Threat Assessment Center found that more than two thirds of attackers in 37 mass school shootings felt persecuted, bullied, threatened, attacked, or injured by others, with revenge as the underlying motive behind their actions. These attackers were twice as likely to have been victims of bullying as their peers.[36] Alarmingly, bullies were more than five times as likely as their peers to carry a weapon to school, and the risk was higher if they engaged in bullying at least weekly.[37]

Epidemiology

Although bullying behavior has long been studied internationally, most US research is recent. The most cited US study from 2001 revealed that in sixth to 10th graders, 13% were classified as bullies, 10.6% were classified as victims, and 6.3% were classified as bully/victims.[1] More than 8.8% of school-aged children reported bullying others at least weekly, and 8.4% reported that they were bullied that often. Gender differences exist in bullying; boys are at least twice as likely as girls to be bullies (13% versus 5%), more than three times as likely to be bully/victims (10% versus 3%), and almost twice as likely to be victims (12% versus 7%).[1,38] Although few data are available about younger children, bullying behavior decreases with age between sixth and 10th grade.[1] To date, studies have not found differences in bullying behavior by urban, suburban, or rural domicile. The age of initiation and the influence of maturation is an important area for future research.

Risk Factors and Characteristics

Bullying most frequently occurs in school when there is minimal adult supervision: during breaks, recess, and lunch. Almost one half of bullied children do not tell their teachers that they have been harassed.[39] Bullies are typically physically strong and impulsive. These persons may have difficulty conforming to rules, sometimes becoming asocial and uncooperative. Bullies often have inflated self-esteem and a positive attitude toward violence. Victims tend to be quiet, cautious, sensitive, insecure, physically weak, and socially isolated. Bully/victims have been described as hyperactive, quick-tempered, and emotionally reactive.[40]

Typical attitudes about bullying in school-aged boys often become less negative over time, reflecting peer group adaptation and normalization, thereby perpetuating bullying behavior.[41] Smoking, alcohol consumption, and poorer academic achievement are more common in youth classified as bullies or bully/victims than in those who do not exhibit these profiles. The parents of victims are more likely to be involved in their children's school than their peers' parents. This may reflect either that victims are more likely to have a lower level of independence than their peers or that the parents of victims are aware of the problems. Both bully/victims and victims, unlike bullies, have poorer relationships with classmates, are lonelier, and find it more difficult to make friends.[1] Victims have been shown to perform better academically than bully/victims,[40] fitting with the notion that "smart children are picked on at school." Obese and disabled children are also known to be targets of victimization.

Families can foster bullying by modeling aggression to their children. Exposure to violence as well as experiencing victimization is associated with increased fighting behavior in children.[42] Furthermore, children who witness violence at home or elsewhere have higher levels of aggression and behavioral problems.[43] Families also encourage antisocial behavior through violent means of discipline such as spanking.[44] Bullies have been found to have more exposure to adult aggression and conflict, yet the home environments of victims do not differ significantly from those of children who are not victimized.[45] Larger societal influences are important in this paradigm as well. The media, for example, can often promote and glorify violence because children are exposed to countless violent acts on television each year. Through the media, children observe that violence is "acceptable" and even necessary in certain circumstances. This message, unfortunately, allows violence to become normative.

Comorbidities

Psychiatric comorbidity is found both in children who engage in bullying behavior and in those who are victims. Bullies have a higher prevalence of ADHD, depression, and oppositional/conduct disorders than those children who do not bully. Bully/victims have a similarly increased prevalence of these mental health disorders; victims are more likely to have anxiety and panic disorder as their risk of ADHD and depression are somewhat increased over the general population.[46] Substance abuse disorders may coexist with both bullying and victimization.[47,48] Suicidal ideation is also increased in both bullies and victims over what is expected in the general population.[49-51]

Clinical Approach

History

Although most physicians do not screen specifically for bullying behavior, they often ask open-ended questions about "how school is going." Children who are being bullied may visit the doctor repeatedly complaining of somatic symptoms including insomnia, abdominal pain, loss of appetite, headaches, new-onset enuresis, depression, loneliness, anxiety, or suicidal ideation.[38,39] They also tend to suffer from irritability, poor concentration, school refusal, substance abuse, academic failure, social problems, or a lack of friends. Heightened awareness of these signs and symptoms in children with chronic medical illnesses, obesity, disabilities, or cognitive impairment will allow the physician to proceed with more direct questioning. A reasonable strategy is to ask whether the child has ever felt "picked on" and then encourage recounting any such events including where and when the incident(s) occurred. Establishing whether an adult was notified and whether the child feels safe allows the physician to understand the acuity of the problem. Asking parents about their concerns about their child's social life may also reveal difficulties.

Identifying that a child is engaging in bullying behavior is much more difficult than detecting victimization. When a patient is identified as a bully, the possibility of current or prior child abuse should be considered. Direct questioning about homicidal or suicidal ideation is appropriate for both bullies and victims.

Physical Examination

When a child is identified as a being bully or a victim, a physical examination is useful to detect injuries and to investigate other possible contributing diagnoses. For example, neurobehavioral disorders such as fetal alcohol syndrome or fragile X syndrome may cause behavioral problems. Signs of neurologic dysfunction may suggest an underlying frontal lobe injury presenting with behavioral or personality changes. A physical examination also assists the physician in discerning whether complaints of insomnia, abdominal pain, loss of appetite, headaches, and new-onset enuresis are primarily medical or psychosomatic in origin.

Diagnostic Tests

Although diagnostic tests are not usually necessary in evaluating bullies and victims, they may be performed when the history or physical examination suggests a comorbid diagnosis. Diagnostic tests may also be used to determine whether a child's presenting symptoms are medical or psychosomatic in origin.

Treatment/Prevention

The physician plays an important role with bullies and victims. To be effective, they should be involved with identification of the problem; counseling the parents, children, and school personnel regarding intervention and prevention of bullying behavior; screening, treating, and referring for mental comorbidities; and advocating for violence prevention.

Victims

Empathetic listening by a physician helps to empower both the child and parent. Victims can be reassured that no one deserves to be a victim of bullying behavior. Because victimization can be extremely distressing to both the child and the family, it is important not to trivialize the problem. A physician's reassurance that many children are victims of bullying may allow the child to develop problem-solving strategies. Children often fear that the bully will retaliate if they tell an adult about the problem. Nonetheless, they should be encouraged to come forward and confront the issue. Explaining that adults tell authority figures, such as the police, when they are threatened may change the child's perception of exposing the bully. This may allow the child to accept the difficult step of telling a teacher, parent, or physician about bullying behavior. Practical advice includes avoiding situations where bullying frequently occurs and seeking social support from adults and friends. Victims may also benefit from the "walk, talk, and squawk" method of dealing with bullying, which encourages children to walk or run away from the scene rather than hang around.[52] Children are told to project an air of confidence and be in control by behaving calmly. Victims are told to talk to the bully in a non-provocative way and say things such as "you do not bother me." The final point is to "squawk," or to go tell a teacher or parent that they are being bullied. Parents of victims are encouraged to engage in role playing with their child to better prepare them to deal with bullying situations. Involvement in extracurricular activities may also prove to be beneficial because this will not only bolster a child's self-esteem, but will also help the child to form new friends and increase the child's social support system.

Bullies

Parents and teachers should be continually educated about the seriousness and severity of bullying behavior. Bullies should be helped to acknowledge the consequences of this behavior including how harmful it is to others. For a treatment plan to be effective, behavioral change must be expected from the bully, and social change must be expected from the school environment. For example, peer bystanders give a bully an audience and therefore further propagate the adverse behavior. Removal of peer support for bullying can help to minimize such behavior. It is important to teach children how to interact socially to resolve conflicts in a nonviolent manner. Schools must maintain adequate adult supervision in lunchrooms and hallways and on playgrounds.

Anti-bullying programs can be effective. A model elementary school program dramatically decreased disciplinary referrals and suspension rates. In this program, there was a zero-tolerance policy for bullying behavior including being a bystander. A discipline plan for modeling appropriate behavior was also instituted. In addition, this program had a physical education component designed to teach self-regulation. There was also a mentoring component in which adults and peers assisted students in preventing bullying.[53] Another researched elementary school violence prevention program, Second Step: A Violence Prevention Curriculum, was designed to prevent aggressive behavior by increasing prosocial behavior. Using a photograph accompanied by a social scenario to facilitate role playing and discussion, students learned to identify their own feelings and the feelings of others. Impulse control and anger management were also taught, and students were presented with problem-solving strategies, coping strategies, and behavioral skills. This program decreased physical aggression and increased prosocial behavior in the intervention group compared with the control group.[54]

It is extremely important that children feel that their world is safe and supportive. Physicians can support families, teachers, and communities in this common goal. Families of school-aged children should receive counseling on guns, the media, and exposure to violence and the possible negative effects that these factors may have on their children. Some of this discussion should happen in the physician's office. Knowledge and education are very powerful when it comes to dealing with bullying behavior.

Prognosis

Bullying is related to long-term negative outcomes. Former bullies have a four-fold increase in criminal behavior by 24 years of age. One third of former bullies with convictions were found to have three or more convictions.[55] Little is known about the long-term prognosis of victims.

Encopresis

Encopresis is defined as the voluntary or involuntary passage of feces in inappropriate places. For diagnosis of this condition, the DSM-IV requires the presence of the symptom for at least 3 months, with at least one episode per month, and it states that encopresis cannot be diagnosed in a patient younger than 4 years of age.[5] To be classified as encopresis, the elimination disorder cannot be due to a general medical condition or the use of a laxative. Encopresis is most often caused by functional constipation but can also occur without constipation, when it is referred to as *functional nonretentive fecal soiling*.

Epidemiology

Encopresis is common, especially in school-aged boys. It is reported to affect 2.8% of 4-year-olds, 1.9% of 6-year-olds, and 1.6% of 10- to 11-year-olds.[56] In a Dutch population-based study, the prevalence was found to be 4.1% in 5- to 6-year-old children and 1.6% in 11- to 12-year-old children, and it was more common in boys than in girls (3.7% versus 2.4%).[4] US clinical studies suggest a higher male-to-female predominance of 3:1.[57]

Etiology

Most commonly caused by functional constipation, encopresis can be due to a low-fiber diet or constipating medications. Some children withhold bowel movements because they have experienced environmental stressors or psychological distress related to toileting. One study found that 63% of children who presented with fecal soiling had a history of painful defecation before the age of 3 years.[58] Withholding bowel movements leads to gradual distention of the rectum. Subsequently, more stool volume is necessary to elicit the urge to have a bowel movement. The retention of stool will also cause rectal sphincter muscles to weaken. Longer transit time in the colon allows for greater fluid reabsorption and causes the stool to become more formed. The soiling seen in encopresis is often due to overflow of liquid feces around the impacted rectum.

Differential Diagnosis

The differential diagnosis for encopresis is vast, encompassing a wide range of diseases. Constipation or fecal soiling can be caused by neurogenic, anatomic, endocrinologic, gastrointestinal, pharmacologic, or developmental processes. Neurogenic causes include Hirschsprung's disease, spina bifida, myelomeningocele, spinal cord injuries, and cerebral palsy. Anal stenosis can cause rectal impaction and overflow incontinence. Leading endocrinologic causes include hypothyroidism and hyperparathyroidism. Constipation can also be caused by metabolic abnormalities such as hypokalemia, hypomagnesemia, hypophosphatemia, and hypercalcemia. Pharmacologic agents that can slow intestinal transit time include opiates, phenothiazine, antidepressants, and anticholinergics. Constipation can also be caused by lead and iron toxicity. Cognitive impairment, autism, depression, oppositional defiant disorder, and ADHD are often associated with chronic constipation and soiling. Although it is important to remember this vast differential diagnosis, the overwhelming majority of children with encopresis have functional constipation.

Clinical Approach

History

The most common presentation of encopresis is underwear soiling. In most cases, symptoms have been present for months to years before they are brought to medical attention. Rarely, a precipitating event is identified. Since the presentation is commonly soiling with liquid stool, the underlying chronic constipation may be missed. The medical history should focus on the frequency, consistency, diameter, and size of the child's stool. Children with encopresis may have long intervals between bowel movements; commonly, the child has experienced abdominal discomfort or appetite changes. Abdominal pain is reported in approximately one half of children with encopresis and may occur daily or just before the evacuation of stool. Attention to urinary symptoms is warranted because approximately 30% of children with encopresis experience daytime and nighttime wetting. Furthermore, 33% of girls and 3% of boys with encopresis develop a urinary tract infection.[59] A thorough history including a complete past medical history, developmental history, meconium passage history, dietary history, medication list, and review of systems should be used to rule out other potential causes of soiling. It is also important to inquire about the child's relationships with peers and family members, as well as investigating any signs of sexual abuse, including sexually acting out, aggression, regression, depression, and eating disturbances.

Physical Examination

A physical examination is often valuable in the evaluation of a child with encopresis. In 50% of cases, an abdominal examination reveals a palpable mass in the left lower quadrant, which is the colon distended by fecal matter[56]; the examiner may also appreciate a dilated rectum on rectal examination. Up to 90% of children with functional constipation have firm, packed stool in the rectum.[56] A rectal examination is also useful for assessing sphincter tone. An examination of the perineum helps to focus on anal placement and the presence of anal fissures. A neurologic examination including lower extremity deep tendon reflexes, the anal wink reflex, and an assessment of lower extremity sensation may detect neurologic causes of constipation. Spina bifida occulta should be considered when examining the back for a sacral dimple or a patch of hair.

Diagnostic Tests

The diagnosis of encopresis relies heavily on the history and physical examination results. In fact, it is usually unnecessary to perform any laboratory or radiographic studies. Nonetheless, plain film abdominal radiographs can be used to document a dilated colon and to assess the extent of stool impaction. They are particularly helpful when the child is obese or unable to cooperate with the physical examination. An x-ray may also be useful when a child does not have an identifiable palpable fecal mass. Serum chemistries, urine cultures, and thyroid function tests are recommended when the clinical history and examination results warrant further investigation. Anorectal manometry, barium enemas, and rectal biopsies are recommended only when there is a high degree of clinical suspicion of a neurologic cause, especially Hirschsprung's disease.

Treatment

The four steps for successful treatment of encopresis are education, disimpaction, maintenance therapy, and gradual removal of medication support. Treatment begins with educating the child and the family, with particular emphasis on the chronic nature of the problem and its typically good prognosis (Table 6-3). Physicians should assure the child and the family that this is not a serious disease and need not become a lifelong problem. Emphasizing the physiologic basis of the disease often alleviates blame, and education demystifies the condition. Family members are the most important persons on the treatment team because they will track symptoms, enforce schedules, and dispense rewards. Complete treatment of encopresis to the point of remission generally requires 6–24 months.[60] Younger patient age at the time of diagnosis typically shortens the necessary treatment time.[61]

Step two, disimpaction, is absolutely essential for successful treatment (Table 6-4). Treatment options can be tailored to family preference. Allowing the child to have input into decisions concerning his medications gives him more power and control. Enemas alone or in combination with suppositories or oral laxatives can be used for disimpaction. High-dose mineral oil is a slower but more effective way to achieve results. High-dose laxatives, including milk of magnesia, are also good alternatives. Osmotic agents can be used in this "clean-out" phase as well.

Once successful disimpaction has been achieved, maintenance therapy is begun (Table 6-5). The primary goal of maintenance therapy is to promote regular stool production and to prevent stool reimpaction. Behavioral training plays a large role in maintenance therapy, while the family monitors and documents stool output. The child practices proper toilet sitting, with the

Table 6-3. Educational Points on Constipation and Soiling for Children and Families

- Functional constipation and soiling are common.
- Functional constipation begins early in life for most children due to:
  - Uncomfortable or painful stool passage
  - Withholding of stool to avoid discomfort
  - Diets higher in constipating foods and lower in fiber and fluid intake
  - The use of medications that are constipating
  - Developmental features (e.g., increasing autonomy and toilet avoidance)
  - Possible family genetic factors for slower colonic transit time
- Chronic impaction causes physiologic changes at the rectum.
  - The rectal vault is dilated and sensation to standard fecal volume is reduced.
  - Dilated rectal musculature may be less able to expel stool effectively.

Many children do not recognize their soiling accidents because of olfactory accommodation.

Low self-esteem and behavioral concerns improve with education/management of constipation.

Effective management requires a substantial commitment of child and family for 6–24 months.

The degree of child and family adherence is a predictor of the child's success.

It is important to work as a team (i.e., child, caretaker, medical provider) in a positive manner.

Adapted from: Felt BT, Brown P, Coran AG, et al: Functional constipation and soiling in children, *Clin Fam Pract* 6(3):709–730, 2004.

upper body flexed slightly forward and with the use of good foot support. Children are asked to routinely sit on the toilet for 5–10 minutes three to four times per day.[60] Praises and small rewards for cooperation are important components of the behavioral plan, and special attention to proper diet must be paid because it is important to ensure adequate daily dietary fiber and nondairy fluid intake. The recommended daily intake of fiber is 5–10 g plus the child's age in years.[62] Chronic medications are used to promote stool regularity including osmotic laxatives, mineral oil, or milk of magnesia. Disimpaction and laxatives are not necessary for the treatment of encopresis without constipation[63]; however, treatment should still entail education, proper toilet usage, and a positive reward system.

Prognosis

Recovery from encopresis is defined as three or more stools per week without soiling, with rates ranging from 30% to 50% after 1 year and from 48% to 75% after 5 years.[56] Treatment failure may occur when there are episodes of reimpaction, which may occur during changes in the child's routine including vacations or with poor treatment adherence. Relapses occur more often in boys than in girls (relative risk, 1.73).[64]

Obesity

A chapter on the health of the school-aged male child would not be complete without addressing obesity, which often begins during childhood and is a serious threat to US public health. Childhood obesity usually leads to adult obesity, and adult obesity creates considerable risk for cardiovascular disease and cancer. Furthermore, obesity that begins in childhood is more likely to be severe and lifelong. Childhood obesity is increasing and is already a problem of epidemic proportions worldwide. It is believed to stem from recent widespread societal changes associated with reductions in energy expenditure and increased caloric intake. Obesity-associated annual hospital costs for children aged 6–17 years increased from $35 million during the period from 1979 to 1981 up to $127 million during 1997 to 1999, based on the 2001 constant US dollar value.[65]

Current adult definitions for *overweight* and *obesity* are based on body mass indices (BMIs) of equal to or greater than 27 and 30, respectively. In children, a BMI equal to or greater than the 95th percentile for age and gender is comparable to an adult BMI at or above 30. However, in children this level is often called "overweight" to avoid the emotionally laden term "obese." Children whose BMI is at or above the 85th percentile have similar body fat to adults with a BMI equal or greater than 27. In children this level is referred to as being "at risk for overweight." *Obesity*, on the other hand, is a surplus of adipose tissue and is defined as a body fat of greater than 17–19% in prepubertal children. Because body fat is not routinely measured in either epidemiologic studies or in clinical work, BMI provides a proxy for body fat composition.

Effective treatment for overweight and obesity is difficult; therefore, prevention is paramount. Physicians can play a role in prevention, identification, and treatment through targeted education efforts. Excess weight gain typically occurs over a long period of time and often goes unnoticed in the early stages. Behavioral change to increase physical activity and to decrease food intake provides a significant challenge both for school-aged boys and their parents.

Table 6-4. Recommended Medications for Clean-Out of Impaction*

Medication	Adverse Effects/Comments
Infants	
Glycerin suppositories	No side effects reported
Children	
Rapid clean-out	
Enemas: 6 mL/kg up to 135 mL every 12–24 hours × 1–3	Invasive, risk of mechanical trauma
	Large impaction: mineral oil enema followed 1–3 hours later by normal saline or phosphate enema
	Small impaction: normal saline or phosphate enema
Mineral oil	Lubricates hard impaction, may not see return after administration
Normal saline	Abdominal cramping, less effective than hypertonic phosphate
Hypertonic phosphate	Abdominal cramping, risk of hyperphosphatemia, hypokalemia, or hypocalcemia if retained, especially with Hirschsprung's disease or renal insufficiency
	Caution with phosphate enema for children younger than 4 years; not advised in those younger than 2 years
Milk-to-molasses, 1:1	For difficult to clear impactions
Combination therapy: enema, suppository, oral laxative	
Day 1: Enema every 12–24 hours	See "enemas"
Day 2: Bisacodyl suppository (10 mg) every12–24 hours	Abdominal cramping, diarrhea, hypokalemia
Day 3: Bisacodyl tablet (5 mg) every 12–24 hours	Abdominal cramping, diarrhea, hypokalemia
Repeat 3-day cycle if needed one or two times	
Oral/nasogastric: Polyethylene glycol solution @ 25 mL/kg/hr up to 1000 mL/hr for 4 hr	Nausea, cramping, vomiting, bloating
	Large volume
Slower clean-out	
Oral high-dosage mineral oil: 15–30 mL per year of age per day up to 240 mL for 3–4 day	Aspiration—lipoid pneumonia
	Give chilled
High-dosage senna: 15 mL every 12 hr × 3	Abdominal cramping
	May not see output until dosage 2 or 3
Magnesium citrate: 30 mL /year of age to maximum of 300 mL /day for 2–3 day	Hypermagnesemia, hypophosphatemia

*Maintenance medications may also be used for cleanout (see Table 6-5).

Adapted from: Felt BT, Brown P, Coran AG, et al: Functional constipation and soiling in children, *Clin Fam Pract* 6(3):709–730, 2004.

Epidemiology

Nationally representative data for the years 1999–2002 reveal that 16.9% of US boys aged 6–11 years were overweight. This prevalence is a large increase from the period of 1971–1974, when only 3.8% of boys in this age range were found to be overweight.[66] An additional 15.6% of boys are in the "at risk" category; thus 32.5% of school-aged boys are either overweight or considered at risk for becoming overweight. Interestingly, boys are slightly more likely to be overweight than girls, prior to adolescence (16.9% versus 14.7%).[67] The prevalence of overweight children is increasing in all racial groups, but the increase in prevalence among minority groups is more dramatic than in white children (rate of increase is 3.2% in white, 4.3% in Hispanic, and 5.9% in African American youth).[68] Overweight children

Table 6-5. Maintenance Medications in the Treatment of Functional Constipation

Medication	Adverse Effects/Comments
Infants	
Oral medications/other	
Juices containing sorbitol	Pear, prune, apple
Lactulose or sorbitol: 1–3 mL/kg/day in two divided dosages	See below
Corn syrup (light or dark): 1–3 mL/kg/day in two divided dosages	Not considered a risk for *Clostridium botulinum* spores
Per rectum	
Glycerin suppository	No side effects reported
Children	
Oral medications	
Lubricants	Softens stool and eases passage
Mineral oil: 1–3 mL/kg/day as one dose or two divided dosages	Risk of aspiration—lipoid pneumonia
	Avoid if vomiting is problematic for the child. Chill or give with juice. Adherence problems may occur.
	If leakage of mineral oil, consider too-high dosage or possibility of impaction
Osmotic	Retains water in stool to aid bulk and softness
Lactulose: 10 g/15 mL, 1–3 mL/kg/day in two divided dosages	Synthetic disaccharide, potentially causes abdominal cramping, flatus
Magnesium hydroxide (milk of magnesia): 400 mg/5 mL, 1–3 mL/kg/day in two divided dosages	Risk of hypermagnesemia, hypophosphatemia, secondary hypocalcemia with overdose and/or renal insufficiency
Polyethylene glycol powder: 17 g/ 240 mL water of juice stock, 1.0 g/kg/day in two divided dosages	Titrate dose at 3-day intervals to achieve mushy stool consistency. May make stock solutions to administer over 1 or 2 days.
	Excellent adherence
Sorbitol: 1–3 mL/kg/day in two divided dosages	Less costly than lactulose
Stimulants[†]	Improves effectiveness of colonic and rectal muscle contractions
Senna syrup: 8.8 g sennoside/ 5 mL 2–5 years: 2.5–7.5 mL/day in two divided dosages. 6–12 years 5–15 mL/day in two divided dosages (tablets and granules available)	Idiosyncratic hepatitis, melanosis coli, hypertrophic osteoarthropathy, analgesic nephropathy, abdominal cramping. Melanosis coli improves after medication stopped
Bisacodyl: 5-mg tablets, 1–3 tablets/dosage 1–2 times daily	Abdominal cramping, diarrhea, hypokalemia
Per rectum	
Glycerin suppository	No side effects reported
Bisacodyl: 10 mg suppositories, 0.5–1 suppository, 1–2 times daily	Abdominal cramping, diarrhea, hypokalemia

[*]A single agent may suffice to achieve daily, comfortable stools.
[†]Stimulants should be reserved for short-term use.
Adapted from: Felt BT, Brown P, Coran AG, et al: Functional constipation and soiling in children, *Clin Fam Pract* 6(3):709–730, 2004.

are very likely to become obese adults, with 69% of 6- to 9-year-old and 83% of 10- to 14-year-old overweight children remaining obese into adulthood.[69] Furthermore, approximately half of obese adults were overweight as children.[70]

Etiology

The etiology of obesity is multifactorial. Energy is stored in adipose tissue, which reflects the balance between food intake and energy expenditure.

Even a small positive balance over a long period of time can lead to substantial weight gain. Hormones and neurochemicals play a role in obesity development by acting on the hypothalamus to increase or decrease appetite and to regulate energy expenditure. The occurrence of single-gene obesity syndromes and obesity-associated conditions such as Prader-Willi syndrome suggests possible genetic mechanisms. Twin and adoption studies also support a possible genetic component to obesity.[71,72] Furthermore, parental obesity is an important risk for child obesity.[69] Shared environment must also be accounted for as a contributor, as the recent increase in the prevalence of obesity suggests a strong environmental component to the etiology of obesity.

Inadequate physical activity plays a significant role in the etiology of obesity. Recent research demonstrated that 20% of school-aged children participate in two or fewer periods of vigorous activity per week.[73] In fact, children are inactive for 75.5% of their day and spend 5.2 hours a day in sedentary activities including television, computer time, or homework. In contrast, these children spend only an average of 12.6 minutes engaged in vigorous activity per day.[68] Television time directly correlates with BMI[73–75] and an increased risk of obesity. The current understanding is that television time is associated with both decreased activity and increased intake of calorie-rich foods.

There are many identified risk factors for childhood obesity. High maternal BMI during pregnancy, increased birth weight, and rapid weight gain during the first 4 months of life have been found to be early risk factors for obesity.[76,77] Formula-fed infants have been found to be at a higher risk for becoming obese compared with breast-fed infants,[78] and children who undergo earlier adiposity rebound have higher rates of obesity later in life, as well.[79] Children of overweight parents appear to prefer foods higher in fat than children of normal-weight parents, which may increase their risk of becoming obese.[80] Sugar-sweetened drinks increase the risk for obesity with a dose-response association.[81]

Differential Diagnosis

Although obesity is largely due to increased caloric balance, endocrine and genetic conditions should be considered as potential causes. Hypothyroidism, Cushing's syndrome, pseudohypoparathyroidism, and growth hormone deficiencies present with increased adiposity and usually short stature. Genetic syndromes, such as Prader-Willi, Laurence-Moon-Biedl, Beckwith-Wiedemann, Cohen, Carpenter, and Alström syndromes are also potential causes of obesity. Hypothetically, childhood depression may be associated with increased eating and decreased activity resulting in increased risk for obesity. Some psychotropic medications cause hyperphagia and weight gain, including risperidone (Risperdal) and olanzapine (Zyprexa).

Comorbidities

Obesity places children at risk for concurrent comorbid conditions as well as future problems in adulthood. Overweight children tend to be taller, have more advanced bone ages, and mature earlier than their non-overweight counterparts.[82] Type 2 diabetes in children is increasing in parallel with the obesity epidemic,[83] and impaired glucose tolerance is quite common in obese children.[84] Hypertension and hyperlipidemia are cardiovascular complications that can be associated with obesity in children. Obstructive sleep apnea, which presents with snoring, fatigue, and daytime somnolence can lead to further decreased physical activity, potentially causing more weight gain. Furthermore, pulmonary hypertension can occur as a result of obstructive sleep apnea. Pseudotumor cerebri may be diagnosed in an obese child presenting with headache and visual impairment. Gastrointestinal complications, including fatty liver disease and cholelithiasis, as well as orthopedic complications such as Blount's disease and slipped capital femoral epiphysis, are also more common in boys who are overweight.

Clinical Manifestations

History

Evaluation of obesity in a school-aged boy begins with a thorough medical history. Documentation of the child's birth weight and past growth points for height and weight allows the clinician to understand when the child developed rapid growth velocity as well as the duration of the problem. The perinatal history should include information regarding the child's early feeding practices. Furthermore, it is useful to assess whether the child experienced normal slowing of appetite during the toddler years. A sudden change in growth velocity may indicate a new medical problem or a change in the child's psychosocial environment. The timing of adiposity rebound can be documented or extrapolated to help in understanding the child's risk. The parent's perception of the child's weight may influence adherence to nutritional and physical activity recommendations.

A complete history should include the child's past medical history, developmental history, medication history, social history, family history, and a review of systems. The past medical history is used to determine other possible causes of the child's obesity, to uncover contributing factors, or to discover comorbid conditions. Evidence of developmental delay suggests underlying genetic or neurodevelopmental problems. The medication history may reveal medications with a potential to alter appetite. A social history contributes to understanding of etiology and helps to define possible barriers to instituting lifestyle changes. For instance, financial barriers may limit the purchasing of healthy food. The family history may determine whether the child's pattern of weight gain is similar to others in the family, including the timing of adiposity rebound and puberty. This is an excellent opportunity to engage the parents by asking whether they have ever "struggled with their weight." Determining whether other family members have difficulty controlling their weight and what treatments and interventions may have been used will reveal a great deal about the family belief system and values concerning body weight. The family history should also include specific questions about diabetes mellitus type 2, hypertension, cardiovascular disease, and obstructive sleep apnea. The review of systems is aimed to uncover any potential causes of the child's weight gain as well as any comorbid conditions. For example, if a child reports polyuria and polydipsia, an evaluation for type 2 diabetes mellitus is warranted. Abdominal pain may prompt an evaluation for gallbladder disease, whereas sleep disturbances and daytime sleepiness may lead to the evaluation for obstructive sleep apnea.

Dietary history is paramount in the evaluation of childhood obesity. A 24-hour recall of meals and snacks allows an estimation of caloric intake. Alternately, a 72-hour food diary can be kept by the parents. Although accuracy is not always perfect, these histories are a good starting place. Identifying eating-associated conditions such as time and place allow for the development of strategies to reduce dietary intake. Eating breakfast has been associated with a lower risk for obesity; consumption of fast food and highly sugared beverages have been associated with an increased risk. Eating together as a family may reduce unhealthy eating behaviors in the child.

However, it may be difficult if there is only one child who needs to restrict caloric intake. Establishing what foods are preferred is also helpful. The physician should ask the parents whether their child has ever engaged in binging or purging behavior. It is also important to ask whether food has ever been used as a reward.

Assessment of the child's physical activity is equally important. Parents are asked about the child's regular physical activity, including sports and physical education classes, as well as walking to school and playing outside. Establishing how often and how long the child engages in these activities is a salient detail. It may be important to determine whether the child lives in an environment where it is safe to be outside. As with the dietary history, a parent can either do a 24-hour recall or a 3-day diary of all of the child's activities (including at least one weekend day and one weekday). This activity history should include homework, television, computer, and video game time. The parents should be asked about the child's eating habits during passive activities. The individual and group physical activity patterns of the family are important determinants of the child's activity patterns. It is also important to establish whether the child's weight impedes desired physical activity or participation in sports.

Lastly, the child's psychological well-being should also be assessed. In some cultures and in some families, shame accompanies obesity. Questions regarding the child's interactions with peers may also be helpful in the assessment of how the child's weight affects his life. Overweight children may be the victims of teasing, leading to low self-esteem. Depression is often associated with obesity, but the causal pathways have not been clearly established.

Physical Examination

A complete physical examination aids the physician in ruling out other potential causes of obesity and allows for the detection of any comorbid conditions. It is important to remember that the child's weight alone does not determine that a child is overweight; the child's age, height, and sex must also be taken into account. Weight, height, and BMI should be plotted on a growth curve specific for the child's age and sex to determine the percentiles for each of these measurements. It is essential to have multiple height and weight measurements to calculate and plot BMI curves and to assess growth velocity. A child who is overweight with a faster rate of weight gain is at an increased risk for complications and problems compared with a child who is overweight with a normal rate of weight gain. Two different children may have the same BMI yet different degrees of fatness or muscle mass. A skinfold thickness measurement can be used to assess subcutaneous fat, yet it is not directly proportional to total body fat and is also not a perfect indicator of obesity.

The recommendations that follow are based on conditions associated with obesity. Blood pressure should be monitored at each visit. A thorough physical examination for findings suggestive of underlying endocrine or genetic disorders is recommended. For example, the presence of dysmorphic features may indicate an associated genetic disorder. Hypogonadism and undescended testes are symptoms of Prader-Willi syndrome. Moon facies, short stature, a buffalo hump, and high blood pressure suggest Cushing's syndrome. Thyroid hypertrophy or nodules may indicate hypothyroidism. Pseudohypoparathyroidism may be suspected if a child has short stature, short metacarpals and metatarsals, and subcutaneous calcifications. A child's Tanner stage assessment may identify early-onset puberty related to obesity.

Comorbidities may also be screened for during the physical examination. For example, hip range of motion is reduced in the condition known as *slipped capital femoral epiphysis.* An inspection of the skin may reveal hirsutism and acne in precocious puberty and androgen disorders. Type 2 diabetes mellitus can lead to examination findings such as acanthosis nigricans in the neck, axilla, and groin. Male genitalia may show signs of balanitis and tinea. After a diagnosis of type 2 diabetes mellitus is established, a funduscopic examination with dilation should be performed annually. An examination of the child's feet including pedal pulses and a peripheral neurologic examination are also important in the case of diabetes or prediabetes to assess long-term foot care.

Diagnostic Tests

Diagnostic tests are unnecessary to confirm a diagnosis of obesity. However, laboratory testing may be considered to determine an endocrine or a genetic cause of obesity suggested by the history or physical examination. Laboratory tests are most important for the assessment of obesity-related medical conditions such as type 2 diabetes mellitus or hyperlipidemia. A fasting plasma glucose concentration greater than 126 mg/dL is diagnostic for diabetes mellitus, and a level between 110 and 126 mg/dL is considered to be prediabetes. A fasting lipid panel, including measurements of total cholesterol, high-density lipoprotein cholesterol, low-density lipoprotein cholesterol (LDL), and triglycerides is recommended by the AAP at least once for an overweight child 3 years of age and older, and more regularly for those with a family history of hyperlipidemia. A total serum cholesterol level equal to or greater than 170 mg/dL and an LDL equal to or greater than 110 mg/dL are considered to be elevated values in childhood and adolescence.[85]

Treatment

The treatment of obesity is complex and requires multiple modalities. It is important that primary care physicians detect childhood obesity early because it is more likely to respond to intervention than adult obesity. An assessment of parental and child willingness to change is the first step in the development of a treatment plan because successful treatment requires behavior change. Using Prochaska's Stages of Change model, individuals and families can be classified as pre-contemplative, contemplative, or ready to change.[86] Once the desire for change has been established, goals for nutrition and physical activity can be developed. Realistic and attainable goals should be set to establish the experience of success and to minimize the child's and family's frustrations. This can begin with a minimal increase in activity and a decrease in passive activity. These goals can be increased as the child successfully meets the previous goal, creating a stepwise process. Guiding the child and family together toward the institution of healthy eating practices and the promotion of physical activity rather than the achievement of ideal body weight is recommended.[87]

Children should begin with an attempt to slow their rapid growth velocity, even before attempting to maintain their baseline weight; maintenance of baseline weight will ultimately lead to a decline in BMI as height increases. For children 7 years of age and older who are "at risk for overweight" (i.e., BMI between the 85th and 95th percentile) prolonged weight maintenance is the goal. For children whose BMI is at or above the 95th percentile, weight loss is recommended after weight maintenance has been achieved. Further changes in diet and physical activity, with the goal of losing 1 pound per month, is often reasonable and achievable.

Families must be involved in the treatment program for weight optimization if the program is to be successful. Although treatment aims for permanent changes in nutrition and physical activity, families should understand that change will be a slow and gradual process. Doctors should encourage families to take a supportive, noncritical approach. Ideally, families will establish regular meal and snack times. Parents should provide mainly healthy options, focusing on eliminating or reducing specific high-calorie foods. It is important that the child does not feel deprived, even though he will experience hunger as calories are reduced. Goals for activity include increasing the child's physical activity level and reducing time spent in sedentary behaviors including television watching and computer time. There are data to support that reducing television time can improve BMI. A comparison study of a classroom intervention to reduce television, video, and video game time in third and fourth graders showed that children in the intervention group who decreased their television time experienced a decrease in their average BMI, whereas that of the comparison group increased. A more recent study of a family intervention to reduce television watching, paired with dance classes, for 8- to 10-year-old African American girls resulted in decreased television viewing and a trend toward decreased BMI after only 12 weeks.[75,88,89]

To date, primary care interventions for childhood obesity have not been well studied.[90] Most research has focused on intensive group- and individual family–based behavioral counseling interventions in multidisciplinary obesity clinics. Bariatric surgery and weight loss medications are not options for school-aged children, although there have been trials examining the role of this procedure in adolescents.

Prognosis

In overweight children who normalize their BMI by adulthood, the prognosis for good health—especially good cardiovascular health—is favorable. The impact of childhood obesity that does not persist into adulthood on socioeconomic, educational, psychological, and social outcomes does not appear to be associated with adult social class, income, years of schooling, educational attainment, relationships, or psychological morbidity in either sex after adjustment for confounding factors.[70] However, childhood obesity persisting into adulthood is associated with poor employment and relationship outcomes in women.[91]

Conclusions

This chapter has focused on four specific health conditions with importance for the proper health of school-aged boys, and this is certainly not a comprehensive list. Although we have focused on health conditions, boys experience educational disparities as well. Boys are more likely than girls to be labeled with an emotional disturbance, learning disability, or speech problem.[92–95] Perhaps some of these educational problems are related to underlying health disparities, including ADHD. Or, perhaps both health and educational disparities are related to social conditions that increase the risk for boys. Some educational and health disparities may relate to social factors including neighborhood safety, income inequality, influences of media, and cultural norms of male success.

Although there are unfortunately more questions than answers, it is clear that school-aged boys and girls have always faced different challenges and still do today. A uniform approach to boys and girls in school or in physicians' offices often neglects gender-defined differences and needs. Physicians can think about the special needs of boys, begin to screen for male-predominant conditions earlier, and strive to identify environmental factors that may predispose boys to ADHD, bullying, and encopresis. Defining these problems is only the first step. Physicians need to consider how early life conditions shape healthy men who will be expected to succeed in cognitive or technical workplaces, and share in the care of a home and nurturing of children. All the while, they must be courageous, loving, and know right from wrong. ADHD, bullying, encopresis, and obesity all create significant risk for the development of low self-esteem and impaired well-being that could last a lifetime.

References

1. Nansel TR, Overpeck M, Pilla RS, et al: Bullying behaviors among US youth: prevalence and association with psychosocial adjustment, *JAMA* 285 (16):2094–2100, 2001.
2. Baker SS, Liptak GS, Colletti RB, et al: Constipation in infants and children: evaluation and treatment. A medical position statement of the North American Society for Pediatric Gastroenterology and Nutrition, *J Pediatr Gastroenterol Nutr* 29(5):612–626, 1999.
3. Levine MD: Children with encopresis: a descriptive analysis, *Pediatrics* 56:412–416, 1975.
4. van der Wal MF, Benninga MA, Hirasing RA: The prevalence of encopresis in a multicultural population, *J Pediatr Gastroenterol Nutr* 40:345–348, 2005.
5. American Psychiatric Association: *Diagnostic and statistical manual of mental disorders*, ed 4, text revision, Washington, DC, 2000, American Psychiatric Association.

6. Committee on Quality Improvement and Subcommittee on Attention-Deficit/Hyperactivity Disorder: Clinical practice guideline: diagnosis and evaluation of the child with attention-deficit/hyperactivity disorder, *Pediatrics* 105:1158–1170, 2000.

7. Brown RT, Freeman WS, Perrin JM, et al: Prevalence and assessment of attention-deficit/hyperactivity disorder in primary care settings, *Pediatrics* 107: e43, 2001.

8. American Psychiatric Association: *Diagnostic and statistical manual of mental disorders*, ed 4, text revision, Washington, DC, 1994, American Psychiatric Association.

9. Dulcan M: Practice parameters for the assessment and treatment of children, adolescents, and adults with attention-deficit/hyperactivity disorder, *J Am Acad Child Adolesc Psychiatry* 36(10 Suppl): 85S–121S, 1997.

10. Subcommittee on Attention-Deficit/Hyperactivity Disorder and Committee on Quality Improvement: Clinical practice guideline: treatment of the school-aged child with attention-deficit/hyperactivity disorder, *Pediatrics* 108:1033–1044, 2001.

11. Green M, Wong M, Atkins D, et al: *Diagnosis of attention deficit/hyperactivity disorder: technical review 3*, Agency for Health Care Policy and Research publication 99–0050, 1999. Rockville, Md, 1999, US Department of Health and Human Services, Agency for Health Care Policy and Research.

12. Barkley RA, Murphy KR: *Attention deficit hyperactivity disorder: a clinical workbook*, ed 2, New York, 1998, Guilford.

13. Wolraich ML, Lambert W, Doffing MA, et al: Psychometric properties of the Vanderbilt ADHD diagnostic parent rating scale in a referred population, *J Pediatr Psychol* 28:559–567, 2003.

14. Bhatara V, Loudenberg R, Ellis R: Association of attention deficit hyperactivity disorder and gestational alcohol exposure: an exploratory study, *J Atten Dis* 9(3):515–522, 2006.

15. O'Malley KD, Nanson J: Clinical implications of a link between fetal alcohol spectrum disorder and attention-deficit/hyperactivity disorder, *Can J Psychiatry* 47(4):349–354, 2002.

16. Cornish KM, Turk J, Wilding J, et al: Annotation: deconstructing the attention deficit in fragile X syndrome: a developmental neuropsychological approach, *J Child Psychol Psychiatry* 45(6): 1042–1053, 2004.

17. Bijur P, Golding J, Haslum M, et al: Behavioral predictors of injury in school-age children, *Am J Dis Child* 142(12):1307–1312, 1988.

18. Swensen A, Birnbaum HG, Ben Hamadi R, et al: Incidence and costs of accidents among attention-deficit/hyperactivity disorder patients, *J Adolesc Health* 35(4):346, e1–e9, 2004.

19. James A, Lai FH, Dahl C: Attention deficit hyperactivity disorder and suicide: a review of possible associations, *Acta Psychiatr Scand* 110(6): 408–415, 2004.

20. Lam LT: Attention deficit disorder and hospitalization owing to intra- and interpersonal violence among children and young adolescents, *J Adolesc Health* 36:19–24, 2005.

21. The MTA Cooperative Group: Multimodal treatment study of children with ADHD: a 14-month randomized clinical trial of treatment strategies for attention-deficit/hyperactivity disorder, *Arch Gen Psychiatry* 56:1073–1086, 1999.

22. Wilens TE, Faraone SV, Biederman J, et al: Does stimulant therapy of attention-deficit/hyperactivity disorder beget later substance abuse? A meta-analytic review of the literature, *Pediatrics* 111(1): 179–185, 2003.

23. Abikoff HB, Jensen PS, Arnold LL, et al: Observed classroom behavior of children with ADHD: relationship to gender and comorbidity, *J Abnorm Child Psychol* 30:349–359, 2002.

24. Gershon J: A meta-analytic review of gender differences in ADHD, *J Atten Dis* 5(3):143–154, 2002.

25. Biederman J, Mick E, Faraone SV, et al: Influence of gender on attention deficit hyperactivity disorder in children referred to a psychiatric clinic, *Am J Psychiatry* 159:36–42, 2002.

26. Graetz BW, Sawyer MG, Baghurst P: Gender differences among children with DSM-IV ADHD in Australia, *J Am Acad Child Adolesc Psychiatry* 44: 159–168, 2005.

27. Barkley RA, Fischer M, Edelbrock CS, et al: The adolescent outcome of hyperactive children diagnosed by research criteria, *J Am Acad Child Adolesc Psychiatry* 29:546–557, 1990.

28. Harpin VA: The effect of ADHD on the life of an individual, their family, and community from preschool to adult life, *Arch Dis Childhood* 90(Suppl 1): i2–i7, 20, 2005.

29. Biederman J, Faraone SV, Spencer TJ, et al: Functional impairments in adults with self-reports of diagnosed ADHD: a controlled study of 1001 adults in the community, *J Clin Psychiatry* 67(4): 524–540, 2006.

30. Mannuzza S, Klein RG: Long-term prognosis in attention-deficit/hyperactivity disorder, *Child Adolesc Psychiatr Clin North Am* 9:711–726, 2000.

31. Elia J, Ambrosini PJ, Rapoport JL: TI Treatment of attention-deficit-hyperactivity disorder, *N Engl J Med* 340:780–788, 1999.

32. Boulton MJ, Underwood K: Bully/victim problems among middle school children, *Br J Educ Psychol* 62:73–87, 1992.

33. Olweus D: *Aggression in the schools: bullying and whipping boys*, Washington, DC, 1978, Hemisphere.

34. Olweus D: *Bullying at school: what we know and what we can do*, Malden, Mass, 1993, Blackwell.

35. Wolke D, Woods S, Stanford K, et al: Bullying and victimization of primary school children in England and Germany: prevalence and school factors, *Br J Psychol* 92:673–696, 2001.

36. Anderson M, Kaufman J, Simon TR, et al: School-associated violent deaths in the United States, 1994–1999, *JAMA* 286:2695–2702, 2001.

37. Nansel TR, Overpeck MD, Haynie DL, et al: Relationships between bullying and violence among

US youth, *Arch Pediatr Adolesc Med* 157:348–353, 2003.

38. Juvonen J, Graham S, Schuster MA: Bullying among young adolescents: the strong, the weak, and the troubled, *Pediatrics* 112:1231–1237, 2003.

39. Fekkes M, Pijpers FI, Verloove-Vanhorick SP: Bullying: who does what, when and where? Involvement of children, teachers and parents in bullying behavior, *Health Educ Res* 20:81–91, 2005.

40. Veenstra R, Lindenberg S, Oldehinkel AJ, et al: Bullying and victimization in elementary schools: a comparison of bullies, victims, bully/victims, and uninvolved preadolescents, *Dev Psychol* 41: 672–682, 2005.

41. Pellegrini AD, Long JD: A longitudinal study of bullying, dominance, and victimization during the transition from primary school through secondary school, *Br J Dev Psychol* 20:259–280, 2002.

42. Durant RH, Pendergrast RA, Cadenhead C: Exposure to violence and victimization and fighting behavior by urban black adolescents, *J Adolesc Health* 15:311–318, 1994.

43. Schuler ME, Nair P: Witnessing violence among inner-city children of substance-abusing and non–substance-abusing women, *Arch Pediatr Adolesc Med* 155:342–346, 2001.

44. Straus MA, Sugarman DB, Giles-Sims J: Spanking by parents and subsequent antisocial behavior of children, *Arch Pediatr Adolesc Med* 151:761–767, 1997.

45. Schwartz D, Dodge KA, Pettit GS, et al: The early socialization of aggressive victims of bullying, *Child Development* 68:665–675, 1997.

46. Kumpulainen K, Rasanen E, Puura K: Psychiatric disorders and the use of mental health services among children involved in bullying, *Aggress Behav* 27:102–110, 2001.

47. Saluja G, Iachan R, Scheidt PC, et al: Prevalence of and risk factors for depressive symptoms among young adolescents, *Arch Pediatr Adolesc Med* 158 (8):760–765, 2004.

48. Smith-Khuri E, Iachan R, Scheidtz PC, et al: A cross-national study of violence-related behaviors in adolescents, *Arch Pediatr Adolesc Med* 158(6):539–544, 2004.

49. Kaltiala-Heino R, Rimpela M, Marttunen M, et al: Bullying, depression, and suicidal ideation in Finnish adolescents: school survey, *Br Med J* 319 (7206):348–351, 1999.

50. Rigby K, Slee P: Suicidal ideation among adolescent school children, involvement in bully-victim problems, and perceived social support, *Suicide Life-Threat Behav* 29(2):119–130, 1999.

51. Ivarsson T, Broberg AG, Arvidsson T, et al: Bullying in adolescence: psychiatric problems in victims and bullies as measured by the Youth Self Report (YSR) and the Depression Self-Rating Scale (DSRS), *Nordic J Psychiatry* 59(5):365–373, 2005.

52. Glew G, Rivara F, Feudtner C: Bullying: children hurting children, *Pediatr Rev* 21:183–190, 2000.

53. Twemlow SW, Fonagy P, Sacco FC, et al: Creating a peaceful school learning environment: a controlled study of an elementary school intervention to reduce violence, *Am J Psychiatry* 158:808–810, 2001.

54. Grossman DC, Neckerman HJ, Koepsell TD, et al: Effectiveness of a violence prevention curriculum among children in elementary school: a randomized controlled trial, *JAMA* 277:1605–1611, 1997.

55. Olweus D: Bullying among school children: intervention and prevention. In Peters RD, McMahon RJ, Quinsey VL, editors: *Aggression and violence throughout the life span*, London, 1992, Sage Publications, pp 100–125.

56. Loening-Baucke V: Encopresis, *Curr Opin Pediatr* 14:570–575, 2002.

57. Felt BT, Brown C, Kochhar AG, et al: Functional constipation and soiling in children, *Clin Fam Pract* 6:709–730, 2004.

58. Partin JC, Hamill SK, Fischel JE, et al: Painful defecation and fecal soiling in children, *Pediatrics* 89(6 pt 1):1007–1009, 1992.

59. Loening-Baucke V: Urinary incontinence and urinary tract infection and their resolution with treatment of chronic constipation of childhood, *Pediatrics* 100(2 pt 1):228–232, 1997.

60. Felt B, Wise CG, Olson A, et al: Guideline for the management of pediatric idiopathic constipation and soiling: multidisciplinary team from the University of Michigan Medical Center in Ann Arbor, *Arch Pediatr Adolesc Med* 153:380–385, 1999.

61. Taubman B, Buzby M: Overflow encopresis and stool toileting refusal during toilet training: a prospective study on the effect of therapeutic efficacy, *J Pediatr* 131:768–771, 1997.

62. Williams CL, Bollella M, Wynder EL: A new recommendation for dietary fiber in childhood, *Pediatrics* 96(5 pt 2):985–988, 1995.

63. van Ginkel R, Benninga MA, Blommaart PJ, et al: Lack of benefit of laxatives as adjunctive therapy for functional nonretentive fecal soiling in children, *J Pediatr* 137:808–813, 2000.

64. van Ginkel R, Reitsma JB, Buller HA, et al: Childhood constipation: longitudinal follow-up beyond puberty, *Gastroenterology* 125:357–363, 2003.

65. Wang G, Dietz WH: Economic burden of obesity in youths aged 6 to 17 years: 1979–1999, *Pediatrics* 1009:e81, 2002.

66. Troiano RP, Flegal KM: Overweight children and adolescents: description, epidemiology, and demographics, *Pediatrics* 101(3 pt 2):497–504, 1998.

67. Hedley AA, Ogden CL, Johnson CL, et al: Prevalence of overweight and obesity among US children, adolescents, and adults, 1999–2002, *JAMA* 291: 2847–2850, 2004.

68. Strauss RS, Pollack HA: Epidemic increase in childhood overweight, 1986–1998, *JAMA* 286: 2845–2848, 2001.

69. Whitaker RC, Wright JA, Pepe MS, et al: Predicting obesity in young adulthood from childhood and parental obesity, *N Engl J Med* 337:869–873, 1997.

70. Freedman DS, Kettel-Khan L, Dietz WH, et al: Relationship of childhood obesity to coronary heart disease risk factors in adulthood: the Bogalusa Heart Study, *Pediatrics* 108:712–718, 2001.

71. Stunkard A, Foch T, Hrubec Z: A twin study of human obesity, *JAMA* 256:51–54, 1986.

72. Stunkard A, Sorensen T, Hanis C: An adoption study of human obesity, *N Engl J Med* 314:193–198, 1986.

73. Anderson RE, Crespo CJ, Bartlett SJ, et al: Relationship of physical activity and television watching with body weight and level of fatness among children: results from the third national health and nutrition examination survey, *JAMA* 279: 938–942, 1998.

74. Gortmaker SL, Must A, Sobol AM, et al: Television viewing as a cause of increasing obesity among children in the United States, 1986–1990, *Arch Pediatr Adolesc Med* 150:356–362, 1996.

75. Robinson TN: Reducing children's television viewing to prevent obesity: a randomized controlled trial, *JAMA* 282:1561–1567, 1999.

76. Eriksson J, Forsen T, Osmond C, et al: Obesity from cradle to grave, *Int J Obes Relat Metab Disord* 27:722–727, 2003.

77. Stettler N, Zemel BS, Kumanyika S, et al: In fact weight gain and childhood overweight status in a multicenter cohort study, *Pediatrics* 109: 194–199, 2002.

78. Toschke AM, Vignerova J, Lhotska L, et al: Overweight and obesity in 6 to 14 year old Czech children in 1991: protective effect of breast-feeding, *J Pediatr* 141:749–757, 2002.

79. Whitaker RC, Pepe MS, Wright JA, et al: Early adiposity rebound and the risk for adult obesity, *Pediatrics* 101:e5, 1998.

80. Fischer JO, Birch LL: Fat preferences and fat consumption of 3 to 5 year old children are related to parental adiposity, *J Am Diet Assoc* 95:759–764, 1995.

81. Ludwig DS, Peterson KE, Gortmaker SL: Relation between consumption of sugar-sweetened drinks and childhood obesity: a prospective, observational analysis, *Lancet* 357:505–508, 2001.

82. Forbes GB: Nutrition and growth, *J Pediatr* 91:40–42, 1977.

83. Pinhas-Hamiel O, Dolan LM, Daniels SR: Increased incidence of non–insulin-dependent diabetes mellitus among adolescents, *J Pediatr* 128:608–615, 1996.

84. Sinha R, Fisch G, Teague B, et al: Prevalence of impaired glucose tolerance among children and adolescents with marked obesity, *N Engl J Med* 346:802–810, 2002.

85. American Academy of Pediatrics, Committee on Nutrition: Cholesterol in childhood, *Pediatrics* 101: 141–147, 1998.

86. Prochaska JO, DiClemente CC: Transtheoretical therapy toward a more integrative model of change, *Psychotherapy* 19(3):276–287, 1982.

87. Barlow SE, Dietz WH: Obesity evaluation and treatment: expert committee recommendations, *Pediatrics* 102:e29, 1998.

88. Epstein LH, Valoski AM, Vara LS, et al: Effects of decreasing sedentary behavior and increasing activity on weight change in obese children, *Health Psychol* 14:109–115, 1995.

89. Robinson TN, Killen JD, Kraemer HC, et al: Dance and reducing television viewing to prevent weight gain in African-American girls: the Stanford GEMS pilot study, *Ethnicity Dis* 13(1 Suppl 1):S65–S77, 2003.

90. US Preventive Services Task Force Screening and Interventions for Overweight in Children and Adolescents: Recommendation statement, *Pediatrics* 116: 205–209, 2005.

91. Viner RM, Cole TJ: Adult socioeconomic, educational, social, and psychological outcomes of childhood obesity: a national birth cohort study, *Br Med J* 330(7504):1354, 2005.

92. Arnot M, Gray J, James M, et al: *Recent research on gender and educational performance*, London, 1998, OFSTED/HMSO.

93. National Institute of Mental Health: Learning disabilities: decade of the brain, NIH95–3611. Electronic document. Available at: http://www.ldonline.org/ld_indepth/general_info/gen-nimh-booklet.html#anchor109836.

94. Pollack WS: *Real boys: rescuing our sons from the myths of boyhood*, New York, 1998, Random House.

95. Prior M, Smart D, Sanson A, et al: Sex differences in psychological adjustment from infancy to 8 years, *J Am Acad Child Adolesc Psychiatry* 32(2):291–304, 1993.

The Adolescent Male

Arik V. Marcell, MD, MPH

Key Points

- Clinicians should provide, at a minimum, tailored clinical preventive service visits to the male throughout adolescence (strength of recommendation: C).
- Clinicians should screen for sexual activity among adolescent male patients; adolescent males should be counseled on sexual activity and contraception routinely (strength of recommendation: B).
- At-risk adolescent males should be screened for HIV (strength of recommendation: A), syphilis (strength of recommendation: A), and gonorrhea (strength of recommendation: C). All adolescent males should be screened for HIV (strength of recommendation: C) and asymptomatic chlamydia (strength of recommendation: C).
- Immunization records should be reviewed and age-appropriate vaccinations administered during routine healthcare visits when appropriate (strength of recommendation: A).
- Table 7-3 provides a detailed comparison of recommendations for adolescent clinical preventive services developed by various national organizations that focuses on aspects of the adolescent male visit, each with appropriate evidence ratings according to the respective organization's standards.

Introduction

Between the ages of 10 and 20 years, boys undergo rapid physiologic, psychological, and social changes. Although adolescent males are typically viewed as being "healthy," a gender differential exists in adolescent morbidity and mortality with adolescent males being in the disadvantaged group.[1] Moreover, most causes of adolescent males' morbidity and mortality are preventable. Both unintentional and intentional injury, including the use of alcohol while driving or swimming, involvement in motor vehicle accidents, lack of use of seatbelts or helmets, access to and use of guns, and completed suicides, contribute to overall higher rates of deaths among adolescent males compared with females. The main causes of morbidity among adolescent males are related to drug use, sexual activity, asthma, behavioral problems, and nonfatal injuries.[1–3] Routine clinical preventive services for all adolescents that allows for screening for high-risk behaviors and health conditions by clinicians could help to identify adolescents at risk earlier and target appropriate interventions. Moreover, during middle adolescence, the typical male's use of healthcare declines and continues to remain low throughout adulthood. Although adherence to traditional masculine beliefs may play a role in this decline, other factors also make important contributions, including a lack of health insurance, a lack of a regular source of primary care, a lack of knowledge about confidential services, a lack of clinical hooks that females have with contraceptive care and Papanicolaou guidelines, and a decreased involvement by parents in appointment making.

A routine office visit provides the clinician with a unique opportunity to connect with an adolescent male who may otherwise have few subsequent interactions with the healthcare system as a young adult. The primary care physician plays an integral role in overall adolescent male health promotion and disease prevention. The goal of this chapter is to review a typical adolescent male clinical encounter, including a review of male puberty and development, components of the adolescent male visit, and a review of common adolescent male health issues. This chapter will help to guide clinicians in their work with adolescent males through an evidence-based approach to preventive healthcare.

Normal Puberty and Development

Although pubertal timing for adolescent males is highly variable, pubertal changes generally follow a predictable sequence and are permanent. Sexual maturity rating (SMR), also known as *Tanner staging,* is an essential sexual maturity scale that can assist in assessing adolescent physical development.[4] The SMR is highly correlated with physical maturity as measured by bone age as opposed to chronologic age. For the adolescent male, changes in SMR are separately described for genitalia (e.g., testes and penis) and pubic hair.

Sexual Maturity Rating

A prepubertal male is staged as genital sexual maturity rating 1 (SMR1) and pubic hair SMR1, whereas an adult male is classified as genital SMR5 and pubic hair SMR5 (Figure 7-1 and Table 7-1). Genital SMR2 is characterized by the

first sign of puberty—testicular enlargement. The hallmark of genital SMR3 is penile lengthening. During genital SMR4, testicular growth continues to final adult size in genital SMR5. Racial and familial hair variation can occur with some males not progressing beyond pubic hair SMR4 (e.g., Asian males). It is also possible for a male to be at different genital and pubic hair SMRs, but typically SMRs are closely correlated with one another. An orchidometer can help the clinician appropriately stage a male's genital SMR in the clinical setting. During an examination, it is common and normal to find a male's left testis to hang slightly lower than the right testis. It is also common for a growing male to be concerned about his genital size. Adolescent males may require reassurance that genital sizes vary during and after pubertal development and depend on whether the penis is flaccid or erect.[5]

Pubertal Timing and Sequence

The male's predictable sequence of puberty begins with the first visible sign of puberty, called *gonadarche,* or testicular enlargement. This occurs, on average, between 11–12 years of age but can occur as early as 9.5 years and is the hallmark of genital SMR2. Approximately 6 months later, pubic hair becomes visible *(pubarche). Adrenarche,* an event independent of puberty, is due mainly to the adrenal production of androgens and can occur as early as 6 years of age. This event can

A guide to the male sexual maturity rating

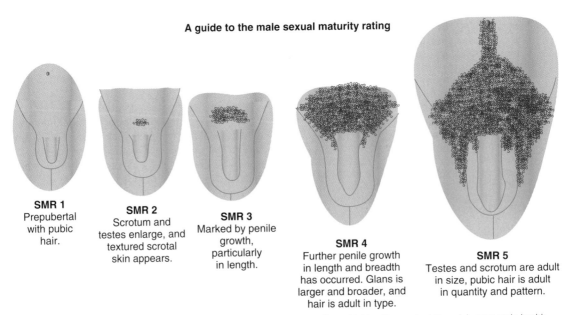

SMR 1
Prepubertal with pubic hair.

SMR 2
Scrotum and testes enlarge, and textured scrotal skin appears.

SMR 3
Marked by penile growth, particularly in length.

SMR 4
Further penile growth in length and breadth has occurred. Glans is larger and broader, and hair is adult in type.

SMR 5
Testes and scrotum are adult in size, pubic hair is adult in quantity and pattern.

Figure 7-1. Tanner stages for adolescent males. (Adapted from: Marcell AV: Making the most of the adolescent male health visit Part 2: the physical exam, *Contemp Peds* 23[6]:38–46, 2006.)

Table 7-1. Classification of Sex Maturity States in Boys

SMR Stage	Pubic Hair	Testes	Penis
1	None or fine nonpigmented hair (adrenarche)	Preadolescent (<4 mL in volume; <2.5 cm in diameter); thick scrotal skin, pink	Preadolescent (<6 cm in length)
2	Scant, long, straight, slightly pigmented at base of symphysis pubis	Testicular enlargement (4–8 mL in volume; 2–3 cm in diameter); enlarged scrotum, skin reddening, texture altered	Minimal change
3	More pigmented, curly, spread across symphysis pubis junction	Larger (8–10 mL in volume; 3.5 cm in diameter); scrotal skin darkens, thins, wrinkles	Penis lengthens
4	Curly, pigmented, fills in pubic triangle; no extension onto thighs or toward umbilicus	Larger (10–15 mL in volume; 4–4.5 cm in diameter); scrotum dark	Larger (11–17 cm length when flaccid); glans and breadth increase in size
5	Extension onto medial surface of thighs and toward umbilicus	Adult size (20–25 mL in volume; >4.5 cm in diameter)	Adult size

SMR, Sexual maturity rating.
Adapted from: Tanner JM: *Growth at adolescence*, ed 2, Oxford, England, 1962, Blackwell Scientific Publications.

contribute to faint body hair growth and underarm odor prior to puberty. The lengthening of the phallus follows pubarche and represents the hallmark of genital SMR3. *Spermarche*, or sperm found in the ejaculate, is evident approximately 12–18 months after the testes enlarge during genital SMR3 when the male may begin to experience two normal events: the onset of nocturnal ejaculatory events during sleep ("wet dreams") and spontaneous erections during the daytime. Rapid enlargement of the larynx, pharynx, and lungs lead to alterations in vocal quality that are typically preceded by vocal instability (i.e., voice cracking) during SMR3–4. The male's growth spurt occurs approximately 2–2.5 years after gonadarche, when testicular volumes reach approximately 9–10 cm^3, representing the hallmark of SMR4.

The typical duration of a male's pubertal sequence is 4–5 years. A medical workup should be considered in a boy who has genital changes before the age of 9.5 years for precocious puberty and for delayed puberty in a male who has had no changes in genital development by age 13.7 years, no hair growth by 15.1 years, or a lapse of more than 4–5 years after genital SMR2 onset with no progression.[6,7] Other pubertal events include growth of axillary, facial, and body hair during SMR4, the ability to grow a beard during SMR5, and the completion of chest and body hair development during the mid 20s.

The original studies that describe sexual maturity development conducted by Reynolds and Wines[8] and later by Tanner and Marshall[9] were predominantly performed among white males. Limited in their generalizability to other racial groups, these studies were longitudinal in design and thus described variations in the pattern of pubertal changes in boys over time. A recent cross-sectional study by Sun and colleagues[10] reported the timing of sexual maturation among a more diverse national sample of adolescent males in the United States. This study sampled non-Hispanic white, non-Hispanic black, and Mexican-American boys as part of the Third National Health and Nutrition Examination Survey (NHANES III) conducted between 1988 and 1994. Findings for males included significant differences in the median age of entry for genital SMR2 between only non-Hispanic black (9.20 years) and Mexican-American (10.29 years) males (age for non-Hispanic white males, 10.03 years). Significant differences were also found in the median age of entry for pubic hair SMR2 among all three groups: 11.98 years for non-Hispanic white, 11.16 years for non-Hispanic black, and 12.30 years for Mexican-American males. The original article also describes the median age of entry into SMR 3, 4, and 5 where fewer racial differences were found as well as the mean ages of timing of males' genital and hair development.

Growth and Development

During puberty, the adolescent male experiences changes in physical growth, including changes in height, weight, relative body compositions, and organ systems. Changes in the male's physical appearance are first evident distally (e.g., hands and feet) followed by arms and legs, and then centrally (e.g., trunk and chest). In total, a male will gain approximately 20% of his adult height during puberty.[7] The growth spurt occurs late in puberty (SMR4) at, on average, 14 years of age. The prepubertal male grows approximately

5 cm/year (2 in/year). During puberty, the male will gain an average of 28 cm (11 in). By the end of pubertal development, males are taller than females because males' growth spurt occurs approximately 2 years later than females', allowing for 2 additional years of growth at prepubertal rates, and males experience greater height gain (approximately 3 cm more than females during peak height velocity).

Weight gain parallels linear growth during puberty but is delayed by several months, with the male gaining approximately 50% of ideal adult weight in total.[7] Lean body mass, approximately 80% in the average prepubertal child, increases in boys to 90% compared with 75% in girls due to accumulation of less subcutaneous fat. An increase in males' muscle mass is followed approximately 6 months later by an increase in muscle strength. Approximately 67% of males' bone density is deposited during adolescence.[11] Other changes include doubling in heart size and vital lung capacity as well as increases in blood pressure, blood volume, and hematocrit.[4,12,13] Stimulation by androgens of sebaceous and apocrine glands results in acne and body odor.

Psychosocial Development

Whereas *puberty* is the biologic process during which a child becomes an adult, *adolescence* is more broadly defined. Adolescence is a period highlighted by the achievement of normal developmental tasks including physical growth, formation of an identity and moral system, formation of sexual identity, and preparation for the future. It is also marked by changing relationships including separation from parents (independence) and intimacy with members of same and/or opposite gender. A summary of the main tasks accomplished by adolescents across three distinct periods—early, middle, and late adolescence—is found in Table 7-2. Males are behind females of the same chronological age, not only in their physical development, but also in their emotional and psychosexual development. Thus, the distinct age ranges for adolescence for males may be considered as 11–14/15 years for early adolescence, 14/15–17 years for middle adolescence, and 17–21 years for late adolescence.[14]

The Health Visit

A number of guidelines including the American Medical Association Guidelines for Adolescent Preventive Services (AMA GAPS), the American Academy of Pediatrics (AAP) Guidelines for Health Supervision III, the Maternal and Child Health Bureau's (MCHB) Bright Futures (BF), the US Preventive Services Task Force's (USPSTF) Guide to Clinical Preventive Services, and the American Academy of Family Practice (AAFP) Summary of Recommendations for Clinical Preventive Services each make significant contributions toward our understanding of adolescent male-specific services as part of the health visit (Table 7-3).[15-19] The different organizations use varying methodologies to determine its guidelines. For example, the USPSTF guidelines are based on the proven ability of screening procedures and interventions to improve clinical outcomes. The AMA GAPS, BF, and AAP guidelines incorporate expert opinion due to limited data from preventive service studies that examine clinical outcomes using adolescent subjects in clinical settings. The AMA GAPS guidelines were released in 1994 and are highlighted by the 1997 addition of the adolescent annual visit as a measurement battery by the National Committee for Quality Assurance through its Health Employer Data and Information System.

Upon comparison of adolescent male clinical preventive service recommendations developed by national organizations (see Table 7-3), one will note great variability in the recommendations as well as the fact that for many content areas there is insufficient research. Despite this, clinicians should not discount the importance of providing adolescent male preventive services in the clinical setting. On the contrary, the AMA GAPS presents an important set of recommendations that can help organize the adolescent male health visit. Overall, the main focus of a routine health visit for an adolescent male aged 11–21 years is to address the biomedical and psychosocial aspects of his health and to focus on the promotion of preventive services. The AMA GAPS guidelines make 24 recommendations, 23 of which are applicable to the adolescent male (Table 7-4), including the following:

- The delivery of health services for adolescents
- The use of health guidance to promote the health and well-being of adolescents and their parents or guardians
- The need to screen for specific conditions that are relatively common to adolescents and that cause significant suffering either during adolescence or later in life
- The use of immunizations for the primary prevention of selected infectious diseases

In 2007, the AAP and MCHB will release an updated version of Bright Futures as a single

Table 7-2. Central Issues in Early, Middle, and Late Adolescence

Variable	Early Adolescence	Middle Adolescence	Late Adolescence
Age (years)	11–14/15	14/15–17	17–21
SMR*	1–2	3–5	5
Somatic	• Secondary sex characteristics • Beginning of rapid growth • Awkward appearance	• Height growth peaks • Body shape and composition change • Advanced secondary sexual characteristics • Acne and odor • Spermarche	• Physically mature • Slower growth
Cognitive and moral	• Concrete operations • Unable to perceive long-term outcome of current decision making • Conventional morality • Frequent daydreaming	• Emergence of abstract thought (formal operations) • May perceive future implications but this may not apply in decision making • Questioning mores	• Future oriented with sense of perspective • Idealism; absolutism • Able to think things through independently
Self-concept/ identity formation	• Preoccupied with changing body • Self-consciousness about appearance and attractiveness • Fantasy and present oriented	• Concern with attractiveness • Increasing introspection; may withdraw under stress • Sense of invincibility • "Stereotypical adolescent"	• More stable body image • Attractiveness may still be of concern • Emancipation complete • Firmer identity
Family	• Increased need for privacy • Increased bid for independence • Less interested in parental activities	• Conflicts over control and independence • Struggle for acceptance of greater autonomy	• Emotional and physical separation from family • Increased autonomy • Adult-adult family interactions
Peers	• Seeks same-sex peer affiliation to counter instability	• Intense peer group involvement • Preoccupation with peer culture • Peers provide behavioral example	• Peer group and values recede in importance • Intimacy/possible commitment takes precedent
Sexual	• Increased interest in sexual anatomy • Normal to compare one's body to others and self-explore • Anxieties and questions about genital changes, size • Limited dating and intimacy	• Testing ability to attract partner • Initiation of relationships & sexual activity • Questions of sexual orientation	• Consolidation of sexual identity • Focus on intimacy & formation of stable relationships • Planning for future & commitment
Relationship to society	• Middle-school adjustment	• Gauging skills and opportunities	• Career decisions (e.g., college, work)

*See Table 7-1.
SMR, Sexual maturity rating.
Adapted from: Marcell AV: Adolescence. In Kliegman RM, Behrman RE, Jenson HB, Stanton BF, editors: *Nelson textbook of pediatrics,* ed 18. Philadelphia, 2007, Saunders.

combined effort that will replace the current two separate guidelines. The USPSTF and AAFP guidelines are updated yearly. The following section reviews components of the health visit for the adolescent male and summarizes key recommendations for service delivery based on the above guidelines. Recommendations from other guidelines are reviewed as appropriate.

Visit Frequency

The periodicity of the healthcare visit for adolescent males varies from one guideline to another. Annual visits are promoted by the AMA GAPS,

AAP, and BF, all of which make a distinction among developmental stages of adolescence, whereas the USPSTF and AAFP promote more tailored visits.

Components of the Healthcare Visit

The AMA GAPS, AAP, and BF discuss the need to perform a comprehensive physical examination as part of the healthcare visit. The AMA GAPS states that a complete physical examination should occur during three of these preventive services visits: once during early (ages 11–14 years), middle (ages 15–17 years), and late (ages 18–21 years)

Table 7-3. Comparisons Among Recommendations for Adolescent Clinical Preventive Services Developed by National Organizations: The Adolescent Male

	AMA GAPS	AAP	BF	USPSTF	AAFP
	PANEL GUIDELINES			EVIDENCE-BASED GUIDELINES	
Target age range (years)[a]	11–21	11–21	11–21	11–24	13–18
Periodicity of visit	Annual	Annual	Annual	Tailored	Tailored
Comprehensive physical examination	Yes	Yes	Yes	ND	ND
Sports physical examination	ND	No[b1]	ND	ND	ND[b2]
History: Screening and Counseling					
School performance/problems[c]	Yes	Yes	Yes	ND	ND
Nutrition[c]	Yes	Yes[d]	Yes	I	ND
Physical activity[c]	Yes	Yes	Yes	I	I
Eating disorders[c]	Yes	Yes	Yes	ND	ND
Sexual activity and contraception[e]	Yes	Yes	Yes	B	ND
STI/HIV counseling[c]	Yes	Yes	Yes	B	B
Tobacco use[c]	Yes	Yes	Yes	I	I[c]
Alcohol use[c]	Yes	Yes	Yes	I	I
Other drug use[c]	Yes	Yes	Yes	I	ND
Depression[c]	Yes	Yes	Yes	I	I
Risk for suicide[c]	Yes	Yes	Yes	I	ND
Abuse[c]	Yes	ND	Yes	I[g]	I
Injury and violence prevention[c,h]	Yes	Yes[i1]	Yes	B[i2]; I[i3]	B (injury)
Physical Exam/Health Guidance					
Hearing and vision[c]	ND	Yes[d]	Yes	I	ND
Hypertension (BP)[c]	Yes	Yes	Yes	I[k]	I[k]
Normal development (including Ht and Wt)[l]	Yes	Yes	Yes	I	ND
Obesity (BMI)[c]	Yes	ND	Yes	I	I
Sexual maturity rating	Yes	Yes	Yes	ND	ND
Testicular cancer screen	No	Yes	Yes	D	D
Teaching of TSE[c]	ND	Yes	Yes	D	D
Scoliosis	ND	Yes	Yes	D	D
Skin protection[c]	ND	Yes	ND	I	I
Dental health[c]	ND	Yes[m1]	Yes	B[m2]; I[m3]	A[m2]
Laboratory Screening Tests					
Cholesterol[e]	Yes	Yes[n]	Yes	ND	ND
Tuberculosis[e]	Yes	Yes[o1]	Yes	Yes[o2]	A
Hematocrit[e]	No	No	Yes	D	ND
Urinalysis	No	Yes[p1]	Yes[p2]	D[p3]	D[p3]
STI (GC, CT)[e]	Yes	Yes[q1]	Yes	I[q2]; D[q3]	I[q2]; D[q3]
STI (HCV, HSV, HBV)	No	No	Yes (HSV)	D	D
Syphilis[e]	Yes	Yes	Yes	A	A
HIV infection[e]	Yes	Yes	Yes	A	A

Table continued on following page

Table 7-3. Comparisons Among Recommendations for Adolescent Clinical Preventive Services Developed by National Organizations: The Adolescent Male (Continued)

	AMA GAPS	AAP	BF	USPSTF	AAFP
		PANEL GUIDELINES		EVIDENCE-BASED GUIDELINES	
Immunizations					
ACIP recommendations	Yes	Yes[r1]	Yes	Yes[r2]	Yes
Health Guidance for Parents[†]	Yes	Yes	Yes	ND	ND

AMA, American Medical Association (data from Elster and Kuznets[17]); AAP, American Academy of Pediatrics (data from AAP[19]); BF, Bright Futures (data from Green and Palfrey[18]); USPSTF, US Preventive Services Task Force (data from USPSTF[16]); AAFP, American Academy of Family Physicians (data from AAFP[15]); ND, not discussed; I, insufficient evidence for or against; A, strongly recommend; B, recommend; D, recommend against; STI, sexually transmitted infection; HIV, human immunodeficiency virus; BP, blood pressure; Ht, height; Wt, weight; BMI, body mass index; TSE, testicular self examination; GC, *Neisseria gonorrhoeae*; CT, *Chlamydia trachomatis;* HCV, hepatitis C virus; HSV, herpes simplex virus; HBV, hepatitis B virus; ACIP, Advisory Committee on Immunization Practices.

[a]The AAP, AMA, and BF make a distinction among developmental stages of adolescence.

[b1]Not to be performed in place of a comprehensive physical examination. [b2]The AAFP recommends against the use of routine electrocardiogram as part of a periodic health or pre-participation physical examination for cardiac disease in asymptomatic children and adults.

[c]Procedure recommended for all adolescents/parents.

[d]Age-appropriate nutrition counseling should be an integral part of each visit per the *AAP Handbook of Nutrition* (1998).

[e]Procedure recommended for selected adolescents who are at high risk for the medical problem.

[f]The AAFP strongly recommends to counsel smoking parents with children in the house regarding the harmful effects of smoking and children's health.

[g]Child abuse is not addressed as a separate screening topic, but it is included in the general screening for family violence.

[h]This includes activities such as promoting the use of safety belts and safety helmets, placing home fire alarms, and reducing the risk of injury from firearms and violence. Organizations differ in the activities they include for injury preventions.

[i1]Violence prevention and management for all patients per AAP Statement "The role of the pediatrician in youth violence prevention in clinical practice and at the community level" (1999); [i2]counseling all patients to use occupant restraints, to wear helmets, and to refrain from driving under the influence; [i3]insufficient evidence for or against counseling to reduce risk of unintentional household and/or recreational injuries.

[j]Objective once in early, middle, and late adolescence; subjective all other times.

[k]Recommended in persons 18 years or older.

[l]This includes providing adolescents with information on normal physical, psychosocial, and sexual development.

[m1]As appropriate per dentist; [m2]fluoride supplementation recommended in children aged 6 months to 16 years; [m3]insufficient evidence to recommend for or against routine risk assessment of preschool children; adolescents are not discussed.

[n]Cholesterol screening for high-risk patients per AAP statement "Cholesterol in Childhood" (1998). If family history cannot be ascertained and other risk factors are present, screening should be at the discretion of the physician.

[o1]TB testing per recommendations of the Committee on Infectious Diseases, published in the current *Red Book.*[71] Testing should be done upon recognition of high-risk factors. [o2]The USPSTF defers to the US Centers for Disease Control and Prevention (CDC) recommendations on tuberculosis control.

[p1]Conduct dipstick urinalysis for leukocytes for sexually active adolescent males; [p2]conduct urinalysis a minimum of once during adolescence; [p3]screen for asymptomatic bacteriuria.

[q1]All sexually active patients should be screened for STIs; [q2]for GC, men at increased risk for infection; for CT, asymptomatic men; [q3]for GC, men who are at low risk for infection.

[r1]Schedule per Committee on Infectious Disease, published annually in the January edition of *Pediatrics.* Every visit should be an opportunity to update and complete a child's immunizations; [r2]The USPSTF defers to the CDC ACIP recommendations on immunization.

Adapted from: Elster AB: Comparison of recommendations for adolescent clinical preventive services developed by national organizations, *Arch Pediatr Adolesc Med* 152(2):193–198, 1998 with updates.

adolescence, respectively, and that more frequent examinations may be warranted based on clinical signs or symptoms. The AAP and BF recommend yearly examinations with the need for older children to be undressed and suitably draped.

The recommendations described above are not inclusive of the pre-participation physical examination (PPE). The goal of the PPE is to identify musculoskeletal and other medical conditions that could be worsened by sports participation or could cause significant morbidity and mortality in an adolescent athlete (see Chapter 26, The Collegiate/Professional Male Athlete).[20] Such an examination is described to include a history and physical examination that focuses on sports involvement, for example, a comprehensive orthopedic examination and a history of and risk for sports injury. Unfortunately, the effectiveness of the PPE is limited[21–24] because these examinations (1) detect a very small proportion of cardiac abnormalities, such as abnormalities that would put an individual at risk for sudden death; (2) do not adequately identify exercise-induced bronchospasm; and (3) are poorly predictive of orthopedic injuries. The PPE is used in place of an annual comprehensive health evaluation by many teens, a practice that is not consistent with the AMA GAPS, AAP, and BF guidelines.[17–19]

Table 7-4. Guidelines for Adolescent Preventive Services with a Total of 24 Recommendations

---

Recommendations for Delivery of Health Services

Recommendation 1. From ages 11–21 years, all adolescents should have an annual preventive services visit.

Recommendation 2. Preventive services should be age and developmentally appropriate, and should be sensitive to individual and sociocultural differences.

Recommendation 3. Physicians should establish office policies regarding confidential care for adolescents and how parents will be involved in that care. These policies should be made clear to adolescents and their parents.

Recommendations for Health Guidance

Recommendation 4. Parents or other adult caregivers of adolescents should receive health guidance at least once during early adolescence, once during middle adolescence, and preferably, once during late adolescence.

Recommendation 5. All adolescents should receive health guidance annually to promote a better understanding of their physical growth, psychosocial and psychosexual development, and the importance of becoming actively involved in decisions regarding their healthcare.

Recommendation 6. All adolescents should receive health guidance annually to promote the reduction of injuries.

Recommendation 7. All adolescents should receive health guidance annually about dietary habits, including the benefits of a healthy diet and ways to achieve a healthy diet and safe weight management.

Recommendation 8. All adolescents should receive health guidance annually about the benefits of physical activity and should be encouraged to engage in safe physical activities on a regular basis.

Recommendation 9. All adolescents should receive health guidance annually regarding responsible sexual behaviors, including abstinence. Latex condoms to prevent sexually transmitted diseases (including HIV infection) and appropriate methods of birth control should be made available with instructions on ways to use them effectively.

Recommendation 10. All adolescents should receive health guidance annually to promote avoidance of tobacco, alcohol and other abusable substances, and anabolic steroids.

Recommendations for Screening

Recommendation 11. All adolescents should be screened annually for hypertension according to the protocol developed by the National Heart, Lung, and Blood Institute's Second Task Force on Blood Pressure Control in Children.

Recommendation 12. Selected adolescents should be screened to determine their risk of developing hyperlipidemia and adult coronary heart disease, following the protocol developed by the Expert Panel on Blood Cholesterol Levels in Children and Adolescents.

Recommendation 13. All adolescents should be screened annually for eating disorders and obesity by determining weight and stature, and asking about body image and dieting patterns.

Recommendation 14. All adolescents should be asked annually about their use of tobacco products, including cigarettes and smokeless tobacco.

Recommendation 15. All adolescents should be asked annually about their use of alcohol and other abusable substances, and about their use of over-the-counter or prescription drugs, including anabolic steroids, for nonmedical purposes.

Recommendation 16. All adolescents should be asked annually about involvement in sexual behaviors that may result in unintended pregnancy and STIs, including HIV infection.

Recommendation 17. Sexually active adolescents should be screened for STIs.

Recommendation 18. Adolescents at risk for HIV infection should be offered confidential HIV screening with the ELISA and confirmatory test.

Recommendation 19. Female-specific recommendation regarding need for regular Papanicolaou testing.

Recommendation 20. All adolescents should be asked annually about behaviors or emotions that indicate recurrent or severe depression or risk of suicide.

Recommendation 21. All adolescents should be asked annually about a history of emotional, physical, or sexual abuse.

Recommendation 22. All adolescents should be asked annually about learning or school problems.

Recommendation 23. Adolescents should receive a tuberculin skin test if they have been exposed to active tuberculosis, have lived in a homeless shelter, have been incarcerated, have lived in or come from an area with a high prevalence of tuberculosis, or currently work in a healthcare setting.

Recommendations for Immunizations

Recommendation 24. All adolescents should receive prophylactic immunizations according to the guidelines established by the federally convened Advisory Committee on Immunization Practices.

HIV, Human immunodeficiency virus; STI, sexually transmitted infection; ELISA, enzyme-linked immunosorbent assay.
Adapted from: Elster A, Kuzsets N: *Guidelines for adolescent preventive services (GAPS)*, Baltimore, MD, 1993, Williams & Wilkins.

Minor Consent and Confidentiality

Physicians should establish office policies to accommodate minors seeking services for which they are able to consent. The age of majority in the United States is 18 years of age. Males and females may be able to consent as minors for reproductive health issues (e.g., pregnancy and prenatal care, sexually transmitted infections [STIs], and human immunodeficiency virus [HIV]-related care), substance abuse, and mental health services in addition to services related to an alleged rape or sexual offense. Laws regarding minor consent vary from state to state and exceptions to the rule, such as the emancipated minor, also exist.[25] The AMA GAPS recommendation #3 (see Table 7-4) also suggests that physicians establish office policies regarding confidential care for adolescents and how parents can be incorporated in this care, and recommends that such policies be made clear to adolescents and their parents.[17]

Clinical services provided to adolescents are confidential with conditional limits based on whether or not the adolescent has been physically or sexually abused and/or is at harm to himself/herself or others. Concern about any physical abuse warrants contacting local or county child protective services. Concern about self-harm or harm to others warrants referral to child crisis or psychiatric services, social workers, and in urgent cases, law enforcement. The Health Insurance Portability and Accountability Act (HIPAA) "Privacy Rule" provides standards to protect the security and privacy of "protected health information" for children and adolescents as it does for adults but should not restrict the ability of a health care provider to share information with other providers needed to treat an adolescent patient."

Taking a History

The medical and psychosocial history should be taken while the adolescent male is clothed to make him feel more comfortable and less distracted. As with any adolescent, clinicians should be sensitive to the adolescent male patient's needs and provide him with an environment that allows for conversation with minimal interruptions. The medical history should be obtained with the parent or guardian in the examination room to ensure accuracy and completeness and should include the review of existing medical health issues, classification of risk for future medical problems such as obesity or diabetes, and a review of current medications, allergies to medications, and vaccination status. Use of a family tree or genogram can help to map family history for significant medical conditions.

Before the initiation of the psychosocial assessment, the parent or guardian should be asked to step out of the examination room so that the clinician can speak with the adolescent male alone and confidentially. During the psychosocial history, the clinician should use a balance of closed- and open-ended questions as well as active listening. The use of self-administered questionnaires before the physician-patient interaction can help in both time-efficiency and direct assessment, although such questionnaires should not be used in place of verbal assessment or interaction on more pressing issues or concerns.

The AMA GAPS and BF have developed screening questionnaires and suggested questions to incorporate as part of the routine psychosocial history.[17,18] Another specific strategy that can help the clinician organize the psychosocial history is called the "HEADSS Assessment."[26,27] *HEADSS* stands for specific content areas that are recommended for assessment: Home, Education, Eating, Activities, Drugs, Sexual identity/activity, Suicide/depression, and Safety. The updated article by Goldenring and Rosen[27] provides a more detailed discussion regarding handling confidentiality in the clinical setting; Marcell and Bell[28] also provide a more detailed discussion regarding how to take a history of an adolescent male patient.

Table 7-3 provides a comparative summary of recommendations by national organizations for the provision of health guidance screening and counseling on various topics as part of an adolescent male clinical visit,[15–19] including guidance on school performance/problems; nutrition; physical activity; eating disorders; sexual activity and contraception; STI counseling; tobacco, alcohol, and other drug use; depression; risk for suicide; abuse; and injury/violence prevention.[29–41] The USPSTF is currently updating recommendations for drug abuse screening and counseling on motor vehicle injuries and has decided not to update recommendations for counseling on household and recreational injuries and youth violence. The USPSTF states that it "recognizes the impact that injuries have on children and adults and the importance of violence as a public health issue and the burden that youth violence has on a community" but believes that, based on the limited evidence on counseling on these topics in clinical settings, a recommendation would have limited impact. The CDC's Community Guide has published recommendations on preventing violence to which the clinician may want to refer (www.thecommunityguide.org). The AMA GAPS,

BF, and AAP also recommend that parents receive health guidance on many of the above topics at least once during their child's early adolescence, again during middle adolescence, and, preferably, again during late adolescence.

The Physical Examination

After the history is taken, the male patient should be asked to change into a gown in private. An examination with an adolescent clothed can miss important physical examination findings, including gynecomastia or acne on the trunk. Before starting the examination, the clinician should review with the patient the components of the physical. As the examination progresses, the clinician should briefly comment on any pertinent findings and what will be conducted next. The comprehensiveness of the examination will depend on the reason for the visit. Lengthy discussions should be avoided while the male patient is in a compromising position, such as during the genital examination or in a gown.

Vital Signs

Current guidelines do not provide recommendations on the effectiveness or frequency needed to check a pulse, temperature, or respiratory rate during non-urgent care visits. The performance of blood pressure screening as part of an adolescent preventive services visit has varying degrees of acceptance (see Table 7-3). Hypertension among older adolescent males is most commonly due to essential hypertension, whereas secondary hypertension among younger males is more commonly due to renovascular disease. Appropriate age and height charts should be used for interpretation of child and adolescent blood pressure readings.[42] Follow-up includes performing multiple readings (at least three) obtained on different occasions before hypertension can be appropriately diagnosed. Hypertension in adolescents is defined as a systolic or diastolic blood pressure reading greater than the 95th percentile for the patient's age, height, and gender.[12,43] *Severe hypertension* is defined as readings greater than 99th percentile, whereas values between the 90th and 95th percentiles are defined as *prehypertension*; appropriate referral to a pediatric cardiologist should be considered for evaluation and management in such cases.

Body Mass Index

Checking body mass index (BMI) as part of an adolescent preventive services visit also has varying degrees of acceptance (see Table 7-3). BMI can help to identify a male who is underweight, at risk for obesity, or obese, but it is somewhat limited in that it does not differentiate well between muscle bulk and fat, nor does it accurately assess a person who has a large frame. Regarding eating disorders, males account for approximately 5–15% of persons with anorexia nervosa and bulimia nervosa,[44] and approximately 7% of adolescent males report disordered eating patterns, including a history of binging, purging, or using a laxative.[45] Additional findings seen among patients with eating disorders include abnormal vital signs (e.g., bradycardia or hypothermia) as well as a history of engagement in activities to modify weight, such as involvement in higher risk sports (e.g., wrestling), excessive power lifting or weight training, or the use of nutritional supplements.

An overweight or obese condition may signal a risk factor for the identification of other medical conditions. Sixty percent of overweight adolescents have at least one medical complication, including sleep apnea, slipped capital femoral epiphysis, hypertension, glucose intolerance, hyperlipidemia, and pseudotumor cerebri.[46] An additional tool to the measurement of BMI includes the assessment of regional fat distribution. Fat that is distributed in the waist area has been shown to be predictive of morbidity in adults, including an elevated risk of cardiac disease and diabetes mellitus. Standardized waist circumference measurements for children and adolescents are currently in development. Any adolescent male who has a BMI greater than the 95th percentile should undergo an in-depth medical assessment.[46,47] A male who is obese and short in stature should undergo evaluation for an endocrine (e.g., growth hormone deficiency, hypothyroidism) or genetic disorder (e.g., Prader-Willi syndrome and Laurence-Moon syndrome).

Vision and Hearing

Recommendations for the routine assessment of vision and hearing are less consistent across guidelines (see Table 7-3). Only the AAP and BF endorse routine vision and hearing screening among adolescents.[18,19] The USPSTF is currently updating its 1996 vision and hearing impairment recommendation that stated there is insufficient evidence to recommend for or against routine screening of asymptomatic adolescents for vision or hearing impairment.[48] Recommendations against hearing impairment screening, except for those exposed to excessive occupational noise levels, may be made on other grounds.

Growth

A separate assessment of height and weight is endorsed by all guidelines except the USPSTF (see Table 7-3). The plotting of height and weight measurements on standardized growth charts and sharing of findings and trends can be an excellent method for the clinician to connect with adolescent male patients, especially pre-teenaged and early teenaged males who will be interested about their growth and final adult height. If childhood trends are not available to estimate final height, this can be done by using mid-parental heights ([mother's height (in) + 5 in] + father's height [in] divided by 2 [or 13 cm instead if heights are provided in centimeters]).[7]

Development

The AMA GAPS, AAP, and BF endorse examination for appropriate development.[17–19] Components include tracking for somatic growth and appropriate progression through Tanner stages by documenting sexual maturity ratings as described above. This should be performed at least annually for adolescents who have not gone through puberty or are in the midst of puberty.

Genital Examination

Periodic genital examination is important for a number of reasons: (1) to reveal problems in a male's development using Tanner stages for hair and genitalia separately, (2) to screen for sexually transmitted infections, (3) to identify previously undiagnosed genetic disease (e.g., Klinefelter's syndrome, late-onset 21-CAH), (4) to identify structural anomalies, some of which may lead to problems with infertility including varicocele, spermatocele, hydrocele, meatal abnormalities (e.g., hypospadias) and signs of testicular trauma, (5) to identify issues related to an uncircumcised penis including phimosis/paraphimosis or issues related to hygiene, (6) to identify hair or skin issues including folliculitis or jock itch, (7) to examine for signs of an absent testes (e.g., cryptorchidism) or testicular atrophy due to either a central etiology or steroid or marijuana abuse, (8) to reassure the male about variations in normal genital findings (e.g., penile pearly papules, sebaceous cysts), and (9) to help the male gain a better understanding of his body.

Specific recommendations about screening for testicular cancer by the clinician are controversial, as is the practice of teaching the patient about testicular self-examination. The AAP and BF recommend that examination of male genitalia for normal development be part of the complete physical examination during early, middle, and late adolescence and the teaching of testicular self-examinations to middle and late adolescent males.[18,19] The American Cancer Society also recommends that a testicular examination be included as part of a routine examination and teaching about the testicular self-examination among men at risk for testicular cancer.[48a] Conversely, in 2004 the USPSTF changed its recommendation from insufficient evidence to recommend for or against screening for testicular cancer to a recommendation *against* routine screening.[49] They also note that "clinicians should be aware that patients who present with symptoms of testicular cancer are frequently diagnosed as having epididymitis, testicular trauma, hydrocele or other benign disorders." Thus for a male presenting with a genital complaint, a genital examination and, specifically, a testicular examination is important and testicular cancer should be a consideration in one's differential. The AAFP now defers to this updated USPSTF recommendation.[15] Risk factors for testicular cancer include Caucasian race, age between 13 and 39, cryptorchidism, testicular atrophy/dysgenesis, testicular trauma, family history of testicular cancer, HIV, and Klinefelter's syndrome. The association between trauma to the testes and testicular cancer may be due to increased cell turnover in an already malignant testicle or to increased awareness of a testicle with an existing tumor.

Whether guideline updates will impact males' genital health is an important area of future research. This is of particular relevance because studies show that young men are unaware of testicular pathology that affects their age group.[50,51] Although one study reports that males with a history of cryptorchidism are able to recall that they have had this condition,[52] no previous study has examined whether males at increased risk for testicular cancer know about their risk.

Genital Examination Pointers

The male patient should stand during the genital examination. While in a gown, he should be instructed to lower his pants and underpants to expose his genitalia and inguinal area. The clinician should begin the examination by inspecting the skin around the genital area—including inspection of pubic hair for crabs, lice, or nits—and Tanner staging should be performed. Next, the inguinal lymph nodes should be palpated bilaterally for swelling or tenderness. Palpation of the scrotal contents includes gentle compression of the testes and epididymis between the clinician's thumb and first two fingers. Any abnormalities, including tenderness upon palpation, abnormal testicle shape or size, masses, swelling, or presence of any nodules, should be noted. Each testis should be evaluated for Tanner stage and each spermatic cord with its connecting vas deferens should be identified and palpated for any tenderness or swelling.

Palpation of the penis should also include inspection of skin on the shaft and glans for ulcers, raised lesions, or signs of inflammation. If a foreskin is present, the patient should be asked to retract it. The glans should be gently compressed between the clinician's thumb and index finger to open the urethral meatus. If no discharge is visible (a sign of urethritis), the shaft of the penis may be stripped/milked from its base to the glans. The meatus should also be inspected for stenosis, lesions, and mal-opening position of the urethra (i.e., hypospadias). Lastly, to evaluate for possible hernia the clinician should insert a digit in the opening of each inguinal canal and ask the patient to cough (Valsalva maneuver). A rectal examination is not routinely recommended for adolescent males unless significant risk factors are present (e.g., a male who is engaging in sex with another male).

The Use of a Chaperone

Using a chaperone for the male genital examination is highlighted by a separate AAP guideline[53] that recommends the physician be "sensitive to the patient's feelings about an examination" and that "physician judgment and discretion must be paramount in evaluating the needs for a chaperone." The discussion of the need for physicians to use a chaperone has generally focused on female patients only. Few studies have examined adolescents' preferences for use of chaperones,[54–56] particularly preferences of the adolescent male. The only study that examined both adolescent male and female preferences found that younger males and females preferred to be accompanied, generally by a family member, whereas with increasing age males preferred to be alone with the physician compared with females, who preferred accompaniment. A history of sexual abuse and the request for a chaperone are situations where the use of a chaperone is definitely warranted. The need to use a chaperone is a separate issue from patient preference regarding the provider's gender; studies remain inconsistent regarding adolescent males' provider gender preference.[57–59]

Laboratory Screening Tests
Non-STI Related Screening Tests

Cholesterol

The GAPS, AAP, and BF guidelines recommend cholesterol screening among adolescents.[17–19] The USPSTF does not discuss evidence regarding screening adolescents for lipid abnormalities, whereas it concludes that the benefits of screening for and treating high-risk young adults outweigh any potential harms.[60] The Executive Summary of the Third Report of the National Cholesterol Education Program Expert Panel on Detection, Evaluation, and Treatment of High Blood Cholesterol in Adults makes recommendations for men aged 20–35 years only and not younger.[61] This panel concludes that "risk factor identification in young adults is an important aim for long-term prevention." This would include measurement of low-density lipoprotein cholesterol as a component of a fasting lipid profile analysis once every 5 years and the identification of accompanying risk determinants. If only nonfasting testing is available, the values for total cholesterol and high-density lipoprotein cholesterol will be useful.

Tuberculosis

All guidelines recommend routine screening for tuberculosis in asymptomatic high-risk persons.[15,17–19] The USPSTF will not update its 1996 recommendations and defers to Centers for Disease Control and Prevention (CDC) guidelines for targeted tuberculosis screening.[62] The CDC also recommends that providers of medical care for children and adolescents should use a questionnaire to screen all new patients for risk factors of latent tuberculosis infection.[63] Persons at high risk include HIV-infected persons, close contacts of persons with known or suspected tuberculosis, immigrants from countries with high tuberculosis prevalence, medically underserved low-income populations, and residents of correctional or mental institutions and long-term care facilities.

Hematocrit

No guideline recommends specific routine hematocrit screening of adolescent males. The AAP describes that screening should only occur among adolescents at risk, defined as those for whom there is a concern about anemia (e.g., a menstruating female).[19]

STI-Related Tests

Urinalysis

The USPSTF and AAFP recommend against conducting a urinalysis to screen for asymptomatic bacteriuria.[15,64] If the clinician is testing for STIs, specifically *Chlamydia trachomatis* and *Neisseria gonorrhoeae*, painless and noninvasive genetic probe urine-based testing techniques are available and easy to use.[65] Although the AAP recommends conducting dipstick urinalysis for leukocytes at least once between 11 and 21 years of age and annually for the sexually active adolescent,[19] and the BF recommends a urinalysis once during adolescence but does not describe a rationale (e.g., screening for asymptomatic bacteriuria or for STIs),[18] recent recommendations by the CDC state that the leukocyte esterase test is not recommended for screening males for *Chlamydia trachomatis*.[65a]

Neisseria gonorrhoeae

The GAPS, AAP, and BF recommend routine screening for STIs, including gonorrhea, among symptomatic adolescents.[17–19] The USPSTF and AAFP state that there is insufficient evidence to recommend for or against routine screening of men for gonorrhea at increased risk for infection.[15,66] High-risk men include those who have a history of previous gonorrheal infection or other STIs; have new or multiple sex partners; inconsistently use condoms; exchange sex for drugs or money; use drugs; are African American; have sex with other men; or live in regions of high gonorrhea prevalence. The USPSTF and AAFP recommend against routine gonorrhea screening in men who are at a low risk for infection.[15,66]

Chlamydia trachomatis

The GAPS, AAP, and BF recommend routine screening of STIs, including chlamydia.[17–19] Although asymptomatic infection is common, the USPTF and the AAFP state that there is insufficient evidence to recommend for or against routine screening of asymptomatic men for *Chlamydia* of any age.[15,67] These guidelines state though that partners of infected individuals should be tested and treated if infected or treated presumptively. Recent new recommendations by the CDC review the evidence in male *Chlamydia* screening and conclude that screening for *Chlamydia* should be performed among males attending STD clinics and Job Corps and among males less than 30 years of age entering jails. Males with *Chlamydia* infection should be re-screened at 3 months for repeat infection and partner services should be offered to partners of males with *Chlamydia*. These new recommendations specifically do not address whether all sexually active men of certain ages should undergo annual *Chlamydia* screening or whether selected high-risk populations of males warrant screening. In addition, theses recommendations promote the use of urine as the specimen of choice for screening asymptomatic men (NAATs are the test of choice) and that pooling of urine specimens should be considered for testing of *Chlamydia* in low prevalence settings.[65a] The CDC STD

Guidelines endorses that males younger than 25 who are sexually active should be screened for STIs, including *Chlamydia* and gonorrhea, using urine-based techniques, especially if the STI prevalence is high in that community.[65]

Hepatitis C Virus

The USPSTF and AAFP recommend against routine screening for hepatitis C virus (HCV) in asymptomatic adult men who are not at increased risk for infection and state that there is insufficient evidence to recommend for or against routine screening for HCV in adult men at high risk for infection.[15,68] Risk factors for the contraction of HCV include any blood-borne exposure via intravenous or intranasal drug use or contaminated blood transfusions; it is thought that the risk of sexual transmission of HCV is very low.

Herpes Simplex Virus

All guidelines recommend against routine screening for herpes simplex virus in asymptomatic adolescents and adults[15,17,18,69] except the BF, which does not specify how to screen for herpes simplex virus (e.g., physical examination versus serologic assay).[19]

Hepatitis B Virus

All guidelines recommend against routine screening of asymptomatic men for hepatitis B virus (HBV).[15,17–19,70] The AAP's *Red Book*[71] does not recommend the need for susceptibility testing before immunization routinely in children or adolescents with unknown or uncertain immunization status. *Red Book* states that "testing for previous infection may be considered for people in risk groups with high rates of HBV infection, such as users of injection drugs, homosexually or bisexually active men, and household contacts of HBsAg-positive people, provided testing does not delay or impede immunizations efforts."[71] *Red Book* also states that "routine postimmunization testing for anti-HBsAb is not necessary but is recommended 1–2 months after the third vaccine dose for the following specific groups: (1) hemodialysis patients, (2) people with HIV infection, (3) people at occupational risk of exposure from sharp injuries, (4) immunocompromised patients at risk of exposure to HBV, and (5) regular sexual contacts of HBsAg-positive people."[71]

Syphilis

All guidelines recommend routine serologic testing (via rapid plasma reagin or venereal disease research laboratory non-treponemal tests) for persons at increased risk for syphilis.[15,17–19,72] Men at increased risk for syphilis include men who have sex with men, are detained, exchange money or drugs for sex, have a history of other STIs including HIV, and are in sexual contact with persons with active syphilis.[72]

Human Immunodeficiency Virus

All guidelines recommend routine HIV screening.[15,17–19,73] The USPSTF specifically recommends screening of adolescents and adults at increased risk for infection.[73] Persons at high risk include men who have engaged in any of the following behaviors: had sex with men after 1975; have unprotected sex with multiple partners; are past or present injection drug users; exchange sex for money or drugs; are past or present sex partners of HIV-infected, bisexual, or injection drug users; are being treated for an STI; have a history of blood transfusion between 1978 and 1985; or who request an HIV test since nondisclosure may be indicative of high-risk behavior.[73] The USPSTF also states that there is good evidence of increased yield from routine HIV screening of persons who report no individual risk factors but are seen in high-risk or high-prevalence clinical settings, such as jails, STI clinics, and teen clinics.[73] Males who continue to engage in high-risk activities are also recommended to be tested periodically.

In September 2006, the CDC released new guidelines that "HIV screening is recommended for patients in all health-care settings after the patient is notified that testing will be performed unless the patient declines (opt-out screening). The CDC recommends that persons at high risk for HIV infection should be screened for HIV at least annually; separate written consent for HIV testing should not be required and general consent for medical care should be considered sufficient to encompass consent for HIV testing; and prevention counseling should not be required with HIV diagnostic testing or as part of HIV screening programs in health-care settings."[74]

Other Issues

Mandatory Physician Notification

Physicians are mandated to report to the public health department in most districts patients who test positive for gonorrhea, chlamydia, syphilis, and HIV and report that these patients have received appropriate treatment and referral when applicable.

Partner Treatment

Physicians are encouraged to discuss with patients who test positive for STIs to contact any partners who may have been exposed within 2–3 months of infection for testing and treatment. This can involve one of three options: (1) immediate involvement of the local health department in tracking, contacting, and treating partners; (2) clinician referral of sexual partners by eliciting the names of sex partners and taking responsibility for seeking them out for treatment; or (3) self-referral that involves giving the patient a card with appropriate information on it (specifics about the disease and where and when partner(s) can obtain medical evaluation) that the patient can give to his partner(s). Expedited partner therapy can reduce rates of persistent or recurrent STIs but is not currently approved by all states.

Immunizations

Current immunization recommendations are based on the CDC's Advisory Committee on Immunization Practices.[75] In brief, the hepatitis B vaccine is recommended for all adolescents not previously immunized. The hepatitis A vaccine is now recommended universally for all children at 1 year of age and for persons at risk, including men who have sex with men; children in states, counties, and communities where rates are at least double the national average (greater than 20 cases per 100,000) during baseline period of 1987–1997; illegal-drug users; persons who have occupational risk for infection, chronic liver disease, or clotting-factor disorders; and persons traveling to or working in countries that have high or intermediate rates. The combined tetanus, diphtheria, and pertussis vaccine (Tdap) is now recommended for adolescents aged 11–12 years of age and those who have completed the recommended childhood diphtheria-tetanus-pertussis/ diphtheria–tetanus–acellular pertussis (DTP/ DTaP) vaccination series and have not received a tetanus and diphtheria (Td) booster dose. Adolescents aged 13–18 years of age who missed the age-11–12 booster dose should also receive Tdap. Subsequent Td boosters are recommended every 10 years. Meningococcal conjugate vaccine (Menactra) is recommended for all children at aged 11–12 years as well as to unvaccinated adolescents at high school entry (age 15 years) and for all college freshmen living in dormitories or other communal settings. Additional vaccinations recommended for adolescents not previously immunized include measles/mumps/rubella and varicella for adolescents not previously infected. Influenza vaccine is now recommended for children aged 6 months or older with certain risk factors, including but not limited to asthma, cardiac disease, sickle cell disease, HIV infection, diabetes, and conditions that compromise respiratory function. Human papillomavirus vaccine (HPV) is now recommended for female adolescents at age 11–12 years. Currently, no HPV immunization schedule is recommended for males. The impact of HPV vaccination in males is currently under investigation.

Common Adolescent Male Physical Examination Findings

Acne

Skin disorders, including acne and eczema, provide the physician clinical "hooks" to engage adolescent males in clinical services. Almost all adolescent males by the SMR4 stage will develop visible acne. During the clinical encounter, it is common for an adolescent male with acne to not raise it as a concern. In the majority of instances, when asked, an adolescent male with acne will be interested in treatment options. Clinicians should review prior treatment histories, including use of products that could be making the acne worse (such as astringents). The specific type (e.g., inflammatory, comedonal/obstructive, or scars/noninflammatory lesions) and severity (e.g., mild, moderate, severe) of acne should then be determined during the physical examination.[76]

Topical retinoids should be included in the management of most patients with acne and are recommended as the first-line therapy for mild to moderate inflammatory acne, comedonal acne, and maintenance therapy.[76] Combination therapy (e.g., topical retinoids and antimicrobial therapy) is considered to be significantly better than antimicrobial agents alone for treatment of inflammatory lesions.[76] The primary indication for systemic antibiotics is the presence of moderate to severe inflammatory acne (i.e., acne on the face, back, or chest).[76] For example, a recent Cochrane database review of the literature found that minocycline is likely to be an effective treatment for moderate acne vulgaris, but the researchers found "no reliable randomized controlled trial evidence to justify its continued use as a first-line agent, especially given the price differential and the concerns that still remain about its safety."[77] Patients with severe acne and scarring most benefit from referral to dermatology.

Gynecomastia

During the SMR2–SMR3 stages, approximately 40–65% of males develop some degree of breast hypertrophy that typically occurs bilaterally due to a relative excess of estrogenic stimulation. On examination, the clinician may be able to visualize a breast bud or palpate breast tissue.

- Type 1 gynecomastia represents a breast bud (equivalent to the female breast at SMR2 stage).
- Type 2 gynecomastia represents a breast nodule.
- Type 3 gynecomastia represents findings equivalent to a stage SMR3 (female) breast.

The majority of males experience bilateral budding usually no larger than female breast size stage SMR2–SMR3. One fifth of adolescent males may experience unilateral gynecomastia. Physiologic gynecomastia sufficient to cause embarrassment and social disability occurs in fewer than 10% of males. Swelling of the breast that is less than 4 cm in diameter has a 90% chance of resolving itself within 3 years.[78]

Gynecomastia that presents in the prepubertal stage, later in puberty, or in the absence of signs of pubertal development may be pathologic and requires a medical workup, including taking a thorough history of medication (e.g., histamine-2 receptor antagonists, psychotropic drugs), drug use (e.g., anabolic steroids), and medical complications (e.g., Klinefelter's syndrome, testicular failure, thyroid disease, tumor) as well as performing a comprehensive examination that includes determination of testicular size, neurologic and adrenal system functioning, and signs of chronic illness. Pathologic gynecomastia typically occurs before pubertal onset or later in adolescence (stage SMR4–SMR5). Breast size may be larger than a stage SMR2–SMR3 female breast.

Pseudogynecomastia should be effectively ruled out; this condition results from fatty infiltration in the breast area that may or may not include breast tissue. It is typically seen in overweight males and may not reduce in size even after weight loss. Surgical correction may be appropriate but should wait until after pubertal development is completed and some volitional weight loss is achieved for best results when corrected (see Chapter 23, Cosmetic Plastic Surgery).

Conclusion

Before evaluating adolescent males, clinicians should address any inherent stereotypes of what it means to be a male in society today. Adolescent males experience an intense culture at school and in the media that creates many stereotypes about what it means to be male. Gender role stereotypes (i.e., beliefs that males and females possess distinctly different psychological and behavioral traits and characteristics) are socially and culturally constructed. In the United States, men are socialized to be emotionally inexpressive, tough, competitive, and homophobic, and to not seek help. Furthermore, adolescent males may be exposed to intense school and sports cultures as well as media images that may exaggerate male role stereotypes. As a result, males may experience shame and humiliation, internalization of low self-esteem, and longer-term emotional and physical consequences in attempts to fulfill prescribed male roles. Clinicians who understand these issues can serve as positive role models and create "safe spaces" for males to talk openly about the explicit and implicit "strains" of growing up male in the United States.

No explicit study has examined the most effective ways to counsel adolescent males in the clinical setting. Nonetheless, the manner in which the clinician phrases questions to a male patient should be carefully considered. Males will express their feelings on various levels, but in contexts that feel "safe" to them. This feeling of safety may be due more to a sense of safety for ego than environment. For example, the clinician can ask a male adolescent, "What do/did you think about what happened to you?" rather than "How did that make you feel?" when exploring a specific situation in the male's experience. Follow-up questions then can be asked to explore choices of the words that best express the emotion. The clinician will also need to take the male's developmental stage into account and use strategies to counsel for behavior change that are developmentally appropriate.[14]

Provision of didactic messages, information only, or use of fear is not effective to change a person's behavior and should not be used in isolation. Approaches that have been successful to change a person's behavior include the use of skills development techniques (e.g., refusal skills)

Table 7-5. Adolescent Male-Friendly Health Education Resources

Brochures	
Office of Population Affairs Clearinghouse http://opa.osophs.dhhs.gov/pubs/publications.html	Reproductive health focused brochures (free and at cost)
ETR Publishing http://www.etr.org/pub/titles/browse.html	Brochures and other health resources on various topics (at cost)
Planned Parenthood http://www.plannedparenthood.org/teens	Reproductive health focused brochures (free and at cost)
Web Sites/Downloadable Brochures	
Cool Nurse http://www.coolnurse.com/male_health.htm	Information about adolescent male-specific topics including athlete's foot, hygiene, "blue balls," circumcision, hair loss, masturbation, penis problems, penis size, performance anxiety, wet dreams, and testicular self-examination
TeensHealth—Nemours Foundation http://www.kidshealth.org/kid/grow	Information for: Younger adolescent males on more general topics including boys and puberty, what's an Adam's apple, acne, and braces; older adolescent males on medical-related topics, including why is my voice changing? Is it normal to get erections? I'm a guy…so how come I'm developing breasts? and shaving
Palo Alto Medical Foundation—A Sutter Health Affiliate http://www.pamf.org/teen/health/malehealth	Information for older adolescent males on medical-related topics, including athlete's foot, foreskin and circumcision, ejaculation, erections, hernia, jock itch, male breasts, prostate health, and testicular health
Youth Resource http://www.youthresource.com/health/men.htm	A website by and for gay, lesbian, bisexual, transgender, and questioning (GLBTQ) young people that takes a holistic approach to sexual health and exploring issues of concern to GLBTQ youth
Videos	
Fight for Your Rights—Kaiser Family Foundation/MTV http://www.kff.org/entpartnerships/mtv.cfm	Videos on reproductive topics in addition to influence of culture on adolescent behavior (free)

Adapted from: Marcell AV, Bell DL: Making the most of the adolescent male health visit part 1: history and anticipatory guidance, *Contemp Peds* 23(5):50–63, 2006.

and client-centered counseling (e.g., personalized risk reduction plans that identify barriers and facilitators of behavior change) because these methods serve to increase a person's self-efficacy and self-esteem.[79,80]

Clinicians and staff should also take the time to evaluate the clinic setting to determine whether it is male friendly. Assuming that the environment is adolescent friendly, clinicians and staff should review the types of posters, brochures, magazines, videos, and other resources to determine whether they are appropriate for male patients (Table 7-5).

All of the general principles of an adolescent visit apply when working with an adolescent male. The clinician should review with the patient and his parents the clinic's hours, best phone number(s) to call, after-hours protocols, and what to expect during initial and subsequent visits. The patient should also be provided expectations about visit frequency and the types of healthcare visits recommended throughout adolescence (e.g., vaccine visits, visits for anticipatory guidance) according to the most recent evidence. The male patient should be encouraged as he approaches adulthood to become more involved in making his own clinic appointments. Finally, clinicians should help transition the male patient to appropriate adult healthcare clinicians when appropriate.

References

1. National Adolescent Health Information Center: *A health profile of adolescent and young adult males,* San Francisco, CA, 2005, University of California. Available at: http://nahic.ucsf.edu/index.php/nahic/article/a_health_profile_of_adolescent_and_young_adult_males.
2. Eaton DK, Kann L, Kinchen S, et al: Youth risk behavior surveillance—United States, 2005, *MMWR Surveill Summ* 55(5):1–108, 2006.
3. Newacheck PW: Adolescents with special health needs: prevalence, severity, and access to health services, *Pediatrics* 84(5):872–881, 1989.
4. Tanner JM: *Growth at Adolescence,* ed 2, Oxford, England, 1962, Blackwell Scientific.
5. Lee PA, Reiter EO: Genital size: a common adolescent male concern, *Adolesc Med State Art Rev* 13(1):171–180, 2002.
6. Mansbach JM, Gordon CM: Demystifying delayed puberty, *Contemp Peds* 4:43, 2001.
7. Neinstein LS, editor, *Adolescent health care: a practical guide,* ed 4, Philadelphia, 2002, Lippincott Williams & Wilkins.
8. Reynolds EL, Wines JV: Physical changes associated with adolescent boys, *Am J Dis Child* 82:529–547, 1951.
9. Marshall WA, Tanner JM: Variations in the pattern of pubertal changes in boys, *Arch Dis Child* 45 (239):13–23, 1970.
10. Sun SS, Schubert CM, Chumlea WC, et al: National estimates of the timing of sexual maturation and racial differences among US children, *Pediatrics* 110 (5):911–919, 2002.
11. Forbes GB: Body composition in adolescent children. In Falkner F, Tanner JM, editors: *Human Growth,* vol 2. New York, 1986, Plenum Press, pp 119–145.
12. Rosner B, Prineas RJ, Loggie JM, et al: Blood pressure nomograms for children and adolescents, by height, sex, and age, in the United States. *J Pediatr* 123(6):871–886, 1993.
13. Bailey DA, Malina RM, Mirwald RL: Physical activity and growth of the child. In Falkner F, Tanner JM, editors: *Human Growth,* vol 2. New York, 1986, Plenum Press, pp 147–170.
14. Marcell AV, Monasterio EB: Providing anticipatory guidance and counseling to the adolescent male, *Adolesc Med State Art Rev* 14(3):565–582, 2003.
15. American Academy of Family Physicians: Summary of Recommendations for Clinical Preventive Services, Revision 6.3, March 2007. Leawood, KS, 2006, American Academy of Family Physicians. Available at: http://www.aafp.org/exam.
16. Agency for Healthcare Research and Quality: The Guide to Clinical Preventive Services, 2005. Recommendations of the US Preventive Services Task Force: U.S. DHHS AHRQ. Pub No. 05–0570, 2005. Available at: http://www.preventiveservices.ahrq.gov.
17. Elster A, Kuzsets N: *Guidelines for Adolescent Preventive Services (GAPS),* Baltimore, MD, 1993, Williams & Wilkins.
18. Green M, Palfrey JS, editors: *Bright Futures: Guidelines for Health Supervision of Infants, Children, and Adolescents,* ed 2, revised, Arlington, VA, 2002, National Center for Education in Maternal and Child Health.
19. American Academy of Pediatrics, Committee on Psychosocial Aspects of Child and Family Health: *Guidelines for Health Supervision III,* Elk Grove Village, IL, 1997, American Academy of Pediatrics.
20. AAFP, AAP, American Medical Society for Sports Medicine, American Orthopedic Society for Sports Medicine, & the Osteopathic Academy of Sports Medicine: *Preparticipation Physical Evaluation,* ed 2, Minneapolis, MN, 1996, Physician & Sports Medicine.
21. Carek PJ, Mainous A: The preparticipation physical examination for athletics: a systematic review of current recommendations, *BMJ* 327:170–173, 2003.
22. Hulkower S, Fagan B, Watts J, et al: Do preparticipation clinical exams reduce morbidity and mortality for athletes? *J Fam Pract* 54(7):628–632, 2005.
23. Wingfield K, Matheson GO, Meeuwisse WH: Preparticipation evaluation: an evidence-based review, *Clin J Sport Med* 14(3):109–122, 2004.
24. Stickler GB: Are yearly physical examinations in adolescents necessary? *J Am Board Fam Pract* 13 (3):172–177, 2000.

25. English A, Kenney K: *State Minor Consent Laws: A Summary*, ed 2, Chapel Hill, NC, 2003, Center for Adolescent Health & the Law.

26. Goldenring JM, Cohen E: Getting into adolescents' HEADS, *Contemp Peds* 5(7):75–90, 1988.

27. Goldenring JM, Rosen DS: Getting into adolescent HEADS: an essential update, *Contemp Peds* 21(64): 64–90, 2004. Available at: http://www.contemporary pediatrics.com.

28. Marcell AV, Bell DL: Making the most of the adolescent male health visit Part 1: history and anticipatory guidance, *Contemp Peds* 23(5):50–63, 2006. Available at: http://www.contemporarypediatrics.com.

29. US Preventive Services Task Force: Behavioral counseling in primary care to promote a healthy diet: recommendations and rationale, *Am J Prev Med* 24(1):93–100, 2003.

30. US Preventive Services Task Force: Behavioral counseling in primary care to promote physical activity: recommendation and rationale, *Ann Intern Med* 137(3):205–207, 2002.

31. Counseling to prevent unintended pregnancy, In *Guide to Clinical Preventive Services*, ed 3, US Preventive Services Task Force. 1996. Available at: http://www.ncbi.nlm.nih.gov/books/bv.fcgi?rid=hstat.

32. Counseling to prevent HIV infection and other sexually transmitted diseases, In *Guide to Clinical Preventive Services*, ed 3, U.S. Preventive Services Task Force. 1996. Available at: http://www.ncbi.nlm. nih.gov/books/bv.fcgi?rid=hstat3.

33. US Preventive Services Task Force: Counseling to prevent tobacco use and tobacco-caused disease 2003. Available at: http://www.ahrq.gov/clinic/uspstf/uspstbac.htm.

34. US Preventive Services Task Force: Screening and behavioral counseling interventions in primary care to reduce alcohol misuse: recommendation statement, *Ann Intern Med* 140(7):554–556, 2004.

35. US Preventive Services Task Force: Screening for drug abuse. 1996. Available at: http://www.ncbi.nlm.nih.gov/books/bv.fcgi?rid=hstat3.section.10931#15313.

36. US Preventive Services Task Force: Screening for depression: recommendations and rationale, *Ann Intern Med* 136(10):760–764, 2002.

37. US Preventive Services Task Force: Screening for suicide risk: recommendation and rationale, *Ann Intern Med* 140(10):820–821, 2004.

38. US Preventive Services Task Force: Screening for family and intimate partner violence: recommendation statement, *Ann Intern Med* 140(5):382–386, 2004.

39. Counseling to prevent motor vehicle injuries, In *Guide to Clinical Preventive Services*, ed 3, US Preventive Services Task Force. 1996. Available at: http://www.ncbi.nlm.nih.gov/books/bv.fcgi?rid=hstat3.

40. Counseling to prevent household and recreational injuries, In *Guide to Clinical Preventive Services*, ed 3, US Preventive Services Task Force. 1996. Available at: http://www.ncbi.nlm.nih.gov/books/bv.fcgi?rid=hstat3.

41. Counseling to prevent youth violence, In *Guide to Clinical Preventive Services*, ed 3, US Preventive Services Task Force. 1996. Available at: http://www.ncbi.nlm.nih.gov/books/bv.fcgi?rid=hstat3.

42. National High Blood Pressure Education Working Group on High Blood Pressure in Children and Adolescents: The fourth report on the diagnosis and evaluation and treatment of high blood pressure in children and adolescents, *Pediatrics* 114 (2):555–576, 2004.

43. National High Blood Pressure Education Program Working Group on Hypertension Control in Children and Adolescents: Update on the 1987 Task Force Report on High Blood Pressure in Children and Adolescents: a working group report from the National High Blood Pressure Education Program, *Pediatrics* 98(4 Pt 1):649–658, 1996.

44. Rosen DS: Eating disorders in adolescent males, *Adolesc Med State Art Rev* 14(3):677–689, 2003.

45. Neumark-Sztainer D, Hannan PJ: Weight-related behaviors among adolescent girls and boys: results from a national survey, *Arch Pediatr Adolesc Med* 154(6):569–577, 2000.

46. Centers for Disease Control and Prevention: Overweight children and adolescents: recommendations to screen, assess and manage. Available at: http://www.cdc.gov/nccdphp/dnpa/growthcharts/training/modules/module1/text/mainmodules.htm.

47. Barlow SE, Dietz WH: Obesity evaluation and treatment: Expert Committee recommendations. The Maternal and Child Health Bureau, Health Resources and Services Administration and the Department of Health and Human Services, *Pediatrics* 102(3):e29, 1998.

48. US Preventive Services Task Force: Screening for hearing impairment, 1996. Available at: http://www.ahrq.gov/clinic/2ndcps/hearing.pdf.

48a. American Cancer Society. Detailed guide: Testicular cancer can testicular cancer be found early? 2007, Revised: July 26, 2006. Available at http://www.cancer.org/docroot/CRI/content/CRI_2_4_3X_Can_Testicular_Cancer_Be_Found_Early_41.asp.Retrieved June 10, 2007.

49. US Preventive Services Task Force: Screening for testicular cancer: recommendation statement, February 2004. Available at: http://www.ahrq.gov/clinic/3rduspstf/testicular/testiculup.htm.

50. Congeni J, Miller SF, Bennett CL: Awareness of genital health in young male athletes, *Clin J Sports Med* 15(1):22–26, 2005.

51. Nasrallah P, Nair G, Congeni J, et al: Testicular health awareness in pubertal males, *J Urol* 164(3 Pt 2): 1115–1117, 2000.

52. Coughlin MT, LaPorte RE, O'Leary LA, et al: How accurate is male recall of reproductive information? *Am J Epidemiol* 148(8):806–809, 1998.

53. American Academy of Pediatrics Committee on Practice and Ambulatory Medicine: The use of chaperones during the physical examination of the pediatric patient, *Pediatrics* 98(6 Pt 1):1202, 1996.

54. Sanders JM Jr, DuRant RH, Chastain DO: Pediatricians' use of chaperones when performing gynecologic examinations on adolescent females, *J Adolesc Health Care* 10(2):110–114, 1989.

55. Buchta RM: Adolescent females' preferences regarding use of a chaperone during a pelvic examination: observations from a private-practice setting, *J Adolesc Health Care* 7(6):409–411, 1986.

56. Phillips S, Friedman SB, Seidenberg M, et al: Teenagers' preferences regarding the presence of family members, peers, and chaperones during examination of genitalia, *Pediatrics* 68(5):665–669, 1981.

57. Kapphahn CJ, Wilson KM, Klein JD: Adolescent girls' and boys' preferences for provider gender and confidentiality in their health care, *J Adolesc Health* 25(2):131–142, 1999.

58. Klein JD, Wilson KM, McNulty M, et al: Access to medical care for adolescents: results from the 1997 Commonwealth Fund Survey of the Health of Adolescent Girls, *J Adolesc Health* 25(2):120–130, 1999.

59. Rosenfeld SL, Fox DJ, Keenan PM, et al: Primary care experiences and preferences of urban youth, *J Pediatr Health Care* 10(4):151–160, 1996.

60. US Preventive Services Task Force: Screening for lipid disorders: recommendations and rationale. Article originally in *Am J Prev Med* 20(3S):73–76, 2001. Agency for Healthcare Research and Quality, Rockville, MD. Available at: http://www.ahrq.gov/clinic/ajpmsuppl/lipidrr.htm.

61. Executive Summary of The Third Report of The National Cholesterol Education Program (NCEP) Expert Panel on Detection, Evaluation, and Treatment of High Blood Cholesterol in Adults (Adult Treatment Panel III), *JAMA* 285(19):2486–2497, 2001.

62. US Preventive Services Task Force: Screening for tuberculosis infection. 2006. Available at: http://www.ahrq.gov/clinic/uspstf/uspstubr.htm.

63. Taylor Z, Nolan CM, Blumberg HM: Controlling tuberculosis in the United States: recommendations from the American Thoracic Society, CDC, and the Infectious Diseases Society of America, *MMWR Recomm Rep* 54(RR-12):1–81, 2005.

64. U.S. Preventive Services Task Force. Asymptomatic bacteriuria: Brief evidence update. 2004. Agency for Healthcare Research and Quality, Rockville, MD. Available at: http://www.ahrq.gov/clinic/3rduspstf/asymbac/asymbacup.htm.

65. Centers for Disease Control and Prevention: Sexually transmitted diseases treatment guidelines, 2006, *MMWR* 55(No.RR-11):1–94, 2006. Available at: http://www.cdc.gov/mmwr/pdf/rr/rr5511.pdf.

65a. Division of STD Prevention (March 28–29, 2006). Male Chlamydia Screening Consultation. Atlanta, Georgia, National Center for HIV/AIDS, Viral Hepatitis, STD and TB Prevention. U.S. Centers for Disease Control and Prevention: http://www.cdc.gov/std/chlamydia/.

66. US Preventive Services Task Force: Screening for gonorrhea: recommendation statement, *Ann Fam Med* 3(3):263–267, 2005.

67. Screening for chlamydial infection: US Preventive Services Task Force recommendation statement, *Ann Intern Med* 174(2):128–133, 2007.

68. Screening for hepatitis C virus infection in adults: recommendation statement, *Ann Intern Med* 140(6):462–464, 2004.

69. Glass N, Nelson HD, Huffman L: Screening for genital herpes simplex: brief update for the USPSTF. March 2005. Available at: http://www.preventiveservices.ahrq.gov. Accessed August 8, 2006.

70. U.S. Preventive Services Task Force. Screening for Hepatitis B Infection: Recommendation Statement. 2004. Agency for Healthcare Research and Quality, Rockville, MD. Available at: http://www.ahrq.gov/clinic/3rduspstf/hepbscr/hepbrs.htm.

71. American Academy of Pediatrics: Hepatitis B: In Pickering LK, Baker CJ, Long SS, McMillan JA, editors: *Red Book: 2006 Report of the Committee on Infectious Diseases*, ed 27, Elk Grove, IL, 2006, American Academy of Pediatrics, p 343.

72. Calonge N: Screening for syphilis infection: recommendation statement, *Ann Fam Med* 2(4):362–365, 2004.

73. Screening for HIV: recommendation statement, *Ann Intern Med* 143(1):32–37, 2005.

74. Centers for Disease Control and Prevention: Revised recommendations for HIV testing of adults, adolescents, and pregnant women in health-care settings, *MMWR* 55(No. RR-14):1–17, 2006.

75. Centers for Disease Control and Prevention: 2007 childhood and adolescent immunization schedules, *MMWR CDC Surveill Summ* 2006; 54(Nos. 51&52): Q1–Q4: 2006. Available at: http://www.cdc.gov/nip/recs/child-schedule.htm#Printable.

76. Gollnick H, Cunliffe W, Berson D, et al: Management of acne: a report from a Global Alliance to Improve Outcomes in Acne, *J Am Acad Dermatol* 49(1 Suppl):S1–S37, 2003.

77. Garner SE, Eady EA, Popescu C, et al: Minocycline for acne vulgaris: efficacy and safety, *Cochrane Database Syst Rev* 1:CD002086, 2003.

78. Nydick M, Bustos J, Dale JH, et al: Gynecomastia in adolescent boys, *JAMA* 178(5):109–114, 1961.

79. Bandura A: *Principles of behavior modification*, New York, 1969, Holt, Rinehart & Winston.

80. Kamb ML, Fishbein M, Douglas JM Jr, et al: Efficacy of risk-reduction counseling to prevent human immunodeficiency virus and sexually transmitted diseases: a randomized controlled trial. Project RESPECT Study Group, *JAMA* 280(13):1161–1167, 1998.

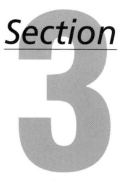

Section

The Adult Male

Cardiology

Joel J. Heidelbaugh, MD

Key Points

Hypertension

JNC 7 Recommendations[7]:

- In persons older than 50 years of age, a systolic blood pressure greater than 140 mm Hg is a much more significant cardiovascular risk factor than elevated diastolic blood pressure (strength of recommendation: A).
- The risk of development of cardiovascular disease with blood pressure readings beginning at 115/75 mm Hg doubles with each increment of 20/10 mm Hg; persons who are normotensive at the age of 55 years have a 90% lifetime risk for developing hypertension (strength of recommendation: A).
- Persons with a systolic blood pressure of 120–139 mm Hg or a diastolic blood pressure of 80–89 mm Hg should be considered prehypertensive and require the integration of health-promoting lifestyle modifications to prevent cardiovascular disease (strength of recommendation: B).
- Thiazide-type diuretics should be used as initial pharmacotherapy for patients with uncomplicated hypertension, either alone or combined with drugs from other classes (e.g., angiotensin-converting enzyme inhibitors, angiotensin receptor blockers, beta-blockers, calcium channel blockers) (strength of recommendation: A).
- Most patients with essential hypertension will at some point require two or more antihypertensive medications to achieve their blood pressure goal (less than 140/90 mm Hg, or less than 130/80 mm Hg for patients with diabetes or chronic kidney disease) (strength of recommendation: A).
- If blood pressure is more than 20/10 mm Hg above the goal blood pressure, consideration should be given to initiating therapy with two agents, one of which should be a thiazide-type diuretic (strength of recommendation: C).
- The most effective pharmacotherapy will control hypertension only if patients are motivated; motivation improves when patients have both positive experiences with and trust in their clinician (strength of recommendation: C).

Hypercholesterolemia

NCEP ATP III Recommendations[28]:

- The NCEP ATP III recommends that cholesterol screening should commence at the age of 20 years in both men and women (strength of recommendation: C).
- Tables 8-8 and 8-9 reflect NCEP ATP III recommendations for treatment goals of hypercholesterolemia (strength of recommendation for all: A).

USPSTF Recommendations[42]:

- The USPSTF recommends against routine screening with resting electrocardiography, exercise treadmill stress testing, or electron-beam computerized tomography scanning for coronary artery calcium scores to determine either the presence of severe coronary artery stenosis or the prediction of CHD events in adults at low or high risk for such events (strength of recommendation: C).

- The USPSTF strongly recommends that clinicians routinely screen men aged 35 years and older and women aged 45 years and older for lipid disorders and treat abnormal lipids in those who are at increased risk of CHD; the USPSTF makes no recommendation for or against routine screening for lipid disorders in younger adults (men aged 20–35 years or women aged 20–45 years) in the absence of known risk factors for CHD (strength of recommendation: B).
- The USPSTF recommends that clinicians routinely screen younger adults (men aged 20–35 years and women aged 20–45 years) for lipid disorders if they have other risk factors for CHD (strength of recommendation: A).
- The USPSTF recommends that screening for lipid disorders should include the measurement of both total cholesterol and HDL-C (strength of recommendation: A).
- The USPSTF concludes that the evidence is insufficient to recommend for or against triglyceride measurement as a part of routine screening for lipid disorders (strength of recommendation: C).

Primary prevention of cardiovascular disease[115]:

- Patients with elevated cholesterol levels should reduce dietary fat consumption, yet this step may lead to only a small reduction in cardiovascular events (strength of recommendation: A).
- Statins are indicated to decrease cardiovascular events and cardiac deaths in patients with elevated cholesterol levels, although a decrease in all-cause mortality has not been demonstrated (strength of recommendation: A).
- Following a Mediterranean diet may reduce all-cause mortality (strength of recommendation: B).

Secondary prevention of cardiovascular disease[115]:

- Statins should be used for aggressive lipid control in patients with CHD to decrease cardiovascular events, cardiovascular mortality, and overall mortality (strength of recommendation: A).
- Cholesterol-lowering medications prevent disease progression and improve symptoms in patients with lower limb atherosclerosis; statins can decrease cardiovascular events and all-cause mortality in these patients (strength of recommendation: A).
- Cholesterol-lowering medications should be used to reduce the risk of stroke in patients with a history of CHD and average-to-high

cholesterol levels (strength of recommendation: A).

Introduction and Epidemiology

Diseases of the heart perennially account for the leading causes of morbidity and mortality in the United States for both men and women of all ethnicities. The most current data available at the time of authorship of the relevant chapter from *Deaths: Preliminary Data for 2004*[1] reveal that 654,092 deaths were attributable to heart disease, with an age-adjusted death rate of 217.5 per 100,000, reflecting a 6.4% decrease from data compiled in 2003. Essential (primary) hypertension and hypertensive renal disease were the 13th leading cause of mortality, accounting for 22,953 deaths and an age-adjusted death rate of 7.6 per 100,000 during the same time period.[1] According to the *National Health Interview Survey* from 2004,[2] approximately 22,040,000 US men had hypertension and approximately 7,934,000 US men had coronary artery disease (CAD). These data highlighted that the men who most commonly experienced hypertension and CAD were white, were aged 45–64 years, lived in the southern United States, had private health insurance, had at least a high school diploma or a general equivalency diploma, and had an annual income of less than $20,000. These data also revealed that whereas 21.9% of both men and women have hypertension, 8.3% of men compared with 4.9% of women have CAD.[2] According to the American Heart Association's (AHA) *Heart Disease and Stroke Statistics—2006 Update*,[3] coronary heart disease (CHD) accounts for $142.5 billion in direct and indirect costs, followed by hypertensive disease ($63.5 billion), stroke ($57.9 billion), and heart failure ($29.6 billion).

Data compiled in 2003 by the Centers for Disease Control and Prevention (CDC) and the National Heart, Lung, and Blood Institute (NHLBI) for the AHA attribute 53% of US deaths from cardiovascular diseases to CHD, 17% to stroke, and 6% each to hypertension and heart failure (Figure 8-1). Trends in age-adjusted prevalence in US adults aged 20–74 years have revealed a steady decrease in the incidence of hypercholesterolemia since the 1970s to 2000 (29% to 18%); a decrease in the incidence of hypertension from the early 1970s to 1994 (40% to 24%) has been followed by a moderate increase to 29% currently. More impressively, US adults in this age range have exhibited a significant increase in

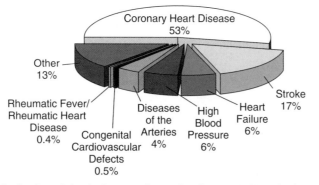

Figure 8-1. Percentage distribution of deaths from cardiovascular diseases, 2003, United States. (Adapted from: Heart Disease and Stroke Statistics—2006 Update. American Heart Association. Available at: http://www.americanheart.org/presenter. jhtml?identifier=3018163.)

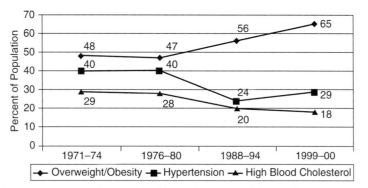

Figure 8-2. Trends in age-adjusted prevalence of health conditions, US adults aged 20–74 years. (Adapted from: Heart Disease and Stroke Statistics—2006 Update. American Heart Association. Available at: http://www.americanheart.org/presenter. jhtml?identifier=3018163.)

the rate of overweight/obesity from the 1970s to 2000 (47% to 65%) (Figure 8-2). Data from the National Household Education Survey and the National Health and Nutrition Examination Survey (NHANES) from the 1960s through 2000 revealed similar trends in the decreases in incidence of hypercholesterolemia and hypertension as well as smoking rates, yet demonstrated steady but consistent increases in the incidence of diabetes (Figure 8-3). Specific data reflecting cardiovascular disease mortality rates between genders reveal that from the late 1970s through the mid 1980s men exceeded women in number of deaths, yet the former have since exhibited fewer deaths annually (Figure 8-4).

These statistics herald an important public health challenge, emphasizing the importance of the primary care clinician's role in educating male patients about the primary and secondary prevention of heart disease. The current lay press is riddled with articles informing the American public of the obesity epidemic, alarming heart disease statistics, and advertisements for healthier foods, exercise options, and lifestyle choices. Despite lower rates of hypertension and hyperlipidemia in the United States, obesity and the metabolic syndrome are dramatically increasing in incidence, and cardiovascular disease still claims the life of approximately 223 in 100,000 persons annually in the United States.[1]

The goals of this chapter are to examine two predominate contributing factors to cardiovascular disease, namely hypertension and hyperlipidemia. Approaches to primary and secondary prevention of CHD will be emphasized through an evidence-based review of the current literature and accepted guidelines. An exhaustive review of the diagnosis and treatment of all relevant cardiovascular diseases affecting men is beyond the limitations of this textbook; therefore, current evidence-based guideline references for congestive heart failure, atrial fibrillation, acute coronary syndrome, unstable angina, and venous thromboembolic disease will be provided for reader review.

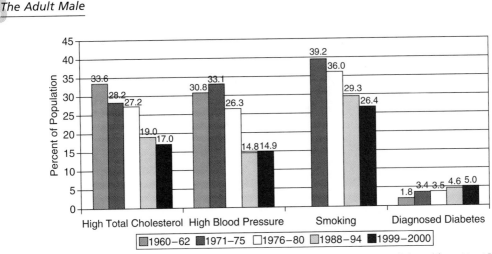

Figure 8-3. Trends in cardiovascular risk factors in the US population aged 20–74 years. (Adapted from: Heart Disease and Stroke Statistics—2006 Update. American Heart Association. Available at: http://www.americanheart.org/presenter.jhtml?identifier=3018163.)

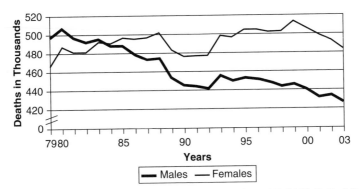

Figure 8-4. Cardiovascular disease mortality trends for males and females, 1979–2003, United States. (Adapted from: Heart Disease and Stroke Statistics—2006 Update. American Heart Association. Available at: http://www.americanheart.org/presenter.jhtml?identifier=3018163.)

Stratification of Risk for Coronary Heart Disease

The most widely accepted guidelines for the risk stratification of CHD are derived from the Framingham Heart Study.[4,5] A separate point scoring system exists for men (Table 8-1) and women that estimates the 10-year risk of CHD based on age, total cholesterol, high-density lipoprotein cholesterol (HDL-C), smoking status, and systolic blood pressure.

Metabolic Syndrome/Insulin Resistance Syndrome

The AHA defines *metabolic syndrome/insulin resistance syndrome* as a constellation of metabolic risk factors existing in one person. These factors include the following[6]:

- Abdominal obesity (i.e., excessive fat tissue in and around the abdomen)
- Atherogenic dyslipidemia
  - Elevated serum triglyceride levels
  - Low HDL-C
  - Elevated low-density lipoprotein cholesterol (LDL-C)
- Elevated blood pressure
- Insulin resistance or glucose intolerance
- A prothrombotic state (e.g., elevated serum fibrinogen or plasminogen activator inhibitor[6])
- A proinflammatory state (e.g., elevated serum C-reactive protein [CRP])

Persons who have the metabolic syndrome are at an increased risk of CHD and other diseases related to atherosclerosis including stroke, peripheral vascular disease, and type 2 diabetes mellitus. In 2005, it was estimated that more than 50 million Americans have the metabolic syndrome.[6] The dominant underlying risk factors for this syndrome appear to be abdominal obesity, defined

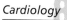
Table 8-1. Estimate of 10-Year Risk for Coronary Heart Disease in Men Using Framingham Point Scores

FRAMINGHAM POINT SCORES BY AGE GROUP	
Age (Years)	Points
20–34	−9
35–39	−4
40–44	0
45–49	3
50–54	6
55–59	8
60–64	10
65–69	11
70–74	12
75–79	13

FRAMINGHAM POINT SCORES BY AGE GROUP (YEARS) AND TOTAL CHOLESTEROL					
Total Cholesterol	Age 20–39	Age 40–49	Age 50–59	Age 60–69	Age 70–79
<160	0	0	0	0	0
160–199	4	3	2	1	0
200–239	7	5	3	1	0
240–279	9	6	4	2	1
280+	11	8	5	3	1

FRAMINGHAM POINT SCORES BY AGE (YEARS) AND SMOKING STATUS					
	Age 20–39	Age 40–49	Age 50–59	Age 60–69	Age 70–79
Nonsmoker	0	0	0	0	0
Smoker	8	5	3	1	1

FRAMINGHAM POINT SCORES BY HDL LEVEL	
HDL	Points
60+	−1
50–59	0
40–49	1
<40	2

FRAMINGHAM POINT SCORES BY SYSTOLIC BLOOD PRESSURE AND TREATMENT STATUS		
Systolic BP	If Untreated	If Treated
<120	0	0
120–129	0	1
130–139	1	2
140–159	1	2
160+	2	3

Table continued on following page

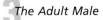

Table 8-1. Estimate of 10-Year Risk for Coronary Heart Disease in Men Using Framingham Point Scores (Continued)

10-YEAR RISK BY TOTAL FRAMINGHAM POINT SCORES	
Point Total	**10-Year Risk**
<0	<1%
0	1%
1	1%
2	1%
3	1%
4	1%
5	2%
6	2%
7	3%
8	4%
9	5%
10	6%
11	8%
12	10%
13	12%
14	16%
15	20%
16	25%
17 or more	30%

HDL, High-density lipoprotein.
Adapted from: National Cholesterol Education Program: Third report of the National Cholesterol Education Program (NCEP) Expert Panel on the Detection, Evaluation, and Treatment of High Blood Cholesterol in Adults (Adult Treatment Panel III): executive summary. NIH Publication no. (NIH) 01–3670. Bethesda, MD, 2001, National Cholesterol Education Program, National Institutes of Health, National Heart, Lung, and Blood Institute.

as an increased hip-to-waist ratio, and insulin resistance. Other conditions associated with the metabolic syndrome include physical inactivity, aging, hormonal imbalance, and a genetic predisposition. The biologic mechanisms occurring at the molecular level between insulin resistance and metabolic risk factors are not fully understood and are the subject of current intense research.

Currently, there are no well-accepted criteria for diagnosing the metabolic syndrome. The AHA and the NHLBI recommend that the metabolic syndrome be identified as the presence of three or more of the following components[6]:
- Elevated waist circumference
  - Men: Equal to or greater than 40 inches (102 cm)
  - Women: Equal to or greater than 35 inches (89 cm)
- Elevated serum triglyceride levels greater than or equal to 150 mg/dL
- Reduced HDL-C
  - Men: Less than 40 mg/dL
  - Women: Less than 50 mg/dL
- Elevated blood pressure greater than or equal to 130/85 mm Hg
- Elevated fasting glucose greater than or equal to 100 mg/dl

According to the AHA, three groups of persons often have metabolic syndrome[6]:
- People with diabetes who cannot maintain a proper level of glucose (glucose intolerance)
- People without diabetes who have high blood pressure and who also secrete large amounts of insulin (hyperinsulinemia) to maintain blood glucose levels
- People who have had a myocardial infarction and who have hyperinsulinemia without glucose intolerance

The primary goal of clinical management of the metabolic syndrome is to reduce the risk for cardiovascular disease and type 2 diabetes. First-line therapy is to reduce the major cardiovascular disease risk factors including smoking cessation and reduction of LDL-C, blood pressure, and serum glucose to the recommended levels. For managing both long- and short-term CHD risks, lifestyle therapies are the first-line interventions toward reduction of metabolic risk factors including the following[6]:

- Weight loss to achieve a desirable weight (body mass index [BMI] less than 25 kg/m^2) (Figure 8-5)
- Increased physical activity, with a goal of at least 30 minutes of moderate-intensity activity on most days of the week
- Healthy eating habits that include the reduced intake of saturated fats, trans fats, and cholesterol

Hypertension

This section builds on the framework of the Seventh Report of the Joint National Committee on Prevention, Detection, Evaluation, and Treatment of High Blood Pressure (JNC 7),[7] as well as data compiled from the AHA, Cochrane reviews, and recent meta-analyses. The JNC 7 report is heralded as the definitive guideline for hypertension, providing recommendations for patients with essential and secondary hypertension, as well as for those with heart failure, diabetes mellitus, chronic kidney disease, cerebrovascular disease, and other chronic conditions among men, women, and minority populations.

Epidemiology

According to *Health, United States, 2006,*[8] data from 2001 to 2004 demonstrate that 28.1% of males and 30.7% of females 20 years of age and older (i.e., age-adjusted) have hypertension. These data also demonstrate that African American males (41.6%) and females (44.7%) have significantly higher rates of hypertension compared with other ethnic groups. In 2004, hypertension accounted for 38 million outpatient office visits or 4.2% of total visits in the ambulatory care setting, consistently ranking as the most common primary diagnosis.[9] The vast majority of these persons have *essential hypertension,* defined as hypertension without any definable cause. Common causes of secondary hypertension include renal artery stenosis (i.e., renovascular hypertension), renal parenchymal disease, coarctation of the aorta, pheochromocytoma, and obstructive sleep apnea.[7]

NHANES data from 1999 to 2002[10] demonstrates that fewer than one half of persons aged 20–39 years were aware of their diagnosis of hypertension, with approximately three quarters of those aged 40 years and above aware of their diagnosis (Figure 8-6). Adequate treatment and control rates for hypertension (defined as blood pressure 140/90 mm Hg or below) were even lower in the 20- to 39-year age group at 28.1% and 17.6%, respectively. There was no significant difference in the awareness and treatment of hypertension in age groups 40- to 59 years and 60 years and above, yet the 40- to 59-year age group had a superior rate of hypertension control compared with the group aged 60 years and older (40.5% and 31.4%, respectively). When examining the parameters of awareness, treatment, and control of hypertension among ethnicities, non-Hispanic blacks were shown to have higher rates of awareness and treatment compared with non-Hispanic whites and Mexican Americans (Figure 8-7). Non-Hispanic whites and non-Hispanic blacks

Body Mass Index Table

	Normal						Overweight					Obese										Extreme Obesity														
BMI	19	20	21	22	23	24	25	26	27	28	29	30	31	32	33	34	35	36	37	38	39	40	41	42	43	44	45	46	47	48	49	50	51	52	53	54
Height (inches)																Body Weight (pounds)																				
58	91	96	100	105	110	115	119	124	129	134	138	143	148	153	158	162	167	172	177	181	186	191	196	201	205	210	215	220	224	229	234	239	244	248	253	258
59	94	99	104	109	114	119	124	128	133	138	143	148	153	158	163	168	173	178	183	188	193	198	203	208	212	217	222	227	232	237	242	247	252	257	262	267
60	97	102	107	112	118	123	128	133	138	143	148	153	158	163	168	174	179	184	189	194	199	204	209	215	220	225	230	235	240	245	250	255	261	266	271	276
61	100	106	111	116	122	127	132	137	143	148	153	158	164	169	174	180	185	190	195	201	206	211	217	222	227	232	238	243	248	254	259	264	269	275	280	285
62	104	109	115	120	126	131	136	142	147	153	158	164	169	175	180	186	191	196	202	207	213	218	224	229	235	240	246	251	256	262	267	273	278	284	289	295
63	107	113	118	124	130	135	141	146	152	158	163	169	175	180	186	191	197	203	208	214	220	225	231	237	242	248	254	259	265	270	278	282	287	293	299	304
64	110	116	122	128	134	140	145	151	157	163	169	174	180	186	192	197	204	209	215	221	227	232	238	244	250	256	262	267	273	279	285	291	296	302	308	314
65	114	120	126	132	138	144	150	156	162	168	174	180	186	192	198	204	210	216	222	228	234	240	246	252	258	264	270	276	282	288	294	300	306	312	318	324
66	118	124	130	136	142	148	155	161	167	173	179	186	192	198	204	210	216	223	229	235	241	247	253	260	266	272	278	284	291	297	303	309	315	322	328	334
67	121	127	134	140	146	153	159	166	172	178	185	191	198	204	211	217	223	230	236	242	249	255	261	268	274	280	287	293	299	306	312	319	325	331	338	344
68	125	131	138	144	151	158	164	171	177	184	190	197	203	210	216	223	230	236	243	249	256	262	269	276	282	289	295	302	308	315	322	328	335	341	348	354
69	128	135	142	149	155	162	169	176	182	189	196	203	209	216	223	230	236	243	250	257	263	270	277	284	291	297	304	311	318	324	331	338	345	351	358	365
70	132	139	146	153	160	167	174	181	188	195	202	209	216	222	229	236	243	250	257	264	271	278	285	292	299	306	313	320	327	334	341	348	355	362	369	376
71	136	143	150	157	165	172	179	186	193	200	208	215	222	229	236	243	250	257	265	272	279	286	293	301	308	315	322	329	338	343	351	358	365	372	379	386
72	140	147	154	162	169	177	184	191	199	206	213	221	228	235	242	250	258	265	272	279	287	294	302	309	316	324	331	338	346	353	361	368	375	383	390	397
73	144	151	159	166	174	182	189	197	204	212	219	227	235	242	250	257	265	272	280	288	295	302	310	318	325	333	340	348	355	363	371	378	386	393	401	408
74	148	155	163	171	179	186	194	202	210	218	225	233	241	249	256	264	272	280	287	295	303	311	319	326	334	342	350	358	365	373	381	389	396	404	412	420
75	152	160	168	176	184	192	200	208	216	224	232	240	248	256	264	272	279	287	295	303	311	319	327	335	343	351	359	367	375	383	391	399	407	415	423	431
76	156	164	172	180	189	197	205	213	221	230	238	246	254	263	271	279	287	295	304	312	320	328	336	344	353	361	369	377	385	394	402	410	418	426	435	443

Figure 8-5. Body mass index. (Adapted from: National Heart, Lung, and Blood Institute: Clinical guidelines on the identification, evaluation, and treatment of overweight and obesity in adults: the evidence report. Available at: http://www.nhlbi.nih.gov/guidelines/obesity/ob_home.htm.)

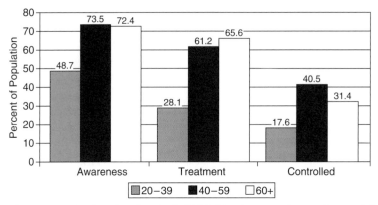

Figure 8-6. Extent of awareness, treatment and control of high blood pressure by age (in years), based on National Health and Nutrition Examination Survey (NHANES) data, 1999–2002. (Adapted from: American Heart Association: Heart disease and stroke statistics—2006 update. Available at: http://www.americanheart.org/presenter.jhtml?identifier=3018163. Source: Centers for Disease Control and Prevention [CDC]: Racial/ethnic disparities in prevalence, treatment, and control of hypertension—United States, 1999–2002, *MMWR* 54[1]:7–9, 2005.)

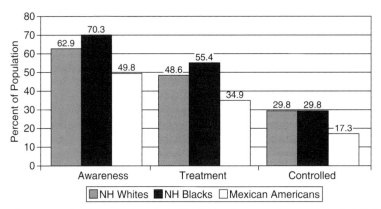

Figure 8-7. Extent of awareness, treatment and control of high blood pressure by race and ethnicity based on National Health and Nutrition Examination Survey (NHANES) data, 1999–2002. NH, Non-Hispanic. (Adapted from: American Heart Association: Heart disease and stroke statistics—2006 update. Available at: http://www.americanheart.org/presenter.jhtml?identifier=3018163. Source: Centers for Disease Control and Prevention [CDC]: Racial/ethnic disparities in prevalence, treatment, and control of hypertension—United States, 1999–2002, *MMWR* 54[1]:7–9, 2005.)

had identical rates of hypertension control. Mexican Americans had significantly lower rates of all three parameters compared with the other groups.

Hypertension is a major risk factor for the development of cardiovascular disease. Others risk factors according to the JNC 7[7] include the following:
- Age older than 55 years for men or 65 years for women
- Family history of premature cardiovascular disease (men younger than 55 years or women younger than 65 years)
- Cigarette smoking
- Obesity (BMI greater than or equal to 30 kg/m^2)
- Physical inactivity

- Hyperlipidemia
- Diabetes mellitus
- Microalbuminuria or estimated glomerular filtration rate less than 60 mL/min

Target organ damage from uncontrolled hypertension includes the following:
- Heart
  - Left ventricular hypertrophy
  - Angina or prior myocardial infarction
  - Prior coronary revascularization
  - Heart failure
- Brain
  - Stroke or transient ischemic attack
- Chronic kidney disease
- Peripheral arterial disease
- Retinopathy

Diagnosis

A patient with a new diagnosis of hypertension deserves special clinical attention. A detailed medical history, physical examination, current blood pressure reading, discussion of family history focusing on significant cardiovascular risk factors, basic laboratory panel including renal function tests (e.g., blood urea nitrogen and serum creatinine), urinalysis, and electrocardiogram should be performed.[7] Abnormalities in any of these categories should prompt the clinician to consider secondary causes of hypertension. It is recommended that patients also receive a written statement of the current blood pressure with specific target goals outlined. Cardiovascular risk factors should also be discussed as outlined above, and strategies for addressing them should be entertained.[11] The current classification and management of hypertension, as outlined by the JNC 7, appears in Table 8-2.

Ambulatory Blood Pressure Monitoring

Campbell and Green's[11] review of the diagnosis and management of hypertension summarizes the JNC 7 guideline recommendation for how ambulatory blood pressure monitoring (ABPM) provides information regarding blood pressure during daily activities and sleep, and is specifically warranted for the evaluation of "white-coat hypertension" in the absence of target organ injury. Given this phenomenon, it is often challenging to determine whether a patient is truly hypertensive and thus ABPM may prove helpful in accurately diagnosing hypertension. Ambulatory blood pressures generally follow a circadian rhythm because persons with hypertension, while awake, have an average blood pressure of greater than 135/85 mm Hg, and during sleep they exhibit values greater than 120/75 mm Hg.[12] It is therefore advisable to assess patients with apparent drug resistance, hypotensive symptoms (in patients who are taking antihypertensive medications), episodic hypertension, and autonomic dysfunction.[11] The JNC 7 discerns that ambulatory blood pressure values are commonly lower than the values obtained in our clinics; however, the level of blood pressure measurement by using ABPM correlates with target organ injury to a greater degree than office measurements.[13] In most persons, blood pressure decreases by a factor of 10–20% during the sleep cycle, and thus it is believed that those in whom such reductions are not present are at increased risk for cardiovascular events.[7]

Treatment

Lifestyle Modifications

A thorough discussion of various dietary guidelines, including the Dietary Approaches to Stop

Table 8-2. Classification and Management of Blood Pressure for Adults

BP Classification	SBP* (mm Hg)	DBP* (mm Hg)	Lifestyle Modification	INITIAL DRUG THERAPY Without Compelling Indication	With Compelling Indications (Refer to Table 8-3.)
Normal	<120	and <80	Encourage	No antihypertensive drug indicated.	Drug(s) for compelling indications.‡
Prehypertension	120–139	or 80–89	Yes		
Stage 1 Hypertension	140–159	or 90–99	Yes	Thiazide-type diuretics for most. May consider ACEI, ARB, BB, CCB, or combination.	Drug(s) for the compelling indications.‡ Other antihypertensive drugs (diuretics, ACEI, ARB, BB, CCB) as needed.
Stage 2 Hypertension	≥160	or ≥100	Yes	Two-drug combination for most† (usually thiazide-type diuretic and ACEI or ARB or BB or CCB).	

BP, Blood pressure, SBP, systolic blood pressure; DBP, diastolic blood pressure; ACEI, angiotensin-converting enzyme inhibitor; ARB, angiotensin receptor blocker; BB, beta-blocker; CCB, calcium channel blocker.
*Treatment determined by highest BP category.
†Initial combined therapy should be used cautiously in those at risk for orthostatic hypotension.
‡Treat patients with chronic kidney disease or diabetes to BP goal of <130/80 mm Hg.
Adapted from: Chobanian AV, Bakris GL, Black HR, et al, for the National High Blood Pressure Education Program Coordinating Committee: The seventh report of the Joint National Committee on Prevention, Detection, Evaluation, and Treatment of High Blood Pressure: the JNC 7 report, *JAMA* 289:2560–2572, 2003.

Hypertension (DASH)[14] diet is provided in Chapter 19, Nutrition. An evidence-based approach to physical activity recommendations for primary and secondary prevention of CHD appears in Chapter 21, Exercise and Fitness. A recent evidence-based summary in the *Journal of Family Practice*[15] based on the JNC 7 report highlights key lifestyle recommendations to aid in the treatment of hypertension. These include the following:

- Reduction of dietary sodium intake lowers systolic blood pressure by up to 5 mm Hg (strength of recommendation: A).[16,17]
- Following the DASH diet can lower systolic blood pressure 4–5 mm Hg (strength of recommendation: A).[17,18]
- Regular aerobic exercise can lower systolic blood pressure by up to 4 mm Hg (strength of recommendation: A).[19,20]
- Reducing alcohol consumption to no more than one drink per day lowers systolic blood pressure 3.3 mm Hg (strength of recommendation: A).[21]
- Smoking cessation provides a 36% relative risk reduction in mortality (strength of recommendation: A).[22]
- Weight loss of 3–9% may allow for a decrease in systolic blood pressure by 3 mm Hg (strength of recommendation: C).[23,24]

Medications

Figure 8-8 outlines a treatment algorithm for hypertension derived from the latest recommendations in the JNC 7 report[7]; Table 8-3 lists the recommended pharmacotherapeutic options for various cardiovascular conditions. A detailed review of the evidence behind each of the recommendations appears in the JNC 7 report. Additional evidence for aggressive antihypertensive therapy from recent trials is summarized below.

The Antihypertensive and Lipid-Lowering Treatment to Prevent Heart Attack Trial (ALLHAT)[25] was a landmark study that sought to determine whether treatment with a calcium channel blocker (amlodipine) or an angiotensin-converting enzyme inhibitor (lisinopril) lowers the incidence of CHD or other cardiovascular disease events vs. treatment with a thiazide diuretic (chlorthalidone). ALLHAT was a randomized, double-blind, active-controlled, intention-to-treat trial of 33,357 subjects older than 55 years, 55% of whom were men, who had either stage 1 or 2 hypertension and one or more additional risk factors for CAD. The primary outcome was combined fatal CHD or nonfatal myocardial infarction; secondary outcomes were all-cause mortality, stroke, combined CHD (primary outcome, coronary revascularization, or angina with hospitalization), and combined cardiovascular disease (combined CHD, stroke, treated angina without hospitalization, heart failure, and peripheral arterial disease). The study concluded that thiazide diuretics are superior in preventing one or more major forms of cardiovascular disease and are less expensive than other pharmacotherapeutic agents. Thus, thiazide diuretics should be considered first-line agents for antihypertensive therapy. Of significant note is that treatment in the group of subjects that was randomly assigned to receive the alpha-adrenergic blocker doxazosin was stopped early because these subjects developed substantially more cardiovascular problems, specifically hospitalizations for heart failure.

The Hypertension Optimal Treatment (HOT) trial[26] examined the impact of treatment with low-dose aspirin in patients with documented hypertension on decreasing cardiovascular mortality. This trial recruited 18,790 patients aged 50–80 years with defined hypertension and an average diastolic blood pressure between 100 and 115 mm Hg. In addition to randomized treatment with various antihypertensive agents, approximately one half of the patients were randomly assigned to receive 75 mg/day of aspirin, and the other half were assigned to receive placebo. The HOT investigators concluded that lowering diastolic blood pressure below 85 mm Hg resulted in reduced cardiovascular mortality because treatment with low-dose aspirin reduced major cardiovascular events by 15% and myocardial infarction by 36%, with no significant effect on the incidence of stroke. Data from a HOT study subanalysis[27] suggest potentially different gender-dependent effects of antihypertensive and anti-platelet therapies: the lowering of diastolic blood pressure to approximately 80 mm Hg in hypertensive women and the administration of 75 mg of aspirin to well-treated hypertensive men appears to effectively reduce the incidence of myocardial infarction in patients with essential hypertension.

In summary, the JNC 7[7] report states "the most effective therapy prescribed by the most careful clinician will control hypertension only if patients are motivated. In presenting these guidelines, the committee recognizes that the responsible physician's judgment remains paramount."

Hypercholesterolemia

The framework for this section builds on the National Cholesterol Education Program (NCEP)

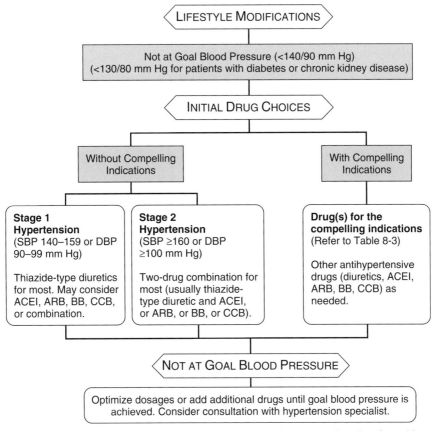

Figure 8-8. Algorithm for the treatment of hypertension. Compelling indications are based on favorable outcome data from randomized controlled clinical trials. DBP, diastolic blood pressure; SBP, systolic blood pressure. ACEI, angiotensin converting enzyme inhibitor; ARB, angiotensin receptor blocker; BB, beta-blocker; CCB, calcium channel blocker. (Adapted from: Chobanian AV, Bakris GL, Black HR, et al, for the National High Blood Pressure Education Program Coordinating Committee: The seventh report of the Joint National Committee on Prevention, Detection, Evaluation, and Treatment of High Blood Pressure: the JNC 7 report, *JAMA* 289:2560–2572, 2003.)

Adult Treatment Panel (ATP) III Guidelines from 2001[28] as well as an overview of the basic components of cholesterol composition and a systematic review of the literature previously summarized by Heidelbaugh and Rion.[29] Newer treatment studies are discussed, as well as the implications of recent clinical trials.[30] Novel biochemical markers for the detection of CHD will also be discussed.

Epidemiology

Primary care clinicians and other healthcare providers frequently encounter patients with unfavorable serum lipid profiles. According to *Health, United States, 2006*,[8] data compiled from 2001–2004 revealed that average serum cholesterol levels for persons in the United States aged 20 years and older were 201 mg/dL for both men and women, with no statistically significant differences among white persons, African Americans, or Hispanics, or among poverty or class status. The average cholesterol level in the United States has decreased significantly from the average of 222 mg/dL in the early 1960s. The percentage of persons aged 20–74 years with high serum cholesterol (defined as greater than 240 mg/dL) dropped from 33.3% during the period of 1960–1962 (30.6% for men, 35.6% for women) to 16.5% during the period of 2001–2004 (16.6% for men, 16.2% for women). According to data from the CDC's Behavioral Risk Factor Surveillance System,[31] in 2005 75.7% of whites, 73.7% of African Americans, and 52% of Hispanic adults reported that they had their cholesterol levels checked within the previous 5 years; approximately 23% reported that they had never had their cholesterol level checked.

Table 8-3. Compelling Indications for Individual Drug Classes for Antihypertensive Therapy

Compelling Indication	RECOMMENDED DRUGS					
	Diuretic	BB	ACEI	ARB	CCB	Aldo ANT
Heart failure	•	•	•	•		•
Postmyocardial infarction		•	•			•
High coronary disease risk	•	•	•		•	
Diabetes	•	•	•	•	•	
Chronic kidney disease			•	•		
Recurrent stroke prevention	•		•			

Compelling indications are based on favorable outcome data from randomized controlled clinical trials.

BB, Beta-blocker; ACEI, angiotensin-converting enzyme inhibitor; ARB, angiotensin receptor blocker; CCB, calcium channel blocker; Aldo ANT, aldosterone antagonist.

Adapted from: Chobanian AV, Bakris GL, Black HR, et al, for the National High Blood Pressure Education Program Coordinating Committee: The seventh report of the Joint National Committee on Prevention, Detection, Evaluation, and Treatment of High Blood Pressure, the JNC 7 report, *JAMA* 289:2560–2572, 2003.

Basic Concepts

Plasma Lipoproteins

Plasma lipoproteins transport essentially all of the cholesterol and esterified lipids in the bloodstream. Four major lipoprotein classes (i.e., chylomicrons, very-low-density lipoproteins [VLDLs], LDLs, and HDLs) and two quantitatively minor lipoprotein classes (i.e., intermediate-density lipoproteins and lipoprotein (a) [Lp(a)]) can be identified based on particle size, chemical composition, physicochemical and flotation characteristics, and electrophoretic mobility.[32] The protein moiety of the lipoproteins is composed of several specific proteins called *apolipoproteins*. Each lipoprotein fraction has a particular and more or less constant apolipoprotein composition. These apolipoproteins play important roles in lipid transport by activating or inhibiting enzymes involved in lipid metabolism, binding lipoproteins to cell surface lipoprotein receptors, or both.[33] The various patterns of lipoprotein elevation in plasma are highlighted in Table 8-4.

Chylomicrons are large particles produced by the intestine, which contain 85–95% triglycerides of exogenous or dietary origin and are relatively poor in free cholesterol and phospholipids. They are estimated to contain approximately 1–2% protein by weight. High chylomicron content in plasma results in a milky appearance.[33] VLDL particles are smaller than chylomicrons, are rich in triglycerides, have a lower lipid-protein ratio, and "float" at a somewhat higher density. When excessive amounts of VLDL are present in plasma, the appearance is also rather turbid. VLDL particles are of endogenous, mainly hepatic origin and constitute roughly one half of the particle mass. Cholesterol

and phospholipids compose approximately 40% of the particle, and 10% of the mass is protein.[33]

LDLs constitute approximately 50% of the total lipoprotein mass in human plasma. LDL particles are much smaller than the triglyceride-rich VLDL particles, and even greatly increased concentrations of LDL do not alter the clarity of plasma. Cholesterol, most of which is esterified, accounts for approximately one half of the LDL mass, and protein composes roughly 25% of the remaining mass.[34] HDLs are small particles secreted from the liver and the intestine and consist of 50% protein (mostly apolipoprotein A-I and A-II), 20% cholesterol, 30% phospholipids, and only traces of triglycerides.[35]

Serum Lipid Profile

General screening of persons for lipid abnormalities includes the quantitative measurements of total serum cholesterol, HDL-C, LDL-C, VLDL cholesterol (VLDL-C), and triglycerides. In addition, Lp(a) has become more widely appreciated as an independent risk factor for CHD in certain populations at risk (e.g., persons with a family history of premature CHD) and may also be assayed.[36] This fraction generally is not reported separately in standard lipid assays because it composes only 2–4 mg/dL.[37]

The most commonly used determination of cholesterol assaying follows the simple formula outlined by Friedewald and colleagues[38]:

$$LDC\text{-}C = \text{total cholesterol} - HDL\text{-}C - VLDL\text{-}C$$

In this equation, VLDL-C is equal to the serum triglyceride value divided by a factor of 5 when

Table 8-4. Patterns of Lipoprotein Elevation

Lipoprotein Pattern	Lipoproteins Elevated	Lipid Elevation
Type 1	Chylomicrons	Triglycerides
Type 2a	LDL-C	Cholesterol
Type 2b	LDL-C, VLDL-C	Cholesterol, triglycerides
Type 3	Chylomicrons, IDL-C	Triglycerides, cholesterol
Type 4	VLDL-C	Triglycerides
Type 5	VLDL-C, chylomicrons	Triglycerides, cholesterol

IDL-C, Intermediate-density lipoprotein cholesterol; LDL-C, low-density lipoprotein cholesterol; VLDL-C, very-low-density lipoprotein cholesterol.

Adapted from: Brown MS, Goldstein JL: The hyperlipoproteinemias and other disorders of lipid metabolism. In Isselbacher KJ, Braunwald E, Wilson JD, et al editors, *Harrison's Principles of Internal Medicine*, ed 13, New York, 1994, McGraw-Hill, pp 2058–2069; with permission.

concentrations are expressed in milligrams per deciliter. If the serum triglyceride value exceeds 400 mg/dL, then the ability to differentiate between chylomicrons and VLDL becomes difficult, and the LDL-C calculation must be derived from direct assay methods.

Ideally, the patient should be requested to fast for a period of 12 hours before venipuncture. Chylomicrons are usually present in postprandial plasma, and depending on the type and amount of food and beverage ingested, they can markedly increase the plasma triglyceride concentration. The concentrations of HDL-C and LDL-C decline transiently, partly because of compositional changes that occur during the catabolism of chylomicrons.[39] Chylomicrons are almost always cleared within 6–9 hours after meal ingestion, therefore their presence after a 12-hour fast is considered to be abnormal. The NCEP ATP III guidelines recommend that all patients fast for 9–12 hours before phlebotomy for lipid analysis.[28] This recommendation accommodates patients who may be unable or unwilling to fast for the complete 12-hour period. The shorter fasting period would be expected to produce only minor variations and, for the most part, only clinically insignificant errors in the estimation of the patient's usual triglyceride, HDL-C, and LDL-C levels.

Numerous factors exist that may influence the various components of a patient's serum lipid profile, including but not limited to posture, venous occlusion, recent myocardial infarction, stroke, cardiac catheterization, trauma, acute infection, and pregnancy.[37] Ideally, venipuncture should only occur after the patient has been seated for at least 5 minutes. When a standing patient reclines, extravascular water transfers into the vascular system and dilutes nondiffusible plasma constituents. Decreases of as much as 10% in the concentrations of total cholesterol, HDL-C, LDL-C, and apolipoproteins have been observed after a 20-minute period of recumbence. The resultant decrease in triglycerides can be up to 50% or greater. These postural changes are reversible when the patient resumes the standing of seated position.[40]

A review by Bachorik and colleagues[37] examined various physiologic factors that influence serum cholesterol levels. They determined that prolonged venous occlusion (e.g., via a rubber tourniquet) before venipuncture can lead to hemoconcentration and total cholesterol increases of 10–15%. Recent myocardial infarction, stroke, and cardiac catheterization are all associated with decreases in total cholesterol and LDL-C; an increase in VLDL-C is frequently observed after an acute coronary event. Decreases in 5–15% in total cholesterol and HDL-C are commonly seen after acute trauma and acute bacterial or viral illness. Lipoprotein measurements should be made no sooner than 8 weeks after a severe bacterial or viral illness. During pregnancy, as in the case of consumption of oral contraceptives or postmenopausal estrogens, total cholesterol and HDL-C levels may be elevated.

Diagnosis

Primary Prevention

The primary prevention of CHD begins with the identification of cardiovascular risk factors, as outlined above. Initially, the clinician must identify the presence of clinical atherosclerotic disease that confers high risk for CHD events, including clinically documented CHD, symptomatic carotid artery disease, peripheral arterial disease, or abdominal aortic aneurysm; these conditions are known as CHD risk equivalents.[28] To date, the NCEP ATP III has determined that an elevated serum LDL-C level serves as the most significant prognosticator for the development

Table 8-5. Coronary Heart Disease Risk Factors (Exclusive of LDL-C) That Modify LDL-C Goals

Major Positive Risk Factors	Minor Positive Risk Factors[*]
Age: men ≥45 years, women ≥55 years or with premature menopause without estrogen therapy	Elevated apolipoprotein B level
Family history of premature CHD, defined as definitive MI or sudden death in a first-degree relative male before 55 years or female before 65 years	Decreased apolipoprotein A-1 level
Hypertension, defined as blood pressure ≥140/90 mm Hg or on current antihypertensive medication	Elevated Lp(a) level
Diabetes mellitus	Elevated homocysteine or decreased folate levels Obesity
Current smoker	Sedentary lifestyle
HDL-C <40 mg/dL; if ≥60 mg/dL, subtract one risk factor from the number of total positive risk factors	Type-A, or "coronary-prone" personality, especially with hostility component
Triglycerides ≥200 mg/dL	Lack of supportive primary relationship

[*]Minor positive risk factors are less well proven and less well studied than those risks in the major list.

CHD, Coronary heart disease; MI, myocardial infarction; LDL-C, low-density lipoprotein cholesterol; HDL-C, high-density lipoprotein cholesterol.

Adapted from: National Cholesterol Education Program: Third Report of the National Cholesterol Education Program (NCEP) Expert Panel on Detection, Evaluation, and Treatment of High Blood Cholesterol in Adults (Adult Treatment Panel III): executive summary. NIH publication no. (NIH) 01–3670. Bethesda, MD, 2001, National Cholesterol Education Program, National Institutes of Health, National Heart, Lung, and Blood Institute.

of atherogenesis and subsequent CHD[41]; both major and minor risk factors for the development of CHD are listed in Table 8-5. The NCEP ATP III guidelines recognize the metabolic syndrome as a secondary target of risk-reduction therapy, after the primary target of lowering LDL-C.[28]

The appropriate age group for screening for primary prevention of CHD via cholesterol level assay remains an area of controversy. The Third US Preventive Services Task Force (USPSTF)[42] recommends screening men between the ages of 35 and 65 years and screening women aged 45–65 years.[43] This extends the recommendations of the second USPSTF recommending that adults be screened until the age of 65 years. Younger adults (men aged 20–35 years and women aged 20–45 years) should be screened if they have other risk factors for heart disease (see Table 8-5). Clinicians should measure total cholesterol, HDL-C, and LDL-C, yet there is currently insufficient evidence to recommend for or against testing measuring triglycerides; most current standard cholesterol assay panels include triglyceride measurements. The Canadian Task Force on the Periodic Health Examination[44] states that there is insufficient evidence for either inclusion or exclusion of universal screening for hypercholesterolemia in a periodic health examination, yet nonfasting serum cholesterol measurements should be considered in men aged 30–59 years of age. The American College of Physicians recommends routine screening of men aged 35–64 and women aged 45–64 years

and states that evidence is insufficient to recommend for or against screening men and women aged 65–75 years. Screening is not recommended for men and women aged 75 years and older.[45] The American Academy of Family Physicians recommends routine screening for men aged 35 years and older and women aged 45 years and older, noting that the upper age limit of screening should be "individualized for each patient."[46]

For the primary prevention screening of hypercholesterolemia, the NCEP ATP III[28] recommends commencement of screening for both men and women at the age of 20 years. Autopsy studies have revealed that atherosclerosis generally begins at adolescence or young adulthood, long before any clinical manifestations. Treating young adults, aside from those identified with familial hypercholesterolemia, has not shown to be of any significant benefit, and given their low absolute risk for CHD, this practice has not been shown to be cost-effective. There is no sufficient evidence to recommend for or against routine screening of asymptomatic persons older than 65 years, but recommendations to screen healthy men and women aged 65–75 years may be made on other grounds depending on their risk factors for having a coronary event. Attributable risk is the highest in elderly persons because elevated cholesterol levels produce a greater number of coronary events in the elderly population compared with a middle-aged population.[47] After the age of 75 years, it is recommended that patients be treated according to their underlying functional status, as well as their own preference for or against screening.[43]

For the primary prevention screening of hypercholesterolemia, the NCEP ATP III recommends that, for all adults aged 20 years or older, a fasting lipoprotein profile (i.e., total cholesterol, LDL-C, HDL-C, and triglycerides) should be obtained once every 5 years.[28] If the testing opportunity performed is nonfasting, only the values for total cholesterol and HDL-C are considered to be accurate. In such a case, if the total cholesterol is greater than or equal to 200 mg/dL or the HDL-C is less than 40 mg/dL, a follow-up lipoprotein profile is required for appropriate management based on the LDL-C value. Patients with borderline levels who do not require any form of initial therapy can be rechecked in 1–2 years.[28] The NCEP ATP III classification of serum lipoprotein levels and treatment goals is listed in Table 8-6.

Secondary Prevention

Patients with documented CHD should also have a complete fasting lipid profile. For patients with normal lipid profile results, this can be

Table 8-6. National Cholesterol Education Program Adult Treatment Panel III Classification of Treatment Goals for LDL-C, Total Cholesterol, HDL-C, and Triglycerides

Agent	Level (mg/dL)	Classification
LDL-C	<100	Optimal
	100–129	Near optimal
	130–159	Borderline high
	160–189	High
	≥190	Very high
HDL-C	<40	Low
	≥60	High
Triglycerides	<150	Normal
	150–199	Borderline high
	200–499	High
	≥500	Very high
Total cholesterol	<200	Desirable
	200–239	Borderline high
	≥240	High

LDL-C, Low-density lipoprotein cholesterol; HDL-C, high-density lipoprotein cholesterol.

Adapted from: National Cholesterol Education Program: Third report of the National Cholesterol Education Program (NCEP) Expert Panel on Detection, Evaluation, and Treatment of High Blood Cholesterol in Adults (Adult Treatment Panel III): executive summary. NIH publication no. (NIH) 01–3670. Bethesda, MD, 2001, National Cholesterol Education Program, National Institutes of Health, National Heart, Lung, and Blood Institute.

performed on a yearly basis; for patients with abnormal profile results, the NCEP ATP III states that treatment and reevaluation should occur every 4–8 weeks until target lipid levels are met.[28] Patients with an acute myocardial infarction should be reassessed within 60 days after the acute event.[28,42]

Treatment

Three main approaches to the treatment of lipid disorders are available and are aimed primarily at the reduction of LDL-C. These approaches are composed of therapeutic lifestyle changes, pharmacotherapy aimed at specific control of the various lipoproteins, and complementary and alternative therapies that may affect various serum lipid levels. The most recently defined NCEP ATP III treatment goals for LDL-C lowering in various risk categories and recommendations for modifications to the previous algorithm are outlined in Tables 8-7 and 8-8, respectively.[30] All recommendations are based on evidence of strength-of-recommendation level A.

The NCEP ATP III treatment guidelines are still the most widely accepted and used, although physicians generally are poorly compliant with the risk factor assessment and counseling guidelines, even in the care of patients at high risk for CHD. One study demonstrated that physicians followed NCEP ATP II algorithms (from 1993) for obtaining an LDL-C value, a key step in evaluating the need for treatment, only 50% of the time.[48] A more recent study assessing compliance with the NCEP ATP III guidelines commented that compliance of primary care physicians with these guidelines, especially in ambulatory care settings, has been shown to be poor and that of cardiologists is less well documented. This particular study revealed that 38% of patients in a cardiology practice who were receiving lipid-lowering statin therapy had a suboptimal lipid profile despite more than 2 years of therapy.[49] A study by the RAND Corporation in 2003 estimated that only 48% of patients are receiving recommended treatment for hyperlipidemia.[50] A summation of the primary and secondary prevention trials that follow is outlined in Table 8-9.

Primary Prevention

One of the first studies to examine the primary prevention of CHD related to serum cholesterol lowering was the Lipid Research Clinics Coronary Primary Prevention Trial from 1984.[51] This study compared the bile acid sequestrant

Table 8-7. Adult Treatment Panel III LDL-C Goals and Cutpoints for Therapeutic Lifestyle Changes and Drug Therapy in Different Risk Categories and Proposed Modifications Based on Recent Clinical Trial Evidence

Risk Category	LDL-C Goal	Initiate TLC	Consider Drug Therapy**
High risk: CHD* or CHD risk equivalents[†] (10-year risk >20%)	<100 mg/dL (optional goal: <70 mg/dL)[‖]	≥100 mg/dL[#]	≥100 mg/dL[††] (<100 mg/dL: consider drug options)**
Moderately high risk: 2+ risk factors[‡] (10-year risk 10–20%)[§§]	<130 mg/dL[¶]	≥130 mg/dL[#]	≥130 mg/dL (100–129 mg/dL; consider drug options)[‡‡]
Moderate risk: 2+ risk factors[‡] (10-year risk <10%)[§§]	<130 mg/dL	≥130 mg/dL	≥160 mg/dL
Lower risk: 0–1 risk factor[§]	<160 mg/dL	≥160 mg/dL	≥190 mg/dL (160–189 mg/dL: LDL-lowering drug optional)

LDL-C, Low-density lipoprotein cholesterol; TLC, therapeutic lifestyle changes; CHD, coronary heart disease; HDL-C, high-density lipoprotein cholesterol; BP, blood pressure.

*CHD includes history of myocardial infarction, unstable angina, stable angina, coronary artery procedures (angioplasty or bypass surgery), or evidence of clinically significant myocardial ischemia.

[†]CHD risk equivalents include clinical manifestations of noncoronary forms of atherosclerotic disease (peripheral arterial disease, abdominal aortic aneurysm, and carotid artery disease [transient ischemic attacks or stroke of carotid origin or >50% obstruction of a carotid artery]), diabetes, and 2+ risk factors with 10-year risk for hard CHD >20%.

[‡]Risk factors include cigarette smoking, hypertension (BP ≥ 140/90 mm Hg or on antihypertensive medication), low HDL-C (<40 mg/dL), family history of premature CHD (CHD in male first-degree relative <55 years of age; CHD in female first-degree relative <65 years of age), and age (men ≥45 years; women ≥55 years).

[§§]Electronic 10-year risk calculators are available at http://www.nhlbi.nih.gov/guidelines/cholesterol.

[§]Almost all people with zero or 1 risk factor have a 10-year risk <10%, and 10-year risk assessment in people with zero or 1 risk factor is thus not necessary.

[‖]Very high risk favors the optional LDL-C goal of <70 mg/dL, and in patients with high triglycerides, non-HDL-C <100 mg/dL.

[¶]Optional LDL-C goal <100 mg/dL.

[#]Any person at high risk or moderately high risk who has lifestyle-related risk factors (eg, obesily, physical inactivity, elevated triglyceride, low HDL-C, or metabolic syndrome) is a candidate for therapeutic lifestyle changes to modify these risk factors regardless of LDL-C level.

**When LDL-lowering drug therapy is employed, it is advised that intensity of therapy be sufficient to achieve at least a 30–40% reduction in LDL-C levels.

[††]If baseline LDL-C is <100 mg/dL, institution of an LDL-lowering drug is a therapeutic option on the basis of available clinical trial results. If a high-risk person has high triglycerides or low HDL-C, combining a fibrate or nicotinic acid with an LDL-lowering drug can be considered.

[‡‡]For moderately high-risk persons, when LDL-C level is 100–129 mg/dL, at baseline or on lifestyle therapy, initiation of an LDL-lowering drug to achieve an LDL-C level <100 mg/dL is a therapeutic option on the basis of available clinical trial results.

Adapted from: Grundy SM, Cleeman JI, Merz, NB, et al: Implications of recent trials for the National Cholesterol Education Program Adult Treatment III Guidelines, *Circulation*, 110:227–239, 2004.

cholestyramine to placebo in 3806 men aged 35–59 years with elevated total cholesterol and LDL-C and demonstrated an 18% absolute risk reduction of CHD events after a period of 7 years. In 1987, the Helsinki Heart Study[52] compared gemfibrozil to placebo in 4081 men aged 40–55 years with elevated total cholesterol and LDL-C levels and noted a 34% risk reduction in CHD events after 5 years.

Two landmark primary prevention trials using statins, the West of Scotland Coronary Prevention Study Group (WOSCOPS) trial[53] and the Air Force/Coronary Atherosclerosis Prevention Study (AFCAPS/TexCAPS) trial[54] have both demonstrated that aggressive lowering of LDL-C can significantly reduce the relative risk for a first coronary event, death resulting from CHD, incidence of revascularization procedures, and total mortality. Before these two trials, cholesterol lowering as a means of primary prevention had never been shown to improve overall mortality. In the

WOSCOPS trial, mortality was reduced by 22%; mortality statistics were not measured in the AFCAPS/TexCAPS trial.

Secondary Prevention

For the secondary prevention of CHD, the NCEP ATP III guidelines recommend lowering LDL-C below 100 mg/dL.[28] Randomized controlled trials including the Scandinavian Simvastatin Survival Study (4S),[55] Long-Term Intervention with Pravastatin in Ischemic Disease (LIPID) Study Group,[56] and Atorvastatin versus Revascularization Treatment Investigators (AVERT) trial[57] all examined the role of pharmacotherapy in the secondary prevention of CHD for men and women. These trials concluded that aggressive reductions in LDL-C can diminish the relative risks or coronary events and death caused by CHD and reduce the need for revascularization procedures and total mortality. The Cholesterol and Recurrent Events (CARE) study[58] found that when

Table 8-8. Recommendations for Modifications to Footnote the Adult Treatment Panel III Treatment Algorithm for LDL-C

• Therapeutic lifestyle changes (TLC) remain an essential modality in clinical management. TLC has the potential to reduce cardiovascular risk through several mechanisms beyond LDL lowering.
• In high-risk persons, the recommended LDL-C goal is <100 mg/dL.
– An LDL-C goal of <70 mg/dL is a therapeutic option on the basis of available clinical trial evidence, especially for patients at very high risk.
– If LDL-C is ≥100 mg/dL, an LDL-lowering drug is indicated simultaneously with lifestyle changes.
– If baseline LDL-C is <100 mg/dL, institution of an LDL-lowering drug to achieve an LDL-C level <70 mg/dL is a therapeutic option on the basis of available clinical trial evidence.
– If a high-risk person has high triglycerides or low HDL-C, consideration can be given to combining a fibrate or nicotinic acid with an LDL-lowering drug. When triglycerides are ≥200 mg/dL, non–HDL-C is a secondary target of therapy, with a goal 30 mg/dL higher than the identified LDL-C goal.
• For moderately high-risk persons (2+ risk factors and 10-year risk 10–20%), the recommended LDL-C goal is <130 mg/dL; and LDL-C goal <100 mg/dL is a therapeutic option on the basis of available clinical trial evidence. When LDL-C level is 100–129 mg/dL, at baseline or on lifestyle therapy, initiation of an LDL-lowering drug to achieve an LDL-C level <100 mg/dL is a therapeutic option on the basis of available clinical trial evidence.
• Any person at high risk or moderately high risk who has lifestyle-related risk factors (e.g., obesity, physical inactivity, elevated triglyceride, low HDL-C, or metabolic syndrome) is a candidate for TLC to modify these risk factors regardless of LDL-C level.
• When LDL-lowering drug therapy is employed in high-risk or moderately high-risk persons, it is advised that intensity of therapy be sufficient to achieve at least a 30–40% reduction in LDL-C levels.
• For people in lower-risk categories, recent clinical trials do not modify the goals and cutpoints of therapy.

LDL-C, Low-density lipoprotein cholesterol; HDL-C, high-density lipoprotein cholesterol.
Adapted from: Grundy SM, Cleeman JI, Merz, NB, et al: Implications of recent trials for the National Cholesterol Education Program Adult Treatment III Guidelines, *Circulation*, 110:227–239, 2004.

examining the relationship between LDL-C levels and coronary event rate, there was no observable incremental benefit in treating LDL-C levels below 125 mg/dL. Post–coronary artery bypass graft (CABG) angiographic studies found that there may not be significant benefit in lowering LDL-C below 135 mg/dL in the prevention of coronary events.[59]

Evidence also exists to support a relationship between low levels of HDL-C and the development of CHD. The Veterans Affairs High-Density Lipoprotein Intervention Trial Study Group (VA-HIT)[60] sought to determine whether treating isolated low HDL-C would reduce the incidence of nonfatal myocardial infarction or coronary death in male subjects with CHD. This trial demonstrated that the fibric acid derivative gemfibrozil reduced the 5-year rate of new CHD events in men with known CHD and low levels of both HDL-C and LDL-C. Overall, HDL-C was raised 6% and triglycerides lowered 31% by gemfibrozil, but only the increased HDL-C predicted the reduction in CHD events. LDL-C concentrations neither predicted the development of new CHD events nor were lowered by gemfibrozil. Ultimately, these parameters were significantly lower, with pharmacotherapy aimed at improving HDL-C, revealing significant mortality benefit from CHD death.[60] The Lopid Coronary Angiography Trial (LOCAT)[61] discovered that specific treatment could reduce the progression of atherosclerosis after CABG in men who had low serum HDL-C levels.

Newer Evidence

Since the publication of the NCEP ATP III guidelines, several major clinical trials using statin therapy and measuring various clinical end points have been published.[30]

The Heart Protection Study[62] examined 20,536 adults living in the United Kingdom aged 40–80 years who were at a high risk for a coronary event given their inclusion criteria of CHD, other occlusive arterial disease, or diabetes. Patients were randomly assigned to receive either simvastatin 40 mg daily or placebo. Primary outcomes included total mortality and fatal or nonfatal vascular events. In patients assigned to receive simvastatin, all-cause mortality was significantly reduced by 13%, major vascular events were reduced by 24%, coronary death rate reduced by 18%, nonfatal myocardial infarction plus coronary death reduced by 27%, nonfatal or fatal stroke reduced by 25%, and cardiovascular

Table 8-9. Summarized Results of Primary and Secondary Prevention Trials of Statins Reflecting LDL-C Reduction and Coronary Heart Disease Prevention

Study (n)	Intervention	Baseline LDL-C (mg/dL)	Reduction in LDL-C (%)	Reduction in Coronary Events (%)	Reduction in CABG/PTCA (%)	Reduction in Total Mortality (%)	NNT
Primary prevention trials							
WOSCOPS[53] (6595 men)	Pravastatin 40 mg/day	192	26	31 (P < .001)	37 (P = .009)	22 (P = .051)	42
AFCAPS/TexCAPS[54] (5608 men, 997 women)	Lovastatin 20–40 mg/day	150	25	42 (P < .001)	33 (P = .001)	0 (P = NS)	83
Secondary prevention trials							
4S[55] (3617 men, 827 women)	Simvastatin 20–40 mg/day	188	35	34 (P < .0001)	37 (P < .0001)	30 (P = .003)	15
CARE[58] (3583 men, 576 women)	Pravastatin 40 mg/day	139	32	24 (P = .003)	27 (P < .001)	9 (P = NS)	33
LIPID[56] (7498 men, 997 women)	Pravastatin 40 mg/day	150	25	24 (P < .0001)	22 (P < .0001)	22 (P < .0001); 19 (P = .024)*	28

*Data for percentage reduction in CABG and PTCA, respectively.

LDL-C, Low-density tipoprotein cholesterol; CHD, coronary heart disease; n, number of patients enrolled in study; CABG, coronary artery bypass grafting; PTCA, percutaneous transluminal coronary angioplasty; NNT, number of patients needed to treat to prevent one major coronary event (100/absolute risk reduction); WOSCOPS, West of Scotland Coronary Prevention Study; AFCAPS/TexCAPS, Air Force Texas Coronary Atherosclerosis Prevention Study; 4S, Scandinavian Simvastatin Survival Study; CARE, Cholesterol and Recurrent Events Trial; LIPID, Long-Term Intervention with Pravastatin in Ischaemic Disease Study; NS, not significant (as reported).

Adapted from: Shepard J, Cobbe SM, Ford I, et al: Prevention of coronary heart disease with pravastatin in men with hypercholesterolemia: West of Scotland Coronary Prevention Study Group, *N Engl J Med* 333:1301–1307, 1995; Downs JR, Clearfield M, Weis S, et al: Primary prevention of acute coronary events with lovastatin in men and women with average cholesterol levels: results of AFCAPS/TexCAPS, *JAMA* 279:1615–1622, 1998; Scandinavian Simvastatin Survival Study Group: Randomized trial of cholesterol lowering in 4,444 patients with coronary artery disease: the Scandinavian Simvastatin Survival Study (4S), *Lancet* 344:1383–1389, 1994; Long-term Intervention with Pravastatin in Ischaemic Disease (LIPID) Study Group: Prevention of cardiovascular events and death with pravastatin in patients with coronary heart disease (CHD) and a broad range of initial cholesterol levels, *N Engl J Med* 339:1349–1357, 1997; Sacks FM, Pfeffer MA, Moye MA, et al: The effect of pravastatin on coronary events after myocardial infarction in patients with average cholesterol levels (CARE), *N Engl J Med* 335:1001–1009, 1996.

revascularization reduced by 24%. Subgroup analysis suggested that simvastatin therapy produced similar reductions in relative risk regardless of the baseline levels of LDL-C, including subgroups with initial or baseline LDL-C levels greater than or equal to 135 mg/dL, less than 116 mg/dL, or less than 100 mg/dL, respectively.

The Prospective Study of Pravastatin in the Elderly at Risk trial[63] examined the effect of pravastatin treatment in older men and women with or at high risk for the development of cardiovascular disease and stroke. Subjects aged 70–82 years who had a history of vascular disease or significant cardiovascular risk factors were randomly assigned to receive either pravastatin 40 mg daily or placebo. The primary end point was a combination of coronary death, nonfatal myocardial infarction, and fatal or nonfatal stroke. Pravastatin was found to reduce LDL-C levels by 34% in this study. Nonfatal myocardial infarction decreased by 19% in the treatment group, and total CHD mortality decreased by 24%. Although

no significant reduction in stroke was observed, the incidence of transient ischemic attacks was found to decrease by 25% in the treatment group. The authors concluded that these results allow statin therapy to be extended to older persons, as treatment may offer some benefit in risk reduction.

The Antihypertensive and Lipid-Lowering Treatment to Prevent Heart Attack Trial—Lipid-Lowering Trial (ALLHAT-LLT)[64] was an arm of a larger trial[25] described above that was designed to assess whether pravastatin therapy compared with usual care could reduce all-cause mortality in older patients with hypertension and moderately elevated cholesterol levels with at least one additional CHD risk factor. This arm of the trial randomly assigned 10,355 patients (51% men) with a mean baseline serum cholesterol level of 224 mg/dL to receive either pravastatin or placebo. By the conclusion of the study, serum cholesterol levels were found to be decreased by 17% in the treatment group and 8% in the placebo group. All-cause mortality was similar for both the treatment and placebo groups (14.9% and 15.3%, respectively) over the 6-year period. CHD event rates were found to not be statistically significant between the two groups (9.3% vs. 10.4%), yet in the African American subgroup, CHD events were significantly reduced in the pravastatin-treated group compared with the placebo group.

Contrasting results were observed in the Anglo-Scandinavian Cardiac Outcomes Trial—Lipid-Lowering Arm study.[65] This study randomly assigned 19,342 patients aged 40–79 years who had hypertension and at least three additional cardiovascular risk factors to receive one of two antihypertensive regimens. Among these subjects, 10,305 were also randomly assigned to receive 10 mg of atorvastatin daily or placebo. In the atorvastatin group, the incidence of fatal and nonfatal stroke was reduced by 27% compared with placebo; total cardiovascular events were reduced by 21%; and coronary events were reduced by 29%. The authors concluded that LDL-C lowering with atorvastatin therapy has great potential to reduce the risk for cardiovascular disease via primary prevention in patients with multiple risk factors.

The Pravastatin or Atorvastatin Evaluation and Infection Therapy—Thrombolysis in Myocardial Infarction 22 trial[66] sought to examine whether intensive LDL-C lowering would reduce major coronary events, including mortality, to a greater degree than "standard" LDL-C lowering with statin therapy in patients at high risk for cardiovascular disease. Prior clinical trials demonstrated that in patients with established CHD, treatment with 40 mg of pravastatin daily will reduce LDL-C levels to near 100 mg/dL and will reduce the risk for coronary events by nearly 27%.[67] This trial examined 4162 patients who had been hospitalized for an acute coronary syndrome within the preceding 10 days and randomly assigned them to receive either 80 mg of atorvastatin daily or 40 mg of pravastatin daily. At the end of 2 years of therapy, the composite cardiovascular end point was reduced by 16% with atorvastatin compared with pravastatin.[30,67] The LDL-C levels attained on 40 mg of pravastatin daily and 80 mg of atorvastatin daily were 95 and 62 mg/dL, respectively. The authors concluded that intensive lipid-lowering therapy reduces major cardiovascular events in patients with acute coronary syndrome compared with those receiving less aggressive lipid-lowering therapy over a period of 2 years.[30,67]

Newer trials entitled Treating to New Targets,[68] Incremental Decrease in End Points Through Aggressive Lipid Lowering,[69] and A Study to Evaluate the Effect of Rosuvastatin on Intravascular Ultrasound-Derived Coronary Atheroma Burden[70] highlight the growing realization that lower LDL-C levels are superior in the secondary prevention of CHD, outlining a goal of lowering LDL-C levels to below 70 mg/dL versus below 100 mg/dL as targeted in previous guidelines.[30]

Therapeutic Lifestyle Changes

Lifestyle modifications are the first step in the treatment of hypercholesterolemia as recommended by the NCEP ATP III guidelines.[28] These changes include dietary modifications, smoking cessation, limitation of alcohol consumption to moderate amounts, weight loss, and exercise, which are similar to recommendations to treat all cardiovascular diseases. These basic interventions may provide sufficient treatment for a number of patients with lipid disorders. As a primary prevention measure, a reduction in the total cholesterol value by 1% may decrease a person's risk for developing CHD by up to 2%.[71]

Diet

The general aim of dietary therapy is to reduce elevated serum cholesterol while maintaining a nutritionally adequate eating pattern. Dietary therapy should reduce the intakes of saturated fats and cholesterol and promote weight loss in patients who are overweight by eliminating excess total calories and increasing physical activity.[28] A more detailed guide to dietary strategies, coupled with evidence-based recommendations, can be found in Chapter 19, Nutrition.

Smoking Cessation

Tobacco smoking continues to contribute to the high morbidity and mortality associated with CHD. Mero and colleagues[72] have demonstrated that even healthy male subjects with normal cholesterol profiles who smoke have altered postprandial HDL-C and apolipoprotein A-1 and E composition. The postprandial increase in triglycerides and the lowering of HDL-C may promote atherogenesis in smokers. Within 1–2 years of smoking cessation, an increase of 5–10% in HDL-C and up to a 50% reduction in coronary event rate in patients with CHD has been observed.

Alcohol Consumption

Population studies suggest lower observed CHD rates when alcohol is consumed in moderate amounts. These amounts are defined specifically by the *Dietary Guidelines for Americans* developed by the US Department of Agriculture and the US Department of Health and Human Services[73] as no more than two drinks per day for men and no more than one drink per day for women. In this definition, a "drink" is defined as 5 oz of wine, 12 oz of beer, or 1½ ounces of 80-proof liquor. Alcohol consumption above this level on a daily basis is not recommended and may lead to such complications as cirrhotic liver disease, dilated cardiomyopathy, hypertension, various adverse psychosocial consequences, and motor vehicle and other accidents.

The ingestion of ethyl alcohol affects lipoprotein metabolism in several ways. Ostrander and colleagues[74] determined that, initially, there is an almost immediate elevation in serum triglycerides, which may be profound in persons with diabetes or existing hypertriglyceridemia; HDL-C levels are also commonly found to be elevated. The effect of alcohol on LDL-C is almost negligible in most persons. The theory that the alcohol-induced rise in HDL-C may afford some cardio-protection is not known, and due to uncertainty about the benefit of alcohol on HDL-C levels and its well-known adverse effects, alcohol intake cannot be recommended for the prevention of CHD.[28]

Weight Loss

According to the American Obesity Association,[75] data from 1999–2002 revealed that 127 million Americans are overweight, a condition defined as a BMI greater than 25 kg/m^2, 60 million are obese (BMI greater than 30 kg/m^2), and 9 million are severely obese (BMI greater than 40 kg/m^2). Obesity is an important contributor to CHD because it adversely affects additional risk factors including serum lipids, blood pressure, and glucose intolerance. Weight reduction must be an integral component of dietary therapy in overweight and obese patients. The ultimate goal is to reach a BMI of 21–25 kg/m^2. Even small degrees of weight loss can greatly enhance decreasing LDL-C lowering; for example, 5–10 pounds of weight loss can double the LDL-C reduction achieved by reducing saturated fats and cholesterol.[76] An added benefit of weight loss is the reduction of triglycerides coupled with an increase in HDL-C.[76,77] Weight reduction and exercise reduce blood pressure and decrease the risk for type 2 diabetes mellitus. The more overweight the patient, the less responsive he or she generally is to dietary therapy if weight loss does not occur concomitantly.

Exercise

Fletcher and colleagues[78] have demonstrated that regular exercise has been shown to raise HDL-C and to lower triglycerides; exercise alone has been shown to have little effect on LDL-C. Exercise in combination with a low-fat diet induces greater reduction in total cholesterol levels, LDL-C, and weight loss than dietary therapy alone. Even mild exercise such as walking performed regularly (30–45 minutes, 4–5 times per week) has been shown to be beneficial in improving serum lipid profiles. Weight training has been shown to increase HDL-C levels. It is believed that the degree of exercise must be tailored in patients with known CHD such that aerobic exercises like walking, swimming, and cycling do not precipitate angina. Chapter 21, Exercise and Fitness, explores the relationship between physical activity and fitness and cardiovascular and all-cause mortality in-depth through a comprehensive review of the literature.

Pharmacologic Treatment

HMG-CoA Reductase Inhibitors/Statins

The 3-hydroxy-3-methylglutaryl coenzyme A (HMG-CoA) reductase inhibitors, or statins, work via the competitive inhibition of HMG-CoA reductase, the rate-limiting enzyme in the synthesis of cholesterol. The statins decrease the production of LDL-C by way of the increase in LDL receptor activity in the liver and the rate of removal of LDL-C from the plasma.[79] More than 20 years of clinical research on this class of medication has demonstrated effectiveness in reducing total cholesterol and LDL-C by 20–60%, decreasing triglyceride levels slightly, and mildly increasing HDL-C in some patients.[80] Examples of the statins as well as their dose-equivalent relative potency in reduction of LDL-C are found in Table 8-10. Pooled results from the landmark statin trials on the primary and secondary prevention of CHD, reflecting percent reductions in LDL-C and various coronary event parameters, including percentage reduction in total mortality, appear in Table 8-9. The statins are generally well tolerated, and the major reported adverse effects are elevations in liver transaminases and occasionally alkaline phosphatase, as well as myopathy, rhabdomyolysis, headache, and gastrointestinal disturbances. Although there is no current recommendation to support the routine testing of serum creatine phosphokinase in asymptomatic patients, this may be necessary in patients with suspected

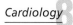

Table 8-10. Dose of Currently Available Statins Required to Attain an Approximate 30–40% Reduction in LDL-C Levels

Drug	Dose, mg/day	LDL Reduction,* %
Atorvastatin	10[†]	39
Lovastatin	40[†]	31
Pravastatin	40[†]	34
Simvastatin	20–40[†]	35–41
Fluvastatin	40–80	25–35
Rosuvastatin	5–10[‡]	39–45

*Estimated low-density lipoprotein (LDL) reductions were obtained from US Food and Drug Administration package inserts for each drug.
[†]All of these are available at doses up to 80 mg. For every doubling of the dose above standard does, an approximate 6% decrease in LDL cholesterol level can be obtained.[79]
[‡]For rosuvastatin, doses available up to 40 mg; the efficacy for 5 mg is estimated by subtracting 6% from the Food and Drug Administration–reported efficacy at 10 mg.[79]
Adapted from: Grundy SM, Cleeman JI, Merz, NB, et al: Implications of recent trials for the National Cholesterol Education Program Adult Treatment III Guidelines, *Circulation* 110:227–239, 2004.

myopathy who complain of myalgias. Although most manufacturers of the statins have slightly different recommendations, it is generally suggested that clinicians obtain baseline serum aspartate aminotransferase and alanine aminotransferase levels before commencement of statin therapy and monitor these levels periodically thereafter.[79]

The choice of which statin to use generally depends on the clinician's judgment for familiarity for the drug, evidence of beneficial clinical outcomes, efficacy for lowering LDL-C, potential for drug-drug interactions, and favorable cost with relation to insurance plan coverage. Although a decade old, the most recently available cost-benefit analyses have demonstrated that the estimated cost per year of life saved as a result of statin therapy ranges from $4500 to $14,000; these figures can be compared with an estimated cost of $70,000 per year of life saved for CABG surgery for one-vessel coronary disease.[81]

Cholesterol Absorption Inhibitors

Ezetimibe blocks the absorption of dietary and biliary cholesterol within the brush-border enzyme system of the small intestine. It is a well-tolerated drug, with angioedema being the most common, albeit quite rare, adverse effect. Current data have not proved that it alters or decreases the absorption of bile acids, fatty acids, fat-soluble vitamins, or triglycerides. Ezetimibe is labeled for use in the treatment of primary hypercholesterolemia, as either monotherapy or in combination with statins. Knopp and colleagues[82] performed a randomized, double-blind placebo-controlled trial on 827 patients with baseline LDL-C levels ranging from 130 to 250 mg/dL and triglycerides

350 mg/dL who were randomized 3:1 to receive 10 mg of ezetimibe or placebo orally once daily in the morning for 12 weeks. Treatment with ezetimibe was found to reduce direct LDL-C by a mean of 17.7% from baseline to end point, compared with an increase of 0.8% with placebo and also significantly improved levels of plasma total cholesterol, apolipoprotein B, HDL-C, and lipoprotein (a), and it elicited a trend toward lower triglyceride levels. Long-term trials comparing ezetimibe to the statins that measure various coronary event outcomes are lacking.

Fibric Acid Derivatives

The fibric acid derivatives, or fibrates, work to increase the clearance of VLDL-C by enhancing lipolysis, as they increase lipoprotein lipase activity, reduce hepatic cholesterol synthesis, and increase cholesterol excretion in the bile. The LOCAT[61] and VA-HIT[60] trials have demonstrated that gemfibrozil and fenofibrate are indicated as first-line treatment for hypertriglyceridemia, with decreases of 20–50% frequently observed. The fibrates are also found to be effective in lowering LDL-C by 5–15% and by raising HDL-C by up to 20%. Rarely, mild elevations in LDL-C are seen. The VA-HIT trial demonstrated a significant reduction in morbidity and mortality from CHD with the use of gemfibrozil, especially in overweight patients.[60] In general, this class of medications is not considered to be first-line or solo therapy for the secondary prevention of CHD because it does not generally achieve maximal reductions in LDL-C compared with the statins. In patients with primary hypertriglyceridemia, gemfibrozil may increase LDL-C levels, whereas in patients with elevations of both total cholesterol and triglycerides, this medication can cause either an increase or a decrease in LDL-C levels.[83] Persons with diabetes or type 3 dyslipoproteinemia are excellent candidates for this class of medication (see Table 8-5). Adverse effects of the fibrates include up to a six-fold increase in cholelithiasis and gastrointestinal disturbances including nausea, abdominal pain, and diarrhea. When used in conjunction with the statins, the risk for development of elevated transaminases and rhabdomyolysis is significantly increased.[28] The fibrates are contraindicated in preexisting gall bladder, renal, or hepatic disease or in pregnancy.

Nicotinic Acid

Nicotinic acid, or niacin (a form of vitamin B_3), diversely affects lipid metabolism by decreasing hepatic synthesis of LDL-C and VLDL-C, increasing synthesis of HDL-C, inhibiting lipolysis in adipose tissue, and increasing lipase activity. Reductions in total cholesterol and LDL-C by 10–25%, decreases in triglycerides by 20–50%, and increases in HDL-C of 15–35% have been observed.[84] Niacin may be considered as a choice in patients with concomitant elevations in LDL-C and triglycerides. There is some evidence in secondary prevention trials that nicotinic acid may reduce cardiac events and total mortality.[85] Its use is often limited by unpleasant adverse effects and the frequent presence of coexisting contraindications. By starting at a low dose of 100–200 mg daily and gradually increasing the dose up to 3–6 g daily, as well as adding a daily aspirin, increased tolerance often develops as do the common adverse effects of cutaneous flushing, rashes, hives, and pruritus. Niacin is relatively inexpensive and is available in over-the-counter formulations. A sustained-release preparation is available that has been shown to minimize adverse effects since it is generally taken at nighttime. Niacin is contraindicated in patients with peptic ulcer disease, liver disease, diabetes mellitus, hyperuricemia, and gout. Although niacin has been proved to have some significant action in modifying lipid abnormalities, statin therapy remains the mainstay of treatment in the vast majority of cases.

Cholesterol Ester Transfer Protein Inhibitors

A review by Nash[86] highlights a new approach to lipid-modifying therapy involving the development of drugs that inhibit cholesterol ester transfer protein (CETP) to increase HDL-C levels. The inverse relationship between HDL-C levels and premature CHD has been demonstrated via numerous studies for decades; in general, a 1%

reduction in HDL-C levels has been associated with a 2% increase in the risk of CHD, and the reverse trend is also true. Torcetrapib is a CETP inhibitor that was thought to have significant promise, given HDL-C elevations of 15–90% in early cohort trials.[87] Trials were halted in December 2006 because of deaths of some individuals taking the drug. A decrease in LDL-C levels was also observed, apolipoprotein A-1 was significantly elevated, and apolipoprotein B was reduced by 26% at doses of 120 mg twice daily. To date, solid evidence from rigorously controlled large-scale trials with adequate follow-up is lacking.

Complimentary and Alternative Therapies

In 2002, the AHA Scientific Statement *Fish Consumption, Fish Oil, Omega-3 Fatty Acids and Cardiovascular Disease*[88] highlighted that omega-3 fatty acids have been shown in epidemiologic and clinical trials to reduce the incidence of cardiovascular disease[89] via lowering triglycerides[90] and blood pressure,[91] decreasing platelet aggregation,[92] and reducing the risk of sudden cardiac death.[93] Large-scale epidemiologic studies suggest that persons at risk for CHD benefit from the consumption of plant- and marine-derived omega-3 fatty acids, although the ideal amount suggested for daily consumption is presently unclear. Evidence from prospective secondary prevention studies suggests that eicosapentaenoic acid and docosahexaenoic acid supplementation ranging from 0.5 to 1.8 g/day, either as fatty fish or supplements, significantly reduces subsequent cardiac and all-cause mortality; regarding alpha-linolenic acid, total intakes of 1.5–3 g/day seem to be beneficial.[88] Collectively, these data are supportive of the recommendation made by the AHA Dietary Guidelines to include at least two servings of fish per week, particularly fatty fish including tuna and salmon. In addition, the data support inclusion of vegetable oils (e.g., soybean, canola, walnut, flaxseed) and food sources (e.g., walnuts, flaxseeds) high in alpha-linolenic acid in a healthy diet for the general population. The fish recommendation must be balanced with concerns about environmental pollutants, in particular polychlorinated biphenyls (PCBs) and methylmercury, described in state and federal advisories. Consumption of a variety of fish is recommended to minimize any potentially adverse effects due to environmental pollutants and, at the same time, to achieve desired cardiovascular disease health outcomes.[89]

A meta-analysis by Ripsin and colleagues[94] found that oat bran, a soluble fiber, can reduce total cholesterol levels by as much as 5 mg/dL and triglyceride levels by up to 5%. No trials to date have supported that garlic supplementation is efficacious in lowering cholesterol. Chinese red yeast rice (*Monascus purpureus*) contains a basic compound similar in function to the statins. In two human studies,[95,96] lower LDL-C, total cholesterol, and triglycerides were observed, and a single study conducted in China suggested that red yeast was as effective as simvastatin in lowering lipids.[97] The concentration of the active ingredient in red yeast rice is often unpredictable, and given that this is a dietary supplement, patients are rarely monitored for potential hepatotoxicity or rhabdomyolysis. Additional herbal supplements that have been thought to have a role in lipid lowering include artichoke leaf (*Cynara scolymus*), curcumin (*Curcuma longa*), fenugreek seed (*Trigonella foenum-graecum*), garlic (*Allium sativa*), and guggulipid (*Commiphora mukul*).[98]

Novel Markers for CHD

High Sensitivity C-Reactive Protein

CRP is a nonspecific serum marker of inflammation; routine measurements cannot accurately predict either the location or extent of inflammation. As it has been well established that an inflammatory component to the development and progression of CAD exists, the high-sensitivity CRP (hs-CRP) assay has been shown to have utility in detecting persons at high risk for plaque rupture. A review by Ridker in 2001[99] summarized that several large-scale prospective studies have demonstrated hs-CRP to be a strong independent predictor of future myocardial infarction and stroke among apparently healthy men and women, and that the addition of hs-CRP to standard lipid screening may improve global risk prediction among those with high as well as low serum cholesterol levels.

This novel marker has received significant attention in recent years as an adjunct test for CHD screening, since up to 50% of persons who experience a myocardial infarction have normal cholesterol profile results.[100] To date, the hs-CRP assay has been shown to be cost-effective and readily available through most medical laboratories, and it may provide additional prognostic benefit in the primary prevention of CHD. It is thought to be an excellent predictor of cardiovascular events regardless of a patient's LDL-C level, with a particularly impressive predictive value in women.[101] Ridker and colleagues[101] demonstrated that although hs-CRP and LDL-C may be minimally correlated, baseline levels of each factor had a strong linear relation with the incidence of cardiovascular events. These data also suggested that the hs-CRP level may be a stronger predictor of cardiovascular events than the LDL-C level and that it adds prognostic information to that conveyed by the Framingham risk score.

The AHA has stated that hs-CRP is best used to facilitate decision making in persons whose estimated 10-year coronary disease risk according to the Framingham Risk Score (see Table 8-1) is in the range of 10–20%.[102] A review by Reamy describes how the current serum assays for hs-CRP are classified into low-risk (less than 1 mg/liter), intermediate-risk (1–3 mg/liter), and high-risk (greater than 3 mg/liter) groups.[100,103] A value greater than 10 mg/liter indicates a primary etiology for inflammatory disease, including cancer or autoimmune disease, and thus would not be accurately predictive of CHD. Unlike routine cholesterol screening, it is not necessary for the patient to be fasting for this assay.

The pravastatin inflammation/CRP evaluation study[104] was a randomized, double-blind, prospective secondary prevention trial that aimed to examine whether pravastatin could effect anti-inflammatory properties as evidenced by hs-CRP reduction over a 24-week period. In this trial, no significant association was observed between baseline CRP and baseline LDL-C levels, end-of-study hs-CRP and end-of-study LDL-C levels, or change in hs-CRP and change in LDL-C levels over time. Modest reductions in hs-CRP levels were observed at 12 and 24 weeks (−14.3% and −13.1%, respectively) in the secondary prevention cohort treated with pravastatin. The authors concluded that pravastatin reduced hs-CRP levels at both 12 and 24 weeks independent of LDL-C, suggesting that statins may have anti-inflammatory effects in addition to lipid-lowering effects.

The Justification for the Use of Statins in Primary Prevention: An Intervention Trial Evaluating Rosuvastatin (JUPITER) trial[105] is a current research effort that seeks to enroll 15,000 men aged 55 years and older and women aged 65 years and older who, on initial screening, have an hs-CRP level greater than or equal to 2 mg/liter, a LDL-C level less than 130 mg/dL, and a triglyceride level less than 500 mg/dL. These prospective subjects also must have no history of myocardial infarction, stroke, arterial revascularization, or coronary risk equivalent as defined by NCEP ATP III guidelines. The primary objective of the JUPITER trial is to determine whether long-term treatment with rosuvastatin (20 mg/day) will reduce the rate of first major cardiovascular events, defined as the combined end point of cardiovascular death, stroke, myocardial infarction, hospitalization for unstable angina, or arterial revascularization among persons meeting the above criteria. Secondary objectives of the JUPITER trial are to evaluate the safety of long-term treatment with rosuvastatin with regard to total mortality, noncardiovascular mortality, and adverse events and to determine whether rosuvastatin reduces the incidence of type 2 diabetes. It has been postulated that the latter objective reflects the fact that hsCRP levels may also predict the onset of diabetes and that inflammation appears to be a critical link between diabetes and atherogenesis. Finally, on the basis of observational evidence regarding statins, osteoporosis, and hypercoagulability, the JUPITER trial will also seek to determine whether rosuvastatin reduces the incidence of bone fractures and venous thromboembolic events.

Lipoprotein (a)

Lipoprotein (a) [Lp(a)], a major inherited risk factor for atherosclerosis, consists of an LDL-like particle containing apolipoprotein B-100 plus the distinguishing component apolipoprotein (a) [apo(a)], which is structurally similar to plasminogen.[106] Lp(a) has gained increasing attention in recent years due to its role as a novel major risk factor for atherosclerosis. Although its precise function remains unclear, it is known that Lp(a) is concentrated in the artery wall by virtue of binding to fibrin, plasminogen receptors, matrix, and other targets that lead to increased thrombosis and inhibition of fibrinolysis.[107]

Several retrospective, case-controlled studies in men have demonstrated an association between elevated serum levels of Lp(a) and an increased risk for CHD, ischemic stroke, and peripheral arterial disease.[108,109] It is currently unclear whether lifestyle modifications including diet, weight loss, and exercise have a positive effect on serum Lp(a) levels that would ultimately minimize cardiovascular risk. To date, pharmacologic treatment with statins has not been shown to have a significant effect on serum levels of Lp(a), yet one study of hyperlipidemic patients with Lp(a) levels greater than 20 mg/dL demonstrated a 14% decrease in Lp(a) while they were taking fenofibrate.[110] The lack of rigorous, prospective case-controlled trials with quantifiable outcomes data limits formal recommendations for routine screening for Lp(a) as well as any current treatment recommendations. It may be reasonable to consider screening for elevated serum Lp(a) levels in patients with premature CHD, those with a strong family history of cardiovascular disease, those who have undergone angioplasty or CABG, and those with documented cardiovascular disease in the absence of traditional risk factors.[111]

Homocysteine

Homocysteine, a by-product of the metabolism of the essential amino acid methionine, is metabolized by a series of enzymes that use B vitamins as cofactors, including folate, cobalamin (i.e., vitamin B_{12}), and pyridoxine (i.e., vitamin B_6). Although numerous studies have suggested an association between elevated plasma homocysteine levels and cardiovascular disease, no conclusive evidence has emerged that dictates routine surveillance. Some evidence suggests that homocysteine may promote atherosclerosis by damaging the inner lining of arteries and promoting thrombosis, yet a definitive causal link has not yet been established.[112]

In observational studies, elevated serum total homocysteine levels have been positively associated with the risk of ischemic stroke; however, the utility of homocysteine-lowering therapy to reduce this risk has not been confirmed by randomized trials. The Vitamin Intervention for Stroke Prevention trial[113] was a double-blind, randomized, controlled trial that sought to determine whether high doses of folic acid, pyridoxine, and cobalamin, if given to patients with lower total homocysteine levels, would reduce the risk of recurrent stroke, CHD events, or death in 3680 subjects over a 2-year period compared with low doses of these vitamins. Overall, decreased serum levels of homocysteine resultant from vitamin therapy had no significant effect on stroke recurrence during the 2 years of follow-up, and it was thus postulated that high doses of these vitamins may not prevent stroke or myocardial infarction.

The Norwegian Vitamin Trial (NORVIT)[114] was a randomized, controlled, double-blinded secondary prevention trial that tested the hypotheses that long-term treatment (3.5 years) with a combination of 0.8 mg of folic acid, 40 mg of vitamin B_6, a combination of both treatments, or placebo would lower the incidence of myocardial infarction and stroke. The NORVIT study included 3749 patients aged 30–84 years with a history of acute myocardial infarction within the last 7 days. After 2 months, plasma homocysteine levels fell in the patients receiving folic acid (irrespective of whether they were also receiving vitamin B_6) and remained 28% lower in those patients compared with vitamin B_6 and placebo groups throughout the study. Plasma folate levels rose six- to seven-fold with folic acid supplementation. This group concluded that lowering plasma homocysteine levels by as much as 28% does not result in any reduction in the risk of myocardial infarction or stroke in secondary prevention of cardiovascular disease. In fact, patients who received folic acid or vitamin B₆ alone were shown to have a small increase in the risk of cardiovascular disease, and among those who took both vitamins, the risk of a cardiovascular event increased by 20%.

Additional Guidelines

The AHA, the American College of Cardiology, and other related organizations have constructed evidence-based guidelines for the evaluation and management of numerous additional cardiovascular diseases that affect men. An in-depth discussion of each of these disorders is beyond the scope and limitations of this chapter. Several cardiovascular disorders that deserve significant attention are listed below with the most recent corresponding guideline references.

- Congestive heart failure
  - Hunt SA, Abraham WT, Chin MH, et al: ACC/AHA 2005 guideline update for the diagnosis and management of chronic heart failure in the adult: a report of the American College of Cardiology/AHA Task Force on Practice Guidelines [trunc], Bethesda, MD, 2005, American College of Cardiology Foundation (ACCF).
  - Heart failure-systolic dysfunction. Available at: http://www.med.umich.edu/i/oca/practiceguides/heart/HF06.pdf.
- Atrial fibrillation
  - Fuster V, Ryden LE, Asinger RW, et al: ACC/AHA/ESC guidelines for the management of patients with atrial fibrillation: a report of the American College of Cardiology/AHA Task Force on Practice Guidelines and the ESC Committee for Practice Guidelines and Policy [trunc], *Eur Heart J* 22(20):1852–1923, 2001.
  - Singer DE, Albers GW, Dalen JE, et al: Antithrombotic therapy in atrial fibrillation: the Seventh ACCP Conference on Antithrombotic and Thrombolytic Therapy, *Chest* 126(3 Suppl):429S–456S, 2004.
- Acute coronary syndrome
  - Acute coronary syndromes. In: 2005 International Consensus Conference on Cardiopulmonary Resuscitation and Emergency Cardiovascular Care Science with Treatment Recommendations, *Circulation* 112(22 Suppl):III55–III72, 2005.
- Unstable angina/Non–ST elevation myocardial infarction
  - American College of Cardiology Foundation, AHA: ACC/AHA guidelines for the management of patients with unstable angina and non–ST-segment elevation myocardial infarction: a report of the American College of Cardiology/AHA Task Force on Practice Guidelines, Bethesda, MD, 2002, American College of Cardiology Foundation (ACCF).
- Venous thromboembolic disease
  - University of Michigan VTE Evidence-Based Guideline Panel: Venous thromboembolism (2004 update). Available at: http://www.guidelines.gov.
  - Geerts WH, Pineo GF, Heit JA, et al: Prevention of venous thromboembolism: the Seventh ACCP Conference on Antithrombotic and Thrombolytic Therapy, *Chest* 126(3 Suppl):338S–400S, 2004.

Conclusion

Cardiovascular disease ranks as the most common cause of morbidity and mortality in developed countries around the globe. Many risks factors for the development of cardiovascular disease can be minimized and potentially prevented through appropriate lifestyle guidelines for diet, exercise, and appropriate weight management. Primary care clinicians are commonly at the forefront of the diagnosis of hypertension and hypercholesterolemia. These conditions can be appropriately managed through cost-effective evidence-based strategies, proper patient-directed education, interval follow-up, and motivation of patients to take the initiative in modifying their risk factors for cardiovascular disease and complying with prescribed medication regimens.

The future will bring new pharmacologic strategies for the treatment of various forms of cardiovascular disease, and newer technologies will allow clinicians to screen for and detect CHD earlier in our patient's lives, both of which have the potential to minimize overall morbidity and mortality risks. One cannot understate the importance of impressing upon patients that cigarette smoking is the single most common preventable risk factor for CHD, and every attempt to discuss smoking cessation and provide options for quitting should be made during medical encounters. The developed world is losing ground on its battle with obesity, as more persons are classified as overweight and obese. Clinicians must not hesitate to provide their patients with appropriate dietary and exercise guidelines for both the primary and secondary prevention of CHD.

References

1. Miniño AM, Herron MP, Smith BL: Deaths: preliminary data for 2004, *National Vital Stat Rep* 54 (19):1–49, 2006.
2. Summary Health Statistics for US Adults: National Health Interview Survey, 2004, *Vital Health Stat* 10 (228): 2006.
3. American Heart Association: Heart disease and stroke statistics—update. 2006. Available at: http://www.americanheart.org/presenter.jhtml? identifier=3018163.
4. The Framingham Heart Study. Available at: http://www.framingham.com/heart/.
5. National Cholesterol Education Program: Third report of the National Cholesterol Education Program (NCEP) Expert Panel on the Detection, Evaluation, and Treatment of High Blood Cholesterol in Adults (Adult Treatment Panel III): executive summary. NIH Publication no. (NIH) 01–3670. Bethesda, Md, 2001, National Cholesterol Education Program, National Institutes of Health, National Heart, Lung, and Blood Institute.
6. American Heart Association: Metabolic syndrome. Available at: http://www.americanheart.org/presenter.jhtml?identifier=4756.
7. Chobanian AV, Bakris GL, Black HR, et al, for the National High Blood Pressure Education Program Coordinating Committee: The seventh report of the Joint National Committee on Prevention, Detection, Evaluation, and Treatment of High Blood Pressure: the JNC 7 report, *JAMA* 289:2560–2572, 2003.
8. National Center for Health Statistics: *Health, United States, 2006: with chartbook on trends in the health of Americans*, Hyattsville, MD, 2006, National Center for Health Statistics.
9. Hing E, Cherry DK, Woodwell DA: *National ambulatory medical care survey: 2004 summary*, no 374, Washington, DC, 2006, US Department of Health and Human Services.
10. Centers for Disease Control and Prevention (CDC): Racial/ethnic disparities in prevalence, treatment, and control of hypertension—United States, 1999–2002, *MMWR* 54(1):7–9, 2005.
11. Campbell DL, Green LA: Hypertension, *Prim Care Clin Office Pract* 32:1011–1025, 2005.
12. Pickering T: Recommendations for the use of home (self) and ambulatory blood pressure monitoring: American Society of Hypertension Ad Hoc Panel, *Am J Hypertension* 9:1–11, 1996.
13. Verdecchia P: Prognostic value of ambulatory blood pressure: current evidence and clinical implications, *Hypertension* 35:844–851, 2000.
14. Sacks FM, Svetkey LP, Vollmer WM, et al: Effects on blood pressure of reduced dietary sodium and the Dietary Approaches to Stop Hypertension (DASH) diet: DASH–Sodium Collaborative Research Group, *N Engl J Med* 344:3–10, 2001.
15. McDonald KC, Blackwell JC: What lifestyle changes should we recommend for the patient with newly diagnosed hypertension? *J Fam Pract* 55(11):991–993, 2006.
16. He FJ, MacGregor GA: Effect of longer-term modest salt reduction on blood pressure, *Cochrane Database Syst Rev* 3:CD004937, 2004.
17. Bray GA, Vollmer WM, Sacks FM, et al, and the DASH Collaborative Research Group: A further subgroup analysis of the effects of the DASH diet and three dietary sodium levels on blood pressure: results of the DASH–Sodium Trial, *Am J Cardiol* 94:222–227, 2004.
18. Appel LJ, Champagne CM, Harsha DW, et al, and the Writing Group of the PREMIER Collaborative Research Group: Effects of comprehensive lifestyle modification on blood pressure control: main results of the PREMIER clinical trial, *JAMA* 289:2083–2093, 2003.
19. Whelton SP, Chin A, Xin X, et al: Effect of aerobic exercise on blood pressure: a meta-analysis of randomized, controlled trials, *Ann Intern Med* 136:493–503, 2002.
20. Kelley GA, Sharpe Kelley K: Aerobic exercise and resting blood pressure in older adults: a meta-analytic review of randomized controlled trials, *J Gerontol A Biol Sci Med Sci* 56:M298–M303, 2001.
21. Xin X, He J, Frontini MG, et al: Effects of alcohol reduction on blood pressure: a meta-analysis of randomized controlled trials, *Hypertension* 38:1112–1117, 2001.
22. Critchley J, Capewell S: Smoking cessation for the secondary prevention of coronary heart disease, *Cochrane Database Syst Rev* 1:CD003041, 2004.
23. Mulrow CD, Chiquette E, Angel L, et al: Dieting to reduce body weight for controlling hypertension in adults, *Cochrane Database Syst Rev* 2:CD000484, 2000.
24. He J, Whelton PK, Appel LJ, et al: Long-term effects of weight loss and dietary sodium restriction on incidence of hypertension, *Hypertension* 35:544–549, 2000.
25. ALLHAT Officers and Coordinators for the ALLHAT Collaborative Research Group: Major outcomes in high-risk hypertensive patients randomized to angiotensin-converting enzyme inhibitor or calcium channel blocker vs. diuretic: the antihypertensive and lipid-lowering treatment to prevent heart attack trial (ALLHAT), *JAMA* 288:2981–2997, 2002.
26. Hansson L, Zanchetti A, Carruthers SG, et al: Effects of intensive blood-pressure lowering and low-dose aspirin in patients with hypertension: principal results of the Hypertension Optimal Treatment (HOT) randomised trial. HOT Study Group, *Lancet* 351:1755–1762, 1998.
27. Kjeldsen SE, Kolloch RE, Leonetti G: Influence of gender and age on preventing cardiovascular

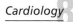

disease by antihypertensive treatment and acetyl-salicylic acid. The HOT study. Hypertension Optimal Treatment, *J Hypertens* 18(5):629–642, 2000.

28. National Cholesterol Education Program: Third report of the National Cholesterol Education Program (NCEP) Expert Panel on the Detection, Evaluation, and Treatment of High Blood Cholesterol in Adults (Adult Treatment Panel III): executive summary. NIH Publication no. (NIH) 01–3670. Bethesda, MD, 2001, National Heart, Lung, and Blood Institute.

29. Heidelbaugh JJ, Rion RJ: Diagnosis and management of lipid disorders, *Clin Fam Pract* 3 (4):757–780, 2001.

30. Grundy SM, Cleeman JI, Merz NB, et al: Implications of recent trials for the National Cholesterol Education Program Adult Treatment III Guidelines, *Circulation* 110:227–239, 2004.

31. Centers for Disease Control and Prevention: Behavioral risk factor surveillance system: 2005 prevalence data. Available at: http://www.cdc.gov/brfss.

32. Bachorik PS, Wood PDS, Albers JJ, et al: Plasma high-density lipoprotein cholesterol concentrations determined after removal of other lipoproteins by heparin/manganese precipitation or by ultracentrifugation, *Clin Chem* 22:1828–1834, 1976.

33. Alaupovic P: Apolipoproteins and lipoproteins, *Atherosclerosis* 13:141–146, 1971.

34. Albers JJ, Hazzard WR: Immunochemical quantification of human plasma Lp(a) lipoprotein, *Lipids* 9:15–26, 1974.

35. Havel RJ: Lipoprotein biosynthesis and metabolism, *Ann NY Acad Sci* 348:16–29, 1980.

36. Berg K, Dahlen G, Borresen AL: Lp(a) phenotypes, other lipoprotein parameters and family history of heart disease in middle-aged males, *Clin Genet* 16:347–352, 1979.

37. Bachorik PS, Rifkind BM, Kwiterovich PO: Lipids and dyslipoproteinemia, In Henry JB, editor: *Clinical diagnosis and management by laboratory methods*, ed 19. Philadelphia, 1996, WB Saunders, pp 208–236.

38. Friedewald WT, Levy RI, Frederickson DS: Estimation of the concentration of low density lipoprotein cholesterol in plasma without the use of the preparative ultracentrifuge, *Clin Chem* 18:499–502, 1972.

39. Cohn JS, McNamara JR, Schaefer EJ: Lipoprotein cholesterol concentrations in plasma of human subjects as measured in the fed and fasted states, *Clin Chem* 34:2456–2459, 1998.

40. Miller M, Bachorik PS, Cloey TA: Normal variation of plasma lipoproteins: postural effects on plasma concentrations of lipids, lipoproteins, and apolipoproteins, *Clin Chem* 38:569–574, 1992.

41. National Cholesterol Education Program: Second report of the National Cholesterol Education Program (NCEP) Expert Panel on the Detection, Evaluation, and Treatment of High Blood Cholesterol in Adults (Adult Treatment Panel II): executive summary. DHSS publication no. (NIH) 93–3095:5. Bethesda, MD, 1993, National Cholesterol Education Program, National Institutes of Health, National Heart, Lung, and Blood Institute.

42. Berg AO: Screening adults for lipid disorders: recommendations and rationale, *Am J Prev Med* 20(3 Suppl):73S–76S, 2001.

43. US Preventive Services Task Force: What's new from the Third US Preventive Services Task Force: screening adults for lipid disorders. AHRQ Publication No. APPIP01–0011 March 2001. Available at: http://www.ahrq.gov/clinic/prev/lipidwh.pdf.

44. Canadian Task Force on the Periodic Health Examination: The periodic health examination, 1993 update: 2. Lowering the blood total cholesterol level to prevent coronary heart disease, *Can Med Assoc J* 148:521–538, 1993.

45. Garber AM, Browner WS, Hulley SB: Cholesterol screening in asymptomatic adults, revisited, *Ann Intern Med* 124:518–531, 1996.

46. Green ML: Management of dyslipidemia in the age of statins, *Prim Care Clin Office Pract* 30(4):641–649, 2003.

47. Malenka DJ, Baron JA: Cholesterol and coronary heart disease: the importance of patient-specific attributable risk, *Arch Int Med* 148:2247–2252, 1988.

48. Frolkis JP, Zyzanski SJ, Schwartz JM, et al: Physician noncompliance with the 1993 National Cholesterol Education Program (NCEP-ATP II) guidelines, *Circulation* 98:851–855, 1998.

49. Aliyu ZY, Yousif SB, Plantholt K, et al: Assessing compliance of cardiologists with the national cholesterol education program (NCEP) III guidelines in an ambulatory care setting, *Lipids Health Dis* 3:9, 2004.

50. McGlynn EA, Asch SM, Adams J, et al: The quality of health care delivered to adults in the United States, *N Engl J Med* 348:2635–2645, 2003.

51. The Lipid Research Clinics Coronary Primary Prevention Trial results: I. Reduction in incidence of coronary heart disease, *JAMA* 251:351–364, 1984.

52. Frick MH, Elo O, Happa K, et al: Helsinki Heart Study: primary-prevention trail with gemfibrozil in middle-aged men with dyslipidemia. Safety of treatment, changes in risk factors: and incidence in coronary heart disease, *N Engl J Med* 317:1237–1245, 1987.

53. Shepard J, Cobbe SM, Ford I, et al: Prevention of coronary heart disease with pravastatin in men with hypercholesterolemia: West of Scotland Coronary Prevention Study Group, *N Engl J Med* 333:1301–1307, 1995.

54. Downs JR, Clearfield M, Weis S, et al: Primary prevention of acute coronary events with lovastatin in men and women with average cholesterol levels: results of AFCAPS/TexCAPS, *JAMA* 279:1615–1622, 1998.

55. Scandinavian Simvastatin Survival Study Group: Randomized trial of cholesterol lowering in 4,444 patients with coronary artery disease. The Scandinavian Simvastatin Survival Study (4S), Lancet 344:1383–1389, 1994.

56. Long-term Intervention with Pravastatin in Ischaemic Disease (LIPID) Study Group: Prevention of cardiovascular events and death with pravastatin in patients with coronary heart disease (CHD) and a broad range of initial cholesterol levels, *N Engl J Med* 339:1349–1357, 1997.

57. Pitt B, Waters D, Brown WV, et al: Aggressive lipid-lowering therapy compared with angioplasty in stable coronary artery disease: Atorvastatin versus Revascularization Treatment Investigators, *N Engl J Med* 341:70–76, 1999.

58. Sacks FM, Pfeffer MA, Moye MA, et al: The effect of pravastatin on coronary events after myocardial infarction in patients with average cholesterol levels (CARE), *N Engl J Med* 335:1001–1009, 1996.

59. The Post Coronary Artery Bypass Graft Trial Investigators: The effect of aggressive lowering of low-density lipoprotein cholesterol levels and low dose anticoagulation on obstructive changes in saphenous vein coronary artery bypass grafts, *N Engl J Med* 336:153–162, 1997 [erratum appears in *N Engl J Med* 337:1859, 1997].

60. Rubins HB, Robins SJ, Collins D, et al: Gemfibrozil for the secondary prevention of coronary heart disease in men with low levels of high-density lipoprotein cholesterol: Veterans Affairs High-Density Lipoprotein Intervention Trial Study Group, *N Engl J Med* 341:410–418, 1997.

61. Frick MH, Syvanne M, Nieminen MN, et al: Prevention of the angiographic progression of coronary and vein-graft atherosclerosis by gemfibrozil after coronary bypass surgery in men with low levels of HDL cholesterol: Lopid Coronary Angiography Trial (LOCAT) Study Group, *Circulation* 96:2317–2343, 1997.

62. Heart Protection Study Collaborative Group: MRC/BHF Heart Protection Study of cholesterol lowering with simvastatin in 20,536 high-risk individuals: a randomized placebo-controlled trial, *Lancet* 360(9326):7–22, 2002.

63. Shepherd J, Blauw GJ, Murphy MB, et al, for the PROSPER study group: Pravastatin in elderly individuals at risk of vascular disease (PROSPER): a randomized controlled trial, PROspective Study of Pravastatin in the Elderly at Risk, *Lancet* 360:1623–1630, 2002.

64. The ALLHAT Officers and Coordinators for the ALLHAT Collaborative Research Group: Major outcomes in moderately hypercholesterolemic hypertensive patients randomized to pravastatin vs. usual care, the Antihypertensive and Lipid-Lowering Treatment to Prevent Heart Attack Trial (ALLHAT-LLT), *JAMA* 288:2998–3007, 2002.

65. Sever PS, Dahlof B, Poulter NR, et al, for the ASCOT investigators: Prevention of coronary and stroke events with atorvastatin in hypertensive patients who have average or lower-than-average cholesterol concentrations, in the Anglo-Scandinavian Cardiac Outcomes Trial—Lipid-Lowering Arm (ASCOT-LLA): a multicentre randomized controlled trial, *Lancet* 361:1149–1158, 2003.

66. Cannon CP, Braunwald E, McCabe CH, et al, for the Pravastatin or Atorvastatin Evaluation and Infection Therapy—Thrombolysis in Myocardial Infarction 22 Investigators: Intensive versus moderate lipid lowering with statins after acute coronary syndromes, *N Engl J Med* 350:1495–1504, 2004.

67. Sacks FM, Tonkin AM, Shepherd J, et al: Effect of pravastatin on coronary disease events in subgroups defined by coronary risk factors: the Prospective Pravastatin Pooling Project, *Circulation* 102:1893–1900, 2000.

68. LaRosa JC, Grundy SM, Waters DD, et al, for the Treating to New Targets (TNT) Investigators: Intensive lipid lowering with atorvastatin in patients with stable coronary disease, *N Engl J Med* 352:1425–1435, 2005.

69. Pedersen TR, Faergeman O, Kastelein JJ, et al, for the Incremental Decrease in End Points Through Aggressive Lipid Lowering (IDEAL) Study Group: High-dose atorvastatin vs usual-dose simvastatin for secondary prevention after myocardial infarction: the IDEAL study, *JAMA* 294:2437–2445, 2005.

70. Nissen SE, Nicholls SJ, Sipahi I, et al: Effect of very high-intensity statin therapy on regression of coronary atherosclerosis: the ASTEROID trial, *JAMA* 295:1556–1565, 2006.

71. Lipid Research Clinics Coronary Primary Prevention Trial Results: I. Reduction in incidence of coronary heart disease. II. The relationship of reduction in incidence of coronary heart disease to cholesterol lowering, *JAMA* 251:351–364, 1984.

72. Mero N, Van Tol A, Scheek LM, et al: Decreased postprandial high density lipoprotein cholesterol and apolipoprotein A-1 and E in normolipidemic smoking men: relations with lipid transfer proteins and LCAT activities, *J Lipid Res* 39:1493–1502, 1998.

73. United States Department of Agriculture and US Department of Health and Human Services: Dietary guidelines for Americans, 2005. Available at: http://www.health.gov/dietaryguidelines/dga2005/document/pdf/DGA2005.pdf.

74. Ostrander LD, Lamphiaer DE, Block WD, et al: Relationship of serum lipid concentrations to alcohol consumption, *Arch Intern Med* 134:451–456, 1974.

75. American Obesity Association: AOA fact sheets Available at: http://www.obesity.org/subs/fastfacts/obesity_US.shtml.

76. Caggiula AW, Christakis G, Ferrand M, et al: The multiple risk factors intervention trial (MRFIT): IV. intervention on blood lipids, *Prev Med* 10:443–475, 1981.

77. Wood PD, Stefanick ML, Williams PT, et al: The effects of plasma lipoproteins of a prudent weight-reducing diet, with or without exercise, in overweight men and women, *N Engl J Med* 325:461–466, 1991.

78. Fletcher GF, Balady G, Blair SN, et al: Statement on exercise: benefits and recommendations for physical activity programs for all Americans, *Circulation* 94:857–862, 1996.

79. Jones P, Kafonek S, Laurora I, et al: Comparative dose efficacy study of atorvastatin versus simvastatin, pravastatin, lovastatin, and fluvastatin in patients with hypercholesterolemia (the CURVES study), *Am J Cardiol* 81(5):582–587, 1998.

80. Knopp RH: Drug therapy: drug treatment of lipid disorders, *N Engl J Med* 341(7):498–511, 1999.

81. Rembold CM: Number-needed-to-treat analysis of the prevention of myocardial infarction and death by antidyslipidemic therapy, *J Fam Pract* 42:577–586, 1996.

82. Knopp RH, Gitter H, Truitt T, et al, for the Ezetimibe Study Group: Effects of ezetimibe, a new cholesterol absorption inhibitor, on plasma lipids in patients with primary hypercholesterolemia, *Eur Heart J* 24(8):729–741, 2006.

83. Grundy SM, Vega GL: Fibric acids: effects on lipids and lipoprotein metabolism, *Am J Med* 83:9–20, 1987.

84. Brown WV, Goldberg IJ, Ginsberg HN: Treatment of common lipoprotein disorders, *Prog Cardiovasc Dis* 27:1–20, 1984.

85. Criqui MH, Heiss G, Cohn R, et al: Plasma triglyceride level and mortality from coronary heart disease, *N Engl J Med* 328:1220–1225, 1993.

86. Nash DT: Role of statins in reducing risk of coronary heart disease, *Drug Benefit Trends* 18:535–544, 2006.

87. Clark RW, Sutfin TA, Ruggeri RB: Raising high density lipoprotein in humans through inhibition of cholesterol ester transfer protein: an initial multidose study of torcetrapib, *Arterioscler Thromb Vasc Biol* 24:490–497, 2004.

88. American Heart Association: Fish consumption, fish oil, omega-3 fatty acids and cardiovascular disease. Available at: http://www.americanheart.org/presenter.jhtml?identifier=4632.

89. Kris-Etherton PM, Harris WS, Appel LJ, for the American Heart Association: Nutrition Committee: Fish consumption, fish oil, omega-3 fatty acids, and cardiovascular disease, *Circulation* 106: 2747–2757, 2002.

90. Harris WS: n-3 Fatty acids and serum lipoproteins: human studies, *Am J Clin Nutr* 65(5 Suppl): 1645S–1654S, 1997.

91. Morris MC, Sacks F, Rosner B: Does fish oil lower blood pressure? a meta-analysis of controlled trials, *Circulation* 88:523–533, 1993.

92. Mori TA, Beilin LJ, Burke V, et al: Interactions between dietary fat, fish, and fish oils and their effects on platelet function in men at risk of cardiovascular disease, *Arterioscler Thromb Vasc Biol* 17:279–286, 1997.

93. Albert CM, Hennekens CH, O'Donnell CJ, et al: Fish consumption and risk of sudden cardiac death, *JAMA* 279:23–28, 1998.

94. Ripsin CM, Keenan JM, Jacobs DR, et al: Oat products and lipid lowering: a meta-analysis, *JAMA* 288:2569–2578, 2002.

95. Heber D, Yip I, Ashley JM, et al: Cholesterol-lowering effects of a proprietary Chinese red-yeast-rice dietary supplement, *Am J Clin Nutr* 69:231–236, 1999.

96. Wang J, Lu Z, Chi J: Multicenter clinical trial of the serum lipid-lowering effects of a *Monascus purpureus* (red yeast) rice preparation from traditional Chinese medicine, *Curr Ther Res Clin Exper* 58:964–978, 1997.

97. Kou W, Lu Z, Guo J: Effect of xuezhikang on the treatment of primary hyperlipidemia [in Chinese], *Chung Hua Nei Ko Tsa Chih* 36:529–531, 1997.

98. Warber SL, Zick SM: Biologically based complementary medicine for cardiovascular disease: help or harm? *Clin Fam Pract* 3(4):945–975, 2001.

99. Ridker PM: High-sensitivity C-reactive protein: potential adjunct for global risk assessment in the primary prevention of cardiovascular disease, *Circulation* 103:1813–1818, 2001.

100. Ridker PM: Clinical application of C-reactive protein for cardiovascular disease detection and prevention, *Circulation* 107:363–369, 2003.

101. Ridker PM, Rifai N, Rose L, et al: Comparison of C-reactive protein and low-density lipoprotein cholesterol levels in the prediction of first cardiovascular events, *N Engl J Med* 347:1557–1565, 2002.

102. Pearson TA, Mensah GA, Alexander RW, et al: Markers of inflammation and cardiovascular disease: applications to clinical and public health practice. A statement for healthcare professionals from the Centers for Disease Control and Prevention and the American Heart Association, *Circulation* 107:499–511, 2003.

103. Reamy BV: Hyperlipidemia: applying the evidence to prevent atherosclerosis, *Fam Pract Recert* 28 (9):49–57, 2006.

104. Albert MA, Danielson E, Rifai N, and the PRINCE Investigators: Effect of statin therapy on C-reactive protein levels: the pravastatin inflammation/CRP evaluation (PRINCE): a randomized trial and cohort study, *JAMA* 286(1):64–70, 2001.

105. Ridker PM, and the JUPITER Study Group: Rosuvastatin in the primary prevention of cardiovascular disease among patients with low levels of low-density lipoprotein cholesterol and elevated high-sensitivity C-reactive protein, *Circulation* 108:2292–2297, 2003.

106. Lawn RM, Boonmark NW, Schwartz K, et al: The recurring evolution of lipoprotein (a): insights from cloning of hedgehog apolipoprotein (a), *J Biol Chem* 270(41):24004–24009, 1995.

107. Kostner G, Krempler F: Lipoprotein(a), *Curr Opin Lipidol* 3:279–284, 1992.

108. Valentine RJ, Grayburn PA, Vega GL, et al: Lp(a) lipoprotein is an independent, discriminating risk factor for premature peripheral atherosclerosis among white men, *Arch Intern Med* 154:801–806, 1994.

109. Genest JJ, McNamara JR, Ordovas JM, et al: Lipoprotein cholesterol, apolipoprotein A-1 and B and lipoprotein(a) abnormalities in men with premature coronary artery disease, *J Am Coll Cardiol* 19:792–802, 1992.

110. Farnier M, Bonnefous F, Debbas N, et al: Comparative efficacy and safety of micronized fenofibrate and simvastatin in patients with primary type IIa or IIb hyperlipidemia, *Arch Intern Med* 154:441–449, 1994.
111. Hackam DG, Anand SS: Emerging risk factors for atherosclerotic vascular disease: a critical review of the evidence, *JAMA* 290(7):932–940, 2003.
112. American Heart Association Science Advisory: Homocysteine, diet, and cardiovascular diseases, #71–0157, *Circulation* 99:178–182, 1999.
113. Toole JF, Malinow MR, Chambless LE, et al: Lowering homocysteine in patients with ischemic stroke to prevent recurrent stroke, myocardial infarction, and death: the Vitamin Intervention for Stroke Prevention (VISP) randomized controlled trial, *JAMA* 291(5):565–575, 2004.
114. Bonaa KH: NORVIT: Randomized trial of homocysteine-lowering with B-vitamins for secondary prevention of cardiovascular disease after acute myocardial infarction. *Program and Abstracts from the European Society of Cardiology Congress 2005.* Stockholm, Sweden, 2005, Hot Line II.
115. Lockman AR, Tribastone AD, Knight KV, Franko JP: Treatment of cholesterol abnormalities, *Am Fam Phys* 71:1137–1142, 1147–1148, 2005.

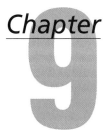
Endocrinology

Naila Goldenberg, MD, and Arno K. Kumagai, MD

Key Points

Hypogonadism

- The diagnostic criteria for partial androgen deficiency of the aging male (PADAM) are based on clinical symptoms and biochemical evidence of hypogonadism, yet most symptoms do not correlate with serum androgen levels, and a minority of elderly and otherwise healthy men with signs of PADAM have a low serum total testosterone level compared with young men (strength of recommendation: B).
- If testicular enlargement has not occurred in a boy by 14 years of age, the possibility of delayed puberty should be considered and further diagnostic evaluation should be performed (strength of recommendation: C).
- In young and otherwise healthy men, screening for male hypogonadism (MHG) is not recommended; however, in persons with certain medical conditions that are associated with an increased risk of MHG, screening along with measurement of serum testosterone concentrations should be considered in symptomatic men suspected to have the disorder (strength of recommendation: C).
- The Endocrine Society currently does not recommend routine screening or treatment of elderly men with low serum testosterone levels, unless they are symptomatic and exhibit consistently low measurements (strength of recommendation: C).
- The goal of replacement testosterone therapy for MHG in men who do not wish fertility is to provide physiologic concentrations of testosterone levels, dihydrotestosterone (DHT) and estradiol,

which would allow optimal virilization and normal sexual function with minimal adverse effects (strength of recommendation: B).

Osteoporosis

- Osteoporosis in men continues to be underdiagnosed, and the majority of men with fragility fractures due to osteoporosis are not being treated (strength of recommendation: B).
- The International Society for Clinical Densitometry recommends bone densitometry in women after the age of 65 years and men after 70 years of age, in patients with secondary causes of osteoporosis, and in those taking medications associated with the potential for low bone mass or bone loss and after any fragility fracture; no consensus regarding screening of older men who were not in high-risk categories was reached (strength of recommendation: C).
- Evidence from large clinical trials in men is lacking for calcium supplementation alone (strength of recommendation: B); vitamin D at a daily dose of 700–800 IU has been found to be associated with a significant reduction of hip fractures and nonvertebral fractures (strength of recommendation: A).
- There are high-quality clinical data on the effectiveness of bisphosphonate therapy on improving bone mineral density (BMD) and reduction of vertebral and nonvertebral fracture risks for primary and secondary osteoporosis in men (strength of recommendation: A).
- Calcitonin and the selective estrogen receptor modulator raloxifene are thought to exhibit some effect on reduction of

vertebral and nonvertebral fractures in men; current data suggest that they are inferior to the bisphosphonates in fracture prevention (strength of recommendation: B).

Diabetes Mellitus

- Type 1 and type 2 diabetes are associated with chronic microvascular and macrovascular complications, including retinopathy, neuropathy, nephropathy, and cerebrovascular and cardiovascular disease (strength of recommendation: A).
- Well-designed multicenter trials have conclusively demonstrated that rigorous metabolic control significantly reduces the development and progression of microvascular complications in both type 1 and type 2 diabetes (strength of recommendation: A).
- Evidence that rigorous control of diabetes decreases the risk of cardiovascular and cerebrovascular disease is less convincing. In type 2 diabetes, intensive metabolic control should be part of a general clinical approach that includes control of blood pressure and cholesterol in the prevention of cardiovascular events (strength of recommendation: A).

Erectile Dysfunction

- Etiologies of erectile dysfunction (ED) in diabetic men are similar to those without diabetes; however, these factors may be compounded by microvascular and neurologic complications of diabetes, as well as associated metabolic or endocrine disorders (e.g., hypertension, hyperlipidemia, obesity, hypogonadism, thyroid disease) and suboptimal metabolic control (strength of recommendation: B).
- Strong clinical evidence supports the effectiveness of the PDE5 inhibitors, including sildenafil, vardenafil, and tadalafil, in diabetic men with ED (strength of recommendation: A).
- Transurethral alprostadil, vacuum devices, and intercavernous injections of vasoactive agents have less convincing evidence supporting their use and should be considered as alternatives in the case of contraindications to (e.g., use of nitrates), or lack of effectiveness of, PDE5 therapy (strength of recommendation: B).

The authors would like to acknowledge Dr. Elana Stolpner for her assistance with the research and writing of the section on osteoporosis. Dr. Kumagai was supported in part by National Institutes of Health Grant RPO60DK-20572, which supports the Michigan Diabetes Research and Training Center.

Introduction

The dynamic symphony of feedback regulation and cellular actions of the circulating hormones of the endocrine system contributes to the internal homeostasis of the human body. In this chapter, we discuss several disease topics in endocrinology of particular importance to men's health, as well as an evidence-based approach to their diagnosis and treatment. In particular, we will focus attention on male hypogonadism (MHG) and its complications, the oft-neglected topic of osteoporosis in men, and an overview of diabetes mellitus with an emphasis on one of its most common complications affecting men's health: erectile dysfunction (ED).

Hypogonadism

Definition

As the physiologic role of sex hormones changes during different stages of male sexual and reproductive development, gonadal hormone deficiency has different implications depending upon age. The Endocrine Society Task Force has defined *male hypogonadism* through a clinical practice guideline to be a clinical syndrome that results from failure of the testis to produce physiologic levels of testosterone (i.e., androgen deficiency) with a resulting failure of spermatogenesis, due to disruption of one or more levels of the hypothalamic-pituitary-gonadal axis.[1] This section will discuss the differential diagnosis, evaluation, and treatment of hypogonadism in men. Congenital abnormalities are well-described causes of gonadal failure in the developing fetus, infant, and child; however, as the primary theme of this textbook is centered on issues in men's health, we will focus our discussion exclusively on disorders that lead to hypogonadism in male adults.

Classification of Male Hypogonadism

MHG is classified according to the locus on the hypothalamic-pituitary-gonadal axis where the causative lesion occurs. A list of disorders associated with primary and secondary hypogonadism, as well as disorders involving combinations of primary and secondary hypogonadism, is presented in Table 9-1.

Primary hypogonadism occurs in conditions that involve a primary gonadal (testicular) abnormality or failure. These disorders may be either

Table 9-1. Disorders of Primary and Secondary Hypogonadism

Primary Hypogonadism (Hypergonadotropic Hypogonadism)	
Congenital	**Acquired**
Klinefelter syndrome	Autoimmune
Cryptorchidism	Viral (e.g., mumps)
Gonadal dysgenesis	Trauma/surgery
"Vanishing testes" syndrome	Radiation
Rare genetic causes of Wolffian duct development	Chemotherapy
Secondary Hypogonadism (Hypogonadotropic Hypogonadism)	
Congenital	**Acquired**
Pituitary hypogenesis or other pituitary abnormality	Pituitary, hypothalamic tumors (e.g., craniopharyngioma, histiocytosis, germinomas, pituitary adenoma, prolactinoma)
Idiopathic (e.g., Kallmann syndrome)	Chronic disease, malnutrition (e.g., celiac disease, inflammatory bowel, chronic renal failure, leukemia, cancers)
Leptin deficiency/resistance	Brain radiation, chemotherapy
Prader-Willi syndrome	Diabetes mellitus, obesity
Combination of Both Primary and Secondary Hypogonadism	
Congential/Metabolic	**Acquired**
Hemochromatosis	Alcoholism
Sickle cell disease, thalassemia	
Target organ resistance to sex steroids	
Testicular feminization (androgen insensitivity syndrome)	

Adapted from: Bhasin S, Cunningham GR, Hayes FJ, et al: Testosterone therapy in adult men with androgen deficiency syndromes: an endocrine society clinical practice guideline, *J Clin Endocrinol Metab* 91(6):1995–2010, 2006.

congenital or acquired later in life and may be associated with multiple causes. Since the lesion involves a primary defect in the production of testosterone and inhibin B and a lack of negative feedback on the hypothalamus and pituitary, this class of MHG is associated with increased levels of gonadotropins and is therefore called *hyper*gonadotropic hypogonadism.

Secondary and *tertiary hypogonadism* are the result of pituitary and hypothalamic failure, respectively. Since hypothalamic causes of hypogonadism are relatively rare, our focus will primarily be on secondary causes. An absence of secretion of gonadotropin-releasing hormone (GnRH) or luteinizing hormone (LH) and follicle-stimulating hormone (FSH) results in the lack of adequate stimulation of testicular development or function. These disorders may be due to congenital pituitary or hypothalamic abnormalities or acquired later in life. Since the inherent defect is due to the lack of hypothalamic or pituitary

gonadotropin production, this class of disorders is associated with low serum levels of LH and FSH and is therefore called *hypo*gonadotropic hypogonadism. Some conditions and disorders are associated with a defect in both pituitary and testicular levels of sex hormones. There are few conditions associated with tissue resistance or insensitivity to testosterone, leading to hypogonadism.

Epidemiology of Hypogonadism in Male Adults

Epidemiologic data from the Massachusetts Male Aging Study reported an overall incidence rate of MHG as 12.3 per 1000 person-years among men aged 40–79 years old, with a statistically significant rise in incidence with age.[2] The prevalence of MHG in this survey was found to be 4.1% among men aged 40–49 years; 4.5–7.1% for ages

49–59 years; 9.4–11.5% for ages 60–69 years; and 22.8 % in men aged 70–79 years.[2]

Hypogonadism is also found among men evaluated for common urologic or fertility disorders. Marberger and colleagues[3] reported that in a study of 4254 men with a mean age of 66 years who had benign prostatic hypertrophy, 27% had a serum testosterone level less than 300 ng/dL. In a separate study among 700 infertile American men with a mean age of 36 years, 6% were found to have hypogonadism.[4]

Signs and Symptoms

The signs and symptoms of MHG vary considerably, depending on the age of onset. If testosterone deficiency starts during early fetal life (e.g., testicular agenesis or androgen insensitivity syndrome,[5] then the male external genitalia fail to develop, and a genotypic XY fetus will present with external female genitalia at birth. In such cases, the true genotype and underlying disorder may not be diagnosed until later in life. Congenital or acquired hypogonadism in prepubertal boys with a normal growth hormone axis leads to delayed or absent puberty associated with tall stature, eunuchoid body habitus, general absence or underdevelopment of secondary male characteristics, and aspermatogenesis.

Common physical signs and symptoms of androgen deficiency are listed in Table 9-2. In addition, decreased energy or motivation, poor

Table 9-2. Signs and Symptoms of Androgen Deficiency

Incomplete sexual development
Eunuchoid body habitus
Reduced libido and sexual activity
Decreased spontaneous erections
Gynecomastia and breast discomfort
Loss of facial, axillary, or pubic hair
Very small (especially < 5 mL) or shrinking testes
Male infertility
Aspermia or severe oligospermia
Evidence of osteoporosis, loss of height, or low-trauma fractures
Reduced muscle bulk and strength
Hot flashes in men

Adapted from: Bhasin S, Cunningham GR, Hayes FJ, et al: Testosterone therapy in adult men with androgen deficiency syndromes: an endocrine society clinical practice guideline, *J Clin Endocrinol Metab* 91(6):1995–2010, 2006.

concentration and memory, depression, sleep disturbances, decreased physical or work performance, or increased body fat or body mass index (BMI) may also be associated with androgen deficiency.[1] These signs and symptoms are, of course, very nonspecific and alone do not indicate androgen deficiency. Specific signs and symptoms that may be associated with MHG are described below according to organ system.

Urogenital System

Changes associated with MHG may include micropenis and small (< 5 mL) or absent testicles if the onset of MHG was prepubertal.[6] A normal-size penis associated with shrinking or small (5–15 mL) testes indicates postpubertal onset of MHG.[6] In a male adult, decreased libido, ED, or infertility are often presenting symptoms of MHG.[7,8]

Constitutional and Psychological

Sleep disturbance, decreased energy, inability to concentrate, and depression may be a part of testosterone deficiency syndrome.[9,10]

Musculoskeletal System

Testosterone clearly has an anabolic effect on muscular development and accrual of bone. Therefore, if MHG begins before the onset of puberty, it may be associated with eunuchoid body habitus and often with decreased bone mineral density (BMD). In adult-onset MHG, the effect on muscle will lead to decreased muscle strength and bulk. Long-standing untreated hypogonadism may present with fragility fractures or osteoporosis, the latter detected by a dual-energy x-ray absorptiometry (DEXA) scan.[11]

Skin and Extremities

Long-standing untreated MHG is associated with thinning of the skin and decreased turgor. Secondary male characteristics including facial hair growth and body hair distribution may change during the course of development of MHG.

Gynecomastia

Gynecomastia relates to the relative excess of estrogen compared with testosterone.[12] Secondary MHG could be present in up to 25% of men with gynecomastia.[13]

Cardiovascular System

It is well known that men have a higher prevalence of cardiovascular disease, with earlier onset, than women.[14] Interestingly, recent data from the Framingham Study have suggested that cardiovascular disease was not associated with the concentration of serum testosterone in 2084 middle aged men monitored for 10 years; however, the prevalence was lower in men with higher levels of estrogen.[15]

Metabolic

Low serum testosterone levels are associated with several cardiovascular risk factors, including dyslipidemia, adverse clotting profiles, obesity, and insulin resistance. It is important to note that these are associations and are not necessarily indicative of causation. Relevant in this regard is a study by Liu and colleagues[16] that found no significant change in insulin resistance after hCG-induced restoration of testosterone in elderly hypogonadal men after the 3 months of treatment.

Hematologic

Testosterone affects hemopoietic function of bone marrow, and a normocytic, normochromic anemia of chronic disease may be a sign of MHG. Hypogonadal men with a pituitary adenoma and associated low testosterone levels were found to have an average hematocrit of 39.9%, in contrast to a hematocrit of 45.6% in men with a normal serum testosterone[17]; of 67 men with MHG in this study, 31 (46.3%) were found to be anemic.[17] The institution of testosterone in boys with constitutional delay of puberty leads to significant increase of hemoglobin/hematocrit levels.[18]

Signs and Symptoms in Older Men

Recently, a controversy has arisen in the diagnosis and treatment of hypogonadism in older men. Serum testosterone concentrations decline, on average, 1–2% per year in adult men.[19,20] With this decline, some fraction of older men will have testosterone concentrations that are less than the normal reference range for young men. Some researchers believe that in older men, a decrease in testosterone leads to a specific symptom complex, the so-called, "andropause." The International Society for the Study of Aging Male (ISSAM) has named this phenomenon the *partial androgen deficiency of the aging male* (PADAM). According to ISSAM, the diagnostic criteria for PADAM are based on the presence of clinical symptoms together with biochemical evidence of hypogonadism.[6] However, most of these symptoms, including those listed in Table 9-1 along with the more nonspecific symptoms described above, do not have a clear correlation with serum androgen levels, and fewer than one quarter of elderly and otherwise healthy men with signs of PADAM have a low serum total testosterone level compared with young men.[21]

Diagnosis

The possibility of MHG may arise during a routine history and physical examination. Initial laboratory evaluation should include a serum testosterone measurement. Serum testosterone concentrations fluctuate, depending on the circadian rhythm of gonadotropins[22]; therefore, screening for MHG should start with a morning serum total testosterone. Furthermore, the finding of a low testosterone concentration should be confirmed by a second measurement since 30% of normal, healthy men have low serum testosterone values as a result of gonadotropin pulsatility.[22] Since any acute changes including weight loss, stress, or illness may lead to abnormal testosterone results, it is important to perform the laboratory evaluation when the patient is not affected by these potential confounders.

The majority of testosterone in circulation is bound to sex hormone–binding globulin (SHBG) and, to a lesser degree, albumin. The level of total testosterone depends on conditions affecting SHBG and albumin concentrations including liver dysfunction, nutritional status, thyroid disease, nephrotic syndrome, and different medications (e.g., glucocorticoids, anticonvulsants, progestins, estrogen, and androgenic steroids) that may affect binding protein synthesis or metabolism in the liver. If one or more of these conditions or medications is present, then the measurement of a free testosterone level should be considered.

The absolute lower limit of the "normal" testosterone concentration below which replacement is necessary is also a matter of a debate among specialists.[1] According to the most recent Endocrine Society Guidelines, a serum total testosterone level of less than 300 ng/dL on at least two different occasions is diagnostic for hypogonadism.[1] When hypogonadism has been confirmed, it should be determined whether the deficiency is primary or secondary hypogonadism, and an evaluation to establish possible etiologies should be conducted (Figure 9-1). Karyotyping and Y-chromosome analysis should be offered to any man with primary hypogonadism of unknown etiology and in men with nonobstructive azoospermia or severe oligospermia before intracytoplasmic sperm injection is performed.[23]

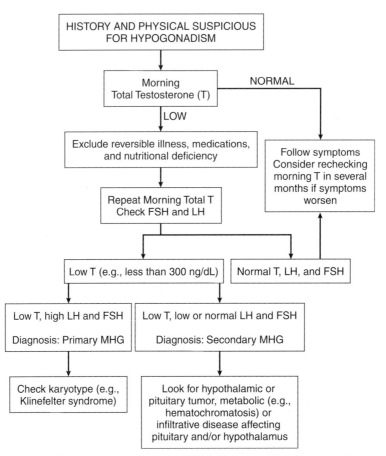

Figure 9-1. Diagnostic evaluation for male hypogonadism. FSH, Follicle-stimulating hormone; LH, luteinizing hormone; MHG, male hypogonadism. (Adapted from: Bhasin S, Cunningham GR, Hayes FJ, et al: Testosterone therapy in adult men with androgen deficiency syndromes: an endocrine society clinical practice guideline, *J Clin Endocrinol Metab* 91[6]:1995–2010, 2006.)

Male Hypogonadism Before and During Puberty

MHG in a young person is often diagnosed due to failure to develop secondary sex characteristics during puberty. Determination of whether an individual patient in puberty is hypogonadal is complicated by the fact that the timing of normal pubertal changes varies greatly in boys. Recent data from the NHANES III survey demonstrate significant variation between the age of pubertal milestones for North American boys based on race and ethnicity.[24,25] For example, the average age of onset of genital growth was measured at 9.5 years of age for African Americans, 10.1 years for white persons, and 10.4 years for Mexican Americans. The onset of pubic hair development is similar, at 11.2, 12, and 12.3 years of age for African American, white, and Mexican American boys, respectively.[25]

If no testicular enlargement (e.g., an estimated volume of more than 5 mL) has occurred in a boy

by 14 years of age, the possibility of delayed puberty should be considered and further diagnostic evaluation should be performed.[6] Most teenage boys with delayed puberty or short stature have a constitutional delay of growth and puberty (CDGP). CDGP is a normal variant and is characterized by delayed bone age, shorter stature than that expected in comparison to the parents' height, and a family history of delayed growth.[26] Dynamic testing with GnRH or beta-human chorionic gonadotropin (β-hCG) has been used frequently to differentiate male children with delayed puberty from patients with disorders of permanent hypogonadism, and these tests are often performed at approximately 14 years of age.[27–29] There is, however, significant overlap of both spontaneous nocturnal concentrations of LH and FSH, as well as concentrations of these gonadotropins after the GnRH stimulation (up to 44%), between male subjects with CDGP and MHG[30,31] providing a sensitivity, specificity, and positive predictive value of only 56%, 94%, and 75%, respectively.[31] A schematic approach to delayed puberty in boys is shown in Figure 9-2.

Male Hypogonadism in Young Men

In young and otherwise healthy men, screening for MHG is not recommended; however, in persons with certain medical conditions that are associated with an increased risk of MHG,

screening along with measurement of serum testosterone concentrations should be considered in symptomatic men suspected with the disorder. Medical conditions in this category include pituitary disorders or a history of head/sella turcica radiation; treatment with medications affecting the testosterone metabolism (e.g., glucocorticoids, opioids, ketoconazole, spironolactone); human immunodeficiency virus (HIV) disease with HIV-associated weight loss; end stage renal disease; moderate to severe chronic obstructive

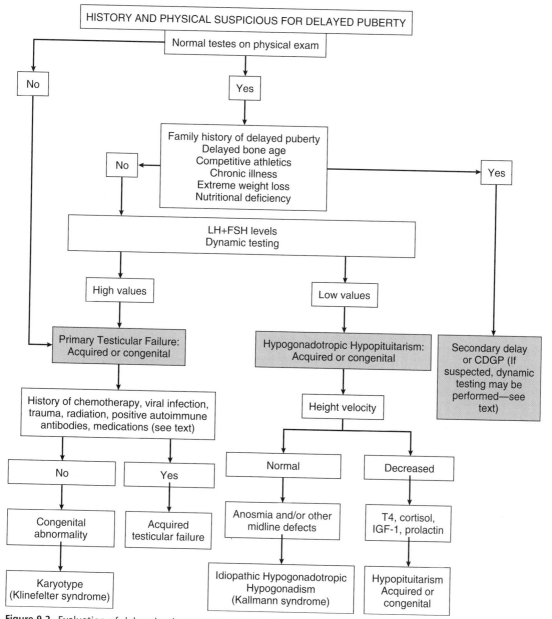

Figure 9-2. Evaluation of delayed puberty. LH, Luteinizing hormone; FSH, follicle-stimulating hormone; CDGP, constitutional delay of growth and puberty; T4, thyroxine; IGF-1, insulin-like growth factor-1.

pulmonary disease; infertility; osteoporosis or low trauma fracture; and type 2 diabetes mellitus.[1]

With regard to evaluations for MHG in the setting of infertility, male factor infertility may be the cause in up to 50% of infertile couples.[32] The evaluation of an infertile couple should be considered if pregnancy has not occurred within 1 year of unprotected intercourse, or earlier if a known infertility risk factor exists. The initial laboratory workup for male factor infertility consists of the analysis of two semen samples. Any abnormalities in initial screening necessitates a further evaluation by a urologist or other specialist in male reproduction. According to the American Urological Association, an initial endocrine evaluation is recommended if there is (1) an abnormally low sperm concentration, especially if it is less than 10 million/mL; (2) impaired sexual function; or (3) other clinical findings suggestive of a specific endocrinopathy.[23] If hypogonadism is suspected, a complete developmental history and thorough physical examination should be performed to look for other clues of possible associated conditions.

Male Hypogonadism in Older Men

There is a lack of evidence supporting the benefit of testosterone replacement in elderly men. As mentioned above, the concept of "andropause" is an extremely controversial one, and symptoms of androgen deficiency do not often correlate with actual serum testosterone concentrations.[21] Consequently, the Endocrine Society currently does not recommend routine screening or treatment of elderly men with low testosterone levels unless they are symptomatic and consistently low measurements have been observed.[1]

Treatment

Treatment options for MHG often depend on several factors including age, type of hypogonadism, fertility issues, and the presence of any significant comorbidities.

Prepubertal/Pubertal

The goals of androgen therapy for adolescents are to promote linear growth and secondary sexual characteristics while permitting the normal accrual of muscle mass and bone mineral content. Secondary goals are mainly in the psychosocial sphere, as boys with pubertal delay often have problems being accepted as peers and cannot participate in sports with the same ability as pubertal boys due to their small size. At present, it is recommended to use an injectable form of testosterone rather than other methods of administration because the small doses of testosterone required in boys may be delivered more accurately by injection.[33] Generally, clinicians may start with small doses (50–75 mg/month) of the long-acting esters enanthate or cypionate for 3–6 months. After 6–12 months, testosterone administration should be held, and reevaluation of possible spontaneous puberty should be performed. If spontaneous puberty has not occurred, then testosterone therapy should be restarted, gradually titrated up to 100–150 mg/month, and changed to twice monthly administration.[33] After achieving full virilization and an adult height, any of the available testosterone formulations may be used.[33–35] In persons with permanent hypogonadism, treatment with testosterone should be lifelong.[35]

Adults

In young men with infertility, testosterone therapy is not recommended because testosterone decreases sperm count and has in fact been investigated as a male contraceptive agent in combination with progesterone.[1] In adult men who do not wish fertility, different formulations of testosterone are available; these will be discussed later in this chapter.

Infertility in hypogonadal men is generally treated by a specialist in male reproductive endocrinology. In primary testicular failure, it is generally not possible to achieve fertility; however, in many of secondary cases of MHG, infertility may be treatable. Depending on the time of development of MHG, the goal is either to restore or to initiate spermatogenesis. Several agents are available to stimulate testosterone synthesis and spermatogenesis. GnRH, hCG, and FSH[36–38] are very expensive and require injections as the mode of administration. Sperm production with these agents approaches 85–100%, depending on underlying pathology and previous pubertal development in patients with hypogonadotropic hypogonadism, and reported pregnancy rates range between 50 and 90%.[38–40] Clomiphene citrate increases endogenous GnRH secretion and promotes intratesticular testosterone concentrations. This mode of treatment is less successful (only 64.3% demonstrated sperm in their semen analyses)[41] but is more convenient and less expensive and may be used as a first-line treatment.

The goal of replacement testosterone therapy for MHG in men who do not wish fertility is to provide physiologic concentrations of testosterone levels, dihydrotestosterone (DHT), and estradiol, which would allow optimal virilization and normal sexual function with minimal adverse effects. Before testosterone replacement, a careful prostate examination and testing for prostate-specific antigen (PSA) should be performed to ensure that there is no significant prostate pathology present. Other comorbidities should be considered and kept in mind during the course of treatment with testosterone. Breast and prostate cancer and severe erythrocytosis (hematocrit, >55%) are absolute contraindications to testosterone treatment, whereas severe obstructive sleep apnea, moderate erythrocytosis (hematocrit, 52–55%), and severe symptomatic benign prostatic hypertrophy are relative contraindications.[1]

Testosterone Preparations

Intramuscular Injections

Before 1990, intramuscular injections of testosterone were the only available form of testosterone replacement in men with hypogonadism. The long-acting testosterone esters make this mode of therapy the most cost-effective choice and consist of intramuscular injections every 1–2 weeks. They are associated with a peak and trough in testosterone concentrations, which may be associated with mood swings and other symptoms. Local skin irritation occurs in one third of the patients. Testosterone and estrogen (not DHT) levels rise to supraphysiologic levels for several days after the injection.[42]

Transdermal Patches

Only the transdermal patch is currently available in the United States. The transdermal patch may cause mild skin irritation in up to 60% of men; however, this approach is otherwise is generally well tolerated and restores testosterone, DHT, and estrogen levels to physiologic ranges.[42]

Testosterone Gel

Testosterone gel provides a very easy and convenient method for testosterone replacement, restoring testosterone and estrogen into the physiologic range, but DHT levels are often moderately elevated. A recent study of therapy with testosterone patches versus 1% testosterone gel demonstrated that nightly application of the transdermal patch yielded serum testosterone profiles mimicking the circadian pattern of healthy men. Morning application of testosterone gel provided a flatter mean profile with occasional variable peaks. DHT was found to be markedly higher in patients who received gel treatment. Otherwise, both preparations met the criteria for bioequivalence.[43]

Transmucosal Administration

Buccal bioadhesive testosterone is applied twice daily and normalizes both testosterone and DHT levels. It is associated with fairly high rate of local irritation (up to 16.3%).[44]

Other Treatment Modalities

Transdermal DHT administration in a 6-month, double-blind, randomized controlled trial involving 114 Finnish men with a mean age 58 years was reported to lead to an improvement of sexual performance and a decrease of estrogen, testosterone, SHBG, LH, and FSH levels. Prostate volume and PSA measurements, as well as liver function test results, did not change appreciably; hemoglobin and hematocrit increased, but not to dangerous levels.[45]

Anastrozole is a potent aromatase inhibitor that decreases estrogen production and increases androgen production in men. In one trial, the treatment of elderly men with mild hypogonadism for a period of 12 weeks led to an increase of total and bioavailable testosterone levels and the decrease of serum estradiol levels.[45]

Adverse Effects of Testosterone Treatment

Urogenital

Excessive frequency and duration of penile erections may require urgent treatment and, therefore, the patient has to be informed about this possibility before the initiation of therapy. Priapism is a rare complication and is more frequently reported in adolescents treated for delayed puberty[46]; however, it still occurs in adults.[47]

Prostate hypertrophy or possible stimulation of growth of preexisting prostate cancer has long been thought to be a risk of testosterone replacement therapy. This suspicion has been raised because of evidence that suppression (or elimination) of endogenous testosterone synthesis is effective in causing regression of many prostate cancers. There is, however, currently no evidence that testosterone replacement is associated with a significantly higher risk of prostate cancer.[48–50] Because this matter is still unsettled, most authorities recommend routine screening for prostate pathology, including an inquiry about urinary problems and an annual digital rectal examination and PSA test, in men taking testosterone replacement therapy.[1,50,51]

Skin and Appendage

Irritative or allergic skin reactions with testosterone treatment are observed frequently, especially in cases of nonscrotal testosterone patches.[50] Gynecomastia is believed to arise as a result of peripheral conversion of testosterone into estrogen, which is in part dependent on the modality of testosterone replacement. A single case report suggests satisfactory response to the aromatase inhibitor anastrozole[52]; however, significant gynecomastia may require withdrawal of treatment.

Gastrointestinal

Nausea, cholestatic jaundice, alterations in liver function test results, and, rarely, hepatocellular neoplasm and peliosis hepatis (i.e., sinusoidal dilatations forming large blood cysts scattered throughout the liver) have been noted in men taking anabolic steroids. These adverse reactions do not occur with testosterone treatment, and therefore the Endocrine Society guidelines do not recommend follow-up liver function tests on a routine basis as part of testosterone replacement therapy.[1]

Hematologic

In a meta-analysis of 19 randomized clinical trials, Calof and colleagues[53] reported that an increase in hematocrit level was the most frequent adverse event associated with testosterone replacement. Men taking testosterone therapy were almost four times more likely to develop an elevation of hemoglobin and hematocrit levels than persons in the placebo group.[53]

Metabolic

Changes in serum cholesterol are common in men taking testosterone therapy. A meta-analysis of 29 randomized controlled trials undertaken by Isidori and colleagues[54] reported that men treated with testosterone have a reduced total serum cholesterol level, with no change in low-density lipoprotein cholesterol levels. High-density

lipoprotein cholesterol changes were not uniform and possibly were related to the mode of administration and the different formulation of testosterone used, especially the effect on aromatization.

Pulmonary

One study determined that testosterone treatment may worsen obstructive sleep apnea without change of upper airway dimension even after short-term testosterone administration.[55]

Miscellaneous

Transfer to children and women may occur with testosterone gels, if close skin-to-skin contact happens shortly after the application of the gel. This is easily prevented by wearing a thin layer of clothing, hand washing, and careful avoidance.[43]

Drug Abuse and Dependence

Testosterone and other anabolic steroids are common drugs of abuse, particularly among male athletes and body builders.[56] For this reason, testosterone preparations are classified as a controlled substance under the Anabolic Steroids Control Act of 1990 and have been assigned to the US Drug Enforcement Administration Schedule III.

Drug/Laboratory Test Interferences

Androgens may decrease levels of thyroxin-binding globulin, resulting in decreased total thyroxine serum levels and increased resin uptake of triiodothyronine and thyroxine. Free thyroid hormone levels remain unchanged, however, and there is no clinical evidence of thyroid dysfunction in reported studies.

Monitoring

Prepuberty

It is important to ensure the proper progression of puberty in hypogonadal boys. Therefore, monitoring of secondary sex characteristics and growth is imperative through the following of standard developmental milestones.

Adults with Fertility Issues

Testicular size is predictive of spermatogenesis, and it is recommended to assess size by palpation or Doppler ultrasound examination every 3–6 months. Testosterone levels and estradiol levels should be monitored every 6–12 months to prevent supraphysiologic levels and to avoid adverse effects. Semen analysis should be monitored every 6 months after normalization of testosterone level.

Testosterone Replacement in Adults

The monitoring of serum testosterone levels depends on the formulation used. The testosterone level should be assessed at the mid point of the injection interval for intramuscular preparations. For patches, testosterone levels should be measured 10–12 hours after application of the patch; for buccal administration, immediately before application of a new pellet; and for gel, after 1–2 weeks of use.[1]

Because testosterone may stimulate erythropoiesis, the hematocrit level should be monitored at 3–6 months after the start of therapy and then annually thereafter. If an elevation of hematocrit of more than 54% is seen, then testosterone treatment should be held until the hematocrit level returns to normal. Afterwards, the administration of testosterone may be restarted at lower dose.[1]

BMD of lumbar spine and total femoral neck should be checked via DEXA scanning at the baseline and 1–2 years after testosterone therapy is initiated. Symptoms of sleep apnea should be formally evaluated at 3–6 months after commencement of therapy, and then annually thereafter.

As mentioned above, a PSA measurement and digital rectal examination should be performed 3–6 months after the initiation of testosterone therapy, and then according to standard guidelines for prostate cancer screening. A referral for further urologic evaluation is indicated if any of the following occur:

- The PSA is greater than 4.0 ng/mL at any point.
- There is an increase of PSA greater than 1.4 ng/mL over any 12-month period.
- The change in the PSA is more than 0.4 ng/mL-year over at least a 2-year period using the baseline value during the first 6 months of testosterone therapy as a reference.[1]

If significant urologic symptoms arise or if a prostatic abnormality is detected during a digital rectal examination, consultation with a urologist should be considered.[51]

Osteoporosis

Introduction

Osteoporosis in men represents an often unrecognized but very serious condition that is associated with high morbidity and mortality resultant from complications, as nearly 2 million men in the United States are affected by this disease.[57] Up to 30% of hip fractures occur in men, and the mortality rate in men is twice as high as in women.[58] Male osteoporosis remains vastly undertreated, even in the population of men with fragility fractures. In one study, only 16% of men with a hip or vertebral fracture received treatment for osteoporosis during the 6 months after discharge for their fracture.[59] Approximately 50% of cases of male osteoporosis have a secondary cause.[60]

Definition

A 2000 National Institutes of Health Consensus Panel on Osteoporosis defines the disorder as "a systemic skeletal disorder characterized by compromised bone strength predisposing to an increased risk of fracture."[61] Bone strength depends on bone size, shape, mineral density, and quality. BMD is measured by a DEXA scan and reflects bone mineralization (measured as gram of calcium hydroxyapatite per square centimeter). The World Health Organization definition of osteoporosis is based on the measurement of BMD,[62] which is expressed as a T-score (i.e., the number of standard deviations from the mean compared with the mean BMD for young adult healthy people) and Z-score (i.e., the number of standard deviations from the mean for people of the same age group) (Table 9-3). A BMD between −1 and −2.5 is considered to be osteopenic, less than −2.5 indicative of osteoporosis, and greater than −1 is in the normal range.[62] A low BMD was found to be the best predictor of hip, vertebral, and other fractures in several studies[63–65] and remains a widely accepted method of diagnosis and follow-up of osteoporosis in the US population and in the world.

There is, however, a certain amount of controversy regarding the diagnosis of osteoporosis by DEXA in men. For any given age, the BMD in the spine is lower in women than in men, and after adjusting for age, the BMD in the femoral neck is higher in men and than women.[64] Consequently, the International Society for Clinical Densitometry[66] currently recommends use of a uniform, non–race-adjusted male normative database for men of all ethnic groups.

With these caveats in mind, osteoporosis can be diagnosed in men age 50 years and older if the T-score of the lumbar spine, total hip, or femoral neck is −2.5 or less. In men younger than 50 years of age, the diagnosis of osteoporosis cannot be made solely on the basis of low BMD; instead, other factors including a history of fragility

Table 9-3. Calculation of T- and Z-Scores for Bone Mineral Density (BMD) and Parameters Used in the Diagnosis of Osteopenia and Osteoporosis

The following equation is used to calculate a T-score: T-score = [(measured BMD − young adult population mean BMD)/young adult population SD].   A Z-score is the number of SDs above or below the mean for a gender-, ethnicity-, and age-matched healthy population.   A Z-score is calculated from the following equation: Z-score = [(measured BMD − age-matched population mean BMD)/age-matched population SD]

SD, Standard deviation.

Adapted from: Assessment of fracture risk and its application to screening for postmenopausal osteoporosis: report of a WHO Study Group, *World Health Organ Tech Rep Ser* 843:1–129, 1994.

fracture or secondary causes of osteoporosis should be present[62] (Table 9-4).

The gold standard of bone-quality assessment is histomorphology, although with technologic developments, other modalities are currently used (e.g., ultrasound and high-resolution magnetic resonance imaging). These approaches provide assessment of the trabecular microarchitecture, which bone densitometry does not offer. The results of histomorphology studies suggest a strong association of trabecular bone microarchitecture with risk of vertebral fractures in men with osteoporosis.[67–69]

Pathophysiology

The skeleton consists of 80% cortical and 20% trabecular bone. The cortex is an external thick and dense layer of calcified bone that surrounds the medullary cavity containing bone marrow. The shafts of the long bones and bones of the appendicular skeleton are examples of cortical bone. Trabecular bone, also known as spongy or calculous bone, consists of a network of thin trabeculae surrounding cavities, which contain hemopoietic cells. Vertebral bodies, pelvis, and ends of long bones are the examples of trabecular bone.

The turnover of the bone is a dynamic process and involves generally two types of cells, namely osteoblasts and osteoclasts. *Osteoclasts* are responsible for the resorption of old, damaged, or underused bone, and *osteoblasts* are responsible for laying down replacement bone tissue, which becomes mineralized and leads to the formation of remodeled bone. As the osteoblast matures, it gradually develops into an *osteocyte* and becomes incorporated into the bone matrix. Bone mineral content provides mechanical rigidity and load-bearing strength and depends on the balance between the actions of the osteoclasts and osteoblasts, that is, between bone resorption and new bone formation. An imbalance in this dynamic relationship leads to bone loss. Histomorphologic studies demonstrate that in osteoporotic bone, trabecular structure changes; and this leads to an overall change of microarchitecture and microfractures.[69,70]

Bone formation and resorption are influenced by multiple hormones, cytokines, and growth factors. The most important regulators are parathyroid hormone (PTH), vitamin D, gonadal and corticosteroids, growth hormone, and insulin-like growth factor-1. Any disruption in the normal physiology of those hormonal systems may lead

Table 9-4. WHO 1994 Diagnostic Criteria for Osteoporosis in Men 20 Years of Age and Older

Age	T-scores	Other Factors
<50 years old	−2.5 or less (male reference database)	Presence of a fragility fracture
50–65 years	−2.5 or less (male reference database)	Other risk factors for fracture are identified
>65 years of age	−2.5 or less (male reference database)	Other factors may be present or absent

Note: This classification was originally designed for white postmenopausal women.[62] According to the latest International Society for Clinical Densitometry Official Position Statement,[67,68] for men younger than 50 years old, a Z-score less than −2 should be considered as "below the expected range for age," and for men older than 50 years old, a T-score should be used with the uniform white (non–race-adjusted) male normative database for men of all ethnic groups.

Adapted from: Assessment of fracture risk and its application to screening for postmenopausal osteoporosis: report of a WHO Study Group, *World Health Organ Tech Rep Ser* 843:1–129, 1994.

to or be associated with bone abnormality and osteoporosis.

The bone matrix contains collagen (predominantly type I), which provides elasticity and bone flexibility. Conditions and disorders affecting collagen formation or structure could be associated with increased fragility and risk of fractures (e.g., osteogenesis imperfecta, Ehlers-Danlos syndrome, scurvy, and homocystinuria).[71–73]

BMD depends on the rate of accrual of bone at a young age; consequently, it depends on the age of puberty, nutritional factors, and exercise.[74–76] For this reason, delayed puberty, nutritional deficiencies (calcium and vitamin D), and lack of exercise at early age may be associated with lower bone density accrual and earlier development of a lower level of BMD.[77]

Clinical Presentation

The most common clinical manifestation of osteoporosis is vertebral compression fractures; low impact fractures, particularly of the hip, are also a common clinical manifestation of osteoporosis. This type of fracture is characterized as occurring from a fall from a height no greater than the patient's standing height. Likewise, osteoporosis may present as a spontaneous fragility fracture occurring from activities such as coughing, sneezing, or abrupt movements. A Colles' fracture of the wrist is also commonly seen in osteoporosis.[78]

Classification and Risk Factors

In most cases, osteoporosis is a multifactorial disorder and may be classified as either primary or secondary. According to Riggs and Melton,[79] primary osteoporosis can be classified as type I or type II. *Type I* osteoporosis predominantly affects women after menopause (female-to-male ratio of 6:1) and is associated with wrist fractures and vertebral compression fractures; cortical bone is primarily affected in this type of osteoporosis. *Type II* osteoporosis is age-related (originally called "involutional" or "senile" osteoporosis) and affects both women and men (female-to-male ratio 2:1) who are generally older than 70 years. This type of osteoporosis is associated with hip fractures and vertebral wedge fractures and affects both trabecular and cortical bone.[80]

Primary osteoporosis includes the osteoporosis of aging and idiopathic osteoporosis, which can present in men of any age. Genetic factors are very important in the development of idiopathic osteoporosis and associated fractures; twin and family studies suggest that between 50% and 80% of the variance in the incidence of osteoporosis is genetically determined, and several quantitative trait loci have been identified on linkage analysis.[81–83]

Recent evidence suggests that estrogen in men also plays an important role in regulation of the male skeleton. In several independent observational studies, increased BMD correlated with total and bioavailable estrogen but not testosterone in men, and decreased serum estradiol levels in men were associated with decreased BMD.[84–86] In addition, a possible association between idiopathic osteoporosis abnormalities in the growth hormone and insulin-like growth factor-1 have been reported.[87]

Secondary osteoporosis is osteoporosis that is caused or exacerbated by illness, medical conditions, medications, or drugs. Secondary causes of osteoporosis are more common among premenopausal women, and in men, up to 64% of cases of severe osteoporosis have a secondary cause.[88] Various factors can contribute to secondary osteoporosis (Table 9-5). Depending on the age of presentation, different comorbidities and secondary causes of osteoporosis have to be considered.[89] Osteoporosis occurring at a younger age may be found in patients with cystic fibrosis, malabsorptive syndromes, congenital or acquired early hypogonadism, and conditions requiring frequent use of corticosteroid preparations.[74,90,91] Prevention and diagnosis of osteoporosis in young men with sickle cell anemia and other hemoglobinopathies is also paramount.[92,93] Although anorexia nervosa is more frequently observed in girls and young women, it may occur in boys and young men as well and should be considered as a possible culprit behind the development of osteoporosis in younger men.[94] In the older male population, glucocorticoid use, hypogonadism, and alcoholism are the most prevalent causes of secondary osteoporosis.[61] The increased prevalence of coexisting disorders with aging, such as chronic renal and hepatic disease, alcoholism, chronic obstructive pulmonary disease, and hyperthyroidism may be associated with secondary osteoporosis and should be considered as well in any older man presenting with decreased BMD. Certain diseases including chronic inflammatory autoimmune conditions, endocrinopathies, malignancies, and malabsorptive states are commonly related to bone loss and should be considered during evaluation of men with osteoporosis.[95]

Table 9-5. Secondary Causes of Osteoporosis

Factors	Examples
Congenital conditions	Homocystinuria; porphyria; hypophosphatasia; osteogenesis imperfecta; Ehlers-Danlos syndrome; Marfan syndrome Congenital hypogonadal states: Turner syndrome; Klinefelter syndrome; androgen insensitivity
Nutritional and gastrointestinal disorders	Anorexia nervosa; inflammatory bowel disease; primary biliary cirrhosis; calcium, magnesium or vitamin D deficiency; malabsorption syndromes (e.g., celiac disease); scurvy; starvation
Drugs	Alcohol; anticonvulsants; cancer chemotherapy; excess thyroid hormone; glucocorticoids; heparin and warfarin; immunosuppressive agents (e.g., cyclosporine and tacrolimus)
Endocrine disorders	Primary and secondary hyperparathyroidism; Cushing's syndrome; growth hormone deficiency; adrenal insufficiency; hyperthyroidism; hypogonadism; diabetes mellitus
Other systemic disorders	Leukemias and lymphomas; hemaglobinopathies (e.g., sickle cell disease and thalassemia); hemochromatosis; systemic mastocytosis; multiple myeloma; renal tubular acidosis; rheumatoid arthritis
Other conditions	Alcoholism; immobility; congestive heart failure; cystic fibrosis; sarcoidosis; amyloidosis; end-stage renal disease

Adapted from: Kelepouris N, Harper KD, Gannon, F et al: Severe osteoporosis in men, *Ann Int Med* 123(6):452–460, 1995; Templeton K: Secondary osteoporosis, *J Am Acad Orthop Surg* 13(7):475–486, 2005.

Risk Factors

Risk factors for fractures and osteoporosis may be considered as modifiable or nonmodifiable. Some risk factors for fractures are also risk factors for osteoporosis, and some are independent of BMD. Nonmodifiable risk factors include advanced age (e.g., older than 65 years), race and ethnicity (Asian and white persons are at higher risk), genetics, and delayed puberty. Modifiable risk factors include vitamin D deficiency, cigarette smoking, sedentary lifestyle or prolonged immobilization, low body weight, excessive alcohol consumption, increased likelihood of falling, glucocorticoid use, solid organ or bone marrow transplantation, and previous fragility fracture.

Another important risk factor for osteoporotic fractures, particularly of the hip, is a low BMI. De Laet and colleagues[96] performed a meta-analysis of 12 prospective population-based cohorts comprising nearly 60,000 men and women and reported that the BMI is a very important independent risk factor for osteoporotic fracture for any age and gender; however, BMI-associated risk was dependent on BMD. The same meta-analysis found a nonlinear relationship between the BMI and osteoporotic fractures, with a greater association between low BMI and fracture risk. For example, when compared with persons with a BMI of 25 kg/m^3, persons with a BMI of 20 kg/m^3 had a nearly two-fold increase in the risk ratio of fracture, whereas the decrease in the risk ratio was only 17% in persons with a BMI of 30 kg/m^3.[96]

Risk factors for osteoporotic fractures are less clearly identified in middle-aged men. A 25-year follow-up from the population-based Framingham study[97] found that few factors, with the exception of alcohol use and a history of previous vertebral fractures, predicted long-term risk of vertebral fractures in men. Factors including age, height, weight, grip strength, physical activity, metacarpal cortical area, and estrogen use (in women) had little or no effect on the cumulative incidence of vertebral fracture.[97] Similarly, the European Prospective Osteoporosis Study, which observed a total of 3173 men (mean age, 63.1 years) and 3402 women (mean age, 62.2 years) for 3.8 years, found that none of the lifestyle factors studied—including smoking, alcohol intake, physical activity, or milk consumption—showed any consistent associations with incidental vertebral fracture.[98] In men and women, increasing body weight and BMI were associated with a reduced risk of vertebral fracture; however, this was only significant with regard to the BMI in men.[98] To clarify the factors underlying fracture risk in older men, an even larger study[99] is in progress with 5995 men of at least 65 years of age. This study is designed to evaluate risk factors for fracture and how fractures affect the quality of life over 4.5 years of observation.

Diagnosis

The International Society for Clinical Densitometry recommends bone densitometry in women after the age of 65 years and men after 70 years in patients with secondary causes of osteoporosis and in those taking medications associated with the potential for low bone mass or bone loss and after any fragility fracture.[66] These recommendations, however, are not universally accepted. A recent National Institutes of Health (NIH) Consensus Panel[61] on osteoporosis reported general agreement that bone densitometry should be considered in all persons taking glucocorticoids for 2 months or more and for persons with other conditions that placed them at high risk for osteoporotic fractures. In addition, this panel concluded that the value of universal screening for osteoporosis, especially in perimenopausal women, was not clearly established by clinical evidence, and interestingly, no consensus regarding screening of older men who were not in high-risk categories was reached.[61]

All patients with osteoporosis or a fragility fracture should undergo a minimal laboratory screening to rule out secondary causes and to establish comorbidities (Table 9-6). It should be emphasized that the laboratory evaluation of possible causes of secondary osteoporosis should be guided by clinical assessment of individual patients and should not be performed in a "cookbook" fashion. Currently, there is no consensus regarding routine use of serum or urine markers of bone turnover for diagnosis and monitoring of osteoporosis, but there are some clinical data to support this approach.[100,101]

Treatment and Prevention

As is true with the diagnosis of osteoporosis, most of the clinical evidence on its prevention and treatment has been gathered in women. In this section, we will discuss general approaches to, and the evidence basis underlying, the prevention and treatment of primary and secondary osteoporosis and will cite specific clinical trials investigating their efficacy in men.

Primary Osteoporosis

Nonpharmacologic Approaches. Although nutritional factors and exercise play important roles in bone remodeling and strength, with the exception of dietary calcium and vitamin D supplementation, there is a paucity of evidence demonstrating a positive role of exercise or nutritional factors (e.g., dietary protein, magnesium, fluoride, or milk) in lowering fracture risk in either women or men.[102,103] A recent meta-analysis by Lock and colleagues[103] investigated the effectiveness of lifestyle interventions including exercise on fracture risk in people at high risk of osteoporosis. In six randomized controlled trials, exercise was found to decrease fracture risk in postmenopausal women (men were not studied); however, the difference was not statistically significant. Likewise, multifactorial interventions, including environmental modifications, exercise, and review of medications and aids, resulted in a non–statistically significant decline in fracture risk in women and men.[103] Lock and colleagues indicated that a clear interpretation of the available clinical evidence is hampered by the small numbers of subjects and the heterogeneity of approaches. Therefore, specific nutritional and exercise interventions cannot be recommended at this time.

Calcium and Vitamin D. The importance of adequate calcium and vitamin D intake for bone health has been recognized for decades. It is of great importance to have sufficient dietary vitamin D and calcium to avoid osteomalacia and to maintain normal bone mineralization. The Food and Nutrition Board of the US Institute of Medicine[104] has recommended a calcium intake of 1000 mg of elemental calcium a day for adults aged 18–50 years old, and 1200 mg/day for adults older than the age of 50 years. The average US diet consists of approximately 600 mg of calcium daily[105] and, therefore, falls far short of the recommended intake.

Calcium supplementation may take two forms, either calcium carbonate (containing 40% elemental calcium) or calcium citrate (containing 23% elemental calcium). Several recent meta-analyses of randomized clinical trials[106–108] concluded that calcium supplementation is associated with slowing bone loss in postmenopausal women. Evidence from large clinical trials in men is lacking for calcium supplementation alone; the evidence from clinical trials investigating use of calcium and vitamin D supplementation in men is discussed below.

There are several options for vitamin D supplementation. Cholecalciferol is a form of vitamin D_3 that is derived from animal sources, and ergocalciferol is a form of vitamin D_2 derived from plant sources. Vitamin D_2 and D_3 formulations

Table 9-6. Recommendations for Ancillary Tests in the Evaluation of Possible Secondary Osteoporosis

A biochemical profile that includes the following:
Renal function
Hepatic function
Serum calcium (important if starting an anti-resorptive or anabolic agent) - Elevated in hyperparathyroidism and decreased in malabsorption, vitamin D deficiency, hypoparathyroidism
Serum alkaline phosphatase - Elevated in Paget's disease, prolonged immobilization, acute fractures and other bone diseases
Serum phosphorus - Decreased in osteomalacia
The following other laboratory evaluations, depending on clinical suspicion:
A complete blood count may uncover bone marrow malignancy or infiltrative process or malabsorption (e.g., anemia, microcytosis, or macrocytosis)
Serum parathyroid hormone - Elevated PTH is diagnostic of hyperparathyroidism (primary, secondary or tertiary), and a low PTH suggests hypoparathyroidism
Serum 25-hydroxy vitamin D - A low serum concentration suggests vitamin D deficiency or osteomalacia
Serum total testosterone in men
FSH, LH, and prolactin if there is evidence of hypogonadotropic hypogonadism
An elevated ESR or CRP level may indicate an inflammatory process or monoclonal gammopathy
Serum TSH
A 24-hour urinary calcium excretion on a high-calcium diet may screen for malabsorption and hypercalciuria, a correctable cause of bone loss - Low 24-hour urine calcium suggests vitamin D deficiency, osteomalacia, or malabsorption due to small bowel diseases, such as celiac sprue
Tissue transglutaminase antibodies, if there is a clinical suspicion for gluten-sensitive enteropathy (celiac disease)
A 24-hour urinary free cortisol or overnight dexamethasone suppression test, if there is clinical suspicion of Cushing's syndrome
Serum and urine protein electrophoresis, if multiple myeloma is suspected

Note: These recommendations should be individually tailored for the individual clinical status of each patient

PTH, Parathyroid hormone; FSH, follicle stimulating hormone; LH, luteinizing hormone; ESR, erythrocyte sedimentation rate; CRP, C-reactive protein; TSH, thyroid-stimulating hormone.

Adapted from: Looker AC, Bauer DC, Chestnut CH 3rd, et al: Clinical use of biochemical markers of bone remodeling: current status and future directions, *Osteoporos Int* 11(6):467–480, 2000; and Bonnick S, Saag KG, Kiel DP, et al: Comparison of weekly treatment of postmenopausal osteoporosis with alendronate versus risedronate over two years, *J Clin Endocrinol Metab* 91(7):2631–2637, 2006.

have been traditionally considered to be equivalent with a half-life of approximately 2–3 weeks. Ergocalciferol is available as a capsule of 50,000 IU, and cholecalciferol is available as 400–1000-IU pills. A study[109] of 30 men who took 50,000 IU of ergocalciferol or cholecalciferol demonstrated that despite good absorption of both compounds, the serum concentration of total 25-hydroxy vitamin D decreased to the pre-study level at day 14 after the ergocalciferol dose, whereas the total serum vitamin D concentrations began to decline slowly after 15 days after cholecalciferol dose and were still 13 nmol/liter above the pre-study level at 28 days.

In some clinical conditions, such as chronic renal insufficiency and hypoparathyroidism, there is a defect in conversion of 25-hydroxy vitamin D into 1,25-dihydroxy vitamin D. For this reason, treatment with vitamin D analogs may be appropriate for replacement. There are three forms of vitamin D analogs: calcitriol, paricalcitol, and doxercalciferol. The mean elimination half-lives for these preparations are 3.5, 5–7, and 11.6 hours, respectively.[110]

With regard to vitamin D therapy, a recent meta-analysis by Bischoff-Ferrari and colleagues[111] of 12 randomized controlled studies in elderly persons involving a total of 3219 men (five studies for hip fracture [n = 9820] and seven for nonvertebral fractures [n = 9294]) reported that vitamin D (cholecalciferol) at a daily dose of 700–800 IU was associated with a 26% risk reduction of hip fractures and a 23% risk reduction of nonvertebral fractures. Trials using lower doses of 400 IU showed no beneficial effect.[111] A subgroup analysis by gender revealed that only one study (men, n = 2037) reported the results on hip fracture risk reduction in men and demonstrated a significant risk reduction for hip and vertebral fractures in men taking vitamin D compared with placebo.[112]

The 1997 recommendation by the Food and Nutrition Board of the Institute of Medicine[104] for vitamin D intake is 10 µg/day (400 IU/day) for persons aged 51–70 years old and 15 µg/day (600 IU/day) for persons older than 70 years. The most recent NIH Consensus Statement[61] recommends a daily amount of vitamin D of 400–600 IU; however, in light of more recent evidence, a higher intake is probably warranted. In terms of therapy, a dose of at least 700 IU is appropriate.[111] In discussing racial and ethnic differences in serum vitamin D levels and BMD, Dawson-Hughes[113] concluded that for improved bone health the serum 25-hydroxy vitamin D level should be 80 nmol/liter, and to achieve that concentration, 800–1000 IU/day of vitamin D is required, regardless of race and ethnicity.

Medical treatment for osteoporosis may be divided into anti-resorptive and anabolic agents; various options are discussed below.

Bisphosphonates. The most effective and commonly used class of anti-resorptive agents is the bisphosphonates. The principal mode of action of these drugs is to serve as potent inhibitors of osteoclast action on bone resorption. There are three approved agents in the United States for the treatment of osteoporosis: alendronate (Fosamax; Merck), risedronate (Actonel; Proctor and Gamble), and ibandronate (Boniva; Roche-GlaxoSmithKline). These are oral agents that should be taken on an empty stomach, and patients are instructed to remain in an upright position for at least 30 minutes to increase absorption and to avoid gastrointestinal adverse effects, such as esophageal inflammation or, rarely, ulceration.[114] An intravenous form of ibandronate was recently approved by the US Food and Drug Administration for the treatment of osteoporosis.

Bisphosphonates have been shown to increase BMD at the spine, hip, and total body and to prevent vertebral and hip fractures in women.[115,116] In men, the majority of the data on osteoporosis treatment are available for alendronate,[117,118] and these demonstrate that once-daily alendronate at a dose of 10 mg results in significant increases in BMD of the spine and hip compared with placebo.[118] The optimal duration of treatment has not yet been established, but longitudinal data in women receiving alendronate are available and suggest that alendronate is effective and well tolerated for up to 10 years of therapy.[119]

One obstacle to successful therapy with the bisphosphonates has been the difficulty of taking a medication with significant adverse effects on a daily basis. Data for once-weekly administration for alendronate and risedronate suggest that once-weekly dosing is comparable to daily dosing in preserving BMD.[120–123] Recently, the results of a 2-year trial[124] of once-monthly (50, 100, or 150 mg) versus daily (2.5 mg) ibandronate have been published and report that the once-monthly regimens result in similar increases in BMD for lumbar spine and hip in postmenopausal women. There are, however, no similar results in men with osteoporosis.

Human Parathyroid Hormone. PTH is a peptide released by the parathyroid glands in response to decreasing serum ionized calcium levels. PTH increases serum calcium by stimulating osteoclast activity (with resultant release of calcium and phosphorus from bone), increasing renal resorption of calcium and stimulation of the conversion of 25-hydroxyvitamin D to 1,25-dihydroxyvitamin D with a subsequent increase in intestinal absorption of calcium. PTH is catabolic to bone with constant exposure; however, with intermittent exposure, it acts as an anabolic agent and stimulates bone formation.[125] Recombinant forms of human PTH (hPTH) comprising fragments 1–34 and 1–84 of the native hormone have been studied, and hPTH (1–34) is currently approved for the use in United States and marketed under the trade name Forteo (teriparatide; Eli Lilly).

Teriparatide has been shown to be effective in improving the BMD in vertebrae and hips in postmenopausal women and men via daily subcutaneous injection[126,127] and in decreasing both vertebral and nonvertebral fracture risk in women.[126] There are currently no clinical data regarding the effectiveness of teriparatide on fracture risk in men.

With regard to combination therapy, the combination of the anabolic hPTH (1–84) and the anti-resorptive agent alendronate in a 2-year trial in 238 postmenopausal women did not show any benefits of combined therapy compared with hPTH (1–84) or alendronate alone.[128] Similar results were reported in 83 men (i.e., 28 receiving alendronate, 20 receiving hPTH [1–34], and 25 in combination therapy groups) over a 30-month treatment period.[129] It has been suggested that the anabolic effects on bone formation by teriparatide is blocked by the actions of the bisphosphonate.[129]

Adverse effects of teriparatide use include nausea, dizziness, and orthostatic hypotension, which may occur early in the course of treatment.[126,127,129] The greatest concern with this agent is the possibility of stimulating the development of an osteosarcoma during prolonged therapy. Observations of a dose-dependent increase in the prevalence of osteosarcomas in rats after 2 years of therapy[130] led to the early termination of clinical trials with this agent.[125] As Compston[125] indicates in his review, however, extrapolation of the animal data to humans is problematic because of the high doses administered to the rats (up to 75 μg/kg/day) and the more rapid bone turnover in rats compared with humans. Nonetheless, it is not recommended to use teriparatide in humans for more than 2 years.

Calcitonin. Calcitonin is a polypeptide hormone secreted by the parafollicular "C" cells of the thyroid in response to elevated serum calcium concentrations; however, it plays no known role of significance in normal calcium metabolism.[131] At pharmacologic doses, calcitonin has been shown to inhibit osteoclast function, and it has occasionally been used for the treatment of hypercalcemia of malignancy, albeit, with limited effect.[132] The major therapeutic role of calcitonin is in the treatment of osteoporosis. Use of calcitonin is generally associated with lower increases in the BMD and very modest risk reductions in vertebral fractures compared with the bisphosphonates[133] and, therefore, it is considered to be a second-line agent and should be reserved for patients who are intolerant of bisphosphonates or who are experiencing acute pain from vertebral fractures.[134] It is indicated for the treatment of osteoporosis in postmenopausal women; however, very few studies exist on its efficacy in men.[135] Calcitonin from salmon is used in most preparations, due to its increased potency (50–60 times greater than the human form of the hormone). Administered via nasal spray or injections, it is generally well tolerated.[131]

Selective Estrogen Receptor Modulators. Selective estrogen receptor modulators carry an anti-resorptive effect through their agonist effects on estrogen receptors. Raloxifene has been proved to be beneficial for the treatment and prevention of osteoporosis and has been shown to produce a reduction of vertebral fracture risk in postmenopausal women[136]; it has been shown to be generally well tolerated in men. Raloxifene's effect on BMD and fracture risk in men has not been reported; however, its effect on bone resorption markers was studied in a 6-week randomized, placebo-controlled, double-blind, crossover study in healthy middle-aged men.[137] The administration of raloxifene led to an increase in serum testosterone and estradiol concentrations; however, raloxifene decreased bone resorption markers only in men with low serum estradiol concentrations at baseline.[137] More studies of selective estrogen receptor modulators in a subgroup of men with low estradiol levels are necessary to investigate its effect on BMD and fracture risk and its possible use in the treatment of osteoporosis in men.

Other Agents. Selective androgen receptor modulators are currently under investigation and appear to improve cortical bone and prevent the loss of trabecular bone in orchiectomized rats.[138] Denosumab, a human monoclonal antibody to the receptor activator of nuclear factor-B (RANK) ligand, interferes with osteoclast differentiation, activation, and survival and has an anti-resorptive effect on bone. A 12-month clinical trial[139] in women with osteoporosis showed increases in BMD at the spine and hip comparable to that produced by alendronate and greater than that by placebo. There is, however, a concern that denosumab may affect the immune system as well as bone, and concerns over possible increased risk of infection, tumors, and adynamic bone have been raised.[140] Almost all of these agents have been studied in osteoporotic women, and data regarding treatment of osteoporosis in men are lacking.

Secondary Osteoporosis

The first step in the treatment of secondary osteoporosis is to eliminate or correct the underlying condition, if possible. Additional treatment strategies are highlighted below.

Hypogonadism: Testosterone Replacement Therapy. Osteoporosis is a well-known complication of hypogonadism.[141] It is recommended to replace testosterone in hypogonadal men with osteoporosis if there are no contraindications to hormone replacement therapy, such as a history of prostate cancer. With respect to osteoporosis, testosterone possesses an anti-resorptive activity, possibly through aromatization and conversion to estrogen. A meta-analysis[142] of eight studies (n = 365 men) revealed that replacement of testosterone via intramuscular injections led to an 8% increase in vertebral BMD; however, effects of intramuscular testosterone on the BMD at the femoral neck were inconclusive. In contrast, transdermal testosterone had no significant impact. There are no available clinical data on the effects of testosterone on fracture risk in hypogonadal men.[142]

Currently, other options for treatment of osteoporosis in hypogonadal men exist. Alendronate (10 mg/day) was studied in a double-blind, randomized, placebo controlled trial in men with long-standing hypogonadism who were receiving standard testosterone replacement. Treatment with alendronate resulted an 8.4% improvement in vertebral and 1.9% in femoral BMD over the course of 1 year.[143] This study included only 24 patients (mean age, 52 years), and none sustained any fractures over the course of study.[143]

Osteoporosis Due to Glucocorticoid Treatment. Glucocorticoid treatment is associated with rapid loss of BMD and high risk for fractures.[144] Generally, vitamin D and bisphosphonates are used as prophylactic and therapeutic agents for this type of osteoporosis. Risedronate has been shown to be beneficial in this type of treatment and produces an 82.4% decrease in the incidence of vertebral fractures over 1 year.[145] Treatment with alendronate was also compared with the vitamin D analog, alfacalcidol, in 163 women (most of whom were postmenopausal) in whom steroid treatment was newly initiated for different rheumatologic conditions. Alendronate was associated with increased BMD in the lumbar spine and reduction of a new vertebral fracture risk, compared with the vitamin D analog.[146] It is not known whether alendronate is a useful agent in the treatment of steroid-induced osteoporosis in men.

Follow-Up Testing After Pharmacologic Intervention. Sequential bone density testing using central DEXA scanning may be useful, and the International Society of Clinical Densitometry recommends monitoring drug therapy for the treatment of osteoporosis within 1 year after initiation or change of therapy, with longer intervals once therapeutic effect is established.[147] In conditions associated with rapid bone loss such as

glucocorticoid therapy, testing more frequently is appropriate.[147] These recommendations are not universally accepted, and the most recent NIH Consensus Statement[148] made no specific recommendations regarding follow-up studies.

Diabetes Mellitus
Classifications and Epidemiology

Diabetes mellitus is a major cause of morbidity and mortality worldwide. Therefore, a discussion of diabetes in the context of men's health should include a general overview of diabetes and its management. The vast majority of persons with diabetes mellitus have one of two major types, which are categorized according to their pathophysiology: type 1 diabetes, formerly known as "juvenile" or insulin-dependent diabetes, and type 2 diabetes, formerly known as "adult-onset" or non–insulin-dependent diabetes. This new nomenclature was established in 1997 by the American Diabetes Association and is based on pathophysiology rather than on use of insulin or age of onset. It is meant to avoid confusion between the two major classes of diabetes and resulting misdiagnosis (e.g., erroneously identifying someone with type 2 diabetes who takes insulin as having "insulin-dependent" diabetes). Type 1 diabetes is caused by autoimmune cell-mediated destruction of pancreatic beta cells and results in an absolute deficiency in insulin; it represents 5–10% of persons with diabetes in the United States. Type 2 diabetes is the result of a variable combination of insulin resistance, abnormally high hepatic glucose production, an inadequate compensatory response in insulin secretion, and represents 90–95% of persons with diabetes.[149]

According to data from the most recent National Health and Nutrition Examination Surveys (NHANES III, 2000–2002), the prevalence of diabetes in the general US population is 8.3% of the US population, or approximately 17 million persons, of whom one third are unaware that they carry the diagnosis.[150,151] According to the 2004 National Ambulatory Medical Care Survey,[152] diabetes accounted for 27.1 million outpatient visits, 2.7 million hospital admissions, and is ranked as the sixth leading cause of mortality, accounting for 72,815 US deaths. There is no discernible difference in prevalence in diabetes according to gender.[150] Among ethnic groups in the United States, however, diabetes prevalence varies greatly and disproportionately affects ethnic minorities.[151,153] Type 2 diabetes is also associated with obesity in most ethnic groups as the prevalence of obesity among persons with diabetes is approximately 85% among white persons, non-white Hispanics, African Americans, Native Americans, and Pacific Islanders[150,153]; however, it is significantly less among Asian Americans.[153]

Diagnosis

The current criteria for the diagnosis of diabetes that are clinically most useful are from the Expert Committee on the Diagnosis and Classification of Diabetes of the American Diabetes Association.[154] Diabetes may be diagnosed by one of the following criteria:

1. A fasting blood glucose of $\geq$ 126 mg/dL (7.0 mmol/liter); or
2. A random (e.g., nonfasting) blood glucose level of $\geq$ 200 mg/dL (11.1 mmol/liter) with symptoms of diabetes (e.g., polyuria, polydipsia, or unexplained weight loss); or
3. A blood glucose of $\geq$ 200 mg/dL (11.1 mmol/liter) 2 hours after an oral glucose tolerance test showing a 75-g glucose load.[154]

In the absence of unequivocal hyperglycemia, these criteria should be confirmed on a subsequent day.

In the 1997 Expert Committee report,[154] an intermediate category of abnormal glucose metabolism was defined, namely *impaired fasting glucose* or *impaired glucose tolerance*. In this category, persons displayed blood glucose concentrations that, while failing to meet the above-mentioned diagnostic criteria of diabetes, exhibited blood glucose levels that could not be considered to be in the normal range. Therefore, the categories for fasting blood glucoses are as follows:

1. *Normal*: fasting glucose level < 100 mg/dL (5.6 mmol/liter);
2. *Impaired fasting glucose*: fasting glucose level $\geq$ 100 mg/dL but < 126 mg/dL;
3. *Provisional diagnosis of diabetes*: fasting glucose level of $\geq$ 126 mg/dL

Similarly, based on the 2-hour post-challenge results of the oral glucose tolerance test, *impaired glucose tolerance* is defined as glucose concentrations greater than 140 mg/dL (7.8 mmol/liter) but less than 200 mg/dL (11.1 mmol/liter). It should be stated, however, that although the diagnosis of diabetes using an oral glucose tolerance test is listed as one of the diagnostic criteria, it is not recommended for routine clinical practice.[154]

The categories of impaired fasting glucose/impaired glucose tolerance, which are also referred to as "prediabetes," are not considered clinical entities per se but should be considered risk factors for the development of clinical diabetes.

Complications

The chronic hyperglycemia associated with long-standing diabetes is associated with tissue and organ-specific complications,[155] which may be generally grouped into microvascular and macrovascular disorders (Table 9-7). Microvascular complications include retinopathy (both nonproliferative and proliferative forms); nephropathy (manifested at the earliest stages by *microalbuminuria*, defined as albumin excretion of greater than 10 but less than 250 mg/g creatinine, and later by gross *proteinuria*, defined as albumin excretion of greater than 250 mg/g creatinine and detectable on standard urine dipsticks); and neuropathy (i.e., peripheral sensory neuropathies and autonomic neuropathies, including gastroparesis and motility disorders, and orthostatic hypotension), peripheral and autonomic diabetic neuropathy, and diabetic nephropathy. Cardiovascular autonomic neuropathies resulting in cardiac arrhythmias have been the subject of intense investigation recently and may account in part for the increased mortality from cardiac sudden death experienced by persons with diabetes.[156–159]

The burden of diabetes and its complications is significant, both on the individual and his family, as well as within the healthcare system as a whole. Currently, diabetes is the leading cause of adult blindness, renal dialysis and transplantation, and nontraumatic lower extremity amputation in the United States, and the annual direct indirect costs of diabetes and its complications is estimated to exceed $92 billion (based on 2002 figures) with an additional $40 billion in indirect costs.[149]

"Metabolic Control Matters": The Evidence Basis for Rigorous Metabolic Control

The risk of development and progression of chronic microvascular and macrovascular complications of diabetes is positively associated with the duration of diabetes and with the hemoglobin A_{1c}, more specifically defined as the degree of metabolic control.[155] The observation that type 1 and type 2 diabetes are two (or more) very different disease processes whose only major pathophysiologic similarities are chronic hyperglycemia and the near-identical chronic microvascular and macrovascular complications that result led to the formulation of the "glucose

Table 9-7. Chronic Complications of Diabetes

Microvascular Complications
- Ophthalmologic
  - Retinopathy
- Nonproliferative retinopathy, including macular edema
- Proliferative diabetic neuropathy
  - Cataracts
  - Glaucoma
- Nephropathy
  - Microalbuminuria
  - Gross proteinuria with renal insufficiency
- Neuropathy
  - Peripheral neuropathies
    - Sensory neuropathies
      - Distal sensory neuropathy
      - Proximal sensory neuropathy
    - Cranial and truncal neuropathy
    - Mononeuropathy multiplex
  - Autonomic neuropathies
    - Gastroparesis
    - Gastroenteropathies—chronic diarrhea or constipation
    - Orthostatic hypotension
    - Cardiovascular autonomic neuropathy
    - Erectile dysfunction

Macrovascular Complications
- Cardiovascular disease
- Cerebrovascular disease
- Peripheral vascular disease

Other
- Musculoskeletal disorders
  - Carpal tunnel syndrome
  - Trigger finger
  - Adhesive capsulitis

Adapted from: Nathan DM: Long-term complications of diabetes mellitus, *N Engl J Med* 328(23):1676–1685, 1993; Maser RE, Lenhard J: Cardiovascular autonomic neuropathy due to diabetes mellitus: clinical manifestations, consequences, and treatment, *J Clin Endocrinol Metab* 90(10):5896–5903, 2005; Ferris FL 3rd, Davis MD, Aiello LM: Treatment of diabetic retinopathy, *N Engl J Med* 341(9):667–678, 1999; Crispin JC, Alcocer-Varela J: Rheumatologic manifestations of diabetes mellitus, *Am J Med* 114 (9):753–757, 2003.

hypothesis." Simply stated, this hypothesis proposed that chronic hyperglycemia itself was responsible for most, if not all, of the organ-specific damage due to long-standing diabetes.[160] The formal testing of the hypothesis required the demonstration that near-normalization of blood glucose levels would result in the prevention of chronic diabetic complications.[160] Although eloquently simple in its formulation, an absence of standardized measures for determining levels of metabolic control, as well as a lack of animal models of diabetic complications, delayed testing of the glucose hypothesis for decades, and data from smaller clinical trials, albeit encouraging, were not conclusive.[161–165]

Over the past 13 years, several large, well-designed clinical trials have provided convincing evidence that rigorous metabolic control in persons with in type 1 and type 2 diabetes results in significantly lower risk of development and progression of microvascular complications. Follow-up and related studies have investigated the effects of "tight control" on cardiovascular and cerebrovascular risks.[166–168]

Type 1 Diabetes

The Diabetes Control and Complications Trial (DCCT),[169] a multicenter, prospective, randomized control trial compared "conventional" therapy versus "intensive" insulin therapy in persons with type 1 diabetes. Conventional therapy consisted of 1–2 injections of long-acting insulin per day with the goal of an absence of symptoms associated with hyperglycemia, normal growth and development and ideal body weight, and avoidance of severe or frequent hypoglycemia. Intensive therapy consisted of multiple-daily insulin injections (three or more injections daily) or insulin delivery via subcutaneous pumps, in conjunction with frequent home blood glucose monitoring and adjustment of insulin doses based on blood glucose readings, diet, and anticipated physical activity. The goals of the "intensive therapy" group were to achieve preprandial blood glucose concentrations between 70 and 120 mg/dL (3.9–6.7 mmol/liter); postprandial concentrations of less than 180 mg/dL (10 mmol/liter); a weekly 3:00 AM blood glucose measurement of greater than 65 mg/dL (3.6 mmol/liter), and a monthly hemoglobin A_{1c} value within the normal range (<6.05%). A total of 1441 participants with type 1 diabetes from 29 centers were enrolled in the trial and randomly assigned into the treatment groups. The primary trial outcomes of the DCCT were the development or progression of diabetic retinopathy (primary and secondary prevention arms, respectively). The impact of intensive therapy on the development or progression of diabetic nephropathy and neuropathy was investigated as a secondary outcome.[169]

The cohort was followed for a mean of 6.5 years (range, 3–9 years) with 99% of the participants completing the trial. A statistically significant difference in hemoglobin A_{1c} appeared within 3 months of the start of the trial and was maintained throughout the study period. Intensive insulin therapy reduced the risk of development of retinopathy by 76% (primary prevention; 95% confidence interval [CI], 62–85%; $P = .002$) and of progression of preexisting nonproliferative retinopathy by 54% (secondary prevention; 95% CI, 39–66%). Similarly, intensive therapy reduced the development of microalbuminuria by 34% (95% CI, 2–56%; $P < .04$) in the primary prevention cohort and by 43% (95% CI, 21–58%; $P = .002$) in the secondary prevention cohort. Likewise, the risk of clinically detectable neuropathy was reduced by 69% (95% CI, 24–87%; $P < .04$) with intensive insulin therapy. Taking these data together, the DCCT provided incontrovertible evidence that intensive insulin therapy, instituted with the aim of achieving near-normal blood glucose concentrations, substantially lessens the risk of some of the most devastating complications of type 1 diabetes.

In addition, a follow-up study of the DCCT, the Epidemiology of Diabetes Interventions and Complications (EDIC) trial,[167,168,170–172] monitored the participants of the DCCT for over a decade since termination of the DCCT. In EDIC, participants of the conventional therapy group were offered intensive insulin therapy, and medical care of all participants was transferred to their own physicians. Follow-up by the DCCT/EDIC investigators was performed annually, and retinopathy was assessed by centrally graded optic fundus photographs at 4 years.[170] Over the follow-up period, the hemoglobin A_{1c} values of the formerly intensively controlled group increased, whereas those of the formerly conventionally controlled group declined such that by the end of year 5 of the study, there was no statistically significant difference between the two groups.[167] Nonetheless, despite the convergence of the hemoglobin A_{1c} measurements, the benefits previously documented for the intensively controlled group with respect to retinopathy and nephropathy have not only persisted but also continued to diverge from that of the group previously under conventional therapy.[170,172] Taken together, data from the DCCT and EDIC convey two important messages with respect to the management of type 1 diabetes mellitus: (1) that "metabolic control matters *and* it has a memory," that is, the benefits of a period of sustained maintenance of rigorous glycemic control may persist even during periods of less-optimal control, and (2) intensive insulin therapy of type 1 diabetes should be established as early in the course of the disease as possible to derive its maximum long-term benefits in reducing the risk of microvascular complications.

Type 2 Diabetes

Over the years, acceptance of the importance of rigorous metabolic control in persons with type 2 diabetes has encountered a number of obstacles, created in part by controversies surrounding early attempts to test the glucose hypothesis. In the late 1960s, the University Group Diabetes Program (UGDP),[173] a large, randomized, prospective trial, was initiated to test whether a specific therapeutic modality was most effective in lowering the risk of cardiovascular outcomes in type 2 diabetes. One thousand subjects with type 2 diabetes were followed up for an average of 5.5 years. The results, published in 1978, reported that there was no evidence that improved glycemic control reduced cardiovascular risk, and furthermore the UGDP reported a statistical increase in cardiovascular deaths in persons treated with an early sulfonylurea, tolbutamide.[173] The results of the study were almost immediately criticized for, among other things, flaws in the study design and a significant discrepancy in the sex ratio in cardiovascular deaths in the placebo group (lower than that found in other studies).[174] Further analysis of the UGDP data also suggested that increased cardiovascular mortality in subjects with diabetes treated with sulfonylureas was limited to a small subset of persons with relatively poor glycemic control.[174] Nonetheless, because of the controversies surrounding the UGDP trial, and in particular the effects of sulfonylureas on cardiovascular mortality, formal prospective studies testing the glucose hypothesis were limited to small clinical trials.[175,176]

To resolve the controversies and test the glucose hypothesis in persons with type 2 diabetes, the United Kingdom Prospective Diabetes Study[177] (UKPDS) was initiated in 1977. The UKPDS was a 10-year, prospective, randomized trial involving 3867 persons with newly diagnosed type 2 diabetes who, after a 3-month period of dietary intervention, had two fasting blood glucose measurements between 6.1 and 15.0 mmol/liter (110–270 mg/dL). Subjects were randomly assigned to receive either intensive management with a sulfonylurea (e.g., glibenclamide, glipizide, or chlorpropamide) or insulin, or "conventional" therapy, consisting of dietary consultation alone.[177] A subset of 342 overweight subjects (>120% of ideal body weight) were recruited to a trial comparing therapy using metformin with the other treatment modalities.[178] All subjects received ongoing dietary consultation. Those subjects in the control arm who were unable to lower their fasting blood glucose concentrations below 15 mmol/liter (270 mg/dL) with dietary consultation were further randomly assigned to receive either insulin or sulfonylureas. Follow-up with all subjects was undertaken every 3 months for the length of the trial. Three predefined aggregate end points were used to compare intensive therapy with "conventional" therapy for type 2 diabetes: any diabetes-related end point, diabetes-related death, and all-cause mortality. Diabetes-related end points included fatal or nonfatal myocardial infarction; angina; heart failure; stroke; renal failure; amputation; severe proliferative or nonproliferative retinopathy requiring photocoagulation, blindness, or cataracts; peripheral vascular disease or hyperglycemia or hypoglycemia; and sudden death. Diabetes-related deaths included deaths from any of the aforementioned causes.

The median follow-up for the subjects of the UKPDS was 11.1 years, and an astonishing 95.2% of participants completed the study. In both conventional and intensive groups, the fasting blood glucose concentrations and hemoglobin A_{1c} levels steadily increased over time; nonetheless, throughout the trial, the hemoglobin A_{1c} remained statistically different between conventional and intensive therapy groups. At end of the trial, the median hemoglobin A_{1c} values were 7.0% (range, 6.2–8.2%) and 7.9% (range, 6.9–8.8%) in the intensive and conventional therapy arms, respectively ($P < .0001$). The median hemoglobin A_{1c} value for each of the sulfonylurea treatment arms and the insulin treatment arm were statistically different from the conventional therapy arm, and there was no statistical difference in hemoglobin A_{1c} between the sulfonylurea and insulin treatment arms. Compared with the conventional treatment group, intensive therapy resulted in a 12% lower risk for any diabetes-related end point (95% CI, 1–21; $P = .029$). Most of this difference was attributable to a 25% reduction in microvascular complications ($P = .0099$), and in particular, the need for laser photocoagulation. There was no significant difference between the groups with respect to diabetes-related deaths or all-cause mortality, and the reduction in risk with respect to myocardial infarction between the groups was of borderline significance ($P = .052$).

In the subgroup of overweight subjects treated with metformin, there was a significant risk reduction in several aggregate end points compared with control subjects, including a 32% lower risk of any diabetes-related end point ($P = .0023$) and a lower risk of diabetes-related death and all-cause mortality. With respect to diabetes-related end points, there was also a statistically significant difference in the risk reduction between the metformin-treated group and those treated with sulfonylurea or insulin. Of note, and unlike the group treated with sulfonylurea or insulin, those treated with metformin had a 39%

lower risk of myocardial infarction than persons in the conventional treatment group.[178]

Analysis of data generated during the UKPDS revealed two other important insights, namely control of hypertension in persons with type 2 diabetes resulted in significant reductions in the risk diabetic microvascular complications and, in particular, retinopathy.[179] Unlike the findings of the less rigorously designed UGDP, the use of sulfonylurea agents in the treatment of type 2 diabetes was not associated with a higher risk of death from cardiovascular events.[177]

Metabolic Control and Cardiovascular Risk

Since cardiovascular events including myocardial infarction and stroke are responsible for the majority of deaths in diabetes,[180–182] an understanding of whether (and how) rigorous glycemic control decreases cardiovascular risk is critical in developing strategies to treat type 1 and type 2 diabetes. With regard to type 1 diabetes, the DCCT was not designed to determine whether intensive insulin therapy of type 1 diabetes lowered the risk of cardiovascular events; the participants were drawn from a younger age group (the average age was between 26 and 27 years old), and the outcomes studied were limited to microvascular complications.[169] Therefore, the importance of metabolic control was until recently limited to evidence that demonstrated a reduction of carotid artery media-intimal thickness and coronary artery calcification with intensive insulin therapy.[183,184] The EDIC study, however, provides convincing proof that with respect to cardiovascular events, "metabolic control matters."[167] Analysis of data from EDIC participants, with a mean follow-up of 17 years after the initiation of the DCCT, revealed a 42% reduction in cardiovascular-related events and a 57% reduction of nonfatal myocardial infarction, stroke, and cardiovascular-related deaths, reductions that were significantly associated with the reduction in hemoglobin A_{1c} in the intensive insulin group.[167]

The answer, however, has not been clear-cut: even in a trial as large and well designed as the UKPDS, intensive therapy produced reduction in cardiovascular risk only in the metformin arm of the study[178]; compared with dietary control, the lower cardiovascular risk seen with treatment with insulin or sulfonylurea was modest (approximately 3%) and approached, but did not achieve, statistical significance ($P = .052$).[177] During the UKPDS, it was noted that hemoglobin A_{1c} values gradually increased over time regardless of group assignment and that none of the intensive treatment modalities were successful at achieving and maintaining glycemic targets over time. These observations have been cited to explain why a clear difference in cardiovascular outcomes was not found between the conventional and intensive groups.[185]

Given that type 2 diabetes is a disease frequently associated with a constellation of metabolic derangements (e.g., hyperglycemia, hyperlipidemia, hypertension, obesity, and insulin resistance), one might justifiably raise the issue of whether intensive therapy of type 2 diabetes should incorporate intensive approaches to multiple cardiovascular risk factors in addition to rigorous glycemic control. Intervention trials that addressed control of individual cardiovascular risk factors have demonstrated the benefits of aggressive management of hypertension and cholesterol on both microvascular and macrovascular complications in persons with type 2 diabetes[186-189]; however, treatment of persons with type 2 diabetes unusually involves combination therapy directed at multiple related disorders and, therefore, a broadly intensive approach to all cardiovascular risk factors is indicated in most patients with type 2 diabetes.[185]

To address this issue, the Steno-2 study randomly assigned 160 subjects with type 2 diabetes and persistent microalbuminuria (which is an independent risk factor for cardiovascular disease) to either treatment using conventional guidelines (those recommended by the Danish Medical Association and revised in 2000) or an intensive protocol involving a stepwise approach that incorporated behavior modification and pharmacologic intervention aimed at controlling diabetes, blood pressure, and cholesterol and avoidance of smoking.[190] By the end of the trial, targets for the intensive treatment group included a hemoglobin A_{1c} value of less than 6.5%, blood pressure of less than 130/80 mm Hg, a fasting total cholesterol level of less than 175 mg/dL (4.5 mmol/liter), and triglycerides of less than 150 mg/dL (1.7 mmol/liter). All subjects in the intensive treatment group were administered an angiotensin-converting enzyme inhibitor, regardless of blood pressure, and by the end of the trial, all subjects in the intensive group were treated with aspirin therapy. Dietary and behavioral modification in the intensive treatment group included a dietary intake of fat and polyunsaturated fats of less than 30% and 10%, respectively, of daily energy intake; at least 30 minutes of moderate exercise 3–5 times weekly; and smoking cessation classes

for study participants and their spouses. In addition, all subjects in the intensive group received a multivitamin daily that consisted of 250 mg of vitamin C; 100 mg of D-alpha-tocopherol, 400 μg of folic acid, and 100 μg of chrome picolinate.

After an average follow-up of 7.8 years, the investigators found that hemoglobin A_{1c}, blood pressure, fasting blood glucose, total cholesterol, triglyceride, and urinary albumin excretion decreased to a significantly greater degree in the intensive treatment group than in the group receiving conventional treatment.[190] Furthermore, during the trial, at least one cardiovascular event including death from cardiovascular causes, nonfatal myocardial infarction and stroke, revascularization procedures, and amputation occurred in 44% of the conventional treatment group versus 24% in the intensive group. The unadjusted hazard ratio of intensive therapy compared with the conventional therapy group was 0.47 for first-time cardiovascular events (95% CI, 0.23–0.91; $P = .02$). A similar reduction in the risk of progression of retinopathy, nephropathy, and autonomic neuropathy was seen, with relative risks of 0.42, 0.39, and 0.37, respectively. Taken together, the data from the Steno-2 trial demonstrate that aggressive control of multiple cardiovascular risk factors over time may produce an approximately 50% reduction in cardiovascular risk and emphasize the need to approach type 2 diabetes as part of a constellation of clinical conditions whose intensive control may result in improved cardiovascular health.

Erectile Dysfunction in Diabetes

A number of excellent reviews[191,192] discuss the general topic of ED in men. This section will discuss the prevalence, etiologies, and evaluation of ED in men with diabetes and current evidence-based treatment options.

Epidemiology

ED has been defined by a NIH Consensus Conference as the inability to achieve or maintain an erection for satisfactory sexual performance.[193] The term *erectile dysfunction* is used to distinguish these disorders from disorders involving libido or ejaculation: a person affected by ED may have normal libido and ability to ejaculate; however, he is not able to achieve and maintain an erection. ED is estimated to affect between 20% and 75% of men with type 1 and type 2 diabetes,[194-197] and the incidence of ED increases with age and duration of diabetes.[195–198] For example, in men with type 1 diabetes, the prevalence of ED increases from 10.2% in men aged 21–29 years to 38.2% for persons aged 40 years or older.[197] In a large observational study from Italy,[194] the incidence of ED in men with type 1 and type 2 diabetes also increased with age, with 45.5% of men aged 60 years or older reporting problems with ED. In a study of men with type 2 diabetes, an estimated 52% of men aged 55–59 years old are affected by ED.[195] When adjusted for age, men with diabetes have an approximately three-fold higher risk of ED, and ED appears at an earlier age, and is of greater severity, than in nondiabetic men.[199,200] The risk of ED in men with diabetes is associated with poor glycemic control, untreated hypertension, the presence of diabetic microvascular and macrovascular complications, and cigarette smoking.[194,197,199,201] Impotence has a major, negative impact on the quality of life of men with diabetes and adds to the psychosocial stress of living with diabetes.[200] Because large surveys of men, both with diabetes and without, reveal that the majority are often reluctant to raise issues of sexual dysfunction with their healthcare providers,[192] it is critical that healthcare providers be cognizant and open regarding discussion of this issue with their male patients with diabetes.

Etiologies

Numerous psychogenic and organic etiologies of ED exist (Table 9-8). Psychogenic causes are often related to interpersonal dynamics between the man with diabetes and his sexual partner, as well as psychosocial factors including life stressors, performance anxiety, depression, and other psychiatric conditions. The organic causes may in turn be further grouped into those related to specific drugs or hormonal, vascular, and neurogenic disorders. In men with diabetes, the pathophysiology of ED is multifactorial. Suboptimal control of diabetes is associated with an increased prevalence of impotence,[197,201] and ED is more common in men with evidence of microvascular or macrovascular complications.[196,197] In addition, since type 2 diabetes is often accompanied by obesity, hypertension, and hyperlipidemia (all of which are associated with a higher risk of ED), men with type 2 diabetes often have multiple risk factors for the development of impotence. Drugs used to treat chronic complications, such as beta blockers for coronary artery disease and thiazide diuretics for hypertension, may contribute to worsening problems with ED. Furthermore, the association of type 1 diabetes with other autoimmune endocrine disorders, such as hypothyroidism or hypergonadotropic hypogonadism (see

Table 9-8. Causes of Erectile Dysfunction

Psychogenic
- Interpersonal issues: "performance anxiety," relationship difficulties, etc.
- Psychological stress
- Depression, anxiety, and other forms of mental illness

Drug-induced
- Ethanol, particularly chronic alcoholism
- Hypertension medications: thiazide diuretics, nonselective beta adrenergic antagonists, alpha receptor antagonists
- Centrally acting drugs: antidepressant agents, including tricyclic antidepressants, selective serotonin reuptake inhibitors, phenothiazines, butyrophenone
- Drugs with anti-androgen or estrogen-like effects: cimetidine, spironolactone

Endocrine Causes
- Poorly controlled diabetes
- Hypogonadism
- Thyroid dysfunction
- Hyperprolactinemia (due to hypogonadotropic hypogonadism)

Neurogenic
- Diabetic neuropathy (peripheral sensory neuropathy, autonomic neuropathy)
- Alzheimer's disease and stroke
- Spinal cord injury
- Trauma or surgical complications involving damage to pudendal nerves (e.g., radical prostatectomy)

Vascular
- Atherosclerosis
- Hypertension
- Microvascular disease (e.g., diabetic microangiopathy)
- Peripheral vascular occlusive disease
- Peyronie's disease

section titled "Hypogonadism," this chapter),[202] may exacerbate difficulties with impotence in men with type 1 diabetes.

Diagnosis and Evaluation

Since discussion of impotence is often difficult and potentially embarrassing, men with diabetes may be reluctant to raise the issue during visits with healthcare providers. Therefore, it is the responsibility of the healthcare provider to address the topic in a sensitive and effective manner. To avoid discomfort, a screening questionnaire on sexual function may be distributed and completed by the patient while he is waiting to be seen by the clinician or in the privacy of his own home,[203] or questions regarding impotence may be routinely incorporated into the review of systems during the clinic visit (e.g., "I need to ask you a personal question. You might know it's very common for men with diabetes to have problems with impotence. Are you having any difficulties in that area?").

If a history of impotence is volunteered or elicited with questioning, a subsequent evaluation should include an assessment of the patient's level of metabolic control, the presence and severity of microvascular and macrovascular complications, and a review of current medications and smoking history. Conversely, men with impotence who have no known history of diabetes should be screened for risk of diabetes, since undiagnosed hyperglycemia, impaired fasting glucose levels, and metabolic syndrome are independently associated with ED.[204] Laboratory testing should be guided by findings elicited on history and physical examination. Because both hypothyroidism and hypogonadism are prevalent among men with diabetes and are potentially treatable, samples to measure serum thyroid-stimulating hormone and total testosterone should be drawn. Other tests, such as carotid or lower extremity Doppler ultrasound, cardiac stress testing, or electromyographic studies may be ordered, if indicated.

Treatment

Given that poor metabolic control, hypertension, obesity, smoking, and hyperlipidemia are significant risk factors for ED, lifestyle changes would be assumed to result in amelioration of ED in men with diabetes. Unlike the situation with microvascular complications,[169,177] however, there is currently no evidence proving that rigorous metabolic control, weight loss, or smoking cessation improves ED. Nonetheless, these

interventions have obvious health benefits apart from their effects on ED. In a recent 2-year, randomized, partially blinded study of nondiabetic, obese (BMI ≥ 30) men with ED, Esposito and colleagues[201] reported that dietary counseling with the aim of loss of 10% or more of body weight resulted in significant improvements in erectile function, as judged by a validated, standardized questionnaire, in comparison with similarly obese men who did not received counseling. Since the presence of diabetes was an exclusion factor in this study, it is not known whether these results can be applied to obese diabetic men with ED. With regard to medications, the decision to discontinue drugs that may worsen ED, including beta adrenergic blockers, antihypertensive agents, and antidepressants, must be carefully weighed against the availability of alternative agents or the benefits these agents possess with regard to cardiovascular or mental health.

Phosphodiesterase Type 5 Inhibitors

There are currently three oral inhibitors of phosphodiesterase type 5 (PDE5) available in the United States. The first, sildenafil (Viagra; Pfizer Inc), was approved for use in men with ED in 1998. Two other agents, vardenafil (Levitra; Bayer Corp) and tadalafil (Cialis, Lilly Pharm) have been introduced in recent years. All PDE5 inhibitors block the hydrolysis of cyclic guanosine monophosphate (GMP) and results in nitric oxide–mediated elevations in penile cyclic GMP concentrations, with increased smooth muscle relaxation and improved erections.

Sildenafil and vardenafil have similar durations of action (4–5 hours); tadalafil's duration is longer, at approximately 17½ hours.[205] The onset of action with sildenafil and vardenafil each have a time of maximum concentration (t_{max}) of 45–60 minutes and should be taken at least 30 minutes before activity; the t_{max} of tadalafil is estimated to be 2 hours, and therefore it should be taken approximately 1–2 hours before activity.[205] Foods high in fat content result in delays to t_{max} and lower peak drug concentrations with both sildenafil and vardenafil; therefore, high-fat meals should be avoided before using either agent. Tadalafil is reportedly not affected by fat.[205]

PDE5 inhibitors undergo hepatic metabolism, principally via the PCY3A4 system, and dosage adjustment is necessary in hepatic cirrhosis. In addition, drug clearance is also affected in severe renal disease (e.g., estimated glomerular filtration rate < 30 mL/min), and the dose and frequency should be kept to a minimum (e.g., 25 mg of sildenafil; 5 mg of vardenafil or tadalafil per

24-hour period).[205] In terms of drug interactions, PDE5 inhibitors potentiate the hypotensive effect of organic nitrates (e.g., nitroglycerin) and may lead to life-threatening hypotension. Therefore, therapy with PDE5 inhibitors is absolutely contraindicated in men who are taking nitrates, either intermittently or regularly, for the treatment of cardiovascular disease.[205,206] In the case of men who are taking PDE5 inhibitors who are emergently treated for myocardial ischemia, a recent American College of Cardiology/American Heart Association consensus panel has recommended avoidance of the use of nitrates if sildenafil has been taken within the previous 24 hours.[206] Given the similar pharmacokinetics, a similar 24-hour drug-free interval is required for vardenafil, and for tadalafil a 48-hour drug-free period is recommended.[205] In the absence of use of nitrates, PDE5 inhibitors are safe to use in persons with coronary artery disease who do not have acute ischemia or severe congestive heart failure[206]; however, given the high incidence of asymptomatic ischemic heart disease in men with diabetes,[207] a thorough evaluation for underlying cardiac disease should be initiated before PDE5 therapy is initiated. Regarding other drug interactions, medications that affect PCY3A4 including cimetidine, erythromycin, or ketoconazole will cause elevated serum concentrations of the PDE5 inhibitors. Protease inhibitors, such as indinavir and ritonavir, have a similar but more marked effect.[205] Dosage adjustments are recommended in patients using these agents as well.

Data from large clinical trials and meta-analyses of the PDE5 inhibitors suggest that they are generally safe and effective agents for the treatment of ED.[208–211] The most common adverse reactions are headache, flushing, dyspepsia, and nasal congestion.[208,211–214] A small percentage of men (e.g., approximately 3% in trials using sildenafil) in clinical trials have also reported visual changes consisting of slightly increased light sensitivity and changes in red-green color perception. These changes are transient and probably due to inhibition of another isoform of phosphodiesterase (i.e., type 6) in the retina.[205]

Randomized, placebo-controlled, double-blinded trials of diabetic men,[210,214] as well as subgroup analyses of diabetic subjects of large clinical trials,[211,213] have demonstrated the effectiveness of PDE5 inhibitors in men with diabetes and ED. In a 12-week, randomized, placebo-controlled, double-blind trial, Rendell and co-workers[214] investigated the effectiveness of sildenafil in 268 diabetic men with ED. Compared with placebo, treatment with sildenafil resulted in a significant improvement in ED, as determined by responses to the International Index of Erectile Function questionnaire, a standardized instrument to assess severity of ED.[214] In this trial, 56% of diabetic men treated with sildenafil reported improved erections and 61% reported at least one successful attempt at sexual intercourse, compared with 10% and 22%, respectively, in the placebo-treated group.[214] Furthermore, improvement in ED was significantly higher for sildenafil regardless of subject age, duration of ED, or duration of diabetes. Similar results were seen with a 12-week, multicenter trial of vardenafil in men with diabetes as well.[210] Of note, however, response rates to PDE5 inhibitors have been[211] generally lower in diabetic men than in men without diabetes.[209,211] This difference may be due to the multifactorial causes of ED.[215] To date, there have been no head-to-head comparative studies involving the three phosphodiesterase type 5 (DPE5) inhibitors; therefore, clinical superiority or incidence of adverse effects of one over the other DPE5 inhibitors cannot be determined.

Given the effectiveness, relative safety, and convenience of PDE5 inhibitors, they are considered to be the first-line therapy in the treatment of ED in men with diabetes.

Transurethral Alprostadil

Alprostadil is a long-acting synthetic analog of the vasoactive prostaglandin E_2 that has been formulated as a transurethral suppository and marketed under the trade name MUSE (Vivus Corp). Immediately after urination, a pellet containing alprostadil (250–1000 µg) is inserted into the urethra via a proprietary applicator, and the shaft is massaged gently to speed dissolution of the drug. Patients are instructed to remain upright during this process. Adverse effects include mild-to-moderate penile pain or burning and hypotension in approximately 36% and 3.3% of men, respectively.[216] To determine the correct dose and to monitor for hypotension, a trial of the MUSE system should be performed in the physician's office, and education of the patient and his partner should be given regarding correct use.

Padma-Nathan and colleagues investigated the MUSE system in a multicenter, randomized, double-blind, placebo-controlled trial of 1511 men with ED of a variety of etiologies. The subjects were aged 27–88 years, and 20% of them had diabetes.[216] During in-clinic testing, 65.9% of men were able to achieve erections sufficient for intercourse, and during a 3-month home-use double-blinded, placebo-controlled extension trial, 64.9% of the men treated with alprostadil successfully achieved sexual intercourse at least once versus 18.6% of control subjects.[216] Significantly more men with diabetes treated with alprostadil also had erectile responses and reported successful intercourse than control subjects.[216] Based on the clinical evidence, intraurethral alprostadil is relatively safe and effective in men with diabetes; however, given that it is more invasive than the oral DPE5 inhibitors, it is considered a second-line agent.

Intracavernous Injections

Injection of vasoactive agents directly into the corpus cavernosum is another effective treatment of ED. Alprostadil is marketed under the trade names Caverject (Pharmacia & Upjohn,) or Edex (Schwarz Pharma), the latter of which is formulated in a complex with alpha-cyclodextrin.[191] As which transurethral alprostadil, intracavernous injections should be initially performed under medical supervision. Adverse effects include penile pain (reported to occur at some time in approximately 50% of men) and priapism—defined as an erection lasting longer than 4 hours—and penile fibrosis, occurring in 1% and 2% of men, respectively.[217]

A parallel-design, randomized double-blinded study with intercavernous alprostadil reported improved erections in a dose-response manner in men receiving the drug compared with placebo, and an open-label, 6-month, home-use extension study reported successful intercourse after 94% of injections.[217] Other vasoactive agents used for intracavernous injections include papaverine, phentolamine, and alprostadil, which in combination are sold as TriMix.[218] The latter requires compounding by a pharmacy and, to the authors' knowledge, there have been no large randomized, double-blind, placebo-controlled trials of this combination in men with diabetes. Given the potential danger of penile ischemia and the lack of popularity of intercavernous injections, this approach should be considered in men who do not achieve satisfactory responses to either oral DPE5 inhibitors or transurethral alprostadil.

Vacuum Devices

Several vacuum devices are commercially available for the treatment of ED and use mechanical induction of negative pressure around the penis to increase blood flow, along with a constrictive elastic band to occlude venous outflow. These devices are relatively inexpensive, safe, and effective in men with diabetes and ED[219] and should be considered an alternative for those men who have contraindications (e.g., nitrate therapy) to oral PDE5 inhibitor therapy or who are unwilling or unable to use transurethral or intracavernous vasoactive agents.

Other Agents

Yohimbine, an alpha adrenergic antagonist, has been used to treat ED of non-organic and organic etiologies. Its action is presumed to involve central pathways controlling erections and libido.[191] A meta-analysis of randomized, double-blind, placebo-controlled trials of yohimbine in ED of various etiologies reported that the agent was superior to placebo[220]; however, its effect in treatment of ED of organic etiologies was modest, and administration was associated with adverse effects, including sweating, dizziness, and anxiety. Androgens have also been considered to enhance sexual functioning, including erections; however, clear evidence of their effectiveness in men who do not have hypogonadism is lacking, and consequently, they are not recommended in the treatment of ED.[191]

Conclusion

This chapter has been devoted to endocrinologic aspects of men's health and focused on three pertinent endocrine disorders affecting men: MHG, osteoporosis in men, and diabetes mellitus. The prevalence of MHG increases with age and results in androgen deficiency. MHG may be classified as *primary*, if a gonadal disorder is the cause of the deficiency, or *secondary*, if the cause is localized to the pituitary. Signs and symptoms depend greatly on the age of onset, and diagnosis depends on the demonstration of a persistently low serum testosterone level. Hypogonadism in older men (the so-called andropause) is the subject of much controversy, and diagnosis and treatment of MHG in this age group currently lacks a clear basis in clinical evidence.

Osteoporosis in men is underdiagnosed and contributes to increased fracture risk, particularly in elderly persons. Unlike the case in women, osteoporosis due to secondary causes, such as hypogonadism or steroid use, accounts for the majority of cases in men. Most of the evidence basis for different therapies to treat osteoporosis is derived from studies in postmenopausal women; however, several important clinical trials have demonstrated the benefits of bisphosphonate therapy in men with osteoporosis.

With regard to both type 1 and type 2 diabetes, there is a very solid basis in clinical evidence that "metabolic control matters" with respect to chronic diabetic microvascular complications, such as retinopathy, neuropathy, and nephropathy. However, the evidence that rigorous glycemic control decreases the risk of cardiovascular or cerebrovascular events is less convincing and suggests that prevention in these areas must be multifactorial, including control of cholesterol and hypertension in addition to diabetes. One of the least recognized chronic complications of diabetes, ED, may affect up to the majority of men with diabetes of long-standing duration. Currently, there is convincing evidence of the efficacy of PDE5 inhibitors, such as sildenafil, in the treatment of ED in men with diabetes.

References

1. Bhasin S, Cunningham GR, Hayes FJ, et al: Testosterone therapy in adult men with androgen deficiency syndromes: an endocrine society clinical practice guideline, *J Clin Endocrinol Metab* 91(6): 1995–2010, 2006.
2. Araujo AB, O'Donnell AB, Brambilla DJ, et al: Prevalence and incidence of androgen deficiency in middle-aged and older men: estimates from the Massachusetts Male Aging Study, *J Clin Endocrinol Metab* 89(12):5920–5926, 2004.
3. Marberger M, Roehrborn CG, Marks LS, et al: Relationship among serum testosterone, sexual function, and response to treatment in men receiving dutasteride for benign prostatic hyperplasia, *J Clin Endocrinol Metab* 91(4):1323–1328, 2006.
4. Costabile RA, Spevak M: Characterization of patients presenting with male factor infertility in an equal access, no cost medical system, *Urology* 58(6):1021–1024, 2001.
5. Poletti A, Negri-Cesi P, Martini L: Reflections on the diseases linked to mutations of the androgen receptor, *Endocrine* 28(3):243–262, 2005.
6. American Association of Clinical Endocrinologists: Medical guidelines for clinical practice for the evaluation and treatment of hypogonadism in adult male patients—2002 update, *Endocr Pract,* 8(6): 440–456, 2002.
7. Darby E, Anawalt BD: Male hypogonadism: an update on diagnosis and treatment, *Treat Endocrinol* 4(5):293–309, 2005.
8. Handelsman DJ, Conway AJ, Boylan LM: Pharmacokinetics and pharmacodynamics of testosterone pellets in man, *J Clin Endocrinol Metab* 71(1): 216–222, 1990.
9. Handelsman DJ, Liu PY: Andropause: invention, prevention, rejuvenation, *Trends Endocrinol Metab* 16(2):39–45, 2005.
10. Kelleher S, Conway AJ, Handelsman DJ: Blood testosterone threshold for androgen deficiency symptoms, *J Clin Endocrinol Metab* 89(8):3813–3817, 2004.
11. Meier C, Liu PY, Handelsman DJ, Seibel MJ: Endocrine regulation of bone turnover in men, *Clin Endocrinol (Oxf)* 63(6):603–616, 2005.
12. Ersoz H, Onde ME, Terekeci H, et al: Causes of gynaecomastia in young adult males and factors associated with idiopathic gynaecomastia, *Int J Androl* 25(5):312–316, 2002.
13. Eversmann T, Moito J, von Werder K: Testosterone and estradiol levels in male gynecomastia. Clinical and endocrine findings during treatment with tamoxifen [German], *Deutsche Medizinische Wochenschrift* 109(44):1678–1682, 1984.
14. Liu PY, Death AK, Handelsman DJ: Androgens and cardiovascular disease, *Endocr Rev* 24(3):313–340, 2003.
15. Arnlov J, Pencina MJ, Amin S, et al: Endogenous sex hormones and cardiovascular disease incidence in men, *Ann Intern Med* 145(3):176–184, 2006.
16. Liu PY, Wishart SM, Celermajer DS, et al: Do reproductive hormones modify insulin sensitivity and metabolism in older men? a randomized, placebo-controlled clinical trial of recombinant human chorionic gonadotropin, *Eur J Endocrinol* 148(1): 55–66, 2003.
17. Ellegala DB, Alden TD, Couture DE, et al: Anemia, testosterone, and pituitary adenoma in men, *J Neurosurg* 98(5):974–977, 2003.
18. Hero M, Wickman S, Hanhijarvi R, et al: Pubertal upregulation of erythropoiesis in boys is determined primarily by androgen, *J Pediatr* 146(2): 245–252, 2005.
19. Feldman HA, Longcope C, Derby CA, et al: Age trends in the level of serum testosterone and other hormones in middle-aged men: longitudinal results from the Massachusetts male aging study, *J Clin Endocrinol Metab* 87(2):589–598, 2002.
20. Harman SM, Metter EJ, Tobin JD, et al: Longitudinal effects of aging on serum total and free testosterone levels in healthy men: Baltimore Longitudinal Study of Aging, *J Clin Endocrinol Metabol* 86(2):724–731, 2001.
21. T'Sjoen G, Goemaere S, De Meyere, Kaufman JM: Perception of males' aging symptoms, health and well-being in elderly community-dwelling men is not related to circulating androgen levels, *Psychoneuroendocrinology* 29(2):201–214, 2004.
22. Spratt DI, O'Dea LS, Schoenfeld D, et al: Neuroendocrine-gonadal axis in men: frequent sampling of LH, FSH, and testosterone, *Am J Physiol* 254(5 Pt 1):E658–E666, 1988.
23. American Urological Association: Report on optimal evaluation of the infertile male. 2001. Available at: http://www.asrm.org/media/practice/infertilemale.pdf. Accessed June 1, 2006.
24. Karpati AM, Rubin CH, Kieszak SM, et al: Stature and pubertal stage assessment in American boys: the 1988–1994 Third National Health and Nutrition Examination Survey. *J Adolesc Health* 30(3):205–212, 2002.
25. Herman-Giddens ME, Wang L, Koch G: Secondary sexual characteristics in boys: estimates from the national health and nutrition examination survey III, 1988–1994 [see comment], *Arch Pediatr Adolesc Med* 155(9):1022–1028, 2001.

26. Sedlmeyer IL, Palmert MR: Delayed puberty: analysis of a large case series from an academic center, *J Clin Endocrinol Metab* 87(4):1613–1620, 2002.

27. Gordon D, Cohen HN, Beastall GH, et al: Hormonal responses in pubertal males to pulsatile gonadotropin releasing hormone (GnRH) administration, *J Endocrinol Invest* 11(2):77–83, 1988.

28. Delemarre-van de Waal HA, Van den Brande JL, Schoemaker J: Prolonged pulsatile administration of luteinizing hormone-releasing hormone in prepubertal children: diagnostic and physiologic aspects, *J Clin Endocrinol Metab* 61(5):859–867, 1985.

29. Dunkel L, Perheentupa J, Sorva R: Single versus repeated dose human chorionic gonadotropin stimulation in the differential diagnosis of hypogonadotropic hypogonadism, *J Clin Endocrinol Metab* 60(2):333–337, 1985.

30. Partsch CJ, Hermanussen M, Sippell WG: Differentiation of male hypogonadotropic hypogonadism and constitutional delay of puberty by pulsatile administration of gonadotropin-releasing hormone, *J Clin Endocrinol Metab* 60(6):1196–1203, 1985.

31. Smals AG, Hermus AR, Boers GH, et al: Predictive value of luteinizing hormone releasing hormone (LHRH) bolus testing before and after 36-hour pulsatile LHRH administration in the differential diagnosis of constitutional delay of puberty and male hypogonadotropic hypogonadism, *J Clin Endocrinol Metab* 78(3):602–608, 1994.

32. Krausz C, Degl'Innocenti S: Y chromosome and male infertility: update, 2006, *Frontiers Biosci* 11:3049–3061, 2006.

33. Rogol AD: Pubertal androgen therapy in boys, *Pediatr Endocrinol Rev* 2(3):383–390, 2005.

34. Amin S, Zhang Y, Felson DT, et al: Estradiol, testosterone, and the risk for hip fractures in elderly men from the Framingham Study, *Am J Med* 119(5):426–433, 2006.

35. Rogol AD: New facets of androgen replacement therapy during childhood and adolescence, *Expert Opin Pharmacother* 6(8):1319–1336, 2005.

36. Liu PY, Turner L, Rushford D, et al: Efficacy and safety of recombinant human follicle stimulating hormone (Gonal-F) with urinary human chorionic gonadotrophin for induction of spermatogenesis and fertility in gonadotrophin-deficient men, *Hum Reprod* 14(6):1540–1545, 1999.

37. Liu PY, Wishart SM, Handelsman DJ: A double-blind, placebo-controlled, randomized clinical trial of recombinant human chorionic gonadotropin on muscle strength and physical function and activity in older men with partial age-related androgen deficiency, *J Clin Endocrinol Metab* 87(7):3125–3135, 2002.

38. Buchter D, Behre HM, Kliesch S, Nieschlag E: Pulsatile GnRH or human chorionic gonadotropin/human menopausal gonadotropin as effective treatment for men with hypogonadotropic hypogonadism: a review of 42 cases, *Eur J Endocrinol* 139(3):298–303, 1998.

39. Liu L, Banks SM, Barnes KM, Sherins RJ: Two-year comparison of testicular responses to pulsatile gonadotropin-releasing hormone and exogenous gonadotropins from the inception of therapy in men with isolated hypogonadotropic hypogonadism, *J Clin Endocrinol Metab* 67(6):1140–1145, 1988.

40. Schopohl J, Mehltretter G, von Zumbusch R, et al: Comparison of gonadotropin-releasing hormone and gonadotropin therapy in male patients with idiopathic hypothalamic hypogonadism, *Fertil Steril* 56(6):1143–1150, 1991.

41. Hussein A, Ozgok Y, Ross L, Niederberger C: Clomiphene administration for cases of nonobstructive azoospermia: a multicenter study, *J Androl* 26(6):787–791, discussion 792–793, 2005.

42. Dobs AS, Meikle AW, Arver S, et al: Pharmacokinetics, efficacy, and safety of a permeation-enhanced testosterone transdermal system in comparison with bi-weekly injections of testosterone enanthate for the treatment of hypogonadal men, *J Clin Endocrinol Metab* 84(10):3469–3478, 1999.

43. Mazer N, Fisher D, Fischer J, et al: Transfer of transdermally applied testosterone to clothing: a comparison of a testosterone patch versus a testosterone gel, *J Sex Med* 2(2):227–234, 2005.

44. Wang C, Swerdloff R, Kipnes M, et al: New testosterone buccal system (Striant) delivers physiological testosterone levels: pharmacokinetics study in hypogonadal men, *J Clin Endocrinol Metab* 89(8):3821–3829, 2004.

45. Kunelius P, Lukkarinen O, Hannuksela ML, et al: The effects of transdermal dihydrotestosterone in the aging male: a prospective, randomized, double blind study, *J Clin Endocrinol Metab* 87(4):1467–1472, 2002.

46. Arrigo T, Crisafulli G, Salzano G, et al: High-flow priapism in testosterone-treated boys with constitutional delay of growth and puberty may occur even when very low doses are used, *J Endocrinol Invest* 28(4):390–391, 2005.

47. Ichioka K, Utsunomiya N, Kohei N, et al: Testosterone-induced priapism in Klinefelter syndrome, *Urology* 67(3):622.e17–e18, 2006.

48. Gould DC, Kirby RS: Testosterone replacement therapy for late onset hypogonadism: what is the risk of inducing prostate cancer? *Prostate Cancer Prostatic Dis* 9(1):14–18, 2006.

49. Rhoden EL, Morgentaler A: Testosterone replacement therapy in hypogonadal men at high risk for prostate cancer: results of 1 year of treatment in men with prostatic intraepithelial neoplasia, *J Urol* 170(6 Pt 1):2348–2351, 2003.

50. Rhoden EL, Morgentaler A: Risks of testosterone-replacement therapy and recommendations for monitoring, *N Engl J Med* 350(5):482–492, 2004.

51. Bhasin S, Singh AB, Mac RP, et al: Managing the risks of prostate disease during testosterone replacement therapy in older men: recommendations for a standardized monitoring plan, *J Androl* 24(3):299–311, 2003.

52. Rhoden EL, Morgentaler A: Treatment of testosterone-induced gynecomastia with the aromatase inhibitor, anastrozole, *Int J Impot Res* 16(1):95–97, 2004.

53. Calof OM, Singh AB, Lee ML, et al: Adverse events associated with testosterone replacement in middle-aged and older men: a meta-analysis of randomized, placebo-controlled trials, *J Gerontol Series A Biol Sci Med Sci* 60(11):1451–1457, 2005.

54. Isidori AM, Giannetta E, Gianfrilli D, et al: Effects of testosterone on sexual function in men: results of a meta-analysis, *Clin Endocrinol* 63(4):381–394, 2005.

55. Liu PY, Yee B, Wishart SM, et al: The short-term effects of high-dose testosterone on sleep, breathing, and function in older men, *J Clin Endocrinol Metab* 88(8):3605–3613, 2003.

56. Brown JT: Anabolic steroids: what should the emergency physician know? *Emerg Med Clin North Am* 23(3):815–826, 2005.

57. Looker AC, Orwoll ES, Johnston CC Jr, et al: Prevalence of low femoral bone density in older U.S. adults from NHANES III, *J Bone Miner Res* 12(11):1761–1768, 1997.

58. Hawkes WG, Wehren L, Orwiq D, et al: Gender differences in functioning after hip fracture, *J Gerontol A Biol Sci Med Sci* 61(5):495–499, 2006.

59. Feldstein AC, Nichols G, Orwoll E, et al: The near absence of osteoporosis treatment in older men with fractures, *Osteoporos Int* 16(8):953–962, 2005.

60. Kamel HK: Male osteoporosis: new trends in diagnosis and therapy, *Drugs Aging* 22(9):741–748, 2005.

61. National Institutes of Health: *NIH Consensus Statement: Osteoporosis Prevention, Diagnosis, and Therapy*, Bethesda, MD, 2000, National Institutes of Health, pp 1–45.

62. Assessment of fracture risk and its application to screening for postmenopausal osteoporosis. Report of a WHO Study Group, *World Health Organ Tech Rep Ser* 843:1–129, 1994.

63. Riggs BL, Wahner HW, Dunn WL, et al: Differential changes in bone mineral density of the appendicular and axial skeleton with aging: relationship to spinal osteoporosis, *J Clin Invest* 67(2):328–335, 1981.

64. The relationship between bone density and incident vertebral fracture in men and women, *J Bone Miner Res,* 17(12):2214–2221, 2002.

65. Johnell O, Kanis JA, Oden A, et al: Predictive value of BMD for hip and other fractures, *J Bone Miner Res* 20(7):1185–1194, 2005.

66. International Society for Clinical Densitometry: Official Positions of the International Society for Clinical Densitometry: 2005 Update. Available at: http://www.iscd.org/visitors/positions/Official-positionstext.cfm. Accessed August 2006.

67. Portero NR, Arlot ME, Roux JP, et al: Evaluation and development of automatic two-dimensional measurements of histomorphometric parameters reflecting trabecular bone connectivity: correlations with dual-energy x-ray absorptiometry and quantitative ultrasound in human calcaneum, *Calcif Tissue Int* 77(4):195–204, 2005.

68. Leslie WD, Adler RA, El-Hajj Fuleihan G, et al: Application of the 1994 WHO classification to populations other than postmenopausal Caucasian women: the 2005 ISCD Official Positions, *J Clin Densitom* 9(1):22–30, 2006.

69. Audran M, Chappard D, Legrand E, et al: Bone microarchitecture and bone fragility in men: DXA and histomorphometry in humans and in the orchidectomized rat model, *Calcif Tissue Int* 69(4):214–217, 2001.

70. Rupprecht M, Pogoda P, Mumme M, et al: Bone microarchitecture of the calcaneus and its changes in aging: a histomorphometric analysis of 60 human specimens, *J Orthop Res* 24(4):664–674, 2006.

71. Viguet-Carrin S, Garnero P, Delmas PD: The role of collagen in bone strength, *Osteoporos Int* 17(3):319–336, 2006.

72. Zeitlin L, Fassier F, Glorieux FH: Modern approach to children with osteogenesis imperfecta, *J Pediatr Orthop B* 12(2):77–87, 2003.

73. Yen JL, Lin SP, Chen MR, Niu DM: Clinical features of Ehlers-Danlos syndrome, *J Formos Med Assoc* 105(6):475–480, 2006.

74. Bachrach LK: Bone mineralization in childhood and adolescence, *Curr Opin Pediatr* 5(4):467–473, 1993.

75. Lanou AJ, Berkow SE, Barnard ND: Calcium, dairy products, and bone health in children and young adults: a reevaluation of the evidence, *Pediatrics* 115(3):736–743, 2005.

76. Linden C, Ahlborg H, Gardsell P, et al: Exercise, bone mass and bone size in prepubertal boys: one-year data from the pediatric osteoporosis prevention study, *Scand J Med Sci Sports* 2006 (in press).

77. Krupa B, Miazgowski T: Bone mineral density and markers of bone turnover in boys with constitutional delay of growth and puberty, *J Clin Endocrinol Metab* 90(5):2828–2830, 2005.

78. Earnshaw SA, Cawte SA, Worley A, Hosking DJ: Colles' fracture of the wrist as an indicator of underlying osteoporosis in postmenopausal women: a prospective study of bone mineral density and bone turnover rate, *Osteoporosis Int* 8(1):53–60, 1998.

79. Riggs BL, Melton LJ 3rd: Involutional osteoporosis, *N Engl J Med* 314(26):1676–1686, 1986.

80. Adler RA: Epidemiology and pathophysiology of osteoporosis in men, *Curr Osteoporos Rep* 4(3):110–115, 2006.

81. Ralston SH, Galwey N, MacKay I, et al: Loci for regulation of bone mineral density in men and women identified by genome wide linkage scan: the FAMOS study, *Hum Mol Genet* 14(7):943–951, 2005.

82. Diaz MN, O'Neill TW, Silman AJ: The influence of family history of hip fracture on the risk of vertebral deformity in men and women: the European Vertebral Osteoporosis Study, *Bone* 20(2):145–149, 1997.

83. Ralston SH: Genetic determinants of osteoporosis, *Curr Opin Rheum* 17(4):475–479, 2005.

84. Khosla S, Melton LJ 3rd, Atkinson EJ, et al: Relationship of serum sex steroid levels and bone turnover markers with bone mineral density in men and women: a key role for bioavailable estrogen [see comment], *J Clin Endocrinol Metab* 83(7):2266–2274, 1998.

85. Khosla S, Melton LJ 3rd, Atkinson EJ, O'Fallon WM: Relationship of serum sex steroid levels to longitudinal changes in bone density in young versus elderly men, *J Clin Endocrinol Metab* 86(8):3555–3561, 2001.

86. Carlsen CG, Soerensen TH, Eriksen EF: Prevalence of low serum estradiol levels in male osteoporosis, *Osteoporosis Int* 11(8):697–701, 2000.

87. Johansson AG, Lindh E, Blum WF, et al: Effects of growth hormone and insulin-like growth factor I in men with idiopathic osteoporosis, *J Clin Endocrinol Metab* 81(1):44–48, 1996.

88. Kelepouris N, Harper KD, Gannon F, et al: Severe osteoporosis in men, *Ann Intern Med* 123(6):452–460, 1995.

89. Templeton K: Secondary osteoporosis, *J Am Acad Orthop Surg* 13(7):475–486, 2005.

90. Stenson WF, Newberry R, Lorenz R, et al: Increased prevalence of celiac disease and need for routine screening among patients with osteoporosis, *Arch Intern Med* 165(4):393–399, 2005.

91. McKenzie R, Reynolds JC, O'Fallon A, et al: Decreased bone mineral density during low dose glucocorticoid administration in a randomized, placebo controlled trial, *J Rheumatol* 27(9):2222–2226, 2000.

92. Miller RG, Segal JB, Ashar BH, et al: High prevalence and correlates of low bone mineral density in young adults with sickle cell disease, *Am J Hematol* 81(4):236–241, 2006.

93. Vogiatzi MG, Autio KA, Mait JE, et al: Low bone mineral density in adolescents with beta-thalassemia, *Ann N Y Acad Sci* 1054:462–466, 2005.

94. Golden NH: Osteopenia and osteoporosis in anorexia nervosa, *Adolesc Med* 14(1):97–108, 2003.

95. Stein E, Shane E: Secondary osteoporosis, *Endocrinol Metab Clin North Am* 32(1):115–134, 2003.

96. De Laet C, Kanis JA, Oden A, et al: Body mass index as a predictor of fracture risk: a meta-analysis, *Osteoporos Int* 16(11):1330–1338, 2005.

97. Samelson EJ, Hannan MT, Zhang Y, et al: Incidence and risk factors for vertebral fracture in women and men: 25-year follow-up results from the population-based Framingham study, *J Bone Miner Res* 21(8):1207–1214, 2006.

98. Roy DK, O'Neill TW, Finn JD, et al: Determinants of incident vertebral fracture in men and women: results from the European Prospective Osteoporosis Study (EPOS), *Osteoporos Int* 14(1):19–26, 2003.

99. Orwoll E, Blank JB, Barrett-Connor E, et al: Design and baseline characteristics of the osteoporotic fractures in men (MrOS) study—a large observational study of the determinants of fracture in older men, *Contemp Clin Trials* 26(5):569–585, 2005.

100. Looker AC, Bauer DC, Chestnut CH 3rd, et al: Clinical use of biochemical markers of bone remodeling: current status and future directions, *Osteoporos Int* 11(6):467–480, 2000.

101. Bonnick S, Saag KG, Kiel DP, et al: Comparison of weekly treatment of postmenopausal osteoporosis with alendronate versus risedronate over two years, *J Clin Endocrinol Metab* 91(7):2631–2637, 2006.

102. Prentice A: Diet, nutrition and the prevention of osteoporosis, *Public Health Nutr* 7(1A):227–243, 2004.

103. Lock CA, Lecouturier J, Mason JM, Dickinson HO: Lifestyle interventions to prevent osteoporotic fractures: a systematic review, *Osteoporosis Int* 17(1):20–28, 2006.

104. Institute of Medicine: *Dietary Reference Intakes for Calcium, Magnesium, Phosphorus, Vitamin D, and Fluoride,* F.a.N.B., Washington, D.C., 1997, National Academy Press.

105. Wright JD, Wang CY, Kennedy-Stephenson J, Ervin RB: Dietary intake of ten key nutrients for public health, United States: 1999–2000, *Adv Data* 334:1–4, 2003.

106. Shea B, Wells G, Cranney A, et al: Meta-analyses of therapies for postmenopausal osteoporosis. VII. Meta-analysis of calcium supplementation for the prevention of postmenopausal osteoporosis, *Endocrine Rev* 23(4):552–559, 2002.

107. Nordin BE: Calcium and osteoporosis, *Nutrition* 13(7–8):664–686, 1997.

108. Mackerras D, LumLey T: First- and second-year effects in trials of calcium supplementation on the loss of bone density in postmenopausal women, *Bone* 21(6):527–533, 1997.

109. Armas LA, Hollis BW, Heaney RP: Vitamin D2 is much less effective than vitamin D3 in humans, *J Clin Endocrinol Metab* 89(11):5387–5391, 2004.

110. Bailie GR, Johnson CA: Comparative review of the pharmacokinetics of vitamin D analogues, *Semin Dial* 15(5):352–357, 2002.

111. Bischoff-Ferrari HA, Willett WC, Wong JB, et al: Fracture prevention with vitamin D supplementation: a meta-analysis of randomized controlled trials, *JAMA* 293(18):2257–2264, 2005.

112. Trivedi DP, Doll R, Khaw KT: Effect of four monthly oral vitamin D3 (cholecalciferol) supplementation on fractures and mortality in men and women living in the community: randomised double blind controlled trial, *BMJ* 326(7387):469, 2003.

113. Dawson-Hughes B: Racial/ethnic considerations in making recommendations for vitamin D for adult and elderly men and women, *Am J Clin Nutr* 80(6 Suppl):1763S–1766S, 2004.

114. de Groen PC, Lubbe DR, Hirsch LJ, et al: Esophagitis associated with the use of alendronate, *N Engl J Med* 335(14):1016–1021, 1996.

115. Stevenson M, Lloyd Jones M, De Nigris E, et al: A systematic review and economic evaluation of alendronate, etidronate, risedronate, raloxifene and teriparatide for the prevention and treatment of postmenopausal osteoporosis, *Health Technol Assess* 9(22):1–160, 2005.

116. Black DM, Thompson DE, Bauer DC, et al: Fracture risk reduction with alendronate in women

with osteoporosis: the Fracture Intervention Trial. FIT Research Group, *J Clin Endocrinol Metab* 85 (11):4118–4124, 2000.

117. Ringe JD, Dorst A, Faber H, Ibach K: Alendronate treatment of established primary osteoporosis in men: 3-year results of a prospective, comparative, two-arm study, *Rheumatol Int* 24(2):110–113, 2004.

118. Orwoll E, Ettinger M, Weiss S, et al: Alendronate for the treatment of osteoporosis in men, *N Engl J Med* 343(9):604–610, 2000.

119. Bone HG, Hosking D, Devogelaer JP, et al: Ten years' experience with alendronate for osteoporosis in postmenopausal women, *N Engl J Med* 350 (12):1189–1199, 2004.

120. Uchida S, Taniguchi T, Shimizu T, et al: Therapeutic effects of alendronate 35 mg once weekly and 5 mg once daily in Japanese patients with osteoporosis: a double-blind, randomized study, *J Bone Mineral Metab* 23(5):382–388, 2005.

121. Rizzoli R, Greenspan SL, Bone G 3rd, et al: Two-year results of once-weekly administration of alendronate 70 mg for the treatment of postmenopausal osteoporosis, *J Bone Min Res* 17(11): 1988–1996, 2002.

122. Schnitzer T, Bone HG, Crepaldi G, et al: Therapeutic equivalence of alendronate 70 mg once-weekly and alendronate 10 mg daily in the treatment of osteoporosis: Alendronate Once-Weekly Study Group, *Aging Clin Exp Res* 12(1):1–12, 2000.

123. Harris ST, Watts NB, Li Z, et al: Two-year efficacy and tolerability of risedronate once a week for the treatment of women with postmenopausal osteoporosis [erratum appears in *Curr Med Res Opin* 20 (10):1690, 2004], *Curr Med Res Opin* 20(5):757–764, 2004.

124. Reid DM: Once-monthly dosing: an effective step forward, *Bone* 38(4 Suppl 1):S18–S22, 2006.

125. Compston J: Recombinant parathyroid hormone in the management of osteoporosis, *Calcif Tissue Int* 77(2):65–71, 2005.

126. Neer RM, Arnaud CD, Zanchetta JR, et al: Effect of parathyroid hormone (1–34) on fractures and bone mineral density in postmenopausal women with osteoporosis [see comment], *N Engl J Med* 344 (19):1434–1441, 2001.

127. Orwoll ES, Scheele WH, Paul S, et al: The effect of teriparatide [human parathyroid hormone (1–34)] therapy on bone density in men with osteoporosis, *J Bone Miner Res* 18(1):9–17, 2003.

128. Black DM, Greenspan SL, Ensrud KE, et al: The effects of parathyroid hormone and alendronate alone or in combination in postmenopausal osteoporosis, *N Engl J Med* 349(13):1207–1215, 2003.

129. Finkelstein JS, Hayes A, Hunzelman JL, et al: The effects of parathyroid hormone, alendronate, or both in men with osteoporosis, *N Engl J Med* 349 (13):1216–1226, 2003.

130. Vahle JL, Sato M, Long GG, et al: Skeletal changes in rats given daily subcutaneous injections of recombinant human parathyroid hormone (1–34)

for 2 years and relevance to human safety, *Toxicol Pathol* 30(3):312–321, 2002.

131. Silverman SL: Calcitonin, *Endocrinol Metab Clin North Am* 32(1):273–284, 2003.

132. Stewart AF: Clinical practice: hypercalcemia associated with cancer, *N Engl J Med* 352(4):373–379, 2005.

133. Cranney A, Tugwell P, Zytaruk N, et al: Meta-analyses of therapies for postmenopausal osteoporosis: VI. meta-analysis of calcitonin for the treatment of postmenopausal osteoporosis, *Endocr Rev* 23(4):540–551, 2002.

134. Knopp JA, Diner BM, Blitz M, et al: Calcitonin for treating acute pain of osteoporotic vertebral compression fractures: a systematic review of randomized, controlled trials, *Osteoporos Int* 16 (10):1281–1290, 2005.

135. Trovas GP, Lyritis GP, Galanos A, et al: A randomized trial of nasal spray salmon calcitonin in men with idiopathic osteoporosis: effects on bone mineral density and bone markers, *J Bone Miner Res* 17(3):521–527, 2002.

136. Seeman E, Crans GG, Diez-Perez A, et al: Anti-vertebral fracture efficacy of raloxifene: a meta-analysis, *Osteoporos Int* 17(2):313–316, 2006.

137. Uebelhart B, Herrmann F, Pavo I, et al: Raloxifene treatment is associated with increased serum estradiol and decreased bone remodeling in healthy middle-aged men with low sex hormone levels, *J Bone Miner Res* 19(9):1518–1524, 2004.

138. Ke HZ, Wang XN, O'Malley J, et al: Selective androgen receptor modulators—prospects for emerging therapy in osteoporosis? *J Musculoskelet Neuronal Interact* 5(4):355, 2005.

139. McClung MR, Lewiecki EM, Cohen SB, et al: Denosumab in postmenopausal women with low bone mineral density, *N Engl J Med* 354(8): 821–831, 2006.

140. Whyte MP: The long and the short of bone therapy, *N Engl J Med* 354(8):860–863, 2006.

141. Meier C, Liu PY, Handelsman DJ, Seibel MJ: Endocrine regulation of bone turnover in men, *Clin Endocrinol (Oxf)* 63(6):603–616, 2005.

142. Tracz MJ, Sideras K, Bolona ER, et al: Testosterone use in men and its effects on bone health: a systematic review and meta-analysis of randomized placebo-controlled trials, *J Clin Endocrinol Metab* 91(6):2011–2016, 2006.

143. Shimon I, Eshed V, Doolman R, et al: Alendronate for osteoporosis in men with androgen-repleted hypogonadism, *Osteoporos Int* 16(12):1591–1596, 2005.

144. van Staa TP, Leufkens HG, Cooper C: The epidemiology of corticosteroid-induced osteoporosis: a meta-analysis, *Osteoporos Int* 13(10):777–787, 2002.

145. Reid DM, Adami S, Devogelaer JP, Chines AA: Risedronate increases bone density and reduces vertebral fracture risk within one year in men on corticosteroid therapy, *Calcif Tissue Int* 69(4): 242–247, 2001.

146. de Nijs RN, Jacobs JW, Lems WF, et al: Alendronate or alfacalcidol in glucocorticoid-induced osteoporosis, *N Engl J Med* 355(7):675–684, 2006.

147. Prince R: International Society of Clinical Densitometry support for screening women over the age of 65 years and men over the age of 70 years using bone density testing has a scientific and medical perspective, not a third-party payer perspective, *J Clin Densitom* 9(1):128, author reply 128–129, 2006.

148. NIH Consensus conference: Optimal calcium intake. NIH Consensus Development Panel on Optimal Calcium Intake, *JAMA* 272(24): 1942–1948, 1994.

149. *Diabetes 411: Facts, Figures, and Statistics at a Glance,* Alexandria, VA, 2005, American Diabetes Association, p 86.

150. Centers for Disease Control and Prevention: Prevalence of diabetes and impaired fasting glucose in adults—United States, 1999–2000, *MMWR Morb Mortal Wkly Rep* 52(35):833–837, 2003.

151. Harris MI, Flegal KM, Cowie CC, et al: Prevalence of diabetes, impaired fasting glucose, and impaired glucose tolerance in U.S. adults: the Third National Health and Nutrition Examination Survey, 1988–1994, *Diabetes Care* 21(4):518–524, 1998.

152. National Center for Health Statistics: Diabetes Available at: http://www.cdc.gov/nchs/fastats/diabetes.htm. Accessed September 16, 2006.

153. McNeely MJ, Boyko EJ: Type 2 diabetes prevalence in Asian Americans: results of a national health survey, *Diabetes Care* 27(1):66–69, 2004.

154. Report of the Expert Committee on the Diagnosis and Classification of Diabetes Mellitus, *Diabetes Care,* 20(7):1183–1197, 1997.

155. Nathan DM: Long-term complications of diabetes mellitus, *N Engl J Med* 328(23):1676–1685, 1993.

156. Manson JE, Nathan DM, Krolewski AS, et al: A prospective study of exercise and incidence of diabetes among US male physicians, *JAMA* 268 (1):63–67, 1992.

157. Manson JE, Rimm EB, Stampfer MJ, et al: Physical activity and incidence of non–insulin-dependent diabetes mellitus in women, *Lancet* 338(8770): 774–778, 1991.

158. Ziegler D: Diabetic cardiovascular autonomic neuropathy: prognosis, diagnosis and treatment, *Diabetes Metab Rev* 10(4):339–383, 1994.

159. Page MM, Watkins PJ: The heart in diabetes: autonomic neuropathy and cardiomyopathy, *Clin Endocrinol Metab* 6(2):377–388, 1977.

160. Nathan DM: The pathophysiology of diabetic complications: how much does the glucose hypothesis explain? *Ann Intern Med* 124(1 Pt 2): 86–89, 1996.

161. Reichard P, Nilsson BY, Rosenqvist U: The effect of long-term intensified insulin treatment on the development of microvascular complications of diabetes mellitus [see comment], *N Engl J Med* 329(5):304–309, 1993.

162. Chase HP, Jackson WE, Hoops SL, et al: Glucose control and the renal and retinal complications of insulin-dependent diabetes, *JAMA* 261(8): 1155–1160, 1989.

163. Brinchmann-Hansen O, Dahl-Jorgensen K, Hanssen KF, Sandvik L: The response of diabetic retinopathy to 41 months of multiple insulin injections, insulin pumps, and conventional insulin therapy, *Arch Ophthalmol* 106(9):1242–1246, 1988.

164. Lauritzen T, Frost-Larsen K, Larsen HW, Deckert T: Two-year experience with continuous subcutaneous insulin infusion in relation to retinopathy and neuropathy, *Diabetes* 34(Suppl 3): 74–79, 1985.

165. Blood glucose control and the evolution of diabetic retinopathy and albuminuria: a preliminary multicenter trial, The Kroc Collaborative Study Group, *N Engl J Med* 311(6):365–372, 1984.

166. Adler AI, Neil HA, Manley SE, et al: Hyperglycemia and hyperinsulinemia at diagnosis of diabetes and their association with subsequent cardiovascular disease in the United Kingdom prospective diabetes study (UKPDS 47), *Am Heart J* 138(5 Pt 1):S353–S3539, 1999.

167. The Diabetes Control and Complications Trial/Epidemiology of Diabetes Interventions and Complications Study Research Group: Intensive diabetes treatment and cardiovascular disease in patients with type 1 diabetes, *N Engl J Med* 353 (25):2643–2653, 2005.

168. Epidemiology of Diabetes Interventions and Complications: Effect of intensive diabetes treatment on carotid artery wall thickness in the epidemiology of diabetes interventions and complications. Epidemiology of Diabetes Interventions and Complications (EDIC) Research Group, *Diabetes* 48 (2):383–390, 1999.

169. The Diabetes Control and Complications Trial Research Group: The effect of intensive treatment of diabetes on the development and progression of long-term complications in insulin-dependent diabetes mellitus, *N Engl J Med* 329(14):977–986, 1993.

170. Epidemiology of Diabetes Interventions and Complications: Sustained effect of intensive treatment of type 1 diabetes mellitus on development and progression of diabetic nephropathy: the Epidemiology of Diabetes Interventions and Complications (EDIC) study, *JAMA* 290(16):2159–2167, 2003.

171. Epidemiology of Diabetes Interventions and Complications (EDIC): Design, implementation, and preliminary results of a long-term follow-up of the Diabetes Control and Complications Trial cohort, *Diabetes Care* 22(1):99–111, 1999.

172. The Diabetes Control and Complications Trial/Epidemiology of Diabetes Interventions and Complications Research Group: Retinopathy and nephropathy in patients with type 1 diabetes four years after a trial of intensive therapy, *N Engl J Med* 342(6):381–389, 2000.

173. Knatterud GL, Klimt CR, Levin ME, et al: Effects of hypoglycemic agents on vascular complications in patients with adult-onset diabetes: VII. mortality and selected nonfatal events with insulin treatment, *JAMA* 240(1):37–42, 1978.

174. Kilo C, Miller JP, Williamson JR: The Achilles heel of the University Group Diabetes Program, *JAMA* 243(5):450–457, 1980.

175. Ohkubo Y, Kishikawa H, Araki E, et al: Intensive insulin therapy prevents the progression of diabetic microvascular complications in Japanese patients with non–insulin-dependent diabetes mellitus: a randomized prospective 6-year study [see comment], *Diabetes Res Clin Pract* 28(2):103–117, 1995.

176. Abraira C, Colwell JA, Nuttall FQ, et al: Veterans Affairs Cooperative Study on glycemic control and complications in type II diabetes (VA CSDM): results of the feasibility trial. Veterans Affairs Cooperative Study in Type II Diabetes, *Diabetes Care* 18(8):1113–1123, 1995.

177. UK Prospective Diabetes Study Group: Intensive blood-glucose control with sulphonylureas or insulin compared with conventional treatment and risk of complications in patients with type 2 diabetes (UKPDS 33) [erratum appears in *Lancet* 354 (9178):602, 1999], *Lancet* 352(9131):837–853, 1998.

178. UK Prospective Diabetes Study Group: Effect of intensive blood-glucose control with metformin on complications in overweight patients with type 2 diabetes (UKPDS 34) [erratum appears in *Lancet* 352(9139):1558, 1998], *Lancet* 352(9131):854–865, 1998.

179. UK Prospective Diabetes Study Group: Tight blood pressure control and risk of macrovascular and microvascular complications in type 2 diabetes: UKPDS 38 [erratum appears in *BMJ* 318 (7175):29, 1999], *BMJ* 317(7160):703–713, 1998.

180. National Diabetes Data Group, National Institute of Diabetes and Digestive and Kidney, National Institutes of Health: *Diabetes in America.* NIH publication; no. 95-1468. Bethesda, Md, 1995, National Institutes of Health, National Institute of Diabetes and Digestive and Kidney Diseases.

181. Brun E, Nelson RG, Bennett PH, et al: Diabetes duration and cause-specific mortality in the Verona Diabetes Study, *Diabetes Care* 23(8):1119–1123, 2000.

182. Schernthaner G: Cardiovascular mortality and morbidity in type-2 diabetes mellitus, *Diabetes Res Clin Pract* 31(suppl):S3–S13, 1996.

183. The Diabetes Control and Complications Trial/Epidemiology of Diabetes Interventions and Complications Research Group: Intensive diabetes therapy and carotid intima-media thickness in type 1 diabetes mellitus, *N Engl J Med* 348(23):2294–2303, 2003.

184. Cleary P, Orchard T, Zinman B: Coronary artery calcification in the Diabetes Control and Complications Trial/Epidemiology of Diabetes Interventions and Complications (DCCT/EDIC) cohort, *Diabetes* 52(Suppl 2):A152, 2003 (abstract).

185. Laakso M: Hyperglycemia and cardiovascular disease in type 2 diabetes, *Diabetes* 48(5):937–942, 1999.

186. Pyorala K, Pedersen TR, Kjekshus J, et al: Cholesterol lowering with simvastatin improves prognosis of diabetic patients with coronary heart disease: a subgroup analysis of the Scandinavian Simvastatin Survival Study (4S) [see comment] [erratum appears in *Diabetes Care* 20(6):1048, 1997], *Diabetes Care* 20(4):614–620, 1997.

187. Ravid M, Lang R, Rachmani R, Lishner M: Long-term renoprotective effect of angiotensin-converting enzyme inhibition in non–insulin-dependent diabetes mellitus: a 7-year follow-up study [see comment], *Arch Intern Med* 156(3):286–289, 1996.

188. Hansson L, Zanchetti A, Carruthers SG, et al: Effects of intensive blood-pressure lowering and low-dose aspirin in patients with hypertension: principal results of the Hypertension Optimal Treatment (HOT) randomised trial, *Lancet* 351 (9118):1755, 1998.

189. Correction: Effects of an angiotensin-converting-enzyme inhibitor, ramipril, on cardiovascular events in high-risk patients, *N Engl J Med* 342 (18):1376, 2000.

190. Gaede P, Vedel P, Larsen N, et al: Multifactorial intervention and cardiovascular disease in patients with type 2 diabetes, *N Engl J Med* 348(5):383–393, 2003.

191. Lue TF: Erectile dysfunction, *N Engl J Med* 342 (24):1802–1813, 2000.

192. Seftel AD, Mohammed MA, Althof SE: Erectile dysfunction: etiology, evaluation, and treatment options, *Med Clin North Am* 88(2):387–416, 2004.

193. NIH Consensus Conference: Impotence. NIH Consensus Development Panel on Impotence, *JAMA* 270(1):83–90, 1993.

194. Fedele D, Coscelli C, Santeusanio F, et al: Erectile dysfunction in diabetic subjects in Italy: Gruppo Italiano Studio Deficit Erettile nei Diabetici, *Diabetes Care* 21(11): 1973–1977, 1998.

195. McCulloch DK, Campbell IW, Wu FC, et al: The prevalence of diabetic impotence, *Diabetologia* 18 (4):279–283, 1980.

196. McCulloch DK, Young RJ, Prescott RJ, et al: The natural history of impotence in diabetic men, *Diabetologia* 26(6):437–440, 1984.

197. Klein R, Klein BE, Moss SE: Ten-year incidence of self-reported erectile dysfunction in people with long-term type 1 diabetes, *J Diabetes Complications* 19(1):35–41, 2005.

198. Bacon CG, Hu FB, Giovannucci E, et al: Association of type and duration of diabetes with erectile dysfunction in a large cohort of men, *Diabetes Care* 25(8):1458–1463, 2002.

199. Feldman HA, Goldstein I, Hatzichristou DG, et al: Impotence and its medical and psychosocial correlates: results of the Massachusetts Male Aging Study, *J Urol* 151(1):54–61, 1994.

200. Penson DF, Latini DM, Lubeck DP, et al: Do impotent men with diabetes have more severe erectile dysfunction and worse quality of life than the general population of impotent patients? Results from the Exploratory Comprehensive Evaluation of Erectile Dysfunction (ExCEED) database, *Diabetes Care* 26(4):1093–1099, 2003.

201. Esposito K, Giugliano F, Di Palo C, et al: Effect of lifestyle changes on erectile dysfunction in obese men: a randomized controlled trial, *JAMA* 291 (24):2978–2984, 2004.

202. Williams RH, Wilson JD, Foster DW: *Williams' Textbook of Endocrinology*, Philadelphia, 1992, W.B. Saunders.

203. Reynolds CF III, Frank E, Thase ME, et al: Assessment of sexual function in depressed, impotent, and healthy men: factor analysis of a brief sexual function questionnaire for men, *Psychiatry Res* 24 (3):231–250, 1988.

204. Grover SA, Lowensteyn I, Kaouache M, et al: The prevalence of erectile dysfunction in the primary care setting: importance of risk factors for diabetes and vascular disease, *Arch Intern Med* 166 (2):213–219, 2006.

205. Setter SM, Iltz JL, Fincham JE, et al: Phosphodiesterase 5 inhibitors for erectile dysfunction, *Ann Pharmacother* 39(7):1286–1295, 2005.

206. Cheitlin MD, Hutter AM Jr, Brindis RG, et al: Use of sildenafil (Viagra) in patients with cardiovascular disease, *J Am Coll Cardiol* 33(1):273–282, 1999.

207. Wackers FJT, Young LH, Inzucchi SE, et al: Detection of silent myocardial ischemia in asymptomatic diabetic subjects: the DIAD study, *Diabetes Care* 27 (8):1954–1961, 2004.

208. Goldstein I, Lue TF, Padma-Nathan H, et al: Oral sildenafil in the treatment of erectile dysfunction, *N Engl J Med* 338(20):1397–1404, 1998.

209. Fink HA, Mac Donald R, Rutks IR, et al: Sildenafil for male erectile dysfunction: a systematic review and meta-analysis, *Arch Intern Med* 162(12): 1349–1360, 2002.

210. Goldstein I, Young JM, Fischer J, et al: Vardenafil, a new phosphodiesterase type 5 inhibitor, in the treatment of erectile dysfunction in men with diabetes: a multicenter double-blind placebo-controlled fixed-dose study, *Diabetes Care* 26(3):777–783, 2003.

211. Brock GB, McMahon CG, Chen KK, et al: Efficacy and safety of tadalafil for the treatment of erectile dysfunction: results of integrated analyses, *J Urol* 168(4 [Part 1 of 2]):1332–1336, 2002.

212. Saenz de Tejada I, Anglin G, Knight JR, Emmick JT: Effects of tadalafil on erectile dysfunction in men with diabetes, *Diabetes Care* 25(12):2159–2164, 2002.

213. Fink HA, MacDonald R, Rutks IR, et al: Sildenafil for male erectile dysfunction: a systematic review and meta-analysis, *Arch Intern Med* 162(12):1349–1360, 2002.

214. Rendell MS, Rajfer J, Wicker PA, Smith MD: Sildenafil for treatment of erectile dysfunction in men with diabetes: a randomized controlled trial, *JAMA* 281(5):421–426, 1999.

215. Fonseca V, Jawa A: Endothelial and erectile dysfunction, diabetes mellitus, and the metabolic syndrome: common pathways and treatments? *Am J Cardiol* 96(12B):13M–18M, 2005.

216. Padma-Nathan H, Hellstrom WJ, Kaiser FE, et al: Treatment of men with erectile dysfunction with transurethral alprostadil, *N Engl J Med* 336(1):1–7, 1997.

217. Linet OI, Ogrinc FG, and the Alprostadil Study Group: Efficacy and safety of intracavernosal alprostadil in men with erectile dysfunction, *N Engl J Med* 334(14):873–877, 1996.

218. Bennett AH, Carpenter AJ, Barada JH: An improved vasoactive drug combination for a pharmacological erection program, *J Urol* 146(6): 1564–1565, 1991.

219. Wiles PG: Successful non-invasive management of erectile impotence in diabetic men, *Br Med J Clin Res Ed* 296(6616):161–162, 1988.

220. Ernst E, Pittler MH: Yohimbine for erectile dysfunction: a systematic review and meta-analysis of randomized clinical trials, *J Urol* 159(2): 433–436, 1998.

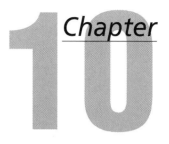

Chapter

10

Gastroenterology

Joel J. Heidelbaugh, MD

Key Points

Peptic Ulcer Disease (PUD)

- A trial of acid suppression therapy and eradication of *H. pylori* (if present) should be considered in the management of functional dyspepsia (strength of recommendation: A).
- The noninvasive *H. pylori* "test and treat" strategy is as effective as upper endoscopy in the initial management of patients with uncomplicated dyspepsia who are younger than 45 years old and do not exhibit alarm signs (strength of recommendation: A).
- Prophylaxis with PPIs should be considered in patients at high risk for NSAID-associated PUD, including patients with a history of PUD, elderly patients, and patients taking corticosteroids or anticoagulants (strength of recommendation: A).

Gastroesophageal Reflux Disease (GERD)

- Although less effective than proton pump inhibitors (PPIs), H2RAs given in divided doses may be effective in some patients with less severe symptoms of GERD. Since GERD is a chronic condition, on-demand (patient-directed) therapy to control symptoms and to prevent complications is appropriate (strength of recommendation: A).

Inflammatory Bowel Disease (IBD)

- Systemic steroids are effective for inducing—but not maintaining—remission in IBD (strength of recommendation: A).
- 5-ASA derivatives are effective in ulcerative colitis (UC) for both therapy induction and maintenance therapy, but largely are ineffective in the treatment of Crohn's disease (strength of recommendation: A).

Irritable Bowel Syndrome (IBS)

- Tegaserod is more effective than placebo at relieving global IBS symptoms in constipation-predominant IBS (strength of recommendation: A). (Note: Evidence reflects studies in women; data regarding men are extrapolated from these studies.)
- Alosetron is more effective than placebo at relieving global IBS symptoms in diarrhea-predominant IBS (strength of recommendation: A). (Note: Evidence reflects studies in women; data regarding men are extrapolated from these studies.)

Diverticular Disease

- Patients who are able to tolerate a diet, who do not have systemic symptoms, and who do not have significant peritoneal signs may be treated on an outpatient basis with oral trimethoprim-sulfamethoxazole or a fluoroquinolone plus metronidazole (strength of recommendation: B).

Pancreatitis

- The two tests that are the most helpful at admission in distinguishing mild from severe acute pancreatitis are the APACHE II score and the serum hematocrit measurement (strength of recommendation: C).

Introduction

The overall impact of gastrointestinal disorders in men is often underestimated from both a biopsychosocial and cost-utilization standpoint. Diseases of the gastrointestinal tract are commonly misdiagnosed, mistreated, and misunderstood ultimately leading to substantial psychological morbidity and direct and indirect expense, estimated to be over $40 billion annually. According to the American Gastroenterological Association,[1] more than 62 million Americans are diagnosed each year with disorders of the digestive tract including peptic ulcer disease (PUD), gastroesophageal reflux disease (GERD), inflammatory bowel disease (IBD), irritable bowel syndrome (IBS), gastrointestinal cancers, motility disorders, hepatitis, cirrhosis, diverticulosis, and food-borne illness. The vast majority of gastrointestinal tract diseases affect male patients between the ages of 15 and 64 years and range from being acute and self-limiting to chronic and relapsing. Loss of work productivity and overall decreases in health-related quality of life can be substantial for male patients with various digestive diseases. This chapter provides an overview of several gastrointestinal disorders commonly encountered in men, highlighting the most recent evidence-based diagnostic and therapeutic guidelines and reviews.

Dyspepsia

Dyspepsia (literally, "bad digestion") refers to an episodic or recurrent pain or discomfort arising from the proximal gastrointestinal tract related to eating and is associated with heartburn, acid reflux, regurgitation, indigestion, bloating, early satiety, or weight loss. The lack of a standardized definition affects any determination of accurate prevalence data, given the challenge of clearly defining dyspepsia as either *functional* or *nonulcer dyspepsia* (NUD). Dyspepsia attributed to structural or biochemical disease accounts for approximately 40% of cases, whereas NUD composes roughly 60% of cases.[2] By definition, patients with functional dyspepsia should have no organic explanation for their symptoms. Uninvestigated dyspepsia includes all symptomatic patients, regardless of whether an etiology has been found. Proposed etiologies for symptoms in patients with functional dyspepsia include disturbances in gastrointestinal motility, gastric accommodation, visceral sensation, intestinogastric reflexes, autonomic nervous system function, and various psychosocial factors.[3]

Dyspepsia accounts for approximately 5% of all primary care visits and is the most common reason for referral to a gastroenterologist in the United States, composing 20–40% of consultations.[4] An estimated 17–25% of adults in the United States and other Western countries experience recurrent dyspepsia; no current data exist to suggest a male versus female predominance. Studies examining factors that determine referral for gastroenterology evaluation of dyspepsia are lacking. Most patients with organic dyspepsia due to GERD, PUD, or even malignancy are managed empirically by their primary care provider.[4] Management strategies for dyspepsia have therefore been designed to reduce the number of endoscopic procedures, and ultimately, direct cost and inconvenience to the patient.

When patients with dyspepsia undergo extensive evaluations and are monitored over time, other related conditions may be identified including nonerosive reflux disease (NERD), lactose intolerance, cholelithiasis, gastroparesis, chronic pancreatitis, pancreatic cancer, celiac disease, giardiasis, and even ischemic heart disease. No single item from the patient history or physical examination has been proved to effectively and clearly establish a diagnosis of dyspepsia. One study demonstrated that epigastric tenderness on physical examination failed to accurately distinguish patients with abnormal endoscopy findings from those with normal findings. In this study, abdominal tenderness to light or deep palpation had a likelihood ratio near 1, signifying that this maneuver had no diagnostic value.[5]

NUD is diagnosed in patients with a negative radiographic or endoscopic evaluation result that failed to suggest an organic lesion such as an ulcer or tumor to explain their upper gastrointestinal symptoms. Potential etiologies for NUD include gastric acid hypersecretion, gastroduodenal dysmotility, visceral hypersensitivity, emotional stress, and other psychological factors. The prognosis of NUD for many patients is discouraging due to chronic relapses. As with other functional gastrointestinal disorders, the potential for underlying psychosocial and lifestyle factors must be addressed. Currently, no evidence-based recommendation exists regarding pharmacologic management of functional dyspepsia, nor is there any solid evidence to support a recommendation of specific diet and lifestyle modifications, or psychosocial interventions.

Peptic Ulcer Disease

PUD is a leading cause of dyspepsia and therefore has numerous etiologies (Table 10-1), with a cumulative lifetime prevalence of approximately 8–14% and a slight male predominance. There are approximately 4.5 million cases of PUD in the United States each year; almost a half

Table 10-1. Causes of Dyspepsia

Common (in Order of Relative Frequency)
GERD (with and without erosive esophagitis)
Functional (nonulcer dyspepsia)
Peptic ulcer disease
Less Common (Alphabetical Order)
Alcohol consumption
Biliary colic
Celiac disease
Gastrointestinal malignancy
Gastroparesis
Infection (viral, bacterial, spirochete, parasitic)
Inflammatory and infiltrative processes involving the esophagus, stomach, or small bowel
Intestinal ischemia
Lactose intolerance
Medications, most commonly aspirin and nonsteroidal anti-inflammatory drugs
Pancreatitis
Pregnancy
Other systemic and metabolic disorders

GERD, Gastroesophageal reflux disease.
Adapted from: Saad R, Scheiman JM: Diagnosis and management of peptic ulcer disease, *Clin Fam Pract* 6(3):569–587, 2004.

a million cases are new, whereas the remainder represents recurrent disease. Although up to 70% of patients with gastric and duodenal ulcers fall between the ages of 25 and 64 years, the peak prevalence of complicated ulcer disease requiring hospitalization is in the 65–74-year age group.[6]

The classic defining symptom of PUD is that of an "aching," "gnawing," or "hunger-like" epigastric pain, although atypical presentations are common. Pain related to gastric ulcers often occurs within minutes after eating and can persist up to several hours until the stomach empties; it is commonly absent during fasting. Pain resultant from duodenal ulcers is often relieved by eating, drinking milk, or taking antacids, and it can return between 90 minutes and 4 hours after eating. Both classifications of ulcers may be associated with nausea and vomiting occurring anytime shortly after eating to several hours later.[6] Complications of PUD often occur without warning symptoms and are frequently seen in elderly patients who routinely take nonsteroidal anti-inflammatory drugs (NSAIDs), aspirin, or both.

Figure 10-1 outlines an algorithm for the evaluation and management of uninvestigated dyspepsia, as well as alarm symptoms concerning advanced disease. The American Gastroenterological Association and the American College of Physicians have endorsed prompt endoscopic evaluation in any patient older than 45 years with a new onset of dyspepsia. The presence of alarm symptoms in men older than 45 years (especially Asian men) should raise immediate concern for a gastric malignancy, necessitating a prompt referral for upper endoscopic evaluation.

The most common complications of PUD include upper gastrointestinal tract bleeding (UGIB), perforation, penetration, and gastric outlet obstruction. UGIB occurs in up to 15% of patients with PUD, most commonly in patients older than 60 years of age, and carries a 10% mortality rate. Gastric perforation occurs in approximately 7% of patients with PUD, again classically in elderly patients taking NSAIDs, aspirin, or both on a chronic basis. Most gastric ulcers perforate along the anterior wall of the lesser curvature of the stomach, whereas most duodenal ulcers perforate anteriorly. Perforation is hallmarked by abdominal pain and rigidity, the absence of bowel sounds, and a reported sense of impending doom by the patient. Confirmation of gastric perforation is accomplished via plain film abdominal radiography, yielding free air under the diaphragm. Barium contrast studies and upper endoscopy are contraindicated if perforation is suspected, and an urgent surgical consultation is mandatory because this condition is life-threatening due to impending hemodynamic instability. Mortality rates range from 30% to 50% in cases of perforation, particularly in elderly and debilitated patients.

Penetration occurs when the ulcer crater erodes through and into adjacent organs including the small bowel, pancreas, liver, or biliary tree, commonly presenting as acute pancreatitis. Gastric outlet obstruction occurs in 1–3% of cases of PUD, resulting from either the effects of acute inflammation or mechanical obstruction due to scarring at the gastroduodenal junction. The presentation of an obstruction is also typically insidious, often presenting with symptoms of GERD, early satiety, weight loss, abdominal pain, and vomiting. If the obstruction is primarily due to acute inflammation, it then commonly responds well to medical therapy, including bowel rest and nasogastric suction, whereas cases resulting from scarring often require endoscopic or surgical therapy.[6]

Approaches to confirm a diagnosis of PUD include double-contrast barium esophagrams (the upper gastrointestinal tract series) and upper endoscopy. Despite a higher procedural cost and a slightly increased risk in procedure-related

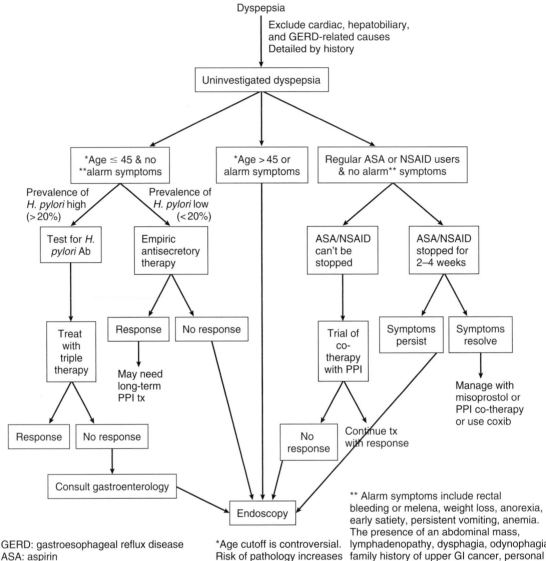

Dyspepsia

Exclude cardiac, hepatobiliary,
and GERD-related causes
Detailed by history

Uninvestigated dyspepsia

*Age ≤ 45 & no
**alarm symptoms

*Age >45 or
alarm symptoms

Regular ASA or NSAID users
& no alarm** symptoms

Prevalence of
H. pylori high
(>20%)

Prevalence of
H. pylori low
(<20%)

Test for *H.
pylori* Ab

Empiric
antisecretory
therapy

ASA/NSAID
can't be
stopped

ASA/NSAID
stopped for
2–4 weeks

Treat
with
triple
therapy

Response

No response

Trial of
co-
therapy
with PPI

Symptoms
persist

Symptoms
resolve

May need
long-term
PPI tx

Manage with
misoprostol or
PPI co-therapy
or use coxib

Response

No response

No
response

Continue tx
with response

Consult gastroenterology

Endoscopy

** Alarm symptoms include rectal
bleeding or melena, weight loss, anorexia,
early satiety, persistent vomiting, anemia.
The presence of an abdominal mass,
lymphadenopathy, dysphagia, odynophagia,
family history of upper GI cancer, personal
history of peptic ulcer, prior gastric surgery,
or malignancy should eliminate
consideration of noninvasive approaches.

GERD: gastroesophageal reflux disease
ASA: aspirin
NSAIDs: nonsteroidal anti-inflammatory drugs
PPI: proton pump inhibitor
H. pylori: Helicobacter pylori

*Age cutoff is controversial.
Risk of pathology increases
slightly with age but older
age (50–55) cutoff in many
guidelines

Figure 10-1. Evaluation of uninvestigated dyspepsia. (Adapted from: Saad R, Scheiman JM: Diagnosis and management of peptic ulcer disease, *Clin Fam Pract* 6[3]:569–587, 2004.)

complications (i.e., bleeding, perforation, and oversedation), the upper endoscopy should be the initial diagnostic study performed in suspected PUD because it provides the advantage of permitting biopsies to potentially identify the presence of underlying pathology and it allows for direct procedural intervention in the event of acute UGIB.

Helicobacter pylori infection is a major risk factor for the development of PUD. Its prevalence and association with PUD is higher in populations where the standard of living is considered to be lower than that of the United States, especially in Africa and Central America. Approximately 90% of patients worldwide with duodenal ulcers are infected with the *H. pylori* pathogen, yet in the United States, its association with PUD ranges from 30% to 60%. The strongest evidence to support the role of *H. pylori* as an etiology of PUD is the elimination of ulcer recurrence when the infection has been successfully eradicated.[7]

Evidence-based guidelines recommend that patients younger than 45 years of age with dyspepsia and without alarm symptoms of advanced gastrointestinal disease should be tested for *H. pylori* infection, then treated if results are positive (the "test and treat" strategy), whereas patients older than 45 years who have alarm symptoms should undergo prompt endoscopy.[8] Biopsy specimens obtained during endoscopy can confirm a diagnosis of *H. pylori* infection with 100% sensitivity and specificity. *H. pylori*–negative patients younger than 45 years and without alarm symptoms should be managed empirically for functional dyspepsia. *H. pylori* testing via nonendoscopic methods includes the quantitative assay for serum immunoglobulin G antibodies, the radio-labeled urea breath test, and the stool antigen test. Comparative studies have shown superiority for urea breath tests in the diagnosis of *H. pylori* infection because they have higher sensitivities and specificities than the serologic assays.[9] The European Helicobacter Pylori Study Group[10] recommends the stool antigen test as the preferred initial noninvasive diagnostic test. The urea breath test is currently the recommended gold standard to determine *H. pylori* eradication,[8] yet it is the most expensive of all tests and is thought to be equal to stool antigen testing in determining eradication. Antibody test results typically remain positive after eradication and should not be used.

When a patient tests positive for *H. pylori* antibodies, treatment should be initiated. Strong evidence suggests that *H. pylori* infection increases the risk of PUD in patients taking concomitant NSAIDs or low-dose aspirin, despite the ongoing controversy regarding the causative roles of *H. pylori* and NSAIDs in ulcer and ulcer complications.[11] Whether persons taking NSAIDs or low-dose aspirin should be routinely tested for *H. pylori* infection and treated if results are positive is still hotly debated, especially in countries where the prevalence of *H. pylori* infection and PUD are both high. Although most *H. pylori*–infected patients do not develop an ulcer, as many as 95% of patients with duodenal ulcers and 80% of those with gastric ulcers are infected. A meta-analysis of randomized controlled trials (RCTs) of *H. pylori* eradication for the treatment of duodenal ulcers found that one ulcer recurrence (evidenced on endoscopy) would be prevented for every 2.8 patients successfully treated.[12]

There are several medication regimens for the treatment of *H. pylori* infection, according to the best data from RCTs and systematic reviews (Table 10-2). Currently, the most effective evidence-based treatment is 14-day triple therapy with a proton pump inhibitor (PPI), clarithromycin, and either amoxicillin or metronidazole, yielding eradication rates from 75% to 90%.[8] Although no studies exist to demonstrate any difference among the available PPIs when used in triple-therapy regimens, the chosen antibiotic has been shown to affect the eradication rates due to various levels of antibiotic resistance. The current resistance rates of *H. pylori* in the United States approximate 33% for metronidazole, 11% for clarithromycin, and almost 0% for amoxicillin. One study revealed that patients who had taken more than five courses of macrolides had an 80% prevalence of clarithromycin-resistant strains of *H. pylori* compared with 7% in patients who had never received macrolides. Patients who had received one course of macrolides had a 28% prevalence of resistant organisms.[13] Risk factors for clarithromycin resistance include older age, female sex, and inactive ulcer disease. Metronidazole resistance has been linked to female sex and Asian ethnicity.[14]

Patients with PUD should have adequate medical follow-up, since further diagnostic testing may be needed to ensure eradication of the *H. pylori* organism, particularly in the cases of treatment failure and relapse. Since eradication therapy cures PUD in most cases, chronic acid suppression is often unnecessary in most patients who have cleared the *H. pylori* infection and who are not currently taking NSAIDs. One study showed that, among patients with a history of PUD and who were taking chronic acid suppressive therapy, 78% of those treated for *H. pylori* were able to discontinue therapy.[15]

The other main etiology of PUD is the increasing and widespread use of both NSAIDs and aspirin. The recommendations for aspirin use for cardiovascular risk prevention are strong, and many men take NSAIDs in addition to aspirin, often without disclosing this practice to their healthcare provider. Approximately 60% of unexplained cases of PUD are attributed to unrecognized NSAID use, as the use and overuse of these medications is the most common cause of PUD in *H. pylori*–negative patients. A meta-analysis of observational studies of gastrointestinal bleeding risk due to various NSAIDs showed that a four-fold increased risk associated with NSAID use persisted throughout therapy and fell to baseline within 2 months of discontinuation of the NSAID.[16] Concomitant NSAID and aspirin use is frequently associated with symptoms of

Table 10-2. Pharmacologic Regimens for *Helicobacter pylori* Eradication

Regimen	Eradication Rates	Comments
PPI*	80–90%	First-line therapy
Clarithromycin 500 mg bid		
Amoxicillin 1000 mg bid		
PPI	80–90%	Only consider in penicillin allergy
Clarithromycin 500 mg bid		Concern for antibiotic resistance
Metronidazole 500 mg bid		
Ranitidine 150 mg bid	75–85%	Conventional regimen
Bismuth subsalicylate 525 mg qid		Cheapest regimen
		High pill count
Metronidazole 250 mg qid		
Tetracycline 500 mg qid		
PPI qd	75–85%	Alternative to first-line therapy
Bismuth subsalicylate 525 mg qid		
Metronidazole 250 mg qid		
Tetracycline 500 mg qid		

PPI, Proton pump inhibitor, bid, twice a day, qid, four times a day, qd, once a day.
*Standard dosages for PPIs are as follows: lansoprazole 30 mg bid, omeprazole 20 mg bid, pantoprazole 40 mg bid, rabeprazole 20 mg bid, esomeprazole 40 mg qd.
Note: Treatment should be for 10 to 14 days for PPI-based triple therapy and 14 days for all other regimens.
Adapted from: Saad R, Scheiman JM: Diagnosis and management of peptic ulcer disease, *Clin Fam Pract* 6(3):569–587, 2004.

dyspepsia, even in the absence of PUD. A recent RCT demonstrated that the PPI esomeprazole is effective in preventing ulcers in long-term users of NSAIDs, including cyclooxygenase-2 inhibitors.[17] Although *H. pylori* infection and aspirin and NSAID use account for the overwhelming majority of cases of PUD, other factors contribute to the remaining minority of cases (Table 10-3).

A thorough evaluation by primary care providers should be conducted to exclude *H. pylori* infection and surreptitious NSAID and aspirin use. The optimal management plan is the avoidance of NSAIDs in high-risk persons (particularly in elderly persons), in patients with a prior history of PUD, and in patients taking chronic corticosteroids or anticoagulants. These agents have been proved to have beneficial effects from their anti-inflammatory and antithrombotic properties, yet in many disease states there may be no other effective alternative medication to treat concomitant medical conditions. Both meta-analyses and large population-based case-controlled studies have demonstrated that patients older than 70 years or those with previous ulcer complications are at the greatest risk for peptic ulcer complications in NSAID users. Evidence suggests that smoking may increase the risk of PUD and ulcer complications by impairing gastric mucosal healing. Alcohol consumption may increase the risk of ulcer complications in NSAID users, but its overall effect in those patients without concomitant liver disease has not been clearly defined. Epidemiologic data have shown an increased risk of duodenal ulcers in patients with chronic obstructive pulmonary disease (a three- to five-fold increase), hepatic cirrhosis (a five- to eight-fold increase), chronic renal failure, and cystic fibrosis.[18] Lastly, it has been recognized that there is an increased familial incidence of PUD, most likely due to the familial clustering of *H. pylori*, and inherited genetic factors reflecting poor host responses to this organism.[6]

Gastroesophageal Reflux Disease

GERD is a common chronic and relapsing condition defined as symptoms or mucosal damage produced by the abnormal reflux of gastric contents into the esophagus. Forty percent of US adults experience heartburn at least once a month, and the age- and sex-adjusted prevalence of either weekly heartburn or acid regurgitation approaches 20%.[19,20] Most patients with symptoms of GERD self-treat with over-the-counter

Table 10-3. Etiologies of Peptic Ulcer Disease

Major Causes
Helicobacter pylori infection
Nonsteroidal anti-inflammatory drugs
Aspirin
Minor Causes
Duodenal obstruction from an annular pancreas
Use of topically injurious drugs (e.g., potassium chloride, nitrogen-containing bisphosphonates)
Immunosuppressants (e.g., mycophenolate)
Infection with *Helicobacter heilmannii*
Mucosal infection with herpes simplex virus type 1, cytomegalovirus, tuberculosis, and/or syphilis
Systemic processes (e.g., systemic mastocytosis, Crohn's disease, lymphoma, or various carcinomas)
Radiation involving the duodenum
Use of cocaine or "crack" cocaine
Zollinger-Ellison syndrome

Heidelbaugh JJ: Peptic ulcer disease. In Rakel RE, editor: *Essential Family Medicine: Fundamentals and Cases with Student Consult Access,* ed 3, Philadelphia, 2006, Elsevier.

Table 10-4. Atypical or Extraesophageal Manifestations of Gastroesophageal Reflux Disease

Aspiration of stomach contents
Asthma/wheezing
Chronic nonproductive cough
Globus sensation
Loss of dental enamel
Noncardiac chest pain
Recurrent laryngitis
Recurrent noninfectious pharyngitis
Subglottic stenosis

Adapted from: Heidelbaugh JJ, Nostrant TT: Medical and surgical management of gastroesophageal reflux disease, *Clin Fam Pract* 6 (3):547–568, 2004.

(OTC) medications and do not initially seek medical attention. Survey studies assessing health-related quality of life report that patients with GERD have lower symptomatic assessment scores than patients with congestive heart failure, coronary artery disease, and diabetes mellitus.[21]

Most patients with GERD who are evaluated in primary care practices have NERD, and over time a small percentage of these cases will progress to erosive esophagitis, and even fewer to more severe disease resulting in esophageal strictures, Barrett's esophagus, and adenocarcinoma of the esophagus. Patients with NERD are prone to develop atypical or extraesophageal manifestations of disease (Table 10-4), yet because of a small risk of disease progression, they generally do not require long-term endoscopic surveillance despite persistent reflux symptoms. Symptom relapse rates in patients with NERD are similar to those in patients with erosive esophagitis. Although many patients will require continuous pharmacologic treatment to control their symptoms, almost all of these patients continue to exhibit no definable erosive esophagitis on upper endoscopy.[22]

An accurate clinical history is imperative in appropriately diagnosing GERD. The 24-hour pH probe is accepted as the standard for establishing or excluding the presence of GERD, but lacks adequate sensitivity and specificity required to be a gold standard and is often impractical and unnecessary. Double-contrast barium radiography has limited usefulness in diagnosing GERD but may be useful in defining the presence of anatomic abnormalities including hiatal hernia and esophageal strictures. Upper endoscopy is the gold standard in assessing esophageal and gastric complications of GERD, yet this modality lacks an appreciable sensitivity and specificity for identifying pathologic reflux.[23]

Treatment goals for GERD include symptom relief and improvement of health-related quality of life, healing erosive esophagitis if present, managing and preventing complications, and avoiding recurrence and progression of disease using acid suppressive medications in a cost-effective fashion. Pharmacologic options for the treatment of GERD include antacids, OTC (1/2 strength) and prescription histamine-2 receptor antagonists (H2Ras), Prilosec OTC and prescription PPIs, and prokinetic agents. Although promotility agents can be used to augment therapy, they are seldom used due to their association with rare fatal cardiac arrhythmias.[23]

Empiric pharmacotherapy consists of either an H2RA or a PPI initially, as the immediate need for diagnostic testing is unnecessary in the majority of cases. Expert opinion supports either step-up or step-down therapy for the initial pharmacologic treatment of patients with GERD (Figure 10-2). In patients who incompletely respond to a trial of either OTC or prescription H2RAs, PPIs taken once daily 30 minutes before the first meal of the day are preferred over continuing H2RA therapy due to their greater efficacy and faster symptom control, as well as the limited additional benefit gained from extending therapy with the same

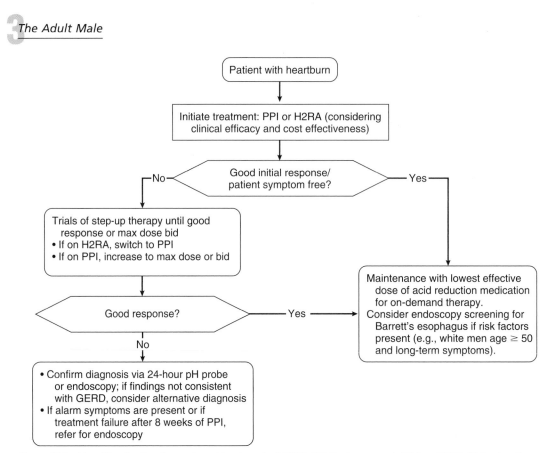

Figure 10-2. Algorithm for the diagnosis and treatment of GERD. PPI, Proton pump inhibitor; H2RA, histamine-2 receptor antagonist; bid, twice a day. (Adapted from: Heidelbaugh JJ, Gill A, Nostrant TT, Harrison RV: Gastroesophageal reflux disease [GERD], Ann Arbor, MI, 2006, Office of Clinical Affairs, University of Michigan Health System. Available at http://www.guideline.gov.)

or higher dose of H2RA.[24] An inadequate response to a 4- or 8-week trial of standard-dose PPI therapy may indicate the need for longer treatment, more severe disease, or an incorrect diagnosis. Since a substantial proportion of patients may remain in remission without maintenance therapy, an attempt to discontinue therapy is considered to be a reasonable option in most patients.[24]

Diagnostic testing is warranted in patients with GERD who (1) have an inadequate response to continuous PPI therapy, (2) have chronic symptoms lasting longer than 5 years and are at risk for development of Barrett's esophagus, (3) have atypical and/or extraesophageal manifestations suggesting complicated disease, or (4) have alarm symptoms suggesting cancer (Table 10-5). Observational studies have suggested that the progression to severe esophagitis has not occurred in patients with an initial normal endoscopy whose symptoms have remained unchanged during a 10-year follow-up period, arguing against the need for repeat endoscopy during that time period in the absence of any alarm symptoms.[25]

Lifestyle modifications should be recommended as adjunctive therapy in all patients with GERD (Table 10-6). Although evidence is lacking to support the use of nonpharmacologic measures as sole initial or long-term therapy for GERD,

Table 10-5. Alarm Symptoms of Gastroesophageal Reflux Disease Suggesting Complicated Disease

Black or bloody stools
Choking
Chronic coughing
Dysphagia
Early satiety
Hematemesis
Hoarseness
Iron-deficiency anemia
Odynophagia
Weight loss

Adapted from: Heidelbaugh JJ, Nostrant TT: Medical and surgical management of gastroesophageal reflux disease, *Clin Fam Pract* 6(3):547–568, 2004.

Table 10-6. Suggested Lifestyle Modifications for the Treatment of Gastroesophageal Reflux Disease (GERD)

Avoiding acidic foods (e.g., citrus and tomato-based products), alcohol, caffeinated beverages, chocolate, onions, garlic, salt*, and peppermint
Avoiding large meals
Avoiding medications that may potentiate GERD symptoms: calcium channel blockers, beta-agonists, alpha-adrenergic agonists, theophylline, nitrates, and sedatives
Avoiding recumbency 3–4 hours postprandially
Avoiding tight clothing around the waist
Decreasing dietary fat intake
Elevating the head of bed 4–8 inches
Losing weight
Smoking cessation

*Dietary fibers and physical exercise may be protective from this contributing factor.

Summarized from: DeVault KR, Castell DO: Updated guidelines for the diagnosis and treatment of gastroesophageal reflux disease: the Practice Parameters Committee of the American College of Gastroenterology, *Am J Gastroenterol* 100:190–200, 2005; Nilsson M, Johnsen R, Ye W, et al: Lifestyle related risk factors in the aetiology of gastro-oesophageal reflux, *Gut* 53:1730–1735, 2004.

expert opinion considers them to be of some potential benefit and no proven harm, yet not sufficiently effective in treatment alone in most cases of NERD.

Endoscopic therapies for the treatment of GERD refractory to pharmacotherapy include endoscopic gastroplasty and radiofrequency ablation (the Stretta procedure). These procedures are aimed at reducing reflux symptomatology, decreasing the use of anti-reflux medications, and improving the patient's overall quality of life without incurring the risks and costs associated with conventional anti-reflux surgery. Preliminary results using these various techniques are promising, yet all procedures described to date are limited by the absence of large, rigorously controlled trials against safe and effective, conventional anti-reflux therapy with PPIs.

The choice regarding whether to consider anti-reflux surgery for the treatment of refractory GERD must be individualized. The basic tenets of anti-reflux surgery include reduction of the hiatal hernia, repair of the diaphragmatic hiatus, strengthening of the gastroesophageal junction–posterior diaphragm attachment, and strengthening of the anti-reflux barrier by adding a gastric wrap around the gastroesophageal junction (the Nissen/Toupet fundoplication).[24] In case-controlled studies comparing anti-reflux surgery to anti-

secretory therapy, surgery has shown marginal superiority as measured by heartburn relief, esophagitis healing, and improved quality of life in patients with erosive esophagitis. Long-term follow-up trials have found that more than half of patients have resumed taking anti-reflux medications 3–5 years after surgery, most likely as a result of poor patient selection and surgical breakdown.[26]

Barrett's Esophagus and Esophageal Adenocarcinoma

Barrett's esophagus is a premalignant condition related to chronic GERD hallmarked by a change in the mucosal lining of the distal esophagus from the normal squamous epithelium to columnar-appearing mucosa resembling that of the stomach and small intestines (i.e., intestinal metaplasia.) The estimated risk of progression to adenocarcinoma of the esophagus with Barrett's esophagus is approximately 0.5% per year, whereas that without Barrett's esophagus is 0.07% per year. Adenocarcinoma of the esophagus has had the fastest rising incidence of any cancer in the United States and Western Europe over the last two decades. Primary care physicians who see the vast majority of patients with GERD in its nonerosive and more complicated forms must suspect and appropriately refer patients with Barrett's esophagus for upper endoscopy. Although risk factors for Barrett's esophagus and adenocarcinoma are not truly evidence-based, epidemiologic data suggest that male gender, white race, older age, smoking, and obesity place patients at a higher risk.[27]

No evidence-based guidelines currently exist regarding the assessment and surveillance of patients with Barrett's esophagus. Recommendations from the American College of Gastroenterology (ACG)[27] state that if no esophageal dysplasia is recognized after two endoscopic evaluations with biopsy, then a patient can undergo repeat upper endoscopy at 3–4-year intervals. If low-grade dysplasia is detected, then a repeat endoscopy is necessary to confirm that only low-grade dysplasia is present in the esophagus. If low-grade dysplasia is once again documented, then the patient should undergo two more endoscopic examinations at 6-month intervals and then yearly until low-grade dysplasia is no longer recognized. If a patient has high-grade dysplasia evidenced on upper endoscopy (highest risk for progression to cancer), then a repeat endoscopic examination is needed to confirm that cancer is not yet present in the esophagus. When adenocarcinoma is detected on biopsy in an appropriate surgical candidate, referral to a cardiothoracic surgeon for evaluation of esophageal resection is deemed appropriate.[27]

Adenocarcinoma of the esophagus is a potentially treatable disease from a palliative standpoint that is rarely curable. The overall 5-year survival rate in patients amenable to surgery ranges from 5% to 20%. The occasional patient who presents very early in the course of the disease has a better chance of survival. Patients with severe dysplasia in distal esophageal Barrett's mucosa often have in situ or even invasive cancer within the dysplastic area. After esophageal resection, these patients usually have an excellent prognosis but may have chronic GERD, nausea, vomiting, and upper gastrointestinal dysmotility. Primary treatment modalities aimed at palliation include surgery alone or in combination with chemotherapy, radiation therapy, or both.

Cirrhosis

Cirrhosis and chronic liver failure rank as the twelfth leading cause of death in the United States, accounting for 26,549 deaths, or 9.0 deaths per 100,000 in the US population in 2004, with a slight male predominance.[28] In the United States, the vast majority of cirrhosis-related morbidity and mortality is a result either of a solitary factor or a combination of excessive alcohol consumption, viral hepatitis (most commonly B and C), or obesity-related nonalcoholic fatty liver disease and is thus, in theory, preventable. *Cirrhosis* refers to a progressive diffuse, fibrosing, and nodular condition that disrupts the entire normal architecture of the liver. As a consequence of hepatic necrosis and inflammation, fibrosis with distortion of the hepatic microcirculation occurs, leading to synthetic dysfunction and increased resistance to portal blood flow. Almost one half of patients with cirrhosis are asymptomatic because the condition is commonly discovered during a routine examination, via laboratory or radiographic studies, or at autopsy. Mortality rates in patients with alcoholic liver disease are considerably higher than in patients with other forms of cirrhosis.

The major complications of cirrhosis that affect survival include the formation of ascites, spontaneous bacterial peritonitis, hepatorenal syndrome, encephalopathy, and gastrointestinal bleeding resulting from portal hypertension and esophageal and gastric varices. Another serious complication of cirrhosis is the development of hepatocellular carcinoma, for which screening protocols with ultrasound and serum alpha fetoprotein testing have been shown to be cost-effective.[29] All patients with ascites should be evaluated for liver transplantation due to poor 5-year survival rate estimated at 30–40%.[30]

The most common indications for liver transplantation include fulminant hepatic failure from alcoholic liver disease and hepatitis C. For each patient, the risks of transplant surgery and post-transplant immunosuppression must be weighed against the potential benefits of improved survival, decreased morbidity, and hope for improved quality of life. Transplant care before and after surgery requires a multidisciplinary approach including primary care providers, medical specialists, and surgeons.[31] In the last few decades, post–liver transplantation outcomes have improved given the use of newer immunosuppressive medications, improvement in surgical techniques, and improvement in organ recipient and donor selection.[32]

Inflammatory Bowel Disease

IBD is a chronic and relapsing condition that often requires long-term maintenance therapy for most of the more than half a million Americans affected. The most common forms of IBD are ulcerative colitis (UC) and Crohn's disease. The incidence of UC and Crohn's disease is approximately 1.5–8 new cases per 100,000 persons per year in the United States, more commonly seen among white persons and with no specific gender predominance, although some reviews have suggested a male predominance in Crohn's disease and a female predominance in UC. Most patients are diagnosed with IBD either between the ages of 15 and 25 years or during a second peak of incidence between 55 and 65 years of age.[33]

Genetic factors have been shown to play an important role in the development of IBD. First-degree relatives of patients with either form of IBD have been shown to have a 10% lifetime risk of developing disease. Environmental factors are also thought to be important in IBD pathogenesis because the risk of IBD has been shown to increase when people migrate to a higher-risk region, such as the United States or Western Europe. It is believed that exposure to endemic parasites in Africa and Asia has a protective effect against development of IBD because an anti-inflammatory immune response is stimulated.[33]

UC involves the mucosal layer of the sigmoid colon and rectum in the vast majority of cases, causing proctitis and proctosigmoiditis. Proximal spread of disease tends to be continuous and symmetric, causing intestinal mucosal inflammation with edema and friability that is visualized from the rectum proximally. Pancolitis is caused by inflammatory exudates producing a "backwash ileitis" through a patent ileocecal valve, leading to involvement of the small intestine. Chronic cycles of flares and healing can produce scarring and ultimately shortening of the colon.

Crohn's disease differs from UC in that it may involve any part of the gastrointestinal tract from the mouth to the anus, including the gallbladder and biliary tree, and involves the entire thickness of the bowel wall. It is most commonly found in the immunologically rich terminal ileum and involves the rectum in fewer than half of cases. In contrast to UC, the mucosal abnormalities are discontinuous and asymmetric "skip lesions" are commonly seen, which account for obstruction, abscesses, and perianal fistulae. Crohn's disease often produces an endoscopic appearance of "rake marks" or "cobblestone patterns." Recurrent disease flares and healing of the disease can result in significant muscular hypertrophy and fibrosis of the intestinal wall leading to small bowel strictures, upstream dilation of intestine and increased fistula formation, and eventual bowel obstruction and the imminent need for surgical resection.[33]

Most patients with UC present with mild to moderate diarrhea and without any constitutional symptoms. Typically, the more severe the illness, the greater the number of bowel movements, and the more likely constitutional symptoms such as fever, fatigue, dehydration, and weight loss will also occur. UC can be intermittent with flare-ups, and remission may occur without therapy. A minority of patients with UC present with severe or fulminant panniculitis, ranging from an acute abdomen to toxic megacolon. Frequent urgent and bloody diarrhea usually suggests rectal disease and is most consistent with UC. During an exacerbation, patients with UC and Crohn's disease can look and feel ill and often require hospitalization, yet if the disease is mild, they can appear quite normal except for the complaint of diarrhea.

In mild cases of Crohn's disease, or when only a few inches of the terminal ileum are involved, abdominal pain may be vague, diarrhea intermittent, and weight loss absent. In cases with more extensive small bowel or colonic involvement, the presentation often consists of significant abdominal pain, frequent diarrhea, and a weight loss of 5–20 lb. Colonic involvement with Crohn's disease may present similar to UC, with predominantly bloody diarrhea. Rectal involvement produces more urgent and frequent

small, bloody stools as a result of an inflamed, nondistensible rectum. Mucus in the stool is nonspecific for any gastrointestinal disease and is found in both IBD and IBS.[33] When Crohn's disease involves primarily the colon, it may be indistinguishable from UC. Since Crohn's disease frequently affects the terminal ileum or the right side of the colon, patients with this condition may have steady right lower quadrant abdominal pain due to transmural inflammation that may worsen with movement. Sometimes, abscesses may develop because of the microperforations in the area of disease, and sometimes acute small bowel obstruction appears because of cicatricial narrowing and the injudicious ingestion of high-residue foods.

Common findings in patients with UC or Crohn's disease include weight loss, anemia, and oral aphthous ulcers. In patients with an acute flare of Crohn's disease, an abdominal examination may reveal mild to severe tenderness or occasionally a tender mass in the right lower quadrant signifying inflamed loops of bowel or an abscess. During remissions, the results of physical examination may be entirely negative. The presence or absence of bowel sounds is not helpful unless the patient presents with severe, cramping abdominal pain and distention, when a lack of bowel sounds should raise concern for intestinal obstruction.

In some cases, extraintestinal manifestations may be the presenting symptoms of UC or Crohn's disease. Uveitis, iritis, or episcleritis often flare concomitantly with intestinal symptoms. Large joint pain and sacroiliitis may be a form of enteropathic arthritis. Common skin manifestations include erythema nodosum, perianal fistulae, and pyoderma gangrenosum. Seventy percent of patients with primary sclerosing cholangitis will have UC that is identifiable on intestinal biopsy.

Patients with diarrhea containing blood or mucus should undergo an appropriate workup including fecal occult blood testing, fecal leukocytes and lactoferrin measurements, stool cultures, and ova and parasite smears. If no pathogen is identified, and functional etiologies and IBS are unlikely, then a diagnosis of IBD should be strongly considered, and a prompt referral to a gastroenterologist for lower endoscopy with biopsy should be arranged. Patients with unexplained diarrhea and hematochezia should undergo colonoscopy to rule out gastrointestinal cancer, as those patients with UC and Crohn's disease have an increased risk of colorectal cancer and should be monitored with surveillance colonoscopy. Extreme caution should be taken during colonoscopy in a patient with a flare-up of IBD given a high risk of iatrogenic perforation.

Laboratory values in the workup of IBD usually include an elevated erythrocyte sedimentation rate and C-reactive protein level and decreased hemoglobin and serum albumin levels, all indicating the chronicity and severity of disease. An elevated alkaline phosphatase level in a patient who has been diagnosed with UC always should raise the question of coexisting primary sclerosing cholangitis.

Pharmacologic treatment of IBD is aimed at inducing remission and maintaining a symptom-free life. Treatment of active flare-ups with systemic steroids has been the mainstay of remission induction therapy and produces remission rates of 70% in Crohn's disease versus 30% with placebo, with similar results seen in the remission of UC. Budesonide, a nonsystemic steroid used in an enema formulation, has been shown to be effective for the induction of remission in Crohn's disease and distal UC flares. Mild flares of UC are commonly treated with 5-aminosalicylic acid (5-ASA) derivatives such as sulfasalazine in the form of suppositories or enemas, yet RCTs have shown only marginal superiority to placebo at controlling flares of Crohn's disease.[33]

The immunosuppressant azathioprine and its metabolite 6-mercaptopurine are often are added to systemic steroids to help induce and maintain remission and to ease steroid tapering in the treatment of Crohn's disease. Patients taking these medications should not be exposed to live vaccines and should receive high priority for annual influenza vaccinations and Pneumovax (pneumococcal vaccine). Methotrexate is also effective for the induction of remission in Crohn's disease. Close monitoring of complete blood counts (CBCs) and serum transaminases are recommended, with monthly testing upon initiation and with dosage changes. Infliximab, an anti–tumor necrosis factor–a antibody, is remarkably effective in treating approximately 60% of steroid-resistant patients with Crohn's disease. It has significant adverse effect risks, however—namely, infusion reactions—yet rarely some patients have experienced worsening of heart failure, activation of latent tuberculosis, serum sickness, and invasive fungal infections.[34]

In patients who are in remission and not receiving maintenance therapy, 50% of patients who have Crohn's disease will have a flare-up within 2 years and approximately 89% of patients who have UC will relapse within 1 year. The risk of undergoing exploratory or bowel resection surgery for complications of Crohn's disease is approximately 60% by 10 years from the diagnosis; this risk increases with an early age at diagnosis and previous surgery for Crohn's disease. In patients with UC, the risk of requiring a total colectomy is approximately 50% after a period of 5 years in those with pancolitis and approximately 10% after 10 years for patients who have only left-sided disease.[35]

Irritable Bowel Syndrome

IBS is one of the most common gastrointestinal conditions, with a prevalence ranging from 5% to 19% in men in the United States and England, characterized by the presence of abdominal pain, bloating, and disturbed defecation in the absence of known structural or biochemical abnormality. The syndrome commonly appears among persons in their late 20s, although it may present in teenagers and in patients as old as 45 years; patients older than 45 years with suspected IBS should be evaluated for organic disease. IBS is responsible for approximately 2.4–3.5 million physician visits per year in the United States and represents 12% of primary care visits and 28% of referrals to gastroenterologists.[36]

Studies have indicated that the health-related quality of life in patients in the United States with IBS is worse than that of patients with clinical depression.[37] Consultations for non-gastrointestinal problems are four times more common in this population compared with patients who do not have IBS. The economic burden of IBS in the United States accounts for approximately $1.7–$10 billion in annual direct medical costs per year, including costs from physician visits, diagnostic testing, and medical treatment. Work absenteeism and decreased productivity attributed to IBS is substantial, equivalent to the leading cause in the United States—viral upper respiratory tract infections.[38]

IBS represents multiple potential pathophysiologic factors, including a genetic predisposition to the disease, disturbed central nervous system pain processing, visceral hypersensitivity, mucosal inflammation, abnormal colonic motility, and emotional stress. Psychosocial stressors likely exacerbate symptoms in patients with functional gastrointestinal disorders. Anxiety disorders, somatoform disorders, and a history of physical or sexual abuse have been identified in 42–61% of patients with IBS who have been referred to gastroenterologists.[39]

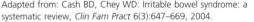
The results of physical examination in patients with IBS are often nonspecific and may demonstrate a normal abdomen examination, a diffusely tender abdomen, or a focally tender abdomen. Diagnostic screening tests including a CBC, erythrocyte sedimentation rate, serum chemistries, thyroid function tests, stool cultures including ova and parasites, fecal occult blood testing, colonoscopy, and hydrogen breath testing specifically to rule out other causes of disease are recommended, depending on the pretest probability of organic disease in each patient. The pretest probability will depend on the presence or absence of alarm symptoms, including hematochezia, fevers, weight loss of more than 10 pounds, chronic severe diarrhea, and family history of colon cancer.[36]

If alarm symptoms are present, then the pretest probability for organic disease is higher, and diagnostic testing including lower endoscopy should be performed. In the absence of alarm symptoms, all diagnostic testing should be limited. Studies have suggested that accurately diagnosing IBS is imperative yet challenging, and protracted negative workup results can negatively affect symptomatology and outcomes.[36] Diagnostic testing may be performed to reassure the clinician as well as the patient, yet the value of reassurance from diagnostic testing has never been examined.[40]

The differential diagnosis of IBS includes IBD, lactose intolerance, acute gastroenteritis, celiac disease, small intestinal bacterial overgrowth, colorectal cancer, and motility-altering metabolic disturbances, for example, from hypo- or hyperthyroidism. Although some consider IBS to be a diagnosis of exclusion, the Rome II criteria are currently the most widely accepted classification (Table 10-7).[40]

There is no single evidence-based consistently successful therapeutic approach for patients with IBS. Largely a chronic condition, the goals of therapy should focus on patient reassurance, education about the natural course of the syndrome, and global symptomatic improvement, rather than on definitive cure of the disease. This is best achieved through a well-developed patient-physician relationship with a clear delineation of realistic goals and expectations and plans for continued follow-up. Treatment for symptoms related to IBS are indicated when the patient and physician believe there has been a significant decrease in quality of life.

Treatment options for IBS include dietary therapy and pharmacotherapy. Dietary therapy is aimed at increasing supplemental fiber to increase

Table 10-7. Rome II Criteria for Diagnosis of Irritable Bowel Syndrome

Abdominal pain or discomfort for at least 12 weeks, although not necessarily contiguous, during the last 12 months
At least 2 out of 3 of the following features:
- Relief with defecation
- Onset associated with change in form of the stool
- Onset with change in the frequency of bowel movements
Additional supporting features include:
- Fewer than 3 bowel movements per week
- More than 3 bowel movements per day
- Hard or lumpy stool

Adapted from: Cash BD, Chey WD: Irritable bowel syndrome: a systematic review, *Clin Fam Pract* 6(3):647–669, 2004.

stool weight and to decrease colonic transit time. Treatment of constipation-predominant IBS can be achieved with fiber-bulking agents, but these have not been shown to improve global IBS symptoms over placebo. Pharmacotherapy includes antidiarrheals and laxatives, antispasmodics, and antidepressants (i.e., tricyclics [TCAs] and selective serotonin reuptake inhibitors [SSRIs]). Treatment of diarrhea-predominant IBS can be achieved with the use of loperamide; however, no advantage over placebo for global IBS symptoms has been reported. The TCAs, SSRIs, and peppermint oil have been shown in some studies to reduce abdominal pain, yet global symptom reduction and health-related quality of life have not been shown to be significantly improved by these agents compared with placebo.[36]

Recent advances in the treatment of IBS include the use of tegaserod, a 5-HT4 receptor agonist (indicated for women, but also used in men) with constipation-predominant IBS that has been shown to be more effective than placebo at relieving global symptoms.[41] Alosetron, a 5-HT3 antagonist (also more widely studied in women, but used in men) indicated for patients with diarrhea-predominant IBS, has also been shown to be more effective than placebo in RCTs. Due to reports of ischemic colitis, the use of alosetron has been limited to physicians participating in the manufacturer's risk-management program.[40]

Cognitive behavioral therapy, interpersonal psychotherapy, group therapy, biofeedback, and hypnosis have been shown to improve individual aspects of diarrhea-predominant IBS but have not been shown to improve global IBS symptoms. Alternative medicine techniques including acupuncture, probiotic therapy, and Chinese herbal medicine are becoming increasingly popular in the treatment of gastrointestinal disorders and have been shown to have some limited symptomatic improvement in select cases of IBS.[40]

Diverticular Disease

Diverticulosis refers to the presence of diverticula, or herniations of the intestinal mucosa and submucosa, most commonly present in the sigmoid colon. More than half of patients older than 50 years of age have incidental colonic diverticula; there is no known gender predominance. *Diverticulitis* is the most common and concerning complication of diverticulosis, occurring in up to 20% of patients, resulting from a microperforation of a diverticulum from inspissated fecal material that often becomes a pericolic or intraabdominal abscess.

The initial assessment of a patient with suspected diverticulitis includes a thorough history and physical examination, highlighting abdominal and rectal examinations. Most patients will have left lower quadrant abdominal pain (93–100%), fever (57–100%), and a leukocytosis (69–83%). Other associated features include nausea, vomiting, constipation, diarrhea, dysuria, and urinary frequency. The differential diagnosis in these patients includes IBS, IBD, colon cancer, ischemic colitis, bowel obstruction, and urologic disorders.[42] Initial examinations of patients with suspected diverticulitis may include a CBC, urinalysis, and flat and upright abdominal radiographs.

The American Society of Colon and Rectal Surgeons Standards Task Force for the Treatment of Diverticulitis[42] states that if the patient's clinical picture clearly suggests acute diverticulitis, then the diagnosis can be made on the basis of clinical criteria alone. The need for additional tests in a patient with suspected diverticulitis is determined by the severity of the presenting signs and symptoms and security of the diagnosis of diverticulitis. In cases where the diagnosis of diverticulitis is in question, water-soluble contrast enema, ultrasound, or abdominal computed tomography (CT) scan may be performed. Due to the risks of extravasation of barium from bowel perforation in persons with acute diverticulitis, barium enemas should be avoided in patients with suspected acute diverticulitis and localized peritoneal signs. Ultrasound may reveal bowel wall thickening, abscess, and rigid

hyperechogenicity of the colon due to inflammation. Use of the CT scan with oral, rectal, or intravenous contrast has become increasingly used as the initial imaging test for patients with suspected diverticulitis, particularly when moderate severity disease or abscess is anticipated. Criteria for diagnosis of diverticulitis include colonic wall thickening, pericolic fat infiltration ("streaky" fat), pericolic or distant abscesses, and extraluminal air.[42] Endoscopy is commonly avoided in the setting of acute diverticulitis on account of the iatrogenic risk of perforating the inflamed colon, either with the instrument itself or by the insufflation of air. In situations where the diagnosis of acute colonic diverticulitis is uncertain, limited flexible sigmoidoscopy with minimum insufflation of air may be performed to exclude other diagnoses.

The decision of whether to proceed with inpatient or outpatient treatment of diverticulitis depends on the clinical judgment of the physician, the severity of the disease process, and likelihood that the patient's condition will respond to outpatient therapy. Patients who are able to tolerate a diet, who do not have systemic symptoms, and who do not have significant peritoneal signs may be treated on an outpatient basis with oral trimethoprim-sulfamethoxazole or a fluoroquinolone plus metronidazole.[43] Conservative treatment of diverticulitis results in resolution in 70–100% of cases.[42] After the patient recovers from an initial episode of diverticulitis, when the inflammation has settled, they should be reevaluated. Appropriate examinations include a combination of flexible sigmoidoscopy and single- or double-contrast barium enema or colonoscopy. Commencement of long-term fiber supplementation after the first episode of diverticulitis has been shown to prevent recurrence in more than 70% of patients followed up for more than 5 years.

The risk of recurrent symptoms after an attack of diverticulitis ranges from 7% to 45%. With each recurrent episode, the patient is less likely to respond to medical therapy (70% chance of response to medical therapy after the first attack compared with a 6% chance after the third). Thus, after two attacks of uncomplicated diverticulitis, colonic resection is commonly recommended.[42]

Patients with abscesses that are not amenable to CT-guided percutaneous drainage or in whom clinical symptoms persist after percutaneous drainage should undergo laparotomy. Except in extraordinary circumstances, initial resection of the diseased segment (rather than drainage and fecal diversion) should be performed. Free perforation of acute diverticulitis with fecal or purulent peritonitis is a surgical emergency that requires immediate resuscitation with intravenous fluids, broad-spectrum antibiotics, cardiovascular support when indicated, and prompt operative therapy. Colovesical fistulae are the most common spontaneously occurring fistulae and compose approximately 65% of diverticular fistulae.[42]

Pancreatitis

Acute Pancreatitis

Acute pancreatitis continues to cause significant morbidity and mortality despite dramatic advances in the understanding of its pathophysiology and its critical care management. Pancreatitis accounts for nearly 210,000 US hospital admissions each year and exhibits no significant gender preference.[44] Thus, it is imperative for primary and emergency care physicians to identify those patients who are affected early in the course of pancreatitis to forestall the potential late adverse effects that are responsible for the high mortality rate, which approaches 10%.[45]

The Atlanta International Symposium on Pancreatitis in 1992 set out to clarify definitions and criteria for acute pancreatitis[46]; the most recent practice guidelines were released in 2006 in conjunction with the Practice Parameters Committee of the ACG.[47] These guidelines highlight that 85% of patients have interstitial pancreatitis whereas 15% have necrotizing pancreatitis, the latter form resulting in a higher rate of complications (e.g., infection, hemorrhage) and ultimately, mortality. Approximately 10% of patients will experience organ failure, and in these patients the overall mortality rate is approximately 5%. In mild acute pancreatitis, recovery is usually rapid (measured in days), and any distal organs affected by the acute event quickly return to their baseline function. In severe acute pancreatitis, parenchymal and fat necrosis ensues, as well as profound multisystem organ failure, infection, and life-threatening hemodynamic instability. As with any paradigm for strict definitions in the clinical setting, most patients fall somewhere in between these categories.[48]

The causes of acute pancreatitis are diverse and demonstrate changing trends over time and variation by geography. Gallstones, biliary sludge, and microlithiasis are recognized as the proximate cause in well over half of reported cases in several studies from around the world.[49]

Ethyl alcohol ingestion is the second most commonly reported cause of acute pancreatitis (approximately 30% of cases), although it is unclear whether alcohol is a toxin or an exacerbating factor in persons who have compromised pancreatic function. Studies suggest a greater shift toward alcohol as the putative cause and, irrespective of the exact pathophysiology, it may reflect increased alcohol consumption worldwide.[50] The remaining causes of acute pancreatitis account for less than 15% of total cases by most accounts, including hypertriglyceridemia, trauma, medications, endoscopic retrograde cholangiopancreatography, neoplasms, perforated PUD, viral infection, and idiopathic causes. Formerly, cases that were labeled as *idiopathic pancreatitis* numbered up to 10% of the total reported cases; recent studies suggest that half of these may be due to unrecognized microlithiasis.[51]

According to the recent ACG guidelines, there is general acceptance that a diagnosis of acute pancreatitis requires two of the following three features: (1) abdominal pain characteristic of acute pancreatitis (i.e., a gnawing, epigastric abdominal pain that often radiates to the back, described as constant and lasting from hours to days, but most often present for more than 24 hours); (2) serum amylase and/or lipase more than three times the upper limit of normal; and (3) characteristic findings of pancreatitis on CT scan, hallmarked by inflammation, edema, fat stranding, necrosis, and, in advanced or chronic cases, pseudocyst formation and hemorrhage.[47]

Serum markers of acute pancreatitis have high sensitivities and specificities but have no direct usefulness in predicting the severity or course of disease. The most common enzymes assayed, amylase and lipase, are released at approximately the same time after the initial insult to the pancreas but are cleared from the bloodstream at different rates. Therefore, relying on total serum amylase alone to make an accurate diagnosis of acute pancreatitis is prone to error because it is cleared almost totally from the blood within 48–72 hours. The sensitivity of pancreatic amylase for the diagnosis of acute pancreatitis decreases to less than 30% between the second and fourth day after the onset of the acute episode. Amylase levels may be elevated in a variety of non-pancreatic conditions; a small bowel obstruction is the most relevant of these when abdominal pain is of an unclear etiology. The clearance of pancreatic amylase is diminished with a decline in renal function, and thus may cloud the clinical picture even further.[45]

Early prognostic factors that can be measured and indicate severity of disease include Ranson's criteria and, more recently, the Acute Physiology and Chronic Health Evaluation II (APACHE II) score. The APACHE II severity of illness classification system includes a variety of physiologic variables, age points, and chronic health points, which can be determined at admission and daily as needed to help identify patients with severe pancreatitis.[49] A variety of reports have correlated a higher APACHE II score at admission and during the first 72 hours with a higher mortality (less than 4% with an APACHE II score of less than 8 and 11–18% with an APACHE II score greater than 8).[52,53] The overall success at prediction of mortality from acute pancreatitis at hospital admission remains at 40%, and even at 48 hours is no better than 80% when all diagnostic strategies of morbidity and mortality prediction are compared.[54]

One factor considered to be significant in the management of patients with acute pancreatitis is intravascular volume status. Many of the factors that are predictors of severity of pancreatitis are directly related to third spacing of fluids and include hemoconcentration and rising creatinine. The hematocrit may be high as a secondary effect of hypovolemia resulting from third spacing of fluids. In many circumstances, patients may be as many as 6 liters intravascularly depleted due to third spacing of fluids. Volume resuscitation during the first 24 hours is believed to be extremely important because this may minimize or even prevent pancreatic necrosis.[55] When rehydrated, patients with a low hematocrit level may be experiencing acute hemorrhagic pancreatitis. Supplemental oxygen should be administered during the first 24–48 hours, bedside oxygen saturation monitored at frequent intervals, and blood gases obtained when clinically indicated, particularly when oxygen saturation is less than 95%.[47] Transfer to an intensive care unit is recommended if there is sustained organ failure or if there are other indications that the pancreatitis is severe including oliguria, persistent tachycardia, and labored respiration.[47]

Contrast-enhanced CT is the most extensively studied modality for the confirmation of acute pancreatitis and provides the highest level of sensitivity and specificity among existing imaging technologies.[54] It may not be as readily available to the clinician as ultrasound, which has the advantages of low cost, rapid result that requires minimal preparation, and ability to be performed without the administration of potentially harmful contrast media. Limitations include overlying gas (often seen with pancreatitis-related ileus), excessive abdominal fat, and distortions of the skin from scarring that can make visualization of the underlying organs less reliable. With this caveat in mind, ultrasound should be a routine part of the initial evaluation of most patients who have suspected acute pancreatitis because it can provide time-critical information about the biliary tree and its neighboring structures.[56] Contrast-enhanced CT may have a lower detection rate for gallstones than ultrasound because of their isoattenuation with the bile in which they are immersed. Overall, sensitivities using ultrasound for the diagnosis of acute pancreatitis ranged between 62% and 95% and probably reflect the failure to visualize the organ as frequently as 30% of the time.[57] Cumulative studies have noted that the milder the disease presentation, the less likely it is that abnormalities will manifest that are detectable on CT examination.

Medical therapy of acute pancreatitis is primarily supportive, with the major objective being hemodynamic stabilization. Nutritional status and maintenance should be considered early in the course of acute pancreatitis to minimize morbidity and mortality risk. Most patients are kept NPO (i.e., given nothing to eat or drink by mouth) until their abdominal pain subsides and appetite returns. Patients who are unlikely to resume oral nutrition within 5 days because of sustained organ failure or other indications require nutritional support, which can be provided via total parenteral nutrition or by enteral feeding.[47] Pain management in the hospital setting is best achieved using morphine derivatives. Seldom, patient-controlled anesthesia may be used in cases of severe abdominal pain, and alternative diagnoses and complications should be considered.

Chronic Pancreatitis

Permanent pathologic damage to the pancreas results in chronic pancreatitis. In addition to exocrine deficiency (with malabsorption, diabetes mellitus, or both), a chronic pain syndrome may evolve that is challenging to manage effectively. Some patients with pancreatitis may practice alcohol or substance abuse and may have additional behavioral problems that require time, patience, compassion, and skill to resolve. Patients who continue to consume alcohol are more likely to have recurrent attacks. In those patients who can cease drinking permanently, the frequency of attacks may decrease. This is an area in which the primary care clinician can apply basic preventive principles to counsel patients, with the hope of reducing the number of future attacks. Exocrine deficiency should be treated with supplementation of pancreatic enzyme preparations with each meal.[58]

Chronic pancreatitis indicates some degree of progressive and permanent damage to the pancreas, usually visualized as calcifications on radiographs and CT imaging. This damage often leads to diabetes and pancreatic insufficiency resulting in malabsorption with chronic diarrhea. Patients with chronic pancreatitis present with repeated attacks of abdominal pain and are commonly admitted for acute on chronic exacerbations. Chronic pancreatitis may be characterized by mild distress due to epigastric pain present for weeks to months that is typically unresponsive to conservative measures including empiric treatment with acid-suppressing medications. For the primary care clinician, late complications of pancreatitis must be surveyed closely because they may present weeks to months after recovery from the initial presentation. Potential complications include pseudocyst and abscess formation, fistula formation between pseudocysts and the gut, persistent pancreatic ascites due to a disrupted pancreatic duct system, communication with the peritoneal cavity, mesenteric venous thrombosis, and arterial pseudoaneurysm.[58]

Conclusion

Diseases of the gastrointestinal tract confer significant disruptions to the health-related quality of life in men of all ages. Acute, chronic, and relapsing, they compose a modest proportion of conditions that will affect or confront almost many men at some point in their lives. In the years to come, clinicians will witness advances in medical technology ranging from more specialized radiographic imaging to improved endoscopic and novel laparoscopic techniques, as well as groundbreaking pharmacologic therapies to aid in the diagnosis and treatment of many gastrointestinal diseases. The primary care clinician's understanding of these commonly presenting illnesses in men becomes imperative, not solely to offer an accurate diagnosis and treatment, but also to facilitate a prompt referral to a gastroenterologist or surgeon when indicated.

References

1. American Gastroenterologic Association (AGA) issue briefs: AGA urges creation of research commission to develop second long-range plan to combat digestive diseases. Available at: http://www.gastro.org/pubPolicy/issueBriefs/urges-Creation.html. Accessed April 25, 2005.
2. Dickerson LM, King DE: Evaluation and management of nonulcer dyspepsia, *Am Fam Phys* 70:107–114, 2004.
3. Tack J, Bisschops R, Sarnelli G: Pathophysiology and treatment of functional dyspepsia, *Gastroenterology* 127:1239–1255, 2004.
4. Jones MP, Lacy BE: Dyspepsia: the spectrum of the problem. In Fass R, editor: *GERD/Dyspepsia: Hot Topics*, Philadelphia, 2004, Hanley and Belfus, pp 285–302.
5. Numans M, van der Graaf Y, de Wit NJ, et al: How much ulcer is ulcer-like? Diagnostic determinates of peptic ulcer in open access gastroscopy, *Fam Pract* 11:382–388, 1994.
6. Saad R, Scheiman JM: Diagnosis and management of peptic ulcer disease, *Clin Fam Pract* 6(3):569–587, 2004.
7. Hopkins RJ, Girardi LS, Turney EA: Relationship between *Helicobacter pylori* eradication and reduced duodenal and gastric ulcer recurrence: a review, *Gastroenterology* 110:1244–1252, 1996.
8. Scottish Intercollegiate Guidelines Network (SIGN): *Dyspepsia: A National Clinical Guideline*, Edinburgh, 2003, Scottish Intercollegiate Guidelines Network (SIGN).
9. Cutler AF, Havstad S, Ma CK, et al: Accuracy of invasive and noninvasive tests to diagnose *Helicobacter pylori* infection, *Gastroenterology* 109:136–141, 1995.
10. European Helicobacter Pylori Study Group (EHPSG): Current European concepts in the management of *Helicobacter pylori* infection: the Maastricht Consensus Report, *Gut* 41:8–13, 1997.
11. Huang JQ, Sridhar S, Hunt RH: Role of *Helicobacter pylori* infection and non-steroidal anti-inflammatory drugs in peptic ulcer disease: a meta-analysis, *Lancet* 359(9300):14–22, 2002.
12. Laine L, Hopkins RJ, Girardi L: Has the impact of Helicobacter pylori therapy on ulcer recurrence in the Unites States been overstated? A meta-analysis of rigorously designed trials, *Am J Gastroenterol* 93:1409–1415, 1998.
13. McMahon BJ, Hennessy TW, Bensler JM, et al: The relationship among previous antimicrobial use, antimicrobial resistance, and treatment outcomes for *Helicobacter pylori* infections, *Ann Intern Med* 139(6):463–469, 2003.
14. Meyer JM, Silliman NP, Wang W, et al: Risk factors for *Helicobacter pylori* resistance in the United States: the surveillance of *H. pylori* antimicrobial resistance partnership (SHARP) study, 1993–1999, *Ann Intern Med* 136(1):13–24, 2002.
15. De Wit NJ, Quartero AO, Numans ME: *Helicobacter pylori* treatment instead of maintenance therapy for peptic ulcer disease: the effectiveness of case-finding in general practice, *Aliment Pharmacol Ther* 13:1317–1321, 1999.

16. Hernandez-Diaz S, Rodriguez LA: Association between nonsteroidal anti-inflammatory drugs and upper gastrointestinal tract bleeding/perforation: an overview of epidemiologic studies published in the 1990s, *Arch Intern Med* 160:2093–2099, 2000.

17. Scheiman JM, Yeomans ND, Talley NJ, et al: Prevention of ulcers by esomeprazole in at-risk patients using non-selective NSAIDs and COX-2 inhibitors, *Am J Gastroenterol* 101:1–10, 2006.

18. Del Valle J: Acid peptic disorders. In Yamada T, Alpers DH, editors: *Textbook of Gastroenterology*, Philadelphia, 2003, Lippincott Williams & Wilkins, pp 1322–1376.

19. The Gallup Organization: *Heartburn Across America*: Princeton, NJ, 1998, Gallup Organization.

20. Locke GR III, Talley NJ, Fett SL, Zinsmeister AR, et al: Prevalence and clinical spectrum of gastroesophageal reflux: a population-based study in Olmstead County, Minnesota, *Gastroenterology* 112: 1448–1456, 1997.

21. Revicki DA, Wood M, Maton PN, Sorenson S: The impact of gastroesophageal reflux disease on health-related quality of life, *Am J Med* 104: 252–258, 1998.

22. Fass R: Gastroesophageal reflux disease revisited, *Gastroenterol Clin North Am* 31:4S, S1–S10, 2002.

23. Heidelbaugh JJ, Nostrant TT, Kim C, Harrison RV: Management of gastroesophageal reflux disease, *Am Fam Phys* 68:1311–1318, 1321–1322 2003.

24. Medical Advisory Panel for the Pharmacy Benefits Management Strategic Healthcare Group: *VHA/DoD Clinical Practice Guideline for the Management of Adults with Gastroesophageal Reflux Disease in Primary Care Practice,* Washington, DC, 2003, Veterans Health Administration, Department of Defense.

25. Heidelbaugh JJ, Nostrant TT: Medical and surgical management of gastroesophageal reflux disease, *Clin Fam Pract* 6(3):547–568, 2004.

26. Lundell L, Miettinen P, Myrvold HE, et al: Continued (5-year) follow-up of a randomized clinical study comparing antireflux surgery and omeprazole in gastroesophageal reflux disease, *J Am Coll Surg* 192:172–181, 2001.

27. Sampliner RE, Practice Parameters Committee ACG: Updated guidelines for the diagnosis, surveillance, and therapy of Barrett's esophagus, *Am J Gastroenterol* 97:1888–1895, 2002.

28. National Center for Health Statistics (NCHS): Chronic liver disease/cirrhosis. Available at: http://www.cdc.gov/nchs/fastats/liverdis.htm. Accessed October 30, 2006.

29. Marrero JA: Screening tests for hepatocellular carcinoma, *Clin Liver Dis* 9:235–251, 2005.

30. Gines P, Cardenas A, Arroyo V, Rodes J: Management of cirrhosis and ascites, *N Engl J Med* 350:1646–1654, 2004.

31. Dove L, Brown R: The emerging role of gastrointestinal organ transplantation, *Clin Fam Pract* 6 (3):775–791, 2004.

32. Haberal M, Dalgic A: New concepts in organ transplantation, *Transplant Proc* 36:1219–1224, 2004.

33. Higgins PDR, Zimmerman EM: An evidence-based approach to inflammatory bowel disease, *Clin Fam Pract* 6(3):671–692, 2004.

34. Feagan BG: Maintenance therapy for inflammatory bowel disease, *Am J Gastroenterol* 98(12):S6–S17, 2003.

35. Sinclair TS, Brunt PW, Mowat NA: Nonspecific proctocolitis in northeastern Scotland: a community study, *Gastroenterology* 85:1–11, 1983.

36. Cash BD, Chey WD: Irritable bowel syndrome: a systematic review, *Clin Fam Pract* 6(3):647–669, 2004.

37. Gralnek IM, Hays RD, Kilbourne A, et al: The impact of irritable bowel syndrome on health-related quality of life, *Gastroenterology* 119:654–660, 2000.

38. Camilleri M, Williams DE: Economic burden of irritable bowel syndrome, *Lancet* 340:1447–1452, 1992.

39. Miller AR, North CS, Clouse RE, et al: The association of irritable bowel syndrome and somatization disorder, *Ann Clin Psych* 13:25–30, 2001.

40. Brandt LJ, Locke GR, Olden K, et al: Evidence-based position statement on the management of irritable bowel syndrome in North America, *Am J Gastroenterol* 97(11 Suppl):S1–S5, 2002.

41. Novick J, Miner P, Krause R, et al: A randomized, double-blind, placebo controlled trial of tegaserod in female patients suffering from irritable bowel syndrome with constipation, *Aliment Pharmacol Ther* 16:877–878, 2002.

42. Standards Task Force. American Society of Colon and Rectal Surgeons: Practice parameters for the treatment of sigmoid diverticulitis, *Dis Colon Rectum* 43(3):289, 2000.

43. Salzman H, Lillie D: Diverticular disease: diagnosis and treatment, *Am Fam Phys* 72:1229–1234, 1241–1242 2005.

44. Swaroop VS, Chari ST, Clain JE: Severe acute pancreatitis, *JAMA* 291:2865–2868, 2004.

45. Orbuch M: Optimizing outcomes in acute pancreatitis, *Clin Fam Pract* 6(3):607–629, 2004.

46. Bradley EL 3rd: A clinically based classification system for acute pancreatitis: summary of the International Symposium on Acute Pancreatitis, Atlanta, GA, September 11 through 13, 1992, *Arch Surg* 128:586–590, 1993.

47. Banks PA, Freeman ML, and the Practice Parameters Committee of the American College of Gastroenterology: Practice guidelines in acute pancreatitis, *Am J Gastroenterol* 101:2379–2400, 2006.

48. Bradley EL III: A clinically based classification system for acute pancreatitis, *Arch Surg* 128:586–590, 1993.

49. Toouli J, Brooke-Smith M, Bassi C, et al: Working party report: guidelines for the management of acute pancreatitis, *J Gastroenterol Hepatol* 17 (Suppl):15–39, 2002.

50. Pandol SJ, Gukovsky I, et al: Emerging concepts for the mechanism of alcoholic pancreatitis from experimental models, *J Gastroenterol* 38:623–628, 2003.

51. Levy MJ: The hunt for microlithiasis in idiopathic acute recurrent pancreatitis: should we abandon the search or intensify our efforts? *Gastrointest Endosc* 55:286–292, 2002.

52. Blum T, Maisonneuve P, Lowenfels AB, et al: Fatal outcome in acute pancreatitis: its occurrence and early prediction, *Pancreatology* 1:237–241, 2001.

53. Lankisch PG, Warnecke B, Bruns D, et al: The APACHE II score is unreliable to diagnose necrotizing pancreatitis on admission to hospital, *Pancreas* 24:217–222, 2002.

54. Papachristou GI, Whitcomb DC: Predictors of severity and necrosis in acute pancreatitis, *Gastroenterol Clin North Am* 33:871–890, 2004.

55. Mayerle J, Simon P, Lerch MM: Medical treatment of acute pancreatitis, *Gastroenterol Clin North Am* 33:855–869, 2004.

56. Merkle EM, Gorich J: Imaging of acute pancreatitis, *Eur Radiol* 12:1979–1992, 2002.

57. Turner MA: The role of US and CT in pancreatitis, *Gastrointest Endosc* 56(6 Suppl):S241–S245, 2003.

58. Apte MV, Keogh GW, Wilson JS: Chronic pancreatitis: complications and management, *J Clin Gastroenterol* 29:225–240, 1999.

Chapter 11

Infectious Diseases

Sandro Cinti, MD, Anurag Malani, MD, and James Riddell, MD

Key Points

- Risk factors should weigh heavily on the decision to admit in patients with suspected community-acquired pneumonia (CAP), including advanced age, comorbid conditions, and physical examination, laboratory, and chest radiograph findings, all of which support the diagnosis (strength of recommendation: C).
- First-line antibiotic therapy for acute bacterial rhinosinusitis should include amoxicillin or trimethoprim/sulfamethoxazole (TMP/SMX) for 7–10 days (strength of recommendation: A).
- High-dose amoxicillin (80–90 mg/kg divided twice daily for 5–7 days) is the antibiotic of choice for the initial treatment of acute otitis media (AOM) (strength of recommendation: B); lack of subjective improvement after 72 hours of treatment with amoxicillin indicates treatment failure, at which point the patient should be switched to amoxicillin/ clavulanate. Patients with persistent symptoms after therapy with high-dose amoxicillin/clavulanate should receive 1–3 doses of intramuscular ceftriaxone (strength of recommendation: B).
- Pharmacotherapy treatment for influenza should be initiated within 48 hours of the start of symptoms, and it has been shown to reduce the duration of symptoms by only 1 day compared with placebo (strength of recommendation: B).
- The American Association for the Study of Liver Diseases recommends that persons at high risk of infection, recipients of transfusions or organ transplants before July 1992 (when HCV screening became standard), healthcare workers after a needlestick injury, and sexual partners of HCV-infected persons be tested for HCV infection (strength of recommendation: C).
- Currently, not all patients with HIV infection require the use of antiretroviral medication. Because of the adverse effects and the risk of the development of resistance associated with treatment, these medications are now initiated only when the CD4 count falls to below 350 cells/mL or in the setting of acute infection (strength of recommendation: B).
- More severe immune compromise occurs in HIV-positive patients at CD4 count levels of less than 200 cells/mL, at which point prophylactic antibiotics such as TMP/SMX are recommended (strength of recommendation: B).
- In cases of traveler's diarrhea (e.g., enterotoxigenic *E. coli*, *Shigella*, *Salmonella*, or *Campylobacter* infection), prompt treatment with a fluoroquinolone or, in children, TMP/SMX has been shown to reduce the duration of the illness from 3–5 days to less than 1–2 days (strength of recommendation: A).
- Patients with fever and bloody diarrhea should be treated empirically with TMP/SMZ or a fluoroquinolone (strength of recommendation: A).
- Recommended treatment regimens for gonococcal urethritis and proctitis include ceftriaxone, cefixime, ciprofloxacin, ofloxacin, or levofloxacin in single doses; if chlamydial infection is not ruled out and suspicion is high, then azithromycin or doxycycline should be given concomitantly (strength of recommendation: A).
- Parenteral administration of penicillin G is the preferred drug for treatment for all stages of syphilis (strength of recommendation: A).

Introduction

Infectious diseases are a leading cause of morbidity and mortality in men in all parts of the world. Given the broad scope of infectious diseases that affect men, we have selected several topics that are especially relevant to this patient population. These topics include community-acquired pneumonia (CAP), sinusitis, otitis media and externa, influenza, viral hepatitis (A, B and C), human immunodeficiency virus (HIV) infection, infectious diarrheas, and sexually transmitted diseases. Our aim in this chapter is not to provide an exhaustive review of these topics, but primarily to present an up-to-date and evidence-based approach to diagnosis and treatment of these common illnesses for primary care physicians in caring for male patients.

Community-Acquired Pneumonia

Epidemiology/Pathogenesis

CAP is a serious illness that affects up to 4.5 million people in the United States annually, resulting in hospitalization in approximately 20% of these cases.[1] With a mortality rate of 5.1%, this disease is the sixth most common cause of death in the United States.[2] Empiric antibiotic therapy is necessary since an etiologic organism is not identified in well over 50% of cases. Further complicating the treatment of CAP is the emergence of antibiotic resistant *Streptococcus pneumoniae*, perhaps the most common organism implicated.[1] The rates of pneumonia are higher in men discharged from the hospital (4.1% in men versus 3.1% in women).[2]

Microaspiration of organisms is the most common mechanism of infection leading to CAP, though hematogenous spread can also occur.[3] Host factors that predispose patients to an increased risk of the development of CAP include smoking, underlying lung disease (e.g., chronic obstructive pulmonary disease [COPD], bronchiectasis), uremia, malnutrition, alcohol abuse, ciliary motility defects (e.g., Kartagener's syndrome), alterations in consciousness, immunosuppression (e.g., HIV/acquired immunodeficiency syndrome [AIDS], corticosteroid use), advanced age, and gastric acid suppression.[4] Both bacterial and viral virulence factors play a significant role in the development of CAP.

More than 100 microorganisms have been implicated as causative agents in CAP.[1] The most common "typical" bacterial etiologies include *S. pneumoniae, Haemophilus influenzae, Staphylococcus aureus, Moraxella catarrhalis*, group A *Streptococcus*, and various anaerobic and gram-negative bacteria. The most common "atypical" bacteria include *Legionella* species, *Mycoplasma pneumoniae,* and *Chlamydia pneumoniae*. Although influenza is the most common cause of viral CAP, adenovirus and parainfluenza virus pneumonias also occur, and respiratory syncytial virus is a significant pathogen in infants. A newly emerged strain of corona virus led to an epidemic outbreak of severe acute respiratory syndrome in China and Canada in 2003. Table 11-1 highlights the most common causes of CAP in three settings: ambulatory care, hospital non–intensive care unit (ICU), and the ICU.

Diagnosis

Pneumonia should be suspected in any patient who presents with cough, productive sputum, and dyspnea, especially if a fever is present. Elderly patients with pneumonia may not have fever or respiratory symptoms and frequently present with failure to thrive or confusion.[2] In these patients, tachypnea and abnormal pulmonary examination results exhibited by rhonchi, abnormal breath sounds, tactile fremitus, and egophony will often aid in the diagnosis.

The American Thoracic Society Guidelines[5] state that the initial diagnostic evaluation of a patient with suspected CAP should include a chest radiograph and a sputum Gram stain and culture. A chest radiograph can be used to determine the extent (unilobar versus multilobar) and character (interstitial infiltrate versus consolidation) of the pneumonia, and sputum studies will guide specific therapy.[1] There is some controversy regarding the use of Gram stain and culture because of poor sensitivity and specificity, but some groups still consider these tests useful in targeting initial therapy.[4] These guidelines recommend the use of sputum Gram stain and culture if the presence of drug-resistant bacteria or an organism not covered by empiric therapy is suspected.[1]

Pulse oximetry, a complete blood count with platelets and differential, serum electrolyte and hepatic enzyme measurements, and renal function tests may be helpful prognostic tools to help identify patients requiring hospitalization. Admitted patients with severe illness or with chronic lung disease should have an arterial blood gas performed to assess for oxygenation

Table 11-1. Major Etiologies of Community-Acquired Pneumonia with Regard to Setting

Organism	Ambulatory	Hospitalized	ICU
Mycoplasma pneumoniae	16%	6%	<1%
Respiratory viruses	15%	10%	4%
Streptococcus pneumoniae	14%	25%	17%
Chlamydia pneumoniae	12%	3%	<1%
Legionella species	2%	3%	10%
Haemophilus influenzae	1%	5%	3%
Gram-negative rods	<1%	<1%	5%
Unknown	44%	37%	41%

Adapted from: Niederman MS, Mandell LA, Anzueto A, et al: Guidelines for the management of adults with community-acquired pneumonia: diagnosis, assessment of severity, antimicrobial therapy, and prevention, *Am J Respir Crit Care Med* 163:1730–1754, 2001.

and hypercapnia.[1] Hospitalized patients should have two sets of blood cultures drawn, and patients with pleural effusions should undergo thoracentesis to assess for empyema or complicated parapneumonic effusions.[4] Serologic antibody testing and cold agglutinin assays are not helpful initially and should only be performed if the patient's condition does not improve or for epidemiologic purposes.[4]

Treatment

Although clinical prediction rules are useful when deciding whether a patient with CAP should be admitted to the hospital for observation and treatment, these rules should not supplant clinical judgment.[2] Generally, the following risk factors should weigh heavily on the decision to admit:[5]

- Age older than 65 years
- Coexisting illness: COPD, diabetes mellitus, renal insufficiency, congestive heart failure, chronic liver disease, alcohol abuse, post-splenectomy status
- Physical findings: respiratory rate > 30 breaths/min, systolic blood pressure < 90 mm Hg, diastolic blood pressure < 60 mm Hg, pulse rate > 125 beats/min, temperature > 40°C, confusion, or decreased consciousness
- Laboratory findings: white blood count < 4×10^9 cells/liter or > 30×10^9 cells/liter, hematocrit < 30%, PaO_2 < 60 mm Hg, $PaCO_2$ > 50 mm Hg, pH < 7.35, creatinine > 1.2 mg/dL, or BUN > 20 mg/dL
- Chest x-ray: cavitation, multilobar pneumonia, pleural effusion

Empiric antibiotics are generally recommended as initial therapy for CAP (Table 11-2).[6]

Complications

A patient with CAP should respond to adequate antibiotic therapy within 4 days of initiation of treatment with decreased fever, improved clinical status (e.g., decreased dyspnea and normalized blood pressure), and a decrease in the white blood cell count.[1] If the patient's condition fails to improve or worsens during therapy, then a workup for complications of pneumonia should be initiated. Pulmonary complications of pneumonia include lung abscess, parapneumonic effusion, and empyema.[1] Although findings on a chest radiograph can remain abnormal for 4 weeks or longer after diagnosis of CAP, repeat imaging via either computerized tomography scan of the chest or follow-up chest radiograph may be helpful in patients whose conditions fail to improve or worsen over time.[1] Other complications, particularly resulting from *S. pneumoniae* bacteremia, include meningitis, endocarditis, and pericarditis. Acute respiratory distress syndrome may also occur with severe illness and may necessitate intubation.[1]

Vaccination

The 23-valent purified capsular polysaccharide pneumococcal vaccine offers protection against 85–90% of invasive strains of bacteria that can cause CAP.[1] Patients with risk factors that place them at a greatly elevated risk of development of CAP should be strongly encouraged to receive the pneumococcal vaccine (Table 11-3). A single vaccine can be given to patients aged 65 years or older, including those who received vaccine more than 5 years before turning 65 years old. Repeat vaccination is indicated after 5 years in immunocompromised patients. A yearly influenza vaccine

Table 11-2. Treatment of Community-Acquired Pneumonia with Regard to Setting

Outpatient	
No recent antibiotics	Erythromycin 1–4 g/day for 7–10 days or clarithromycin 1 g/day for 7–10 days or azithromycin 500 mg on first day then 250 mg for 4 days
	Doxycycline 100 mg bid for 7–10 days
Recent antibiotics (within 3 months) or comorbidities (e.g., COPD, diabetes, liver or renal disease, heart failure)	Levofloxacin (Levaquin) 750 mg/day or gatifloxacin (Tequin) 400 mg/day or moxifloxacin (Avelox) 400 mg/day or gemifloxacin (Factive) 320 mg/day for 7–10 days
	Telithromycin (Ketek) 800 mg/day for 7–10 days
	Amoxicillin (Amoxil; Trimox) 3–4 g/day or Amoxicillin/clavulanate (Augmentin) 4 g/day + advanced macrolide (clarithromycin, azithromycin) or doxycycline (see above) for 7–10 days
	Cefpodoxime (Vantin) 200 mg bid or cefuroxime (Ceftin) 200 mg bid + advanced macrolide (clarithromycin, azithromycin) or doxycycline (see above) for 7–10 days
Hospitalized, non-ICU	
Ceftriaxone (Rocephin) 2 g/day IV or cefotaxime (Claforan) 1 g IV every 8 hours + azithromycin 500 mg/day IV until clinically improved then oral antibiotics (see above) for a total of 7–10 days	
Levofloxacin (Levaquin) 750 mg/day or gatifloxacin (Tequin) 400 mg/day or moxifloxacin (Avelox) 400 mg/day or gemifloxacin (Factive) 320 mg/day for 7–10 days	
Ampicillin/sulbactam (Unasyn) 1.5–3 g every 6 hours IV until clinically improved then oral antibiotics (see above) for a total of 7–10 days	
Ertapenem (Invanz) 1 g/day until clinically improved then oral antibiotics (see above) for a total of 7–10 days	
ICU	
No penicillin allergy	Ceftriaxone (Rocephin) 2 g/day IV or cefotaxime (Claforan) 1 g IV every 8 hours + azithromycin 500 mg/day IV or fluoroquinolone PO or IV (see above for dosing) until clinically improved then oral antibiotics (see above) for a total of 7–10 days
	If patient is severely ill or staphylococcal infection is suspected, add vancomycin 1 g every 12 hours IV or linezolid (Zyvox) 600 mg every 12 hours IV until culture results and susceptibility testing are known
Penicillin-allergic	Levofloxacin (Levaquin) 750 mg/day or gatifloxacin (Tequin) 400 mg/day or moxifloxacin (Avelox) 400 mg/day or gemifloxacin (Factive) 320 mg/day ± clindamycin (Cleocin) 600–1200 mg/day IV for 7–10 days
	If patient is severely ill or staphylococcal infection is suspected, add vancomycin 1 g every 12 hours IV or linezolid (Zyvox) 600 mg every 12 hours IV until culture results and susceptibility testing are known
Drug-Resistant *Streptococcus pneumoniae*	
Reduced susceptibility to penicillin (MIC ≥ 2 μg/mL) but MICs to cefotaxime or ceftriaxone of ≤ 2 μg/mL without meningitis	Ceftriaxone or cefotaxime (see above)
	Alternative: fluoroquinolones (see above) although not effective in meningitis
MIC ≥ 4 μg/mL to cefotaxime and ceftriaxone	Fluoroquinolones (see above) although not effective in meningitis
	Alternative: vancomycin, linezolid, telithromycin (outpatients), (see above)

bid, Twice a day; COPD, chronic obstructive pulmonary disease; ICU, intensive care unit; IV, intravenous; PO, per os; MIC, mean inhibitory concentration.

Adapted from: Mandell LA, Bartlett JG, Dowell SF, et al: Update of practice guidelines for the management of community-acquired pneumonia in immunocompetent adults, *Clin Infect Dis* 37(11):1405–1433, 2003.

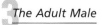

Table 11-3. Risk Factors for the Development of Community-Acquired Pneumonia

- Age 65 years or older
- Alcoholism
- Asplenia
- Cerebrospinal fluid leaks
- Chronic obstructive pulmonary disease
- Chronic renal disease
- Diabetes mellitus
- Immunosuppressed patients, including patients taking corticosteroids and those with hematologic malignancies
- Liver disease

Adapted from: Niederman MS, Mandell LA, Anzueto A, et al: Guidelines for the management of adults with community-acquired pneumonia: diagnosis, assessment of severity, antimicrobial therapy, and prevention, *Am J Respir Crit Care Med* 163:1730–1754, 2001.

Table 11-4. Microbiology and Incidence of Acute Sinusitis

	Percentage (%)
Viruses	
Rhinovirus	15
Influenza virus	5
Parainfluenza virus	3
Adenovirus	—
Bacteria	
Streptococcus pneumoniae	31
Haemophilus influenzae	21
Alpha-streptococci	9
Gram-negative bacteria	9
Moraxella catarrhalis	8
Anaerobes	6
S. pneumoniae + H. influenzae	5
Staphylococcus aureus	4
Streptococcus pyogenes	2

Adapted from: Gwaltney JM: Sinusitis. In Mandell GL, Bennett JE, Dolan R, editors: *Mandell, Douglas, and Bennett's Principles and Practice of Infectious Diseases*, ed 5, Philadelphia, 2000, Churchill Livingstone, pp 676–686.

should be administered concomitantly to patients with any of the above risk factors.[1]

Acute Sinusitis

Epidemiology/Pathogenesis

There are approximately 20 million cases of acute bacterial sinusitis annually in the United States,[7] most of which result from the common colds and influenza-like illnesses occurring an average of two to three times per year in adults. It is estimated that 0.5–2% of all acute respiratory illnesses result in sinusitis. Viral, bacterial, and fungal causes of acute sinusitis have all been implicated (Table 11-4). The healthcare costs related to the diagnosis and management of sinusitis are estimated to be close to $4 billion annually.

The most common predisposing condition associated with bacterial sinusitis is a viral infection that results in thickening of the sinus mucosa and subsequent obstruction of the ostia.[7] The resultant accumulation of secretions allows for bacterial colonization of the normally sterile sinus mucosa. The maxillary sinus is the most commonly involved (87%), followed by the ethmoidal (65%), sphenoid (39%), and frontal (32%) sinuses.[8] Other risk factors include swimming (e.g., microaspiration of contaminated water), allergies, nasal obstruction (e.g., polyps, tumors), decreased mucociliary activity (e.g., cystic fibrosis, smoking), granulomatous disease (e.g., Wegener's granulomatosis), and immunosuppression (e.g., HIV/AIDS, chronic corticosteroid use). Dental infections of the upper teeth, particularly the second bicuspids and first and second molars, are responsible for 5–10% of cases of maxillary sinusitis. Environmental factors including high altitude, air pollution, and living in the Midwest or southern United States increase the risk of acute bacterial sinusitis. Females seem to be at higher risk than males; overall, elderly persons are at an increased risk of development of sinusitis.[8]

Clinical Presentation

Symptoms of acute sinusitis, particularly maxillary sinusitis, include congestion, purulent nasal discharge, facial pain, and maxillary tooth discomfort for less than 4 weeks.[9] It is often reported that facial pain is exacerbated by bending forward. Less specific symptoms including headache, fever, fatigue, and halitosis may also occur. A high fever, acute facial pain, periorbital edema, diplopia, or a change in mental status warrant an immediate evaluation for potential neurologic complications of acute sinusitis.

Diagnosis

The diagnosis of acute bacterial sinusitis is imprecise and, although most cases are likely to be viral rhinosinusitis, primary care physicians prescribe an antibiotic in 85–98% of cases.[10] The Centers for Disease Control and Prevention endorse antibiotic treatment of acute sinusitis in patients who have persistent nasal discharge for longer than 7 days, maxillary sinus pain, and facial or tooth tenderness.[10] Sinus radiography is not recommended in uncomplicated acute sinusitis because it is thought to be inaccurate.[10] Sinus transillumination has limited value as a diagnostic tool because it does not distinguish bacterial from viral sinusitis. Sinus aspiration should not be used for routine evaluation of uncomplicated acute sinusitis because it is both invasive and expensive. Computerized tomography scanning of the sinuses should be limited to refractory or chronic cases of sinusitis because this modality does not accurately distinguish between bacterial and viral causes.[10]

Treatment

Symptoms of acute sinusitis resolve within 2 weeks without antibiotic therapy in 70% of cases and with antibiotics in 85% of cases.[11] Recent guidelines by the Sinus and Allergy Health Partnership recommend treatment for acute bacterial sinusitis in patients who have symptoms of sinusitis and have not improved in 10 days or in those whose conditions worsen after 5–7 days.[12] First-line antibiotic therapy for acute bacterial rhinosinusitis should include amoxicillin or trimethoprim/sulfamethoxazole (TMP/SMX) for 7–10 days. These agents have been proved to be superior to placebo and are as effective as other agents that are more expensive, have a greater risk of adverse effects, and should be reserved for more serious infections that require treatment with amoxicillin-clavulanate, cefuroxime, or cefpodoxime.[11] For partial but incomplete resolution of symptoms after an initial course of antibiotics, the duration of initial therapy should be extended to complete a course for 21 days. In patients with moderate disease or in those with minimal to no improvement with initial therapy, high-dose amoxicillin-clavulanate or levofloxacin should be used.[11] In areas of the United States where there is a high level of penicillin-resistant *S. pneumoniae*, resistance to macrolides and TMP/SMX will also be prevalent, and second-generation cephalosporins (e.g., cefuroxime) should be used as initial therapy.[7] More recently, high-dose short-course regimens (3–5 days) have been used to improve adherence and to decrease drug exposure.[7] Clinical outcomes using these regimens compare favorably to more traditional 10–14-day regimens.[13] Table 11-5 highlights examples of both long- and short-course treatments.

Complications

Complications of acute sinusitis include orbital cellulitis (most common), Pott puffy tumor (a cellulitis over the frontal sinus), intracranial abscesses, meningitis, and cavernous sinus thrombosis.[7] These complications often require surgical drainage and intravenous antibiotics. Nasal culture specimens should be obtained to

Table 11-5. Empiric Therapy of Acute Bacterial Sinusitis

Mild Disease
Amoxicillin/clavulanate (Augmentin) 1.75–4 g/day for 10 days
Amoxicillin* (Amoxil; Trimox) 1.5–4 g/day for 10 days
Cefpodoxime (Vantin) 200 mg every 12 hours for 10 days
Cefuroxime (Ceftin) 200 mg every 12 hours for 10 days
Cefdinir (Omnicef) 600 mg/day for 10 days
Mild Disease in Patients with Beta Lactam Allergy
Trimethoprim/sulfamethoxazole* (Bactrim) DS every 12 hours for 10 days
Doxycycline (Vibramycin) 100 mg every 12 hours for 10 days
Azithromycin (Zithromax) 500 mg/day for 5 days; clarithromycin (Biaxin) 500 mg every 12 hours for 14 days; erythromycin 250 mg qid for 10 days
Telithromycin (Ketek) 800 mg/day for 10 days
Mild to Moderate Disease in Patients with Recent Antibiotic Therapy
Gatifloxacin (Tequin) 400 mg/day; levofloxacin (Levaquin) 500 mg/day; moxifloxacin (Avelox) 400 mg/day for 10–14 days
Amoxicillin/clavulanate (Augmentin) 4 g/day for 10 days
Ceftriaxone (Rocephin) 1–2 g IV/IM once a day for 10 days
Amoxicillin 4 g/day + rifampin (Rifadin) 600 mg/day for 10 days
Clindamycin (Cleocin) 150–300 mg qid + rifampin 600 mg/day for 10 days
Short-course Regimens
Telithromycin (Ketek) 800 mg/day for 5 days
Azithromycin 500 mg/day for 3 days
Gatifloxacin (Tequin) 400 mg/day for 5 days

DS, Double strength; qid, four times a day; IV, intravenous; IM, intramuscular.
*Considered to be first-line therapy.

Adapted from: Anon JB, Jacobs MP, Poole MD: Antimicrobial treatment guidelines for acute bacterial rhinosinusitis: executive summary of the Sinus and Allergy Health Partnership (SAHP), *Otolaryngol Head and Neck Surg* 130:1–45, 2004; and Sher LD, McDoo MA, Bettis RB, Turner MA, Li NF, Pierce PF: A multicenter, randomized, investigator-blinded study of 5- and 10-day gatifloxacin versus 10 day amoxicillin/clavulanate in patients with acute bacterial sinusitis, *Clin Ther* 24:269–281, 2002.

guide therapy in complicated or refractory cases, but initial treatment with broad-spectrum antibiotics, including ceftriaxone with or without an aminoglycoside given intravenously, is often warranted until cultures are proved to be positive.[14] Acute sinusitis is a precursor to chronic sinusitis; in addition to aerobic bacteria, fungi and anaerobic bacteria play a significant role in chronic sinusitis.

Acute Otitis Media/Otitis Externa

Acute Otitis Media

Acute otitis media (AOM) is predominantly a disease of infants and children with the highest incidence occurring between the ages of 6 and 24 months and is less commonly seen in adults. The cost of treating AOM in the United States was estimated at $3.8 billion in 1995 (the most recent accurate estimate).[15] In childhood, boys are affected more frequently than girls. AOM is characterized by a middle ear effusion demonstrated via pneumatic otoscopy, tympanometry, an air fluid level, or a bulging tympanic membrane; evidence of acute inflammation with an opaque, white, yellow, or erythematous tympanic membrane or purulent effusion; and symptoms of otalgia, irritability, or fever.[16] Otitis media with effusion presents in a similar fashion, and a purulent collection of fluid behind the tympanic membrane can be visualized. Unless drainage from the external auditory canal exists, microbiologic diagnosis is usually not feasible and only rarely necessary. The most common organisms that cause AOM include *S. pneumoniae*, *H. influenzae*, and *M. catarrhalis*.

Patients who have no improvement in subjective symptoms, especially fever, after 48–72 hours of observation should be considered for antibiotic treatment. Although it is universally held that many physicians still overtreat AOM with antibiotics, expert opinion states that antibiotic therapy can be deferred for many asymptomatic patients and for most cases of otitis media with effusion.[16] Children younger than 2 years of age and those with recurrent bouts of AOM are more likely to be appropriately treated with antibiotic therapy.[17] High-dose amoxicillin, 80–90 mg/kg divided twice daily for 5–7 days, is the antibiotic of choice for the initial treatment of AOM.[16] Lack of subjective improvement after 72 hours of treatment with amoxicillin suggests treatment failure, and the patient should be switched to amoxicillin/clavulanate; patients with persistent symptoms after administration of high-dose amoxicillin/clavulanate should receive 1–3 doses of intramuscular ceftriaxone.[16] In cases of suspected resistant organisms, macrolides (e.g., azithromycin), TMP/SMX, cephalexin, cefaclor, loracarbef, and cefdinir can also be used. Multiple courses of broad-spectrum antibiotics should be avoided; routine prophylactic therapy is not recommended for recurrent AOM.[16] Complications of AOM include hearing loss, chronic otitis media, tympanic membrane perforation, and mastoiditis. Rare complications include brain/epidural/subdural abscesses, meningitis, and lateral sinus or cavernous vein thrombosis.

Otitis Externa

Otitis externa (OE) is an infection of the external auditory canal that primarily affects children but is not uncommon among adults, particularly in persons with diabetes and immunocompromised patients.[18] Up to 10% of the population will develop OE at some point during their lifetime; risk factors include excessive cleaning of the ear canal via cotton swabs or aggressive itching of the ear canal, swimming ("swimmer's ear"), increased humidity, and wearing ear canal devices such as hearing aids, headphones, or diving caps. Skin conditions including psoriasis, eczema, seborrheic dermatitis, and acne can increase the risk of OE if the ear is involved.[18]

Patients with OE typically present with otalgia and otorrhea.[18] Pain is commonly exacerbated by pulling on the ear lobe or sometimes, while chewing. If the auditory canal is occluded by fluid discharge, then the patient may complain of fullness and hearing loss. Fever and other systemic signs are uncommon in uncomplicated cases of OE. On physical examination, a serous or purulent exudate is commonly seen in the auditory canal, and pulling on the pinna elicits pain. Mastoid tenderness or crepitus suggests a more complicated infection; in these cases, mastoiditis should be strongly considered and a referral to an otolaryngologist promptly facilitated. An erythematous tympanic membrane indicates a concomitant otitis media.

The most common organisms causing OE include *Pseudomonas aeruginosa* (41%) and *S. aureus* (15%). Fungal organisms (*Aspergillus* species) are recovered in 6.5% of cases and one third of cases are polymicrobial, including anaerobes such as *Bacteroides fragilis* and *Peptostreptococcus* species.[19]

Cleansing the involved auditory canal with room temperature tap water should be attempted to optimize topical therapy and should be performed with low suction under direct visualization.

Alternatively, a cotton swab can be used to gently mop secretions from the canal. Flushing of the external auditory canal should not be attempted unless an intact tympanic membrane is visualized. If the tympanic membrane has perforated, flushing may cause significant cochlear damage.

Therapies for the treatment of OE are listed in Table 11-6; topical antibiotics are the treatment of choice for uncomplicated OE. It is recommended that drops be given for 3 days after symptoms resolve, and most patients require a total of 5–7 days of treatment. The addition of steroids to ear drop solutions may help to decrease canal inflammation more quickly. If canal edema is severe, a wick placed in the canal may be required, and drops should be applied more frequently (6–10 times daily) until the canal is opened. Systemic antibiotics are rarely needed but are useful when OE is persistent or when concomitant OM is present.

Complications of OE include necrotizing OE, focal furuncles, mastoiditis, and chronic OE, which can lead to hearing loss.[18] Necrotizing OE is the life-threatening extension of OE into the mastoid and temporal bones. The most common etiologic agent is *P. aeruginosa,* and treatment often requires parenteral antibiotics and, periodically, surgery. An otolaryngologist should be consulted early when necrotizing OE is suspected. Those at highest risk include elderly persons, particularly those with diabetes and immunocompromised patients (e.g., HIV/AIDS).

Influenza

Most human epidemics of influenza are caused by the type A and B influenza viruses.[20] Influenza A viruses, which also cause pandemics, are named by their hemagglutinin (H) and neuraminidase (N) surface antigens. Influenza B viruses are not categorized into subtypes and do not cause pandemics. Since 1977, influenza A H1N1, influenza A H3N2, and influenza B viruses have been circulating worldwide. In the last century there have been three pandemics of influenza A that occurred in 1918, 1957, and 1968. The most devastating of these pandemics was the 1918 outbreak of "Spanish flu," which killed 40–50 million people worldwide and 500,000 in the United States. The outbreak of avian influenza (H5N1) in Southeast Asia that started in 2003 and caused 70 deaths as of January 2006 has raised concern about a seemingly overdue pandemic.[21]

Epidemiology

On average, approximately 36,000 people die from influenza-related complications and 226,000 are admitted to the hospital for influenza each year in the United States.[20] Very young children (0–4 years) and elderly persons (older than 65 years) compose the majority of these cases. The mortality rate in the 1990s for persons older than 65 years was 98.3/100,000 and was

Table 11-6. Treatment of Otitis Externa

Topical treatment	2% acetic acid otic solution (VoSoL) • with hydrocortisone (VolSoL HC Otic) • with aluminum acetate (Otic Domeboro)
	Neomycin otic solution • with polymyxin B-hydrocortisone (Cortisporin) • with hydrocortisone-thonzonium (Coly-Mycin S)
	Polymyxin B-hydrocortisone (Otobiotic)
	Ophthalmic solutions • Ofloxacin 0.3% (Ocuflox) • Ciprofloxacin 0.3% (Ciloxan) • Gentamicin sulfate 0.3% (Garamycin) • Tobramycin sulfate 0.3% (Tobrex)
Systemic antibiotics (IV or PO) • If OM present • Immunocompromised • Persistent OE • Disease beyond auditory canal • Necrotizing OE	• Cephalosporins: ceftazidime, cefepime • Anti-pseudomonal penicillins: piperacillin, ticarcillin • Fluoroquinolones: ciprofloxacin, levofloxacin • Best oral option (covers pseudomonas species) • Necrotizing OE should be treated with IV therapy and an otolaryngology consult should be called early for possible debridement

IV, Intravenous; PO, per os; OM, otitis media; OE, otitis externa.
Adapted from: Sanders R: Otitis externa: a practical guide to treatment and prevention, *Am Fam Pract* 63:927–936, 2001.

7.5/100,000 in those aged 50–64 years. Influenza complications are also much more common in men with high-risk conditions including COPD, coronary heart disease, diabetes mellitus, immunodeficiency (e.g., HIV/AIDS), chronic corticosteroid use (e.g., >7.5 mg/day), hematologic cancers (e.g., leukemia), and chronic renal failure. Males may be disproportionately affected by influenza risk and contracture because they have a higher rate of many of these high-risk conditions.

Clinical Presentation

Influenza is spread via person-to-person contact and, during an epidemic, 25–40% of unvaccinated susceptible persons will get infected and develop symptoms.[20] The incubation period is 1–4 days with an average of 2 days. Viral shedding occurs 1–2 days before the start of symptoms and continues for an average of 5–7 days thereafter; immunocompromised patients can shed the influenza virus for a period of weeks.

Uncomplicated influenza presents as an abrupt onset of fever, chills, headache, myalgias, nonproductive cough, sore throat, and rhinitis.[22] During influenza season, particularly if an epidemic is occurring, the specificity of clinical symptoms can be as high as 71%. Influenza usually resolves within 3–7 days, but cough and malaise may persist for several weeks. Complications of influenza in adults and adolescents include primary viral pneumonia, secondary bacterial pneumonias (e.g., *S. aureus*), bacterial sepsis, myositis, myocarditis and pericarditis, encephalitis, and transverse myelitis. Most deaths are a result of either viral or bacterial pneumonia.[22]

Diagnosis

During influenza season, the diagnosis of the disease is made on the basis of clinical suspicion. The sensitivity and specificity of an influenza-like illness with fevers, myalgias, malaise, nonproductive cough, rhinitis, and headache are approximately 70% and 60%, respectively.[20] Available diagnostic tests for influenza include viral cultures, viral serologic assays, rapid antigen testing, and polymerase chain reaction (PCR) and immunofluorescence assays. Rapid influenza tests require nasopharyngeal swabs and are more than 70% sensitive and 90% specific. They are most useful at the start of the influenza season to confirm an epidemic (positive predictive value, 89–95%) and during non-influenza seasons when influenza is suspected (negative predictive value,

99%).[23] These tests can differentiate between influenza A and B but cannot identify specific influenza A subtypes (e.g., H3N2 versus H1N1). Other diagnostic tests have no clinical value at this time.

Vaccination

The best way to prevent influenza and its complications is through vaccination. Vaccination of healthy adults older than 65 years of age prevents influenza in 70–90% of vaccinated persons and significantly decreases work absenteeism and use of healthcare resources.[20] Among persons older than 65 years, vaccination is 50–60% effective in preventing influenza-related hospitalizations and 80% effective in preventing influenza-related death. A cost-benefit analysis estimated an average annual savings of $13.66/person vaccinated.[24] Unfortunately, vaccination rates vary from 30% to 66% depending on the risk category, and healthcare worker vaccination rates are generally below 40%. Many people refuse influenza vaccination claiming that it has "given them the flu" or they "know someone who has gotten the flu from the vaccine." These perceptions persist regardless of much evidence to the contrary. Healthcare workers are often "too busy" to get vaccinated despite ample opportunity and education.

Two influenza vaccines are currently endorsed by the US Food and Drug Administration (FDA). The inactivated (killed virus) influenza vaccine is most commonly used and is given as an intramuscular injection. The live, attenuated influenza vaccine is administered intranasally as a spray. Both vaccines are equally effective for protection against influenza A and B, both are grown in egg albumin, and both are administered yearly. The live vaccine is more expensive than the inactivated vaccine and is not approved for use in children younger than 5 years old. Since it is a live virus, it should not be administered to immunosuppressed patients. Site reactions and fever have occurred with the inactivated vaccine, whereas very few adverse affects have been associated with the live formulation. The current Advisory Committee on Immunization Practices recommendations for vaccinating against influenza are summarized in Table 11-7.

Treatment

Antiviral medications can be used as either treatment or chemoprophylaxis of influenza A and B[20] (Table 11-8), and there are currently four

Table 11-7. ACIP Influenza Vaccination Recommendations (July 2005)

High risk for influenza complications
- Persons aged ≥65 years
- Residents of nursing homes and other chronic-care facilities that house persons of any age who have chronic medical conditions
- Adults and children who have chronic disorders of the pulmonary or cardiovascular systems, including asthma (hypertension is not considered a high-risk condition)
- Adults and children who have required regular medical follow-up or hospitalization during the preceding year because of chronic metabolic diseases (including diabetes mellitus), renal dysfunction, hemoglobinopathies, or immunosuppression (including immunosuppression caused by medications or by human immunodeficiency virus [HIV])
- Adults and children who have any condition (e.g., cognitive dysfunction, spinal cord injuries, seizure disorders, or other neuromuscular disorders) that can compromise respiratory function or the handling of respiratory secretions or that can increase the risk for aspiration
- Children and adolescents (aged 6 months to 18 years) who are receiving long-term aspirin therapy and, therefore, might be at risk for experiencing Reye's syndrome after influenza infection
- Children aged 6–23 months

Persons aged 50–64 years

Healthcare workers

Persons who can transmit influenza to those at risk

Travelers (e.g., on cruise ships)

General population—if vaccine supplies are adequate

The following groups should not be vaccinated with live, attenuated influenza vaccine (LAIV)
- Persons aged < 5 years or those aged ≥ 50 years
- Persons with asthma, reactive airways disease, or other chronic disorders of the pulmonary or cardiovascular systems; persons with other underlying medical conditions, including such metabolic diseases as diabetes, renal dysfunction, and hemoglobinopathies; or persons with known or suspected immunodeficiency diseases or who are receiving immunosuppressive therapies
- Children or adolescents receiving aspirin or other salicylates (because of the association of Reye's syndrome with wild-type influenza infection)
- Persons with a history of GBS
- Persons with a history of hypersensitivity, including anaphylaxis, to any of the components of LAIV or to eggs

ACIP, Advisory Committee on Immunization Practices; GBS, group B *Streptococcus*.
Adapted from: Harper SA, Fukuda K, Uyeki TM, Cox NJ, Bridges CB: Prevention and control of influenza: recommendations of the Advisory Committee on Immunization Practices, *MMWR* 54:1–40, 2005.

licensed drugs in two classes. Amantadine and rimantadine are only active against influenza A and are FDA approved for both treatment and prophylaxis in adults. Adverse effects include central nervous system (CNS) toxicity (e.g., anxiety, dizziness, insomnia, difficulty concentrating) and gastrointestinal toxicity (e.g., nausea, vomiting). These symptoms are usually mild and resolve with drug discontinuation. Severe adverse effects including delirium, seizures, and hallucinations are rare and only seen with high serum levels of the medications.

The neuraminidase inhibitors, oseltamivir (Tamiflu) and zanamivir (Relenza), were FDA approved in 1999 for treatment of adults with influenza A and B, and oseltamivir was approved for chemoprophylaxis in 2000. The most frequent adverse effects with oseltamivir include nausea and vomiting. Zanamivir is administered as an aerosol inhalant and, in addition to nausea and vomiting, some patients have experienced wheezing and a decline in pulmonary function.

Pharmacotherapy treatment for influenza should be initiated within 48 hours of the start of symptoms, and it been shown to reduce the duration of symptoms by only 1 day compared with placebo.[20] In addition to decreasing duration of symptoms, oseltamivir and zanamivir have been shown to decrease hospitalizations and the use of antibiotics.[20,25] Chemoprophylaxis has been useful in preventing influenza in certain high-risk populations (see Table 11-8).[20] Unfortunately, the use of antiviral agents as treatment and chemoprophylaxis has led to resistance, especially to amantadine and rimantadine.

Viral Hepatitis
Hepatitis A

Hepatitis A is one of the most common vaccine-preventable diseases in the United States. It is caused by a picornavirus and produces both symptomatic and asymptomatic disease. Hepatitis A virus (HAV) infection is most often acquired through fecal-oral spread by either person-to-person transmission or from ingestion of a contaminated food or water source. Children often get asymptomatic disease and, thus, play an important role in transmission of the disease among family members and day care center staff.[26] The most frequently reported source of infection is a household member or sexual partner. Although 10% of those infected with hepatitis A have a history of one of the above exposures, up to 50% do not have an identifiable source. The case-fatality rate for hepatitis A in the United States is 0.3% but is higher among adults older than 50 years of age (1.8%) and in those with chronic liver disease. Groups at a higher risk for hepatitis A disease include international

Table 11-8. Recommendations for Treatment and Prophylaxis of Influenza

Treatment Indications	Medication
• Symptoms (e.g., fever, nonproductive cough, malaise, myalgias) for < 48 hours • Unvaccinated high-risk patient (see Table 11-7)	• Amantadine (Symmetrel) 100 mg bid PO × 3–5 days (reduce dose in elderly, in those with renal hepatic dysfunction); influenza A only • Rimantadine (Flumadine) 100 mg bid PO × 5–7 days (reduce dose in elderly, in those with renal hepatic dysfunction); influenza A only • Oseltamivir (Tamiflu) 75 mg bid PO × 5 days (reduce dose in those with renal hepatic dysfunction); influenza A and B • Zanamivir (Relenza) two inhalations (10 mg) bid × 5 days; influenza A and B
Chemoprophylaxis Indications	
• High-risk persons vaccinated after influenza activity has begun. Treat for 2 weeks after vaccine is given. • Unvaccinated persons, including healthcare workers, who provide care to high-risk persons during an outbreak. Treat for duration of outbreak or 2 weeks after vaccination. • Unvaccinated persons who have immunodeficiencies during an outbreak. Treat for duration of outbreak or 2 weeks after vaccination • Close unvaccinated contacts of persons with influenza. Treat for 7 days. • Residents of institutions (e.g., nursing homes) regardless of vaccination status. Treat for the duration of the outbreak.	• Amantadine (Symmetrel) 100 mg bid PO (reduce dose in elderly, in those with renal hepatic dysfunction); influenza A only • Rimantadine (Flumadine) 100 mg bid PO (reduce dose in elderly, in those with renal hepatic dysfunction); influenza A only • Oseltamivir (Tamiflu) 75 mg qd PO (reduce dose in those with renal hepatic dysfunction); influenza A and B

bid, Twice a day; PO, per os; qd; once a day.

Adapted from: Harper SA, Fukuda K, Uyeki TM, Cox NJ, Bridges CB: Prevention and control of influenza: recommendations of the Advisory Committee on Immunization Practices, *MMWR* 54:1–40, 2005.

travelers, men who have sex with men (MSM), intravenous drug users, day care staff, and those who work with infected primates. Patients with clotting-factor disorders are also considered to be at a high risk through clotting factor transfusions. Healthcare workers and food handlers do not have a higher risk of disease but may be a source of transmission.

Hepatitis A has an average incubation period of 28 days (range, 15–50 days).[26] Symptoms including fever, malaise, nausea, abdominal pain, jaundice, scleral icterus, and dark urine last generally less than 2 months, but 10–15% of persons may have a prolonged or relapsing syndrome lasting up to 6 months. There is no chronic infection with hepatitis A; treatment is supportive because the infection is self-limited. The diagnosis of HAV infection is based on a combination of symptoms and the presence of serum transaminase (i.e., alanine aminotransferase and aspartate aminotransferase) and bilirubin elevations. Definitive diagnosis requires serologic evidence of acute disease via the presence of immunoglobulin M (IgM) anti-HAV. The presence of only IgG anti-HAV is not sufficient to diagnose acute

hepatitis A, as approximately 33% of the US population has had exposure at some time.[26]

Prevention of HAV infection can be achieved through vaccination or passive immunization.[26] Inactivated whole-virus HAV vaccine is used in the United States and confers protection in 94–100% of adults. The two formulations used in the United States include Havrix and VAQTA. Adverse events from vaccination are rare and are usually limited to local irritation at the site of intramuscular injection. Twinrix, a combination vaccine containing HAV and hepatitis B components, should be administered in three doses at 0, 1, and 6 months. Complete seroprotection generally occurs 4 weeks after the first dose is received, and a second dose provides long-term protection (up to 7 years). International travelers, MSM, persons who use intravenous or intranasal illicit drugs, persons who have clotting-factor disorders, persons with occupational risk, and persons with chronic liver disease should be strongly encouraged to receive the HAV vaccine.

Immunoglobulin (IG) provides protection against HAV infection through passive transfer of antibodies from pooled human plasma.[24] IG is administered intramuscularly at a dose of 0.02 mL/kg and it provides up to 3 months of seroprotection. Hepatitis A IG should be administered prophylactically to unvaccinated exposed high-risk persons and should be administered simultaneously with HAV vaccine. Other eligible persons include those with close contact with a person with a confirmed case, staff at child care centers where an HAV infection outbreak has occurred, persons exposed to food prepared by an HAV-infected food handler, and travelers going to high-risk areas who have received HAV vaccine less than 2 weeks before traveling.

Hepatitis B

Hepatitis B virus (HBV) is a DNA virus that replicates primarily in the liver.[27] Like HAV, it is a vaccine-preventable disease; however, unlike HAV, a chronic disease state can occur with hepatitis B that can eventually lead to end-stage liver disease. HBV is primarily transmitted by percutaneous or mucosal exposure to infectious blood or body fluids that contain HBV. Persons at high risk of becoming infected with HBV include intravenous and intranasal drug users, persons engaging in unprotected sex with multiple partners, infants born to infected women, and healthcare workers. Recommendations to vaccinate infants and adolescents against HBV have resulted in a plummeting incidence of the disease in the United States—from 8.5/100,000 population in 1990 to 2.1/100,000 population in 2004. The prevalence of HBV infection in the United States is currently approximately 5%, and 1.5 million persons are chronic carriers of the virus. The incidence of infection in men is twice that in women (3.0/100,000 versus 1.5/100,000).[27]

The incubation period for HBV is 90 days (range, 60–150 days) from exposure to jaundice. Clinical symptoms of acute disease include anorexia, malaise, nausea, vomiting, and jaundice.[27] The fatality rate is up to 1.5% and is highest among persons older than 60 years of age. Asymptomatic disease also occurs and is more common in children younger than 5 years. Approximately 10% of acutely infected adults become chronic persistent carriers (i.e., hepatitis B surface antigen [HBsAg] positive), and 25–30% of these persons develop chronic active hepatitis.[27] Chronic HBV carriers are at an increased risk for hepatocellular carcinoma, cirrhosis, membranous glomerulonephritis, polyarteritis nodosum, and chronic serum sickness–like syndrome.

The diagnosis of acute HBV infection is based on clinical symptoms and serologic markers, particularly HBsAg.[27] Patients who eventually develop hepatitis B surface antibody (HBsAb) have cleared infection (or have been successfully vaccinated). If HBsAg does not clear by 4 months, then the patient is considered to be a chronic carrier. The presence of hepatitis B core IgG antibody (HBcAb) by itself is not adequate to confirm clearing of HBV, nor is it protective against the disease and its sequelae. Thus, persons who are HBcAb positive, HBsAb negative, and HBsAg negative should not be considered immune to HBV infection. Persons who are HBeAg positive are considered to be highly infective and are more likely to transmit the virus to others through unprotected sex or from an accidental needle stick. More recently, a PCR test has been used to quantify HBV DNA and to guide treatment for chronic disease. Immunocompromised patients (e.g., persons with HIV/AIDS) are less likely to clear virus from the blood.

No specific therapy exists for the treatment of acute HBV infection. However, several antiviral drugs including lamivudine (3TC), emtricitabine (Emtriva), adefovir (Hepsera), tenofovir (Viread), entecavir (Baraclude), and alpha-interferon (Cellferon) have been used in chronically infected patients to decrease HBV viral loads. Only entecavir, alpha-interferon, lamivudine, and adefovir have been approved by the FDA for treatment of HBV.

Prevention of HBV infection is best achieved through vaccination; however, hepatitis B immunoglobulin (HBIG) is also used in postexposure prophylaxis.[27] HBsAg is the antigen used for vaccination and is produced in the United States using recombinant DNA technology. The vaccine is available as a single-antigen formula (Recombivax HB, Engerix-B) or in combination with HAV vaccine (Twinrix). Since March of 2000, HBV vaccines do not contain thimerosal; all formulations are safe with minor site reactions being the most common adverse effect. Vaccination consists of three intramuscular injections at 0, 1, and 6 months for adults and children. In immunocompetent adults, vaccination is likely to be protective for 15–20 years. HBV vaccine is currently recommended in childhood and mandated by many states before children are allowed to enter school. Immunocompromised patients (e.g., persons with HIV/AIDS), patients receiving dialysis, persons receiving clotting factors via transfusion, healthcare workers and persons coming into contact with blood in the workplace, injection/intranasal drug users, persons with multiple sex partners, inmates and workers in correctional facilities, and international travelers should all strongly consider prophylactic vaccination.

Postexposure prophylaxis involves giving both HBIG and HBV vaccine.[28] HBIG is prepared from the plasma of donors with high concentrations of anti-HBs. Postexposure prophylaxis can be offered to persons who experience percutaneous or permucosal exposure to HBV. Unvaccinated persons should receive the hepatitis B vaccine and HBIG (0.06 mL/kg IM × 1 dose). If the person has been vaccinated and is a known responder, then no postexposure prophylaxis is required; if the person has been vaccinated but response status is unknown, then a serum antibody test should be performed. Patients with an adequate response (>10 IU/mL) do not require postexposure prophylaxis, whereas those with an inadequate response should receive both HBIG and hepatitis B vaccine.

Hepatitis C

Hepatitis C virus (HCV) is a single-stranded RNA virus that causes chronic liver disease and is the most common reason for liver transplantation in the United States.[29] The prevalence of HCV antibody (anti-HCV) in the United States is 1.4%, and approximately 36,000 new infections occur every year. Thus, 3.9 million persons are anti-HCV positive, and between 8000 and 13,000 die each year from end-stage liver disease. The highest incidence of infection is among 20–39 year olds, and males and African Americans are more likely to develop chronic infection.[29]

HCV is transmitted through contact with infected blood or mucosal secretions.[30] Those at increased risk of acquiring HCV infection include intravenous and intranasal drug users, healthcare workers, persons having unprotected sex with multiple partners, and persons undergoing body piercing or tattoos; data on acquisition of the virus through sexual contact and tattooing have been inconsistent. Acquiring HCV infection through the blood supply or from blood products is unlikely today in the United States given current blood and blood product testing. Sexual transmission of HCV is reportedly lower than HBV, especially among monogamous couples, and transmission through casual contact is not believed to occur. Perinatal transmission occurs in 5% of infants born to anti-HCV–positive mothers.[30] Quite alarming is that 44% of newly diagnosed cases have no risk factors identified over the previous 6 months.[30]

Unlike HAV and HBV, acute infection with HCV is usually asymptomatic, and jaundice is present in fewer than 25% of cases.[31] Eighty percent of persons acutely infected with HCV remain anti-HCV positive, and 60–80% will have persistently elevated serum transaminase levels. Most patients with chronic HCV infection are asymptomatic and the only clue to disease is the elevated serum transaminase levels. Cirrhosis eventually develops in 7–17% of patients with chronic infection after an average of 20–25 years[31]; immunocompromised patients (e.g., persons with HIV/AIDS) and alcoholics may progress to cirrhosis more quickly. The development of cirrhosis is silent, but end-stage liver disease eventually occurs at a rate of 3.9% per year. These patients will eventually develop jaundice, ascites, anasarca, and esophageal varices and the mortality rate is 43% at 34 months unless liver transplant is performed.[31] Hepatocellular carcinoma develops at a rate of 3% per year in patients with cirrhosis.[31]

The diagnosis of HCV infection is difficult because few persons present symptomatically with acute disease[32]; many clinicians discover the infection on further investigation of incidental elevated serum transaminase levels. Given the success of newer treatments for HCV infection, an early diagnosis is essential. Currently, the American Association for the Study of Liver Diseases recommends that persons at high risk of infection (see above), recipients of transfusions or organ transplants before July 1992 (when HCV screening became standard), healthcare workers after a needlestick injury, and sexual partners of HCV-infected persons be tested.[32]

Persons who are found to be HCV positive should be counseled to avoid sharing dental and shaving equipment with others, to cover any bleeding wounds, and to avoid donating blood or blood products. In addition, HCV-infected persons should be counseled that the risk of sexual transmission is low and that infection is no reason to change sexual practices in a long-term relationship.[32] Diagnosis of HCV infection is achieved via serologic assays for anti-HCV. Those persons with a positive anti-HCV should undergo HCV PCR testing to quantify viral load and genotype testing to determine HCV type (e.g., type 1, 2). Selected patients should undergo a liver biopsy to determine the extent of hepatic disease.[32]

Treatment decisions should be individualized and are based on the severity of liver disease, the potential of serious adverse effects, the likelihood of treatment response, and the presence of comorbid conditions.[32] Thus, HCV-infected persons should be monitored by an expert in infectious diseases or hepatology. The current treatment of choice is pegylated interferon plus ribavirin for a period of 6–12 months.[32] Success of therapy depends on HCV genotype (genotype 1 is the most refractory to treatment), underlying comorbidities, and the extent of hepatic injury. A sustained viral response, defined as the absence of HCV virus in the blood 6 months after treatment, is achieved in 25–40% of treated persons. Re-treatment is sometimes necessary for nonresponders or in the case of relapse.[32]

Human Immunodeficiency Virus and Acquired Immunodeficiency Syndrome

Epidemiology/Pathogenesis

HIV is a human retrovirus that infects and destroys CD4-positive T cells (lymphocytes) that, over time, leads to severe immunodeficiency and allows for the development of opportunistic infections and neoplasms. HIV is transmitted from person to person through sexual intercourse, from mother to child via child birth or breast milk, or through infected blood products (including needlestick injuries). Since 1981, there have been approximately 25 million deaths attributable to HIV/AIDS worldwide.[33] Forty million people are estimated to be living with HIV infection globally in 2005, with 5 million people becoming newly infected and 3 million deaths yearly. In the United States, there are more than 1 million people currently living with HIV infection and more than 40,000 people with AIDS. In 2004, it was estimated that there were more than 15,000 AIDS-related deaths in the United States. In the early 1980s, MSM constituted the majority of new infections. More recently, in 2004, women accounted for 30% of new infections in the United States as heterosexual transmission rates have continued to rise.[34] Despite efforts at prevention focusing on condom use, HIV infection has remained a significant public health concern both globally and in the United States. In 2004, there were 15,737 deaths attributable to AIDS, 75% of which occurred in men.

Clinical Presentation

Many people who are infected with HIV are unaware of their status since there often are no symptoms associated with chronic infection. Therefore, performing HIV antibody screening tests in patients who have high-risk exposures is of critical importance both for the health of the patient and to prevent HIV transmission to others. Conversely, up to 89% of patients who acutely are infected with HIV will have a constellation of symptoms consisting of fever, rash, myalgias, headache, and anorexia.[35] They also may develop laboratory abnormalities including thrombocytopenia and transaminitis. Unfortunately, these signs and symptoms are quite nonspecific and may be confused with other viral infections. Therefore, a high index of suspicion must be maintained and HIV testing must be performed if any risk factors are discovered after careful evaluation (Table 11-9). Identifying patients with acute HIV infection is important since people are most highly infectious to others at the time of initial infection, and since the virus is multiplying at a very high rate before an organized immune response. It remains unclear whether initiating antiretroviral therapy during this time is of clinical benefit, although this issue remains a subject of ongoing study since decreasing the rate of HIV replication early in the course of infection may theoretically preserve specific CD4 cell responses.[36]

Diagnosis

The standard method of screening for HIV infection is the HIV 1/2 enzyme-linked immunosorbent assay (ELISA). This test screens for antibodies that react against both HIV-1 and HIV-2 antigens. Although the test has very high sensitivity and specificity, false-positive results can occasionally occur when nonspecific cross-reacting antibodies

Table 11-9. Risk Factors for Acquisition of HIV Infection*

Unprotected sexual intercourse: • Men who have sex with men   • Heterosexual intercourse
Perinatal transmission from HIV-infected mother to child: • At time of child birth   • Through breast milk
Exposure to contaminated blood or blood products: • Injection drug users who share contaminated needles   • Healthcare worker needlestick injury   • Healthcare worker blood product exposure to open wound or mucous membrane   • Transfusion of contaminated blood or blood product

*HIV cannot be transmitted through casual contact.

are present. Therefore, confirmatory testing via the Western blot is essential for diagnosis because this test detects specific host antibody responses against certain HIV-1 epitopes. An HIV-1 Western blot analysis result is interpreted as positive when at least two of three bands are present: p24, gp41, and gp120/160. When a false-positive ELISA result is encountered, there is often only one of three bands present, or bands are present that do not correspond to known HIV-1 antigens.

The screening ELISA test result may be negative during the first 2 weeks after acute HIV infection, the "window period," since anti-HIV antibodies require time to develop. During an acute infection, as HIV is often replicating at very high levels, the diagnosis can be made by performing either a quantitative PCR assay for HIV RNA (viral load) or a qualitative proviral HIV DNA PCR assay. Confirmatory testing with a repeat ELISA at a later time remains mandatory.[37]

Treatment

An enormous amount of research effort has been directed toward developing effective therapeutic strategies for HIV infection over the past 20 years. Since 1996, when multiple antiretroviral medications became available that acted at different stages of the viral life cycle, the long-term prognosis for patients living with HIV infection has improved dramatically. Pharmacotherapy is now available in four different classes that act to disrupt viral replication at the level of HIV RNA to DNA transcription (nucleoside reverse transcriptase inhibitors and non-nucleoside reverse transcriptase inhibitors), HIV capsid assembly (protease inhibitors), and HIV fusion to the CD4 positive T cell (fusion inhibitors). These drugs are used in certain combinations under the guidance of an HIV specialist to create highly active antiretroviral therapy that fully suppresses HIV replication and allows the regeneration of CD4 cells that reconstitute the patient's immune system to improved levels of functioning.[38]

When the immune system is successfully reconstituted, patients are no longer at a high risk for the opportunistic infections associated with the morbidity and mortality that occurs with AIDS. Currently, not all patients with HIV infection require the use of antiretroviral medication. Because of the adverse effects and the risk of the development of resistance associated with treatment, these medications are now initiated only when the CD4 count falls to below 350 cells/mL or in the setting of acute infection.[38]

Complications

The morbidity and mortality associated with HIV infection are due to the consequences of immune suppression (i.e., AIDS) and to the sometimes serious adverse effects of antiretroviral medications. If viral replication is left unmonitored in patients who are not diagnosed early in the course of HIV infection or in patients who develop resistance to antiretroviral medications, then the CD4 count inexorably declines over time in most cases. The end result is a loss of appropriate functioning of the immune system, which allows for the development of both opportunistic infections and neoplasms (Table 11-10).

Different opportunistic infections may be observed at various levels of immune suppression depending on the CD4 count level. With relatively normal CD4 counts (500 cells/mL or greater), patients with HIV infection encounter a greater risk of bacterial infections, including pneumonia and soft tissue infections.[39] Reactivation of herpes virus infections such as herpes simplex virus (HSV) and varicella zoster may also occur in this range. Patients become at a high risk for Kaposi sarcoma and tuberculosis when CD4 counts fall between 200 and 400 cells/mL. More severe immune compromise occurs at

Table 11-10. Selected AIDS-associated Opportunistic Infections and Neoplasms

Central nervous system toxoplasmosis
Cervical cancer
Cryptococcosis (including meningitis)
Cytomegalovirus (CMV) retinitis
Esophageal candidiasis
HIV encephalopathy
Histoplasmosis (including disseminated disease)
Kaposi sarcoma
Lymphoma
Mycobacterium avium complex (including disseminated infection)
Mycobacterium tuberculosis
Oral thrush
Pneumocystis jerovici pneumonia
Progressive multifocal leukoencephalopathy
Recurrent bacterial pneumonia

Adapted from: Centers for Disease Control and Prevention: 1993 revised classification system for HIV infection and expanded surveillance case definition for AIDS among adolescents and adults, *MMWR Morb Mortal Wkly Rep* 41(No. RR-17):1–18, 1992.

CD4 count levels of less than 200 cells/mL, at which point prophylactic antibiotics such as TMP/SMX are recommended.[39] Patients in this range are at risk for *Pneumocystis jerovici* (formerly *Pneumocystis carinii*) pneumonia, cryptococcosis, and toxoplasmosis reactivation. Patients are considered to be profoundly immune compromised when the CD4 count drops below 50 cells/mL, at which point they are at risk for other severe infections including disseminated *Mycobacterium avium* complex, cytomegalovirus reactivation, and lymphoma.[40]

Over the past 10 years, HIV specialists have learned that although antiretroviral medication can dramatically alter the natural history of HIV and AIDS, they also carry the risk for adverse effects and drug interactions.[38] Each individual medication and class of medication has a unique set of potential adverse effects, some of which are irreversible. For example, protease inhibitors and some nucleoside reverse transcriptase inhibitors have been linked to the development of fat redistribution syndromes (peripheral lipodystrophy). Glucose intolerance and hyperlipidemia can occur with the use of some protease inhibitors as well including lopinavir/ritonavir (Kaletra).[38] Mitochondrial toxicity leading to lactic acidosis can be caused by any of the nucleoside reverse transcriptase inhibitors and has been particularly linked to the use of stavudine (Zerit) and didanosine (Videx), especially when used together.[38] The non-nucleoside reverse transcriptase inhibitors such as nevirapine (Viramune) can cause a drug-induced hepatitis and sometimes severe cutaneous drug eruptions.[38] Although antiretroviral therapy has significantly reduced the morbidity and mortality associated with HIV infection and has been of great benefit to many patients, these drugs must be used judiciously to minimize the risk of severe toxicity.

Prevention

Until an effective vaccine is developed, the key to eliminating the threat of the spread of HIV is through prevention efforts.[41,42] Educating patients about the importance of condom use to prevent the spread of sexually transmitted diseases such as HIV is of paramount importance. Intravenous drug users can minimize their risk through needle-exchange programs. In the case of occupational exposures (e.g., needlestick injuries) or sexual assault, postexposure prophylaxis with antiretroviral drugs can significantly reduce the risk of infection.[43,44] Lastly, it is important that physicians work closely with their local health departments so that sexual partners of HIV-infected patients can be notified and tested and the chain of ongoing risk of HIV transmission to others can be broken.

Infectious Diarrheas

Epidemiology/Microbiology

In the United States, nearly 400 million episodes of diarrheal illness occur each year or, on average, one diarrheal episode per person per year.[45] Food-borne diarrhea accounts for one fifth of these cases (80 million) and is the cause of 5000 deaths per year. Although the highest mortality worldwide occurs among children, in the United States most of those who die from diarrheal disease are elderly.[45]

Since many different microorganisms can cause infectious diarrhea, it is useful to divide them into three groups: community-acquired or traveler's diarrhea, nosocomial diarrhea, and persistent diarrhea (diarrhea lasting for greater than 7 days) (Table 11-11).[45] The most common community-acquired organisms include viruses such as Norovirus, Enterovirus, and Rotavirus and bacteria including *Campylobacter*, *Salmonella* species (non-*typhi*), *Shigella* species, *Escherichia coli*, and enterotoxigenic *S. aureus*. A new vaccination is available for rotavirus and is administered to children at 2, 4, and 6 months of age; the previous version of the vaccination was taken off the market several years ago as a result of numerous fatal cases of intussusception. Traveler's diarrhea is most likely to be caused by *E. coli*, but *Entamoeba histolytica* and *Salmonella typhi* must also be included. Nosocomial diarrhea is almost exclusively caused by *Clostridium difficile*, although *S. aureus* has been implicated in some cases. Both of these diarrheas are associated with antibiotic use. Although clindamycin is classically associated with *C. difficile* infection, any antibiotic (particularly broad-spectrum antibiotics) can cause the disease. Persistent diarrheas are most commonly caused by protozoal organisms including *Giardia lamblia*, *Cryptosporidium*, *Cyclospora*, and *Isospora belli*.

Populations at increased risk of developing infectious diarrheas include young children, immunocompromised patients, and patients taking antibiotics. HIV-positive patients are at a particular risk of acquiring protozoal diarrheal infections such as *Entamoeba histolytica* and *Cryptosporidium*. The low gastric pH in children younger than 5 years places them at a significantly increased risk for *Salmonella* infections.

Table 11-11. Common Causes of Infectious Diarrhea

Organism	Mode of Transmission	Treatment
Viruses		
Rotavirus	Transmitted person to person; transmitted through contaminated food or liquid	Viral gastroenteritis is self-limited and does not require antibiotic treatment
Norovirus		
Enteroviruses		
Bacteria		
Shigella species	Person to person; food (rare)	TMP-SMZ (160/800 mg); fluoroquinolone (e.g., ciprofloxacin 500 bid PO); ceftriaxone IM/IV; azithromycin 500 mg qd PO × 3 days. Use IV if patient not taking PO
Non-*typhi Salmonella*	Food associated (e.g., chicken, eggs)	Generally no treatment. Treat severe disease, younger than 6 months or older than 50 years, compromised (see Shigella) × 5–7 days
Campylobacter species	Food (e.g., chicken), milk	Erythromycin 500 mg bid × 5 days
Escherichia coli species	Food (e.g., beef, fresh produce), water, raw milk	TMP-SMZ (160/800 mg); fluoroquinolone (e.g., ciprofloxacin 500 bid PO); ceftriaxone IM/IV; azithromycin 500 mg qd PO × 3 days
Enterotoxigenic		
Enteropathogenic		
Enteroinvasive		
Escherichia coli 0157 enterohemorrhagic	Food (e.g., beef), water	Avoid antimotility drugs; Avoid antibiotics
Aeromonas, Plesiomonas	Water	TMP-SMZ (160/800 mg); fluoroquinolone (e.g., ciprofloxacin 500 bid PO); ceftriaxone IM/IV; azithromycin 500 mg qd PO × 3 days
Yersinia species (not pestis)	Food (e.g., pork), milk	No treatment
Staphylococcus aureus	Food (e.g., egg salad, ham, poultry, pastries)	No treatment
Bacillus cereus	Food (e.g., fried rice, meats)	No treatment
Clostridium perfringens	Food (e.g., beef, poultry, gravy)	No treatment
Clostridium difficile	Antibiotic associated	Stop antibiotic; metronidazole 250 mg PO qid to 500 mg tid × 10 days
Parasites		
Giardia	Water	Metronidazole 250–750 mg PO tid × 10 days
Entamoeba histolytica	Water, food (fresh produce)	Metronidazole 750 mg PO tid × 5–10 days + paromomycin 500 mg tid × 7 days
Cryptosporidium	Water	Usually self-limited

TMP-SMZ, trimethoprim/sulfamethoxazole; bid, twice a day; PO, per os; IM, intramuscular; IV, intravenous; qid, four times a day; tid, three times a day; qd, once a day.

Adapted from: Guerrant RL, Van Gilder T, Steiner TS, et al: Practice guidelines for the management of infectious diarrhea, *Clin Infect Dis* 32:331–351, 2001.

Clinical Evaluation

A thorough history should be the first step in determining the source of an infectious diarrhea. In patients who have recently traveled overseas (within 2 weeks) *E. coli, Entamoeba,* and *S. typhi* should be considered.[46] Endemic food-associated diarrheas are caused by organisms including *Campylobacter, S. aureus, Salmonella typhimurium, Shigella, Listeria,* and noroviruses (see Table 11-11). Seasonal diarrhea might implicate enteroviruses or Rotavirus. Diarrhea occurring after consumption of untreated water is suggestive of *Giardia* or *E. coli* infection. A complete exposure history is particularly critical in food-associated diarrheas that have public health implications; all documented infections should be reported to respective counties for epidemiologic surveillance.

The timing and character of the diarrhea often helps in establishing an etiology.[46] Rapid onset (within 2–6 hours) is characteristic of toxin-mediated diarrheas such as *S. aureus* and *Bacillus cereus.* A somewhat longer period from exposure to onset of symptoms (8–16 hours) is commonly seen in *Clostridium perfringens* toxin-mediated diarrhea. *Salmonella, Shigella,* and *Campylobacter* generally have incubation periods of 16–48 hours. Chronic diarrheas lasting 1–3 weeks are typical of *Cryptosporidium* and *Giardia* infections. Bloody diarrhea with fever and tenesmus is referred to as *dysentery* and indicates an invasive process. Although this presentation is characteristic of *Entamoeba* and *Shigella,* it is sometimes seen with *Campylobacter* and *Salmonella.* A profuse secretory diarrhea (i.e., "rice water diarrhea") that can lead to rapidly fatal dehydration is caused by *Vibrio cholera.* Diarrhea associated with upper gastrointestinal signs such as bloating and belching is typical of *G. lamblia.* Diarrhea with fevers and a high white blood cell count in a hospitalized patient should raise concern for *C. difficile* infection. Bloody diarrhea without fever that is associated with renal failure (hemolytic uremic syndrome) suggests enterohemorrhagic *E. coli* (EHEC 0157) infection.

Laboratory Diagnosis

Selective fecal testing is useful in the following situations: (1) community-acquired or traveler's diarrhea, especially if accompanied by fever and bloody stools; (2) nosocomial diarrhea occurring 3 days after hospitalization; and (3) persistent diarrhea lasting longer than 1 week.[45] Fecal leukocyte testing may help to identify an inflammatory diarrhea but is a neither specific nor sensitive. Stool culture and assessment for ova and parasites should be used for investigation of community-acquired and traveler's diarrheas. Because most infectious diarrheas are self-limited, these tests should be used for epidemiologic studies and for those patients who present with bloody diarrhea and fever. In patients hospitalized for more than 3 days, stool cultures for community-acquired organisms (e.g., *Campylobacter, S. aureus, S. typhimurium, Shigella, Listeria*) and ova and parasites are unlikely to be helpful and

should not be performed.[45] These patients should, however, be tested for *C. difficile* toxin.[45] In patients with continued diarrhea with no identified pathogen, a colonoscopy may be helpful in identifying noninfectious causes of diarrhea, such as inflammatory bowel disease.

Management and Treatment

Treatment of dehydration is the cornerstone of therapy of community-acquired infectious diarrheas because most of these infections are self-limited.[45] Oral hydration with an electrolyte solution (e.g., Pedialyte, World Health Organization rehydration solution) is preferred, but if the patient cannot sustain oral rehydration, then parenteral hydration may be necessary. Although traveler's diarrhea is usually self-limited, TMP-SMZ or a fluoroquinolone can reduce the duration of illness from 3–5 days to 1–2 days.[45] Patients with fever and bloody diarrhea should be treated empirically with TMP-SMZ or a fluoroquinolone.[45] These patients are most likely to have invasive disease with *Shigella* or *Campylobacter* species. Antimotility agents can be used for uncomplicated traveler's diarrhea but should be avoided in patients with fever and bloody diarrhea or those with fecal leukocytes.[45] Treatment of EHEC 0157 with antimicrobial agents has been associated with an increased risk of hemolytic uremic syndrome and should therefore be considered carefully. Table 11-11 details various treatment regimens for infectious diarrhea commensurate with each pathogen.

Complications

The most devastating complication of an infectious diarrhea is toxic megacolon and bowel perforation.[47] This should be suspected in patients who have a sudden increase in pain, decreased bowel sounds, and a septic appearance. Rebound pain or guarding on palpation of the abdomen are characteristic findings and should prompt immediate surgical evaluation. Invasive organisms are most likely to cause this complication and include *Entamoeba, Shigella, C. difficile, C. perfringens,* and enteropathogenic *E. coli* infection. Enterohemorrhagic *E. coli* infection is associated with hemolytic uremic syndrome in children but rarely occurs in adults. *Entamoeba* infection can lead to amoebic liver abscesses, which require additional antibiotic treatment and sometimes drainage. Dehydration is the leading cause of death in developing countries from infectious diarrheas, particularly via *V. cholera.*

Bacteremia can occur with *S. typhimurium* in immunocompromised patients (e.g., persons with HIV/AIDS).

Sexually Transmitted Diseases

Urethritis

Urethritis is defined as the presence of urethral inflammation. It is clinically characterized by the discharge of mucopurulent or purulent material and by dysuria or urethral pruritus. The classic bacterial pathogen of acute urethritis is *Neisseria gonorrhoeae*. Urethral infection of all other causes is referred to collectively as nongonococcal urethritis (NGU). The organism most clearly associated with NGU is *Chlamydia trachomatis* (15–55% of cases).[48] The pathogens responsible for *Chlamydia*-negative NGU include *Ureaplasma urealyticum, Trichomonas vaginalis, Mycoplasma genitalium*, and HSV. The etiology of most cases of non-chlamydial NGU is unknown.

Urethritis can be documented on the basis of any of the following signs: mucopurulent or purulent discharge, a Gram stain of urethral secretions demonstrating 5 or more white blood cells per high power field, microscopic examination demonstrating 10 or more white blood cells per high power field, or a positive leukocyte esterase test on first-void urine.[48] The Gram stain is a highly sensitive and specific test for evaluating urethritis and the presence or absence of gonococcal infection. Gonococcal infection is established by documenting the presence of white blood cells containing intracellular gram-negative diplococci.

Gonococcal Urethritis

The rate of gonorrhea infection in males in the United States is most common in African American men aged 20–24 years.[49] Historically, the reported rates of gonococcal infection in men is higher than in women, differences attributable to the higher incidence of asymptomatic disease in women and the occurrence of infection among MSM, as the incidence of gonococcal infection has been increasing in the latter population.[49] Gonorrhea in MSM is associated with an approximately three-fold increase in the risk of acquisition of HIV infection.[50]

Acute urethritis is the predominant manifestation of gonorrhea in men. The incubation period is typically 2–5 days, but recent studies suggest that this may be increasing.[51] Dysuria is usually more prominent and the discharge is generally more profuse and purulent than NGU. Epididymitis, proctitis, and pharyngitis are less common complication of *N. gonorrhoeae* infection. Anorectal gonorrhea is frequently the only site of infection in MSM and is uncommon in heterosexual men. Symptoms of proctitis include a mucopurulent rectal discharge, anal pruritus, tenesmus, pain, and rectal bleeding. Oropharyngeal infections with *N. gonorrhoeae* are frequently asymptomatic. First-line treatment for gonococcal pharyngeal infection is either intramuscular ceftriaxone or oral ciprofloxacin.[48]

Disseminated gonococcal infection results from gonococcal bacteremia and is often highlighted with petechial or pustular acral skin lesions, asymmetrical arthralgia, tenosynovitis, or septic arthritis.[48] It is a relatively common cause of infective arthritis in young adults. Gonococcal bacteremia often is intermittent, so that a minimum of three blood cultures should be obtained when disseminated disease is suspected. Approximately one half of patients with a disseminated gonococcal infection will have positive cultures of blood or synovial fluid.[52] Hospitalization is recommended for initial therapy, especially for patients who may not comply with treatment. Patients should be examined for clinical evidence of endocarditis and meningitis. The recommended regimen for disseminated gonococcal infection is intramuscular or intravenous ceftriaxone (1 g every 24 hours).[48]

Culture for *N. gonorrhoeae* remains the gold standard for diagnosis. Urethral, rectal, and pharyngeal specimens can be obtained using cotton swabs plated on Thayer-Martin agar. Nucleic acid amplification tests offer noninvasive, rapid results on both urine and urethral specimens and are the most commonly used assays in practice today. The sensitivity and specificity of nucleic acid amplification tests via both specimens is similar, and in some studies greater, than via standard culture.[48] Recommended treatment regimens for gonococcal urethritis and proctitis include ceftriaxone, cefixime, ciprofloxacin, ofloxacin, or levofloxacin in single doses (Table 11-12). Quinolone-resistant *N. gonorrhoeae* is common in Hawaii, California, and parts of Asia and the Pacific and among MSM,[44] and thus quinolones are no longer recommended for the treatment of gonorrhea in these areas or in MSM; the first-line therapy for these groups is ceftriaxone.[48] A detailed travel history for the patient and his or her partners is recommended before a therapy is chosen. If chlamydial

Table 11-12. Treatment of Sexually Transmitted Diseases

Organism	Primary Therapy	Alternative Therapy
Treponema pallidum (syphilis)	Primary, secondary, and early latent: benzathine PCN G 2.4 million units IM Late latent or latent of unknown duration, tertiary (excluding neurosyphilis): benzathine PCN G 7.2 million units IM, 2.4 million units/week × 3 weeks IM Neurosyphilis: Aqueous crystalline PCN G 18–24 million units/day (3–4 million units every 4 hours IV) for 10–14 days	PCN allergy: Doxycycline 100 mg bid × 14 days or tetracycline 500 mg qid × 14 days or azithromycin 2 g PO single dose ± PCN allergy: Doxycycline 100 mg bid × 28 days or tetracycline 500 mg qid × 28 days Procaine PCN G 2.4 million units IM qd + probenecid 500 mg PO qid, both for 10–14 days
Neisseria gonorrhoeae (gonococcal urethritis)	Single doses: Ceftriaxone 125 mg IM or cefixime 400 mg PO or ciprofloxacin 500 mg PO or ofloxacin 400 mg PO or levofloxacin 250 mg PO	Single doses: Cefotaxime 500 mg IM or cefoxitin 2 g IM with probenecid 1 g PO or spectinomycin 2 g IM
Chlamydia trachomatis (non-gonococcal urethritis)	Azithromycin 1 g PO single dose or doxycycline 100 mg PO bid for 7 days	Erythromycin 500 mg PO for 7 days or ofloxacin 300 mg bid for 7 days or levofloxacin 500 mg PO for 7 days
Chlamydia trachomatis (lymphogranuloma venereum)	Doxycycline 100 mg PO bid × 21 days	Erythromycin 500 mg PO qid × 21 days
Haemophilus ducreyi (chancroid)	• Azithromycin 1 g PO × 1 • Ceftriaxone 250 mg IM × 1	• Ciprofloxacin 500 mg PO bid × 3 days • Erythromycin 500 mg PO qid × 7 days
Human papilloma virus (HPV)	• Podophyllin solution topically qod × 3–4 weeks • Imiquimod (Aldara) cream 3×/week for 10–16 weeks • Benzoin tincture every week × 4 weeks • Trichloroacetic acid every week × 4 weeks • 5-flourouracil cream qd × 5–7 days • Intralesional alpha-interferon qod × 8–12 weeks • Removal-cryosurgery, electrosurgery, laser surgery, surgical excision	
Herpes simplex virus (HSV) (genital ulcers)	**Treatment** • Acyclovir 400 mg PO tid × 7–10 days • Famciclovir 250 mg PO tid × 7–10 days • Valacyclovir 1 g PO bid × 7–10 days **Suppression** • Acyclovir 400 mg PO bid • Famciclovir 250 mg PO bid • Valacyclovir 500 mg PO qd	**Treatment** • Acyclovir 200 mg PO 5×/day × 7–10 days **Suppression** • Acyclovir 200 mg PO 2–5×/day

IM, Intramuscular; bid, twice a day; qid, four times a day; PO, per os; qd, once a day; qod, every other day.

Adapted from: Centers for Disease Control and Prevention: Sexually transmitted diseases treatment guidelines 2002, *MMWR Recomm Rep* 51(No. RR-6):1–78, 2002.

infection is not ruled out and suspicion is high, then azithromycin or doxycycline should be given concomitantly.[48]

Nongonococcal Urethritis

The prevalence of *C. trachomatis* differs by age group, with a lower prevalence seen among older men; the number of cases due to this pathogen appears to be decreasing.[53] Most cases of NGU are sexually acquired. The incubation period of NGU is variable, but is typically 5–10 days after exposure. Patients with NGU have a less acute onset than gonorrhea, with symptoms increasing over several days. Patients typically present with a mucoid or watery discharge. Many men who are infected with *C. trachomatis* or *N. gonorrhoeae* are asymptomatic. The diagnosis of chlamydial urethritis is best made by nucleic acid amplification tests using PCR. Treatment for NGU is azithromycin or doxycycline (see Table 11-12).[48]

C. trachomatis can also cause proctitis, epididymitis, prostatitis, and reactive arthritis or Reiter syndrome. Asymptomatic chlamydial infection has not been associated with infertility in men. Chlamydial proctitis, defined as inflammation of the distal rectal mucosa, is relatively uncommon and occurs almost exclusively in MSM. Acute epididymitis is most commonly caused by *N. gonorrhoeae* or *C. trachomatis* among sexually active men younger than 35 years old. Symptoms include unilateral testicular pain and tenderness, hydrocele, and palpable swelling of the epididymis. Treatment for acute epididymitis caused by *N. gonorrhoeae* or *C. trachomatis* is ceftriaxone (250 mg intramuscular as a single dose) plus doxycycline (100 mg orally twice daily for 10 days).[48]

Follow-up for Gonococcal Urethritis and Nongonococcal Urethritis

Patients should be instructed to return for evaluation if symptoms persist or recur after completion of therapy. Patients should be instructed to abstain from sexual intercourse until 7 days after therapy is initiated. Patients should refer for evaluation and treatment all sex partners they have had within the preceding 60 days. Sexual partners are often asymptomatic and, unless treated, will reinfect the index patient or spread infection to other partners. Patients who have persistent or recurrent urethritis should be re-treated with the initial regimen if they did not comply with the treatment regimen or if they were re-exposed to an untreated sex partner.[48] Persistent gonococci that are isolated should be tested for antibiotic susceptibility. Persistent urethritis may also be caused by other organisms including *U. urealyticum* and *T. vaginalis.*

Syphilis

Syphilis is a spirochetal disease caused by *Treponema pallidum* and is most often acquired sexually. The incidence of primary and secondary syphilis increased between 2001 and 2004, with the increases observed only among men.[49] The rate of primary and secondary syphilis among males rose 81% between 2000 and 2004.[49] The natural history of syphilis is divided into several stages that sometimes overlap:

- Primary syphilis: After an incubation period of 10–90 days (usually 3 weeks), a painless papule appears at the site of inoculation, usually the external genitalia, anal area, lips, oral cavity, breasts, or fingers. This lesion ulcerates within a few days, producing the classic painless chancre, which usually resolves in 3–6 weeks.
- Secondary syphilis: Weeks to months later, the majority of untreated patients will develop symptoms and signs of secondary syphilis including diffuse lymphadenopathy, focal alopecia, mucosal lesions, and condyloma lata. A classic rash, characterized as a symmetric red and papular eruption involving the entire trunk and extremities including the palms and soles where it can become squamous, is the most characteristic finding of secondary syphilis, occurring in approximately 90% of patients. Nonspecific symptoms include fever, headache, malaise, anorexia, sore throat, myalgias, and weight loss.
- Latent syphilis: If untreated, clinical manifestations of secondary syphilis last for 2–6 weeks. Latent syphilis starts after the resolution of secondary syphilis and is defined by a positive serologic test result in an asymptomatic patient. Infection of less than 1 year is defined as early latent (infectious) and of more than 1 year as late latent (noninfectious).[48]
- Tertiary syphilis: After a variable level of latency, tertiary syphilis develops in about one third of untreated patients presenting as gummatous (i.e., nodules found anywhere in the body, most often in the skin and bones), cardiovascular, or neurosyphilis manifestations.[54]

Neurologic involvement can occur during all stages of syphilis. Acute asymptomatic or symptomatic meningitis can be seen during primary or secondary syphilis. The most fearful manifestations of CNS involvement occur during tertiary syphilis including meningovascular syphilis (leading to cerebrovascular accidents) and parenchymatous syphilis (general paresis or tabes dorsalis).

The diagnosis of syphilis is made by microscopy or serologic tests. Darkfield examinations and direct fluorescent antibody tests of lesion exudates or tissue are the definitive methods for diagnosing early syphilis.[48] Serologic tests for syphilis are classified into nontreponemal and treponemal assays. Nontreponemal tests include the Venereal Disease Research Laboratory (VDRL) and Rapid Plasma Reagin tests. Treponemal tests include the fluorescent treponemal antibody absorbed and *T. pallidum* particle agglutination tests. The use of only one type of serologic test is insufficient for diagnosis because false-positive nontreponemal test results may occur as a result of various medical conditions (e.g., autoimmune diseases). The nontreponemal tests are recommended as screening tools, and the treponemal tests are required for confirmation. Nontreponemal tests usually correlate with disease activity and usually become nonreactive with time, which can provide a false-negative result if they are the sole test performed in a patient with a previous infection. Reactive treponemal tests usually remain reactive regardless of treatment or disease activity. Some HIV-infected patients can have atypical serologic tests results (unusually high, unusually low, or fluctuating titers).[48] Positive cerebrospinal fluid (CSF) VDRL results are diagnostic of neurosyphilis, if the specimen is not contaminated with blood. CSF leukocytosis and increased CSF protein levels are common in cases of neurosyphilis.

Parenteral administration of penicillin G is the preferred drug for treatment for all stages of syphilis.[48] The preparations used (e.g., benzathine, aqueous procaine, or aqueous crystalline), the dosage, and the length of treatment depend on the stage and clinical manifestations of disease (see Table 11-12).

Chancroid

Chancroid is a sexually transmitted disease caused by the bacteria *Haemophilus ducreyi*. It is rare in the United States, with a steady decline in cases from a high of 5000 in 1987 to 39 cases in 2004. Men are more commonly infected than women, and 60% of all cases occur in persons aged 35 years or older.[55] *H. ducreyi* is highly infectious, and having only 100 colony-forming units leads to disease in 90% of exposed persons. Because it is difficult to grow, disease may be underestimated. Chancroid presents as a painful genital papule after 4–10 days of incubation. The papule becomes a 1–2-cm ulcer with an erythematous base and a clear, undermined border. The lesions most commonly occur on the prepuce, corona, or glans of the penis, and one half of infected men will progress to develop painful inguinal lymphadenitis.

The diagnosis of chancroid is challenging and depends on clinical presentation, a negative result in a test for HSV, and a Gram stain revealing small gram-negative rods in chains.[56] Culture of *H. ducreyi* is difficult and beyond the capability of most labs in the United States. Treatment is successful in 90% of cases, and the drugs of choice include azithromycin or ceftriaxone (see Table 11-12). Fluctuant inguinal buboes (severe lymphadenitis) should be drained by needle aspiration or they may develop draining fistulas. Sex partners should be treated, regardless of signs or symptoms, if they have had sexual contact with the infected person within 10 days of symptom presentation.

Lymphogranuloma Venereum

C. trachomatis infection can also lead to lymphogranuloma venereum.[48] This disease is most common in tropical and subtropical areas, represents less than 1% of all genital ulcers in the United States, and is more common among MSM. Clinically, it is characterized by a painless genital ulcer that initially heals but is followed in 2–6 weeks by painless inguinal lymphadenopathy. Untreated lymphogranuloma venereum progresses to inguinal buboes with chronic fistulous tracts. Diagnosis is often challenging and is based on a high degree of clinical suspicion and a positive IgG test for chlamydia (>1:256). Antibiotic treatment for lymphogranuloma venereum is outlined in Table 11-12.

Human Papilloma Virus

Human papilloma virus (HPV) is a DNA virus that causes penile and perirectal warts in men.[48] The prevalence of anal HPV (i.e., PCR positive) in MSM is approximately 57% and the most common genotype seen is HPV-16, a high-risk type associated with anal cancer. Nineteen percent of men attending sexually transmitted disease clinics in the United States have been found to be seropositive for HPV-16.[48] The most consistent risk factor for HPV acquisition is unprotected sexual activity and is directly related to the number of sexual partners a patient has had. In men, HPV most commonly presents as a painless, cauliflower-like anogenital wart (i.e., condyloma acuminatum) that grows over time. Although the diagnosis of HPV is most often made on a clinical basis, definitive diagnosis can be obtained via biopsy. There is currently no antiviral medication available for HPV eradication; however, ablative treatment is useful (see Table 11-12). HPV can be transmitted even when lesions are not present, and condom use does not guarantee protection because the virus is often transmitted through nonpenetrative sexual contact. Males who practice anal receptive intercourse should have yearly examinations for anal warts and, if lesions are present, a biopsy should be performed to evaluate for anal cancer. A vaccine against many serotypes of HPV (Gardasil) has shown success in various trials and was approved by the FDA in 2006, but it currently only has an indication in females aged 9–26 years.

Herpes Simplex Virus Types 1 and 2

Herpes simplex virus types 1 (HSV-1) and 2 (HSV-2) were linked to more than 200,000 genital infections in 2003, and it is estimated that more than 30 million persons in the United States currently have genital HSV. Although HSV-2 is responsible for most cases of genital infection, the prevalence of HSV-1 is rising, especially among women. The highest rates of HSV-2 seroprevalence in the United States have been reported among female prostitutes and homosexual males (83%).[57] Males are only one half as likely as females to be infected with both HSV-1 and HSV-2.[57] There is a wide spectrum of HSV genital disease, ranging from asymptomatic shedding to a painful genital ulcer with dysuria, painful inguinal adenopathy, and fever. In men, a vesicular penile ulcer with an erythematous base and dysuria are the most common presenting symptoms. Recurrent genital lesions are common, especially with HSV-2 (60%).[57] Nineteen days is the average duration of lesions seen in primary infection, and this decreases by up to 10 days with recurrences. Although transmission to sexual partners is higher with active lesions, 70% of transmissions are attributed to asymptomatic viral shedding. Transmission is greater with male versus female source patients (17% versus 4%). Diagnosis is usually suggested by a painful, shallow, genital ulcer, but viral culture, direct fluorescent antibody testing, and PCR can be used as confirmatory tests.[57] PCR is especially useful in the diagnosis of asymptomatic carriage. Serologies are most helpful for epidemiologic studies and are not useful acutely to diagnose infection. Various treatment options for HSV genital infection are outlined in Table 11-12.[48]

Conclusion

We have provided an evidence-based summary of several of the most important infections in men. A more exhaustive rendition of each infection can be found in the associated references. Education regarding minimizing communicable transmission of infectious diseases as well as early testing and treatment remain the standard in the movement toward minimizing morbidity and mortality.

References

1. Niederman MS, Mandell LA, Anzueto A, et al: Guidelines for the management of adults with community-acquired pneumonia: diagnosis, assessment of severity, antimicrobial therapy, and prevention, *Am J Respir Crit Care Med* 163:1730–1754, 2001.
2. File TM: Community-acquired pneumonia, *Lancet* 362:1991–2001, 2003.
3. Mason CM, Nelson S: Pulmonary host defenses and factors predisposing to lung infection, *Clin Chest Med* 26:11–17, 2005.
4. Laheij RJ, Sturkenboom MC, Hassing RJ, et al: Risk of community-acquired pneumonia and use of gastric-acid suppressive drugs, *JAMA* 292(16): 1955–1960, 2004.
5. Bartlett JG, Dowell SF, Mandell LA, et al: Practice guidelines for the management of community-acquired pneumonia in adults, *Clin Infect Dis* 31:347–382, 2000.
6. Mandell LA, Bartlett JG, Dowell SF, et al: Update of practice guidelines for the management of community-acquired pneumonia in immunocompetent adults, *Clin Infect Dis* 37(11):1405–1433, 2003.
7. Lauer J: Acute community-acquired sinusitis: a review of epidemiology and management, *Infect Med* 20:44–48, 2003.
8. Gwaltney JM: Acute community-acquired sinusitis, *Clin Infect Dis* 23:1209–1225, 1996.
9. Snow V, Mottur-Pilson C, Hickner JM: Principles of appropriate antibiotic use for acute sinusitis in adults, *Ann Intern Med* 134:495–497, 2001.
10. Hickner JM, Bartlett JG, Besser RE, et al: Principles of appropriate antibiotic use for acute rhinosinusitis in adults: background, *Ann Intern Med* 134(6): 498–505, 2001.
11. University of Michigan Health System: Guidelines for clinical care: acute rhinosinusitis. Available at: http://cme.med.umich.edu/pdf/guideline/rhino05.pdf. Accessed July 30, 2006.
12. Anon JB, Jacobs MP, Poole MD: Antimicrobial treatment guidelines for acute bacterial rhinosinusitis: executive summary of the Sinus and Allergy Health Partnership (SAHP), *Otolarygol Head Neck Surg* 130:1–45, 2004.
13. Sher LD, McDoo MA, Bettis RB, et al: A multicenter, randomized, investigator-blinded study of 5- and 10-day gatifloxacin versus 10 day amoxicillin/clavulanate in patients with acute bacterial sinusitis, *Clin Ther* 24:269–281, 2002.
14. Gwaltney JM: Sinusitis. In Mandell GL, Bennett JE, Dolan R, editors: *Mandell, Douglas, and Bennett's Principles and Practice of Infectious Diseases*, ed 5, Philadelphia, 2000, Churchill Livingstone, pp 676–686.
15. Daly KA, Giebink GS: Clinical epidemiology of otitis media, *Pediatr Infect Dis J* 19:S31–S36, 2000.
16. University of Michigan Health System: Guidelines for clinical care: otitis media. Available at: http://www.cme.med.umich.edu/pdf/guideline/om.pdf. Accessed July 30, 2006.

17. Lieberthal AS, Ganiats TG, Cox EO, et al: Diagnosis and management of acute otitis media, *Pediatrics* 113:1451–1466, 2004.

18. Sanders R: Otitis externa: a practical guide to treatment and prevention, *Am Fam Pract* 63:927–936, 2001.

19. Hughes E, Lee JH: Otitis externa, *Pediatr Rev* 22:191–198, 2001.

20. Harper SA, Fukuda K, Uyeki TM, et al: Prevention and control of influenza: recommendations of the Advisory Committee on Immunization Practices, *MMWR* 54:1–40, 2005.

21. World Health Organization: Cumulative number of confirmed human cases of avian influenza A/(H5N1) reported to WHO. Available at: http://www.who.int/csr/disease/avian_influenza/country/cases_table_2006_08_14/en/index.htmL.

22. Nicholson KG: Clinical features of influenza, *Semin Respir Infect* 7:26–37, 1992.

23. Ebell MH: Diagnosing and treating patients with suspected influenza, *Am Fam Physician* 72:1789–1792, 2005.

24. Nichol KL: Cost-benefit analysis of a strategy to vaccinate healthy working adults against influenza, *Arch Intern Med* 161:749–759, 2001.

25. Kaiser L, Wat C, Mills T, et al: Impact of oseltamivir treatment on influenza-related lower respiratory tract complications and hospitalizations, *Arch Intern Med* 163:1667–1672, 2003.

26. Centers for Disease Control and Prevention: Prevention of hepatitis A through active or passive immunization: recommendations of the Advisory Committee on Immunization Practices (ACIP), *MMWR* 48(RR-12):1–37, 1999.

27. Centers for Disease Control and Prevention: A comprehensive immunization strategy to eliminate transmission of hepatitis B virus infection in the United States: recommendations of the Advisory Committee on Immunization Practices (ACIP), *MMWR* 54(RR-16):1–35, 2005.

28. Centers for Disease Control and Prevention: Updated U.S. Public Health Service guidelines for the management of occupational exposures to HBV, HCV, and HIV and recommendations for postexposure prophylaxis, *MMWR* 50(No. RR-11):1–52, 2001.

29. Alter MJ, Margolis HS: Recommendations for prevention and control of hepatitis C virus (HCV) infection and HCV-related chronic disease, *MMWR Morb Mortal Wkly Rep* 47(RR–19):1–13, 15, 1998.

30. Murphy EL, Bryzman SM, Glynn SA, et al: Risk factors for hepatitis C virus infection in United States blood donors, *Hepatology* 31:756, 2000.

31. Liang TJ, Rehermann B, Seeff LB, Hoofnagle JH: Pathogenesis, natural history, treatment, and prevention of hepatitis C, *Ann Intern Med* 132:296, 2000.

32. Strader DB, Wright T, Thomas DL, Seeff LB, and the American Association for the Study of Liver Diseases: Diagnosis, management, and treatment of hepatitis C, *Hepatology* 39(4):1147–1171, 2004.

33. Joint United Nations Programme on HIV/AIDS (UNAIDS), World Health Organization (WHO) *AIDS Epidemic Update*, December 2005, pp 1–97.

34. Centers for Disease Control and Prevention. HIV/AIDS Surveillance Report, 2004 2005; 16:1–46. Also available at: http://www.cdc.gov/hiv/stats/hasrlink.htm.

35. Schacker T, Collier AC, Hughes J, et al: Clinical and epidemiologic features of primary HIV infection, *Ann Intern Med* 125:257–264, 1996.

36. Smith DE, Walker BD, Cooper DA, et al: Is antiretroviral treatment of primary HIV infection clinically justified on the basis of current evidence? *AIDS* 18:709–718, 2004.

37. Centers for Disease Control and Prevention: Revised guidelines for HIV counseling, testing, and referral, *MMWR* 50(RR-19):1–58, 2001.

38. Department of Health and Human Services (DHHS): Guidelines for the use of antiretroviral agents in HIV-1–infected adults and adolescents, April 7, 2005, Available at: http://www.aidsinfo.nih.gov/contentfiles/AdultandAdolescentGL.pdf.

39. Kovacs JA, Masur H: Prophylaxis against opportunistic infections in patients with human immunodeficiency virus infection, *N Engl J Med* 342:1416–1429, 2000.

40. Department of Health and Human Services (DHHS): Treating opportunistic infections among HIV-infected adults and adolescents, December 2004. Available at: http://www.aidsinfo.nih.gov/contentfiles/TreatmentofOI_AA.pdf.

41. Aberg JA, Gallant JE, Anderson J, et al: Primary care guidelines for the management of persons infected with human immunodeficiency virus: recommendation of the HIV Medicine Association of the Infectious Diseases Society of America, *Clin Infect Dis* 39:609–629, 2004.

42. Centers for Disease Control and Prevention, Health Resources and Service Administration, National Institutes of Health, HIB Medicine Association of the Infectious Diseases Society of America, and the HIV Prevention in Clinical Care Working Group: Recommendations for incorporating human immunodeficiency virus (HIV) prevention into the medical care of persons living with HIV, *Clin Infect Dis* 38:104–121, 2004.

43. Centers for Disease Control and Prevention: Antiretroviral postexposure prophylaxis after sexual, injection-drug use of other nonoccupational exposure to HIV in the United States: recommendations from the U.S. Department of Health and Human Services, *MMWR* 54(No. RR-2):1–19, 2005.

44. Centers for Disease Control and Prevention: Updated U.S. public health service guidelines for the management of occupational exposures to HBV, HCV, and HIV and recommendations for postexposure prophylaxis, *MMWR* 50(No. RR-11): 1–53, 2001.

45. Guerrant RL, Van Gilder T, Steiner TS, et al: Practice guidelines for the management of infectious diarrhea, *Clin Infect Dis* 32:331–351, 2001.

46. Guerrant RL, Shields DS, Thorson SM, et al: Evaluation and diagnosis of acute infectious diarrhea, *Am J Med* 78:91–98, 1985.
47. Mead PS, Slutsker L, Dietz V, et al: Food-related illness and death in the United States, *Emerg Infect Dis* 5:607–625, 1999.
48. Centers for Disease Control and Prevention: Sexually transmitted diseases treatment guidelines 2002, *MMWR Morb Mortal Wkly Rep* 51(No. RR-6): 1–78, 2002.
49. Centers for Disease Control and Prevention: Sexually transmitted diseases. Available at: http://www.cdc.gov/std.
50. Schwarcz SK, Kellog TA, McFarland W, et al: Characterization of sexually transmitted disease clinic patients with recent human immunodeficiency virus infection, *J Infect Dis* 186:1019–1022, 2002.
51. Sherrard J, Barlow D: Gonorrhoea in men: clinical and diagnostic aspects, *Genitourin Med* 72:422–426, 1996.
52. Handsfield HH, Sparling PF: *Neisseria gonorrhoeae*. In Mandell GL, Bennett JE, Dolin R, editors: *Principles and Practice of Infectious Diseases*, ed 6, New York, 2005, Churchill Livingstone, pp 2519–2526.
53. Burstein GR, Zenilman JM: Nongonococcal urethritis—a new paradigm, *Clin Infect Dis* 28(Suppl 1): S66–S73, 1999.
54. Hook EW III, Marra CM: Acquired syphilis in adults, *N Engl J Med* 326:1060–1067, 1992.
55. Mertz KJ, McQuillan GM, Levine WC, et al: A pilot study of the prevalence of chlamydial infection in a national household survey, *Sex Trans Dis* 25: 225–228, 1998.
56. Marrazzo JM, Handsfield HH: Chancroid: new developments in an old disease. In Remington JS, Swartz MN, editors: *Current Clinical Topics in Infectious Diseases*, Blackwell Science, 1995, Cambridge, MA, pp 129–140.
57. Whitley RJ, Kimberlin DW, Roizman B: Herpes simplex viruses, *Clin Infect Dis* 26:541–553, 1998.

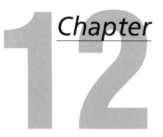

Chapter 12

Nephrology

Masahito Jimbo, MD, PhD, MPH

Key Points

- Current guidelines recommend annual urine microalbumin testing in diabetic patients for the early detection of diabetic nephropathy (strength of recommendation: A).
- Screening for albuminuria in patients with diabetes and for proteinuria in patients with hypertension and those aged 60 years and older is cost-effective (strength of recommendation: B).
- Serum creatinine and calculated creatinine clearance by means of the Cockcroft-Gault or MDRD equations, with an understanding of their limitations, can effectively assess renal function in most cases (strength of recommendation: C).
- Blood pressure and blood glucose control should be optimized in patients with chronic kidney disease (CKD) (strength of recommendation: A).
- Angiotensin-converting enzyme (ACE) inhibitors or angiotensin-receptor blockers (ARBs) should be considered in the treatment of patients with CKD, especially when patients also have diabetes mellitus (strength of recommendation: A).
- Daily aspirin should be recommended for patients with CKD who also have hypertension or diabetes or who smoke (strength of recommendation: A).
- Patients with CKD should be encouraged to stop smoking (strength of recommendation: A) and should be immunized for influenza and pneumococcus (strength of recommendation: B).
- Cholesterol control, hemoglobin concentration, and calcium/phosphate balance should be optimized in patients with CKD, particularly those whose disease is at

stage 3 or higher (strength of recommendation: C).
- To prevent renal deterioration in patients with CKD, nephrotoxic medications, malnutrition, and dehydration should be avoided, and treatment of infection should be promptly considered (strength of recommendation: C).

Introduction

It can be argued that the most important task for a primary care clinician in managing renal disease in men is to identify chronic kidney disease (CKD) early enough and to devise an appropriate follow-up and management strategy to minimize its progression to end-stage renal disease (ESRD). CKD is increasing in morbidity and mortality, particularly among men. Furthermore, primary care clinicians may not only be failing to find patients CKD early enough, but also may be unnecessarily delaying appropriate treatment, including referral to renal specialists.

This chapter will address the important issue of CKD and how it affects men, rather than attempting to cover the vast spectrum of renal, fluid, and electrolyte problems that one encounters in nephrology. First, the current epidemiology of renal disease and CKD in the United States will be discussed. Second, the similarities and differences between men and women regarding renal disease and CKD will be addressed. Third, the common symptoms and signs attributable to CKD (e.g., edema, proteinuria) will be described. Fourth, the common evaluative tools available to a primary care clinician (e.g., urinalysis, serum creatinine) will be reviewed. Finally, the management of CKD, including the timing of referral from the primary care provider to the nephrologist, will be summarized.

To avoid confusion regarding terminology, the definition of CKD and ESRD will be clearly stated here. As defined by the National Kidney Foundation (NKF) Kidney Disease Outcomes Quality Initiative (K/DOQI), *chronic kidney disease* is manifested by either or both of the following for at least 3 months:

- Kidney damage, ascertained by markers of kidney damage including persistent proteinuria, abnormalities in urine sediment, abnormalities in blood and urine chemistry measurements, abnormal findings in imaging studies, and abnormalities in renal histology
- Glomerular filtration rate (GFR) of less than 60 mL/min/1.73 m^2, which represents a loss of half or more of the adult level of normal kidney function, typically GFR of 120–130 mL/min/1.73 m^2

CKD is classified in stages from 1 to 5 depending on the GFR, as illustrated in Table 12-1.[1]

End-stage renal disease is defined by the US Renal Data System as advanced CKD requiring renal replacement therapy (RRT) such as dialysis and renal transplant.[2] Although 98% of patients with stage 5 CKD will begin dialysis, ESRD is not synonymous with stage 5 CKD.[3] For instance, patients who have received renal transplant with resultant improvement in GFR are no longer classified as having stage 5 CKD, but continue to be classified as ESRD. These definitions for CKD and ESRD will be used throughout the chapter.

Epidemiology of Renal Disease

The incidence and prevalence of CKD and other renal diseases are clearly on the rise. Current prevalence of CKD in the United States is estimated to be nearly 20 million, or 11% of the adult population. The great majority of adult Americans with CKD have mild to moderate disease, with 5,900,000 (3.3%), 5,300,000 (3.0%), and 7,600,000 (4.3%) in stages 1, 2, and 3, respectively. The number of adult Americans with more advanced CKD is much smaller, with those in stage 4 and 5 being 400,000 (0.2%) and 300,000 (0.1%), respectively.[1]

The incidence of ESRD jumped from 198 new cases per million in 1991 to 338 per million in 2003. The prevalence of ESRD during the same time increased from 209,000 to 453,000.[2] (Note that this approximates the sum of the number of adult Americans with stage 5 CKD and renal transplant recipients, which total almost 130,000. The prevalence of ESRD includes children, in contrast to just the adults in CKD, so the total number for the prevalence of ESRD is higher.) The cost of RRT, which is covered by Medicare, was $23 billion in 2001. Hemodialysis costs per person currently average approximately $63,000 per year.[2] Diabetes is the most common cause of ESRD, followed by hypertension; additional etiologies of ESRD are listed in Table 12-2.[2]

Mortality rates due to ESRD are also increasing. Kidney diseases (e.g., nephritis, nephrotic syndrome, and nephrosis), which were the twelfth leading cause of death in 1991, rose to the ninth leading cause in 2003.[4] Since 50% of patients with ESRD die from cardiovascular disease, with mortality 3–100 times the rate of the general population, it is likely that the above figure underestimates the actual impact of renal disease on overall mortality.[2,5] Indeed, CKD with a GFR of less than 60 mL/min/1.73 m^2 is now

Table 12-1. Staging of Chronic Kidney Disease

Stage	Definition	GFR (mL/min per BSA 1.73m^2)
1	Kidney damage with normal or increased GFR	90 or greater
2	Mildly decreased GFR	60–89
3	Moderately decreased GFR	30–59
4	Severely decreased GFR	15–29
5	Kidney failure	Less than 15 (or dialysis)

GFR, Glomerular filtration rate; BSA, body surface area.

Adapted from: Levey AS, Coresh J, Balk E, et al: National Kidney Foundation practice guidelines for chronic kidney disease: evaluation, classification, and stratification, *Ann Intern Med* 139:137–147, 2003.

Table 12-2. Etiologies of End-Stage Renal Disease

Disease	Percentage (%)
Diabetes mellitus	44.8
Hypertension	27.1
Primary glomerulopathy (e.g., IgA nephropathy)	8.5
Interstitial nephropathy (e.g., analgesic abuse)	3.6
Hereditary/cystic disease (e.g., polycystic kidney disease)	3.2
Secondary glomerulopathy (e.g., lupus nephritis, hepatitis C)	2.2

IgA, Immunoglobulin A.

Adapted from: United States Renal Data System: *USRDS 2005 annual data report: atlas of end-stage renal disease in the United States*, Bethesda, MD, 2005, National Institutes of Health, National Institute of Diabetes and Digestive and Kidney Diseases.

considered to be an independent risk factor for cardiovascular disease.[6] Survival in patients who experience ESRD while receiving dialysis remains dismal. The expected remaining lifetimes of persons aged 30–34, 50–54, and 70–74 years on dialysis are 10.5, 5.9, and 3.1 years, respectively, compared with age-comparable general population at 46.8, 23.6, and 13.4 years, respectively.[2]

Impact of Male Gender on Renal Disease

Renal Structure and Function

Most of the differences in renal structure and function between men and women arise from the larger size of men because, on average, male kidneys are larger than female kidneys. Male kidneys contain approximately the same number of glomeruli as female kidneys, but male kidneys have larger glomeruli and thus have greater total glomerular volume. These differences are all attributable to the larger body surface area of men compared with women, and gender is not an independent determinant.[7] Men have slightly higher GFR than women: young men have an average GFR of 130 mL/min/1.73 m^2 compared with an average 120 mL/min/1.73m^2 in women.[8] However, when healthy kidney donors were evaluated with inulin and para-amino hippurate, the gold standards for determination of GFR, there was no difference between men and women.[9]

Renal Diseases

The size advantage of men does not translate to advantages in the incidence, prevalence, and progression of renal disease. In the Third National Health and Nutrition Examination Survey, the prevalence of an elevated serum creatinine concentration was greater in adult men (3.3%) than in women (2.7%).[10] The prevalence of kidney disease, defined as GFR less than 60 mL/min/1.73 m^2 and persistent proteinuria, showed no difference by gender when age adjustment was made.[11]

More men than women develop ESRD each year. In 2003, 55,584 men (54.2% of total) and 46,955 women (45.8% of total) initiated RRT for ESRD.[2] The prevalence of ESRD is higher for men than for women (1670 per million versus 1163 per million), adjusted for age, race, and ethnicity.[12] The rate of progression of CKD is more rapid in men than women, requiring RRT at a rate 59% higher than women.[13] This difference is evident across a spectrum of renal diseases, including polycystic kidney disease, immunoglobulin A (IgA) nephropathy, membranous nephropathy, and hypertensive renal disease.[2,12,14] In contrast, the incidence of ESRD is higher in women with vasculitis, lupus nephritis, and scleroderma, and data are conflicting regarding rates of ESRD in men and women for diabetic nephropathy.[2]

The impact of gender on renal disease progression may reflect differences in environmental, socioeconomic, genetic, and hormonal factors. Estrogen may protect against the progression of renal disease by decreasing the accumulation of matrix proteins that cause glomerulosclerosis, increasing nitric oxide synthesis, and decreasing renin-angiotensin system activity. Conversely, testosterone may increase renin-angiotensin system and endothelin activity, both implicated in renal damage and disease progression.[12]

Mortality

Because of the higher prevalence of ESRD among men, more men with ESRD die in any given year than women. For example, in 2003, 41,570 men (53% of total) with ESRD died compared with 36,912 women (47% of total).[2] However, when these figures are adjusted, there was no mortality difference between genders.[2,13]

Common Symptoms and Signs Attributable to Chronic Kidney Disease and Other Renal Diseases

One of the challenges in diagnosing renal disease, particularly CKD, is the subtle and insidious nature of the symptoms. Many of the uremic symptoms do not appear until the GFR falls below 15 mL/min, by which time the patient will require urgent RRT. Thus, it would be important for the clinician to look for symptoms of renal disease before ESRD develops, such as edema and hypertension. Urinary abnormalities including proteinuria and hematuria provide the earliest signs of renal disease, and efficient follow-up of these abnormalities is crucial in the early identification of renal disease.

Uremic Symptoms

Uremia is a multisystem abnormality, particularly involving fluid, electrolytes, and hormonal imbalance, due to the accumulation of toxins not adequately removed by the failing kidney.

Uremic symptoms are varied and are relatively nonspecific, reflecting the multiple organs and systems affected by advanced renal disease. General symptoms such as fatigue and weakness may arise from renal anemia due to lack of erythropoietin and metabolic acidosis.[15,16] Cardiovascular symptoms including dyspnea, edema, and pericarditis may occur due to a combination of fluid retention from anemia and decreased GFR; myocardial depression from metabolic acidosis and other uremic toxins; and myocardial ischemia from accelerated atherosclerosis due to abnormal lipid metabolism and increased vasoconstrictors.[17] Gastrointestinal symptoms such as anorexia, nausea, and vomiting may be caused by metabolic acidosis, other uremic toxins, and autonomic neuropathy.[16,18] Neuropathy may also involve sensorimotor neurons through the accumulation of uremic toxins and ischemia of vasa nervosum, causing numbness and restless legs syndrome.[18] Renal osteodystrophy, which is caused by secondary hyperparathyroidism and hypovitaminosis D, results in osteomalacia and osteitis fibrosa.[19] Secondary hyperparathyroidism can also cause chronic, recalcitrant itching of the skin.[16]

Edema

Edema may occur relatively early in the course of renal disease, particularly in patients with nephrotic syndrome, which is manifested by significant proteinuria and hypoalbuminemia. However, the differential diagnosis is not confined to renal disease and includes heart failure, cirrhosis, and other causes of hypoalbuminemia such as malabsorption syndrome. The degree of edema in renal disease generally correlates with GFR (i.e., the lower the GFR, the greater the fluid retention and, thus, edema) and hypoalbuminemia (i.e., the lower the plasma albumin, the greater in the shift of fluid from intravascular to extravascular space and, thus, edema). Because of its association with fluid retention, intravascular volume tends to be greater in patients with decreased GFR; thus, in patients who have nephrotic syndrome but relatively normal renal function and GFR, the intravascular volume may actually be decreased.[20] This phenomenon will have implications in the management of edema in these patients, since overdiuresis may lead to further intravascular volume loss, hypotension, and renal ischemia. The edema from nephrotic syndrome and other renal diseases has been traditionally thought to occur periorbitally and peripherally (e.g., pretibial), although empiric evidence to support this is lacking in the literature.[21]

Hypertension

Between 90% and 95% of patients who present with chronically elevated blood pressure (BP) have essential hypertension. Since hypertension is second only to diabetes as the most common cause of CKD, most patients who present with hypertension and renal disease have the former preceding the latter. However, of the patients with secondary hypertension, renal disease is the most common etiology. Thus, any BP elevation, once confirmed, should entail an evaluation for renal disease, which is most commonly performed by urinalysis, serum creatinine measurement, and calculation of GFR, which will be discussed later in this chapter.[22]

Proteinuria

The normally excreted urinary protein contains approximately 20% low-molecular-weight protein of about 20,000 Daltons (e.g., immunoglobulins), 40% high-molecular-weight albumin of about 65,000 Daltons, and 40% Tamm-Horsfall protein, which is secreted by the distant tubule. Proteins smaller than 20,000 Daltons pass easily across the glomerular capillary wall but are then reabsorbed in the proximal renal tubule. *Proteinuria* is defined as urinary protein excretion of greater than 150 mg/day (10–20 mg/dL).[23] It is arguably the most important sign of renal disease and begins early in the course of the disease. Its degree and duration correlate with renal damage. Thus, the greater the magnitude and longer the duration of proteinuria, the greater the renal damage. Furthermore, the greater the magnitude of proteinuria, the greater the rate of renal disease progression. This correlation is accelerated in the presence of hypertension. These observations, combined with the studies that show reductions in proteinuria in patients administered angiotensin-converting enzyme (ACE) inhibitors leading to a delay in renal disease progression, suggest that proteinuria itself is a cause of progressive renal damage.[24,25]

Despite the increasing incidence and prevalence of CKD, no organization currently advocates screening of the general population for proteinuria as a marker of CKD.[26] The NKF, which is currently making a concerted effort to educate the general public and physicians about CKD, also does not advocate general screening. However, it recommends that all persons should be assessed as part of routine health maintenance examination to determine whether they are at increased risk for developing CKD.[1] A recent cost-effectiveness analysis concluded that annual urine dipstick testing for proteinuria in patients with diabetes or hypertension and those with neither disease but aged 60 years and older was cost-effective.[27] Age is an independent risk factor for CKD: after peaking at 120–130 mL/min/1.73 m^2 at age 30 years, the GFR declines by 1 mL/min/1.73 m^2 per year. Seventeen percent of persons older than 60 years have a GFR below 60 mL/min/1.73 m^2.[28] In persons with diabetes, screening for microalbuminuria has been shown to be more sensitive and thus is recommended annually.[24]

The urine dipstick is the most common tool used to detect proteinuria. The color indicator is tetrabromophenol blue in a citric acid buffer, which changes color in the presence of negatively charged urinary proteins.[29] The change in color from yellow (negative) to darker shades of green, and finally blue (4+), correlates with the degree of proteinuria, as shown in Table 12-3. A result of 1+ or greater is considered abnormal. For detection of significant proteinuria of 3+ or greater, the sensitivity and specificity are 96% and 87%, respectively.[23] False-positive and false-negative results can occur, which are summarized in Table 12-4.[29]

Transient proteinuria may occur when a temporary change in glomerular hemodynamics causes the protein excess. These conditions include dehydration, stress, exercise, fever, and prolonged standing.[23] Thus, when proteinuria is detected, one or two samples of first-void, morning urine should be checked over the next 1–3 months to confirm persistent proteinuria.[25,30] This may be performed via repeat urine dipstick, but a more accurate method would be to assess the total urine protein-creatinine ratio. Values above 200 mg/g are considered to be abnormal. The ratio of total protein to creatinine in an untimed

Table 12-4. Causes of False-Positive and False-Negative Results in Urine Dipstick Test for Proteinuria

False-Positive	False-Negative
Specific gravity 1.030 or greater	Specific gravity less than 1.015
Urine pH 8 or greater	Light chains (e.g., Bence-Jones protein)
Prolonged immersion of dipstick in urine	
Blood, pus, semen, vaginal secretions	
Radiocontrast agents	
Drugs (e.g., penicillin, sulfonamides, tolbutamide)	

Adapted from: Ahmed Z, Lee J: Asymptomatic urinary abnormalities, *Med Clin North Am* 81:641–652, 1997.

(spot) urine specimen has replaced the timed (overnight or 24-hour) urine collection as the preferred method for measuring proteinuria.[1,31]

Once persistent proteinuria is confirmed, an effort should be made to quantify the degree of proteinuria and to determine whether it is overflow, glomerular, or tubular in nature. Overflow proteinuria occurs when increased production of low-molecular-weight proteins (e.g., light chains) that freely pass through the glomeruli overwhelm the ability of the proximal tubules to reabsorb them. Examples of this include multiple myeloma and amyloidosis. The diagnosis of overflow proteinuria is typically made by documenting the pathologically increased protein in the serum. Glomerular proteinuria occurs when the glomerular capillary permeability to protein is increased; this is the most common cause of pathologic proteinuria and may result in large protein losses. Typically, urinary protein excretion of more than 2 g per 24 hours is glomerular, and nephritic-range proteinuria (3.5 g per 24 hours or greater) is almost always glomerular in origin. Examples include the primary glomerulopathies including minimal change disease and IgA nephropathy; secondary glomerulopathies such as diabetes, lupus, and human immunodeficiency virus infection; and drugs including heroin, nonsteroidal anti-inflammatory drugs (NSAIDs), gold, penicillamine, lithium, and heavy metals. Tubular proteinuria occurs when tubulointerstitial disease prevents the proximal tubule from reabsorbing low-molecular-weight proteins that were freely filtered through the glomeruli. Examples include hypertensive nephrosclerosis, analgesics, sickle cell disease, and uric acid

Table 12-3. Correlation of Urine Dipstick with Proteinuria

Urine Dipstick	Urine Protein Concentration (mg/dL)
Negative	Less than 5–10 mg/dL
Trace	10–20 mg/dL
1+	30 mg/dL
2+	100 mg/dL
3+	300 mg/dL
4+	1000 mg/dL

Adapted from: Carroll MF, Temte JL: Proteinuria in adults: a diagnostic approach, *Am Fam Physician* 62:1333–1340, 2000.

nephropathy.[30] Figure 12-1 illustrates these three mechanisms.

Since albumin, at 55,000 Daltons, is larger than the low-molecular-weight proteins (<20,000 Daltons) that freely pass through the glomeruli, its excretion into urine is not increased unless a glomerular disease causes an increase in glomerular capillary permeability. Thus, albuminuria is a more sensitive marker of glomerular disease, such as diabetic nephropathy.[25] Indeed, current guidelines recommend annual urine microalbumin testing in diabetic patients for the early detection of diabetic nephropathy.[32] This is usually performed by measuring the urine microalbumin-creatinine ratio in a spot urine sample. *Microalbuminuria* is defined as a urine microalbumin-creatinine ratio ranging from 30 to 299 mg/g. The term *microalbuminuria* is used to describe urine albumin excretion that is indicative of glomerular disease but not detected by the typical urine dipstick test for proteinuria. Once the ratio gets to or above 300 mg/g, the urine dipstick will detect albumin, and thus, it is termed *overt albuminuria*. Untreated patients with overt albuminuria may see a decline in GFR of 1 mL/min/month or 10–12 mL/min/year.[24]

Hematuria

Hematuria is a less reliable indicator of renal disease, since the source of bleeding may be in the extrarenal urinary tract, such as the pelvis, ureter, bladder, or urethra. Extrarenal sites are responsible for more than 60% of the causes of hematuria.[29] Approximately 5% of patients with microscopic hematuria may have a urinary tract malignancy, commonly of the bladder and prostate.[33] Even when excluding prostate cancer, urinary tract malignancies are more common in men, with an incidence twice that of women.[34] In particular, gross hematuria, which may occur with as little as 1 mL of blood in 1 liter of urine, is associated with urinary tract malignancy in up to 20% of patients, and a full urologic workup with cystoscopy and upper urinary tract imaging is indicated.[23]

The definition of *microscopic hematuria* varies from 1 to more than 10 red blood cells (RBCs) per high-power field (×400 magnification). Thus, making a clear-cut recommendation in its evaluation based on past studies is difficult.[33] Here, the definition by the American Urological Association is used: the presence of three or more RBCs per high-power field in two of three urine samples.[35] Its prevalence in the general population ranges from 0.18% to 16.1%, with two of six studies showing lower prevalence among men.[33] Currently, routine screening for microscopic hematuria is not advocated by any organizations.[26] Transient microscopic hematuria may occur in as many as 39% of men, depending on the study population,[36] and may be caused by vigorous exercise, sexual intercourse, and mild trauma.[33]

Typically, the urine dipstick test for blood initially identifies patients with microscopic hematuria. It detects the peroxidase activity of RBCs; thus, hemoglobin and myoglobin may elicit a false-positive response. Other causes of false-positive and false-negative results are listed in Table 12-5.[29]

The sensitivity and specificity of urine dipstick test for blood vary from 91% to 100% and from 65% to 99%, respectively.[23] Due to its high

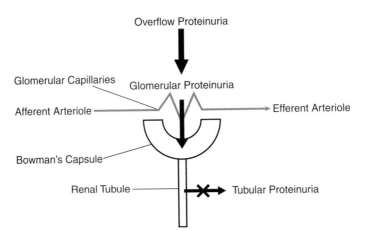

Figure 12-1. Mechanism of proteinuria. (Adapted from: Carroll MF, Temte JL: Proteinuria in adults: a diagnostic approach, *Am Fam Physician* 62:1333–1340, 2000.)

Table 12-5. Causes of False-Positive and False-Negative Results in Urine Dipstick Test for Blood

False-Positive	False-Negative
Dehydration	Vitamin C
Exercise	Air exposure
Hemoglobinuria	
Myoglobinuria	
Povidone-iodine	
Oxidizing agents	

Adapted from: Ahmed Z, Lee J: Asymptomatic urinary abnormalities, *Med Clin North Am* 81:641–652, 1997.

sensitivity, urine dipstick test is generally sufficient to rule out hematuria. However, to confirm the presence of RBCs in persons who test positive for blood, it is crucial to look at the urine microscopically. This would not only confirm hematuria but also may differentiate glomerular from nonglomerular sources of bleeding by the morphology of the RBCs. In glomerular hematuria, the RBCs, as they travel through the renal tubules, are exposed to large changes in pH and osmotic pressure.[37] Thus, they are dysmorphic, with various shapes and sizes, in contrast to nonglomerular hematuria, in which RBCs are homogeneous and normal in shape. Accompaniment of proteinuria greater than 2+ by dipstick also suggests glomerular hematuria, since hematuria alone would never result in such a large protein excretion.[23] Blood clots do not occur in glomerular hematuria because of the presence of urokinase and tissue-type plasminogen activators in glomerular filtrate.[29] RBC casts are virtually pathognomonic for glomerular hematuria, since the matrix of the cast is Tamm-Horsfall protein, which is secreted by the distal tubule; thus, bleeding would have to be proximal to the renal tubule for the cast to be created, for example, at the glomerular level (Figure 12-2). The differences between glomerular and nonglomerular hematuria are summarized in Table 12-6.

The most common cause of isolated glomerular hematuria (without significant proteinuria) is IgA nephropathy, followed in descending order by thin basement membrane disease, hereditary nephritis (Alport's syndrome), and mild focal glomerulonephritis of other causes. More common renal causes of nonglomerular hematuria include nephrolithiasis, pyelonephritis, polycystic kidney disease, and renal cell carcinoma. The most common extrarenal causes of nonglomerular hematuria are infections such as cystitis, prostatitis, and urethritis, followed by prostate and bladder cancers.[33]

Common Evaluative Tools in Ambulatory Care

Urinalysis

Urinalysis is a simple yet efficient tool to diagnose renal disease. Its role in the evaluation of

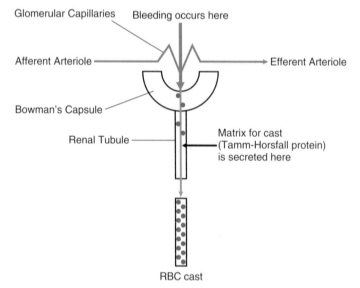

Figure 12-2. Mechanism of red blood cell (RBC) cast formation. (Adapted from: Silkensen JR, Kasiske BL: Laboratory assessment of kidney disease: clearance, urinalysis, and kidney biopsy. In Brenner BM, editor: *Brenner and Rector's The Kidney*, ed 7, Philadelphia, 2004, Saunders, pp 1107–1150.)

Table 12-6. Characteristics of Glomerular and Nonglomerular Hematuria

Glomerular	Nonglomerular
Dysmorphic RBCs	Normal RBCs
RBC casts	Blood clots
Proteinuria 2+ or greater	
Brown, "coca-cola" urine	

RBC, Red blood cell.
    Adapted from Simerville JA, Phira JJ: Urinalysis: a comprehensive review, *Am Fam Physician* 71:1153–1162, 2005; Ahmed Z, Lee J: Asymptomatic urinary abnormalities, *Med Clin North Am* 81:641–652, 1997; Silkensen JR, Kasiske BL: Laboratory assessment of kidney disease: clearance, urinalysis, and kidney biopsy. In Brenner BM, editor: *Brenner and Rector's The Kidney*, ed 7, Philadelphia, 2004, Saunders, pp 1107–1150.

proteinuria and hematuria has been discussed in the previous section. A midstream clean-catch technique is adequate in men.[23] When performing urine microscopy, proper care should be exercised in preparing the sample. A fresh sample of 10–15 mL of urine should be centrifuged at 1500–3000 rpm for 5 minutes. The supernatant is then decanted and the sediment agitated in the remaining supernatant. A single drop is applied to a clean glass slide, and a cover slip is applied.[23,38]

Serum Creatinine and Calculation of Glomerular Filtration Rate

GFR is the most reliable estimate of renal function and is the foundation of the CKD definition and staging by the NKF-K/DOQI.[8] GFR cannot be measured directly and is estimated from the urinary clearance of a filtration marker. *Clearance* is defined as the rate at which it is cleared from the plasma by excretion in the urine (Table 12-7). When an ideal filtrate is used, characteristics of which are described in Table 12-8, the clearance of the filtrate (C_F) approximates GFR.[8,31] Inulin, a 5200-Dalton uncharged polymer of fructose, meets the characteristics of an ideal filtrate and is thus the gold standard filtration marker, yet it is not readily available and is difficult to assay. Other exogenous filtration markers have been tried, but all of them require a complicated measurement protocol.[8]

Table 12-7. Calculation of Clearance of a Filtrate

$$C_F = \frac{U_F \times V}{P_F}$$

C_F, Clearance of the filtrate; U_F, urinary concentration of the filtrate; V, urine flow rate; P_F, average plasma concentration of the filtrate.
    Adapted from: Stevens LA, Levey AS: Measurement of kidney function, *Med Clin North Am* 89:457–473, 2005.

Table 12-8. Characteristics of an Ideal Filtration Marker

Freely filtered by the glomerulus
Not secreted, reabsorbed, synthesized, or metabolized by the renal tubule
Inert
No effect on the renal function

Adapted from: Stevens LA, Levey AS: Measurement of kidney function, *Med Clin North Am* 89:457–473, 2005.

Of the endogenous filtration markers, serum creatinine is currently use most often. Creatinine is an amino acid derivative with a molecular mass of 113 Daltons that is freely filtered by the glomerulus. It has all the characteristics of an ideal filtrate, except that it is actively secreted in the renal tubule, which proportionately increases as renal function declines.[8] Thus, its clearance overestimates GFR, particularly as the renal dysfunction progresses. Also, serum creatinine is affected by factors such as age, sex, and lean body mass, with greater levels at similar GFR seen in those who are younger, male, and more muscular.

Equations that estimate GFR from serum creatinine at least partially overcome the inaccuracy of creatinine clearance and the inconvenience of collecting urine over 24 hours. The two most often used equations are the Cockcroft-Gault equation and the Modification of Diet in Renal Disease Study Group (MDRD) equation (Table 12-9).[39,40]

The MDRD equation has slightly greater advantage in that it is adjusted for body size and accounts for race. However, whereas the Cockcroft-Gault equation overestimates GFR, the MDRD equation underestimates GFR, particularly in healthy subjects.[41] Also, both equations are less accurate in extremes of ages, body size,

Table 12-9. Formulas for Calculating GFR from Creatinine

Cockcroft-Gault equation
$$\text{GFR (mL/min)} = \frac{[140 - \text{Age (years)}] \times \text{Weight (kg)}}{72 \times \text{serum creatinine (mg/dL)}} \times 0.85 \text{ (if female)}$$
MDRD study equation
$$\text{GFR (mL/min/1.73m}^2) = 186 \times \text{creatinine}^{-1.154} \times \text{Age}^{-0.203} \times 0.742 \text{ (if female)} \times 1.212 \text{ (if African American)}$$

GFR, Glomerular filtration rate; MDRD, Modification of Diet in Renal Disease Study Group.
    Adapted from Cockcroft D, Gault M: Prediction of creatinine clearance from serum creatinine, *Nephron* 16:31–41, 1976; Levey A, Bosch J, Lewis J, et al: A more accurate method to estimate glomerular filtration rate from serum creatinine: a new prediction equation, *Ann Intern Med* 130:461–470, 1999.

and lean body mass, and in pregnancy, where a 24-hour urine collection to estimate creatinine clearance may be preferable.[8] In most situations, however, either equation would suffice, and a 24-hour urine collection to estimate clearance is no longer recommended.[1] The NKF has a link on its Web site where the GFR can be quickly calculated using either equation: http://www.kidney.org/professionals/kdoqi/gfr_calculator.cfm.

Recently, cystatin C, a nonglycosylated basic protein of 13,000 Daltons, has received increasing attention as a potential endogenous filtration marker to replace creatinine. Its generation appears to have less individual variability than creatinine, and studies have shown a better correlation between cystatin C and myocardial infarction, heart failure, stroke, and death than creatinine.[42,43] However, there are still unresolved issues before it can be unequivocally considered as a superior alternative to creatinine and creatinine-derived equations in the measurement of renal function.[44,45]

Imaging Studies

Numerous radiographic methods are available for both anatomic and functional assessment of the kidneys and urinary tract.[46] For the evaluation of renal disease, ultrasound offers an accurate, noninvasive approach to rule out obstructive uropathy, determine renal size and cortical thickness, and look for presence of masses and cysts. It is the first choice among the imaging studies to evaluate a patient with deterioration in renal function.[47] Computed tomography of the kidneys and urinary tract is superior to ultrasound in detecting stones in patients who present with hematuria.[33] Because of these and other rapidly developing technologies including radionuclide and magnetic resonance imaging, intravenous urography is used less often in the evaluation of renal diseases.

Management of Chronic Kidney Disease

In the previous sections, definition, epidemiology, symptoms and signs, and evaluative tools for CKD have been discussed. In this section, management issues of CKD will be reviewed. Key issues in the management of CKD are to diagnose and treat underlying conditions, slow the progression of renal deterioration, reduce cardiovascular disease risk, and manage complications of renal disease. It is particularly important to diagnose and manage CKD at its early stages, for two reasons. First, CKD that is at stage 3 or worse is an independent risk factor for cardiovascular disease.[43] Second, once CKD progresses to stage 4 or 5, significant complications are increased.[45]

Treatment of Underlying Conditions

Strict control of serum blood glucose levels (hemoglobin A_{1c} < 7%) in both type 1 and type 2 diabetes mellitus reduces the development of diabetic nephropathy and its progression.[48–50] Diligent BP control (BP < 130/80 mm Hg; BP < 120/75 mm Hg in overt albuminuria) reduces renal disease progression and cardiovascular morbidity and mortality.[22] Once CKD progresses to stage 4 or worse, loop diuretics to control volume-dependent hypertension are usually required.

Of the antihypertensive agents, ACE inhibitors and angiotensin-receptor blockers (ARBs) are particularly effective in slowing disease progression in both diabetic and nondiabetic CKD.[22,51] The mechanism is multifactorial, including the effect on renal hemodynamics, local growth factors, and glomerular permselectivity.[51] Angiotensin causes greater vasoconstriction of efferent arterioles than afferent arterioles, leading to increases in intraglomerular pressure.[52] This subsequently leads to hyperfiltration, which when prolonged leads to glomerular structural changes and functional deterioration. By reversing this process, renal disease progression is delayed. However, although the reduction of intraglomerular pressure has long-term benefit, it may cause a small rise in serum creatinine levels in the short term, since GFR is directly correlated to intraglomerular pressure. A rise of up to 35% above the baseline is acceptable and not a reason to withhold treatment unless hyperkalemia develops.[53] In conditions such as bilateral renal artery stenosis, in which angiotensin serves the critical role of preserving the intraglomerular pressure and GFR, its blockade could lead to acute renal failure. Figure 12-3 illustrates the mechanism of angiotensin inhibition.

Delaying of Renal Deterioration

In addition to ACE inhibitors and ARBs, statins may decrease proteinuria and preserve GFR in patients with CKD, an effect that may be separate from blood cholesterol reduction.[54] Smoking is an independent risk factor for the development of ESRD in men with CKD and should be strongly

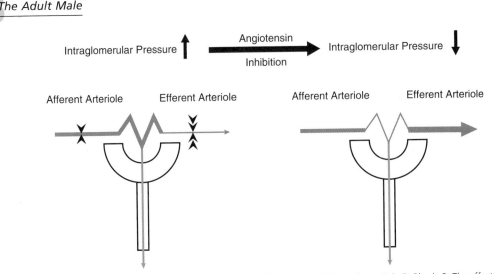

Figure 12-3. Mechanism of angiotensin inhibition. (Adapted from: Lewis E, Hunsicker L, Bain R, Rhode R: The effect of angiotensin converting enzyme inhibition on diabetic nephropathy, *N Engl J Med* 329:1456–1462, 1993; Navis G, de Jong PE, de Zeeuw D: specific pharmacologic approaches to clinical renoprotection. In Brenner BM, editor: *Brenner and Rector's The Kidney*, ed 7, Philadelphia, 2004, Saunders, pp 2453–2490.)

discouraged.[55] Indeed, smoking cessation may reduce the risk of renal disease progression by 30% in patients with type 2 diabetes.[56] The role of protein restriction in CKD remains controversial.[57]

Many commonly used drugs are nephrotoxic. They may exacerbate renal function by causing decreased renal perfusion (e.g., NSAIDs), tubular dysfunction (e.g., lithium, aminoglycosides, radiocontrast dye), interstitial nephropathy (e.g., penicillins, cephalosporins), or tubular obstruction (e.g., acyclovir).[58] Each drug the patient receives should always be scrutinized for this possibility, including over-the-counter medications.

Generally, patients with CKD do not experience fluid overload until they are at stage 4 or even stage 5. Rather, since patients with CKD may not be able to concentrate their urine as much as persons with healthy kidneys, dehydration becomes a concern. Dehydration may worsen renal ischemia by decreasing renal perfusion and should be avoided. Urinary tract infections should be promptly treated and potential exacerbating factors, such as benign prostate hypertrophy, addressed.

Decreasing Cardiovascular Risk

As stated in previous sections, CKD significantly increases the risk of cardiovascular disease. Smoking cessation should be strongly encouraged.[26] Men who smoke, have diabetes or hypertension, or are older than 40 years of age should be prescribed daily aspirin.[26] In addition, aggressive cholesterol management should be instituted.[26]

Addressing Complications

As stated previously, once CKD progresses to stage 3 or worse, metabolic and other complications commonly appear. The most common complications include anemia, renal osteodystrophy, and malnutrition. Primary care physicians can manage most of these complications. Hemoglobin levels should be kept at 11–12 g/dL. Serum ferritin should be obtained to assess iron deficiency; if it is below 100 ng/mL, iron supplementation should be given. When hemoglobin levels decrease below 10 g/dL, the administration of erythropoietin at the dose of 50–100 units/kg administered subcutaneously or intravenously three times a week should be initiated.[59] Calcitriol, a synthetic vitamin D analog, should be prescribed at 0.25–1 μg/day to suppress secondary hyperparathyroidism and the consequent renal dystrophy.[59] To avoid malnutrition, daily meals should contain protein at 0.8–1.0 g/kg/day and 30–35 calories per kg/day. Nutritional counseling with a dietitian knowledgeable in diets appropriate for patients with CKD should be arranged.[59] The Centers for Disease Control and Prevention recommend that patients with CKD receive influenza and pneumococcal vaccines.[60]

When to Refer

Once patients with CKD reach stage 4 or worse, a nephrologist should be consulted to co-manage the patient. Patients receiving comprehensive care by the nephrology team have shown slower renal disease progression, greater likelihood of starting dialysis with higher hemoglobin, better calcium control, a permanent access, and a greater likelihood of choosing peritoneal dialysis.[57] Unfortunately, 25% of patients initially see a nephrologist within a month of beginning dialysis, leading to greater mortality. African American men, patients without insurance, and patients with severe comorbid illnesses have been shown to be less likely to receive timely referral.[61] Even before the development of stage 4, patients with CKD may be referred for particularly difficult control of anemia, osteodystrophy, and malnutrition. Other indications include a possible indication for renal biopsy (e.g., persistent proteinuria 2+ or greater by urine dipstick, hematuria with persistent proteinuria, persistent isolated glomerular hematuria for greater than 1 year); an unclear underlying etiology; management of underlying cause (e.g., primary glomerulopathy); and rapid deterioration.[62]

Conclusion

Men have higher disease burden from CKD than women. Its early symptoms and signs are subtle. Because early initiation of treatment could slow the progression of renal disease and delay RRT, early detection is crucial. Simple office-based tests, such as urinalysis and serum creatinine measurements to calculate GFR, are adequate in most cases. Treatment in the early stages of CKD targets the underlying disease, slowing the progression of renal disease and lowering cardiovascular risk. Once CKD advances, careful monitoring for complications and prompt initiation of treatment is important. Early referral to a nephrologist for co-management increases the likelihood of successful management.

References

1. Levey AS, Coresh J, Balk E, et al: National Kidney Foundation practice guidelines for chronic kidney disease: evaluation, classification, and stratification, *Ann Intern Med* 139:137–147, 2003.
2. United States Renal Data System: *USRDS 2005 Annual Data Report: Atlas of End-Stage Renal Disease in the United States*, Bethesda, MD, 2005, National Institutes of Health, National Institute of Diabetes and Digestive and Kidney Diseases.
3. Obrador GT, Arora P, Kausz AT, et al: Level of renal function at the initiation of dialysis in the U.S.end-stage renal disease population, *Kidney Int* 56:2227–2235, 1999.
4. Hoyert DL, Heron MP, Murphy SL, Kung HS: Deaths: final data for 2003, *Natl Vital Stat Rep* 54:1–120, 2006.
5. Foley RN, Parfrey PS, Sarnak MJ: Clinical epidemiology of cardiovascular disease in chronic renal disease, *Am J Kidney Dis* 32:S112–S119, 1998.
6. Shlipak MG, Fried LF, Cushman M, et al: Cardiovascular mortality risk in chronic kidney disease, *JAMA* 293:1737–1745, 2005.
7. Neugarten J, Kasiske B, Silbiger SR: Effects of sex on renal structure, *Nephron* 90:139–144, 2002.
8. Stevens LA, Levey AS: Measurement of kidney function, *Med Clin North Am* 89:457–473, 2005.
9. Slack TK, Wilson DM: Normal renal function: CIN and CPAH in healthy donors before and after nephrectomy, *Mayo Clin Proc* 51:296–300, 1976.
10. Coresh J, Wei GL, McQuillan G, et al: Prevalence of high blood pressure and elevated serum creatinine level in the United states: findings from the Third National Health and Nutrition Examination Survey (1988–1994), *Arch Intern Med* 161:1207–1216, 2001.
11. Coresh J, Astor BC, Greene T, et al: Prevalence of chronic kidney disease and decreased kidney function in the adult US population: third national health and nutrition examination survey, *Am J Kidney Dis* 41:1–12, 2003.
12. Reyes D, Lew SQ, Kimmel PL: Gender differences in hypertension and kidney disease, *Med Clin North Am* 89:613–630, 2005.
13. Evans M, Fryzek JP, Elinder CG, et al: The natural history of chronic renal failure: results from an unselected, population-based, inception cohort in Sweden, *Am J Kidney Dis* 46:863–870, 2005.
14. Neugarten J, Acharyna A, Silbiger A: Effect of gender on the progression of nondiabetic renal disease: a meta-analysis, *J Am Soc Nephrol* 11:319–329, 2000.
15. Remuzzi G, Schieppati A, Minetti L: Hematologic consequences of renal failure. In Brenner BM, editor: *Brenner and Rector's The Kidney*, ed 7, Philadelphia, 2004, Saunders, pp 2165–2188.
16. Bailey JL, Mitch WE: Pathophysiology of uremia. In Brenner BM, editor: *Brenner and Rector's The Kidney*, ed 7, Philadelphia, 2004, Saunders, pp 2139–2164.
17. McMahon LP, Parfrey PS: Cardiovascular aspects of chronic kidney disease. In Brenner BM, editor: *Brenner and Rector's The Kidney*, ed 7, Philadelphia, 2004, Saunders, pp 2189–2226.
18. Arieff AI: Neurologic complications or renal insufficiency. In Brenner BM, editor: *Brenner and Rector's The Kidney*, ed 7, Philadelphia, 2004 Saunders, pp 2227–2254.
19. Martin KJ, Gonzalez EA, Slatopolsky E: Renal osteodystrophy. In Brenner BM, editor: *Brenner and Rector's The Kidney*, ed 7, Philadelphia, 2004 Saunders, pp 2255–2304.
20. Anderson S, Komers R, Brenner BM: Renal and systematic manifestations of glomerular disease. In Brenner BM, editor: *Brenner and Rector's The Kidney*, ed 7, Philadelphia, 2004 Saunders, pp 1927–1955.

21. Stigant C, Stevens L, Levin A: Nephrology: strategy for the care of adults with chronic kidney disease, *CMAJ* 168:1553–1560, 2003.
22. The Seventh Report of the Joint National Committee on Prevention, Detection, Evaluation, and Treatment of High Blood Pressure: the JNC 7 report, *JAMA* 289:2560–2572, 2003.
23. Simerville JA, Phira JJ: Urinalysis: a comprehensive review, *Am Fam Physician* 71:1153–1162, 2005.
24. Bennett PH, Haffner S, Kasiske BL, et al: Screening and management of microalbuminuria in patients with diabetes mellitus: recommendations to the Scientific Advisory Board of the National Kidney Foundation from an ad hoc committee of the Council on Diabetes Mellitus of the National Kidney Foundation, *Am J Kidney Dis* 25:107–112, 1995.
25. Keane WF, Eknoyan G: Proteinuria, albuminuria, risk, assessment, detection, elimination (PARADE): a position paper of the National Kidney Foundation, *Am J Kidney Dis* 33:1004–1010, 1999.
26. United States Preventive Services Task Force. Available at: http://www.ahrq.gov/clinic/uspstfix.htm.
27. Boulware LB, Jaar BG, Tarver-Carr ME, et al: Screening for proteinuria in US adults: a cost-effectiveness analysis, *JAMA* 290:3101–3114, 2003.
28. Epstein M: Aging and the kidney, *J Am Soc Nephrol* 7:1106–1122, 1996.
29. Ahmed Z, Lee J: Asymptomatic urinary abnormalities, *Med Clin North Am* 81:641–652, 1997.
30. Carroll MF, Temte JL: Proteinuria in adults: a diagnostic approach, *Am Fam Physician* 62:1333–1340, 2000.
31. Perrone RD: Means of clinical evaluation of renal disease progression, *Kidney Int* 41:S26–S32, 1992.
32. American Diabetes Association: Standards of medical care in diabetes—2006, *Diabetes Care* 29:S4–S42, 2006.
33. Cohen RA, Brown RS: Microscopic hematuria, *N Engl J Med* 348:2330–2338, 2003.
34. Jemal A, Siegel R, Ward E, et al: Cancer statistics, 2006, *CA Cancer J Clin* 56:106–130, 2006.
35. Grossfeld GD, Litwin MS, Wolf JS, et al: Evaluation of asymptomatic microscopic hematuria in adults: the American Urological Association best practice policy—part I: definition, detection, prevalence, and etiology, *Urology* 57:599–603, 2001.
36. Fromm P, Ribak J, Benbassat J: Significance of microhaematuria in young adults, *Br Med J* 288:20–22, 1984.
37. Silkensen JR, Kasiske BL: Laboratory assessment of kidney disease: clearance, urinalysis, and kidney biopsy. In Brenner BM, editor: *Brenner and Rector's The Kidney*, ed 7, Philadelphia, 2004, Saunders, pp 1107–1150.
38. Fogazzi GB, Garigali G: The clinical art and science of urine microscopy, *Curr Opin Nephrol Hypertens* 12:625–632, 2003.
39. Cockcroft D, Gault M: Prediction of creatinine clearance from serum creatinine, *Nephron* 16:31–41, 1976.
40. Levey A, Bosch J, Lewis J, et al: A more accurate method to estimate glomerular filtration rate from serum creatinine: a new prediction equation, *Ann Intern Med* 130:461–470, 1999.
41. Rule AD, Larson TS, Bergstralh EJ, et al: Using serum creatinine to estimate glomerular filtration rate: accuracy in good health and in chronic kidney disease, *Ann Intern Med* 141:929–937, 2004.
42. Sarnak MJ, Katz R, Stehman-Breen CO, et al: Cystatin C concentration as a risk factor for heart failure in older adults, *Ann Intern Med* 142:497–505, 2005.
43. Shlipak MG, Sarnak MJ, Katz R, et al: Cystatin C and the risk of death and cardiovascular events among elderly persons, *N Engl J Med* 352:2049–2060, 2005.
44. Levin A: Cystatin C, serum creatinine, and estimates of kidney function: searching for better measures of kidney function and cardiovascular risk, *Ann Intern Med* 142:586–588, 2005.
45. Stevens LA, Coresh J, Greene T, Levey AS: Assessing kidney function—measured and estimated glomerular filtration rate, *N Engl J Med* 354:2473–2483, 2006.
46. Kellert MJ: The genitourinary tract: methods of investigation. In *Grainger & Allison's Diagnostic Radiology: A Textbook of Medical Imaging*, ed 4, New York, 2001, Churchill Livingstone, pp 1489–1497.
47. Webb JAW, Maisey MN, Reidy JF: Renal failure and transplantation. In *Grainger & Allison's Diagnostic Radiology: A Textbook of Medical Imaging*, ed 4, New York, 2001, Churchill Livingstone, pp 1671–1692.
48. The Diabetes Control and Complications Trial (DCCT) Research Group: Effect of intensive therapy on the development and progression of nephropathy in the DCCT, *Kidney Int* 47:1703–1720, 1995.
49. UK Prospective Diabetes Study Group: Tight blood pressure control and risk of macrovascular and microvascular complications in type 2 diabetes, UKPDS 38, *Br Med J* 317:703–713, 1998.
50. Wang P, Lau J, Chalmers T: Meta-analysis of the effects of intensive blood-glucose control on late complications of type I diabetes, *Lancet* 341:1306–1309, 1993.
51. Lewis E, Hunsicker L, Bain R, Rhode R: The effect of angiotensin converting enzyme inhibition on diabetic nephropathy, *N Engl J Med* 329:1456–1462, 1993.
52. Navis G, de Jong PE, de Zeeuw D: specific pharmacologic approaches to clinical renoprotection. In Brenner BM, editor: *Brenner and Rector's The Kidney*, ed 7, Philadelphia, 2004, Saunders, pp 2453–2490.
53. Bakris GL, Weir MR: Angiotensin-converting enzyme inhibitor-associated elevations in serum creatinine, *Arch Intern Med* 160:685–693, 2000.
54. Fried LF, Orchard TJ, Kasiske BL: Effect of lipid reduction on the progression of renal disease: a meta-analysis, *Kidney Int* 59:260–269, 2001.
55. Orth S, Stockmann A, Conradt C, et al: Smoking as a risk factor for end-stage renal failure in men with primary renal disease, *Kidney Int* 54:926–931, 1998.
56. Ritz E, Ogata H, Orth SR: Smoking a factor promoting onset and progression of diabetic nephropathy, *Diabetes Metab* 26:S54–S63, 2000.

57. Parmar MS: Chronic renal disease, *Br Med J* 325:85–90, 2002.
58. Taber SS, Mueller BA: Drug-associated renal dysfunction, *Crit Care Clin* 22:357–374, 2006.
59. Snivley CS, Gutierrez C: Chronic kidney disease: prevention and treatment of common complications, *Am Fam Physician* 70:1921–1928, 2004.
60. Centers for Disease Control and Prevention: Recommended adult immunization schedule—United States, October 2005–September 2006, *MMWR* 54: Q1–Q4, 2005. Available at: http://www.cdc.gov/mmwr/PDF/wk/mm5440-Immunization.pdf.
61. Kinchen KS, Sadler J, Fink N, et al: The timing of specialist evaluation in chronic kidney disease and mortality, *Ann Intern Med* 137:479–486, 2002.
62. Snyder S, Pendergraph B: Detection and evaluation of chronic kidney disease, *Am Fam Physician* 72:1723–1732, 2005.

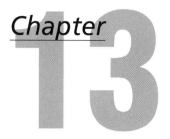

Chapter 13

Neurology

Raman Malhotra, MD, and Alon Y. Avidan, MD, MPH

Key Points

Stroke

- Intravenous recombinant tissue plasminogen activator (r-TPA), if given within 3 hours of stroke onset, and if specific inclusion and exclusion criteria are met, provides better neurologic outcome in patients (strength of recommendation: A).
- Use of intravenous fractionated or unfractionated heparin is not recommended for treatment of acute stroke (strength of recommendation: B).
- Aspirin (160–325 mg) is recommended for patients with acute stroke who are not given thrombolytics (strength of recommendation: A).
- If more than 70% stenosis of the carotid artery on the symptomatic side is found, carotid endarterectomy is recommended to reduce the risk of subsequent stroke (strength of recommendation: A).
- Aspirin (50–325 mg/day), aspirin and extended-release dipyridamole (Aggrenox) twice a day, or clopidogrel (Plavix; 75 mg/day) is recommended for secondary prevention of ischemic stroke (strength of recommendation: A).
- The use of clopidogrel (Plavix) and aspirin in combination for secondary prevention of stroke is not recommended since increased risk of life-threatening or major bleeding events has been shown without any benefit in reducing recurrent stroke (strength of recommendation: A).

Parkinson's Disease

- Levodopa/carbidopa and dopamine agonists are recommended for initial therapy to improve motor function and activities of daily living disability in patients with Parkinson's disease (strength of recommendation: B).

Alzheimer's Disease (AD)

- Donepezil, galantamine, and rivastigmine are recommended for the treatment of mild to moderate AD to stabilize or delay cognitive and behavioral problems associated with the disease (strength of recommendation: B).
- Memantine is recommended for patients with moderate to severe AD since it has been shown to help slow progression of the disease (strength of recommendation: B).
- Vitamin E (1000 IU twice a day) can be considered to help slow the progression of AD (strength of recommendation: C).

Obstructive Sleep Apnea (OSA)

- There is a strong correlation between sleep apnea and the development of cardiovascular heart disease, systemic and pulmonary hypertension, ischemic heart disease, myocardial infarction, cerebrovascular accidents, nocturnal cardiac arrhythmias, and congestive heart failure (strength of recommendation: B).
- Positive airway pressure improves nocturnal oxygenation and quality of sleep in patients with OSA (strength of recommendation: A).
- Oral appliances and surgical interventions have also shown effectiveness as treatments for OSA in patients who cannot tolerate positive airway treatment (strength of recommendation: B).

Restless Legs Syndrome (RLS)

- Dopamine agonists, such as ropinirole and pramipexole, have been shown to be effective in treating RLS (strength of recommendation: A).

- Opiates, benzodiazepines, and certain anticonvulsants (e.g., carbamazepine, gabapentin) can also be used as treatments for RLS (strength of recommendation: B).

Insomnia

- Cognitive-behavioral therapy can be effective in the treatment of chronic insomnia (strength of recommendation: B).
- Newer hypnotic agents (e.g., zaleplon, zolpidem, and eszopiclone) and a melatonin-receptor agonist (ramelteon) have been shown to improve symptoms of chronic insomnia and have an advantage over other hypnotics by having fewer adverse effects and a lower incidence of tolerance and rebound insomnia (strength of recommendation: B).

Circadian Rhythm Sleep Disorders

- Light therapy and melatonin have both been shown to be effective in treating circadian rhythm disorders such as jet lag and shift-work sleep disorder (strength of recommendation: B).
- Modafinil (Provigil) can also help with symptoms of shift-work sleep disorder and is FDA approved for use in this condition (strength of recommendation: B).

Introduction

Neurologic diseases are commonly encountered but frequently unrecognized in the outpatient and inpatient setting by primary care clinicians. Furthermore, the number of patients with neurologic symptoms will increase as our population ages, since many neurologic diseases are more prevalent in elderly persons. In this chapter, we address some of these common neurologic disorders that are frequently seen in male patients, describing the epidemiology, clinical features, diagnosis, treatment, and follow-up. We discuss stroke, Parkinson disease, and Alzheimer's disease (AD), and the last section covers sleep disorders, such as obstructive sleep apnea (OSA), restless legs syndrome (RLS), insomnia, and circadian rhythm disorders that can also regularly affect males. As will be described below, knowledge and evidence-based practice in the specialty of neurology and sleep disorders has greatly expanded in recent years and will likely continue to develop. Recognizing the disorder and initiating prompt treatment can be vital to the final outcome of the patient.

Stroke

Epidemiology

Cerebrovascular accident, commonly referred to as *stroke,* is the third leading cause of death in the United States. On average, every 45 seconds someone in the United States has a stroke. Of the people living in this country, each year approximately 700,000 will have a stroke, 500,000 of which are new attacks and 200,000 of which are recurrent attacks.[1] In 2005, the estimated direct and indirect cost of stroke was $56.8 billion.[2] The incidence rate of stroke in men is 1.25 times greater than that for women; this difference is larger at younger ages and disappears after the age of 80 years, when equal incidence rates are seen.[2] African Americans have almost twice the risk of having a first stroke compared with white Americans.[1] Hispanic Americans and Native Americans also carry a higher incidence of stroke compared with whites—almost twice the relative risk.[3] Risk factors for stroke include older age, positive family history of stroke, hypertension, diabetes mellitus, hypercholesterolemia, and heavy tobacco and alcohol use.[2] Of all strokes, 84% are ischemic and 16% are hemorrhagic in nature.[2] Hemorrhagic strokes consist of intracerebral and subarachnoid bleeds from various causes. Ischemic strokes, which will be the focus of this section below, are classified as atherothrombotic/embolic (44% of total), cardioembolic (21% of total), or secondary to small vessel disease (19% of total) (Figure 13-1).

Clinical Features

Symptoms associated with a stroke are usually sudden in onset and correspond to the location of the central nervous system that is being affected by an abnormality in the blood supply. Symptom severity may not peak until several days after the event as a result of cerebral edema from the infarction. Classically, the duration of fixed neurologic symptoms for a period longer than 24 hours is suggestive of a stroke, whereas any reversible deficits that last less than 24 hours are more likely to represent a transient ischemic attack (TIA). This labeling system is arbitrary for several reasons, as there is a known association between future stroke risk and TIAs, which will necessitate a complete workup to rule out a stroke.[4] Secondly, many neurologic symptoms that last less than 24 hours demonstrate abnormalities visible on magnetic resonance imaging (MRI) consistent with acute ischemia.[5]

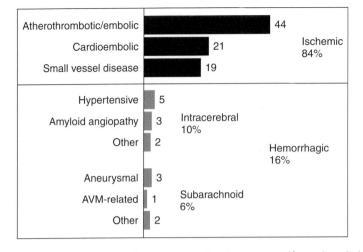

Figure 13-1. Classification of cerebrovascular disease. AVM, Arteriovenous malformation. (Adapted from: Zivin J: Approach to cerebrovascular diseases. In Goldman L, editor: *Cecil Textbook of Medicine*, ed 22, Philadelphia, 2004, W.B. Saunders, pp 2280–2287.)

Ischemic strokes and TIAs are frequently classified into two separate categories based on vascular distribution; namely, the anterior circulation, which is supplied by the carotid artery, and the posterior circulation, which is supplied by the vertebrobasilar system. Eighty percent of ischemic strokes involve the anterior circulation, yet a stroke in either the anterior or posterior territory can exhibit symptoms of focal weakness, sensory loss, dysarthria, or dysphagia. A stroke in the anterior circulation can also produce aphasia, gaze deviation, visual neglect, and monocular visual loss. In contrast, strokes involving the posterior circulation typically cause clinical manifestations of vertigo, diplopia, binocular visual field deficits, ataxia, altered levels of consciousness, ipsilateral cranial nerve deficits, and motor and sensory deficits contralateral to the lesion.

Diagnosis

The diagnosis of an ischemic stroke can be made clinically on the basis of the history and physical examination results and can be confirmed with findings seen on neuroimaging using either a computed tomography (CT) scan of the head or a brain MRI scan. A brain MRI scan using diffusion-weighted imaging has a much higher sensitivity for an acute ischemic stroke compared with a CT scan of the brain, which may not show changes due to an ischemic event until 12–24 hours later, if at all.[6] Diffusion-weighted MRI can demonstrate an abnormal signal in the affected area within minutes of the event[6] (Figure 13-2). A CT scan of the brain may not be as sensitive

for detecting strokes in the brainstem or cerebellum due to artifact from surrounding bony calvarium. However, emergent imaging with a head CT should be performed when a stroke is suspected to distinguish an ischemic stroke from a hemorrhagic stroke or intracranial bleeding, as bleeding in the brain may demand immediate management via craniotomy due to the potential of herniation.

Routine laboratory studies in the evaluation of a patient with a suspected stroke should include a complete blood count and measurements of serum glucose, electrolytes, platelets, prothrombin time, and partial thromboplastin time. Hypoglycemia can mimic the clinical presentation of a stroke. It is also important to evaluate for any hypercoagulable states that may place the patient at an increased risk for stroke. A routine electrocardiogram and cardiac monitoring may be performed to evaluate for paroxysmal atrial fibrillation or other arrhythmias, which also may place the patient at higher risk of stroke from a cardiac source of embolus.[2]

The other major aim of the diagnostic workup for ischemic stroke is to determine the underlying cause to assist in secondary prevention of another ischemic event, since many patients (up to 12%) who experience one stroke have another within the next year.[7] Ischemic strokes can be caused by local vascular occlusion (thrombus), occlusion from intravascular material that originates elsewhere (embolism), or poor perfusion (e.g., shock, hypotension, heart failure). Thrombosis primarily originates from atherosclerotic disease but can also result from other prothrombotic states (e.g., sickle cell disease, fibromuscular dysplasia, dissection,

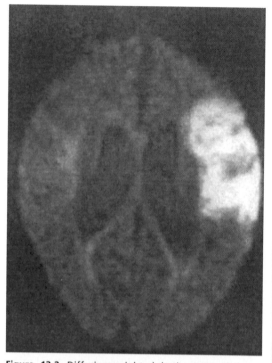

Figure 13-2. Diffusion-weighted brain magnetic resonance image demonstrating decreased signal in the left middle cerebral artery distribution from an acute stroke. (Adapted from: Koenigsberg RA, Faro SH, Hershey BL, et al: Neuroimaging. In Goetz CG, editor: *Textbook of Clinical Neurology*, ed 2, Philadelphia, 2003, Saunders, An Imprint of Elsevier, pp 427–464.)

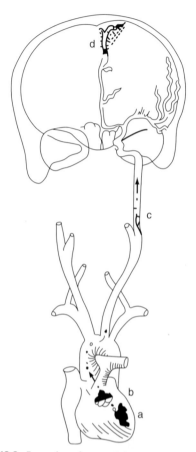

Figure 13-3. Examples of potential sources of embolism in stroke. *a,* Cardiac mural thrombus; *b,* vegetation on a heart valve; *c,* emboli from a carotid plaque; *d,* infarcted cortex in an area supplied by the terminal anterior cerebral artery due to embolism. (Adapted from: Chung CS, Caplan LR: Neurovascular disorders. In Goetz CG, editor: *Textbook of Clinical Neurology*, ed 2, Philadelphia, 2003, Saunders, An Imprint of Elsevier, pp 991–1016.)

and arteritis). Potential sources of embolism may include the heart (e.g., intracardiac shunt), aorta, large vessels, or the deep venous system (Figure 13-3). Stenosis in the internal carotid artery or other large arteries can lead to a watershed infarction in the zones between the anterior, middle, and posterior cerebral arteries if there is a sudden and profound reduction in blood pressure.

Transthoracic or transesophageal echocardiography can be performed to help investigate a cardiac source of the embolism. The use of either modality is likely to be of low yield (identification of potential management alters findings in fewer than 10% of patients studied), unless the patient is young or there is known cardiac disease.[8] Compared with transthoracic echocardiography, transesophageal echocardiography may be cost-effective, and it has improved capability to detect clots in the left atrial appendage or a patent foramen ovale that transthoracic echocardiography may not visualize.[8]

Imaging of the carotid vessels is also of importance to evaluate for significant stenosis. Carotid

Doppler and magnetic resonance angiography (MRA) are safe, noninvasive screening tests for this purpose compared with the gold standard of a cerebral angiogram, which may have some risks associated with the procedure, such as stroke. The accuracy of the results, in comparison with the conventional cerebral angiogram, is reliant on imaging equipment and the technologist acquiring the data. Studies comparing the accuracy of each noninvasive testing relative to the gold standard of angiography are inconclusive and are still being investigated, with early evidence showing better concordance rates with MRA in combination with carotid Doppler scans. One study showed misclassification rates of stenosis at 28% for carotid duplex, 18% for MRA, and 8% for both used concordantly.[9,10] CT angiography has also shown promise as a noninvasive testing alternative,[11] but carries a risk of anaphylactic reaction and renal impairment resulting from iodinated contrast.

Treatment

Treatment of ischemic stroke can be divided into acute management and secondary prevention. Intravenous recombinant tissue plasminogen activator (r-TPA) is a proven medical therapy for patients who have experienced an acute stroke if given within 3 hours of the onset of symptoms and if specific inclusion and exclusion criteria are met. Some important exclusion criteria include an international normalized ratio greater than 1.7, platelets less than 100,000 per microliter, stroke within the last 3 months, major surgery in the previous 14 days, and rapidly improving neurologic deficits.[12] The dose of r-TPA for ischemic stroke is 0.9 mg/kg (maximum of 90 mg) with the initial 10% of the dose delivered as a bolus, and the remaining 90% delivered intravenously over a period of 1 hour.[12] In a double-blinded control study, the correct use of r-TPA has been associated with better neurologic outcomes compared with placebo.[12] At 3 months, the group treated with r-TPA for acute stroke had a 30% greater chance at having minimal to no neurologic disability on clinical assessment compared with the group who did not receive r-TPA treatment.[12] Patients must be monitored closely for at least 24 hours, preferably in a specialized stroke unit, for risk of intracranial hemorrhage (approximately 6%) and blood pressure fluctuations after administration.[12] Despite widespread use of empiric treatment with intravenous fractionated or unfractionated heparin for acute stroke in the past, several prospective, double-blinded trials have not shown an effect on overall mortality or functional outcome.[13]

It is not unusual for blood pressure to be transiently elevated after a stroke and for the next several days thereafter.[14] The most current guidelines recommend avoiding antihypertensive treatment unless systolic blood pressure is greater than 220 mm Hg or if there are other clinical indications for decreasing blood pressure.[14] There are no definitive data from controlled clinical trials nor clinically proven benefit for lowering blood pressure among patients with acute ischemic stroke.[14] A variety of other neurologic and medical complications can occur after an ischemic stroke, including cerebral edema, pneumonia, deep venous thrombosis due to immobility, seizures, cardiac arrhythmias, myocardial infarction, electrolyte disturbances, decubitus ulcers, falls, and urinary tract infections.[15] Appropriate nutritional support and physical rehabilitation targeted at improving deficits have also been implicated as important factors in long-term recovery from stroke.[16]

Secondary prevention of ischemic stroke should begin with identifying known risk factors for cerebrovascular disease, as mentioned above, and appropriately modifying them.[2] One important factor in reducing the risk of another stroke is finding the underlying cause for the current ischemic event. Carotid endarterectomy may be indicated for carotid stenosis greater than 70% on the symptomatic side, which in randomized, blinded, controlled studies had shown a 19% absolute risk reduction in the patient's chance of recurrent stroke at 2 years compared with maximal medical treatment of antiplatelet therapy and risk factor modification alone.[17]

Antiplatelet therapy has also been recommended for the secondary prevention of ischemic stroke.[14,18] For patients with non-cardioembolic strokes, acceptable initial treatments include aspirin 50–325 mg daily,[14] the combination of aspirin 325 mg and extended-release dipyridamole 200 mg twice daily,[18] or clopidogrel 75 mg daily.[19] The addition of aspirin to clopidogrel in high-risk patients with ischemic stroke or TIA has not been associated with a difference in reducing major vascular events, but it has shown an increased risk of life-threatening or major bleeding events and is therefore not recommended for secondary stroke prevention.[20] Evidence supports the use of warfarin over aspirin for secondary stroke prevention in some instances, if the patient is found to have paroxysmal atrial fibrillation and has had a stroke.[21]

Follow-up

Patients who continue to experience neurologic deficits after a stroke may benefit from inpatient or outpatient physical, occupational, and speech therapy. Patients with a history of ischemic strokes also need to be closely monitored by their primary care providers for management of their risk factors for cardiovascular disease. Close monitoring of hypercholesterolemia or initiation of pharmacotherapy for cholesterol lowering should be strongly considered, with a goal of lowering the low-density-lipoprotein cholesterol level below 100 mg/dL. Hypertension should be controlled through dietary modifications, exercise, and antihypertensive agents. Diabetes mellitus and glucose control are also important issues that need to be monitored. Tobacco cessation, if not addressed already, is also another risk factor that can be modified. Education of the patient and family members regarding follow-up care in the case of another event suspicious for a stroke can also prove to be helpful in improving outcomes.

Parkinson's Disease

Epidemiology

Parkinson's disease is a neurodegenerative disorder of unknown etiology that most often begins in the sixth decade of life.[22] Excluding essential tremor, Parkinson's disease is the most common movement disorder and affects approximately 500,000 people in the United States.[22] Lifetime risk tables report the risk of developing Parkinson's disease to be 2% for men and 1.3% for women.[23] Numerous population studies have documented that Parkinson's disease is more common in highly industrialized countries than in agricultural societies and more frequent in Europe and North America than in the Far East.[24] Epidemiologic studies have confirmed that smoking and caffeine consumption are less frequent among subjects who develop Parkinson's disease.[25]

Clinical Features

Parkinson's disease is a clinical diagnosis based on the signs of resting tremor, bradykinesia or slowness of movement, cogwheel rigidity, and loss of postural reflexes seen on neurologic examination.[26] In the early months of Parkinson's disease, these classic "parkinsonian" signs may be particularly subtle, and patients may only complain of slowness, stiffness, and trouble with handwriting.[27] Physicians are often tempted to diagnose arthritis, depression, or normal aging unless a resting tremor is evident. Particular attention to the history of tremor (even if not visible in the office), poor fine motor control, a hunched and slightly flexed posture, and micrographia may permit the clinician to diagnose Parkinson's disease in its early phase.[27] The resting tremor is the most frequent presenting symptom and usually begins in one limb before slowly progressing to involve the other side as well. The tremor is commonly 4–5 Hz in frequency as measured on an electromyelogram, and has been described as a "pill-rolling" tremor, which often improves or disappears with movement of the affected limb.[26]

Patients with Parkinson's disease commonly have a masked facies and a decreased blink rate of 5–10 blinks per minute, compared with the normal 12–20 blinks per minute.[26] Bradykinesia, or slowness of voluntary movements, usually causes common motor tasks such as dressing and writing to become much slower. "Freezing episodes," in which patients have difficulties initiating movement, can also occur. Accidental falls may become quite common as the disease progresses.[26] As a result of postural instability and rigidity, patients tend to turn "en bloc" when walking, defined as making several angular adjustments while standing in one place instead of pivoting 180 degrees in a single step.

Among the behavioral and cognitive troubles experienced by persons with Parkinson's disease, depression occurs in approximately one third of patients.[28] Dementia also occurs in one third of Parkinson's disease patients[29] and was six times more prevalent in a diagnostic group compared with a control population.[30] Tests that involve maintenance of attention, procedural learning, executive function, and working memory are particularly affected in Parkinson's disease. Excessive daytime somnolence and fatigue are common in patients with Parkinson's disease and, from the patient's perspective, are frequently some of the most disabling initial features.[31] Rapid eye movement (REM) sleep behavior disorder is a common sleep disorder seen persons with Parkinson's disease, wherein patients can have abnormal motor activity during sleep (e.g., acting out their dreams).[32]

Urologic problems including urgency and nocturia can significantly affect the overall function of patients with Parkinson's disease and may require pharmacologic interventions.[33] Autonomic dysfunction in the form of orthostatic hypotension and progressive cardiac sympathetic denervation can develop.[34] Constipation is a frequent symptom, as persons with Parkinson's disease have slow colonic transit, decreased rectal contractions, and weak abdominal straining.[35]

Diagnosis

A history of the aforementioned symptoms, as well as the classic signs of Parkinson's disease evident on neurologic examination, can help to establish an accurate the diagnosis.[26] Cogwheel rigidity, resting tremor, shuffling gait, en bloc turning, reduced blink rate, masked facies, and slowed fine finger movements are all supportive of Parkinson's disease. A response of these signs and symptoms to empiric treatment with dopamine agonists is also supportive of the diagnosis.

Essential tremor is the movement disorder most frequently confused with Parkinson's disease. This tremor is usually worse with action or postural in nature, rather than a resting tremor. In essential tremor, the head and voice are often involved and family history is suggestive of an autosomal dominant mode of inheritance.[36] Patients commonly comment that the use of alcohol often improves the tremor, which should prompt the clinician to consider alternative diagnoses other than Parkinson's disease.

Another difficulty in obtaining an accurate diagnosis is to distinguish idiopathic Parkinson's disease from other parkinsonian syndromes caused by other neurodegenerative diseases, medications or toxins, and trauma. Among subjects diagnosed with early Parkinson's disease by movement disorder specialists in a large cohort of untreated patients, 8.1% were later found to have another diagnosis after 7.6 years of follow-up.[37] Several neurodegenerative diseases also cause parkinsonian features in their patients. In these conditions, collectively termed "parkinsonism-plus" syndromes, additional neurologic signs are present including conjugate gaze paresis in progressive supranuclear palsy; ataxia, dyssynergia, and kinetic tremor in multiple system atrophy; pyramidal signs in striatonigral degeneration; marked dysautonomia in Shy-Drager syndrome; or early dementia and hallucinations in diffuse Lewy body disease.

Many drugs can either cause or aggravate parkinsonism.[38] Metoclopramide (Reglan), calcium channel blockers, antidepressants, and neuroleptic drugs can all cause symptoms and signs indistinguishable from idiopathic Parkinson's disease. Standard MRI evaluations of the brain typically have normal results in patients with Parkinson's disease, although more specialized images focusing on the basal ganglia have been helpful in distinguishing parkinsonism-plus syndromes from idiopathic Parkinson's disease.[39]

Treatment

As of yet, there are no proven disease-modifying treatments that exist for Parkinson's disease. Available therapy is aimed at symptomatic improvement and does not address the underlying disease pathology or delay the natural progression of the disease. Therefore, if a patient's symptoms are relatively mild and do not cause impairment in their activities of daily living, delay of treatment may be the appropriate choice. Levodopa and other dopamine agonists have been shown to be moderately effective in improving motor disorders, activities of daily living, and disability in patients with Parkinson's disease; levodopa has been shown to be the most effective drug.[40] Treatment is associated with decreased morbidity and mortality in comparison with the pre-levodopa era.[41] Levodopa is routinely administered in combination with the decarboxylase inhibitor carbidopa to prevent the peripheral conversion of levodopa to dopamine and the resultant nausea and vomiting, which are its most unpleasant adverse effects. In general, it is better to begin therapy at low doses of levodopa/carbidopa and to increase the dose gradually to minimize the risk of acute adverse effects including nausea, vomiting, hypotension, and pathologic sleepiness.[41]

The dopamine agonists cabergoline (Dostinex), ropinirole (Requip), and pramipexole (Mirapex) have been shown to result in fewer motor complications than levodopa/carbidopa after 2.5 years of follow-up.[40] Motor complications are common and can occur in as many as 50–90% of patients after 5–10 years of use.[41] Examples of motor complications include "wearing off," "on-off" motor fluctuations, and dyskinesias. With advancing Parkinson's disease, patients taking levodopa therapy begin to experience a "wearing off" effect in which the length of time of treatment effect of the each dose shortens with use. Eventually, patients may begin to experience rapid and unpredictable fluctuations between "on" and "off" periods, known as the "on-off" phenomenon. Levodopa-induced dyskinesias, or involuntary movements, also develop, and are usually choreiform or dystonic in nature. Although dopamine agonists seem to result in fewer motor complications than levodopa replacement, they are significantly more expensive and are associated with more frequent adverse effects such as hallucinations, sleepiness, and edema.[40]

Medications including anticholinergic agents, amantadine, and selegiline can also be used to treat mild to moderate symptoms of Parkinson's disease. Anticholinergics are helpful in the treatment of resting tremor, and amantadine is helpful for early bradykinesia, yet eventually, levodopa or dopamine agonists are required for progressive disability in most patients.[42] Surgical procedures including pallidotomy and deep brain stimulation have been used for treatment of Parkinson's disease. Surgical treatments can be considered in patients with Parkinson's disease who are responsive to dopamine but are having difficulties with motor fluctuations and dyskinesias. Fetal tissue and stem cell transplants are also being considered as a treatment option, but these are still experimental and quite controversial at this time.

Follow-up

Parkinson's disease is known to be a slowly progressive disorder, and certain patient subgroups may have a more indolent course than others. Studies have suggested that patients who present at a young age of onset, with marked asymmetry, and tremor-predominant disease tend toward milder declines.[43] Patients must be followed up closely by their primary care providers to plan for problems related to their worsening neurologic function. Fall precautions, driving safety, medical and financial decision making, as well as ensuring proper nutrition, are just a few issues that must be addressed on a routine basis.

Medication-related adverse effects must be monitored closely. Most symptomatic treatments can lead to severe sleepiness, hallucinations, nausea, and vomiting.[41] Several forms of motor fluctuations exist, most commonly a predictable decline in motor performance that occurs near the end of each medication dose (i.e., "wearing off").[39] This problem can be managed in a variety of ways, including more frequent dosing of levodopa, the use of controlled-release levodopa, or the addition of a dopamine agonist such as ropinirole or pramipexole.[40] In addition, catechol

O-methyltransferase inhibitors such as entacapone (Comtan) prolong the action of levodopa and can reduce the "off" time phenomena.[43]

Alzheimer's Disease

Epidemiology

Dementia represents a decline in cognitive function, especially memory, of a gradual nature from a previously higher level. The major causes of dementia include AD, vascular dementia, dementia with Lewy bodies, Parkinson's disease with dementia, and frontotemporal dementia.[44] The prevalence of dementia is 1% at 65 years of age, doubling every 5 years to a prevalence of 32% at 85 years of age.[44] It is estimated that, worldwide, 24.3 million people have dementia today, with 4.6 million new cases of dementia being discovered each year. The number of people with dementia is expected to double every 20 years to reach 81.1 million by 2040.[45]

AD is the most common form of dementia in elderly persons, accounting for up to 90% of dementia in the United States.[46] It is characterized pathologically by generalized cerebral cortical atrophy with widespread cortical neuritic (or senile) plaques and neurofibrillary tangles. It is estimated to currently affect more than 4 million Americans,[47] and there is an exponential increase of incidence with advancing age (Figure 13-4).

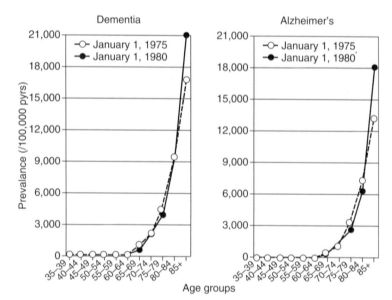

Figure 13-4. Prevalence rates of dementia in Olmstead County, Minnesota, by age for two prevalence dates, January 1, 1975, and January 1, 1980 (reflects most currently available data). pyrs, Patient-years. (Adapted from: Caselli R, Boeve BF: The degenerative dementias. In Goetz CG, editor: *Textbook of Clinical Neurology*, ed 2, Philadelphia, 2003, Saunders, An Imprint of Elsevier, pp 681–712.)

The incidence in men and women seems to be equivalent. Patients with an earlier age of onset (younger than 70 years of age) are more likely to have a positive family history.[48] The cost of caring for one person with this disorder at home or in a nursing home is more than $47,000 per year.[49]

Clinical Features

The most common initial sign exhibited in AD is memory impairment that typically affects short-term memory, causing patients to have difficulties incorporating new memory. Early in the course of the disease, well-learned material from the past is preserved, although specific dates and timing of events can often be forgotten.[50] Progressive disorientation in time and place may occur. Later in the disease process, memory can be severely impaired, which causes difficulties in recalling of family members, friends, and even one's address.[50] Language is also commonly impaired in patients with AD. Initially, pauses in spontaneous speech and reduced vocabulary are noted. With progression of the disease, fluency of speech, anomia, and impaired comprehension are apparent.[51] Apraxia, or difficulties in performing skilled movement despite normal strength and coordination, is common and often causes difficulties with eating and dressing.[51] Spatial disorientation, left-right confusion, and difficulties with calculation (i.e., acalculia) are present in many patients with AD and are likely associated with neurodegenerative changes in the temporoparietal lobes.

Executive dysfunction and difficulties with judgment, planning, and abstract thought, are also prominent clinical symptoms noted in AD. Socially inappropriate behavior and disinhibition can be present, although these can be more characteristic of frontotemporal dementias, such as Pick's disease. Apathy, social withdrawal, and depression are present in more than 70% of patients, sometimes up to 2 years before the initial diagnosis of AD.[52] Other psychiatric disturbances seen in patients with AD include agitation, delusions, and hallucinations, usually occurring in the later stages of disease.[53]

Diagnosis

The diagnosis of AD should be made by taking a detailed history and a careful and complete neurologic and mental status examination. Sometimes, a formal neuropsychiatric assessment may be needed to fully evaluate cognition. The National Institute of Neurologic and Communicative Disorders and Stroke and Alzheimer Disease and Related Disorders Association has set criteria for the diagnosis of AD.[51] The presence of dementia, and deficits in two or more of the following areas are needed to establish the diagnosis of probable AD: cognition, progressive worsening of cognition, onset between 40 and 90 years of age, and absence of an underlying systemic disease to help explain the syndrome. Other supportive criteria include a positive family history, normal cerebrospinal fluid examination results, and normal electroencephalography and brain neuroimaging results.[51] If a patient presents with a sudden onset of memory disturbances, focal neurologic signs, seizures, or gait difficulties early in the course of the disease, an alternative diagnosis must be entertained. Neuropathologic confirmation of AD was found in up to 90% of patients who were diagnosed using the above criteria.[54]

Other diseases and conditions that should be considered in the differential diagnosis of AD include metabolic disturbances, depression, illicit drug use, and medication-related adverse effects. Reversible causes of dementia such as hypothyroidism, vitamin B_{12} deficiency, vasculitis, neurosyphilis, and human immunodeficiency virus infection also must be ruled out with their respective serum assays, although they are usually seen in fewer than 10% of cases.[55] Other central nervous system disorders that can be easily mistaken for AD include frontotemporal dementia (Pick's disease), Lewy body dementia, normal pressure hydrocephalus, and multi-infarct dementia. Imaging with either brain CT or MRI should be performed to evaluate for these other possible etiologies, including large ventricles or numerous infarcts. Depending on the clinical picture, further testing with a lumbar puncture to evaluate for infectious or neoplastic disease, or electroencephalography to evaluate for seizures, may be considered in specific cases but need not be performed routinely (Table 13-1).

Treatment

The acetylcholinesterase inhibitors tacrine (Cognex), donepezil (Aricept), galantamine (Reminyl), and rivastigmine (Exelon) have been approved for use as cognitive enhancers in the treatment of mild to moderate AD.[56] These medications work by reducing degradation of acetylcholine in the brain, and thus enhancing cholinergic transmission in the central nervous system. Tacrine administration is often problematic because of adverse effects consisting of hepatotoxicity and the need to administer the drug at frequent

Table 13-1. Laboratory Evaluation of the Patient with Dementia

Routine	When Indicated
Complete blood count	Erythrocyte sedimentation rate
Chemistry panel	Urinalysis
Thyroid function tests	Toxicology
Vitamin B_{12} level	Chest radiograph
Computed tomography/ magnetic resonance imaging	Heavy metal screen
	Human immunodeficiency virus assay
	Syphilis serology
	Cerebrospinal fluid examination
	Electroencephalogram
	Positron emission tomography/single-photon emission computed tomography

Adapted from: Cory-Bloom J: Alzheimer's disease. In Rakel RE, editor: *Conn's Current Therapy 2006,* ed 58, Philadelphia, 2006, Saunders, pp 1071–1077.

dosing intervals.[56] The other three agents have all been shown to be effective in promoting stabilization or to delay deterioration of cognitive or behavioral problems in AD compared with placebo. No head-to-head studies have been performed to display superiority of one agent over the other; none of these medications have been effective in preventing the eventual progression of the disease.[56]

Memantine has been approved for the treatment of moderate to severe AD. This drug is an N-methyl-D-aspartate receptor antagonist and is thought to selectively block the excitotoxic effects that glutamine plays at these receptors in the brain. A benefit relative to placebo was observed for at least 6 months in patients with moderate to severe AD.[57] One study suggests a possible benefit of vitamin E or possibly selegiline for slowing the progression of AD.[58] Antidepressants, specifically selective serotonin reuptake inhibitors, can be helpful in combating social withdrawal, depressed mood, and sleep disturbances that are commonly seen in patients with AD.[59] Antipsychotic medications are often needed to treat symptoms of delusions or hallucinations, which are often very disabling in AD. Short-term programs directed toward educating family caregivers about AD should be offered to improve caregiver satisfaction. Intensive long-term education and support services (when

available) should be offered to caregivers of patients with AD to delay time to institutionalization in a nursing home or skilled care facility.[56]

Follow-Up

The average survival of patients who are diagnosed with AD is 4–6 years, but the range can be as long as 15 years.[60] These patients most often experience complications such as urinary tract infections, decubitus ulcers, pneumonia, and dehydration that lead to significant morbidity and, ultimately, mortality.[60] Acute confusion or delirium can be common in any demented patient as a result of a metabolic, toxic, or infectious disease. Unfamiliar surroundings, such as a new environment or the sleeping quarter (e.g., hospital) can also worsen disorientation and confusion. It is therefore prudent to ensure safety by surveying the patient's living environment during the course of the disease. The patient may be safe living at home, managing expenses, bathing, and driving early on, but the situation almost always needs to be reassessed later in the course of the disease (Figure 13-5).

Sleep Disorders
Obstructive Sleep Apnea
Epidemiology

OSA is one of the most important and frequently encountered sleep disorders in primary care practices, and it has adverse effects on almost every organ system. Reports from a large epidemiologic study in the United States found that the prevalence of reported sleep apnea is 13% in men (compared with 4% in women), whereas the prevalence of reported snoring was even higher at 33% for men compared with 19% for women.[61,62]

Clinical Features

OSA is characterized by repetitive airway obstructions. The major symptoms include daytime sleepiness, snoring, and impairment of cognition. Sleep apnea is associated with a variety of disturbances ranging from hypersomnolence to concentration and memory disturbances, nocturnal hypertension, nighttime arousals, confusion, and impairment in the neuropsychological functioning. The principle symptom of OSA, sleepiness, results from repeated nighttime arousals. Several large epidemiologic studies have also reported a strong correlation between sleep apnea and cardiovascular heart disease, systemic

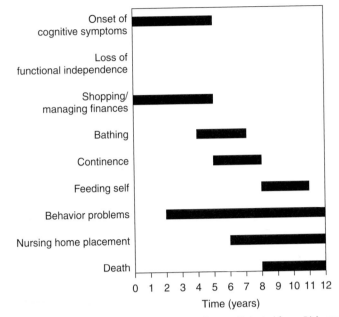

Figure 13-5. Typical occurrence of manifestations of Alzheimer's disease. (Adapted from: Dickman R: Care of the elderly. In Rakel RE, editor: *Textbook of Family Practice*, ed 6, Philadelphia, 2002, W.B. Saunders, pp 88–130.)

and pulmonary hypertension, ischemic heart disease, myocardial infarction, cerebrovascular accidents, nocturnal cardiac arrhythmias, and congestive heart failure.[63–67]

Diagnosis

A diagnosis of OSA should be suspected based on the clinical history of excessive daytime sleepiness, snoring, and nocturnal apneic episodes (reported by the bed partner). Some patients will also present with memory problems, whereas some will describe impotence and nocturia. The clinical encounter serves as a way to establish the possibility of sleep-disordered breathing and to inquire about other possible causes of daytime sleepiness including insufficient sleep time, depression, and other sleep disorders including disorders of motor control during sleep, circadian rhythm disorders, and narcolepsy. Important information to obtain from patients includes bed time, rise time, sleep latency, number of awakenings during the night, length of naps, and sleep pattern on the weekends. The Epworth Sleepiness Scale is an eight-point questionnaire that asks patients about the propensity to fall asleep in various situations on a scale from 0 to 3, where 24 is the maximum score. Patients with a total score of 10 or higher should be considered to have significant daytime sleepiness, and those with a score over 15 are defined as having severe daytime sleepiness.[68]

Obesity, a thick neck, a crowded oropharyngeal inlet, and the presence of retrognathia or micrognathia are consistent physical examination findings associated with the presence of sleep apnea. Midsagittal and axial MRIs of a normal subject compared with a patient with OSA demonstrate significant airway obstruction in the OSA patient. The Mallampati Classification is helpful in rating the severity of oropharyngeal occlusion.[69] Intranasal examination to evaluate for the possibility of a nasoseptal deviation and signs of allergic rhinitis are important in anticipation of positive pressure therapy. If a patient has a significant stenosis of the nasal passages due to an anatomic occlusion, then a referral to an otolaryngologist is advisable. Patients at risk for having OSA should also be evaluated for the systemic consequences of the disease, and physicians should record pulse rate and blood pressure and conduct a thorough cardiopulmonary examination. In patients with dementia, a neurologic examination is warranted with particular emphasis on the Folstein Mini-Mental Status Examination.

The nocturnal polysomnogram is critical in the evaluation of OSA and the assessment of other specific sleep stage abnormalities, leg movements, unusual behaviors, and the presence of an underlying sleep-related breathing disorder. The multiple sleep latency test may also provide an objective assessment of sleepiness and is important in the evaluation of narcolepsy.

Treatment

Management of OSA can be divided into conservative and nonconservative approaches. Conservative approaches include modification of behavioral factors such as weight loss, avoidance of alcohol, limiting the use of sedating compounds, and smoking cessation. Weight reduction in obese patients with OSA improves the upper airway cross-sectional area[70] and may decrease the number of respiratory disturbances and sleep disruption and improve nocturnal oxygen saturation. Although significant weight loss is often difficult to obtain, even moderate weight loss can improve the severity of the underlying sleep apnea.

Assuming the supine position during sleep places the patient at an increased risk of OSA, and sleep position adjustment may be a viable treatment for some non-obese patients.[71,72] Patients may be asked to use tennis balls, sewn into the back part of pajamas, to make it uncomfortable for the patient to lie in the supine position. Sometimes, special mattresses can also be used to encourage the patient to avoid sleeping on his back. Positional therapy may be particularly beneficial for patients with mild and strictly positional sleep apnea.

The most commonly accepted and first-line mode of therapy is nasal continuous positive airway pressure (CPAP). CPAP is the most widely used treatment for OSA and has been shown to improve the nocturnal oxygen saturation and quality of sleep in younger adults, yet compliance rates vary from as low as 46–80%.[73,74] Some of the compliance problems stemming from adverse effects attributable to this treatment modality include claustrophobia, nasal congestion, and dryness. CPAP therapy should be viewed as a symptomatic rather than curative therapy, and patients must use it on a nightly basis as long as they have sleep apnea, which for many patients is an indefinite period.[61]

Oral appliances are considered by many as very useful for the treatment of snoring and mild to moderate sleep apnea. Appliances that are fabricated and fitted by dentists work by repositioning the mandible and improving the upper airway space at the hypopharyngeal level. They can be particularly advantageous because they require minimal upkeep and are relatively simple to use. These oral appliances are attractive for many patients because they are also much more mobile than a CPAP apparatus, and they are smaller and less expensive.[75] They are also a nice alternative to patients who become very claustrophobic when using the CPAP masks. Adverse effects of the appliances may include temporal mandibular joint dysfunction, tooth and gum pain, proprioceptive malocclusion, disturbed salivation, and at times, gum disease.

Surgical treatment options for OSA target potential sites of airway obstruction. Surgical techniques involve extirpation of soft tissue, secondary soft tissue repositioning through primary skeletal mobilization, or bypass of the pharyngeal airway. There are three sides of obstruction, which include the nasopharynx, oropharynx, and hypopharynx. Surgical procedures for the management of OSA are chosen when there is a clear anatomic airway obstruction or when management with nasal CPAP is not achieved. Patients need to be evaluated by an otolaryngologist and often an oral-maxillofacial surgeon and must undergo extensive presurgical evaluation with cephalometric radiography and fiber-optic endoscopy of the nasopharyngeal passages. Surgery may be targeted at the level of the upper airways preventing their collapse. Frequent surgical treatment approaches include uvulopalatopharyngoplasty, genioglossus advancement and hyoid myotomy, bimaxillary advancement, and maxillomandibular advancement, which aim to enlarge the pharyngeal space and prevent airway collapse. Success rates range from 30% for the less aggressive interventions up to 90% for the more aggressive procedures.[76–79] Common adverse effects include pain, alteration in taste, nasal regurgitation, and loss of sensation at the site of surgery.

Sleep-Related Movement Disorders

The most common movement disorders during sleep are RLS and periodic limb movement disorder (PLM). Both RLS and PLM consist of nocturnal involuntary limb movements causing sleep disruption. Unlike PLM, which is diagnosed by polysomnography, the diagnosis of RLS is made by meeting established clinical criteria.[80,81] In addition, PLM can occur in RLS and with other sleep disorders as well as in patients with no sleep disorder, and is therefore a nonspecific finding.[80]

Restless Legs Syndrome

Epidemiology

Symptoms of RLS have been identified in 5–15% of healthy subjects, 15–20% of uremic patients, and in up to 30% of patients with rheumatoid arthritis. RLS symptom prevalence in the general population varies significantly among countries. The highest prevalence seen is in Western European countries, with rates as high as 10%, whereas studies from Asia-India, Singapore, and Turkey have reported lower prevalence rates (0.8%, 0.6%, and 3.2% respectively).[82–85] Of patients with clinically significant RLS symptoms, which can occur more than 15 times per month, only one quarter to one third may benefit most from therapy.[86]

Clinical Features

The most recent diagnostic criteria developed at a National Institutes of Health workshop with members of the International Restless Legs Syndrome Study Group require four essential criteria for the diagnosis of RLS[87]:

- Disagreeable leg sensations that usually occur before sleep onset
- An irresistible urge to move the limbs
- Partial or complete relief of the discomfort with leg movement
- Return of the symptoms upon cessation of leg movements

The most disabling complaint in RLS is the irresistible and profound urge to move the lower limbs. Patients often describe a building of this sensation to the point they must give in and move their legs. RLS has been described as quiesogenic (i.e., arising from rest), and the symptoms are present only at rest and just before the patient's sleep period. The symptoms sometimes usually interfere with sleep onset and may induce insomnia and prolonged awakenings leading to significantly reduced sleep time; patients often report averaging less than 4 hours sleep per night.[88] The sensory complaints are typically difficult to describe and are left to subjective interpretation by patients who may use multiple terms such as "creepy-crawly," "burning," "creeping," "crawling," "tingling," or "itching" to describe the discomfort. RLS symptoms improve when patients engage in challenging activities such as playing a mentally consuming game or even arguing. Getting out of bed and ambulating typically provides immediate relief, which is short lived and abates soon after the activity ceases.

Typical symptoms involve the ankle and knee but, when RLS is severe, the upper extremities can also become involved. The symptoms are typically bilateral, can be asymmetric in both severity and frequency, but are rarely unilateral. RLS can occur at other times of the day, but they become much more pronounced during times of prolonged inactivity, particularly when in an airplane or driving long distances. The symptoms usually last for a few minutes or several hours. New evidence suggests that patients with RLS may have symptoms consistent with anxiety and depression and may have lower scores on quality of life measures,[89,90] suggesting that the sleep disturbances associated with RLS is probably the "tip of the iceberg."

RLS has a clearly established circadian tendency for symptoms to be much worse in the evening and increasing in intensity toward the early sleep period. The majority of patients with RLS describe that their best sleep quality is generally earlier in the morning with a relatively "protected" time between 6:00 and 10:00 AM, which is relatively free of RLS symptoms.

Both PLM and RLS show a maximal severity in timely coincidence with the falling phase of the core temperature circadian cycle. There is some evidence that the amplitude of circadian rhythm of dopaminergic function is increased in RLS, with a hypofunction at night.[91] This finding, in addition to the fact that RLS responds to dopaminergic agents (e.g., ropinirole and pramipexole) and is exacerbated by dopamine antagonists (e.g., metoclopramide and haloperidol) fuels the hypothesis that the underlying pathophysiology may be related to dopamine dysfunction. Another hypothesis postulates brain iron-storage deficiency in RLS[92] and the fact that patients with RLS have reduced cerebrospinal fluid iron content compared with normal control subjects.[93]

RLS has two forms with separate etiologies and age of onset. The early-onset form of RLS begins before the age of 45 years, tends to cluster in families, has a slower progression, and has approximately a 2:1 female to male ratio. Late-onset RLS begins after the age of 45 years and has an equal male to female ratio, has a more rapid progression, is more severe with more frequent daily symptoms, has little or no associated family history, and is more commonly associated with underlying medical conditions such as neuropathy, radiculopathy or myelopathy.[90]

RLS can be associated with anemia and uremia. Patients with renal failure requiring hemodialysis have a prevalence rate of RLS ranging between 20% and 50% but may be even greater in some cohorts.[94,95] Higher prevalence rates of RLS have also been reported in other neurologic conditions such as Parkinson's disease[85,96] spinocerebellar ataxia (SCA-3),[97,98] chronic low back pain, myelopathy, and arthropathy.[99] Medications that may exacerbate RLS and PLM include dopamine antagonists (particularly antiemetic agents), antihistamines (H_1 antagonists), antidepressants including the tricyclic antidepressants and serotonin-selective reuptake inhibitors, and neuroleptic drugs.[100–103]

Most patients with RLS have PLM, whereas PLM is less common in patients with RLS. Patients may experience features of intense anxiety and depression in association with RLS. In some patients, the emotional distress may be severe and associated with psychosocial dysfunction. RLS occurs with waxing and waning cycles of symptoms. RLS is most often seen as an isolated case, but a definitive familial pattern has been reported assuming an autosomal dominant mode of transmission. RLS may cause severe insomnia, psychological disturbance, and depression, sometimes producing severe social dysfunction.

Diagnosis

All patients need to fulfill the diagnostic criteria for RLS and have a screening neurologic evaluation to rule out an underlying neuropathy. Although a sleep study is not indicated when the clinical diagnostic criteria have been met,[104,105] it can be helpful to exclude other underlying primary sleep disorders such as OSA or in cases when the RLS does not respond to conventional therapy. All patients with RLS should have a serum ferritin sample drawn because patients in whom the serum ferritin level is in a low range (less than 45 µg/liter) are at a higher risk of having RLS. Iron plays a role in the pathophysiology of the RLS as iron-deficiency states (e.g., frequent blood donation, menstruation, pregnancy) provoke RLS, and iron level normalization helps to improve RLS symptoms.[106–112]

Treatment

Pharmacotherapeutic options for treatment of RLS are outlined in Table 13-2. Patients with serum ferritin levels less than 45 µg/liter should begin iron-replacement therapy with oral iron

Table 13-2. Pharmacotherapy for Treatment of Restless Leg Syndrome

Drug (Generic/Brand)	Dose	Potential Adverse Effects
Iron		
Ferrous sulfate	325 mg bid/tid with vitamin C 100–200 mg Recommended for ferritin < 45 µg/liter	Constipation
Dopamine agonists		
Pramipexole (Mirapex)*	0.125–0.5 mg 1 hour prior to bedtime Start low and increase slowly	Severe sleepiness, nausea
Ropinirole (Requip)*	0.5–4 mg 1 hour prior to bedtime Divided doses, gradually increase As needed	
Dopaminergic agents		
Levodopa/Carbidopa (Sinemet)	25/200 mg 0.5–3 tablets 30 minutes before to bedtime	Nausea, sleepiness, augmentation of daytime symptoms, insomnia, sleepiness, gastrointestinal disturbances
Anticonvulsants		
Gabapentin (Neurontin)	300–2700 mg/day Divided tid	Daytime sleepiness, nausea
Clonidine		
Catapres	0.1 mg bid May be helpful in patients with hypertension	Dry mouth, drowsiness, constipation, sedation, weakness, depression (1%), hypotension
Opiate		
Darvocet (Darvocet-N)	300 mg/day	Nausea, vomiting, restlessness, constipation; addiction and tolerance are possible
Darvon (Propoxyphene)	65–135 mg at bedtime	
Codeine	30 mg	

bid, Twice daily; tid, three times daily.
* Only agent with US Food and Drug Administration approval as of June 2007.

sulfate.[112] Dopamine (D3) agonists such as ropinirole (Requip) and pramipexole (Mirapex) may also be used. At the time of submission of this chapter, the only medication with a clear approval from the US Food and Drug Administration (FDA) for the treatment of RLS is ropinirole. Dopamine agonists as a category are the preferred treatment because they have been shown to control most RLS symptoms throughout the night.[113]

If symptoms persist despite these therapies, other medications including benzodiazepines (e.g., clonazepam or temazepam) may be added,[114] and the dopamine agonist levodopa/carbidopa[115] may be considered. Both levodopa and dopamine agonists ameliorate RLS symptoms, decrease PLM, and improve sleep.[116,117] The drawback of levodopa therapy is the potential for augmentation of symptoms, characterized by the development of an increased symptom severity earlier in the day.[118] Of the anticonvulsants, both carbamazepine (Tegretol) and gabapentin (Neurontin) have been proposed, with gabapentin being effective in controlling the leg movements as well.[119] For refractory and severe cases of RLS, opiates (especially methadone) have a proven efficacy.[120]

Insomnia

Epidemiology

In the United States, the prevalence of insomnia in a given year is between 50% and 60%. Using a more strict definition, defined by persistent sleep disturbance for a period of at least 2 weeks in the previous year, the prevalence in the general population drops to approximately 10–15%.[121,122] In primary care settings, more than one half of patients may report insomnia, although two thirds of these patients will not spontaneously report sleep problems to their doctors.[123,124] Epidemiologic data has demonstrated a higher prevalence of insomnia in older persons compared with younger persons.[125] Up to 40% of patients older than 60 years of age may experience insomnia, frequent awakening, and disrupted sleep.[126] In a recent study from Thailand, nearly half of patients over 60 years had insomnia[127]; poor perceived health and depression were factors found to be strongly associated with insomnia in this cohort.[127] In a survey completed a decade ago by the National Institute on Aging of more than 9000 patients aged 65 years or older, 28% reported difficulties initiating sleep and 42% reported symptoms of both difficulties in sleep initiation and maintenance.[128]

Reports of problems with sleep in this cohort were associated with multiple comorbidities including an increasing number of respiratory symptoms, physical disabilities, use of nonprescription medications, depressive symptoms, and poorer self-perceived health status[128]

Clinical Features

It is important to remember that insomnia is a symptom, not a diagnosis, and it is by far the most common sleep-related problem reported. Insomnia is marked by subjective symptoms regarding quantity or quality of sleep that result in daytime impairment. Commonly encountered symptoms include sleep initiation difficulty, sleep maintenance difficulties, early morning awakening and being unable to reinitiate sleep, and the perception of non-restorative or poor-quality sleep. Patients with insomnia commonly report that their sleep is "unrefreshing" or "non-restorative" and that they wake up in the morning feeling tired. Polysomnographic studies demonstrate that patients with insomnia have prolonged latency to sleep onset, increased time awake during the sleep period, decreased total sleep time, and reduced amounts of slow-wave sleep.[129]

A number of different approaches have been used to classify insomnia based on symptoms, frequency, duration, severity, and presumed etiology. Symptom-based classifications, such as sleep initiation or maintenance insomnia, are generally not useful since symptoms tend to change over time for individual patients and may not have useful clinical utility.[130,131] More recently proposed clinical definitions for insomnia established by the American Academy of Sleep Medicine include the requirement of daytime impairment resulting from the sleep disturbance.[132] Commonly encountered daytime symptoms include fatigue, cognitive impairment causing difficulty functioning in school or at work, and worries about sleep.

Insomnia classifications based on frequency, duration, and severity vary considerably across different nosologies and may have limited diagnostic utility; however, insomnia duration is likely the best indicator for diagnosis. Patients with insomnia are generally classified in the acute form, lasting days to weeks, and the chronic form, lasting weeks to months.[133] Acute (short-term) insomnias are usually due to psychosocial stressors including stressful life events, surgery, examinations, and divorce, whereas chronic insomnia is frequently associated with a variety of comorbid conditions as well as behavioral factors that seem to perpetuate the insomnia.

Another commonly used definition of insomnia divides it further into primary or secondary forms. *Secondary insomnia* assumes an etiologic perspective that is triggered by another disorder, yet the limited understanding of mechanistic pathways in chronic insomnia precludes drawing conclusions about the causality.[132] A major concern is that the term *secondary insomnia* may promote undertreatment, and it is therefore suggested that the term *comorbid insomnia* may be a more accurate and appropriate label.[132] Common comorbidities include psychiatric disorders (particularly mood disorders); cardiopulmonary disorders; and conditions associated with chronic somatic complaints (e.g., musculoskeletal syndromes such as rheumatoid arthritis or lower back pain) that may disrupt sleep. Underlying sleep disorders may also contribute to insomnia, particularly RLS, OSA, and PLM. The term *primary insomnia* should therefore be used when no coexisting disorder has been identified.[132]

Evaluation

Since insomnia is not a "diagnosis" it may be evaluated but not actually diagnosed. The evaluation of insomnia should begin with a detailed medical and sleep history. Particular attention should be directed toward the underlying comorbidities such as medical conditions (e.g., heart disease, diabetes), medication use or misuse (e.g., polypharmacy), and substance use (e.g., alcohol, caffeine, tobacco, illicit drugs). Sleep history should focus on the sleep hygiene (e.g., bedtime, sleep time, wake time). Sleep diaries or sleep logs are crucial in the evaluation, as these self-reported subjective measures allow for easy calculation of total time spent in bed, total sleep time, and sleep efficiency.[134] Polysomnograms are often not necessary as a first step in the evaluation of most cases of insomnia. A single polysomnogram may not be representative of a patient's sleep at home and may not detect insomnia that is not present on a nightly basis. However, polysomnography may be indicated if the clinician suspects an underlying sleep disorder such as RLS, PLM, or OSA.[135] Others have advocated a formal polysomnographic evaluation when traditional therapy of insomnia fails and the possibility of an underlying primary sleep disorder persists.[136]

Underlying psychiatric conditions are important contributors to disruption of the sleep architecture; up to 90% of patients with depression have an abnormal sleep architecture.[137] The most striking polysomnographic features of depression include a decreased REM latency and early morning awakening.[138] In the sleep practice, it is

not uncommon to see alcohol being used as a sleeping aid. Although initially it does decrease the sleep latency, it produces arousals, sleep fragmentation, REM deprivation, and REM rebound later during the night. Stimulants (e.g., caffeine and medications containing stimulants) are notorious causes of insomnia.[139] Caffeine is associated with increased sleep latency, reduced sleep efficiency, and spontaneous arousals. Caffeine withdrawal is associated with depression, irritability, and hypersomnolence. Nicotine induces insomnia and sleep fragmentation.

Treatment

Hypnotics. All hypnotic agents will, if given in appropriate doses, improve insomnia. The goal is to use the medication with the fewest adverse effects at the lowest dose and for the shortest period of time that can be clinically effective. Potential adverse effects of hypnotics include anterograde amnesia and rebound insomnia, which are commonly seen in conjunction with hypnotic drugs with short to intermediate half-lives. Hypnotic agents, when prescribed to patients with underlying OSA, may produce further nocturnal hypoxemia.[140] Withdrawal from hypnotics may actually produce a worsening of insomnia and heightened anxiety. This is especially true with abrupt cessation from longer-acting medications. The newer short-acting hypnotic drugs do not have these same adverse effects and seem to be much safer. Examples of newer medications include the benzodiazepine-receptor agonists (e.g., zaleplon [Sonata], zolpidem [Ambien], and eszopiclone [Lunesta]) and a melatonin-receptor agonist called ramelteon (Rozerem).

Sleep Hygiene. Drug therapy alone is not appropriate if one aims to eradicate chronic insomnia because it must be combined with educational, behavioral, and cognitive interventions aimed at introducing adaptive behaviors. One of the most important educational approaches for insomnia includes modifying disadvantageous sleep hygiene habits that patients may have adopted over the years.[141] Originally developed by Hauri and Wisbey,[141] the basic elements of better sleep hygiene include limiting naps to less than 30 minutes per day, avoiding stimulants and sedatives, limiting liquids at bedtime, keeping a regular sleep schedule, and incorporating light exposure and exercise into the daily routines. Stimulus-control therapy, originally proposed by Bootzin and Engle-Friedman,[142] proposes that sleep disturbances are behaviorally conditioned and thus need to be reconditioned. The aim of this intervention is to recondition the bed and bedroom as cues for sleep. Patients are instructed to go to bed only when tired, to get out of bed after 20 minutes of being unable to fall asleep, and to return to bed when sleepy. They are also instructed to avoid looking at the clock, to shorten daytime naps, to use the bed only for sleep, and to get out of bed at a consistent time each morning.[139]

Sleep restriction therapy proposed by Spielman and colleagues[143] has in its merits the need to restrict time in bed to provide for better sleep efficiency. This technique involves curtailing time in bed and total sleep time, which may initially lead to a state of sleep deprivation. It works by preventing patients from becoming frustrated by restricting the time spent in bed. Other common therapeutic modalities for insomnia include cognitive intervention, which helps patients gain insight into maladaptive beliefs and attitudes toward sleep, and relaxation techniques and biofeedback, which help patients lower the degree of anxiety and arousal associated with insomnia.[142]

Circadian Rhythm Sleep Disorders

Clinical Features

Circadian rhythm sleep disorders are a distinct class of sleep disorders. Abnormalities in circadian function are caused by a misalignment between the internal circadian rhythm and the external environment. These disorders may be caused by an alteration in the functioning of the circadian timing system or may be due to changes in the external environment. Physiologic, behavioral, and environmental factors all affect the severity of these disorders, which may present as reports of insomnia and excessive daytime sleepiness.

Circadian-based sleep disorders can occur for two main reasons:

1. Alteration of the external environment relative to the internal circadian timing system. Circadian rhythm sleep disorders, such as shift-work sleep disorder (SWSD) and jet lag, occur when the physical environment is altered relative to the internal circadian clock. Highlights of these two disorders are explained below.
2. Circadian sleep phase disorders consist of alteration of the endogenous circadian system itself. These conditions are characterized by an alteration in the timing of the major consolidated sleep period, with

sleep being either delayed or advanced in relation to conventional sleep and wake times. Examples include delayed sleep phase syndrome and advanced sleep phase syndrome. The clinical presentation of most of the circadian rhythm sleep disorders is influenced by a combination of physiologic, behavioral, and environmental factors.

Shift-Work Sleep Disorder

Shift work disrupts the sleep-wake cycle by moving the opportunity for sleep to a time when the internal clock and societal cues are out of phase (i.e., telling a person to be awake when, conventionally, he or she would be asleep). Approximately one quarter of persons scheduled to work at night present with SWSD. Night-shift workers in the transportation industry are one of the most vulnerable groups to the consequences of the adverse effects of shift work. The degree that shift work affects sleep and daily functioning varies, and not all shift workers have difficulties in obtaining adequate and quality sleep.[144] Several internal and external factors exist that can influence an individual's ability to cope with shift work including age,[145] domestic responsibilities,[146, 147] commute times, diurnal preference, type of work schedule, and other underlying sleep disorders (e.g., OSA, narcolepsy).

SWSD typically presents as insomnia or hypersomnia that occurs transiently with the work schedule. The hypersomnia should be differentiated from that due to other primary sleep disorders such as narcolepsy or OSA. The relationship between the sleep disturbance and the shift-work schedule should be evident from a thorough history. Two to four weeks of a sleep diary, when appropriate, actigraphy (wearing a device on the wrist to record movement during sleep), and a work history may be useful to determine the degree of circadian disruption and sleep curtailment. The inclusion of a work diary may be particularly useful for persons who work irregular schedules; this can help to determine the relationship between work and sleep and may aid in developing a treatment plan for the patient.

Patients with SWSD commonly report feeling unrefreshed on awakening. This feeling can persist despite good sleep hygiene practices and optimizing the sleep environment. In addition, patients with this condition often report feeling sleepy because they are awake when the circadian propensity for sleep is high.

Treatment of Shift-Work Sleep Disorder

Treatments for SWSD fall into two main categories: (1) treatment aimed at improving sleep via good sleep hygiene and short-term use of sleeping medications, and (2) treatment aimed at realigning circadian rhythms, specifically the use of bright light and melatonin.[148] Bright light and melatonin administration are useful agents to improve sleep disruption in shift workers by matching the circadian rhythm of sleep propensity with desired sleep time.[149–151] Both continuous and intermittent light exposure[152, 153] have been used to successfully increase phase adjustment in shift workers.[154] In addition to the phase-shifting properties, bright light has acute alerting effects that have been shown to improve cognitive performance.[154] It is important to start light treatment early in the shift to achieve a maximum potential benefit. Treatment should begin with the first night shift, and bright light exposure should stop approximately 2 hours before the end of the shift. It is also important to avoid light exposure at the wrong circadian time.

Reports of melatonin taken at bedtime after a night shift have shown improvements in daytime sleep duration and limited increase in nocturnal alertness.[148] The use of other pharmacologic agents such as caffeine and modafinil (Provigil), recently approved by the FDA for the treatment of SWSD, are additional strategies for improving alertness and performance in a shift-work setting.[155,156]

Treatment of SWSD requires multimodal strategies. Several factors can make treatment of SWSD a challenge, including individual differences in tolerance to shift work, motivation of the patient, social/family support, and an increasingly diverse number of shift-work schedules. Therefore, to achieve maximum success, the treatment plan needs to be individualized to address the multiple factors involved.

Jet Lag

Jet lag is the result of the external environment being temporarily altered in relation to the internal clock by traveling across several time zones. Although symptoms are generally temporary, they can be disruptive and may range from a difficulty sleeping, excessive daytime sleepiness, general malaise, impaired performance, and gastrointestinal upset.[154] The severity of jet lag symptoms and the ability to adapt to the new time zone is typically influenced by the direction of travel (slower adaptation when traveling east) and the number of time zones crossed. Eastward travel generally results in difficulty falling asleep and westward travel results in difficulties maintaining sleep.[154] Not all travelers crossing time zones suffer from jet lag to the same degree. These differences probably result from individual variation, similar to those reported for adaptation to shift work.

Treatment of Jet Lag. Treatments aimed at speeding up retraining of circadian rhythms to a new time zone are typically the most effective treatments for jet lag. Bright light[154,157] and or melatonin treatment[158] can be used to effectively to retrain circadian rhythms and improve sleep. Alterations to the timing of the sleep-wake cycle and light exposure should be modified depending on the direction of travel and the number of times zones crossed. On an eastward flight, patients should remain awake and avoid bright light in the morning, but get as much light as possible in the afternoon.[159] Conversely, on westward flights, patients should try to stay awake while it is daylight at the destination and try to sleep when it gets dark. Melatonin in doses of 1–3 mg (commonly available in over-the-counter preparations) can be taken at bedtime in the new location to reduce symptoms of jet lag.[159] Zolpidem (Ambien), in a dose of 10 mg taken for 3 consecutive nights starting with the first night's sleep after travel, has been shown to improve sleep in some seasoned travelers.[160]

Other strategies that may aid in reducing the impact of jet lag include improving sleep hygiene by getting enough sleep, eating meals according to local time, and achieving light exposure at the appropriate clock times.[161,162] For some persons it may be useful, when practical, to gradually shift the sleep-wake cycle to match the location of travel before departure, thereby reducing the time required to adjust to the new time zone upon arrival.

Conclusion

Many different neurologic diseases are commonly seen in the primary care setting. As more evidence-based treatments and prevention strategies become available for these diseases, it becomes increasingly important for the physician to quickly recognize and manage the conditions to ameliorate the final clinical outcome for the patient. As our knowledge about the nervous system continues to grow, our management and treatment strategies will also evolve.

References

1. Broderick J, Brott T, Kothari R, et al: The Greater Cincinnati/Northern Kentucky Stroke Study: preliminary first-ever and total incidence rates of stroke among blacks, *Stroke* 29(2):415–421, 1998.
2. American Heart Association: Heart disease and stroke statistics—2005 update. Available at: http://www.americanheart.org/downloadable/heart/1105390918119HDSStats2005Update.pdf. Accessed January 23, 2006.
3. Morgenstern LB, Smith MA, Lisabeth LD, et al: Excess stroke in Mexican Americans compared with non-Hispanic Whites: the Brain Attack Surveillance in Corpus Christi Project, *Am J Epidemiol* 160(4):376–383, 2004.
4. Johnston SC, Gress DR, Browner WS, Sidney S: Short-term prognosis after emergency department diagnosis of TIA, *JAMA* 284(22):2901–2906, 2000.
5. Kidwell CS, Alger JR, Di Salle F, et al: Diffusion MRI in patients with transient ischemic attacks, *Stroke* 30(6):1174–1180, 1999.
6. Gonzalez RG, Schaefer PW, Buonanno FS, et al: Diffusion-weighted MR imaging: diagnostic accuracy in patients imaged within 6 hours of stroke symptom onset, *Radiology* 210(1):155–162, 1999.
7. Petty GW, Brown RD Jr, Whisnant JP, et al: Survival and recurrence after first cerebral infarction: a population-based study in Rochester, Minnesota, 1975 through 1989, *Neurology* 50(1):208–216, 1998.
8. McNamara RL, Lima JA, Whelton PK, Powe NR: Echocardiographic identification of cardiovascular sources of emboli to guide clinical management of stroke: a cost-effectiveness analysis, *Ann Intern Med* 127(9):775–787, 1997.
9. Johnston DC, Goldstein LB: Clinical carotid endarterectomy decision making: noninvasive vascular imaging versus angiography, *Neurology* 56(8):1009–1015, 2001.
10. Johnston DC, Eastwood JD, Nguyen T, Goldstein LB: Contrast-enhanced magnetic resonance angiography of carotid arteries: utility in routine clinical practice, *Stroke* 33(12):2834–2838, 2002.
11. Josephson SA, Bryant SO, Mak HK, et al: Evaluation of carotid stenosis using CT angiography in the initial evaluation of stroke and TIA, *Neurology* 63(3):457–460, 2004.
12. The National Institute of Neurological Disorders and Stroke rt-PA Stroke Study Group: Tissue plasminogen activator for acute ischemic stroke, *N Engl J Med* 333(24):1581–1587, 1995.
13. Coull BM, Williams LS, Goldstein LB, et al: Anticoagulants and antiplatelet agents in acute ischemic stroke: report of the Joint Stroke Guideline Development Committee of the American Academy of Neurology and the American Stroke Association (a division of the American Heart Association), *Stroke* 33(7):1934–1942, 2002.
14. Adams HP Jr, Adams RJ, Brott T, et al: Guidelines for the early management of patients with ischemic stroke: a scientific statement from the Stroke Council of the American Stroke Association, *Stroke* 34(4):1056–1083, 2003.
15. Langhorne P, Stott DJ, Robertson L, et al: Medical complications after stroke: a multicenter study, *Stroke* 31(6):1223–1229, 2000.
16. Van Peppen RP, Kwakkel G, Wood-Dauphinee S, et al: The impact of physical therapy on functional outcomes after stroke: what's the evidence? *Clin Rehabil* 18(8):833–862, 2004.
17. Barnett HJ, Taylor DW, Eliasziw M, et al: Benefit of carotid endarterectomy in patients with symptomatic moderate or severe stenosis. North American Symptomatic Carotid Endarterectomy Trial Collaborators, *N Engl J Med* 339(20):1415–1425, 1998.
18. Diener HC, Cunha L, Forbes C, et al: European Stroke Prevention Study: 2. dipyridamole and acetylsalicylic acid in the secondary prevention of stroke, *J Neurol Sci* 143(1–2):1–13, 1996.
19. CAPRIE Steering Committee: A randomized, blinded, trial of clopidogrel versus aspirin in patients at risk of ischaemic events (CAPRIE), *Lancet* 348(9038):1329–1339, 1996.
20. Diener HC, Bogousslavsky J, Brass LM, et al: Aspirin and clopidogrel compared with clopidogrel alone after recent ischaemic stroke or transient ischaemic attack in high-risk patients (MATCH): randomised, double-blind, placebo-controlled trial, *Lancet* 364(9431):331–337, 2004.
21. EAFT (European Atrial Fibrillation Trial) Study Group: Secondary prevention in non-rheumatic atrial fibrillation after transient ischaemic attack or minor stroke, *Lancet* 342(8882):1255–1262, 1993.
22. Tanner CM, Aston DA: Epidemiology of Parkinson's disease and akinetic syndromes, *Curr Opin Neurol* 13(4):427–430, 2000.
23. Elbaz A, Bower JH, Maraganore DM, et al: Risk tables for Parkinsonism and Parkinson's disease, *J Clin Epidemiol* 55(1):25–31, 2002.
24. Woo J, Lau E, Ziea E, Chan DK: Prevalence of Parkinson's disease in a Chinese population, *Acta Neurol Scand* 109(3):228–231, 2004.
25. Checkoway H, Powers K, Smith-Weller T, et al: Parkinson's disease risks associated with cigarette smoking, alcohol consumption, and caffeine intake, *Am J Epidemiol* 155(8):732–738, 2002.
26. Sethi KD: Clinical aspects of Parkinson disease, *Curr Opin Neurol* 15(4):457–460, 2002.
27. Becker G, Muller A, Braune S, et al: Early diagnosis of Parkinson's disease, *J Neurol* 249(Suppl 3):III/40–48, 2002.
28. McDonald WM, Richard IH, DeLong MR: Prevalence, etiology, and treatment of depression in Parkinson's disease, *Biol Psychiatry* 54(3):363–375, 2003.
29. Elmer L: Cognitive issues in Parkinson's disease, *Neurol Clin* 22(3 Suppl):S91–S106, 2004.
30. Aarsland D, Andersen K, Larsen JP, et al: Risk of dementia in Parkinson's disease: a community-based, prospective study, *Neurology* 56(6):730–736, 2001.

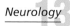
31. Fabbrini G, Barbanti P, Aurilia C, et al: Excessive daytime sleepiness in de novo and treated Parkinson's disease, *Mov Disord* 17(5):1026–1030, 2002.

32. Gagnon JF, Bedard MA, Fantini ML, et al: REM sleep behavior disorder and REM sleep without atonia in Parkinson's disease, *Neurology* 59(4): 585–589, 2002.

33. Araki I, Kitahara M, Oida T, Kuno S: Voiding dysfunction and Parkinson's disease: urodynamic abnormalities and urinary symptoms, *J Urol* 164(5):1640–1643, 2000.

34. Micieli G, Tosi P, Marcheselli S, Cavallini A: Autonomic dysfunction in Parkinson's disease, *Neurol Sci* 24 Suppl 1:S32–S34, 2003.

35. Sakakibara R, Odaka T, Uchiyama T, et al: Colonic transit time and rectoanal videomanometry in Parkinson's disease, *J Neurol Neurosurg Psychiatry* 74(2):268–272, 2003.

36. Jankovic J, Contant C, Perlmutter J: Essential tremor and PD, *Neurology* 43(7):1447–1449, 1993.

37. Jankovic J, Rajput AH, McDermott MP, Perl DP: The evolution of diagnosis in early Parkinson disease: Parkinson Study Group, *Arch Neurol* 57 (3):369–372, 2000.

38. Lang AE, Lozano AM: Parkinson's disease: first of two parts, *N Engl J Med* 339(15):1044–1053, 1998.

39. Yekhlef F, Ballan G, Macia F, et al: Routine MRI for the differential diagnosis of Parkinson's disease, MSA, PSP, and CBD, *J Neural Transm* 110(2): 151–169, 2003.

40. Miyasaki JM, Martin W, Suchowersky O, et al: Practice parameter: initiation of treatment for Parkinson's disease: an evidence-based review: report of the Quality Standards Subcommittee of the American Academy of Neurology, *Neurology* 58 (1):11–17, 2002.

41. Olanow CW, Watts RL, Koller WC: An algorithm (decision tree) for the management of Parkinson's disease (2001): treatment guidelines, *Neurology* 56 (11 Suppl 5):S1–S88, 2001.

42. Lang AE, Lozano AM: Parkinson's disease: second of two parts, *N Engl J Med* 339(16): 1130–1143, 1998.

43. Elbaz A, Bower JH, Peterson BJ, et al: Survival study of Parkinson disease in Olmsted County, Minnesota, *Arch Neurol* 60(1):91–96, 2003.

44. White LR, Cartwright WS, Cornoni-Huntley J, Brock DB: Geriatric epidemiology, *Annu Rev Gerontol Geriatr* 6:215–311, 1986.

45. Ferri CP, Prince M, Brayne C, et al: Global prevalence of dementia: a Delphi consensus study, *Lancet* 366(9503):2112–2117, 2005.

46. Lim A, Tsuang D, Kukull W, et al: Clinico-neuropathological correlation of Alzheimer's disease in a community-based case series, *J Am Geriatr Soc* 47(5):564–569, 1999.

47. Bachman DL, Wolf PA, Linn R, et al: Prevalence of dementia and probable senile dementia of the Alzheimer type in the Framingham Study, *Neurology* 42(1):115–119, 1992.

48. Li G, Silverman JM, Smith CJ, et al: Age at onset and familial risk in Alzheimer's disease, *Am J Psychiatry* 152(3):424–430, 1995.

49. Whitehouse PJ: Pharmacoeconomics of dementia, *Alzheimer Dis Assoc Disord* 11(Suppl 5):S22–S32: discussion S32–S23, 1997.

50. Storandt M, Kaskie B, Von Dras DD: Temporal memory for remote events in healthy aging and dementia, *Psychol Aging* 13(1):4–7, 1998.

51. Knopman DS, DeKosky ST, Cummings JL, et al: Practice parameter: diagnosis of dementia (an evidence-based review). Report of the Quality Standards Subcommittee of the American Academy of Neurology, *Neurology* 56(9):1143–1153, 2001.

52. Jost BC, Grossberg GT: The evolution of psychiatric symptoms in Alzheimer's disease: a natural history study, *J Am Geriatr Soc* 44(9):1078–1081, 1996.

53. Bassiony MM, Lyketsos CG: Delusions and hallucinations in Alzheimer's disease: review of the brain decade, *Psychosomatics* 44(5):388–401, 2003.

54. Galasko D, Hansen LA, Katzman R, et al: Clinical-neuropathological correlations in Alzheimer's disease and related dementias, *Arch Neurol* 51(9): 888–895, 1994.

55. Clarfield AM: The decreasing prevalence of reversible dementias: an updated meta-analysis, *Arch Intern Med* 163(18):2219–2229, 2003.

56. Doody RS, Stevens JC, Beck C, et al: Practice parameter: management of dementia (an evidence-based review). Report of the Quality Standards Subcommittee of the American Academy of Neurology, *Neurology* 56(9):1154–1166, 2001.

57. Reisberg B, Doody R, Stoffler A, et al: Memantine in moderate-to-severe Alzheimer's disease, *N Engl J Med* 348(14):1333–1341, 2003.

58. Sano M, Ernesto C, Thomas RG, et al: A controlled trial of selegiline, alpha-tocopherol, or both as treatment for Alzheimer's disease: the Alzheimer's Disease Cooperative Study, *N Engl J Med* 336 (17):1216–1222, 1997.

59. Alexopolos G, Silver J, Kahn D: *The Expert Consensus Guideline Series: Treatment of Agitation in Dementia. A Postgraduate Medicine Special Report*, Minneapolis, 1998, McGraw-Hill.

60. Larson EB, Shadlen MF, Wang L, et al: Survival after initial diagnosis of Alzheimer disease, *Ann Intern Med* 140(7):501–509, 2004.

61. Shochat T, Pillar G: Sleep apnoea in the older adult: pathophysiology, epidemiology, consequences and management, *Drugs Aging* 20(8): 551–560, 2003.

62. Enright PL NA, Wahl PW, et al: Prevalence and correlates of snoring and observed apneas in 5201 older adults, *Sleep* 19(7):531–538, 1996.

63. Shepard JWJ: *Cardiorespiratory Changes in Obstructive Sleep Apnea*, Philadelphia, 1989, W.B. Saunders.

64. Weiss JW, Launois SH, Anand A, Garpestad E: Cardiovascular morbidity in obstructive sleep apnea, *Prog Cardiovasc Dis* 41(5):367–376, 1999.

65. Shamsuzzaman ASM, Gersh BJ, Somers VK: Obstructive sleep apnea implications for cardiac and vascular disease, *JAMA* 290(14):1906–1914, 2003.

66. Hamilton GS, Solin P, Naughton MT: Obstructive sleep apnoea and cardiovascular disease, *Intern Med J* 34(7):420–426, 2004.

67. Lavie P, Herer P, Hoffstein V: Obstructive sleep apnoea syndrome as a risk factor for hypertension: population study, *BMJ* 320(7233):479–482, 2000.

68. Johns MW: A new method for measuring daytime sleepiness: the Epworth sleepiness scale, *Sleep* 14(6):540–545, 1991.

69. Friedman M, Tanyeri H, La Rosa M, et al: Clinical predictors of obstructive sleep apnea, *Laryngoscope* 109(12):1901–1907, 1999.

70. Rubinstein I, Colapinto N, Rotstein LE, et al: Improvement in upper airway function after weight loss in patients with obstructive sleep apnea, *Am Rev Respir Dis* 138(5):1192–1195, 1988.

71. Cartwright RD: Effect of sleep position on sleep apnea severity, *Sleep* 7(2):110–114, 1984.

72. Oksenberg A, Silverberg DS, Arons E, Radwan H: Positional vs nonpositional obstructive sleep apnea patients: anthropomorphic, nocturnal polysomnographic, and multiple sleep latency test data, *Chest* 112(3):629–639, 1997.

73. Pepin JL, Krieger J, Rodenstein D, et al: Effective compliance during the first 3 months of continuous positive airway pressure: a European prospective study of 121 patients, *Am J Respir Crit Care Med* 160(4):1124–1129, 1999.

74. Kribbs NB, Pack AI, Kline LR, et al: Objective measurement of patterns of nasal CPAP use by patients with obstructive sleep apnea, *Am Rev Respir Dis* 147(4):887–895, 1993.

75. Quinnell TG, Smith IE: Obstructive sleep apnoea in the elderly: recognition and management considerations, *Drugs Aging* 21(5):307–322, 2004.

76. Pillar G SR, Lavie P: Sleep apnea and surgery, *Curr Opin Anesthesiol* 9:536–541, 1996.

77. Powell NB, Riley RW, Robinson A: Surgical management of obstructive sleep apnea syndrome, *Clin Chest Med* 19:77–86, 1998.

78. Riley RW, Powell N, Li KK, et al: *Surgical Therapy for Obstructive Sleep Apnea-Hypopnea Syndrome*, vol 3, Philadelphia, 2000, WB Saunders.

79. Sher A, Gould GA: *Upper Airway Surgery for Obstructive Sleep Apnea*, New York, 2002, Marcel Dekker.

80. Lesage S, Earley CJ: Restless legs syndrome, *Curr Treat Options Neurol* 6(3):209–219, 2004.

81. Lesage S, Hening WA: The restless legs syndrome and periodic limb movement disorder: a review of management, *Semin Neurol* 24(3):249–259, 2004.

82. Rothdach AJ, Trenkwalder C, Haberstock J, et al: Prevalence and risk factors of RLS in an elderly population: the MEMO study. Memory and Morbidity in Augsburg Elderly, *Neurology* 54(5):1064–1068, 2000.

83. Tan EK, Seah A, See SJ, et al: Restless legs syndrome in an Asian population: a study in Singapore, *Mov Disord* 16(3):577–579, 2001.

84. Sevim S, Dogu O, Camdeviren H, et al: Unexpectedly low prevalence and unusual characteristics of RLS in Mersin, Turkey, *Neurology* 61(11):1562–1569, 2003.

85. Krishnan PR, Bhatia M, Behari M: Restless legs syndrome in Parkinson's disease: a case-controlled study, *Mov Disord* 18(2):181–185, 2003.

86. Hening WA, Walters AS, Allen RP, et al: Impact, diagnosis and treatment of restless legs syndrome (RLS) in a primary care population: the REST (RLS epidemiology, symptoms, and treatment) primary care study, *Sleep Med* 5(3):237–246, 2004.

87. Allen RP, Picchietti D, Hening WA, et al: Restless legs syndrome: diagnostic criteria, special considerations, and epidemiology: a report from the restless legs syndrome diagnosis and epidemiology workshop at the National Institutes of Health, *Sleep Med* 4(2):101–119, 2003.

88. Allen RP, Earley CJ: Defining the phenotype of the restless legs syndrome (RLS) using age-of-symptom-onset, *Sleep Med* 1:11–19, 2000.

89. Saletu M, Anderer P, Saletu B, et al: EEG mapping in patients with restless legs syndrome as compared with normal controls, *Psychiatry Res* 115(1–2):49–61, 2002.

90. Berger K, Luedemann J, Trenkwalder C, et al: Sex and the risk of restless legs syndrome in the general population, *Arch Intern Med* 164(2):196–202, 2004.

91. Garcia-Borreguero D, Larrosa O, de la Llave Y: Circadian aspects in the pathophysiology of the restless legs syndrome, *Sleep Med* 3:S17–S21, 2002.

92. Earley CJ, Allen RP, Beard JL, Connor JR: Insight into the pathophysiology of restless legs syndrome, *J Neurosci Res* 62(5):623–628, 2000.

93. Earley CJ, Connors JR, Allen RP: RLS patients have abnormally reduced CSF ferritin compared to normal controls, *Neurology* 52(Suppl 2):A111–A112, 1999.

94. Hui DS, Wong TY, Ko FW, et al: Prevalence of sleep disturbances in Chinese patients with end-stage renal failure on continuous ambulatory peritoneal dialysis, *Am J Kidney Dis* 36(4):783–788, 2000.

95. Hui D, Wong T, Li T, et al: Prevalence of sleep disturbances in Chinese patients with end stage renal failure on maintenance hemodialysis, *Med Sci Monit* 8(5):CR331–CR336, 2002.

96. Ondo WG, Vuong KD, Jankovic J: Exploring the relationship between Parkinson disease and restless legs syndrome, *Arch Neurol* 59(3):421–424, 2002.

97. Abele M, Burk K, Laccone F, et al: Restless legs syndrome in spinocerebellar ataxia types 1, 2, and 3, *J Neurol* 248(4):311–314, 2001.

98. Schols L, Haan J, Riess O, et al: Sleep disturbance in spinocerebellar ataxias: is the SCA3 mutation a cause of restless legs syndrome? *Neurology* 51(6):1603–1607, 1998.

99. Banno K, Delaive K, Walld R, Kryger MH: Restless legs syndrome in 218 patients: associated disorders, *Sleep Med* 1(3):221–229, 2000.

100. Agargun MY, Kara H, Ozbek H, et al: Restless legs syndrome induced by mirtazapine, *J Clin Psychiatry* 63(12):1179, 2002.

101. Bakshi R: Fluoxetine and restless legs syndrome, *J Neurol Sci* 142(1–2):151–152, 1996.

102. Hargrave R, Beckley DJ: Restless leg syndrome exacerbated by sertraline, *Psychosomatics* 39(2): 177–178, 1998.

103. Sanz-Fuentenebro FJ, Huidobro A, Tejadas-Rivas A: Restless legs syndrome and paroxetine, *Acta Psychiatr Scand* 94(6):482–484, 1996.

104. Chesson AL Jr, Ferber RA, Fry JM, et al: The indications for polysomnography and related procedures, *Sleep* 20(6):423–487, 1997.

105. Littner M, Hirshkowitz M, Kramer M, et al: Practice parameters for using polysomnography to evaluate insomnia: an update, *Sleep* 26(6):754–760, 2003.

106. Sadrzadeh SM, Saffari Y: Iron and brain disorders, *Am J Clin Pathol* 121:S64–S70, 2004.

107. Sun ER, Chen CA, Ho G, et al: Iron and the restless legs syndrome, *Sleep* 21(4):371–377, 1998.

108. Akyol A, Kiylioglu N, Kadikoylu G, et al: Iron deficiency anemia and restless legs syndrome: is there an electrophysiological abnormality? *Clin Neurol Neurosurg* 106(1):23–27, 2003.

109. Berger K, von Eckardstein A, Trenkwalder C, et al: Iron metabolism and the risk of restless legs syndrome in an elderly general population—the MEMO-Study, *J Neurol* 249(9):1195–1199, 2002.

110. Krieger J, Schroeder C: Iron, brain and restless legs syndrome, *Sleep Med Rev* 5(4):277–286, 2001.

111. Haba-Rubio J, Staner L, Petiau C, et al: Restless legs syndrome and low brain iron levels in patients with haemochromatosis, *J Neurol Neurosurg Psychiatry* 76(7):1009–1010, 2005.

112. O'Keeffe ST, Gavin K, Lavan JN: Iron status and restless legs syndrome in the elderly, *Age Ageing* 23(3):200–203, 1994.

113. Silber MH, Girish M, Izurieta R: Pramipexole in the management of restless legs syndrome: an extended study, *Sleep* 26(7):819–821, 2003.

114. Mitler MM, Browman CP, Menn SJ, et al: Nocturnal myoclonus: treatment efficacy of clonazepam and temazepam, *Sleep* 9:385–392, 1986.

115. Kaplan P, Allen RP, Buchholz DW, Walters JK: A double-blind, placebo-controlled study of the treatment of periodic limb movements in sleep using carbidopa/levodopa and propoxyphene, *Sleep* 16(8):717–723, 1993.

116. Hening W, Allen R, Earley C, et al: The treatment of restless legs syndrome and periodic limb movement disorder: an American Academy of Sleep Medicine review, *Sleep* 22(7):970–999, 1999.

117. Hening WA, Allen RP, Earley CJ, et al: An update on the dopaminergic treatment of restless legs syndrome and periodic limb movement disorder: an American Academy of Sleep Medicine Interim Review, *Sleep* 27:560–583, 2004.

118. Allen RP, Earley CJ: Augmentation of the restless legs syndrome with carbidopa/levodopa, *Sleep* 19(3):205–213, 1996.

119. Garcia-Borreguero D, Larrosa O, de la Llave Y, et al: Treatment of restless legs syndrome with gabapentin: a double-blind, cross-over study, *Neurology* 59(10):1573–1579, 2002.

120. Kavey N, Walters AS, Hening W, Gidro-Frank S: Opioid treatment of periodic movements in sleep in patients without restless legs, *Neuropeptides* 11(4):181–184, 1988.

121. Ford DE, Kamerow DB: Epidemiologic study of sleep disturbance and psychiatric disorders: an opportunity for prevention? *JAMA* 262(11): 1479–1484, 1989.

122. Ohayon MM, Roth T: What are the contributing factors for insomnia in the general population? *J Psychosom Res* 51(6):745–755, 2001.

123. Ancoli-Israel S, Roth T: Characteristics of insomnia in the United States: results of the 1991 National Sleep Foundation Survey, *Sleep* 22(Suppl 2): S347–S353, 1999.

124. Shochat T, Umphress J, Israel AG, Ancoli-Israel S: Insomnia in primary care patients, *Sleep* 22(Suppl 2):S359–S365, 1999.

125. Klink ME, Quan SF, Kaltenborn WT, Lebowitz MD: Risk factors associated with complaints of insomnia in a general adult population: influence of previous complaints of insomnia, *Arch Intern Med* 152(8):1634–1637, 1992.

126. Miles L, Dement WC: Sleep & aging, *Sleep* 3: 119–220, 1980.

127. Sukying C, Bhokakul V, Udomsubpayakul U: An epidemiological study on insomnia in an elderly Thai population, *J Med Assoc Thai* 86(4):316–324, 2003.

128. Foley DJ, Monjan AA, Brown SL, et al: Sleep complaints among elderly persons: an epidemiologic study of three communities, *Sleep* 18(6):425–432, 1995.

129. Benca RM, Obermeyer WH, Thisted RA, Gillin JC: Sleep and psychiatric disorders: a meta-analysis, *Arch Gen Psychiatry* 49:651–668, 1992.

130. Hohagen F, Kappler C, Schramm E, et al: Sleep onset insomnia, sleep maintaining insomnia and insomnia with early morning awakening—temporal stability of subtypes in a longitudinal study on general practice attenders, *Sleep* 17(6): 551–554, 1994.

131. Ohayon MM: Epidemiology of insomnia: what we know and what we still need to learn, *Sleep Med Rev* 6(2):97–111, 2002.

132. National Institutes of Health State of the Science Conference statement on manifestations and management of chronic insomnia in adults, June 13–15, 2005, *Sleep,* 28(9):1049–1057, 2005.

133. Lichstein KL, Durrence HH, Taylor DJ, et al: Quantitative criteria for insomnia, *Behav Res Ther* 41 (4):427–445, 2003.

134. Gillin JC, Byerley WF: The diagnosis and management of insomnia, *N Engl J Med* 322:239–248, 1990.

135. Edinger JD, Hoelscher TJ, Webb MD, et al: Polysomnographic assessment of DIMS: empirical evaluation of its diagnostic value, *Sleep* 12(4):315–322, 1989.

136. Lichstein KL, Reidel BW: Behavioral assessment and treatment of insomnia: a review with an emphasis on clinical application, *Behav Ther* 15:659–688, 1994.

137. Reynolds CFI: *Sleep in Affective Disorders,* Philadelphia, 1989, Saunders.

138. Benca RM, Obermeyer WH, Thisted RA, Gillin JCSleep and psychiatric disorders: a meta-analysis, *Arch Gen Psychiatry* 49(8):651–668; discussion 669–670, 1992.

139. Espie CA: *The Psychological Treatment of Insomnia,* Chichester, UK, 1991, John Wiley.

140. Gillin JC, Ancoli-Israel S: *The Impact of Age on Sleep and Sleep Disorders,* Baltimore, MD, 1992, Williams & Wilkins.

141. Hauri PJ, Wisbey J: Wrist actigraphy in insomnia, *Sleep* 15(4):293–301, 1992.

142. Morin CM, Hauri PJ, Espie CA, et al: Nonpharmacologic treatment of chronic insomnia. An American Academy of Sleep Medicine review, *Sleep* 22(8):1134–1156, 1999.

143. Spielman AJ, Saskin P, Thorpy MJ: Treatment of chronic insomnia by restriction of time in bed, *Sleep* 10:45–56, 1987.

144. Åkerstedt T, Torsvall L: Shiftwork: shift dependent well being and individual differences, *Ergonomics* 24:265–273, 1981.

145. Harma M, Hakola T, Åkerstedt T, Laitinen J: Age and adjustment to night work, *Occup Environ Med* 51:568–573, 1994.

146. Folkard S, Monk T, Lobban M: Short and long-term adjustment of circadian rhythms in 'permanent' night nurses, *Ergonomics* 21:785–799, 1978.

147. Paik IH, Lee C, Choi BM, et al: Mianserin-induced restless legs syndrome, *Br J Psychiatry* 155:415–417, 1989.

148. Burgess HJ, Sharkey KM, Eastman CI: Bright light, dark and melatonin can promote circadian adaptation in night shift workers, *Sleep Med Rev* 6(5): 407–420, 2002.

149. Campbell SS, Dawson D: Bright light treatment of sleep disturbance in older subjects, *Sleep Res* 20:448, 1991.

150. Dawson D, Encel N, Lushington K: Improving adaptation to simulated night shift: timed exposure to bright light versus daytime melatonin administration, *Sleep* 18(1):11–21, 1995.

151. Sharkey KM, Fogg LF, Eastman CI: Effects of melatonin administration on daytime sleep after simulated night shift work, *J Sleep Res* 10(3): 181–192, 2001.

152. Baehr EK, Fogg LF, Eastman CI: Intermittent bright light and exercise to entrain human circadian rhythms to night work, *Am J Physiol* 277(6 Pt 2): R1598–R1604, 1999.

153. Boivin DB, James FO: Circadian adaptation to night-shift work by judicious light and darkness exposure, *J Biol Rhythms* 17(6):556–567, 2002.

154. Campbell SS, Terman M, Lewy A, et al: Light treatment for sleep disorders: consensus report. V. age-related disturbances, *J Biol Rhythms* 10(2):151–154, 1995.

155. Akerstedt T, Ficca G: Alertness-enhancing drugs as a countermeasure to fatigue in irregular work hours, *Chronobiol Int* 14(2):145–158, 1997.

156. Lavidor M, Libman E, Babkoff H, et al: Good and poor sleepers in an aged population, *Sleep* 21(S3): 269, 1998.

157. Burgess HJ, Crowley SJ, Gazda CJ, et al: Preflight adjustment to eastward travel: 3 days of advancing sleep with and without morning bright light, *J Biol Rhythms* 18(4):318–328, 2003.

158. Beaumont M, Batejat D, Pierard C, et al: Caffeine or melatonin effects on sleep and sleepiness after rapid eastward transmeridian travel, *J Appl Physiol* 96(1):50–58, 2004.

159. Herxheimer A, Waterhouse J: The prevention and treatment of jet lag, *BMJ* 326(7384):296–297, 2003.

160. Jamieson AO, Zammit GK, Rosenberg RS, et al: Zolpidem reduces the sleep disturbance of jet lag, *Sleep Med* 2(5):423–430, 2001.

161. Waterhouse J, Reilly T, Atkinson G: Jet-lag. *Lancet* 350(9091):1611–1616, 1997.

162. Daan S, Lewy AJ: Scheduled exposure to daylight: a potential strategy to reduce "jet lag" following transmeridian flight, *Psychopharmacol Bull* 20(3): 566–568, 1984.

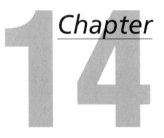

Oral Health

Samuel Zwetchkenbaum, DDS, MPH, and L. Susan Taichman, RDH, MPH, PhD

Key Points

- Many systemic medications have been shown to have important oral health implications and have been associated with oral tissue complications (strength of recommendation: B).
- The recognition and treatment of periodontal disease may be important due to the possible association with systemic conditions such as diabetes, cardiovascular diseases, and stroke (strength of recommendation: B).
- The effects on oral health and the economic impact of altering the recall interval between dental checkups (i.e., the time period between one dental checkup and the next) are unclear; dental examinations are recommended annually if there is no significant disease and more frequently if the patient is prone to dental disease (strength of recommendation: C).
- Currently, no acceptable studies exist to provide evidence to support the efficacy of early oral cancer detection programs, yet routine evaluation is recommended in high-risk patients (strength of recommendation: C).

Introduction

Abnormalities in oral health can significantly affect the general health of the male patient because many systemic diseases exhibit their

The authors thank Russell Taichman, DMD, DMSc, for his assistance in preparation of this chapter.

clinical signs in the tissues and dentition of the oral cavity. Epidemiologic research has delineated associations between oral infections and systemic conditions including diabetes mellitus, respiratory infections, and cardiovascular, autoimmune, and gastrointestinal diseases. Adult males are more likely than women to develop oral cancer and use alcohol and tobacco products, yet they are less likely to seek preventive dental care services.[1] Furthermore, with the dramatic increase in the use of medications that can potentially affect the oral environment, and the knowledge that many of the effects of oral disease are cumulative, additional burden has been placed on healthcare providers for early identification of oral diseases.

Standard medical school education includes only minimal discussion of the oral cavity and dentition, often limited to basic information such as the various types and numbers of infant and adult teeth. Often overlooked are the normal physiologic variations of dentition, both developmental and acquired, and how to distinguish normal from pathologic conditions. Including an oral and dental examination as part of the office- or hospital-based history and physical examination can provide insight into the overall health of an individual patient and can occasionally help to solve mysteries. Hospital-based dental programs receive consultations daily to assess the dentition as a potential source of infection, but it is a small percentage of medical centers that have dentistry programs or even dentists on staff. Requesting a consultation from a dentist outside the hospital may be challenging, but when recognized as part of the overall care, should be pursued.

For the primary care clinician, the recognition of salient signs and symptoms of oral diseases, as well as the identification of systemic disorders and conditions, may assist in the early diagnosis and prompt referral for appropriate specialist treatment. Since many of the most common oral diseases including periodontal disease and caries are largely preventable, disease detection and prevention needs to be established as a high priority by the medical community. The effects on oral health and their economic impact are unclear; nonetheless, dental examinations are recommended annually if there is no significant disease and more frequently if the patient is prone to dental disease.[2] The goal of this chapter is to provide clinicians with an increased knowledge of the signs and symptoms of common oral conditions and the possible links between oral and systemic health for their male patients.

Overview of Dentition

The Normal Dentition

The *enamel* is the hard outer substance of the tooth and should not demonstrate significant breaks of its integrity. Exposure of underlying dentin can occur for a number of reasons, some physiologic, and some pathologic. Physiologic exposure of dentin may occur through tooth wear against another tooth or substance or erosion typically from a chemical (e.g., stomach acid in the case of gastroesophageal reflux disease). This process usually takes long enough that the odontoblasts of the tooth have built up reparative dentin and sensitivity rarely occurs. Notching in the cervical portion or neck of the tooth can result in great sensitivity. The cause of these lesions can either be via abfraction (i.e., the chipping of tooth structure) or abrasion, caused by mechanical contact such as aggressive toothbrushing. Although the nature of these lesions is still not fully understood, in clinical practice they seem to occur in males more frequently.

Restored Dentition

Dental caries is the most ubiquitous infectious process in man, so it is not surprising that most people have had their teeth restored to some degree. The molars are the most commonly restored teeth; however, a Cochrane review[3] found that preventive measures including fluoride supplementation via toothpaste and mouthwash rinses as well as occlusal sealants have significantly reduced the rate of decay. Materials that are used today differ from those used 50 years ago, so the restored dentition of an older patient may appear significantly different than that of a younger person. Use of gold with acrylic resin facings, silicates, and silver amalgam typically look less tooth-like and discolor easily—to the unfamiliar eye, these may appear more like a disease process than treatment of disease. Current practice produces restorations that would challenge even the most trained eye in detection. Stain and discoloration take away from the youthful appearance of the teeth, yet they are not pathologic and are commonly the result of cigarette smoke, coffee, wine, and other foods that contain darkly pigmented staining chemicals. Staining can increase the roughness of the teeth, making plaque more retentive and accelerating periodontal disease.

Dental Caries

Although still considered the infection of mankind with the highest prevalence, dental caries is significantly less likely to occur in a young man coming of age in the 21st century than in his father. *Smooth surface caries,* those occurring on the cheek side or between the teeth, have reduced significantly in number due to the widespread use of systemic fluoride. *Pit* and *fissure caries,* or those occurring in the grooves of the teeth, have experienced reduction thanks to the use of occlusal sealants, which are composed of an unfilled composite resin that dentists or hygienists can place on an eruption of the tooth. Thus, the norm for adolescent and adult men should be little to no tooth decay.

Where there is significant decay, one must take a close look at the underlying cause. A number of conditions lead to *xerostomia,* or decreased salivation, and it is common to see rampant caries on the teeth of patients who are undergoing radiation therapy, who are taking psychiatric medications, or who have Sjögren's syndrome. Significant consumption of sugar-containing carbonated beverages can also result in a large number of teeth experiencing decay (Figure 14-1).

A more recently described pattern of decay has been reported on the teeth of users of methamphetamine, commonly referred to as "meth mouth." This decay is noted on the buccal surfaces of the teeth near the gum line and can wrap around the tooth, resulting in amputation of the crown. The rampant caries associated with methamphetamine use is attributed to the acidic nature of the drug, the drug's xerostomic effect, its propensity to cause cravings for high-calorie carbonated beverages, tooth grinding and

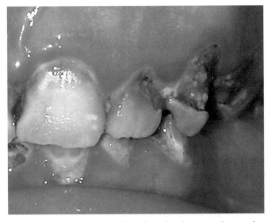

Figure 14-1. Advanced dental caries in a patient who reports daily consumption of a 2-liter bottle of Mountain Dew. (Photograph courtesy of Kathryn Thornton, DDS.)

clenching, and its long duration of action leading to extended periods of poor oral hygiene.[4-6]

Although advanced caries are easy to diagnose, detection of early caries and knowing when to restore them is a matter of great controversy and lacks acceptable standards of evidence. The emergence of expensive high-technology equipment including laser-assisted tooth preparation and computer-aided design/computer-aided manufacturing milling of restorations may contribute to supplier-induced demand for these procedures. The presence of dental insurance often hides the cost of such procedures from patients.

Dental Trauma

Contact sporting activities (e.g., hockey, basketball, football, baseball) and non-sporting activities (e.g., falls, accidents, altercations) can result in dental trauma. Trauma may result in the displacement of teeth, defined as *luxation* (i.e., tooth displacement) and *avulsion* (i.e., completely displaced or knocked out of the dental socket), as well as fractures. Tooth fractures are categorized by the layer of tooth exposed (e.g., enamel, dentin or pulp) and the level (e.g., coronal or root). Ellis class I fractures consist of an enamel-only fracture and can be treated by either smoothing the tooth or simple restoration with a composite resin restoration. Ellis Class II fractures indicate exposure of underlying dentin, likely result in sensitivity to air, and may be simply covered. An Ellis class III fracture results in exposure of the pulp, and often root canal therapy is required. The use of protective mouthguards is encouraged by both professional and amateur sporting organizations to reduce the risk of trauma to the teeth during contact sports, yet a systematic review examining the use of mouthguards in contact sports found insufficient evidence to support their widespread use.[7]

Although early attention is important in tooth fractures to assist in pain control and to prevent microbial invasion of the pulp, it is the luxation or avulsion injury for which immediate attention can affect the long-term prognosis of the tooth. The avulsed tooth can be stored in milk, saliva, or in a Hank's balanced solution (e.g., Save-a-Tooth Emergency Kit [Phoenix-Lazerus, Inc., Pottstown, PA]). Early access to a dentist within 1 hour of injury should be expedited to ensure proper reimplantation and splinting. In some cases, root canal therapy within 1 week is necessary to maintain viability of the damaged tooth. Luxation injuries are treated in a similar fashion. Fractures in the enamel or dentin are typically not urgent and can be followed up in the coming days by a dentist. Fractures into the pulp require early access to a dentist for coverage, or possible root canal or extraction.[8]

Oral Cancer

Approximately 30,000 new cases of oral cancer are diagnosed in the United States every year, and prognosis is closely related to the stage of disease at the time of detection. In 2006, it was estimated that oral cancers accounted for 3% of total cancers in men and 2% in women, with African American men having almost double the cancer death risk (7.1 compared with 3.9).[9] A male's lifetime probability of developing a cancer of the oral cavity is estimated to be 1 in 73.[9] Aggressive treatment is needed for advanced disease, including surgery, chemotherapy, and radiation therapy, and these can greatly affect quality of life. The high-risk patient population includes users of tobacco as well as heavy alcohol, a population that is less likely to seek regular dental visits. Currently, only 13% of adult men older than 40 years report having had an oral and pharyngeal examination to detect cancer within the past year.[7] This places increasing importance on physicians to include an oral examination as a part of their routine annual health maintenance examination, which should include visual inspection of the buccal mucosa, the floor of mouth, the tongue, and palate, and palpation of submandibular glands and cervical lymph nodes. Patients with suspicious lesions should be promptly referred to either an oral surgeon for further evaluation including possible toluidine blue staining or biopsy of any suspicious lesions. The brush-biopsy technique is showing increasing acceptability among dentists for early cytologic evaluation of potential malignant disease.

Periodontal Diseases

The Periodontium

The *periodontium* is defined as the tissues that surround and support the teeth (Figure 14-2) and comprises the following:

- *The gingival tissues* (or gingiva, frequently called *gums* in laypersons' terms) are the soft tissues that cover the alveolar bone of the jaws and the teeth up to the exposed crown of the teeth. In good health, the gingiva are generally pale pink and firm with a stippled surface texture, although considerable heterogeneity exists among individuals based on skin pigmentation and ethnicity. The *interdental gingival* lays between the teeth and typically fills the embrasures between the teeth, functioning to deflect food away from these areas. Between the anterior teeth, the gingiva are typically wedge-shaped, and in the posterior teeth they assume a saddle-shaped configuration. Further away from the crowns, the gingival epithelium is heavily keratinized and attached to the underlying structures including the hard palate termed *attached* or *keratinized gingival* tissue. These tissues transition sharply into a non-keratinized epithelium covering the cheeks, floor of the mouth and posterior pharynx and are termed *alveolar mucosa*.

- *The gingival crevice* (a cuff-like space between the gingiva and the teeth) is a blinded cul-de-sac. This area is bounded laterally on the tooth side by a specialized epithelium called the *sulcular epithelium*. The sulcular epithelium transitions into a tissue termed *junctional epithelium* that is positioned at the base of the crevice. In health, it is thought that through an active desquamation process of epithelial cells the underlying tissues are protected from bacterial invasion.

- The root surface is called the *cementum*.

- Connective tissue attachments are present between the alveolar bone and cementum.

- *Alveolar bone* is attached to the teeth through the periodontal ligament fibers, which form the tooth socket. The crest of the alveolar supporting bone, often viewed on typical dental radiographs, is approximately 2 mm below the point where the enamel of the crown of the tooth meets the root cementum (the *cementoenamel junction*).[10]

Periodontal Disease

The generic term *periodontal disease* refers to a variety of clinical manifestations characterized by the inflammatory process of the tooth's

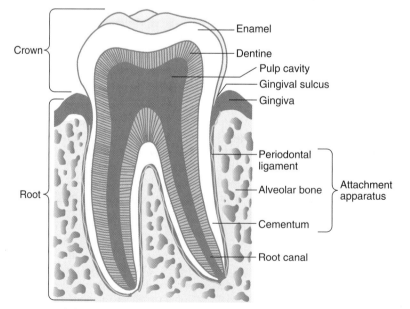

Figure 14-2. Cross-section of the periodontium in health. (Marx J, Hockberger R, Walls R: *Rosen's Emergency Medicine: Concepts and Clinical Practice*, ed 6, St. Louis, MO, 2006, Mosby.)

supporting structures. Periodontal diseases are generally divided into two groups:

- *Gingivitis*, or inflammation affecting the gums.
- *Periodontitis*, or inflammation and damage of the bone and connective tissue that supports the teeth.

Epidemiology

More than 70% of adults have some form of periodontal disease,[11] most typically composed of gingivitis. Research has demonstrated that nearly one in three US adults aged 30–54 years and 50% of adults aged 55–90 years have some form of periodontitis. In males, the incidence ranges from 34% to 56% in these age categories and from 23% to 44% in women, highlighting that periodontitis is more prevalent in males than females.[12] Research has also shown that, among adults, males are at a higher risk of developing chronic periodontitis with advanced periodontal destruction than females.[13–15] Present knowledge regarding the pathogenesis of periodontal disease indicates that there are no inherent differences between men and women in their genetic susceptibility to periodontitis. Most existing data suggest the differences between genders may be related to poorer oral hygiene practices, less positive attitudes toward oral health, and decreased use of professional dental services. Typically, women perform better oral hygiene measures and use professional dental services more frequently.[13]

Gingivitis

Gingivitis is an inflammatory response of the gingival tissues to the metabolic products and pathogenic toxins of bacteria found in oral plaque. Plaque-associated gingivitis most commonly presents as erythematous, edematous tissue that halos the teeth (Figure 14-3). Patients may present with reports of gingival bleeding on tissue manipulation, such as during a dental examination or routine tooth brushing.

The primary risk factor for gingivitis is bacterial plaque resulting from poor oral hygiene. Supra- and subgingival removal of plaque eliminates the inflammatory response and, in most cases, the gingival lesions will heal with a full restoration of tissue form and function. Although gingivitis does not always progress to periodontitis, periodontitis is always preceded by gingivitis.[16,17]

Periodontitis

Periodontitis is the destruction of the supporting structures housing the tooth. If a sufficiently large amount of supporting bone and ligamentous attachment is lost, then the patient may present with a chief symptom of tooth migration or movement, loose teeth, and even tooth loss. The transition from gingivitis to periodontal disease with the associated loss of the connective tissue attachment usually goes undetected. Since periodontitis is generally not painful, it may display few, if any, outward signs initially.

Chronic periodontitis, formerly referred to as *adult periodontitis*, is the most commonly occurring form of periodontitis in men older than 35–44 years.[18] The term *chronic* indicates that the disease progresses slowly and results in the progressive destruction of the supporting tissues of the tooth (i.e., periodontal ligament and alveolar bone) from the margins of the gingiva toward the apices of the roots of the teeth (Figure 14-4). Although the cumulative effects of the disease make it appear chronic in nature, the disease may occur as a series of acute episodes separated by quiescent periods of indeterminate duration. Periodontitis is not a natural consequence of the

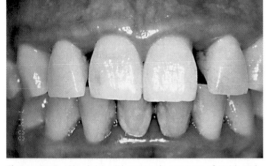

Figure 14-3. Gingivitis. (Photograph courtesy of Keith Kirkwood, DDS, PhD.)

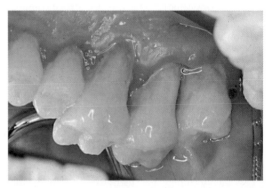

Figure 14-4. Severe periodontitis. (Photograph courtesy of Russell Taichman, DMD, DMSc.)

aging process[19]; however, as repeated bouts with the disease results in cumulative damage and loss of tooth support, it is most frequently detected in middle-aged to older persons. Research indicates that chronic periodontitis in elderly persons is characterized by slow progression and usually does not lead to tooth loss. In cases in which periodontitis is reported as a leading cause of tooth loss in the elderly, it is most likely that the majority of teeth extracted have been seriously diseased for many years, rather than becoming diseased during old age.[20]

A smaller percentage of the population, estimated at 5–15%, are afflicted with generalized aggressive periodontitis that rapidly results in the loss of connective tissue support for the teeth.[11,18] Such aggressive forms of periodontal disease are generally found in circumpubertal adolescents and young adults, yet it is important to note that older persons are not immune from these forms of disease. Most typically, aggressive periodontitis is localized to one or several teeth but may also be more widespread to be characterized as "generalized." As with the "chronic," or the most typical form of periodontal disease, the etiology is due to plaque-derived organisms but are also more frequently found in persons with an altered host resistance to the infections.[21]

Clinical Presentation and Diagnosis

Typical symptoms of periodontal disease include swelling, erythema, bleeding, and recession of gingival tissue (see Figure 14-3). The gums may bleed during brushing, but the teeth are usually not mobile[22]; tooth mobility and pain are often seen in the later stages.[23] Many patients have periodontal inflammation without being aware of any changes in their teeth or gums. By the time these symptoms are present, treatment alternatives are often limited. Therefore, it is imperative for the clinician to look for signs of and symptoms of periodontal disease in asymptomatic patients during the examination of the oral cavity and refer them appropriately and expeditiously for evaluation and treatment.

In cases of severe periodontal disease, more than 30% of the attachment apparatus is lost, and the gingiva is receded, exposing the roots of the teeth (see Figure 14-4). The interdental papillae are often absent, and the gingivae are swollen, red, and boggy in character. Large amounts of calculus and food debris are present along the gum line. The teeth are mobile and the gums bleed easily when the teeth are brushed; the patient may report having "sensitive teeth." Halitosis is a common presentation associated with periodontal disease. Suppurative material may exude from the periodontal pocket, which is often considered a sign that the infection has undergone a transition to a more active stage. Gingival and periodontal abscesses are frequently caused by infections within the tooth pulp and occur in some patients with long-standing periodontal conditions, usually occurring when the entrance to the gingival crevice becomes occluded, limiting the outward flow of the fluids from the gingiva into the oral cavity. These acute and exacerbated conditions are often best treated by obtaining an accurate differential diagnosis and by instituting broad-spectrum antibiotics and immediate tissue debridement.[22]

Etiologies

Bacterial Plaque. Both gingivitis and periodontitis are the result of a complex interaction between pathogenic bacteria, host response, and systemic and local risk factors. Typically there are 300–500 specific species of microorganisms inhabiting the oral cavity at any one time.[24] Both gingivitis and chronic periodontitis are believed to be caused by gram-negative bacteria in the dental plaque that lie in close proximity to the necks of the teeth and marginal gingival tissues, namely *Porphyromonas gingivalis*, *Prevotella intermedia*, *Bacteroides forsythus*, and *Campylobacter rectus*.[25] Thus, subgingival plaque found within the gingival crevice or the sulcus around the necks of the teeth is thought to house the etiologic agent(s).[26]

There is some evidence that the causative agents in the more aggressive forms of periodontitis may differ from those associated with gingivitis or chronic periodontitis. In the condition known as *localized aggressive periodontitis*, the small capnophilic (carbon dioxide–requiring) gram-negative rod *Actinobacillus actinomycetemcomitans* has been implicated.[27,28]

Tobacco Use. Epidemiologic and clinical studies have shown that smokers have a two- to six-fold greater risk of developing periodontal disease than nonsmokers, depending on the criteria used to define periodontal disease.[29] The risk of periodontal disease appears to increase with the number of cigarettes smoked per day as well as duration of pack-years.[30–32] Although a clear relationship exists between smokeless tobacco and oral carcinoma,[33,34] a definitive relationship between smokeless tobacco and generalized periodontitis has not been demonstrated.

The exact mechanism that places smokers at greater risk for periodontal diseases remains unclear.[35] Most evidence points to local and possibly systemic alterations in granulocyte function. Studies have demonstrated that smoking and nicotine increase the inflammation possibly by reducing oxygen in the gingival tissue and by triggering an overproduction of cytokines, which lead to destruction of the cells and tissues. Periodontal therapy, both surgical and nonsurgical, is less likely to be effective in smokers as well as increased risk of dental implant failure. In addition, periodontal disease is more likely to recur than in nonsmokers.

Genetics. Current evidence suggests that severe forms of periodontal disease (i.e., aggressive periodontitis) have a strong genetic component. Rare syndromes that affect neutrophil function, leukocyte adhesion deficiencies, as well as other inherited phagocyte disorders including collagen and enzyme defects, can produce periodontal manifestations. In chronic periodontitis, evidence for a genetic component has been demonstrated in data on concordant twins suggesting that half of population variance for periodontitis may be due to genetic factors.[36,37] Increasing evidence indicates that a combination of two polymorphisms in the interleukin-1 gene is associated with susceptibility to chronic periodontitis.[38,39] Although there is little doubt that periodontitis has a genetic component, insufficient evidence exists to warrant the widespread use of genetic testing to assess for risk of development of periodontal disease.

Compromised Host Defense. Almost any alteration of the adaptive or innate immune responses, or any condition that impedes normal tissue turnover, is thought to place persons at a greater risk for periodontal disease. Recent attention has focused on human immunodeficiency virus (HIV) and acquired immunodeficiency syndrome (AIDS)-associated periodontal conditions, but nearly any process that alters tissue metabolism including stress, trauma, endocrine alterations, and hematologic dyscrasias may result in periodontal diseases that can be exacerbated by the systemic conditions. Particular attention by primary care physicians should be directed in consideration that any limitation of the ability to fight infection or during the repair process might result in more severe forms of periodontal disease. Dental care is indicated for these patients to prevent and treat intra-oral infections, restore dental function, and improve quality of life.[40]

Treatment. The role of the primary care physician in treating periodontal disease consists chiefly of diagnosis and referral of the symptomatic or asymptomatic patient for treatment. Mild periodontal diseases are typically treated by a general dentist; patients with severe forms of the disease are often best referred to a periodontist. Treatment of periodontal disease includes a wide range of modalities including patient education and care instructions, scaling, root planing, surgery, local and systemic antibiotic therapies, and occlusal adjustment.

Prevention of Periodontal Diseases

Prevention is the cornerstone of treatment of periodontal disease and it begins with patient education. Patients should be informed about the causes, treatment and methods used to prevent periodontal disease (Table 14-1). The American Dental Association and the American Dental Hygienists' Association have a variety of patient education materials that are readily accessible, and many local and state organizations are suitable providers for high-quality educational materials, as well.[41,42]

Periodic examinations to screen for periodontal diseases and oral health conditions should be a high priority among healthcare professionals. The timing of these visits depends on whether disease is present and whether the patient complies with care instructions. Physicians can aid in primary prevention by reviewing with their patients the need for good oral hygiene and periodic dental examinations. Physicians may also play an important role in prevention by looking for signs of periodontal disease when they examine the oral cavity because early diagnosis and treatment can significantly reduce the morbidity associated with periodontal disease. Although the common recommendation for dental recall visits is every 6 months, the systematic review by Beirne and others[2] found no evidence to support this traditional recall schedule. As noted previously, adult males have a higher prevalence of periodontal disease, most likely the result of poor oral home care and lower dental care utilization. At the present time, there is no literature to support an increased routine dental recall for adolescent or adult males.

Gingival Recession

Gingival recession is the apical migration of the marginal tissue from the crown of the tooth resulting from destructive periodontal disease, periodontal surgery, or trauma from forceful tooth brushing exposing the underlying root surface.[10] It may also be the result of periodontal treatment in which regenerative therapies were

Table 14-1. Preventive Strategies Against Periodontal Disease

Preventive Action	Mechanism	Effectiveness	Recommendation
Toothbrushing[123–126]	Prevents the accumulation of plaque and disrupts the bacterial colonies on teeth and in the gingival crevice	Toothbrushing is effective in preventing gingivitis. Brushing may prevent periodontitis.	Brush 2–3 times a day. Use a soft-bristle toothbrush.
Flossing[124,127]	Prevents the accumulation of plaque and disrupts the bacterial colonies on teeth and in the gingival crevice	Flossing is effective in preventing gingivitis. Flossing may prevent periodontitis.	Floss daily using waxed or unwaxed floss. Floss aids may help persons who have difficulty with the mechanics of flossing.
Use of oral rinses as adjunct to toothbrushing (e.g., over-the-counter Listerine oral rinse[130,131] prescription CHX [Peridex])[128,129]	These mouthrinse contain a mixture of phenolic compounds with bactericidal properties and anti-inflammatory effects. Peridex is a 0.12% solution of CHX, a bis-biguanide antiseptic	More effective on gingivitis than dental plaque reduction Effective in reducing gingivitis	
Toothbrushing with anticalculus toothpaste[132]	Various anticalculous agents containing crystal growth inhibitors which prevent the development of mineralized plaque	Effective in reducing supragingival calculus	No evidence to recommend to general population; may benefit patients who are at high risk of calculus development

OTC, Over the counter; CHX, chlorhexidine.

not effective. The exposed root surfaces are often of concern due to enhanced risk of carious lesions and reduced esthetics. Gingival recession is associated with age, yet this association does not reflect a physiologic effect but rather a cumulative effect of toothbrush trauma for longer periods of time.[43]

Presentation

Patients may report gingival recession accompanied by dentinal hypersensitivity consisting of a transient sharp pain with varying levels of intensity. It has been estimated that approximately 50% of the general population complains of acute or chronic dentinal hypersensitivity, with the highest incidence between the ages of 30–40 years.[44]

Treatment

Referral to a dentist for instruction of proper tooth-brushing technique and for plaque control can reduce both the sensitivity and risk for root caries. Professional treatments for dentinal hypersensitivity include reduce flow into the dentin tubules by occluding or sclerosing the tubules with dentin sealers (i.e., resins), stannous fluoride, strontium chloride hexahydrate, sodium citrate, and sodium monofluorophosphate, as well as others.[45] Invasive procedures may include gingival surgery, application of resins, pulpectomy, or laser treatment.

In addition, over-the-counter toothpastes containing 5% potassium nitrate have been suggested as a conservative treatment (Table 14-2).[46–48] Antihypersensitivity toothpastes act by depolarizing the nerves located at the dentin-pulpal interface. Potassium ions in the toothpaste prevent the repolarization of the sensory nerve endings, interrupting the transmission of pain-causing nerve impulses associated with dentin hypersensitivity.[49] To date, systematic reviews have not supported the efficacy of potassium nitrate toothpaste for the treatment of dentine hypersensitivity.[50]

Pericoronitis

Pericoronitis is defined as an oral abscess of the soft tissues typically surrounding the crown of a tooth, commonly a mandibular third molar that has partially erupted into the oral cavity.[10] Patients with pericoronitis often present with acute pain ranging from mild to intense that may radiate to the external neck, throat, ear, or the oral floor and swelling in the tissues around the partially erupted third molar (Figure 14-5) resulting in limited jaw opening (trismus). Cervical lymphadenopathy, fever, leukocytosis, and malaise may also be present, as well as concurrentipsilateral tonsillitis or upper respiratory tract infections. Patients presenting with chronic pericoronitis

Table 14-2. Over-the-Counter Toothpastes Designed to Treat Dentinal Hypersensitivity

Product Name	Manufacturer	Active Ingredient
Aquafresh Sensitive	GlaxoSmithKline	5% potassium nitrate
Colgate Sensitive Plus	Colgate-Palmolive	5% potassium nitrate
Crest Sensitivity Protection	Procter and Gamble	5% potassium nitrate
Natural Toothpaste for Sensitive Teeth	Tom's of Maine	5% potassium nitrate
Oral-B Rembrandt Extra Whitening Toothpaste Sensitive Teeth	Oral-B	5% potassium nitrate
Sensodyne	GlaxoSmithKline	5% potassium nitrate

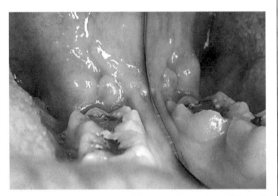

Figure 14-5. Pericoronitis. (Photograph courtesy of Russell Taichman, DMD, DMSc.)

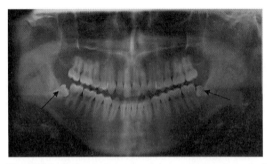

Figure 14-6. Orthopantomogram demonstrating impacted third molars *(arrows)*. (Photograph courtesy of Darnell Kaigler, Jr, DDS, Ph.D.)

may have acute episodes or may present with moderate discomfort around the region of the third molar or complain of a bad taste. Occasionally, pericoronitis may progress to a fascial space abscess or cellulitis. An impacted third molar may lead to caries or resorption of adjacent teeth, or cyst development. Pericoronitis is often obvious from intraoral examination, but an orthopantomogram may be helpful to further delineate an etiology that cannot be readily identified (Figure 14-6).

Etiology

Eruption of the mandibular second or third molars, which generally occurs between the ages of 17 and 25 years, may occur partially or not at all. Infection can occur in the soft tissues partly covering the crown and may spread into the oropharyngeal area, or to the tongue or may progress to an abscess or cellulitis. Risk factors associated with pericoronitis include poor oral hygiene, trauma from the opposing tooth on the soft tissues, smoking, and concurrent upper respiratory tract infections.

Treatment

Chronic pericoronitis may be alleviated by the use of chlorhexidine mouthwashes, warm salt water rinses, or by measures taken to improve oral hygiene. Referral to a dentist should occur as quickly as possible for evaluation to determine if symptomatic treatment can suffice until eruption is complete or if surgical therapy to remove the gum flap or the underlying tooth is necessary. Treatment considerations for acute pericoronitis include debridement, saline irrigation of the undersurface of the peri-coronal flap, and when indicated, systemic antibiotics. A 1980 NIH (National Institutes of Health) consensus[51] and extensive literature reviews[52,53] support the removal of wisdom teeth when associated with symptoms of pain or pathologic conditions. However, the routine removal of asymptomatic third molars in adults has recently been challenged because the benefits may not outweigh the potential complications of removal.[54,55]

Necrotizing Periodontal Diseases

Etiology

The clinical presentation and clinical course of *necrotizing ulcerative gingivitis* (NUG) is completely different from gingivitis. NUG, previously known as *acute necrotizing ulcerative gingivitis,* is related to a diminished systemic resistance to bacterial infection in the periodontal tissues. It is chiefly characterized by clinical appearance of necrotic gingival tissues resulting in a white pseudomembranous surface, significant pain, bleeding, loss of the tips of the interdental papilla (described as "punched out"), halitosis, and occasionally fever and malaise (Figure 14-7). NUG is a relatively uncommon condition (0.1–10% of the population) and is commonly a disease of young adults aged 18–30 years; however, in developing countries, it can also affect young children. Patients with NUG generally seek treatment due to the significant intraoral pain associated with the condition.[56]

As with gingivitis and periodontitis, the etiology of NUG is a mixed floral infection via *Streptococcus intermedia* (alpha-hemolytic streptococci), *Actinomyces* species, and a number of different oral spirochetes.[57] In fact, several studies have shown that the spirochetes may actually infiltrate into the surrounding tissues.[52,55,58–60] At-risk persons include those who have recently undergone stressful events including new military recruits, students during examinations, and persons experiencing major life-transition events. Other factors include poor oral hygiene and diet, and tobacco and alcohol use. During World War I, NUG was described as *Vincent's infection* or "trench mouth." For immediate relief of symptoms, NUG can be treated with systemic antibiotics such as metronidazole and topical antimicrobials such as chlorhexidine; however, resolution is dependent on the patient receiving a professional cleaning of the teeth and implementation of good home dental care.[61,62] NUG generally responds well to treatment if the host defenses remain intact but may require more aggressive therapy in persons with persistent immune deficiencies.

Necrotizing ulcerative periodontitis (NUP) occurs when NUG extends to involve the surrounding and underlying bone and connective tissues supporting the teeth.[62] This form of the disease may cause severe and rapid destruction along with a distinctive fetid odor, loss of the tips of the interdental papilla (seen clinically as a "punched out" papilla), and spontaneous gum tissue bleeding (Figure 14-8). NUP is associated with systemic immune suppression as seen during HIV infection. NUP may indicate deterioration of the immune system and in some cases may be useful in the diagnosis of AIDS and in patients with severe nutritional deficiencies.[63,64]

Treatment

Patients with acute NUG and NUP often require systemic and topical analgesic therapy for pain management and to maintain adequate nutrition. The standard of care is gradual, gentle local debridement of the inflamed areas during the initial visit, supplemented with subgingival povidone-iodine irrigation, if possible. Chlorhexidine gluconate 0.12–0.2% mouthrinse twice daily or saline rinses can help to speed resolution. Oral rinses with a 3% hydrogen peroxide solution also may also be of benefit. For the treatment of ulcers, metronidazole administered in a 500-mg loading dose and followed by 250 mg four times daily until ulcers are healed can be used; penicillin or tetracycline can be used alternatively or in patients who cannot tolerate metronidazole. Topical antifungal medications such as clotrimazole troches can be given for patients with a history of oral candidiasis. Use of nystatin rinse is not encouraged in dentate patients due to the high sugar content. Recommendations to reduce current physical or mental stressors should be used, as well

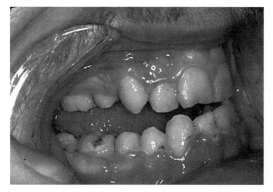

Figure 14-7. Necrotizing ulcerative gingivitis. (Photograph Courtesy of Russell Taichman, DMD, DMSc.)

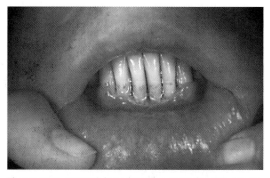

Figure 14-8. Necrotizing ulcerative periodontitis. (Photograph courtesy of Russell Taichman, DMD, DMSc.)

as proper oral hygiene instructions. Most patients are reevaluated within 3 days to ensure improvement. Deep scaling and root planing after cessation of spontaneous bleeding and pain from periodontal lesions is recommended.[65,66]

Oral Manifestations of Systemic Disease

The oral manifestations of certain systemic diseases can mimic the signs and symptoms of periodontitis or gingivitis. Such diseases include immunologic, infectious, neoplastic, and metabolic disorders. In comparison to periodontitis and gingivitis, these disorders are considerably less common, yet since their diagnosis and management differ significantly, a high index of suspicion is required when evaluating a patient who presents with gingival or periodontal disease.

Diabetes Mellitus

Epidemiologic studies have reported consistent results of an association between periodontitis and both type I and type II diabetes mellitus.[67] In general, persons with diabetes have a much greater likelihood of experiencing severe periodontitis than non-diabetics. The majority of studies investigating type I diabetes and periodontal disease have reported a greater prevalence, extent, and severity of periodontal disease among persons with type I diabetes mellitus compared with non-diabetics of the same age.[68–70] A epidemiologic cross-sectional study of the Pima Indians of Arizona showed that persons with type II diabetes had a 2.8- to 3.4-fold increase in odds of having periodontitis compared with non-diabetic subjects after adjusting for the effects of confounding variables such as age, gender, and oral hygiene measures.[71,72]

Studies suggest that the most critical issue in managing periodontitis a patient with diabetes is the degree of glycemic control achieved.[73] Persons with well-controlled diabetes have the same periodontal risk as non-diabetics; however, those with poorly controlled diabetes have a two to three times greater risk of periodontitis and progressive bone loss.[74] The mechanisms by which diabetes may mediate the increased severity of periodontal disease expression include vascular changes, impaired wound healing, impaired collagen metabolism and bone matrix component production, advanced glycosylation end products, and altered subgingival microflora.[75]

Herpes-related Gingivitis

Primary herpetic gingivostomatitis occurs primarily in children, although the condition may occur at any age. The onset is often very painful and debilitating. The lesions appear as small punctuate vesicular lesions that may coalesce with indurated and slightly raised borders. Secondary herpetic gingivostomatitis occurs primarily on the tongue, buccal mucosa, and keratinized gingiva. Occurrence of these lesions is commonly of a rapid onset, usually in response to trauma or stress; the condition is generally self-limited and resolves within 7–10 days. Treatment of either primary or secondary herpetic gingivostomatitis is primarily palliative because the intense oral pain can make maintaining adequate nutrition difficult. Oral rinses with 2% viscous Xylocaine (lidocaine hydrochloride) before eating may prove to be palliative. Several local anesthetic-based compounds that can be obtained as over-the-counter preparations may provide some transient relief but have not been shown to decrease time to resolution. Along with antiviral medications such as acyclovir, analgesics and antipyretics are often recommended to reduce fever (if present) and pain.

Human Immunodeficiency Virus and Acquired Immunodeficiency Syndrome

In early studies, the relationship of HIV-positive status and periodontal disease was unclear. Current evidence now suggests that HIV-related disease has a relatively minor effect on the progression of chronic periodontitis because patients who are HIV-positive and immunosuppressed can present with distinctive forms of the previously described necrotizing gingivitis and periodontitis.[76] It has been suggested that the risk of chronic periodontitis among HIV-positive patients may vary due to factors such as oral hygiene measures, smoking habits, medications being taken, and preexisting periodontal disease. In addition, NUP in HIV-infected persons can present with a clinical appearance similar to Burkitt's lymphoma, cytomegalovirus infection, or herpes zoster infection of the periodontal tissues.[77–79] These similarities can often make accurate diagnosis difficult. The wide variation in prevalence data from epidemiologic studies has brought about the call for standardized evaluation criteria to define periodontal diseases seen in HIV-positive persons. Furthermore, with the introduction of highly active antiretroviral therapies, it has been suggested that the presence of necrotizing periodontal problems associated with HIV has been reduced in populations with access to this therapy.[80,81]

Various hematologic disorders such as leukemia, thrombocytopenia, and leukocyte disorders including agranulocytosis, cyclic neutropenia, and leukocyte adhesion deficiency can be associated with increased severity of periodontal disease. Persons with gastrointestinal diseases including hepatitis and Crohn's disease, connective tissue and other autoimmune disorders including systemic lupus erythematosus and scleroderma, pulmonary disorders such as chronic obstructive pulmonary disease, and genetic disorders such as Down syndrome are at a higher risk for periodontal disease.

Oral Side Effects of Systemic Disease Treatment

Medications may affect the dentition through several mechanisms, leading to either extrinsic (Table 14-3) or intrinsic (Table 14-4) discoloration, whereas others may result in damage to the tooth structure (Table 14-5). Several medications prescribed to treat systemic conditions have been shown to be associated with gingival hyperplasia and xerostomia. Educating patients about the potential for oral side effects of these medications is critical in reducing medication-related periodontal conditions.

Gingival Hyperplasia

Gingival hyperplasia has been most frequently associated with the use of oral anticonvulsants

Table 14-3. Drugs That Can Cause Extrinsic Tooth Discoloration

Drug	Discoloration Caused
Chlorhexidine	Yellow/brown
Oral iron salts	Black
Amoxicillin-clavulanate	Yellow or grey-brown
Essential oils	Yellow/brown

Adapted from: Tredwin CJ, Scully C, Bagan-Sebastian JV: Drug-induced disorders of teeth, *J Dental Res* 84(7):596–602, 2005.

Table 14-4. Drugs That Can Cause Intrinsic Tooth Discoloration

Drug	Discoloration Caused
Fluoride	White/brown discoloration
Tetracycline	Yellow to brown/grey
Minocycline	Green-gray/blue-grey
Ciprofloxacin	Greenish

Adapted from: Tredwin CJ, Scully C, Bagan-Sebastian JV: Drug-induced disorders of teeth, *J Dental Res* 84(7):596–602, 2005.

(e.g., phenytoin), calcium channel blockers (e.g., nifedipine), and immunosuppressants (e.g., cyclosporine). Although the molecular mechanisms of action are different for each drug class, most evidence suggests that the mechanism relates to inhibition of collagenolytic activity and buildup of fibrous tissue.[82] Precise estimates of the prevalence of gingival enlargement associated with each class of drug are difficult to accurately obtain, given the different indices of gingival overgrowth, differing populations, and lack of control over comedication. However, reported prevalence of phenytoin-associated overgrowth was found to be

Table 14-5. Drugs That Can Cause Damage to Tooth Structure

Drug	Examples	Possible Damage to Tooth Structure
Sugar-containing oral (liquid) medication	Various liquid medications (e.g., nystatin)	Dental caries
Drugs that result in decreased salivary secretion (i.e., xerostomia)	See Table 14-7.	Dental caries
Drugs with a pH low enough to cause tooth erosion	Aspirin, anti-asthmatic drugs (e.g., terbutaline or fluticasone inhalers)	Dental erosion
Drugs that may increase susceptibility to gastroesophageal reflux disease	Theophylline, anticholinergics, progesterone, calcium channel blockers	Dental erosion
Drugs used for internal tooth bleaching	Hydrogen peroxide and sodium perborate	Cervical root resorption
Drugs used for treatment of childhood cancer and leukemia	Cytotoxic agents	Abnormal tooth development

Adapted from: Tredwin CJ, Scully C, Bagan-Sebastian JV: Drug-induced disorders of teeth, *J Dental Res* 84(7):596–602, 2005.

50% in one particular study of a noninstitutionalized population.[83] Twenty to thirty percent of adults taking cyclosporine have reported gingival overgrowth,[84] as have 6–15% of adults taking calcium channel blockers, including nifedipine.[85,86] Risk factors known to contribute to gingival hyperplasia include the presence of established dental plaque, the depth of the periodontal pocket, male gender, and the dose and duration of drug therapy.[87–89]

Presentation

Gingival hyperplasia usually begins in the interdental papilla and is located in the anterior segment of the mouth. Inflammatory enlargements are characterized by swelling or edema, redness, and a tendency to bleed during tissue manipulation (Figures 14-9 and 14-10). Long-standing gingival enlargements have a significant fibrotic component as well. Chronic enlargements are generally painless and slowly progressing, whereas acute enlargements are characterized by an acute, painful onset. Generalized enlargements may be disfiguring and may impair nutri-

tion intake and oral hygiene resulting in increased caries, periodontal disease, and other oral infections.[88]

In general, gingival hyperplasia associated with phenytoin and other drugs is most common in children and young adults. Overgrowth usually begins within 3–6 months of initiation of therapy. Gingival enlargement is exacerbated by dental plaque decreasing a person's ability to maintain good oral hygiene; therefore, excellent oral hygiene is necessary.[90]

Treatment

Meticulous patient self-care combined with frequent professional dental care can slow the development of gingival hyperplasia and the need for surgical recontouring of the gingiva. Patients scheduled to receive a medication associated with a potential for gingival overgrowth should be referred to a dentist for a baseline periodontal evaluation before the initiation of drug therapy and for future evaluations of periodontal tissues.

The most effective treatment for gingival hyperplasia is medication substitution or withdrawal.[88] Introductions of a new generation of anticonvulsants such as levetiracetam (Keppra) and topiramate (Topamax) have made phenytoin substitution more feasible.[91] It has also been suggested that changing a patient's antihypertensive treatment from nifedipine to another class of medications such as thiazide diuretics, beta blockers, or angiotensin-converting enzyme inhibitors may result in regression of gingival enlargement.[92] Switching from cyclosporine to tacrolimus has been shown to cause significant resolution or complete regression of the gingival enlargement in renal transplant recipients.[92–94] If gingival overgrowth occurs and leads to subsequent increased dental plaque accumulation, then surgical treatment may be indicated.[95]

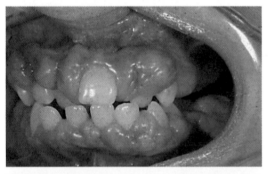

Figure 14-9. Phenytoin-induced gingival enlargement. (Photograph courtesy of Russell Taichman, DMD, DMSc.)

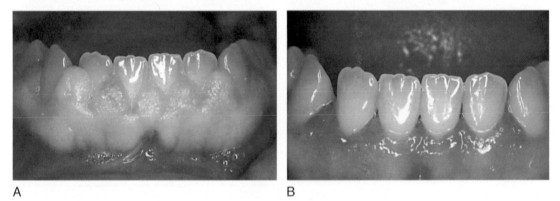

A   B

Figure 14-10. Cyclosporine-induced gingival hyperplasia. Presentation of a patient before (A) and 1–2 weeks after (B) corrective surgery to reshape the gingival tissues. (Photograph courtesy of Rodrigo Neiva, DDS, MS.)

Bisphosphonate-Induced Osteonecrosis

Recent reports of osteonecrosis in the jaws of patients receiving intravenous bisphosphonate therapy for bone cancers, such as multiple myeloma and metastatic prostate cancer, have caused great concern (Figure 14-11). These drugs, including pamidronate and zoledronic acid, work by inhibiting osteoclast action and result in an impairment of the normal bone repair mechanism. The repetitive microtrauma of mastication routinely results in bone remodeling, but this is significantly impaired in these patients.[96,97] Although painless, the exposed bone is alarming to the patient and his physician. Patients who have been treated with intravenous bisphosphonates are advised to avoid surgical procedures such as extractions to minimize the risk of osteonecrosis.

Xerostomia

The presence of saliva is typically taken for granted and is often not appreciated until it is either altered or reduced in quantity. Men who are taking medications that induce dry mouth, or those who have undergone head and neck radiation therapy, often report a reduced quality of life and constantly carry water to sip and lubricate their mouths. Adequate and appropriate saliva is important for oral homeostasis; any significant derangements can lead to pathologic conditions of the oral cavity.

The Functions of Saliva

Saliva is composed predominantly of water and mucins, making a good oral lubricant and buffer for the many acidic foods that we consume. It carries a large number of enzymes and salivary amylases that break down proteins and carbohydrates as the first stage of digestion. The major salivary glands, the parotid, submandibular, and sublingual glands, produce saliva that differs in its mucous and serous nature due to different glandular components (Table 14-6). Minor salivary glands line the lips, palate, and buccal mucosa for additional lubrication. Saliva not only buffers the acids in the foods we eat, but it also buffers the acids produced by bacteria that metabolize the sugars on our gums and teeth. Patients with decreased salivary flow are therefore at a greater risk of tooth decay. The lubricating properties of saliva are important for speech, swallowing, food manipulation, and the use of dentures. As the fluid that lines the main portal of entry and the start of the digestive tract, saliva contains antimicrobial agents to maintain homeostasis of the normal oral flora, in addition to immunoglobulin A, lactoferrin, lysozyme, and peroxidases.

Salivary flow and composition may differ based on stimulation or lack thereof. Stimulated saliva is brought on not just by the ingestion of food but also the sight, smell, or anticipation of it (i.e., pavlovian response). Salivary flow is controlled predominantly through the parasympathetic nervous system as a part of a series of activities geared toward maintaining homeostasis. Changes that inhibit the parasympathetic nervous system, such as the "fight or flight" response, or various anticholinergic medications will cause a reduction in salivary flow. Decreased

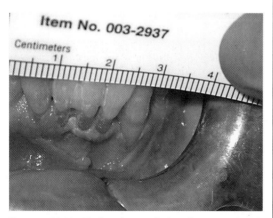

Figure 14-11. Bisphosphonate-induced osteonecrosis associated with the mandibular anterior alveolus. (Photograph courtesy of Brent Ward, DDS, MD.)

Table 14-6. Functions of Salivary Molecules

Functional Property	Salivary Molecule
Antibacterial	Amylase, cystatins, histatins, mucins, peroxidases
Antiviral	Cystatins, mucins
Antifungal	Histatins
Buffering	Histatins, carbonic anhydrases
Digestion	Amylases, mucins
Mineralization	Cystatins, histatins, proline-rich proteins, satherines
Lubrication	Mucins, satherines
Tissue coating	Amylase, cystatin, mucins, proline-rich proteins, satherines

Adapted from: Humphrey SP, Williamson RT: A review of saliva: normal composition, flow, and function, *J Prosthet Dent* 85 (2):162–169, 2001.

salivary flow while sleeping is due in part to reduced oromotor functions but is also thought to be due to circadian rhythms.[98]

Xerostomia, the reduction in salivary flow, may be due to medications with anticholinergic side effects (Table 14-7). Patients who take medications for psychiatric illnesses including depression or schizophrenia are also less likely to demonstrate positive oral health habits, such as good oral hygiene, avoidance of a cariogenic diet, and routine dental care. Radiation therapy to the head and neck of doses greater than 2000 rads can produce permanent damage to salivary glands and result in chronic dry mouth. Rampant tooth decay can result within 12 months of completing treatment.[99]

Prevention

Recognition of the importance of saliva has led to innovations intended to prevent xerostomia where it most often occurs. Radiation therapy regimens can now use computer technology to spare the parotid gland while delivering adequate treatment limited to cancerous tissue. Pharmacologic advances have resulted in antipsychotic and antidepressant medications with less negative effect on salivary flow. Communicating the availability and benefit of these advances to primary care practitioners is of paramount importance.

Attention toward good oral health habits, including brushing, flossing, and avoidance of cariogenic foods, is necessary to prevent tooth decay in this high-risk population. Also recommended is the daily use of a highly concentrated fluoride product, either 1.0% sodium fluoride or 0.4% stannous fluoride in a gel form.[100] Some oral lubricants and saliva substitutes are available, many of which are formulated to match the biochemical properties of saliva; however, most patients still rely on carrying a bottle of water for continued oral lubrication.

Systemic Effects of Oral Disease

Periodontitis Associated with Systemic Conditions

Recent evidence suggests that there are two sides to the relationship between periodontal diseases and systemic health. For some time it has been known that systemic factors (e.g., smoking, diabetes, immunodeficiencies, blood dyscrasias) have a negative impact on periodontal health.[101,102] More recently, an appreciation that chronic oral infections may have an adverse

Table 14-7. Drug Classes Associated with Xerostomia

Class	Examples
Analgesic narcotics	Codeine, morphine
Anti-asthmatics/ bronchodilators	Beclomethasone, tiotropium
Anticholinergics	Scopolamine
Antidepressants	Fluoxetine, doxepin, MAOIs
Antihistamines	Cetirizine, hydroxyzine, clemastine
Antihypertensives	Diuretics, atenolol
Anxiolytics	Triazolam
Anti-Parkinson agents	Benztropine
Antipsychotics	Thioridazine, clozapine
Decongestants	Ephedrine
Anti-acne medications	Isotretinoin
Muscle relaxants	Tizanidine
Anticonvulsants	Carbamazepine
Antiarrhythmics	Disopyramide
Anorexiants	Phentermine
Antidiarrheals	Loperamide
Antiemetics	Droperidol, thiethylperazine, ondansetron
Chemopreventive agents	Phenetidin, transretinoic acid

MAOIs, Monoamine oxidase inhibitors.
Adapted from: *USP DI Drug Information for the Healthcare Professional*, ed 24, Englewood, CO, 2004, Micromedix Inc. Table based on Sreebny LM, Schwartz SS: A reference guide to drugs and dry mouth—2nd edition. Gerodontology 14(1):33–47, 1991; Wynn RL, Meiller TF, Crossley HL: *Drug Information Handbook for Dentistry, 2002–2003*, ed 8, Hudson, OH, 2002, Lexi-Comp.

effect on a person's systemic health has been recognized. This concept is not entirely new, yet greater appreciation for the health consequences of controlling dental and oral conditions by the healthcare community is most welcome. This is a rapidly expanding field in dental research and has received considerable attention in the lay and scientific press. For example, coronary occlusive diseases, diabetes, aspiration pneumonias, and cerebrovascular events including stroke have all been linked in cross-sectional studies to periodontal disease.[73,103–106] The critical component is that few of these conditions have been definitively proven as causative of periodontal disease. Nevertheless, it seems prudent to treat infections promptly and adequately independent of whether oral infections are causative for systemic conditions.

Diabetes Mellitus

A substantial body of evidence suggests a bidirectional relationship between diabetes and periodontal disease. The scientific evidence is strongest for the association of type I diabetes mellitus being related to periodontal disease, yet patients with type II diabetes mellitus also appear to be at a greater risk for severe periodontal disease.[107] Increasing evidence suggests that the treatment of periodontal infections through mechanical therapy combined with systemic antibiotics may improve glycemic control.[108–111] However, other studies in which scaling and root planing were performed without the use of systemic antibiotics showed no effect on glycemic control.[112] Also, a recent meta-analysis attempting to quantify the effects of periodontal treatment on hemoglobin A_{1c} (HbA1c) level among persons with diabetes found that periodontal therapy with antibiotics appeared to decrease HbA1c levels by a statistically nonsignificant 0.71% among patients with type 2 diabetes.[113] Additional research is necessary to firmly establish that treating periodontal infections can contribute to glycemic control management and possibly to the reduction of type 2 diabetes complications.[114] Regardless of causation, prompt diagnosis of periodontitis and aggressive therapy targeted at lowering glycosylated hemoglobin levels in a patient with diabetes is likely to be of benefit for persons at risk for periodontal disease.

Cardiovascular Disease

Several epidemiologic studies and systematic reviews have suggested an association between periodontal disease, coronary heart disease, and stroke.[111,115,116] Other epidemiologic studies have found no relationship between periodontal disease and cardiovascular diseases.[105,117]

Chronic inflammation has been associated with atherosclerosis.[118] Periodontal disease inflammation has been suggested to play a role in the initiation or progression of coronary artery disease and stroke.[116] Current evidence links C-reactive protein as the common association between periodontal disease and cardiovascular diseases. Another suggested linking mechanism is the gram-negative bacteria itself, whereby antibodies to the bacteria are produced, resulting in arterial injury.[119]

The treatment of periodontitis to eliminate infection has not been shown to reduce cardiovascular disease.[120] Several authors have suggested that the evidence does not support a causal relationship between periodontitis and atherosclerosis and its sequelae; rather, periodontitis and cardiovascular disease share risk factors including tobacco smoking, male gender, race/ethnicity, stress, and aging.[117,121] Longitudinal studies with large numbers of participants will be required if causality is to be established.

Respiratory Diseases

The role of oral pathogens in the development of respiratory diseases has been studied extensively but is not fully understood. Both decayed teeth and the periodontium can serve as a reservoir for bacteria, which can seed the lungs and result in aspiration pneumonia. This is a significant concern in alcoholics, bed-bound elderly persons, and others who are dependent on caregivers to provide oral hygiene.[104,105]

Bacterial Endocarditis

The workup for patients with bacterial endocarditis typically includes a dental evaluation and often extraction of diseased teeth as a prophylactic measure. This is performed to rule out the dentition as a potential source of infection and to address the finding of oral pathogens in the bloodstream and on heart valves. In a review of the literature on bacterial endocarditis and oral health, Lockhart[122] finds little evidence that dental procedures can be conclusively linked as causative. Patients with endocarditis are often found to be intravenous drug users, and such behavior often goes hand in hand with poor dental habits such as a cariogenic diet and poor routine dental care.

Conclusion

This chapter has attempted to expose readers to the topic of oral health and disease with the vision of increasing observation of the oral cavity during routine health examinations as an integral component of systemic health. Various medical conditions and therapies can cause oral pathology, and increasingly it is found that oral health can significantly affect systemic conditions. As our society divides further along socioeconomic strata into those who seek dental care and those who do not, primary care physicians may find it necessary to include an oral examination as part of their physical examination and to make appropriate referrals for dental care when they discover significant findings. As the field of dentistry has just begun to examine its data from an evidence-based practice standpoint, dental and medical professionals will be able to communicate well in seeking cost-effective and beneficial care for their patients.

References

1. Sweet M, Damiano P, Rivera E, et al: A comparison of dental services received by Medicaid and privately insured adult populations, *J Am Dent Assoc* 136(1):93–100, 2005.
2. Beirne P, Forgie A, Clarkson J, Worthington HV: Recall intervals for oral health in primary care patients, *Cochrane Database Syst Rev* 2:CD004346, 2005.
3. Marinho VC, Higgins JP, Logan S, Sheiham A: Topical fluoride (toothpastes, mouth rinses, gels or varnishes) for preventing dental caries in children and adolescents, *Cochrane Database Syst Rev* 4:CD002782, 2003.
4. Shaner JW: Caries associated with methamphetamine abuse, *J Mich Dent Assoc* 84(9):42–47, 2002.
5. Howe AM: Methamphetamine and childhood and adolescent caries, *Aust Dent J* 40(5):340, 1995.
6. McGrath C, Chan B: Oral health sensations associated with illicit drug abuse, *Br Dent J* 198(3):159–162, 2005.
7. Truman BI, Gooch BF, Sulemana I, et al: Reviews of evidence on interventions to prevent dental caries, oral and pharyngeal cancers, and sports-related craniofacial injuries, *Am J Prev Med* 23(1 Suppl):21–54, 2002.
8. American Association of Endodontists: Recommended guidelines of the American Association of Endodontists for the treatment of traumatic dental injuries. 2004. Available at: http://www.aae.org/NR/rdonlyres/9232084C-DD96-4459-98B6-33A17A3FEA10/0/2004TraumaGuidelines.pdf. Accessed July 30, 2006.
9. American Cancer Society: Cancer statistics 2006: a presentation from the American Cancer Society. Available at: http://www.cancer.org/downloads/STT/Cancer_Statistics_2006_Presentation.ppt. Accessed July 23, 2006.
10. Newman M, Takei H, Carranza F: *Carranza's Clinical Periodontology*, Philadelphia, 2002, Saunders.
11. Oliver RC, Brown LJ, Loe H: Periodontal diseases in the United States population, *J Periodontol* 69(2):269–278, 1998.
12. Albandar JM, Brunelle JA, Kingman A: Destructive periodontal disease in adults 30 years of age and older in the United States, 1988–1994, *J Periodontol* 70(1):13–29, 1999.
13. US Public Health Service: *Oral Health of United States Adults: National Findings*, NIH Publication number 87–2868, Bethesda, MD, 1987, National Institute of Dental Research.
14. Oral health of US adults: NIDR 1985 national survey, *J Public Health Dent* 47(4):198–205, 1987.
15. Brown LJ, Brunelle JA, Kingman A: Periodontal status in the United States, 1988–1991: prevalence, extent, and demographic variation, *J Dent Res* 75 Spec No:672–683, 1996.
16. Machtei EE, Hausmann E, Dunford R, et al: Longitudinal study of predictive factors for periodontal disease and tooth loss, *J Clin Periodontol* 26(6):374–380, 1999.
17. Listgarten MA, Schifter CC, Laster L: 3-year longitudinal study of the periodontal status of an adult population with gingivitis, *J Clin Periodontol* 12(3):225–238, 1985.
18. Brown LJ, Oliver RC, Loe H: Evaluating periodontal status of US employed adults, *J Am Dent Assoc* 121(2):226–232, 1990.
19. Burt BA: Epidemiology of dental diseases in the elderly, *Clin Geriatr Med* 8(3):447–459, 1992.
20. Burt BA: Periodontitis and aging: reviewing recent evidence, *J Am Dent Assoc* 125(3):273–279, 1994.
21. Burt B: Position paper: epidemiology of periodontal diseases, *J Periodontol* 76(8):1406–1419, 2005.
22. Armitage GC: The complete periodontal examination, *Periodontol 2000* 34:22–33, 2004.
23. Armitage GC: Periodontal diseases: diagnosis, *Ann Periodontol* 1(1):37–215, 1996.
24. Kroes I, Lepp PW, Relman DA: Bacterial diversity within the human subgingival crevice, *Proc Natl Acad Sci U S A* 96(25):14547–14552, 1999.
25. Listgarten MA: Pathogenesis of periodontitis, *J Clin Periodontol* 13(5):418–430, 1986.
26. Page RC: The etiology and pathogenesis of periodontitis, *Compend Contin Educ Dent* 23(5 Suppl):11–14, 2002.
27. Tsai CC, McArthur WP, Baehni PC, et al: Extraction and partial characterization of a leukotoxin from a plaque-derived gram-negative microorganism, *Infect Immunol* 25(1):427–439, 1979.
28. Taichman NS, Wilton JM: Leukotoxicity of an extract from *Actinobacillus actinomycetemcomitans* for human gingival polymorphonuclear leukocytes, *Inflammation* 5(1):1–12, 1981.
29. Bergstrom J, Preber H: Tobacco use as a risk factor, *J Periodontol* 65(5 Suppl):545–550, 1994.
30. Haber J, Wattles J, Crowley M, et al: Evidence for cigarette smoking as a major risk factor for periodontitis, *J Periodontol* 64(1):16–23, 1993.
31. Grossi SG, Zambon JJ, Ho AW, et al: Assessment of risk for periodontal disease: I. risk indicators for attachment loss, *J Periodontol* 65(3):260–267, 1994.
32. Grossi SG, Genco RJ, Machtei EE, et al: Assessment of risk for periodontal disease: II. risk indicators for alveolar bone loss, *J Periodontol* 66(1):23–29, 1995.
33. Wray A, McGuirt WF: Smokeless tobacco usage associated with oral carcinoma: incidence, treatment, outcome, *Arch Otolaryngol Head Neck Surg* 119(9):929–933, 1993.
34. Robertson PB, Walsh M, Greene J, et al: Periodontal effects associated with the use of smokeless tobacco, *J Periodontol* 61(7):438–443, 1990.
35. Soder B, Jin LJ, Wickholm S: Granulocyte elastase, matrix metalloproteinase-8 and prostaglandin E2 in gingival crevicular fluid in matched clinical sites in smokers and non-smokers with persistent periodontitis, *J Clin Periodontol* 29(5):384–391, 2002.

36. Michalowicz BS, Aeppli D, Virag JG, et al: Peri-odontal findings in adult twins, *J Periodontol* 62 (5):293–299, 1991.

37. Michalowicz BS, Diehl SR, Gunsolley JC, et al: Evidence of a substantial genetic basis for risk of adult periodontitis, *J Periodontol* 71(11):1699–1707, 2000.

38. Kornman KS, Crane A, Wang HY, et al: The interleukin-1 genotype as a severity factor in adult periodontal disease, *J Clin Periodontol* 24(1):72–77, 1997.

39. D'Aiuto F, Parkar M, Brett PM, et al: Gene polymorphisms in pro-inflammatory cytokines are associated with systemic inflammation in patients with severe periodontal infections, *Cytokine* 28 (1):29–34, 2004.

40. Beltran-Aguilar ED, Beltran-Neira RJ: Oral diseases and conditions throughout the lifespan: II. systemic diseases, *Gen Dent* 52(2):107–114, 2004.

41. American Dental Association Web site. Available at: http://www.ada.org/. Accessed August 7, 2006.

42. American Dental Hygienists' Association Web site. Available at: http://www.adha.org. Accessed August 6, 2006.

43. Joshipura KJ, Kent RL, DePaola PF: Gingival recession: intra-oral distribution and associated factors, *J Periodontol* 65(9):864–871, 1994.

44. Gillam DG, Aris A, Bulman JS, et al: Dentine hypersensitivity in subjects recruited for clinical trials: clinical evaluation, prevalence and intra-oral distribution, *J Oral Rehabil* 29(3):226–231, 2002.

45. Walters PA: Dentinal hypersensitivity: a review, *J Contemp Dent Pract* 6(2):107–117, 2005.

46. Schiff T, Zhang YP, DeVizio W, et al: A randomized clinical trial of the desensitizing efficacy of three dentifrices, *Compend Contin Educ Dent Suppl* 27:4–10, 2000.

47. Sowinski JA, Battista GW, Petrone ME, et al: A new desensitizing dentifrice—an 8-week clinical investigation, *Compend Contin Educ Dent Suppl* 27:11–16, 2000.

48. Jacobsen PL, Bruce G: Clinical dentin hypersensitivity: understanding the causes and prescribing a treatment, *J Contemp Dent Pract* 2(1):1–12, 2001.

49. Consensus-based recommendations for the diagnosis and management of dentin hypersensitivity, *J Can Dent Assoc,* 69(4):221–226, 2003.

50. Poulsen S, Errboe M, Hovgaard O, Worthington HW: Potassium nitrate toothpaste for dentine hypersensitivity, *Cochrane Database Syst Rev* 2: CD001476, 2001.

51. National Institute of Health: Removal of third molars, *NIH Consensus Statement Online* 2(11): 65–68, 1979. Available at: http://www.consensus.nih.gov/1979/1979Molars021html.htm. Accessed August 3, 2006.

52. Pasqualini D, Erniani F, Coscia D, et al: Third molar extraction: current trends, *Minerva Stomatol* 51(10):411–419, 2002.

53. Precious DS, Mercier P, Payette F: Risks and benefits of extraction of impacted third molars: a critical review of the literature, 2, *J Can Dent Assoc* 58 (10):845–852, 1992.

54. Mettes TG, Nienhuijs ME, van der Sanden WJ, et al: Interventions for treating asymptomatic impacted wisdom teeth in adolescents and adults, *Cochrane Database Syst Rev* 2:CD003879, 2005.

55. Song F, Landes DP, Glenny AM, Sheldon TA: Prophylactic removal of impacted third molars: an assessment of published reviews, *Br Dent J* 182 (9):339–346, 1997.

56. Rowland RW: Necrotizing ulcerative gingivitis, *Ann Periodontol* 4(1):65–73, 1999.

57. Loesche WJ, Syed SA, Laughon BE, Stoll J: The bacteriology of acute necrotizing ulcerative gingivitis, *J Periodontol* 53(4):223–230, 1982.

58. Fives-Taylor P, Meyer D, Mintz K: Characteristics of *Actinobacillus actinomycetemcomitans* invasion of and adhesion to cultured epithelial cells, *Adv Dent Res* 9(1):55–62, 1995.

59. Lamont RJ, Chan A, Belton CM, et al: Porphyromonas gingivalis invasion of gingival epithelial cells, *Infect Immunol* 63(10):3878–3885, 1995.

60. Lamont RJ, Yilmaz O: In or out: the invasiveness of oral bacteria, *Periodontol 2000* 30:61–69, 2002.

61. Hartnett AC, Shiloah J: The treatment of acute necrotizing ulcerative gingivitis, *Quintessence Int* 22(2):95–100, 1991.

62. Winkler JR, Murray PA, Grassi M, Hammerle C: Diagnosis and management of HIV-associated periodontal lesions, *J Am Dent Assoc* Suppl: 25S–34S, 1989.

63. Glick M, Muzyka BC, Salkin LM, Lurie D: Necrotizing ulcerative periodontitis: a marker for immune deterioration and a predictor for the diagnosis of AIDS, *J Periodontol* 65(5): 393–397, 1994.

64. Winkler JR, Robertson PB: Periodontal disease associated with HIV infection, *Oral Surg Oral Med Oral Pathol* 73(2):145–150, 1992.

65. Johnson TC, Winkler JR: Diagnosis and treatment of HIV-associated periodontal disease, *Dentistry* 10(4):9–13, 1990.

66. Robinson PG: Treatment of HIV-associated periodontal diseases, *Oral Dis* 3(Suppl 1):S238–S240, 1997.

67. Stegeman CA: Oral manifestations of diabetes, *Home Healthc Nurse* 23(4):233–240, 2005.

68. Hugoson A, Thorstensson H, Falk H, Kuylenstierna J: Periodontal conditions in insulin-dependent diabetics, *J Clin Periodontol* 16(4):215–223, 1989.

69. Sznajder N, Carraro JJ, Rugna S, Sereday M: Periodontal findings in diabetic and nondiabetic patients, *J Periodontol* 49(9):445–448, 1978.

70. Tervonen T, Knuuttila M, Pohjamo L, Nurkkala H: Immediate response to nonsurgical periodontal treatment in subjects with diabetes mellitus, *J Clin Periodontol* 18(1):65–68, 1991.

71. Nelson RG, Shlossman M, Budding LM, et al: Periodontal disease and NIDDM in Pima Indians, *Diabetes Care* 13(8):836–840, 1990.

72. Taylor GW: Bidirectional interrelationships between diabetes and periodontal diseases: an epidemiologic perspective, *Ann Periodontol* 6(1): 99–112, 2001.

73. Committee on Research, Science and Therapy, American Academy of Periodontology: Diabetes and periodontal diseases, *J Periodontol* 71(4): 664–678, 2000.

74. Emrich LJ, Shlossman M, Genco RJ: Periodontal disease in non–insulin-dependent diabetes mellitus, *J Periodontol* 62(2):123–131, 1991.

75. Mealey BL, Oates TW: Diabetes mellitus and periodontal diseases, *J Periodontol* 77(8):1289–1303, 2006.

76. Mulligan R, Phelan JA, Brunelle J, et al: Baseline characteristics of participants in the oral health component of the Women's Interagency HIV Study, *Commun Dent Oral Epidemiol* 32(2):86–98, 2004.

77. Glick M, Cleveland DB, Salkin LM, et al: Intraoral cytomegalovirus lesion and HIV-associated periodontitis in a patient with acquired immunodeficiency syndrome, *Oral Surg Oral Med Oral Pathol* 72(6):716–720, 1991.

78. Dodd CL, Winkler JR, Heinic GS, et al: Cytomegalovirus infection presenting as acute periodontal infection in a patient infected with the human immunodeficiency virus, *J Clin Periodontol* 20 (4):282–285, 1993.

79. Hernandez VG, Garcia MD, Lopez A, et al: Unusual periodontal findings in an AIDS patient with Burkitt's lymphoma: a case report, *J Periodontol* 60(12):723–727, 1989.

80. Ramirez-Amador V, Esquivel-Pedraza L, Sierra-Madero J, et al: The changing clinical spectrum of human immunodeficiency virus (HIV)-related oral lesions in 1,000 consecutive patients: a 12-year study in a referral center in Mexico, *Medicine (Baltimore)* 82(1):39–50, 2003.

81. Patton LL, McKaig R, Strauss R, et al: Changing prevalence of oral manifestations of human immuno-deficiency virus in the era of protease inhibitor therapy, *Oral Surg Oral Med Oral Pathol Oral Radiol Endod* 89(3):299–304, 2000.

82. Hyland PL, Traynor PS, Myrillas TT, et al: The effects of cyclosporin on the collagenolytic activity of gingival fibroblasts, *J Periodontol* 74(4):437–445, 2003.

83. Brunet L, Miranda J, Roset P, et al: Prevalence and risk of gingival enlargement in patients treated with anticonvulsant drugs, *Eur J Clin Invest* 31 (9):781–788, 2001.

84. Boltchi FE, Rees TD, Iacopino AM: Cyclosporine A–induced gingival overgrowth: a comprehensive review, *Quintessence Int* 30(11):775–783, 1999.

85. Miranda J, Brunet L, Roset P, et al: Prevalence and risk of gingival enlargement in patients treated with nifedipine, *J Periodontol* 72(5):605–611, 2001.

86. Ellis JS, Seymour RA, Steele JG, et al: Prevalence of gingival overgrowth induced by calcium channel blockers: a community-based study, *J Periodontol* 70(1):63–67, 1999.

87. Casetta I, Granieri E, Desidera M, et al: Phenytoin-induced gingival overgrowth: a community-based cross-sectional study in Ferrara, Italy, *Neuroepidemiology* 16(6):296–303, 1997.

88. Marshall RI, Bartold PM: A clinical review of drug-induced gingival overgrowths, *Aust Dent J* 44 (4):219–232, 1999.

89. Seymour RA, Ellis JS, Thomason JM: Risk factors for drug-induced gingival overgrowth, *J Clin Periodontol* 27(4):217–223, 2000.

90. Addy M, Dowell P: Dentine hypersensitivity—a review: clinical and in vitro evaluation of treatment agents, *J Clin Periodontol* 10(4):351–363, 1983.

91. Dongari-Bagtzoglou A: Drug-associated gingival enlargement, *J Periodontol* 75(10):1424–1431, 2004.

92. Westbrook P, Bednarczyk EM, Carlson M, et al: Regression of nifedipine-induced gingival hyperplasia following switch to a same class calcium channel blocker, isradipine, *J Periodontol* 68 (7):645–650, 1997.

93. James JA, Marley JJ, Jamal S, et al: The calcium channel blocker used with cyclosporin has an effect on gingival overgrowth, *J Clin Periodontol* 27(2):109–115, 2000.

94. James JA, Jamal S, Hull PS, et al: Tacrolimus is not associated with gingival overgrowth in renal transplant patients, *J Clin Periodontol* 28(9):848–852, 2001.

95. Khocht A, Schneider LC: Periodontal management of gingival overgrowth in the heart transplant patient: a case report, *J Periodontol* 68(11): 1140–1146, 1997.

96. Woo SB, Hellstein JW, Kalmar JR: Systematic review: bisphosphonates and osteonecrosis of the jaws, *Ann Intern Med* 144(10):753–761, 2006.

97. Ruggiero SL, Mehrotra B, Rosenberg TJ, Engroff SL: Osteonecrosis of the jaws associated with the use of bisphosphonates: a review of 63 cases, *J Oral Maxillofac Surg* 62(5):527–534, 2004.

98. Thie NM, Kato T, Bader G, et al: The significance of saliva during sleep and the relevance of oromotor movements, *Sleep Med Rev* 6(3):213–227, 2002.

99. Dreizen S, Daly TE, Drane JB, Brown LR: Oral complications of cancer radiotherapy, *Postgrad Med* 61(2):85–92, 1977.

100. Epstein JB, van der Meij EH, Lunn R, Stevenson-Moore P: Effects of compliance with fluoride gel application on caries and caries risk in patients after radiation therapy for head and neck cancer, *Oral Surg Oral Med Oral Pathol Oral Radiol Endod* 82(3):268–275, 1996.

101. Genco RJ, Loe H: The role of systemic conditions and disorders in periodontal disease, *Periodontol 2000* 2:98–116, 1993.

102. Genco RJ: Current view of risk factors for periodontal diseases, *J Periodontol* 67(10 Suppl): 1041–1049, 1996.

103. Mealey BL, Rethman MP: Periodontal disease and diabetes mellitus: bidirectional relationship, *Dent Today* 22(4):107–113, 2003.

104. Scannapieco FA, Bush RB, Paju S: Associations between periodontal disease and risk for nosocomial bacterial pneumonia and chronic obstructive pulmonary disease: a systematic review, *Ann Periodontol* 8(1):54–69, 2003.

105. Scannapieco FA: Systemic effects of periodontal diseases, *Dent Clin North Am* 49(3):533–550, 2005.

106. Southerland JH, Taylor GW, Moss K, et al: Commonality in chronic inflammatory diseases: periodontitis, diabetes, and coronary artery disease, *Periodontol 2000* 40:130–143, 2006.

107. American Academy of Periodontology: Position paper: epidemiology of periodontal diseases, *J Periodontol* 67(9):935–945, 1996.

108. Grossi SG, Skrepcinski FB, DeCaro T, et al: Treatment of periodontal disease in diabetics reduces glycated hemoglobin, *J Periodontol* 68(8):713–719, 1997.

109. Miller LS, Manwell MA, Newbold D, et al: The relationship between reduction in periodontal inflammation and diabetes control: a report of 9 cases, *J Periodontol* 63(10):843–848, 1992.

110. Soskolne WA, Klinger A: The relationship between periodontal diseases and diabetes: an overview, *Ann Periodontol* 6(1):91–98, 2001.

111. Taylor GW, Burt BA, Becker MP, et al: Glycemic control and alveolar bone loss progression in type 2 diabetes, *Ann Periodontol* 3(1):30–39, 1998.

112. Aldridge JP, Lester V, Watts TL, et al: Single-blind studies of the effects of improved periodontal health on metabolic control in type 1 diabetes mellitus, *J Clin Periodontol* 22(4):271–275, 1995.

113. Janket SJ, Wightman A, Baird AE, et al: Does periodontal treatment improve glycemic control in diabetic patients? a meta-analysis of intervention studies, *J Dent Res* 84(12):1154–1159, 2005.

114. Taylor GW: Periodontal treatment and its effects on glycemic control: a review of the evidence, *Oral Surg Oral Med Oral Pathol Oral Radiol Endod* 87 (3):311–316, 1999.

115. Beck J, Garcia R, Heiss G, et al: Periodontal disease and cardiovascular disease, *J Periodontol* 67(10 Suppl):1123–1137, 1996.

116. Scannapieco FA, Bush RB, Paju S: Associations between periodontal disease and risk for atherosclerosis, cardiovascular disease, and stroke: a systematic review, *Ann Periodontol* 8(1):38–53, 2003.

117. Hujoel PP, Drangsholt M, Spiekerman C, DeRouen TA: Periodontal disease and coronary heart disease risk, *JAMA* 284(11):1406–1410, 2000.

118. Paoletti R, Gotto AM Jr, Hajjar DP: Inflammation in atherosclerosis and implications for therapy, *Circulation* 109(23 Suppl 1):III20–III26, 2004.

119. Beck JD, Eke P, Heiss G, et al: Periodontal disease and coronary heart disease: a reappraisal of the exposure, *Circulation* 112(1):19–24, 2005.

120. Hujoel PP, Drangsholt M, Spiekerman C, DeRouen TA: Examining the link between coronary heart disease and the elimination of chronic dental infections, *J Am Dent Assoc* 132(7):883–889, 2001.

121. Nakib SA, Pankow JS, Beck JD, et al: Periodontitis and coronary artery calcification: the Atherosclerosis Risk in Communities (ARIC) study, *J Periodontol* 75(4):505–510, 2004.

122. Lockhart PB: The risk for endocarditis in dental practice, *Periodontology 2000* 23:127–135, 2000.

123. Lang NP, Cumming BR, Loe H: Toothbrushing frequency as it relates to plaque development and gingival health, *J Periodontol* 44(7):396–405, 1973.

124. Loe H, Anerud A, Boysen H, Morrison E: Natural history of periodontal disease in man. Rapid, moderate and no loss of attachment in Sri Lankan laborers 14 to 46 years of age, *J Clin Periodontol* 13(5):431–445, 1986.

125. Lang NP, Lindhe J, van d, V: Advances in the prevention of periodontitis. Group D consensus report of the 5th European Workshop in Periodontology, *J Clin Periodontol* 32(Suppl 6):291–293, 2005.

126. Axelsson P, Lindhe J: Effect of controlled oral hygiene procedures on caries and periodontal disease in adults. Results after 6 years, *J Clin Periodontol* 8(3):239–248, 1981.

127. Graves RC, Disney JA, Stamm JW: Comparative effectiveness of flossing and brushing in reducing interproximal bleeding, *J Periodontol* 60(5):243–247, 1989.

128. Baehni PC, Takeuchi Y: Anti-plaque agents in the prevention of biofilm-associated oral diseases, *Oral Dis* 9(Suppl 1): 23–29, 2003.

129. Zimmer S, Kolbe C, Kaiser G, et al: Clinical efficacy of flossing versus use of antimicrobial rinses, *J Periodontol* 77(8):1380–1385, 2006.

130. Sharma NC, Charles CH, Qaqish JG, et al: Comparative effectiveness of an essential oil mouthrinse and dental floss in controlling interproximal gingivitis and plaque, *Am J Dent* 15(6):351–355, 2002.

131. Mandel ID: Antimicrobial mouthrinses: overview and update, *J Am Dent Assoc* 125(Suppl 2):2S–10S, 1994.

132. Netuveli GS, Sheiham A: A systematic review of the effectiveness of anticalculus dentifrices, *Oral Health Prev Dent* 2(1):49–58, 2004.

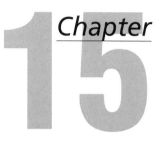

Chapter

15

Sexual Health

Brian D. Zamboni, PhD

Key Points

- Hypoactive sexual desire among men should be assessed by examining their medication regimen, free and total serum testosterone levels, and overall health status. Treatment should involve addressing these medical issues and collaborating with an experienced sex therapist who practices cognitive-behavioral therapy (strength of recommendation: C).
- Assessment of MED should include a review of health and medical risk factors, including vascular disease. Oral medication (e.g., sildenafil) may be helpful in most cases and is the best first-line of medical intervention, but in refractory cases this should be combined with treatment from a trained sex therapist (strength of recommendation: B).
- Men who are concerned about PE may find it helpful to take clomipramine, paroxetine, sertraline, or fluoxetine. Treatment may be enhanced by assistance from a sex therapist (strength of recommendation: C).
- Cases of delayed ejaculation or male orgasmic disorder (MOD) require a thorough evaluation by a medical doctor and a sex therapist. Men who are already taking medication may need a change in the dosage of their medicine or a change in regimen (strength of recommendation: C).
- Reports of men experiencing pain during sexual activity are relatively uncommon and varied, making it difficult to generate treatment guidelines. A multidisciplinary approach to assessment and treatment is paramount (strength of recommendation: C).
- Men with compulsive sexual behavior may need medication for a mood disorder or medication for obsessive-compulsive-type tendencies (e.g., fluoxetine). Medication can be a critical component of treatment in these cases, but an appropriate sex therapist should be involved (strength of recommendation: C).

Introduction

Men's sexual health is a broad topic that can encompass a wide range of sex-related issues. The focus of this chapter will be on sexual dysfunction with some additional attention to compulsive sexual behavior and paraphilias. There are four general categories of sexual dysfunction, largely based on the Masters and Johnson sexual response cycle[1]: sexual desire disorders, sexual arousal disorders, orgasmic disorders, and sexual pain disorders. For men, the corresponding diagnoses include hypoactive sexual desire disorder (HSDD), sexual aversion disorder, male erectile disorder (MED), premature ejaculation (PE), male orgasmic disorder (MOD), and dyspareunia. Most research on male sexual dysfunction focuses on MED or PE, presumably because these are the most common sexual problems among men. Yet, a sizable number of men experience low sexual desire and more and more men are reporting problems related to orgasm.

In addition to the symptoms for each specific sexual dysfunction, the standard definition of any sexual dysfunction using the diagnostic criteria in the fourth edition of the *Diagnostic and Statistical Manual of Mental Disorders* (DSM-IV)[2] includes a notation that (1) "the disturbance causes marked personal distress or interpersonal difficulty" and (2) "the sexual dysfunction is not better accounted for by another disorder, except another sexual dysfunction, and is not due to the direct effects of a substance (e.g., drugs of abuse, medication) or a general medical condition." Situational or acquired sexual problems can have important implications for the diagnosis and treatment of sexual dysfunction, making the need for clinical judgment critical.[3] The DSM-IV definition makes provisions for these instances by including four types of sexual dysfunction: (1) *lifelong type*, in which the person has always experienced the problem; (2) *acquired type*, in which the problem developed after a period of normal sexual functioning; (3) *generalized type*, in which the problem occurs in all situations and with all partners; and (4) *situational type*, in which the difficulty occurs in some situations and/or with some partners.[2,4] A client may receive two of these criteria (i.e., lifelong or acquired type and generalized or situational type). Clinicians may indicate whether the condition originates from psychological factors or a combination of primary psychological factors and a secondary medical condition or substance use.[2] These broad labels hint of a complex and multifaceted etiology in sexual dysfunction.

Brief Overview of History, Theory, and Research of Sex Therapy

The short history of sex therapy[5] started with psychoanalytic perspectives in the late 1960s and changed to a mix of behavioral, social, and cognitive perspectives over the following two decades.[4,6,7] Advances in medicine, increasingly complex clinical presentations, and a bias toward medical interventions have led to a medical focus in treating almost any type of sexual dysfunction.[3,7–10] The psychological versus medical debate of etiology represents a false dichotomy, however, and most scholars recognize the need to take an integrated and multidisciplinary approach to sexual health.[11] In other words, rather than focus on purely psychosocial causes or purely medical causes of sexual dysfunction, healthcare providers should conceptualize, assess, and treat all medical and psychological factors relevant to the sexual difficulty in men.[12] An interdisciplinary team approach to treating sexual dysfunction should include family physicians, psychiatrists, sex therapists, and physical therapists, depending on the nature of the problem.

Unfortunately, regardless of theoretical orientation or treatment approach, there is only modest evidence for empirically validated treatments of sexual dysfunction.[13] Many studies of sexual problems do not use rigorous research methodology, making it difficult to determine the efficacy of the intervention techniques. Typically, outcome data are compared with baseline data to determine treatment efficacy, and comparisons are not made between groups.[14] The challenge of conducting research in clinical settings continues to be formidable, particularly for a sensitive issue such as sexual dysfunction (e.g., limitations in monetary support for staff and resources, obtaining adequate numbers of participants, ethical issues in obtaining a control group). Thus, sex therapy research tends to lack large, well-designed outcome studies that include treatment manuals and waiting list or placebo control groups.[7,13] The lack of funding for adequate sex therapy research is a major contributing factor to this empiric stagnation, leading to a large number of modest outcome studies.[13] Wiederman[7] suggests that integrating sex therapy into other clinical domains, where issues of sexuality are generally ignored, may lead to greater research support and empirically validated outcome studies, which could also lead to better clinical outcomes.

This brief overview of the history of sex therapy research and treatment should serve as a backdrop for each sexual dysfunction highlighted in this chapter. In short, there are many theoretical and therapeutic orientations, but very few data to substantiate empirically validated treatments. The tension between medical and psychosocial causes and treatment of sexual problems needs to mature into a multidimensional, interdisciplinary approach to assessment and treatment of sexual dysfunction.

Hypoactive Sexual Desire Disorder and Sexual Aversion Disorder

The study of HSDD has been limited to the last three decades, having been first identified and described by Kaplan and Lief independently in 1977.[3] Persons with HSDD do not seek sexual gratification, behave as if they have no sex drive, and may fail to initiate or respond to sexual expressions.[15] Sexual aversion disorder is related to HSDD but involves an extreme distaste or avoidance of any sexual activity. There is less research on sexual aversion disorder, but it is often diagnosed among women, particularly those with histories of trauma.[16] Men with a history of trauma may become averse to sex, but the paucity of data on this topic precludes any definitive conclusions. Therefore, this section will focus exclusively on HSDD among men.

Although the incidence of HSDD in the general population is unknown, 31–55% of couples at sex therapy clinics report HSDD.[15] The disorder currently appears to be one of the most common presenting complaints in sex therapy clinics[17-20] and has often been linked to other sexual dysfunctions.[21] Historically, more women than men have been diagnosed with HSDD.[18,22,23] Previous studies show variable frequencies of sexual desire disorders, ranging from 31% to 49% in women and 1% to 38% in men.[24] Population-based studies suggest that 30% of women and 15% of men experience low sexual desire.[25] The number of men with HSDD has grown markedly, with some clinicians reporting nearly equal numbers of men and women presenting with low sexual desire.[18,22,23]

Definitions

The concept of sexual desire remains vague and difficult to define, plagued by such imprecise terms as *libido* and *sexual drive*.[23] Sexual desire has been difficult to study due to societal discomfort with sexuality, a preoccupation with sexual intercourse, and the sheer complexity of sexual desire.[22,23] The standard definition of HSDD using the diagnostic criteria in the DSM-IV[2] is "persistently or recurrently deficient (or absent) sexual fantasies and desire for sexual activity. The judgment of deficiency is made by the clinician, taking into account factors that affect sexual functioning, such as age and the context of the person's life." Researchers have criticized this definition because it offers vague and general criteria, avoids a statement of normal and abnormal sexual desire, and relies on subjective clinical judgment.[26] The lack of normative data on basic sexual desire contributes to the subjectivity of HSDD.

The DSM-IV denotation of HSDD appears to recognize how interpersonal dynamics can relate to the disorder and that persons who are not currently in a relationship can experience a low sexual desire. Although systemic factors are highly important in cases of discrepant sexual desire since interpersonal dynamics can influence interest in sex,[3] HSDD can also interfere with a person's sexuality and sexual activities (e.g., masturbation), causing significant personal distress. Finally, this definition does not include the frequency of sexual intercourse as criteria. A person with HSDD can have sex due to self-inflicted pressure or a partner's pressure, which may be overt or covert. Also, one may have infrequent and satisfying sex. In short, frequency of sexual intercourse alone may not represent sexual desire.[17,23,27,28]

Etiologies

Due to the complex and ambiguous nature of sexual desire, a wide variety of etiologic factors have been suggested to explain HSDD. The proposed etiologic factors can be succinctly summarized, recognizing that HSDD may consist of multiple causes and exists as a multidimensional construct.[3,17,22]

Organic or medical problems related to HSDD have been explored, including illness, medications, and hormone levels, especially low levels of androgens.[9,29,30] Environmental or psychosocial problems such as stress, work, and lack of opportunity have been emphasized.[18] Traumatic events including rape and sexual abuse have also been cited,[28,31] and sociocultural factors have also been stressed.[32] Relationship problems include conflicts, intimacy issues, power imbalance, and negative feelings.[18,20,23,33] Behavioral deficiencies may involve communication skills and sexual skills.[19,21,34,35] Developmental and cognitive factors include negative attitudes toward sex and unhealthy or unrealistic sexual expectations.[21,35] Psychological or emotional states such as fear, depression, anxiety, and anger have been shown to interfere with sexual desire in men.[18,22,36]

Several potential etiologic factors for HSDD have been identified, but clinicians and researchers need to organize and characterize these agents properly. Consideration should be given to which causal factors are most common, for which individuals and couples, under what circumstances and conditions. Furthermore, rigorous, multidimensional models must be built to reflect the various potential pathways in the development of HSDD. Complex statistical techniques, such as structural equation modeling, may help organize and test the relationships between these hypothesized variables. A thorough understanding of the features and course of these etiologic agents should improve treatment strategies for this common sexual disorder.

Treatment

Currently, there are no effective pharmacologic agents available to effectively treat HSDD.[37] Medically, testosterone is the only substance that has been shown to promote sexual desire in men in general,[38] particularly among men with hypogonadism.[39] It is important to assess both the free and total testosterone levels in men with low sexual desire. Testosterone replacement can involve buccal mucosa preparations, intramuscular injections, and scrotal and nonscrotal patches. Dosage and overall treatment should be individualized because androgen replacement can have negative effects on a man's liver function, lipid profile, cardiovascular functioning, prostate, sleep, and emotions.[40]

Although testosterone supplementation can help to promote sexual desire, among men it is primarily mediated by cognitive factors.[41] Many men with a low sexual desire do not have abnormal hormone levels, and men with low testosterone do not necessarily experience HSDD.[42] The small number of double-blind, placebo-controlled studies to date indicate that the correlation between hormones and sexual desire is rather weak.[42] Despite these findings, it is important to rule out low testosterone levels and, more specifically, pituitary problems by gaining a complete hormone profile from male clients. This involves serum assays for morning levels of both free and total testosterone and estradiol, when these hormone levels peak in men.

Perhaps the only other medical intervention for low sexual desire among men would be to consider changing the dosage or regimen of a man's current medications, such as lowering the dosage of an antidepressant or switching the type of cardiovascular medication (e.g., beta-blockers or calcium channel blockers) he takes.[43] Although sexual side effects including low sexual desire are a common adverse effect of selective serotonin reuptake inhibitors (SSRIs), there are no controlled studies that examine SSRI-induced sexual dysfunction and its management.[44] Bupropion (Wellbutrin) is often prescribed for depression or other clinical issues in part because it has a low risk of sexual side effects.[45] Combining medical and psychotherapy becomes critical for the treatment of low sexual desire.[43,46]

In terms of psychotherapy, conceptualizing low sexual desire as a problem in the relationship and including the man's partner (if applicable) has been shown to improve treatment success.[15] Various types of therapy have been used to treat low sexual desire, albeit the existing data often focus on HSDD among women rather than men. These therapeutic approaches include a basic systems approach,[47] Minuchin's structural family therapy,[48] and Haley's strategic therapy.[15] Given the long history of applying behavioral therapies

to sexual dysfunctions,[49] it is not surprising that cognitive-behavioral approaches have been developed and applied to the treatment of HSDD. For example, a cognitive-behavioral treatment program described by LoPiccolo[49] includes effectual awareness of one's attitudes toward sex, insight into negative attitudes toward sex, identifying self-statements that interfere with sexual desire, and generating coping statements to address emotional responses to sex (e.g., a cognitive tactic), and a variety of behaviorally oriented homework assignments are practiced (e.g., assertion, communication, and sexual skills training). Scholars other than LoPiccolo have described cognitive-behavioral models of treating HSDD including McCarthy,[50] who has highlighted various strategies and techniques for the treatment of inhibited sexual desire.

As noted earlier, most studies of HSDD and other sexual dysfunctions do not use rigorous research methodology, making it difficult to determine the efficacy of the intervention techniques. In a review of the literature, O'Carroll[29] concluded that no controlled treatment studies of HSDD using a homogenous sample of patients had been conducted. Using more relaxed criteria, Beck[17] described seven studies of HSDD treatment but concluded that a clear statement of treatment efficacy could not be made. Two controlled outcome studies of HSDD treatment have been reported by Hurlbert and colleagues[19,34] using strict criteria of random assignment to a treatment condition and a control group.[14] Although both studies were targeting women with low sexual desire, the results may be extrapolated to men with low sexual desire. This research warrants some degree of detailed attention because of the scientific rigor involved.

Hurlbert and colleagues have presented the most methodologically sound studies of HSDD treatment to date. The treatment package appears to be influenced by a combination of theories and techniques: cognitive, behavioral, and social exchange theory. In the initial study,[19] women with partner-specific HSDD and their partners were randomly assigned to receive a standard treatment package (n = 28) or standard treatment with orgasm consistency training (n = 11). Standard treatment involved a combination of sex and marital therapy with social exchange theory.[19] The intervention uses LoPiccolo's techniques (described above) and stresses mutual exchange as well as the interdependence of positive reinforcement in a relationship. The treatment increases the ratio of positive to negative reinforcement, enhances communication and conflict-resolution skills, and decreases dysfunctional beliefs.

Orgasm consistency training is a cognitive-behavioral intervention that postulates that HSDD results from sexual technique deficits.[19] The intervention includes directed masturbation, sensate focus exercises, and coital alignment exercises. The exercises stress that men can reach orgasm only after the women do and that the experience of orgasm be due to partner-related sexual activities. This approach emphasizes the importance of rewards via mutual exchange and interdependence of reinforcement in a relationship.[19] At post-treatment, women in both groups reported significantly positive sexual changes on two of four measures (e.g., increased sexual desire and arousal). Compared with those in the standard treatment group, women receiving combined treatment reported greater sexual arousal and assertiveness at post-treatment, 3-month follow-up, and 6-month follow-up as well as greater sexual satisfaction at 6-month follow-up. The fact that significant findings were found despite low numbers of participants in each group may speak to the utility of this treatment approach. Original participants randomly assigned to each group were lost due to military obligations, but analyses showed no significant difference between the groups after the loss.[19]

In a second treatment study for women with HSDD,[34] three groups received the standard treatment combined with orgasm consistency training: a women-only group (n = 19), couples-only group (n = 19), and a waiting list control group (n = 19). The groups were assessed before treatment, after the intervention, and at a 6-month follow-up. Five participants in the women-only group were lost at follow-up. Both treatment groups improved after treatment, but positive change increased with time and was greater for the couples-only group. Thus, this treatment for HSDD was found to be more effective than no treatment at all.[34]

These results indicate that this treatment can be effectively applied to an individual, suggesting that a couples approach is not essential. Nonetheless, the results seen in the couples-only group was superior to the women-only group, suggesting that HSDD involves a strong interpersonal component. Focusing on female sexuality, cognitive factors, and behavioral factors as they relate to sexual desire are strengths of this approach. A theoretically analogous but technically modified approach for males may aid men with HSDD, but this remains an open question as comparable research has not been conducted in male subjects. Rewards via mutual exchange and interdependence of reinforcement in a relationship may be important in treating men with HSDD, but the forms of reinforcement may be different for men than women (e.g., appreciation from a sex partner rather than orgasm consistency training per se).

Hurlbert's[34] standard cognitive-behavioral treatment with orgasm consistency training has been shown to be successful in treating HSDD. Thus, integrating cognitive-behavioral sex therapy and possible medical interventions may provide the most efficacious treatment of low sexual desire among men.

Male Erectile Disorder

MED involves the persistent or recurrent inability to attain or maintain an adequate erection until the completion of sexual activity.[51] Although the "completion of sexual activity" might be presumed to mean ejaculation and orgasm for the man, satisfactory or completed sex need not involve these responses. To make an accurate diagnosis of MED, the erection problem must cause personal distress, interpersonal difficulty, or both. Like other sexual dysfunctions, the diagnosis of MED is only given when it is not better accounted for by another axis I disorder, medication/drugs, or general and potentially reversible medical condition. When a significant comorbid diagnosis (e.g., major depression, alcoholism) is causing the MED, the major condition needs to be treated rather than the MED. It is considered to be normal for a male to lose his erection during sexual activity on occasion, and many times the erection will return if sexual activity is continued. MED reflects consistent and persistent difficulties with erections.

Health professionals have criticized the term impotence when discussing MED because it can be an imprecise and pejorative term.[52] Sometimes a man will say that he has problems with impotence, but on further inquiry, the clinician may learn that he is talking about PE or sexual desire problems. *Impotence* is a term that has been used to describe a wide variety of sexual problems, and its true meaning can become lost.

MED is often cited as one of the most common sexual dysfunctions among men, second only to PE. According to the National Institutes of Health Consensus Panel on Impotence,[53] 10–20 million men have some type of MED. Many outpatient visits, hospital admissions, and presenting complaints at sex therapy clinics have been related to MED.[54,55] MED becomes more common as men age. The Massachusetts Male Aging Study[56] showed that 52% of men 40–70 years old had some degree of MED. Although MED is not life threatening, it is associated with negative mood states (e.g., depression, anxiety, shame, embarrassment). MED can negatively affect a man's self-esteem and interpersonal relationships, sexual happiness, and life happiness.[54] To some degree, MED has become a more socially acceptable problem to discuss and treat, but there is still stigma attached to the condition. Despite the availability of medication and use of medical interventions, the number of cases of MED has not seemed to decrease in the last several years.

Etiology

In the 1960s, scholars assumed that MED was mostly due to psychological factors.[52] Although medical and surgical interventions started in the 1970s, they have flourished over the past 15 years. The advent of sildenafil (Viagra) has certainly played a large role in what Rosen[54] and others have called the "medicalization of male sexuality." Medical treatments are now seen as more efficient and effective than psychological treatments, despite the fact that psychological or psychosocial issues are frequently involved.[52] Currently, most experts agree that a multidisciplinary approach is needed to evaluate and treat erectile disorder.[11,12] A case of MED that seems to have a primarily organic etiology may still have psychosocial factors involved in the evaluation and treatment.[52] Similarly, a case of MED that may have primarily psychosocial causal factors might still benefit from medical evaluation and treatment.

There is a long list of physiologic factors that can influence MED, but there are few data to support the specific prevalence of any particular causal factor. The most common physiologic factors include medications, health status, and advancing age.[37] Other physiologic etiologic factors include diabetes mellitus, heart disease, hypertension, arteriosclerosis, traumatic injury, surgical complications, cigarette smoking, and drug/alcohol use.[57] A detailed account of erectile dysfunction in the setting of diabetes mellitus is highlighted in Chapter 9, Endocrinology. MED can be also associated with some types of cancer, such as testicular or prostate cancer.[58–61] In one meta-analysis of available studies on testicular cancer,[59] the authors concluded that erectile dysfunction and other sexual problems occur in conjunction with, but are not always related to, disease or treatment processes; instead, erectile dysfunction may be associated with

psychological adjustment to the testicular cancer. Statistics concerning the incidence of MED in men after radical prostatectomy vary widely and have been estimated to range from 16% to 82%.[60] The likelihood of MED depends on several factors, such as the man's age, the severity of the cancer, comorbid issues, and the degree to which the surgery has affected the corpus cavernosa.[60]

Having one or multiple risk factors for MED does not necessarily lead to MED. For example, having diabetes does not guarantee that men will have erectile dysfunction. In contrast to prior studies, one comprehensive review of basic research and controlled studies suggests that only 26–35% of men with diabetes will have erectile dysfunction.[62] This is only a slight increase in risk for erectile disorder compared with men without diabetes. Spontaneous remission can occur for some men with erectile disorder.[62] In short, it is important to be aware of medical risk factors for MED and screen men for them. Medications do not necessarily lead to sexual dysfunction like erectile problems, and some medications may be less likely to cause sexual side effects (e.g., Wellbutrin, trazodone, Remeron, angiotensin-converting enzyme inhibitors).

Psychosocial etiologic factors for MED include sociocultural influences, psychosexual trauma, sexual skills or techniques (e.g., changing positions too often; inadequate foreplay), emotional factors, relationship problems, psychological conflicts, performance anxiety, irrational beliefs, intimacy dysfunction (e.g., family of origin), and sexual attitudes and knowledge. Assessment is used for diagnosis, case formulation, and treatment. Because of the long history and high degree of interest in MED, several assessment techniques have been developed.

Ackerman and Carey[52] have provided a thorough review of various assessment strategies for MED. They note that health professionals often rely on client self-report and ask a few clinical questions, but various queries can be organized into a semi-structured clinical interview. They concluded from existing research that semi-structured clinical interviews can be constructed to provide a reliable and valid assessment of erectile function, an assessment that correlates highly with more expensive and intensive biomedical evaluations.[52] Physicians may not have the time, interest, or skill to conduct such clinical interviews; thus, a qualified sex therapist can help with this assessment. In terms of self-administered questionnaires, global measures of personality or sexuality (e.g., Minnesota Multiphasic Personality Inventory, Derogatis Sexual

Functioning Inventory) may be useful for case formulation and planning, but questionnaires with items specific to MED (e.g., Sexual Self-efficacy Scale-Erectile Functioning, Leiden Impotence Questionnaire, Miami Sexual Dysfunction Protocol) are superior for diagnosing the degree and patterns of erectile dysfunction.[52] These types of specific questionnaires are not commonly used except in research and in some sexual therapy clinics. The assessment and treatment of MED might be enhanced if measures specific to erectile functioning are routinely included in practice.

Physiologic assessment approaches to erectile dysfunction can be useful because men can underestimate their erections and their sexual partners can provide contradicting information. Ackerman and Carey[52] also reviewed various physiologic measures for MED, including nocturnal penile tumescence, RigiScan diagnostic monitor, and visual sexual stimulation. These procedures can be expensive for patients, are not readily available for use, and may not be adequately reliable. The authors note, "...[E]ven a perfect measure of tumescence and rigidity should not be regarded as anything more than a single, albeit significant, component in a comprehensive biopsychosocial formulation."[52]

Treatment

There are a wide variety of medical and surgical treatment choices for MED.[37] Semi-rigid surgical prostheses, inflatable prostheses, venous ligation surgery, intracavernosal injections (e.g., papaverine, alprostadil), topical creams, and oral medications have all been used with success.[54] Vascular surgery has been shown to help restore erectile functioning in some men whose MED is related to vascular problems.[51] Penile implant surgery is not reversible, and consequently, it is reserved for cases of MED that have not responded to less invasive forms of therapy.[54] Although there are data to show that implant surgery has been effective, past studies have methodologic flaws that masked some of the problems and concerns of implant surgery (e.g., mechanical problems, suboptimal quality of erections).[51] Advanced technology has improved penile implants, but less invasive and less expensive treatments for MED have decreased the popularity of this treatment option.[51,54]

Injection therapy has been shown to be effective in treating MED in 79–91% of cases, but approximately 50% of men discontinue the injections because of pain or minor bruising.[57] Prolonged erections, fibrotic nodules, liver function problems, vasovagal incidents, and infection can be other adverse effects of injection therapy.[57] The vacuum erection or constriction devices are nonsurgical instruments (e.g., a plastic cylinder) that draw blood into the penis, causing an erection that is maintained with a rubber constriction ring placed at the base of the penis. Despite the strong efficacy of these devices, the dropout rate of men using them can be substantial due to inconvenience and discomfort.[51,54]

Sildenafil (Viagra) is a selective type-5 phosphodiesterase inhibitor that has been shown to be effective in treating MED in randomized double-blind, placebo-controlled trials.[63] Men with cardiac problems need to be evaluated before taking Viagra—specifically, men taking nitrates should not take Viagra.[64] Vardenafil and tadalafil are other similar medications that have been shown to help improve men with MED,[64,65] whereas other oral agents (e.g., yohimbine, apomorphine) have not been as efficacious in treating MED.[57,64] Oral medication can be highly successful in resolving erection problems among men after radical prostatectomy, and any of the main three oral medications (i.e., sildenafil, vardenafil, and tadalafil) are considered the first line of therapy in these cases.[60,61]

Psychological interventions in sex therapy have been shown to be effective in treating MED. These therapy techniques include sex education, sensate focus exercises, systematic desensitization, and sexual communication skills in various therapeutic combinations.[37] In six comparison controlled studies, systematic desensitization was shown to be superior to psychoanalytic therapy or an attention placebo.[13] These therapeutic techniques help to increase comfort with sexuality and to reduce anxiety about sex while teaching sexual skills to maximize erectile functioning and sexual enjoyment (e.g., learning how to touch and provide stimulation, learning new ways of being sexual and intimate). Changing unhealthy thinking patterns (e.g., cognitive distortions) and changing interpersonal or systemic dynamics can be an important part of therapy as well.

Male Orgasmic Disorder

MOD is a challenging sexual dysfunction to explore because there are empiric, conceptual, terminologic, and scientific shortcomings in the literature. The DSM-IV[2] describes MOD as a "persistent or recurrent delay in, or absence of, orgasm following...normal sexual excitement..." Yet, this description does not appear to capture the full range of possible presenting complaints. Case studies and this author's own clinical experience suggest that there is considerable diversity in clinical presentations of MOD. For example, some men have reported ejaculating without an adequate feeling of orgasm. In other cases, men have difficulty ejaculating during vaginal sex or masturbation.

Perhaps the most common clinical scenario involves a man who can ejaculate and experience orgasm via masturbation without problems, but he has difficulty ejaculating and experiencing orgasm via vaginal intercourse. These are very different clinical scenarios that fall under the essentially the same diagnostic category of MOD. It is not clear whether these cases reflect problems with ejaculation, orgasm, or both. The answer likely depends on the specifics of the presenting complaint, but the diversity of clinical presentations clearly challenges our current understanding of ejaculation and orgasm among men. Ejaculation and orgasm are separate events that usually occur closely together.[66] Moreover, orgasm is both a subjective and a physiologic occurrence.

Laypersons and professionals alike tend to simplify men's sexuality and assume that if a man ejaculates, his orgasm is inevitable. Similarly, we might make the questionable assumption that all orgasms for men are easy to obtain, adequate, and subjectively feel the same. There is more research on orgasms among women and, unlike for women, there is no typology of orgasms for men.[62] Clearly, more research is needed on orgasm and orgasmic disorders among men. A potential question for future research could explore whether orgasms with retrograde ejaculation as subjectively pleasurable as orgasms with anterograde ejaculation.

The language used to describe these clinical phenomena appears to be imprecise and pejorative, further complicating our knowledge of MOD, as it is perhaps most commonly referred to as *retarded ejaculation*. Several other terms have been used to describe this condition, including *inhibited ejaculation, delayed ejaculation, ejaculatory incompetence, ejaculatory impotence, ejaculatio retardate, impotentia ejaculandi, absent ejaculation, "blue balls," impotence, ejaculatory anhedonia,* and *incomplete/partial retarded ejaculation*.[67-69] MOD should not be confused with retrograde ejaculation, in which a man's ejaculate is deposited into the bladder rather than exiting via the urethral meatus. A more complete review of retrograde ejaculation is available in Chapter 16, Urology. The professional literature is littered with case

studies and review articles on MOD, yet the majority typically do not add any conceptual or empirical depth to our current understanding of MOD.

Due to the lack of adequate data in the clinical and in general populations, accurate prevalence rates for MOD are difficult to accurately determine. Early studies suggested prevalence rates of 3.37–3.79% among men presenting with sexual dysfunction.[6,70] More recently, Rowland and colleagues[71] estimated the prevalence rate to range from 2% to 5%, depending how MOD is classified, and the overall prevalence of MOD is probably greater than reported.[72,73] Some men may not be bothered by a delayed ejaculation or varying subjective experience of orgasm, if any. Other men may be too embarrassed by these types of sexual difficulties and may avoid seeking treatment. Men with sexual partners may actually like having an absent or delayed ejaculation; thus, interpersonal conflict related to this sexual dysfunction does not occur. Nonetheless, some heterosexual men do seek treatment because of personal distress or, more commonly, because MOD interferes with his ability to conceive.

Etiology

The somewhat esoteric nature of this topic makes it difficult to conduct accurate research because few men actually present with MOD, and large-scale studies of even a descriptive nature are lacking. Consequently, conclusions regarding etiology and treatment are challenging to extrapolate from existing studies. Because of the complexity of this sexual problem, it is critical for health professionals to identify and employ the basic specifiers in each case of MOD: lifelong versus acquired, situational versus generalized, and that due to psychological factors versus that due to combined factors. A man who has never ejaculated via masturbation or other forms of sexual activity is different from a man who has ejaculated via masturbation but not via vaginal intercourse. A careful assessment can give clues to etiologic factors and thus can inform the overall treatment plan.

Pharmacologically induced MOD has become more commonplace.[37] Delayed ejaculation is a common adverse effect of SSRIs, but several medications have been implicated including other types of antidepressants and antipsychotic medications.[37,74,75] Some medical conditions have been linked to MOD, such as diabetes mellitus, spinal cord injury, and genital-urinary problems.

Perelman[72] has suggested that MOD results from an idiosyncratic masturbation style. A man's unique masturbation habits could make it difficult for him or others to reproduce the style and degree of stimulation in any other way. Cultural or religious scripts toward masturbation and sexuality in general could lead to idiosyncratic masturbation habits (e.g., masturbating in a way that makes him feel as if he is not masturbating and thus not violating his values) or personality characteristics that make it difficult for him to feel relaxed and comfortable with his sexual behavior. These possible etiologic factors point toward the importance of conducting a thorough assessment of a man's masturbation habits, sexual fantasies, and personality characteristics. This kind of assessment is sometimes completed over time because a man might reveal more of his sexual history and habits when he becomes more comfortable with a health professional. Such an evaluation is best conducted by a qualified health professional who can take the time for a thorough assessment.

Treatment

Campden-Main and Sara[76] have written, "The only cases of retarded ejaculation that are easy to treat are those secondary to medication that can be promptly discontinued." Although this is a vast overgeneralization, every man's medication regimen should be closely examined at the time of the initial evaluation. If a change in his medications cannot be made, perhaps the dosage can be altered or an adjunct prescription (e.g., bupropion in place of an SSRI) can ameliorate the MOD[77]; however, this strategy will not work for all clients.[78] These treatment approaches are based on modest research, anecdotal clinical evidence, and case studies, rather than empirically based research.

Psychotherapy can offer several options for therapy of MOD, but empirically validated treatment options are, again, lacking. Brief forms of therapy using standard sex therapy techniques appear to be more useful than psychoanalytic, long-term therapy; clients with more severe mental health issues require more therapy.[67,68,73] Cognitive-behavioral tasks with a well-trained sex therapist are important for treatment success. General treatment goals involve desensitizing the man to sexuality, de-emphasizing the symptom, focusing on his lack of psychological arousal, increasing his flexibility or variety in sex, and integrating this into sexual intercourse with his partner. As a part of therapy, men likely need to decrease various forms of shame or guilt about sexual topics and address any anger, anxiety, fear, or other emotional conflicts. Specific tasks vary but might include temporarily abstaining from masturbation and other forms of sexual activity and teaching the man various relaxation techniques. In terms of increasing his comfort with sexuality and exploring ways he can increase his mental or psychological sexual arousal, men with MOD need to ask themselves: What can make sex more fun, safe, or pleasurable? For example, he can explore various activities that might feel sensual or that make him feel sexy, without engaging in sexual behavior. Masturbating alone in a new way (e.g., using the opposite hand, not using any hands) and later involving his partner can be other therapeutic options.[72] Some men may need to learn how they can feel a greater sense of control and other men will need to decrease rigidity or obsessive-compulsive tendencies. As always, addressing relationship conflicts and improving sexual and nonsexual communication will be an important part of successful therapy.

Premature Ejaculation

PE has been a topic concern for men and, thus, a common theme in scholarly papers for many years.[79] Generally speaking, PE occurs when a man ejaculates sooner than he would like to, without any definitive time factor built into the definition. PE has also been referred to as *rapid ejaculation*,[80] among other terms. Typically, men would like to forestall ejaculation or "last longer" to prolong their physical and subjective enjoyment of sexual activity, to prolong their sex partner's enjoyment, or both. Although there are significant numbers of men who present with erectile dysfunction and increasing numbers who present with low sexual desire, several scholars suggest that PE is the most common sexual dysfunction among men.

Prevalence estimates vary considerably[81] but Laumann et al.'s[82] methodologically strong survey in the United States suggests a prevalence rate of 29%. It is important to note that most conceptualizations of PE, like most of the sexual dysfunctions, are heterosexist in that the referent is almost always penile-vaginal intercourse between a man and a woman.[80] In addition, when discussing PE, there is generally a questionable assumption that men should control the pacing of sexual activity and timing of ejaculation.

Assessing PE can be challenging because the diagnostic criteria are vague and subjective, and men may not have accurate perceptions of how long they engage in sexual activity before ejaculating. Grenier and Byers[83] found that several commonly used criteria for PE are only modestly correlated: ejaculatory latency, perceived ejaculatory control, concern over ejaculating more rapidly than desired, satisfaction with ejaculatory control, and involuntary ejaculation before intercourse. Similar findings were reported in a later study by the same authors.[84] These studies show that a man's conception and experience of PE can vary considerably. Although time from intromission to ejaculation is not necessarily a quality indicator of PE, it remains a common method of assessment. Schover and Jensen[85] have reported that healthy young males have a median latency of 7–10 minutes.

Etiology

Several etiologic factors have been theoretically linked to PE, yet little empiric research supports any of these ideas.[80] For example, early sexual experiences in which men masturbate quickly because of shame, guilt, or lack of privacy have often been cited as causing a predisposition to PE. Anxiety has been etiologically linked to PE by either activating the sympathetic nervous system (which causes the emission phase of ejaculation) or by interfering with a man's awareness of his sexual responses and ability to regulate his sexual behavior.[80] In the latter situation, the anxiety causes him to think about his sexual performance and he ejaculates before realization of the event.

Other factors that could contribute to PE include being highly aroused sexually, failing to use sexual techniques that forestall ejaculation, and having a penis that is more sensitive to stimulation (e.g., a man with a more sensitive penis reaches the point of ejaculatory inevitability more quickly). Grenier and Byers[80] argue that there is little empiric research to show that men with PE are different from a control group on these dimensions. As men age, symptoms and concerns about PE diminish.[86] It is unclear whether this suggests a change in biology over time (pointing toward a biologic predisposition to ejaculate quickly) or a change in sexual experience (e.g., learned behavior in a man's sexual development over time).

Treatment

At one time, the psychological and behavioral approaches to treating PE were popular and

apparently successful, with post-treatment success rates of 60–95%.[6] The utility of pharmacotherapy was de-emphasized and behavioral methods were viewed as superior.[87] These therapeutic gains were not necessarily maintained, however, and the success rates for psychological and behavioral treatment approaches to PE have fallen over time.[88] Despite this shift, sex therapy techniques like the "squeeze technique," used in conjunction with other therapeutic work, remain popular. The squeeze technique involves stimulating the penis until the man feels he might ejaculate, stopping before the point of ejaculatory inevitability, and squeezing the penis firmly at the base or below the glans for several seconds.[37] This process is repeated until the man allows himself to ejaculate. This technique is typically practiced by the man alone via masturbation for several trials before he repeats the exercise with his sex partner. In the only controlled study using this procedure, Heiman and LoPiccolo[89] reported longer durations of foreplay and intercourse. Other studies have reported similar results, but these studies lack controls and long-term follow-up data.[13]

Several studies involving the pharmacologic treatment of PE have shown that medication can be useful in ameliorating the symptom.[90] Waldinger and colleagues[91] conducted a review and meta-analysis of drug treatment studies published between 1943 and 2003. Of 79 publications, 35 studies examined the effects of serotonergic antidepressants on PE; eight of these studies were prospective, double-blind investigations that used timed assessments of ejaculation at baseline and during the drug trial.[91] Despite these stringent criteria, there are other studies that use a placebo-controlled design.[92] In general, this body of research suggests that clomipramine, paroxetine, sertraline, and fluoxetine are effective in treating PE.[91] Waldinger and colleagues[91] found the efficacy of paroxetine to be greater than the other agents, which had comparable levels of efficacy with one another. Once a client ceases to take the medication, however, the symptoms of PE typically return. The long-term effects of using pharmacotherapy to treat PE are unclear, and the viability of using medication on an as-needed basis is also unclear. More research is needed to address these topics. Topical anesthetics and herbal medications have also been used to treat PE, but the efficacy of these approaches are unclear because of the few and methodologically inconsistent studies in this area.[93]

Dyspareunia

Dyspareunia, a general diagnosis describing pain during sexual activity, has rarely been diagnosed among men and is not typically discussed in routine reviews of sexual dysfunction.[37] According to a large survey of the general population, 3% of men reported "pain during sexual activity" as a problem in their sexual activity in the past 12 months.[82] When a man presents with pain during sexual activity, the etiology may be related to anatomic features of his genitals, including penile angle, or it may be psychological in origin.[94-96]

Rosser and colleagues[97,98] conducted research that examines *anodyspareunia*, or pain during receptive anal sex among gay/bisexual men. In one study, 61% of gay/bisexual men (n = 197) reported painful receptive anal sex as the most frequent lifetime sexual difficulty,[97] but in another study only 24% of gay/bisexual men (n = 277) reported always experiencing some degree of pain during anal sex.[98] Not all gay/bisexual men practice anal intercourse, but Rosser and colleagues[98] suggest, based in part on subjective reports, that adequate lubrication, bodily relaxation, and preparatory digital anal massaging were important factors in avoiding anodyspareunia. Depth and rate of penile thrusting are other critical factors in predicting (and thus avoiding) pain, which can be rectified via adequate communication between sexual partners.[98] Damon and Rosser[99] found that psychological factors can be primary contributors to the experience of pain during anal intercourse, dispelling the idea that pain is inevitable during anal sex and highlighting the importance of assessing and treating psychological factors in anodyspareunia.

Compulsive Sexual Behavior and Paraphilias

Compulsive sexual behavior, also known as *sexual addiction*, is both a complex and controversial topic that is becoming a common problem among men, and it is important for physicians to be aware of the syndrome. The two types of compulsive sexual behavior include nonparaphilic and paraphilic.[100] Nonparaphilic compulsive sexual behavior involves typical sexual behavior that feels out of control, is causing personal or interpersonal distress, or is otherwise causing problems in some area of a man's life (e.g., work-related problems, social difficulties, financial problems). This sexual behavior often stems from something other than sexual desire, such as anxiety.[100] Some examples of these types of behaviors include excessive masturbation, multiple love affairs or sexual partners, and use of sexually explicit material (e.g., frequent use of pornography on the Internet or in magazines).

A paraphilia is an atypical sexual behavior, and such behaviors can be compulsive in nature for some men. Examples of paraphilic compulsive sexual behavior include using women's undergarments or diapers for sexual purposes and giving or receiving pain or humiliation for purposes of sexual excitement. There are a variety of forms of nonparaphilic and paraphilic sexual behavior, but the degree to which the behavior is problematic requires good clinical judgment by a trained healthcare provider. Sexual behavior that appears to be compulsive should not be confused with normal developmental processes, value differences within a couple, or situational variables.[100] Compulsive sexual behavior also can be overpathologized by professionals with restrictive attitudes about sexuality.[100]

The sexual behaviors in question can start slowly and escalate until the sexual behavior causes problems in some area of a man's life.[101] For example, the man may be so preoccupied by the sexual behavior that he is not getting work or completing domestic tasks in a timely manner. Clients often feel ashamed and have difficulty discussing the problematic sexual behavior and resulting negative effects on their lives. Compulsive sexual behavior can be an ongoing recurrent issue or an episodic problem.[100,101] The prevalence of compulsive sexual behavior has been estimated to be 3–6% of the US population, but these statistics may not be completely reliable.[101]

Empiric research does not support any particular set of etiologic factors for compulsive sexual behavior, but the etiology is likely to be multifaceted. Despite the assumption that men with compulsive sexual behavior have a history of trauma, this may not be a casual factor in all cases.[101] Men with compulsive sexual behavior may have substance abuse problems, mood disorders (e.g., depression or anxiety), obsessive-compulsive disorder–type characteristics, or personality-disorder characteristics such as narcissistic, antisocial, or dependent traits.[102,103] Treatment for this syndrome centers upon the 12-step, self-help approach, more formalized treatment, or both.[101] Group therapy is a common mode of treatment regardless of the setting, although individual therapy and couples therapy are important parts of the treatment process.[100,102] Physicians should know that medication can be a crucial piece of treatment for compulsive sexual behavior, as it may also be used to treat an existing axis I disorder and used to minimize urges for compulsive sexual behavior. Fluoxetine (Prozac), sertraline (Zoloft), and paroxetine (Paxil) are some of the more commonly prescribed medications to treat this condition.[100,102] There are several studies that report these various treatments to be effective, and a comprehensive or integrated approach may be particularly efficacious.[100–102] Unfortunately, empirically based evidence of treatments for compulsive sexual behavior is lacking.[101]

Conclusion

What conclusions can be drawn regarding the evidence for empirically validated treatments for men's sexual health concerns? The results are mixed and arguably modest. Because the treatment for sexual dysfunction needs to involve a combination of factors, it is challenging to quantify the overall quality of the current treatment approaches. Using the strength of recommendation taxonomy classification described by Ebell and colleagues,[104] the treatment for most sexual problems among men reach a B-level strength of recommendation. The need for a multidisciplinary approach to treatment is a C-level recommendation. Using pharmacotherapy to treat MED may be a specific A-level recommendation, but long-term follow-up studies are needed and men will likely need more than medication to achieve long-term amelioration of their symptoms. The treatments for HSDD, PE, and compulsive sexual behavior appear to involve B-level treatment recommendations. In these cases, physicians can consider the need for medication or the need for a change in a patient's medication regimen. Working with a sex therapist who can use carefully planned sex therapy techniques, including cognitive-behavioral methods, will be paramount. In contrast, the treatment for MOD and dyspareunia continue to involve C-level strength of recommendations. These cases tend to be individualized and need careful assessment by a medical professional, a sex therapist, and possibly other health professionals (e.g., a physical therapist). In summary, health professionals have a decent guidebook with which to work when it comes to assessing and treating sexual health concerns among men. Nonetheless, there is a clear need for strong research programs that can empirically test our current treatment paradigms.

References

1. Masters WH, Johnson VE: *Human Sexual Response,* Boston, 1966, Little, Brown.
2. American Psychiatric Association: *Diagnostic and Statistical Manual of Mental Disorders,* ed 4, Washington, DC, 1994, American Psychiatric Association.
3. Rosen RC, Leiblum SR: Hypoactive sexual desire, *Psychiatric Clin North Am* 18:107–121, 1995.
4. Kaplan H: *Disorders of Sexual Desire and Other New Concepts and Techniques in Sex Therapy,* New York, 1979, Brunner/Mazel.
5. Leiblum SR, Rosen RC: Sex therapy in the age of Viagra. In Leiblum SR, Rosen RC, editors: *Principles and Practice of Sex Therapy,* New York, 2000, Guilford Press, pp 1–13.
6. Masters WH, Johnson VE: *Human Sexual Inadequacy,* Boston, 1970, Little, Brown.
7. Wiederman MW: The state of theory in sex therapy, *J Sex Res* 35:88–99, 1998.
8. Leiblum SR, Rosen RC: The changing focus of sex therapy. In Rosen RC, Leiblum SR, editors: *Case Studies in Sex Therapy,* New York, 1995, Guilford, pp 3–17.
9. Schiavi RC, Segraves RT: The biology of sexual dysfunction, *Psychiatric Clin North Am* 18:7–23, 1995.
10. Schover LR, Leiblum SR: Commentary: the stagnation of sex therapy, *J Psychol Human Sex* 6:5–30, 1994.
11. Perelman M: Combination therapy for sexual dysfunction: integrating sex therapy and pharmacotherapy. In Balon R, Segraves RT, editors: *Handbook of Sexual Dysfunction,* New York, 2005, Taylor & Francis, pp 13–41.
12. Basson R: Integrating new biomedical treatments into the assessment and management of erectile dysfunction, *Can J Human Sex* 7:213–229, 1998.
13. Heiman JR, Meston CM: Empirically validated treatment for sexual dysfunction, *Annu Rev Sex Res* 8:148–194, 1997.
14. Baucom DH, Shoham V, Mueser KT, et al: Empirically supported couple and family interventions for marital distress and adult mental health problems, *J Consult Clin Psychol* 66:53–88, 1998.
15. Fish LS, Busby D, Killian K: Structural couple therapy in the treatment of inhibited sexual drive, *Am J Fam Ther* 22:113–125, 1994.
16. Finch S: Sexual aversion disorder treated with behavioural desensitization, *Can J Psychiatry* 46:563–564, 2001.
17. Beck JG: Hypoactive sexual desire disorder: an overview, *J Consult Clin Psychol* 63:919–927, 1995.
18. Donahey KM, Carroll RA: Gender differences in factors associated with hypoactive sexual desire, *J Sex Marital Ther* 19:25–40, 1993.
19. Hurlbert DF: A comparative study using orgasm consistency training in the treatment of women reporting hypoactive sexual desire, *J Sex Marital Ther* 19:41–55, 1993.

20. MacPhee DC, Johnson SM, Van der Veer MMC: Low sexual desire in women: the effects of marital therapy, *J Sex Marital Ther* 21:159–182, 1995.

21. Trudel G, Aubin S, Matte B: Sexual behaviors and pleasure in couples with hypoactive sexual desire, *J Sex Educ Ther* 21:210–216, 1995.

22. Mohl B, Pedersen BL: Men with inhibited sexual desire: the price of women's lib? *Nordisk Sex* 9:243–247, 1991.

23. Trudel G: Review of psychological factors in low sexual desire, *Sex Marital Ther* 6:261–272, 1991.

24. Segraves KB, Segraves RT: Hypoactive sexual desire disorder: prevalence and comorbidity on 906 subjects, *J Sex Marital Ther* 17:55–58, 1991.

25. Rosen RC: Prevalence and risk factors of sexual dysfunction in men and women, *Curr Psychiatry Rep* 2:189–195, 2000.

26. Trudel G, Ravart M, Matte B: The use of multiaxial diagnostic system for sexual dysfunctions in the assessment of hypoactive sexual desire, *J Sex Marital Ther* 19:123–130, 1993.

27. Hurlbert DF, Apt C: Female sexual desire, response, and behavior, *Behav Mod* 18:488–504, 1994.

28. McCabe MP: A program for the treatment of inhibited sexual desire in males, *Psychotherapy* 29: 288–296, 1992.

29. O'Carroll R: Sexual desire disorders: a review of controlled treatment studies, *J Sex Res* 28:607–624, 1991.

30. Schubert DSP: Reversal of doxepin-induced hypoactive sexual desire by substitution of nortriptyline, *J Sex Educ Ther* 18:42–44, 1992.

31. Kinzl JF, Traweger C, Biebl W: Sexual dysfunctions: relationship to childhood sexual abuse and early family experiences in a nonclinical sample, *Child Abuse Neglect* 19:785–792, 1995.

32. Mansfield PK, Voda A, Koch PB: Predictors of sexual response changes in heterosexual midlife women, *Health Values* 19:10–20, 1995.

33. Trudel G, Boulos L, Matte B: Dyadic adjustment in couples with hypoactive sexual desire, *J Sex Educ Ther* 19:31–36, 1993.

34. Hurlbert DF, White LC, Powell RD, Apt C: Orgasm consistency training in the treatment of women reporting hypoactive sexual desire: an outcome comparison of women-only groups and couples-only groups, *J Behav Ther Exp Psychiatry* 24:3–13, 1993.

35. McCarthy BW: Bridges to sexual desire, *J Sex Educ Ther* 21:132–141, 1995.

36. Radin MM: Preoedipal factors in relation to psychogenic inhibited sexual desire, *J Sex Marital Ther* 15:255–268, 1989.

37. Heiman JR: Sexual dysfunction: overview of prevalence, etiological factors, and treatments, *J Sex Res* 39:73–78, 2002.

38. Vignozzi L, Corona G, Petrone L, et al: Testosterone and sexual activity, *J Endocrinol Invest* 28: 39–44, 2005.

39. Albrecht-Betancourt M, Hijazi RA, Cunningham GR: Androgen replacement in men with hypogonadism and erectile dysfunction, *Endocrine* 23:143–148, 2004.

40. Wespes E, Schulman CC: Male andropause: myth, reality, and treatment, *Int J Impotence Res* 14(Suppl 1):S93–S98, 2002.

41. Rochira V, Zirilli L, Madeo B, et al: Sex steroids and sexual desire mechanism, *J Endocrinol Invest* 26:29–36, 2003.

42. LoPiccolo J: Diagnosis and treatment of male sexual dysfunction, *J Sex Marital Ther* 11:215–232, 1985.

43. Baldwin DS: Sexual dysfunction associated with antidepressant drugs, *Expert Opin Drug Safety* 3:457–470, 2004.

44. Woodrum ST, Brown CS: Management of SSRI-induced sexual dysfunction, *Ann Pharmacother* 32:1209–1215, 1998.

45. Zimmerman M, Posternak MA, Attiullah N, et al: Why isn't bupropion the most frequently prescribed antidepressant? *J Clin Psychiatry* 66: 603–610, 2005.

46. Tolman DL, Diamond LM: Desegregating sexuality research: cultural and biological perspectives on gender and desire, *Annu Rev Sex Res* 12: 33–74, 2001.

47. Regas SJ, Sprenkle DH: Functional family therapy and the treatment of inhibited sexual desire, *J Marital Fam Ther* 10:63–72, 1984.

48. Fish LS, Fish RC, Sprenkle DH: Treating inhibited sexual desire: a marital therapy approach, *Am J Fam Ther* 12:3–12, 1984.

49. LoPiccolo J: Sexual dysfunction. In Craighead LW, Craighead WE, Kazdin AF, Mahoney MJ, editors: *Cognitive and Behavioral Interventions: An Empirical Approach to Mental Health Problems*, Boston, 1994, Allyn & Bacon, pp 183–196.

50. McCarthy BW: Strategies and techniques for the treatment of inhibited sexual desire, *J Sex Marital Ther* 10:97–104, 1984.

51. Coleman E: Erectile dysfunction: a review of current medical treatments, *Can J Human Sex* 7: 231–244, 1998.

52. Ackerman MD, Carey MP: Psychology's role in the assessment of erectile dysfunction: historical precedents, current knowledge, and methods, *J Consult Clin Psychol* 63:862–876, 1995.

53. NIH Consensus Panel on Impotence: Impotence, *JAMA* 270:83–90, 1993.

54. Rosen RC: Erectile dysfunction: the medicalization of male sexuality, *Clin Psychol Rev* 16:497–519, 1996.

55. Spector IP, Carey MP: Incidence and prevalence of the sexual dysfunctions: a critical review of the empirical literature, *Arch Sex Behav* 19:389–408, 1990.

56. Feldman HA, Goldstein I, Hatzichristou DG, et al: Impotence and its medical and psychosocial correlates: results of the Massachusetts Male Aging Study, *J Urol* 151:54–61, 1994.

57. Althof SE, Seftel AD: The evaluation and management of erectile dysfunction, *Psychiatric Clin North Am* 18:171–192, 1995.
58. Nazareth I, Lewin J, King M: Sexual dysfunction after treatment for testicular cancer: a systematic review, *J Psychosom Res* 51:735–743, 2001.
59. Jonker-Pool G, Van de Wiel HB, Hoekstra HJ, et al: Sexual functioning after treatment for testicular cancer—review and meta-analysis of 36 empirical studies between 1975–2000, *Arch Sex Behav* 30:55–74, 2001.
60. Kendirci M, Hellstrom WJ: Current concepts in the management of erectile dysfunction in men with prostate cancer, *Clin Prost Cancer* 3:87–92, 2004.
61. Montorsi F, McCullough A: Efficacy of sildenafil citrate in men with erectile dysfunction following radical prostatectomy: a systematic review of clinical data, *J Sex Med* 2:658–667, 2005.
62. Weinhardt LS, Carey MP: Prevalence of erectile disorder among men with diabetes mellitus: comprehensive review, methodological critique, and suggestions for future research, *J Sex Res* 33:205–214, 1996.
63. Eardley I, Morgan R, Dinsmore W, et al: Efficacy and safety of sildenafil citrate in the treatment of men with mild to moderate erectile dysfunction, *Br J Psychiatry* 178:325–330, 2001.
64. Pryor J: Vardenafil: update on clinical experience, *Int J Impot Res* 14(Suppl 1):S65–S69, 2002.
65. Fazio L, Brock G: Erectile dysfunction: management update, *Can Med Assoc J* 170:1429–1437, 2004.
66. Meston CM, Levin R, Sipski ML, et al: Women's orgasm, *Annu Rev Sex Res* 8:173–257, 2004.
67. Munjack DJ, Kanno PH: Retarded ejaculation: a review, *Arch Sex Behav* 8:139–150, 1979.
68. Shull GR, Sprenkle DH: Retarded ejaculation reconceptualization and implications for treatment, *J Sex Marital Ther* 6:234–246, 1980.
69. Vandereycken W: Towards a better delineation of ejaculatory disorders, *Acta Psychiatrica Belgica* 86:57–63, 1986.
70. Mann J: *Retarded Ejaculation and Treatment*, Presented at the International Congress of Sexology, Montreal, Canada, 1976.
71. Rowland DL, Keeney C, Slob AK: Sexual response in men with inhibited or retarded ejaculation, *Int J Impot Res* 16:270–274, 2004.
72. Perelman MA: FSD partner issues: expanding sex therapy with sildenafil, *J Sex Marital Ther* 28:195–204, 2002.
73. Zgourides GD, Warren R: Retarded ejaculation: overview and treatment implications, *J Psychol Human Sex* 2:139–150, 1989.
74. Meston CM, Frohlich PF: The neurobiology of sexual function, *Arch Gen Psychiatry* 57:1012–1030, 2000.
75. Rosen RC, Lane RM, Menza M: Effects of SSRIs on sexual function: a critical review, *J Clin Psychopharmacol* 19:67–85, 1999.
76. Campden-Main BC, Sara ML: Retarded ejaculation, *Med Aspects Human Sex* 19:21–29, 1985.
77. Modell JG, May RS, Katholi CR: Effect of bupropion-SR on orgasmic dysfunction in nondepressed subjects: a pilot study, *J Sex Marital Ther* 26:231–240, 2000.
78. Martinez-Raga J, Sabater A, Cervera G: Anorgasmia in a patient treated with Bupropion SR for smoking cessation, *J Clin Psychopharmacol* 24:460–461, 2004.
79. Waldinger MD: The neurobiological approach to premature ejaculation, *J Urol* 168:59–67, 2002.
80. Grenier G, Byers ES: Rapid ejaculation: a review of conceptual, etiological, and treatment issues, *Arch Sex Behav* 24:447–472, 1995.
81. Metz ME, Pryor JL., Nesvacil LJ, et al: Premature ejaculation: a psychophysiological review, *J Sex Marital Ther* 23:3–23, 1997.
82. Laumann EO, Gagnon JH, Michael RT, et al: *The Social Organization of Sexuality*, Chicago, 1994, University of Chicago Press.
83. Grenier G, Byers ES: The relationships among ejaculatory control, ejaculatory latency, and attempts to prolong heterosexual intercourse, *Arch Sex Behav* 26:27–47, 1997.
84. Grenier G, Byers ES: Operationalizing premature or rapid ejaculation, *J Sex Res* 38:369–378, 2001.
85. Schover LR, Jensen SB: *Sexuality and Chronic Illness: A Comprehensive Approach*, New York, 1988, Guilford Press.
86. Bartlik B, Goldstein MZ: Men's sexual health after midlife, *Psychiatric Serv* 52:291–293, 2001.
87. Ruff GA, St. Lawrence JS: Premature ejaculation: past research progress, future directions, *Clin Psychol Rev* 5:627–639, 1985.
88. Althof SE: Pharmacologic treatment of rapid ejaculation, *Psychiatric Clin North Am* 18:85–94, 1995.
89. Heiman JR, LoPiccolo J: Clinical outcome of sex therapy, *Arch Gen Psychiatry* 40:443–449, 1983.
90. Moreland AJ, Makela EH: Selective serotonin-reuptake inhibitors in the treatment of premature ejaculation, *Ann Pharmacother* 39:1296–1301, 2005.
91. Waldinger MD, Zwinderman AH, Schweitzer DH, et al: Relevance of methodological design for the interpretation of efficacy of drug treatment of premature ejaculation: a systematic review and meta-analysis, *Int J Impot Res* 16:369–381, 2004.
92. Evanoff A, Newton WP: Treatment of premature ejaculation, *J Fam Pract* 46:280–281, 1998.
93. Morales A: Developmental status of topical therapies for erectile and ejaculatory dysfunction, *Int J Impot Res* 12(Suppl 4):S80–S85, 2000.
94. Crenshaw TL, Kessler JM: Male dyspareunia due to anatomical defects produced by anxiety over nonerect penis size, *Med Asp Human Sex* 19:93–107, 1985.
95. Gruver GG: Functional male dyspareunia: a case study, *Am J Psychother* 31:450–455, 1977.
96. Wabrek AJ, Wabrek CJ: Dyspareunia, *J Sex Marital Ther* 1:234–241, 1975.
97. Rosser BRS, Metz ME, Bockting WO, et al: Sexual difficulties, concerns, and satisfaction in homosexual

men: an empirical study with implications for HIV prevention, *J Sex Marital Ther* 23:61–73, 1997.

98. Rosser BRS, Short BJ, Thurmes PJ, et al: Anodyspareunia, the unacknowledged sexual dysfunction: a validation study of painful receptive anal intercourse and its psychosexual concomitants in homosexual men, *J Sex Marital Ther* 24:281–292, 1998.

99. Damon W, Rosser BRS: Anodyspareunia in men who have sex with men: prevalence, predictors, consequences and the development of DSM diagnostic criteria, *J Sex Marital Ther* 31:129–141, 2005.

100. Coleman E: Treatment of compulsive sexual behavior. In Rosen RC, Leiblum SR, editors: *Case Studies in Sex Therapy*, New York, 1995, Guilford Press, pp 333–349.

101. Gold SN, Heffner CL: Sexual addiction: many conceptions, minimal data, *Clin Psychol Rev* 18: 367–381, 1998.

102. Coleman E: Is your patient suffering from compulsive sexual behavior? *Psychiatric Ann* 22:320–325, 1992.

103. Montaldi DF: Understanding hypersexuality with an axis II model, *J Psychol Human Sex* 14:1–23, 2002.

104. Ebell MH, Siwek J, Weiss BD, et al: Strength of recommendation taxonomy (SORT): a patient-centered approach to grading evidence in the medical literature, *Am Fam Phys* 69:548–556, 2004.

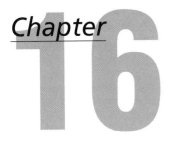

Urology

*Jerilyn M. Latini, MD, Gary J. Faerber, MD, Timothy G. Schuster, MD, and
William W. Roberts, MD*

Key Points

- Pelvic floor muscle training (PFMT) and biofeedback may have some usefulness in the treatment of stress incontinence (strength of recommendation: C).
- The artificial urethral sphincter is the most commonly used surgical procedure for the treatment of urethral sphincteric incontinence in men; although no randomized controlled trials (RCTs) exist to date, outcomes after surgery with this device show high continence rates (80% or greater) and high patient satisfaction rates (strength of recommendation: C).
- An RCT demonstrated that combination therapy with doxazosin and finasteride reduces the rate of progression of BPH more than either drug alone; combination therapy or finasteride alone decreased the rate of acute urinary retention and the future need for invasive therapy better than doxazosin or placebo (strength of recommendation: A).
- For asymptomatic men with varicocele and without testicular atrophy, there are no RCTs to demonstrate benefit from treatment versus expectant management. Although large RCTs are lacking for men with infertility and a varicocele, experimental data have shown deleterious effects of a varicocele on spermatogenesis (strength of recommendation: C).
- RCTs evaluating androgen supplementation for infertile men have not demonstrated a significant benefit in pregnancy rates with androgen supplementation versus placebo (strength of recommendation: B).

- Vitamin E, potassium aminobenzoate, calcium channel blockers, tamoxifen, steroids, and penile implants may have some benefit in the treatment of Peyronie's disease (strength of recommendation: C).
- Phimosis can be treated via topical steroids or circumcision. Paraphimosis requires urgent urologic evaluation and can be treated via manual reduction of or injection of hyaluronidase into the surrounding edema, or performance of an emergent dorsal slit or circumcision (strength of recommendation: C).
- Calcium channel blockers and alpha-1–blockers have demonstrated some benefit in facilitating ureteral stone passage, resulting in decreased narcotic use, quicker passage of stone from the time of diagnosis, and possibly passage of stones that have not passed spontaneously without surgical intervention (strength of recommendation: B).
- Men with clinically localized prostate cancer with median follow-up of 6.2 and 23 years found no significant difference in death due to any cause between radical prostatectomy and watchful waiting in men with clinically detected disease; radical prostatectomy was shown to reduce the risk of treatment failure compared with external-beam radiation (strength of recommendation: A).
- Watchful waiting is a valid alternative to various available treatment modalities in men with prostate cancer, as studies have demonstrated long survival in men with low Gleason scores (strength of recommendation: B).
- Early androgen suppression has been shown to increase survival at 10 years compared

with deferred treatment in men with locally advanced prostate cancer but not at 5 years (strength of recommendation: A); there is limited evidence that immediate androgen suppression reduced complications compared with deferred androgen suppression (strength of recommendation: C).

Introduction

Urology is the specialty that focuses on the male and female urinary tract and on the male genital tract and reproductive system. Although a comprehensive and all-inclusive review of men's urologic health, conditions, and their treatment is beyond the scope of this textbook, in this chapter we aim to provide an evidence-based guideline for the general evaluation and management of common urologic conditions that affect the adult male. Various additional pertinent urologic conditions that are evaluated and managed by urologists and other medical practitioners alike are discussed in Chapter 15, Sexual Health.

The American Urological Association (AUA) has developed peer-reviewed clinical practice guidelines for many urologic conditions and their management. All such reports are available from the AUA, and most have accompanying patient informational guides. These are available through the AUA, both in print and online at http://www.auanet.org/guidelines/. Topics, followed by the year each guideline was published, include the following:

- Staghorn calculi (2005)
- Erectile dysfunction (2005)
- Premature ejaculation (2004)
- Management of priapism (2003)
- Management of benign prostatic hypertrophy (BPH) (2003)
- Antibiotic prophylaxis for urologic patients with total joint replacements (2002)
- Optimal evaluation of the infertile male (2001)
- Evaluation of the azoospermic male (2001)
- Management of obstructive azoospermia (2001)
- Varicocele and infertility (2001)
- Microscopic hematuria (2001)
- Prostate-specific antigen (PSA) (2000)
- Bladder cancer (1999)
- Ureteral calculi (1997)
- Prostate cancer (1995)

In addition to the evidence-based review provided herein, there is a wealth of reliable and increasingly peer-reviewed information available on the Internet, providing updated information according to contemporary clinical urologic practice and ongoing research. The following Web sites are not all inclusive, but they are excellent resources for investigation of urologic health-related issues:

- UrologyHealth.org: http://www.urology-health.org
- AUA Foundation: http://www.auafoundation.org
- Urology Channel: http://www.urology-channel.org

Both medical providers and patients increasingly use these and other pertinent Web sites for dissemination of information, the use of which will only increase with time.

Hematuria

Hematuria, defined as blood in the urine, is a very common symptom reported in primary care practices as well as one of the most common reasons for urologic consultation. Whether gross or microscopic, hematuria can originate from any site in the urinary system and can be the earliest sign of underlying disease (Table 16-1). A Best Practice Policy Panel convened by the AUA[1] does not offer specific recommendations regarding routine screening for patients with microscopic hematuria. The presence of significant proteinuria, red cell casts, renal insufficiency, or a predominance of dysmorphic red blood cells revealed by urinalysis should prompt an evaluation for renal parenchymal (medical renal) disease; all other patients with non-glomerular microscopic hematuria should be evaluated. Gross hematuria (blood in the urine seen with the naked eye) warrants a thorough diagnostic evaluation including an upper urinary tract radiologic examination, urine for cytology, and a urologic evaluation including diagnostic cystoscopy or ureteroscopy.

The prevalence of asymptomatic hematuria varies widely from 0.19% to 16.1%,[2] based on study differences with relation to length of follow-up, age and sex differences, and the number of screenings in the different study cohorts. Older men have a significant prevalence of microscopic hematuria with reported rates as high as 21%.[1] Even if intermittent, hematuria may be associated with significant urologic disease, and clinicians should consider seeking further evaluation.

Diagnosis

Given the limited specificity of the standard urinalysis, an initial finding of microscopic hematuria

Table 16-1. Urologic Causes of Hematuria[7]

Life-threatening	Significant, Requiring Treatment	Significant, Requiring Observation	Insignificant
Bladder cancer	Renal/ureteral calculus	Radiation cystitis	Trigonitis
Renal cell cancer	Vesicoureteral reflux	Bladder diverticulum	Renal cyst
Prostate cancer	Bacterial cystitis	Atrophic kidney	Duplicated system
Urothelial cancer	Bladder calculus	Bladder neck stricture	Bladder neck polyps
Metastatic carcinoma	Renal parenchymal disease	Asymptomatic BPH	Bladder varices
Urethral cancer	Symptomatic BPH	Papillary necrosis	Scarred kidney
Penile cancer	Urethral stricture	Renal arteriovenous fistula	Trabeculated bladder
Renal lymphoma	Bladder papillomas	Renal contusion	Urethral caruncle
Ureterovascular/ vesicovascular fistula	Tuberculous cystitis	Polycystic kidney	Urethritis
	Pyelonephritis	Prostatitis	Pelvic kidney
	Hydronephrosis	Cystocele	Caliceal diverticulum
	Renal artery stenosis	Cystitis cystica/glandularis	Exercise hematuria
	Renal parenchymal disease	Ureterocele	
	Renal vein thrombosis	Eosinophilic cystitis	
		Phimosis	

BPH, Benign prostatic hypertrophy.

Adapted from: Mariani AJ, Mariani MC, Macchioni C: The significance of adult hematuria: 1,000 hematuria evaluations including a risk-benefit and cost-effectiveness analysis, *J Urol* 141(2):350–355, 1989.

on a urinary dipstick should be confirmed by microscopic evaluation. Significant false-positive results associated with using dipsticks alone include exercise, contamination of the urine specimen with menstrual blood in females, and ingestion of large amounts of ascorbic acid (vitamin C) and food products with high concentrations of oxidants.[3] *Microscopic hematuria* is defined as urine that has three or more red blood cells per high-power field from two or three properly collected urine specimens. Urinalysis to detect microscopic hematuria should be performed on a freshly voided, clean-catch, midstream urine. The standard technique involves centrifugation of 10 mm of urine for 5 minutes at approximately 200 rpm. The supernatant should be discarded and the sediment resuspended in 0.5–1.0 mL of the remaining urine, then a drop should be examined with the high-power microscope objective. The presence of squamous epithelial cells is indicative of an improperly obtained specimen, and it may be necessary to collect a new specimen or a catheterized specimen.

The presence of dysmorphic erythrocytes, red blood casts, and proteinuria is highly suggestive of hematuria of renal origin. Immunoglobulin A nephropathy, or Berger's disease, is the most common cause of glomerular hematuria. Other common glomerular nephropathies include mesangioproliferative, focal segmental glomerulosclerosis, membranous and postinfectious glomerulonephritis, familial nephritis (Alport's syndrome), systemic lupus erythematosus, and subacute bacterial endocarditis. Other medical renal diseases that can be associated with hematuria include papillary necrosis (e.g., commonly seen in persons with diabetes, patients with sickle cell disease or sickle cell trait, and analgesic abusers), anticoagulant therapy, exercise, and renal vascular disease.[3]

Cytology

Voided urinary cytology is recommended in all patients who have risk factors for urothelial carcinoma (Table 16-2). The sensitivity of voided urine cytology for detection of urothelial neoplasm ranges from 18% to 76% and is dependent on factors such as tumor grade, the number of specimens examined, and the expertise of the cytopathologist. Specificity of urine cytology specimens have been reported to be as high as 93%.[1] Recently, a multitude of urine-based bladder tumor markers (UBBTM) have been described, yet to date there has not been a consensus regarding the use of these markers in clinical practice. UBBTMs appear to be more sensitive but less

Table 16-2. Risk Factors for Urothelial Carcinoma in Patients with Microscopic Hematuria

Smoking history
History of gross hematuria
Solitary kidney
Age greater than 40 years
History of urologic disorder or disease
History of irritative voiding symptoms
History of urinary tract infection
History of pelvic irradiation
Analgesic abuse
Occupational exposure to chemicals or dyes (e.g., benzenes, aromatic amines)

Adapted from: Grossfeld GD, Litwin MS. Wolf JS, et al: Evaluation of asymptomatic microscopic hematuria in adults: the American Urological Association best practice policy—part I: definition, detection, prevalence, and etiology, *Urology* 57(4):599–603, 2001.

specific than urine cytologies in diagnosing urothelial neoplasms.[4] At present, urine cytology testing and UBBTMs should be considered useful adjuncts but not a substitute for cystoscopy in the evaluation of high-risk patients with microscopic hematuria.

Radiologic Imaging for the Evaluation of Hematuria

Ultrasonography, intravenous pyelography (IVP), and computed tomography (CT) are common radiographic modalities for the evaluation of hematuria (Table 16-3). The IVP was the gold standard for evaluation of the upper urinary system but has now been supplanted by CT because the latter is clearly the best imaging modality for the evaluation of urinary stones and renal and perirenal infections. In the evaluation of suspected urinary stones, the noncontrast spiral CT is superior to either IVP or ultrasonography. CT has a sensitivity of 94–98% compared with 52–59% for IVP and 19% for ultrasonography.[5] IVP is superior to ultrasonography for the detection of urothelial carcinoma of the ureter or kidney. CT urography is comparable to IVP for detection of upper tract urothelial neoplasms.[6]

Cystoscopy

Cystoscopy is recommended as an essential component of the evaluation of microscopic hematuria in all adult patients older than 40 years and

Table 16-3. Evaluation of the Urinary Tract Imaging Modalities

Modality	Advantages	Disadvantages
Intravenous pyelography (IVP)	Widely available	Cannot distinguish solid from cystic masses
	Cost-efficient	Limited sensitivity in detecting small renal masses
	Can detect collecting system abnormalities (e.g., transitional cell carcinoma)	Requires intravenous contrast
	Is both a functional and anatomic study	Requires bowel prep for optimal study
Ultrasonography (US)	Excellent for detection and characterization of renal cysts	Limited in detecting small (less than 3 cm) renal lesions
	Does not require a prep	Is not a functional study
	Does not require intravenous contrast	Limited in detecting ureteral or bladder pathology
Computed tomography (CT)	Preferred modality for detection and characterization of renal masses	Requires intravenous contrast
	Widely available	Expensive imaging modality
	Best modality for evaluation of urinary stones, renal and perirenal infections, and associated complications	
Magnetic resonance imaging (MRI)	Similar detection rate for renal masses to computed tomography	Most expensive of the imaging modalities
		Poor at detecting renal stones

Adapted from: Grossfeld GD, Litwin MS. Wolf JS, et al: Evaluation of asymptomatic microscopic hematuria in adults: the American Urological Association best practice policy—part I: definition, detection, prevalence, and etiology, *Urology* 57(4):599–603, 2001.

in patients younger than 40 years with risk factors for bladder cancer. This includes patients whose upper urinary tract radiographic imaging study reveals a potentially benign etiology of the hematuria. Flexible cystoscopy appears to be equivalent in diagnostic accuracy and significantly more tolerable for patients than rigid cystoscopy.

Follow-Up

Up to 75% of patients will have an apparent reason for their hematuria. In at least 8–10% of cases, no cause for the hematuria is revealed during the initial evaluation. The Best Practice Policy Panel of the AUA[1] suggests a follow-up regimen, which is outlined in Figure 16-1.

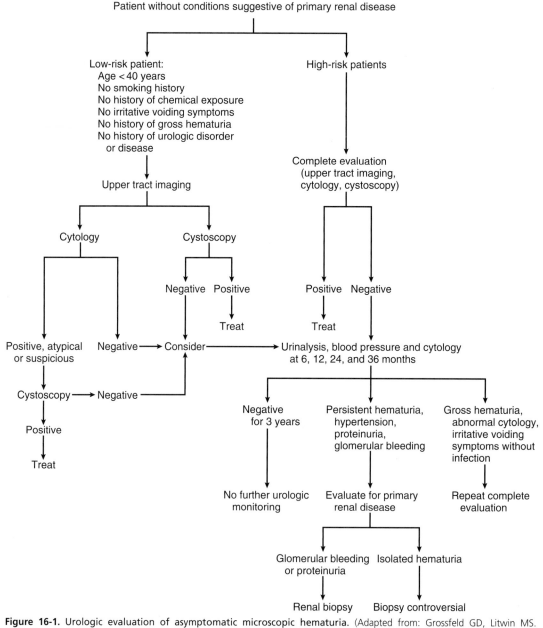

Figure 16-1. Urologic evaluation of asymptomatic microscopic hematuria. (Adapted from: Grossfeld GD, Litwin MS. Wolf JS, et al: Evaluation of asymptomatic microscopic hematuria in adults: the American Urological Association best practice policy—part I: definition, detection, prevalence, and etiology, *Urology* 57(4):599–603, 2001.)

Epididymitis

Inflammation of the epididymis is categorized as acute or chronic based on duration of symptoms. *Acute epididymitis* consists of inflammation with associated pain and swelling of less than 6 weeks' duration. *Chronic epididymitis* is generally the result of scarring and fibrosis from a severe or recurrent acute epididymitis. Epididymitis is most commonly the result of bacterial infection, although epididymal inflammation can also occur as a result of tuberculosis, mumps, the use of amiodarone, and other less common causes.[8]

Incidence

Based on a National Ambulatory Medical Care survey,[9] it was reported that epididymo-orchitis accounted for 0.29% of visits for ambulatory care and was the fifth most common urologic diagnosis among men 18–50 years of age, behind prostatitis, urinary tract infection, renal stones, and sexually transmitted infections. In a study of 610 cases occurring in soldiers enlisted in the US Army, acute epididymitis was found to occur with equal incidence on the right and the left side, with bilateral involvement occurring 9% of the time.[10] Although acute epididymitis can occur in any age group, 70.1% of cases occur in men aged 20–39 years.[10]

Etiology

Acute epididymitis commonly results from the spread of infection from the urethra to the epididymis. In young men aged 20–35 years, this is commonly associated with a sexually transmitted urethritis. In children and in older men, the most common source is bacteriuria associated with lower urinary tract obstruction, abnormal voiding patterns, neurogenic bladder, congenital anomalies, or recent instrumentation or urologic surgery.

Presentation

Patients with acute epididymitis present with scrotal pain resulting from epididymal swelling and inflammation, typically beginning in the vas deferens or tail of the epididymis and spreading to the remainder of the epididymis and ipsilateral testicle. A study of 121 men with acute epididymitis found that 62% exhibited a warm and erythematous scrotum.[11] The spermatic cord is also commonly tender and swollen. Associated symptoms included dysuria (33%), fever (74%), and chills (21%), with leukocytosis noted in 64%.[11]

Evaluation and Diagnosis

The first and most critical step in assessing patients with acute scrotal pain is to distinguish between epididymitis and testicular torsion. Testicular torsion is a urologic emergency requiring surgical exploration to prevent ischemia and testicular loss. Although symptomatically similar to epididymitis, testicular torsion more commonly occurs in adolescents and young adults and has an acute onset. On physical examination, the testicle is often elevated within the scrotum in a transverse rotated position. With epididymitis, the testicle should have a normal orientation and the tail of the epididymis is frequently palpably swollen.

An evaluation of presumed epididymitis begins with a careful history and genitourinary examination. Gram stain and culture of a midstream urine and urethral swab should also be performed. If the Gram stain result is negative or if suspicion for testicular torsion is high, then an emergent urologic evaluation should be obtained. If the Gram stain result is positive but the patient has equivocal findings for testicular torsion on history or physical examination, then a Doppler ultrasonography or radionuclide scan may further clarify the diagnosis. Color Doppler ultrasonography is considered the study of choice when imaging of the acute scrotum is indicated. With torsion, color Doppler ultrasonography demonstrates a reduced or absent vascular signal within the testicle; with epididymitis, hypervascularity is demonstrated.[12] If the Gram stain result is positive and there is no evidence of testicular torsion based on initial history and examination, then treatment for epididymo-orchitis is appropriate without further imaging.

Treatment

The treatment of epididymitis consists of antibiotic therapy directed at the causative organism. Conservative measures such as bed rest, scrotal elevation, and analgesic drugs are generally prescribed. Several studies have demonstrated symptomatic benefit from use of oral nonsteroidal anti-inflammatory drugs (NSAIDs).[13] Steroid administration in addition to antibiotic treatment provides no benefit over antibiotic therapy alone.[14]

Epididymitis with associated urethritis or with suspicion of a sexually transmitted infectious source should include antibiotics to cover *Neisseria gonorrhea* as well as *Chlamydia trachomatis*. Additionally, treatment of sexual partners and testing for syphilis and human immunodeficiency virus

(HIV) is appropriate. The most commonly used antibiotic regimen consists of 250 mg of ceftriaxone given intramuscularly and 100 mg of doxycycline given orally twice daily for 10 days.

Epididymitis associated with bacteriuria can frequently be treated with an oral fluoroquinolone for 14 days.[15] Patients with this condition should be referred for a urologic evaluation to assess for a structural urologic abnormality or lower urinary tract obstruction. Patients with bacteremia or systemic symptoms should be admitted for observation and intravenous antibiotic therapy. If improvement is not seen within 72 hours, or if evidence of abscess or sepsis is present, then a urologic evaluation is indicated. Complications of acute epididymitis include chronic epididymitis, chronic pain, infertility, abscess, and testicular infarction.

Prostatitis

Prostatitis is a collection of interrelated symptom complexes that are thought to arise from bacterial- and non–bacterial-induced prostatic inflammation. The National Institutes of Health (NIH) consensus definition[16] subdivides prostatitis into four categories (Table 16-4). Prostatitis is a common condition affecting 10–14% of men of all ages.[17,18] Data from 1991 revealed that 5.3% of all visits to urologists were for inflammatory disease of the prostate[19]; subsequent studies have found similar prevalence, yet accurate data from visits to primary care practices are lacking.

Acute Prostatitis

Etiology

Acute bacterial prostatitis accounts for fewer than 5% of all cases of prostatitis. This condition is the result of bacterial infection of the prostate, generally occurring from the common urogenital pathogens (e.g., *Escherichia coli, Klebsiella* species, *Proteus mirabilis,* and *Enterobacter* species). Symptoms at presentation are generally not subtle because patients typically demonstrate systemic manifestations of fever, chills, and myalgias. Suprapubic and perineal pain is common. Often, LUTS of frequency, urgency, dysuria, and urinary obstruction are present as well.

Evaluation and Diagnosis

Digital rectal examination classically demonstrates a boggy, exquisitely tender prostate. More than the minimal palpation of the prostate needed to confirm the diagnosis should be avoided in this setting. A complete blood count, urinalysis, urine culture, and blood cultures (if sepsis is suspected) should be performed. A bladder ultrasound scan can be obtained to noninvasively assess for urinary retention.

Treatment

The mainstay of treatment for acute prostatitis is appropriate antibiotic therapy. Patients who are acutely ill or septic or who exhibit urinary retention should be admitted to the hospital for observation and treatment. Urinary retention, if present, should be managed with a suprapubic catheter because urethral instrumentation should be avoided in the acute setting. Analgesics, antipyretics, and stool softeners are also recommended. Once the acute phase has resolved, parenteral antibiotic therapy should be continued for 4 weeks. If patients fail to improve within 1–2 days of the institution of antibiotic therapy, further assessment for a prostatic abscess should be performed via CT or ultrasonographic imaging.

Chronic Prostatitis/Chronic Pelvic Pain Syndrome

Etiology

Chronic prostatitis/chronic pelvic pain syndrome (CP/CPPS) as a disease state is poorly understood. True bacterial prostatitis due to a recurrent bacterial infection (category II) represents less than 10% of CP/CPPS and is thought to represent ascending bacterial spread from the urethra.[20] Additionally, the intraprostatic fibrosis and scarring frequently seen may result in poor drainage of prostatic secretions from the peripheral zone of the prostate and thus may result in chronic infection. In the 90% of men with CPPS where

Table 16-4. NIH Consensus Definition of Prostatitis

Category	Description
I	Acute infection of prostate gland
II	Chronic infection of prostate gland
III	Chronic prostatitis/chronic pelvic pain syndrome
IIIA	Inflammatory
IIIB	Noninflammatory
IV	Asymptomatic inflammatory prostatitis

Adapted from: Krieger JN, Nyberg LJ, Nickel JC: NIH consensus definition and classification of prostatitis, *JAMA* 282:236–237, 1999.

an infectious source is not identified, proposed causes include autoimmune conditions, stress, hormonal factors, dysfunctional voiding, and neuromuscular pain. Patients with CP/CPPS category II and III generally report episodic pain of the perineum, lower abdomen, testicles, groin, penis, scrotum, lower back, or anus and rectum. Pain after ejaculation, dysuria, and obstructive urinary symptoms are common, as is sexual dysfunction.

Evaluation and Diagnosis

Diagnosis and classification of cases of CP/CPPS into the NIH-defined categories is based on three factors: presentation, presence of white blood cells in expressed prostatic secretions, and presence of bacteria in expressed prostatic secretions.[21]

Treatment

For patients with chronic bacterial prostatitis (category II), appropriate antibiotic therapy is indicated. Typically, this consists of 4–6 weeks of a lipid-soluble antibiotic capable of achieving high prostatic concentrations (e.g., fluoroquinolones, trimethoprim/sulfamethoxazole, and doxycycline).[22] At the end of the initial antibiotic course, if symptoms are improved but still present, a lengthy course of suppressive-dose antibiotic therapy is appropriate for 3–6 months. In patients with recurrent episodes of chronic bacterial prostatitis, prophylactic low-dose antibiotics may be used, depending on microbial culture sensitivity results.

Patients with inflammatory nonbacterial prostatitis (category IIIA) should also be started on a 6-week course of antibiotic therapy (same as for category II) based on the possibility of a non-culturable bacterial source. If reassessment reveals no improvement at 2 weeks, then antibiotic therapy should be discontinued and treatment with an alpha-blocker (e.g., terazosin) and NSAIDs is commonly used clinically, although there is limited evidence to support use of alpha-blockers in this setting.[23] Prostatic massage, finasteride, and phytotherapy have also been used. The use of pentosan polysulfate also appears promising in an initial randomized trial.[24]

Patients with noninflammatory chronic prostatitis (category IIIB) should be treated with alpha-blockers for at least 3 months, as well as NSAIDs and muscle relaxant medications such as benzodiazepines or baclofen if sphincter dyssynergia or pelvic floor/perineal muscle spasm is present. If this approach fails, biofeedback, psychotherapy, relaxation exercises, pelvic muscle

physical therapy, and lifestyle changes are other options that can be used.[22]

Urinary Incontinence

Definition

Urinary incontinence is a symptom, defined as the report of any involuntary leakage of urine that results in a social or hygienic problem. The social, physical, and economic impact of urinary incontinence in men is considerable and increasing in incidence. Incontinence is also a physical sign and can be objectively demonstrated as urine leakage seen during examination. Urinary incontinence is caused by abnormalities with the bladder, the urethral sphincter, or both. Problems within the bladder include detrusor overactivity (i.e., involuntary bladder contractions) and low bladder compliance. These abnormalities result in urge incontinence or involuntary loss of urine associated with or immediately preceded by urgency (i.e., a strong desire to void). This phenomenon occurs in men with urinary tract infection, bladder outlet obstruction, bladder cancer, neurogenic disease or injury, and various other causes. De novo urge incontinence can occur after various types of abdominal, pelvic, or back surgery. The most common cause of urgency and urge incontinence in adult males is BPH.

Sphincter abnormalities are primarily caused by anatomic disruption that can occur with all types of prostate surgery, whether performed via transurethral/endoscopic, open, laparoscopic, or robotic methods. Additionally, sphincteric incontinence can be due to trauma or neurologic abnormalities or disease. These abnormalities results in stress incontinence as a result of sphincter or pelvic floor muscle weakness. *Stress incontinence* is a condition involving involuntary loss of urine with physical activity that increases intra-abdominal pressure (e.g., any exertion such as coughing, laughing, sneezing, lifting, exercise, bending).

Overflow incontinence describes urinary leakage in combination with urinary retention; elevated post-void urine residuals in conjunction with urinary incontinence are commonly seen and are usually the result of either an obstructive or neuropathic lesion, alone or in combination with a hypotonic/atonic bladder. Referral to a urologist for evaluation of this condition is important. Treatment is aimed at relieving the obstruction; however, men with impaired bladder contractility will benefit from intermittent catheterization. Caution should be used in treating incontinent men with anticholinergic medications (e.g., tricyclic antidepressants) before ruling out overflow incontinence because these medications can worsen the urinary retention.

Functional incontinence involves limitations or disability (e.g., physical, mental) that prevents one from getting to the toilet in time to void. Identifying and correcting environmental factors and the use of assistive devices, behavioral interventions, bedside commodes, and protective undergarments should be considered. *Continuous incontinence* is a condition involving continuous urinary leakage throughout the day and night. The differential diagnosis includes fistulae (e.g., bladder, prostate, urethra to the skin, perineum, or rectum), ectopic ureters, and severe intrinsic urethral sphincter deficiency. Referral to a urologist for evaluation is of paramount importance. *Nocturnal incontinence* is urinary loss that occurs only during sleep and is usually considered within one of the categories described above.

Epidemiology

Incontinence affects men less commonly than women and is usually a consequence of an underlying illness, injury, or surgery. An estimated 17 million community-dwelling and 1 million institutionalized adults in the United States are incontinent.[25] In a study of pooled data from 21 international population-based surveys stratified for age, sex, and incontinence frequency, 11–34% of older men have incontinence with 2–11% experiencing daily leakage, whereas 3–5% of middle-aged and younger men have incontinence.[26] According to the 2001 National Health and Nutrition Examination Survey data,[27] 17% of the 3.4 million men older than 60 years in the United States have incontinence, with 7% reporting daily leakage. The prevalence of incontinence increases with increasing age, especially in men older than 65 years. This trend may be due to age-related physical and functional changes of the bladder, unstable bladder contractions, residual urine, bladder contractility, multifactorial elements of aging, modified pharmacokinetics, and comorbid conditions. Urge incontinence is the most common form of incontinence (40–80%), followed by mixed (combination of urge and stress; 10–30%) and stress (10%). Ethnicity appears to play less of a role in incontinence in men compared with women. The economic impact of incontinence and overactive bladder symptoms on healthcare resource use and cost is substantial and increasing; total costs in 2000 were $19.5 billion for adults with incontinence

and an additional $12.6 billion for overactive bladder.[25]

Risk Factors

Risk factors for incontinence in adults are many, but the primary risk factors for urge and stress urinary incontinence in men are most commonly benign and malignant prostate diseases and their respective treatments. The most common cause of overactive bladder, urgency, and urge incontinence in adult males is BPH. All therapies for prostate malignancy are recognized to confer an increased risk of incontinence, including radiation (i.e., external beam or brachytherapy), surgery (all types of prostatectomy), and cryotherapy. Radiation of all types can affect the bladder neck and external sphincter, causing stress incontinence and affecting the bladder itself, leading to both urgency and urge incontinence. Prostatectomy (e.g., open, laparoscopic, and robotic) involves extensive dissection around the bladder neck and external sphincter, potentially causing stress incontinence. Transurethral resection of the prostate (TURP) and all types of minimally invasive BPH treatments can affect the bladder neck and external sphincter, causing stress incontinence. Reported frequency of postprostatectomy incontinence varies depending on the type of surgery and surgical technique; definition and quantification of incontinence; timing of the evaluation relative to surgery; and who rates the presence or absence of incontinence—the patient or the physician.

Diagnosis

Evaluation of an incontinent adult male involves reaching a working diagnosis of stress, urge, or mixed urinary incontinence or overflow incontinence. Adequate history taking should ascertain the type of incontinence (e.g., stress, urge, mixed, overflow), onset, duration, prior therapies and response to therapy, inciting events (e.g., surgery, trauma, neurologic event), severity (e.g., pad use—number, type, threshold for changing), degree of bother (e.g., various quality of life instruments, the AUA symptom score), medications (e.g., sympatholytic drugs can weaken sphincter tone, sympathomimetics can cause retention and overflow incontinence, can cause increased urine production that can worsen incontinence), LUTS (e.g., urgency, frequency, nocturia, hesitancy, straining, decreased force of stream, intermittency, pain with urination, suprapubic pain or pressure, sensation of incomplete emptying), surgical history, neurologic disorder (e.g., back surgery/injury, spinal cord injury, cerebrovascular accident, Parkinson's disease, multiple sclerosis, diabetes, myelodysplasia), gastrointestinal disorder (e.g., diarrhea, constipation, fecal incontinence), or other pertinent genitourinary history (e.g., urine infection, hematuria, kidney/bladder stones, urethral stricture, urinary retention, pediatric history). Frequency volume charts (i.e., voiding diaries) are invaluable as an objective method for determining urinary frequency, voided volumes, associated symptoms, and fluid intake (e.g., type, amount). Pads and diapers can be used to collect urine that has leaked over a 24-hour period, and the pads can be weighed (in grams) to quantify the amount of urine leakage.

Physical examination should include a complete abdominal and genitourinary examination, including digital rectal exam to identify benign prostatic enlargement that may be causing obstruction. The neurologic examination should focus on perineal sensation, lumbosacral deep tendon reflexes, and sacral cutaneous reflexes (bulbocavernosus). The evaluation should include urinalysis or urine culture to exclude infection; serum creatinine to assess renal function; cystourethroscopy to exclude bladder calculi, tumors, or fistulae; and ultrasonography or catheterized post-void urine volume to exclude urinary retention. Incontinent men with mixed incontinence, failure of prior treatment, inconsistent history with respect to clinical findings, young age, neurologic disease, or prior prostate surgery should undergo urologic evaluation and urodynamic studies. These may include noninvasive uroflowmetry, cystometrogram, voiding pressure study, leak point pressure testing, electromyography, voiding cystourethrogram, and video fluorourodynamics.

Treatment

The management of urinary incontinence in adult males includes behavioral modification, medication, electronic stimulation, and surgical procedures. The management of stress incontinence during the first year after prostate surgery or treatment for prostate cancer is generally conservative because there can be improvement without intervention during this time. If stress incontinence persists, periurethral injection of a bulking agent (e.g., collagen, carbon coated beads, biocompatible copolymers) or surgical placement of a perineal sling or artificial urinary sphincter is recommended. The long-term continence rates for artificial urinary sphincter (the gold standard procedure for male stress incontinence) vary between 64% and 76%, with continence defined as 0–1 pads per day. Treatment efficacy depends on the etiology and severity of the incontinence. There are only a few randomized controlled trials (RCTs) to date that address the management of men with urinary incontinence. Generally, current recommendations are based on clinical experience, usual practice, and patient-oriented evidence in terms of symptoms, quality of life, morbidity, and healthcare economics.

Nonsurgical Treatments for Urge and Stress Urinary Incontinence

Behavioral modification through a patient education–based program for the treatment of urge and stress incontinence include fluid and dietary modification (e.g., reduction of dietary bladder irritants including caffeine, alcohol, artificial sweeteners), weight reduction, lifestyle changes, bladder retraining/timed voiding, urge inhibition, physical therapy including pelvic muscle training and strengthening, and biofeedback. Compressive devices that block urine leakage from the urethra (e.g., penile clamps) and urine-collection devices (e.g., liners, pads, briefs, diapers, and condom catheters) are available. Therapies involving electrical stimulation and extracorporeal magnetic innervation have been reported, but not in men with incontinence, so outcomes data are not available for recommendation in practice.

The Cochrane group[28] reviewed various conservative approaches to the management of postprostatectomy incontinence and discovered that symptoms tend to improve over time irrespective of the type of conservative treatment. There are few data on men with incontinence after TURP. For men after radical prostatectomy for cancer, pelvic floor muscle training (PFMT) and biofeedback may be better than either sham or no treatment in the short term. The relative risk of incontinence with pelvic muscle training and biofeedback versus no treatment was 0.74 (95% confidence interval, 0.60–0.93). Available evidence for PFMT alone, transcutaneous electrical nerve stimulation, and rectal stimulation alone or in combination is inconclusive. Sacral neuromodulation has been documented as effective and safe in patients with refractory urge incontinence; however, RCTs have included primarily women thus far, and it is unclear whether these data can be extrapolated to men.[28]

This review found that there was no difference in the occurrence of postprostatectomy incontinence between men who had preoperative PFMT and those who did not. There is no current RCT that has examined the role of PFMT for non-postoperative men. No trials involving other conservative interventions such as lifestyle changes were found. Overall, the value of nonpharmaceutical and nonsurgical treatments remains uncertain; however, they tend to carry a low risk of adverse effects and do not preclude subsequent treatment. In an RCT of 102 men after prostatectomy with a 1-year follow-up, there was a more rapid resolution of incontinence in the treatment group (88% versus 56% at 3 months), defined as improved incontinence severity as measured by pad weights, yet the development of incontinence requiring further treatment was not affected.[29] Many studies fail to adequately demonstrate the effectiveness of PFMT exercises in preventing postprostatectomy incontinence. PFMT exercise and education appear to be less effective in continuous or severe incontinence.[30-32]

The Cochrane group[33] attempted to determine the effectiveness of adrenergic agonists in the treatment of urinary incontinence in adults. Twenty-two eligible randomized trials were identified, of which 11 were crossover trials. The trials included 1099 women, 673 of whom received an adrenergic drug; no trials included men. There was weak evidence to suggest that the use of an adrenergic agonist was better than placebo treatment, yet there was not enough evidence to assess the effects of adrenergic agonists when compared with or combined with other treatments. Further larger trials, especially those including male subjects, are needed to identify when adrenergic agents may be useful.[33]

Bladder training aims to increase the interval between voids. Timed voiding is defined as fixed-time-interval toileting. Habit retraining is essentially toileting assistance given by a caregiver and involves the identification of an incontinent person's natural voiding pattern and the development of an individualized toileting schedule that preempts involuntary bladder emptying. Prompted voiding is a behavioral therapy used mainly in nursing homes that aims to improve bladder control using verbal prompts and positive reinforcement. The limited evidence available reviewed by the Cochrane Group[34-36] suggests that these behavioral therapies may be helpful for the treatment of urinary incontinence, but there was insufficient evidence to reach firm conclusions for practice recommendations.

Surgical Treatments for Stress Urinary Incontinence

The most appropriate candidates for treatment with periurethral injectable materials (e.g., Macroplastique, a bulking agent) are those with normal bladder capacity and compliance, sphincteric incontinence, and good anatomic pelvic support. Men with mild to moderate postprostatectomy incontinence who use three pads or fewer per day, who have urodynamic evidence for sphincteric incontinence, and who have not had postoperative radiation, cryotherapy, or bladder neck incision are thought to be the most appropriate patients. Although controlled long-term follow-up studies are not available, large case series report 45–80% improvement in incontinence at 6–12 months; however, this tends to decrease to 38–60% at 2 years. Typically, three to four injections (20–35 mL total injected volume) are required for effectiveness.[37]

A comparison of artificial urinary sphincter (AUS) implantation and endourethral Macroplastique injection for the treatment of postprostatectomy incontinence was conducted as a prospective RCT that included 45 patients with such incontinence resulting from radical retropubic prostatectomy, transvesical prostatectomy, or TURP. The patients were divided into two groups defined as minimal (group I) and total (group II), according to the severity of their incontinence. Patients were randomly assigned to undergo either AUS implantation or Macroplastique injection. Endourethral injection was found to be the treatment of choice for patients with minimal incontinence, whereas AUS implantation was the first choice for patients with total incontinence.[38]

The current version of the male perineal bone-anchored sling was introduced in 2001 by Madjar[39] for postprostatectomy incontinence. It creates fixed compression of the bulbar urethra, is relatively inexpensive, is nonmechanical, and allows physiologic voiding without significant obstruction. Short-term (1-year) follow-up reports a 76–87% cure rate with 7–19% improved and 0–5% failures. The long-term surgical revision and failure rates remain to be seen.[39]

AUS implantation is the gold standard and most commonly used surgical procedure for the treatment of urethral sphincteric incontinence in men, and its effective use is well reported. Contraindications include poor bladder compliance, uninhibited bladder contractions, detrusor sphincter dyssynergia, unstable recurrent urethral stricture or diverticula, or any urologic problem that requires frequent instrumentation. The risk of urethral cuff erosion may be increased in men with a history of pelvic radiation, although this is not necessarily an absolute contraindication. Although no RCTs exist to date, outcomes after AUS surgery show high

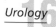

continence rates (80% or greater) and high patient satisfaction rates. Complications necessitating revision or explantation may occur early or late and include infection (0–10%), erosion (0–20%), and mechanical failure (0–25%); a 40% revision rate has been reported.[37]

The future of male urinary incontinence will involve better understanding of the etiology of incontinence, better prevention and treatment strategies, improved pharmaceuticals, improved reconstructive/surgical techniques, pharmacogenetics, gene therapy, and tissue engineering.

Benign Prostatic Hyperplasia

BPH is a pathologic diagnosis of prostatic cellular proliferation. Clinically, this syndrome manifests as poor bladder emptying and lower urinary tract symptoms (LUTS) that are bothersome and disruptive for the patient. BPH can also lead to overactive bladder and urinary retention and can predispose the patient to urinary tract infections, hematuria, and renal insufficiency.[40]

Incidence

BPH is strikingly common in men after the fifth or sixth decade of life. Eighty percent of men by the eighth decade of life have clinical evidence of BPH.[41] Symptoms will produce significant loss of quality of life in 25% of men, warranting medical or surgical treatments.[42]

Etiology

The mechanism by which BPH produces symptoms is not completely understood and is more complex than simply increased urethral resistance from expansion of the prostate. Bladder dysfunction from aging and neural alteration resulting from bladder outlet obstruction are also believed to be contributing factors.

Presentation

Men with symptomatic BPH typically present with LUTS of urinary frequency, urgency, dysuria, nocturia, decreased force of stream, hesitancy, intermittency, dribbling, incomplete emptying, and straining to void. Patients can also present with later manifestations of BPH including urinary retention, recurrent urinary tract infections, hematuria, bladder calculi, and renal insufficiency. It is important to remember that LUTS are not specific to BPH and may be due to other etiologies.

Evaluation and Diagnosis

The initial evaluation of BPH consists of history, physical examination, and urinalysis to exclude nonprostatic causes of symptoms. A careful review of voiding symptoms and severity should be obtained. A frequency volume chart (i.e., bladder or voiding diary) may also provide insight into the extent of the symptoms. The AUA symptom score is a useful validated tool for characterizing and quantifying LUTS (Figure 16-2).[43] Each question is scored 0–5, producing a total score of 0–35. Symptoms are classified as mild (0–7), moderate (8–19), or severe (20–35) based on this total score. An additional question assesses a patient's "bother score" on a scale of 0–6.

Digital rectal examination results frequently demonstrate an enlarged prostate; however, prostate size does not correlate with the severity of symptoms. A focused neurologic examination should also be performed. Urinalysis is used to screen for hematuria and urinary tract infection. PSA should also be checked in men with at least a 10-year life expectancy in cases when knowledge of prostate cancer would change clinical management.

Treatment

Treatment options for patients with BPH cover a broad therapeutic spectrum and include watchful waiting, medical therapy, minimally invasive ablative techniques, and surgery. Appropriate treatment is generally selected based on the severity of disease and the degree of bother as assessed by the AUA symptom score and quality-of-life questionnaire. However, urinary retention, renal insufficiency, bladder calculi, recurrent urinary tract infection, recurrent or persistent hematuria, or severe bothersome symptoms are indications for urologic evaluation and surgical treatment.

Patients with mild to moderate symptoms but minimal bother are candidates for watchful waiting. In this patient group, decreasing alcohol and caffeine intake, instituting a timed voiding regimen, and limiting fluid intake before bedtime may produce some symptom relief. These patients should be examined yearly and additional treatment options discussed if symptoms worsen. Patients exhibiting moderate to severe bothersome symptoms need to be counseled regarding the complete range of therapeutic options. In general, the most invasive treatment options yield the greatest symptom relief; however, many patients are able to achieve

Figure 16-2. The American Urological Association (AUA) Symptom Index for Benign Prostatic Hyperplasia (BPH) and the Disease-Specific Quality-of-Life Question

Patient Name: _____ DOB: _____ ID: _____ Date of assessment: _____

Initial Assessment ( ) Monitor during: _____ Therapy ( ) after: _____ Therapy/surgery( ) _____

AUA BPH Symptom Score

	Not at all	Less than 1 time in 5	Less than half the time	About half the time	More than half the time	Almost always	
1. Over the past month, how often have you had a sensation of not emptying your bladder completely after you finished urinating?	0	1	2	3	4	5	
2. Over the past month, how often have you had to urinate again less than two hours after you finished urinating?	0	1	2	3	4	5	
3. Over the past month, how often have you found you stopped and started again several times when you urinated?	0	1	2	3	4	5	
4. Over the past month, how often have you found it difficult to postpone urination?	0	1	2	3	4	5	
5. Over the past month, how often have you had a weak urinary stream?	0	1	2	3	4	5	
6. Over the past month, how often have you had to push or strain to begin urination?	0	1	2	3	4	5	
	None	1 time	2 times	3 times	4 times	5 or more times	
7. Over the past month, how many times did you most typically get up to urinate from the time you went to bed at night until the time you got up in the morning?	0	1	2	3	4	5	
						Total Symptom Score	

Adapted from: Roerborn CG, McConnell JD, B et al: *AUA Guideline on the Management of Benign Prostatic Hyperplasia (BPH)*, 2003, American Urological Association Education and Research, Inc.

sufficient benefit from medical therapy or minimally invasive ablative procedures.

Medical management of BPH is centered on the use of alpha-blockers (e.g., doxazosin) to reduce smooth muscle tone in the bladder neck and prostate and 5-alpha reductase inhibitors (e.g., finasteride) that decrease prostate volume by causing prostate atrophy. Both alpha-blockers and 5-alpha reductase inhibitors have been shown to improve LUTS. A recent RCT demonstrated that combination therapy with doxazosin and finasteride reduces the rate of progression more than either drug alone.[44] Furthermore, combination therapy

or finasteride alone decreased the rate of acute urinary retention and the future need for invasive therapy better than doxazosin or placebo.[44] In summary, for men with moderate to severe LUTS who elect medical therapy, treatment with an alpha-blocker and 5-alpha reductase inhibitor is the best medical regimen for decreasing risk of progression of BPH. It should be noted that use of a 5-alpha reductase inhibitor artificially lowers the PSA level. For the purposes of prostate cancer screening, the measured value should be doubled in patients taking 5-alpha reductase inhibitors.[45]

Varicocele

Definition

A varicocele is a dilation of the veins in the pampiniform plexus in the spermatic cord. Varicoceles are often graded using the following scale:

- Grade 0: only detected using Doppler ultrasonography
- Grade 1: palpable only by Valsalva maneuver when patient is standing in upright position
- Grade 2: detectable by palpation but not visible when patient is standing in upright position
- Grade 3: visible when patient is standing in upright position

Incidence

It is estimated that approximately 10–15% of the general population has a varicocele, but limited data exist on actual prevalence rates.

Etiology and Risk Factors

A varicocele occurs because of incompetence of the valves in the spermatic veins. Approximately 85% of varicoceles are on the left side of the scrotum because of the asymmetric drainage of the veins, whereas the remainder, in general, are bilateral. There is no epidemiologic evidence for risk factors for varicoceles.

Presentation

Most men with varicoceles are asymptomatic, yet occasionally they can present with a dull ache in the scrotum that worsens when the patient assumes the upright position. Long-standing, large varicoceles may induce testicular atrophy. Many healthcare providers believe there is an association with varicoceles and male factor infertility; only a few RCTs to date have been performed on men with infertility and varicoceles. The best described trials had different inclusion criteria, duration of infertility, size of varicoceles treated, and methods of repair, which may explain the discrepancy in results.[46,47] Madgar and colleagues[46] demonstrated a 44–60% improvement in pregnancy rates in the partners of men undergoing varicocele repair during their first year of follow-up, whereas Nieschlag and colleagues[47] failed to demonstrate a benefit in pregnancy rates.

Patient Evaluation

The scrotal contents should be inspected in a warm room with the patient in an upright position. The spermatic cord should be palpated initially and then again with the patient performing a Valsalva maneuver. The spermatic cord should be reexamined with the patient in the supine position to verify collapse of the veins. For men with continued prominence of the varicocele in the supine position, suspicion should be raised for mechanical obstruction to the venous outflow and additional retroperitoneal imaging should be ordered. Doppler ultrasonographic scan of the scrotum may be used for diagnosis of a varicocele if the physical examination is difficult due to the patient's body habitus or in equivocal examinations.

Treatment

For asymptomatic men without testicular atrophy, there are no RCTs to demonstrate benefit from treatment versus expectant management. It is generally recommended to follow up with adolescents with periodic (every 1–2 years) monitoring to examine for testicular size discrepancy. For men demonstrating ipsilateral testicular atrophy, intervention should be considered. Although large RCTs are lacking for men with infertility and a varicocele, an extensive amount of experimental data has shown deleterious effects of a varicocele on spermatogenesis.[48] For men with unexplained infertility, abnormal semen parameters, and the presence of a varicocele, intervention should be considered.

Treatment of varicoceles includes angioembolization and surgical ligation. Surgical intervention can be performed with or without magnification using various methods including laparoscopy, retroperitoneal, inguinal, and subinguinal approaches. We found no large RCTs to demonstrate the superiority of any of the various treatment options.

Male Infertility

Definition

The classically defined *infertile* couple is one that has failed to conceive after 1 year of unprotected intercourse. Approximately 15% of couples will be unable to conceive after 1 year of unprotected intercourse. A male factor is identified in 20% of cases as the sole factor, whereas another 30–40% of the time it is a contributing factor.[49]

Evaluation

Although a comprehensive review of the infertile male is beyond the scope of this chapter, a description of a basic history and physical examination as well as suggested laboratory testing is provided. The general history of a male patient relative to the evaluation for male factor infertility should ascertain the duration of the couple's attempts at achieving pregnancy, whether they have had children or a positive pregnancy test together or prior to their relationship, and the results of any semen analyses before the current encounter. The clinician should also inquire about any previous evaluation and treatment for male or female factor infertility, a discussion of any systemic illness, as well as recent weight changes. The review of systems should specifically ascertain whether any fevers, colds, sinus infections, anosmia, peripheral field visual problems, breast pain or secretions, and scrotal pain are present. The history should establish that puberty started in the early or middle teens to confirm normal physiologic male development. The evaluation should also include any potential exposure to environmental toxins, either through occupation or hobbies, including such factors as excessive heat, radiation, heavy metals, and glycol ethers or other organic solvents because these may each have an effect on spermatogenesis.

The clinician should then focus the history on any condition that would potentially affect the genitalia or reproductive endocrine system. Pertinent findings would include a history of cryptorchidism, significant genital trauma, and previous diagnosis of varicocele, hypothyroidism, or known pituitary malfunction. It will also include a review of any additional medical conditions for which the patient is being monitored, including any condition that would require radiotherapy or chemotherapy. Diabetes mellitus, chronic obstructive pulmonary disease, sleep apnea, renal insufficiency, and hepatic insufficiency are possible contributors to male subfertility.[50] Any history of genitourinary surgeries including orchidopexy, V-Y plasty to the bladder neck, inguinal hernia repair, correction of epispadias or hypospadias, prostate surgery, bladder reconstructions, bladder surgeries, or testicular surgeries should be noted. Additionally, the examiner should inquire about previous treatment for testicular or other urologic malignancies (either via surgery, chemotherapy, or radiation) and, if appropriate, history of vasectomy and when it was performed.

The history should include the overall pattern of sexual activity, specifically in relation to ovulation. The examiner should inquire about any previously fathered children as well as any evaluation or treatment of the female partner that may have preceded the patient's visit, such as the use of ovulation predictor kits or medications. The optimal timing for sexual intercourse is 24 hours before and after ovulation. The timing of sexual intercourse in relation to ovulation should be noted because simply adjusting the timing of intercourse can result in an increased chance for pregnancy. Both partners should also be asked about a history of sexually transmitted infections.

Each male patient should be queried regarding erectile function, ejaculation, and libido because these issues can contribute to infertility. Typically, erectile difficulties from an organic cause are insidious and progressive and may span the course of several years. Alternatively, the patient may provide a history of relatively rapid or recent onset of a decline in erectile function that may be associated with the history of recently starting new medication (e.g., antihypertensive or antidepressant drugs [especially serotonin specific reuptake inhibitors]) or the stress of the fertility difficulties. The history should include several points specific to the patient's sexual functioning including the precise nature of the dysfunction (e.g., whether the problem is attaining or sustaining an erection, insufficient rigidity, difficulty with penetration); the presence or absence of nocturnal and morning erections and their quality; and any treatments (pharmacologic and nonpharmacologic) that the patient has tried.

If ejaculatory problems exist, the patient should be questioned regarding what type of dysfunction he is experiencing. Problems can be classified into complete lack of ejaculation (i.e., anejaculation), retrograde ejaculation, or delay in ejaculation. Additionally, the examiner should inquire whether there is any pain with ejaculation or any hematospermia present. Ejaculatory difficulties can be the result of a variety of surgical procedures, progressive neurologic disease, or a variety of medications. The couple must also be asked about the use of lubricants during sexual intercourse. Saliva, K-Y Jelly, Surgilube, and hand lotions are all known to impair sperm motility.[50] If lubricant is needed during sexual intercourse, recommendations include Astroglide, egg whites, or vegetable oil, although no RCTs have been performed to evaluate their impact on sperm motility.

A careful review of the medication list must also be part of the initial evaluation of the infertile male. Prescription drugs can affect sperm count, motility, and morphology, and the dose and duration of use should be documented. Common antibiotics can temporarily contribute to a decline in the semen analysis quality (e.g., sulfa drugs). Calcium channel blockers and spironolactone can contribute to a decreased fertilization capacity and a decline in spermatogenesis, respectively.[51] Anabolic steroid use can also result in profound decline in sperm count. The patient must also be asked about the ingestion of nutraceuticals and other over-the-counter medications. Smoking, alcohol consumption, and marijuana use have all been implicated as gonadotoxins.[50]

Physical examination of an infertile male patient should focus primarily on the genitalia, with consideration of the overall body habitus. The patient should be examined about age-appropriate development of male secondary sex characteristics, gynecomastia, or hirsutism. He should be examined for lesions or scarring to the abdomen or groin, any discoloration to the scrotum, asymmetry of testicles, and the location and size of the opening of the meatus. The physical examination may demonstrate some regression of secondary sexual characteristics such as hair loss and possible loss of muscle bulk. Patients using anabolic steroids may have skeletal muscle hypertrophy, acne, gynecomastia, striae, and testicular atrophy on examination. The penis and meatus should be examined to verify that no deformity or urethral stenosis is present. The scrotum should be carefully and thoroughly palpated, and the presence of all scrotal structures should be confirmed, along with their size and consistency. The size and location of each testicle should be noted. The patient may have a testicle that is palpable in the inguinal canal or that cannot be palpated at all. Masses may arise from the surface of the testicle, adjacent to or separate from the testes. The epididymis should also be examined for the presence of induration, cysts, or masses. One should also note the presence or absence of each vas deferens and should examine the patient for the presence of a varicocele (discussed above).

In addition to the history and physical examination, the clinician should evaluate two separate semen analyses ordered after 2–3 days of abstinence. If abnormalities are identified within the semen analysis or history and physical examination suggesting male factor infertility, an evaluation of serum gonadotropins (i.e., follicle-stimulating hormone, luteinizing hormone, free testosterone, and prolactin) should be performed to verify a functioning hypothalamic-pituitary axis. Genetic testing may also be considered for men with severe oligozoospermia or azoospermia, including evaluation of the karyotype and Y chromosome microdeletion testing. Screening for cystic fibrosis should be considered for men with congenital absence of the vas deferens.

Treatment

Treatment of an infertile male requires identification of reversible causes of infertility. For men with gonadotropin deficiency (hypogonadotropic hypogonadism), replacement with gonadotropin-releasing hormone or human chorionic gonadotropin can initiate spermatogenesis. Before this therapy is initiated, the pituitary should be imaged to rule out an underlying pituitary tumor[52] and, if identified, neurosurgical consultation is warranted for further evaluation and treatment.

Although testosterone is required for spermatogenesis to occur in the testicle, exogenous testosterone can cause suppression of sperm production. Despite this, there have been nine RCTs evaluating androgen supplementation for infertile males.[53] None of these trials have demonstrated a benefit in pregnancy rates with androgen supplementation over placebo. Antiestrogens (e.g., clomiphene citrate and tamoxifen) and aromatase inhibitors have also been evaluated in multiple RCTs.[53] Although several studies demonstrated improvements in semen parameters, the vast majority of these trials have not increased fertility in men with idiopathic oligoasthenospermia.[54]

For men presenting with obstructive azoospermia, treatment options include surgical correction of the obstruction or sperm retrieval from the male reproductive system for in vitro fertilization with intracytoplasmic sperm injection. Several techniques have been described to retrieve sperm from the testicle or epididymis both percutaneously and via open surgical extraction with or without the use of an operating microscope. Insufficient evidence exists to recommend any one technique for sperm retrieval.[55] Similarly, for men with nonobstructive azoospermia, spermatozoa can often be retrieved from the testicle using the techniques above, although no RCTs have been performed to demonstrate an optimal procedure.

Peyronie's Disease

Definition

Peyronie's disease is an acquired inflammatory condition of the penis resulting in penile curvature. Additionally, it can be associated with penile pain or erectile dysfunction. In general, the disease progresses through two phases, which include an initial phase consisting of pain and gradual penile deformity followed by resolution of the pain with stabilization of the penile plaque and deformity. It is estimated that the incidence of symptomatic Peyronie's disease is approximately 1%.[56] In white men, the average age of onset is 53 years.

Etiology and Risk Factors

It is generally believed that Peyronie's disease results from trauma that results in abnormal stimulation of the wound-healing process and subsequent scar formation in the tunica albuginea. Several disease entities are also associated with Peyronie's disease, including Dupuytren's contractures, plantar fascial contractures, tympanosclerosis, diabetes mellitus, gout, and Paget's disease, as well as use of phenytoin and beta-blockers.[57]

Evaluation

For men presenting with Peyronie's disease, the history should include disease duration, degree of curvature, whether penetration with intercourse is still possible, and whether concomitant pain or erectile dysfunction is present. Additionally, one should inquire about any history of trauma or other risk factors present above. The physical examination should focus on evaluation of the patient's hands and feet for contractures as well as palpation of the penile plaque. Typically, the plaque will be located on the dorsum of the penis, although plaques can also be lateral or ventral.

Treatment

There are few RCTs that have examined therapies for Peyronie's disease. In general, medical therapy is the first-line treatment for men with newly diagnosed disease. Surgical intervention is reserved for men with a stable plaque/penile deformity for at least 6 months who are unable to engage in intercourse or have concomitant erectile dysfunction unresponsive to nonsurgical therapies.

Multiple medical therapies have been used to treat Peyronie's disease. Vitamin E, given as 800 IU/day, may be effective. It is commonly given because of its antioxidant properties and general tolerability, but no RCT has been performed to demonstrate efficacy over placebo. Potassium aminobenzoate (Potaba), given at 12 g/day (divided in 4–6 doses), has been demonstrated to be efficacious in a small blinded study[58]; however, gastrointestinal upset and the large quantity of oral pills limits its widespread use. Other agents that have been used include colchicine, but results are only anecdotal. A small RCT evaluated tamoxifen versus placebo and found no difference in symptomatic outcomes.[59] Several investigators have reported successful treatment of Peyronie's disease by injecting calcium channel blockers,[60] steroids,[61] and interferons[62] into the penile plaques, although no RCTs on the topic have been performed to date. A small RCT comparing intralesional collagenase and placebo demonstrated improvement in mild to moderate Peyronie's plaques, although there was not a statistically significant improvement for more severe curvature.[63]

Several surgical options exist to correct the penile curvature from Peyronie's disease, although no RCTs have been performed to compare these treatments. Plication of the tunica albuginea on the contralateral side of the corpora cavernosa bend is effective in straightening the penis; however, men will lose some penile length from this procedure. To avoid this, an alternative option is incision or excision of the plaque with grafting using either autologous or synthetic materials. The drawback to this approach is that oftentimes the neurovascular bundle on the dorsum of the penis must be mobilized, which can cause penile numbness and may be permanent. Finally, for men with concomitant erectile dysfunction, a penile prosthesis can be placed and the penis straightened with intraoperative molding.[64]

Priapism

Definition

Priapism is defined as a persistent penile erection that continues hours beyond, or is unrelated to, sexual stimulation. Priapism can be classified as either ischemic (low flow) or nonischemic (high flow). Ischemic priapism is due to decreased inflow of blood to the penis. It typically presents with a painful and engorged corporal cavernosum with a soft glans and requires emergent intervention. In contrast, nonischemic priapism typically presents with painless partial erection due to unregulated arterial inflow. The true incidence of priapism is unknown. For men using intracavernosal injection of medications for erectile dysfunction, the incidence has been reported to range from 1% to 11%.[65]

Etiology and Risk Factors

Although approximately one half of patients with priapism have an unknown etiology, multiple risk factors and diseases have been associated with the entity. The most common cause of ischemic priapism in adults is injectable intracavernosal agents used for erectile dysfunction.[66] Several classes of medications including most classes of antipsychotics, antidepressants (e.g., trazodone), and less commonly, some antihypertensives (e.g., alpha-blockers) have been associated with priapism. Priapism has been reported with the use of phosphodiesterase inhibitors (e.g., vardenafil, sildenafil, tadalafil), although infrequently. Less common causes of ischemic priapism include discontinuation of anticoagulants, use of a high concentration of lipids in total parenteral nutrition, and recreational drugs including alcohol and cocaine. Leukemia and sickle cell disease are hematologic disorders associated with ischemic priapism. Nonischemic priapism typically occurs after perineal trauma causing injury to the cavernosal artery with resultant uncontrolled arterial inflow into the penis.

Evaluation

In men presenting with priapism, a history detailing the duration of the erection, the presence or absence of pain, and the presence of risk factors should be obtained. Physical examination should evaluate for evidence of perineal or pelvic ecchymosis as well as inguinal lymphadenopathy. In differentiating ischemic from nonischemic priapism, examination of the erection should focus on the degree of penile rigidity as well as the presence or absence of pain.

Treatment

Urologic consultation is appropriate to direct management for men with priapism. To differentiate ischemic from nonischemic priapism, a penile blood gas assay is usually obtained. For patients presenting with underlying hematologic disorders, concomitant treatment of the priapism and underlying disorder should occur.[67] For prompt treatment of ischemic priapism, irrigation of the corpora cavernosum with or without instillation of 100–500 μg/mL phenylephrine every 3–5 minutes over 1 hour is first-line therapy. If this fails to resolve the erection, surgical shunts should be performed. Several types of shunts have been described, the details of which are beyond the scope of this chapter; it is recommended that distal shunts be performed first, followed by proximal shunts.[67]

For men diagnosed with nonischemic priapism, initial treatment with observation is recommended.[67] This can be safely undertaken without risk of long-term erectile dysfunction or penile damage since the penile tissue is well oxygenated. For men whose conditions fail to respond to conservative therapy, selective angioembolization of the cavernosal artery is recommended, with open surgical repair reserved for those that fail angiographic intervention.

Phimosis and Paraphimosis

Definition

Phimosis is defined as the inability to retract the foreskin. *Paraphimosis* is the painful swelling of the retracted foreskin distal to the phimotic ring of tissue. At birth, the majority of males will have physiologic phimosis.[68] As the child ages, the preputial opening gradually opens, allowing the foreskin to be retracted. The incidence of phimosis decreases to 10% in 3-year-old males and to 1% in 14-year-old males.[69] The true incidence of paraphimosis is unknown.

Etiology and Risk Factors

Recurrent *balanitis*, defined as either a bacterial or fungal infection of the foreskin, can predispose an uncircumcised male to phimosis due to chronic inflammation with subsequent scarring of the preputial opening. Paraphimosis occurs from leaving the retracted foreskin behind the glans penis, which results in vascular engorgement and edema of the retracted skin. Although patient hygiene may be responsible for this, this condition is often iatrogenic from a healthcare worker forgetting to reduce the foreskin after examination of the penis or via the insertion of a urethral catheter.

Evaluation

For men presenting with phimosis, a history and physical examination evaluating for the presence or absence of underlying infections is important.

The examiner should also inquire whether the foreskin balloons with voiding. In contrast to phimosis, paraphimosis is considered a urologic emergency. A detailed history regarding the duration of foreskin retraction should be obtained. Physical examination should involve inspection of the glans and penile shaft for evidence of necrosis.

Treatment

In men presenting with phimosis and balanitis, treatment with topical antibiotic/antifungal ointments or oral agents with gram-positive coverage is appropriate as a first-line measure. Once this condition is resolved, options for treatment of the phimosis include topical steroids or circumcision. Success rates for topical steroids have been reported up to 67–95%.[69] Although circumcision is an overall safe and effective procedure, potential complications include damage to the urethra, bleeding, infection, and meatal stenosis. There are no RCTs to demonstrate superiority of the various treatment options available for phimosis.

Men diagnosed with paraphimosis need to be treated immediately. Treatment involves reduction of the foreskin to its normal anatomic position or surgical release of the constricting band of tissue. Often, patients have severe pain necessitating pain medications or topical or injectable anesthetics. Several treatment options exist for paraphimosis, although no RCT has been performed comparing the different treatments. Manual reduction can be performed to reduce the paraphimosis. The edema within the penile skin can be manually reduced by circumferential compression. Addition of ice packs or compressive dressings may aid in reducing the edema. Alternative treatment options for reducing edema before manual reduction of the foreskin include injection of hyaluronidase into the edematous tissue[70] or liberally applying granulated sugar on the tissue, which decreases the edema by osmosis.[71] Once the edema in the tissue is resolved, the foreskin can be pulled down over the glans by placing both thumbs on the glans penis and forefingers around the phimotic ring and applying gentle pressure. If this is unsuccessful, an emergent dorsal slit or circumcision can be performed.

Renal Stone Disease

Introduction

Approximately 13% of men and 7% of women in the United States will develop renal stones at

some point during their lifetimes. The prevalence of stones appears to be increasing because over the past two decades the prevalence of stones has increased by 37%.[72] The annual healthcare expenditure in 2001 for treatment of urolithiasis was $2.1 billion, which represents a 150% increase since 1980 and a 45–50% increase in expenditures compared with 1994.[73]

Epidemiology

Lithogenic factors include gender, age, and geography. The frequency of calculi by gender continues to show a higher prevalence of stones in males versus females. The male-to-female ratio of stone prevalence nationwide appears to be between 2:1 and 3:1 and has remained stable over time.[72,74,75] In addition, stone prevalence increases with age in both men and women. Historically, the incidence of stone disease has been reported to be three to four times more common in white persons than in nonwhite persons,[76,77] whereas other studies have suggested that lifestyle and diet may play a more significant role in stone formation than ethnicity.[78] Geography also appears to be a significant risk factor because epidemiologic studies have found age-adjusted stone prevalence to be highest in the South followed subsequently by the East, Midwest, and Western United States.

Additional lithogenic factors include modern sedentary lifestyle, obesity, dietary habits, family history of stone disease, metabolic disorders (e.g., gout, hyperparathyroidism, type 1 renal tubular acidosis), and gastrointestinal diseases (e.g., malabsorption, Crohn's disease, ulcerative colitis). Obesity is a significant risk factor in stone formation because significant positive correlations were found with increasing body mass index (BMI) and increased urinary excretions of uric acid, sodium, phosphate, and ammonium and decreased urinary pH—all of which are associated with stone crystal formation.[79] The relative risk of stone formation in males with BMI greater than 30 compared with those with a BMI less than 23, after adjusting for age, dietary factors, fluid intake, and thiazide use, was 1.33, whereas in females the effect of BMI was even more pronounced; the relative risk of stone formation in females with a BMI greater than 30 compared with BMI less than 23 was 1.90.[80] Experimental studies have demonstrated a higher incidence of renal stone formation in animals that were fed a high-fat diet. Patients who are significantly overweight and who embark on a weight-loss dietary program consisting of high protein or high fat concentrations should be counseled regarding the potential risk of stone formation as a result of these diets. Diets high in sodium chloride intake are directly associated with significant increases in renal calcium excretion. The effect of this increased intake, coupled with low levels of citrate and relative oliguria, further increase the risk of stone formation.

Presenting Signs and Symptoms

Patients with renal lithiasis present with a wide variation ranging from symptoms of severe, agonizing pain to being completely asymptomatic. Typical renal stone pain is manifested by chronic, episodic, flank discomfort. Ureteral colic due to an acutely obstructing stone is commonly manifested as flank pain that is abrupt in onset, severe, colicky, and often associated with nausea and emesis and can mimic an acute gastrointestinal malady. Patients may also complain of ipsilateral radiating groin pain. Approximately 10% of patients will present with gross hematuria, whereas virtually 90% will have microscopic hematuria.

Radiologic Imaging of Renal Stones

Plain abdominal radiographs are an excellent screening modality and are the most common radiologic means by which to follow patients with known stone disease. IVP was the study of choice for patients before noncontrast spiral CT, which has virtually supplanted IVP for the evaluation of a patient presenting with signs and symptoms consistent with renal lithiasis, especially in the emergency department. The advantages of the noncontrast spiral CT include no need for bowel preparation or intravenous contrast administration, speed of the examination, ability to diagnose nonurologic pathology, and superior accuracy in the diagnosis of renal stones independent of composition.[81] The disadvantages are predominately centered on anaphylactic risks of iodinated contrast used in the study.

Medical Management of Symptomatic Stone Disease

Standard medical treatment of acute renal colic consists of vigorous hydration (intravenous, if necessary) and narcotic analgesics for pain relief. NSAIDs used in the acute setting appear to be equal or superior in alleviating renal or ureteral pain.[82] Several investigators have reported that calcium channel blockers and alpha-1–blockers appear to be beneficial in facilitating ureteral stone passage. These agents result in decreased narcotic use and quicker passage of stone from the time of diagnosis, and in some cases they may allow passage of stones that may not have typically passed spontaneously without surgical intervention.[83,84] These agents may also facilitate stone fragment passage after shock wave lithotripsy.

Surgical Management of Stone Disease

Shock wave lithotripsy continues to be the predominant surgical treatment for renal lithiasis. The newer-generation lithotriptors provide a noninvasive, effective, relatively "painless" method of stone treatment. The mechanism of stone fragmentation has not been completely elucidated, but it appears that cavitation is the primary means. The most appropriate stones for shock wave lithotripsy treatment appear to be those less than 1.5 cm in diameter outside of the lower pole, proximal ureteral stones less than 10 mm in diameter, or distal ureteral stones; stone-free resolution rates of 74–90% have been reported.[85] Percutaneous nephrolithotomy with or without intracorporeal lithotripsy is recommended for patients with renal or lower pole stones less than 1.5 cm in diameter or staghorn or struvite stones. Stone-free resolution rates of 75–90% can be achieved even in patients with large stone burdens or complex collecting system anatomy.[86,87] The advent of fiber-optic technology and the miniaturization of endoscopic instrumentation including laser energy via fiber have greatly facilitated direct access to stones in the ureter and renal collecting system. Ureteroscopic stone treatment is the treatment of choice for distal ureteral calculi, with success rates of 87–100%. Stone-free rates for mid and proximal ureteral stones and intrarenal stones are 70–92%.[88] All of these technologies can be transferred to the pediatric age group with comparable success and morbidity.[89]

Urologic Consultation

First-time and recurrent stone formers should be encouraged to undergo urologic evaluation. Patients who present with stones who have known genitourinary abnormalities (e.g., solitary kidney, duplicated collecting system, hydronephrosis) or a concomitant urinary tract infection should also undergo urologic consultation. Such consultation should be strongly considered in patients who have not had progression of a ureteral stone or who continue to be symptomatic after 3–4 weeks of expulsive medical therapy.

Stone Composition

Fifty to seventy percent of renal stones in the United States are composed of calcium oxalate, calcium phosphate, or a combination of these three components. Struvite (infection stones) and uric acid stones are the next most common compositions, followed by cystine and other miscellaneous components, which compose less than 4% of all stones (Table 16-5). The pathophysiology of stone formation within the kidney has not been fully elucidated, yet it appears clear that a prerequisite is urinary crystal formation. Chemical and physical factors that play a role in crystal formation include supersaturated urine (i.e., overabundance of solute in a solution), which is affected by urinary pH and temperature, the presence or lack of urinary stone inhibitors (e.g., citrate, magnesium, zinc, macromolecules, and pyrophosphate), and matrix (i.e., a mucoprotein associated with stone formation).

Metabolic Evaluation and Treatment

First and foremost, it is imperative to attempt to determine renal stone composition. For that reason, patients should have retrieved stones (especially their first stone) sent for analysis. Urinalysis (including urinary pH, specific gravity, and the presence of leukocytes, hematuria, and crystalluria) and serum chemistries (including creatinine, calcium, phosphorus, electrolytes, uric acid, and parathyroid hormone if serum calcium is high) should all compose the initial evaluation.

Not every patient that has passed a stone requires additional evaluation other than what

has been previously mentioned. More than 50% of all patients who form renal stones have an additional recurrence during their lifetime,[90] but if patients follow the general dietary recommendations, then the risk of repeated stone formation decreases to 10–15% (Table 16-6).[91] Approximately 10% of all stone formers have more than three recurrences, and about 15% will require specific metabolic measures for recurrence prevention.[92] For patients who have recurrent stones or for those who are deemed to be at high-risk for stone formation (Table 16-7), additional metabolic evaluation including a 24-hour urine collection (including urine pH, and concentrations of oxalate, phosphorus, calcium, oxalate, uric acid, magnesium, creatinine, citrate, and sodium) and a cystine spot urine test is warranted.

Recommended pharmacologic therapies for specific types of stones are listed in Table 16-8. Dietary calcium restriction as a general means of reducing stone recurrence is not recommended. Several studies have indicated that dietary calcium supplementation may actually serve as a protectant for further stone formation.[93–95] Ascorbic acid and cranberry juice may increase the risk of stone formation in calcium oxalate stone formers.[96,97]

Table 16-5. Composition of Urinary Calculi

Pure calcium oxalate stones: 36–70%
Pure calcium phosphate stones: 6–20%
Mixed calcium oxalate and phosphate: 11–31%
Struvite: 6–20%
Uric acid: 6–17%
Cystine: 0.5–3.0%
Miscellaneous: 1–4%

Adapted from: Straub M, Hautman RE: Developments in stone prevention, *Curr Opin Urol* 15:119–126, 2005.

Table 16-6. Measures to Prevent Renal Stone Formation

Fluid intake, "drinking advice"
Fluid intake should be roughly balanced with urine output
Amount: 2.5–3.0 liters fluid intake per day
Urine volume: 2.0–2.5 liters/day
Specific gravity of urine: <1.010
Neutral beverages (water)
Circadian drinking
Balanced diet, "nutrition advice"
Rich in vegetable fiber
Rich in alkaline potassium
Normal calcium content: 1000–1200 mg/day
Limited sodium chloride content: 4–5 g/day
Limited animal protein content: 0.8–1.0 g/kg/day
Limited fat, oxalate, and sugar intake
Normalized general risk factors, "lifestyle advice"
Adequate physical activity
Balancing excessive fluid loss
Body mass index between 18 and 25 kg/m^2

Adapted from: Straub M, Hautman RE: Developments in stone prevention, *Curr Opin Urol* 15:119–126, 2005.

Table 16-7. Risk Factors for Recurrent Renal Stone Disease

Family history of stone disease
Bilateral or multiple stone disease
Solitary kidney
Highly recurrent stone disease (i.e., more than three stones in 3 years)
Nephrocalcinosis
Infection (struvite) stones
Calcium phosphate stones

Medical conditions
• Hyperparathyroidism
• Gastrointestinal disorders (e.g., ulcerative colitis, Crohn's disease, malabsorption)
• Vitamin D toxicity
• Gout
• Genetically determined stones
  • Cystinuria
  • Primary oxaluria
• Renal tubular acidosis type 1

Children and teenagers

Testicular Cancer

Definition

Any solid testicular mass identified by the patient or incidentally discovered on physical examination requires a thorough evaluation to rule out a testicular tumor. The finding of any lump or firm area on the testis should be considered to be a tumor until proven otherwise. The classic presentation is painless testicular enlargement or swelling, testicular mass (firm lump or nodule), testicular pain (heaviness, aching sensation, acute pain), gynecomastia, or a history of trauma. Acute trauma is not believed to be a causative factor but may heighten awareness of a testicular mass. Uncommonly, testicular cancer presents with systemic disease with abdominal mass or pain, back or bone pain, or pulmonary symptoms (all are sites of potential metastasis). The differential diagnosis includes epididymo-orchitis, testicular torsion, or tumor.[98]

Incidence

Testicular cancer is rare and accounts for only 1–2% of all malignant tumors in males,[99] but it is the most common cancer in males aged 15–34 years.[100] There were an estimated 8010 new cases and 390 deaths in the United States in 2005.[101] There has been a 100% rise in incidence in testicular germ cell tumors every 20 years,[102] and the incidence has been increasing since the middle of the 20th century. Germ cell tumors are the most frequent malignant testicular tumor, with more than 7000 cases diagnosed each

Table 16-8. Medical Therapies for Stone-Forming Patients

Stone Type	Lithogenic Abnormality	Preventive Treatment
Calcium oxalate	Hypercalciuria	Potassium citrate 30–60 mEq/day divided into 3–4 doses
		Alternative: sodium bicarbonate 1.5 g/day divided into 3 doses
	Hypocitraturia	Potassium citrate 30–60 mEq/day divided into 3–4 doses
	Hyperoxaluria	Calcium 500 mg/day with meals
	Hypomagnesuria	Magnesium 200–400 mg/day (Caution: no replacement in renal insufficiency)
Calcium phosphate	Hypercalciuria	Hydrochlorothiazide 25–50 mg/day
Uric acid	Urinary pH < 6	Potassium citrate 30–60 mEq/day divided into 3–4 doses
		Alternative: sodium bicarbonate 1.5 g/day divided into 3 doses
	Hyperuricosuria	Allopurinol 100 mg/day
	Hyperuricosuria/ Hyperuricemia	Allopurinol 300 mg/day
Cystine		Daily fluid intake 3.5–4 liter/day for urinary output 2.5–3.0 liter/day
		Potassium citrate 30–120 mEq/day titrated for urine pH of 7.5–8.5
		Penicillamine 1–4 g/day divided into 4 doses
		Captopril 25–50 mg/day

year and an overall lifetime risk of 1 in 500. The incidence of testicular cancer in white persons is four times more than that in black persons.[103,104]

Etiology, Risk Factors, and Epidemiology

The etiology of testicular cancer is not known. Most established risk factors relate to early life events, the most important being cryptorchidism. It has been hypothesized that testicular atrophy is a common pathway whereby several etiologic factors may be involved. Risk factors for testicular cancer include maternal exposure to androgens during pregnancy, testicular atrophy, history of previous testicular tumor, carcinoma in situ or intraepithelial germ cell neoplasia, and cryptorchidism. Socioeconomic, lifestyle, and occupational risk factors have mixed associations and may be involved in promoting the disease rather than initiating it.[105]

Ten percent of testicular cancers have a history of cryptorchidism; a male with a history of cryptorchidism has a 5–15-fold higher risk for the development of testicular cancer. Interestingly, testicular cancer is more common on the right side, in keeping with the higher incidence of cryptorchidism on that side. An intra-abdominal testis is at greater risk than an undescended testis in the inguinal position. Orchiopexy does not prevent tumor development but may reduce the risk if performed before early puberty (age 8 years)[105] and allows for easier examination of the testis.

An undescended testis (i.e., cryptorchidism), contralateral testicular germ cell tumor, and familial testicular cancer are established risk factors with high levels of evidence. In a meta-analysis of 21 studies, a relative risk of 4.8 (95% confidence interval, 4.0–5.7) was reported for these risk factors.[105] A contralateral testicular tumor confers a 25-fold increased relative risk of the development of a germ cell tumor. Familial testicular cancer involves a relative risk of 3–10.[105] Infertility, testicular atrophy, and twin-ship confer risk with lesser levels of evidence. Scrotal trauma is probably not a risk factor for the development of testicular cancer; HIV may be a predisposing factor. There is conflicting evidence that excess maternal estrogen presents risk.[106] There is a familial tendency toward testicular tumors. A relative risk of 1.96–4.3 to the father and 9.8–12.3 to the brother of a male with testicular cancer has been reported.[107–109]

Diagnosis

A thorough evaluation in a patient with suspected testicular cancer includes a complete examination of the chest, abdomen, pelvis, and genitalia. The examination should begin with palpation of the normal testis, and both should be examined for size, consistency, texture, mobility, nodule, or mass. If the testis is tender or if there is a concomitant hydrocele, examination of the testis may be difficult. Physical examination should assess for lymphadenopathy, gynecomastia, abdominal mass, hepatomegaly, pleural effusion, and lower extremity edema.

Scrotal ultrasonography with Doppler should be obtained as the next step after the physical examination, *but only if time permits*. Ultrasound is highly reliable in differentiating between intratesticular/extratesticular lesions such as epididymitis, hydrocele, inguinal hernia, spermatocele, or testicular torsion. Microlithiasis is a frequent finding in normal testes and is of uncertain significance. However, if a high index for suspicion of a testicular tumor exists on the basis of history and physical examination results, definitive treatment must not be delayed to wait for radiologic imaging.

Testicular cancer is one of the few cancers with accurate serum tumor markers: beta-human chorionic gonadotropin (0–3.5 mIU/mL), alpha-fetoprotein (0–10 ng/mL), and lactate dehydrogenase. These markers are all well established in the diagnosis, staging, prognosis, monitoring of therapeutic response, and prediction of relapse. Serum tumor markers should be obtained if a high index of suspicion exists for a testicular tumor on the basis of history and physical examination results, but *definitive treatment must not be delayed* to wait for serum tumor marker results. In men with testicular cancer, serum markers with chest radiograph and CT thorax scans are important elements of monthly follow-ups in patients after definitive treatment for testicular cancer. Markers may allow detection of a tumor that is too small to be found on physical examination or via radiographs. The absence of detectable markers does not mean the absence of tumor.

After the diagnosis of testicular cancer, the disease should be appropriately staged with a CT scan of the abdomen and pelvis and a chest radiograph. If the results of either are suspicious or positive for disease, then a CT scan of the chest should also be performed. Any clinical suspicion for brain metastases indicates a need for CT scan or magnetic resonance imaging (MRI) of the brain. An essential part of the treatment regimen is evaluation of the retroperitoneal lymph nodes with CT scanning. Patients with negative CT scan results have a 25–30% chance of microscopic nodal involvement. Lymphangiograms had been used instead of and in combination with CT scanning, but these are much less used in common practice today.

Management

If the evaluation of a patient with a suspected testicular mass suggests epididymo-orchitis, then a trial of antibiotics (e.g., ceftriaxone and doxycycline) is reasonable because infectious epididymitis and orchitis are more common than testicular tumors. If signs and symptoms persist after appropriate antibiotic therapy, a testicular tumor must be highly suspected and effectively ruled out. The physical evaluation and scrotal ultrasonography should be repeated within 2 weeks of presentation.

Radical inguinal orchiectomy with initial high ligation of the spermatic cord is the procedure of choice for the definitive diagnosis and initial treatment of a malignant testicular mass, even in the setting of metastatic disease.[110] Radical orchiectomy is performed through an inguinal incision to allow for surgical control of the spermatic cord. Trans-scrotal orchiectomy or trans-scrotal testicular biopsy is contraindicated because of potential tumor contamination of scrotal lymphatics and dissemination of disease into the scrotum.[111] Before orchiectomy, sperm banking must be discussed and is generally recommended for those interested in preserving future fertility, but this should not delay orchiectomy. After orchiectomy, clinicians should obtain follow-up tumor marker and liver function tests and should stage the disease radiographically.

Testicular cancer has become one of the most curable solid neoplasms and serves as the paradigm for the multimodal treatment of malignancies. There has been a decrease in mortality from more than 50% before 1970 to less than 5% in 1997,[103] with the development of effective diagnostic techniques, accurate tumor markers, effective multidrug chemotherapeutic and radiotherapy regimens, and modifications of surgical techniques.

The optimal therapy after orchiectomy must be individualized based on the histology of the primary tumor, the presence or absence of metastases, and relative values of the various serum tumor markers. These factors are all considered in the TNM (i.e., tumor, lymph nodes, metastasis) staging system, which is now widely accepted. The American Joint Committee on Cancer (AJCC)

has designated staging by TNM classification, but the Memorial Sloan-Kettering staging system for testicular cancer is frequently preferred because of its increased clinical utility[112]:

- Stage I: Confined to the testis, epididymis, spermatic cord, scrotum
- Stage II: Confined to retroperitoneal nodes below the diaphragm
- Stage IIA: Nodes less than 2 cm in diameter
- Stage IIB: Nodes 2–5 cm in diameter
- Stage IIC: Nodes more than 5 cm in diameter
- Stage III: Metastases to visceral organ(s) or nodes above the diaphragm

Testicular tumors are divided into two groups: germ cell and non–germ cell tumors. Germ cell tumors are composed of seminomas (40%) and nonseminomatous germ cell tumors (NSGCTs) for the purposes of treatment because seminomas are more sensitive to radiation therapy. NSGCTs include embryonal cell carcinoma (20–25%), teratocarcinoma (25%), teratoma (5%), choriocarcinoma (1%), and yolk sac tumor (<1%). Non–germ cell tumors include gonadoblastomas, Leydig cell tumors, and Sertoli cell tumors. Other secondary tumors are rare and include lymphoma, leukemia, and metastatic tumors (e.g., prostate, melanoma, and lung).

Fewer than 50% of malignant testicular germ cell tumors have a single cell type, whereas the remainder has more than one cell type. The relative proportion of each cell type within a given tumor should be specified because cell type is important for estimating the risk of metastases and response to treatment. (The reader is referred to the World Health Organization for histologic classification of malignant testis tumors.[113])

Testicular cancer is highly curable. Nevertheless, in an effort to improve cure rates and to decrease treatment morbidity, all newly diagnosed patients are appropriately considered candidates for clinical trials. An international prognostic classification for germ cell tumors based on a retrospective analysis of 5202 patients with metastatic nonseminomatous and 660 patients with metastatic seminomatous germ cell tumors was agreed on in 1997 by all major clinical trial groups around the world. This classification should be used for reporting clinical trails of patients with testicular germ cell tumors.[114]

If clinical staging results are positive for disease or if tumor markers remain elevated after orchiectomy, then systemic disease is suspected and adjuvant therapy is indicated. Seminomas are very radiosensitive. Platinum-based chemotherapy (e.g., bleomycin, etoposide, cisplatin) is used for bulky, advanced, and metastatic semi-noma. Nonseminomas are less radiosensitive but are highly responsive to platinum-based chemotherapy. After either chemotherapy or radiation, if para-aortic or para-caval lymph nodes remain enlarged, a retroperitoneal lymph node dissection (RPLND) may be curative. RPLND involves removing the lymph nodes where testicular cancer is likely to spread. This procedure carries the risk of ejaculatory and erectile dysfunction, although this is relatively uncommon with nerve-sparing techniques commonly used in such surgical approaches today. RPLND remains an essential component in the treatment and cure of men with testicular cancer.[115] For men with low-stage nonseminomatous germ cell tumors, primary RPLND is an important staging maneuver and is curative in up to 90% of men with low-volume retroperitoneal disease. In the post-chemotherapy setting, the current inability to exclude the presence of residual teratoma or viable germ cell tumor in the retroperitoneum mandates that post-chemotherapy RPLND be performed in all patients with NSGCTs who have residual masses.[116] RPLND has minimal short- and long-term morbidity in the hands of experienced surgeons in dedicated centers. Treatment of non–germ cell tumors depends on both clinical staging and pathology and involves a combination of orchiectomy and RPLND. The indications for and efficacy of radiation and chemotherapy are not well defined.

A recent European consensus statement[102] on the treatment of testicular germ cell tumors outlines treatment options for testicular germ cell tumors, including platinum-based chemotherapy, with radiation and RPLND. This review provides a summary of the highest level evidence available.[102]

Surveillance

Once a patient has had a testicular tumor, he is at increased risk of developing a second tumor, and thus it is important that he continue to perform monthly testicular self-examinations, often best performed after a warm bath or shower when the scrotal skin is relaxed. In men definitively treated and cured of testicular cancer, there is a 2–5% cumulative risk of developing a tumor in the contralateral testicle over the next 25 years after the initial diagnosis.[117,118] Most tumor recurrences occur within the first 2 years; however, late relapses have been reported. Patients with testicular cancer can expect to be monitored very closely for at least 5 years with periodic

chest radiographs, abdominal and pelvic CT scans, and serum tumor markers. Lifelong serum marker, physical, and radiologic examinations have also been recommended.[119]

Fertility Issues

The removal of one testicle should not impair a patient's sexual potency or fertility. Most men are able to have normal erections after RPLND. A brief decrease in sperm production may occur, but the remaining testis should produce adequate amounts of testosterone. Sperm abnormalities or oligospermia are common before therapy. Additionally, since many patients experience low sperm counts after various treatment modalities, sperm banking before chemotherapy is recommended. Almost all men will become oligospermic during chemotherapy; however, many will recover sperm production and go on to father children. Numerous studies[120–123] have demonstrated that children of men with testicular cancer do not appear to have increased risk of congenital malformations. Radiation scatter to the remaining normal testis during treatment of retroperitoneal lymph nodes may lead to decreased fertility. Shielding techniques can reduce the radiation scatter and, depending on the radiation dose, sperm counts can fall after radiation but may recover over 1–2 years. Children conceived after radiation therapy have been reported and, thus far, have not been found to have a higher risk of congenital malformations.[124] It is important to be aware of these issues, since most cases of testicular cancer are curable.

Prognosis

An optimal definition of risk factors for testicular cancer will likely bring about the development of risk-adjusted treatment modalities and lead to increased treatment efficacy and less toxicity. Ongoing research into the molecular biology of testicular tumors will hopefully allow for improved diagnosis, staging, and targeted treatment in the years to come.

Penile Cancer
Definition

Penile cancer can be thought of as squamous cell cancer of the penile skin. Primary lesions typically occur on the glans or inner foreskin. The most common clinical presentation is a nonhealing penile lesion. Ulceration, erythema, induration, or an inability to retract the foreskin may occur. Invasion of the penile corpora and urethra is more common than metastatic disease. Tumor spread occurs via regional lymphatics to the inguinal and iliac lymph nodes. Distant metastases occur in fewer than 10% of patients and involve the lungs, liver, and bone. Penile cancer mortality usually occurs from local growth causing sepsis, bleeding, or wasting. Patients with a local penile recurrence have a mean survival of 7 years, whereas those with inguinal nodal recurrence have a mean survival of less than 2 years.

Incidence

Penile cancer is rare in the United States, accounting for fewer than 0.5% of cancers in adult males or less than 1 per 100,000 men per year. It is more common in less developed countries including Asia, Africa, and South America, with a 10–20-fold higher incidence, and may represent 10–30% of cancers diagnosed in men in these areas. The average age of presentation is between 50 and 70 years, and the disease rarely occurs in persons younger than 40 years of age.

Etiology, Risk Factors, and Epidemiology

Penile cancer is almost never seen in neonatally circumcised men.[125–127] The incidence of penile cancer is higher when circumcision is delayed until after puberty. Adult circumcision does not confer protection against penile cancer. Chronic irritation from smegma, poor hygiene, and balanitis may contribute to the higher incidence of penile cancer in uncircumcised males. Studies suggest an association between human papilloma virus type 16 infection and penile cancer.[128,129] Premalignant lesions include leukoplakia (associated with chronic irritation and often located adjacent to penile cancer), balanitis xerotica obliterans (severe, chronic inflammatory lesion of the meatus, glans, and foreskin), and giant condyloma acuminata (verrucous carcinoma or Buschke-Lowenstein tumor). Interestingly, tobacco smoking has also been correlated with an increased risk of penile cancer.

Diagnosis

A thorough evaluation for cancer screening includes complete examination of the chest, abdomen, pelvis, and genitalia. The examination should begin with inspection and palpation of the penis. Lesions commonly present on the glans or prepuce and can be papillary or ulcerative in appearance. Although most lesions are not painful, a penile discharge or dysuria may be present. Men typically present at an average of 10–12 months after the lesion is noted, a waiting period often attributed to embarrassment and denial. Physical examination should also specifically assess for the presence of palpable inguinal lymphadenopathy. Approximately 50% of men present with palpable inguinal lymph nodes, typically inflammatory rather than malignant. The differential diagnosis of penile lesions includes syphilitic chancre, chancroid, circinate balanitis (e.g., Reiter's syndrome), and condylomata acuminata. Diagnosis is made on the basis of the results of punch or excisional biopsy performed in the operating room.

Squamous cell carcinoma is the most common and most aggressive penile cancer, accounting for 95% of cases. Basal cell carcinoma, melanoma, sarcoma, and Kaposi sarcoma can also occur, though less commonly. Lesions may start on the glans or foreskin and may extend throughout the glans and foreskin and into the corpora of the penis or urethra. Carcinoma in situ or a malignant change without invasion through the basement membrane is termed *erythroplasia of Queyrat* when it appears as a painful, velvety, erythematous lesion on the glans. Twenty percent of cases of erythroplasia of Queyrat progress to invasive penile cancer. When carcinoma in situ appears as an erythematous plaque on the penile shaft, it is termed *Bowen's disease*. Fifty percent of cases of Bowen's disease progress to invasive penile cancer, and 25% are associated with visceral malignancy. Metastatic tumors to the penis are rare, but 75% are genitourinary in origin; specifically, bladder and prostate followed by colorectal cancer. Symptoms of metastatic tumors to the penis include priapism and local swelling.

Primary tumor diagnosis is performed on the basis of tissue biopsy results. Regional (inguinal and iliac) lymph nodes are assessed via CT scan or lymphadenectomy. Distant metastases are assessed using chest radiographs, CT and MRI scans of the abdomen and pelvis, radionuclide bone scan, and assessment of serum liver function test results and calcium levels.

Management

Therapy for penile cancer is selected based on the size, location, invasiveness, and stage of the tumor. The Jackson staging system is commonly used clinically[130]:

- Stage I: Limited to the glans and foreskin; does not involve the shaft of the penis or the corpora cavernosa
- Stage II: Tumor invades the corpora cavernosa of the penis but is not revealed to have spread to lymph nodes on clinical examination
- Stage III: Tumor has clinical spread to regional lymph nodes in the groin; cure is related to the number and extent of nodes involved
- Stage IV: Invasive cancer that causes extensive and inoperable involvement of lymph nodes in the groin or distant metastases

(The reader is also referred to the AJCC staging system designated by TNM classification.[131])

Penile cancer is highly curable when diagnosed early and at early stages (stages I and II). Chances of cure decrease sharply for higher stage and advanced disease (stages III and IV). Clinical trials for penile cancer are uncommon in the United States due to the rarity of the tumor in this country.

Treatment

The clinical introduction of penile-sparing treatment modalities has spurred an evolution in the treatment of men with penile cancer. Because penile cancers begin as superficial lesions, radical surgery can often be avoided if diagnosed early. Stage I penile cancer is curable. Lesions limited to the foreskin can be cured by wide local excision with circumcision, as long as there is a 2-cm negative surgical margin. The patient must be followed up postsurgically because the recurrence rate can be as high as 50% after circumcision for treatment of a preputial tumor. Small, superficial, noninvasive cancers and carcinoma in situ on the glans can be treated effectively with topical 5-fluorouracil cream, neodymium:yttrium-aluminum-garnet laser excision,[132-134] or Mohs' surgery.[135] Recurrent cases can be retreated with the laser, Mohs' surgery, or partial penectomy. For tumors that infiltrate the glans, with or without adjacent skin involvement, treatment may include partial penectomy,[136] external-beam radiation or brachytherapy,[137,138] or Mohs' surgery.

Regardless of inguinal node status, partial or total penectomy with disease-free proximal margins of 2 cm is the first-line treatment for invasive penile cancer (stages II, III, and IV). Radiation therapy with surgical salvage is an alternative.[138-141] If a 2-cm margin cannot be obtained or if the remaining penile shaft is too short for the patient to urinate standing up, total penectomy with perineal urethrostomy in performed. Sexual function can be achieved with 6 cm of remaining penile corporal length. In cases in which the entire shaft or base of the penis in involved, total penectomy and perineal urethrostomy are necessary.

If a patient with penile cancer has palpable inguinal lymph nodes, treatment with penicillin or cephalosporin antibiotic is prescribed for 6 weeks to decrease nodal inflammation. If palpable lymphadenopathy does not regress after appropriate antibiotic therapy, then bilateral inguinal lymph node dissection is necessary. If the patient has no palpable inguinal lymphadenopathy, then close follow-up is necessary since up to 20% of men will have histologic evidence for nodal disease; this is highly dependent on tumor stage. Lymph node involvement worsens prognosis and decreases 5-year survival from 20% to 50%. Because of the high incidence of microscopic node metastases in patients with larger tumors (>5 cm in diameter) or stage II or III disease, prophylactic bilateral inguinal lymph node dissection is necessary regardless of whether the inguinal lymph nodes are clinically palpable. The incidence of lymph node involvement approaches 50% with invasive disease. In cases of proven inguinal lymph node metastasis without distant spread, bilateral inguinal lymph node dissection is indicated.[136,139,142,143] Many patients with positive lymph node test results are not cured, however, so clinical trials may be appropriate. Possible complications of ilioinguinal lymph node dissection include skin sloughing, wound breakdown, infection, bleeding, nerve injury, deep vein thrombosis, lymphocele, and lymphedema.[142-145]

No standard curative treatment exists for stage IV penile cancer. Palliation is achieved with either surgery or radiation, with the goals of controlling the local penile lesion; preventing necrosis, infection, and hemorrhage from regional nodal disease; and addressing symptoms from bony metastases.

Alternative Therapy

For select men with a small (<3 cm in diameter) superficial, noninvasive lesion on the glans or coronal sulcus, radiation therapy is an alternative to partial penectomy. The advantage of radiation in selected cases of minimally invasive lesions is preservation of penile anatomy and maintenance of sexual function. Total penectomy is indicated for local recurrence after radiation. Radiation is not effective for larger, invasive lesions, and the associated morbidity is high. Radiation therapy for node-positive disease results in cure rates of only 10% for all stages of disease. However, in men with metastatic disease or inoperable inguinal lymph nodes, in those who refuse surgery, or in men who are not candidates for surgery, palliative radiation is an option. With regard to disease that has spread to the lymph nodes, postoperative radiation may decrease incidence of inguinal nodal recurrence.

Most men experience urethritis and edema during radiation therapy for penile cancer. Late complications include meatal stenosis, urethral stricture, fistulae, and discoloration of the penile skin. Brachytherapy protocols with iridium-192 have been used for local control of superficial lesions with a 90% response rate; however, the recurrence rate is 63% at 2 years and 80% at 5 years.[145a] Before any type of radiation therapy is instituted, circumcision must be performed to reduce local morbidity.

Clinical trials using radiosensitizers, cytotoxic drugs, and new biologic and chemotherapeutic agents are ongoing. Chemotherapeutic regimens using vincristine, bleomycin, methotrexate, cisplatin, and 5-fluorouracil as neoadjuvant and adjuvant therapy have shown varying benefit.[146–151] Information about ongoing clinical trials is available from the National Cancer Institute Web site at http://cancer.gov/clinicaltrials.

Prognosis

Prognostic indicators for penile cancer include the size and location of the primary tumor, the degree of nodal involvement, and the 5-year rate of no evidence of disease after initial treatment. The 5-year survival rate for localized disease without metastasis ranges from 60% to 90%. The survival rate falls to 30–50% for inguinal nodal involvement and to 20% when iliac nodes are involved. There is currently no report of 5-year survival in men with distant metastases.[142–145]

Prostate Cancer

Definition

Nonmetastatic prostate cancer can be divided into clinically localized disease (thought to be confined to the prostate gland after clinical examination) and locally advanced disease (that which has spread outside the capsule of the prostate but has not yet spread to other organs). Prostate cancer grows very slowly in some men and moderately rapidly in others. Men with localized disease can often be cured, and men with widespread disease can respond well to treatment. Given that prostate cancer is predominantly a tumor affecting older men, those men especially with localized disease tend to die of other comorbid illnesses without experiencing disability from their cancer. Management of prostate cancer must take a number of issues into consideration: age, comorbid conditions, adverse effects of various treatments, most appropriate staging evaluation, and the value of screening. As diagnostic screening methods have changed with time, there has been an increasing diagnosis of nonlethal tumors. This trend complicates the analysis of management strategies, survival after treatment, and demographic analyses.

Incidence

Prostate cancer is the most common malignancy of adult males. The likelihood of a man acquiring prostate cancer during his lifetime is 15%; estimates indicate that 1 in 10 men will develop prostate cancer during their lifetime.[101] Although the incidence of prostate cancer increases with age, currently the mean age at diagnosis is 65 years, the median age is 72 years, and men younger than 50 years are rarely affected.[101] The probability prostate cancer developing in a man younger than 40 years is approximately 1 in 10,000.[101] The American Cancer Society[101] estimates that 232,090 new cases were diagnosed in 2005 and that 30,350 men will die of prostate cancer. In the United States, prostate cancer is second only to lung cancer as a cause of cancer-related death. Mortality from prostate cancer appears to be declining since 1995. The age-adjusted prostate cancer–specific mortality in the United States for men aged 65 years or older decreased by 15% between 1991 and 1997[152] and is thought to be resultant from aggressive prostate cancer screening, earlier treatment, more intensive treatment via all modalities, or inaccurate death certification.

Etiology, Risk Factors, and Epidemiology

The cause of prostate cancer is unknown, but there have been several associations recognized. About 10% of cases of prostate cancer are believed to be inherited. Men with one first-degree male relative with prostate cancer have a two-fold risk of developing the disease. Men with two or three affected first-degree relatives have a 5- or 10-fold risk, respectively. Prostate cancer is relatively uncommon in Asian men; men of Scandinavian descent have an increased risk of prostate cancer. There is a 50–60% greater incidence of prostate cancer in African Americans than in white persons, and the former also have a higher mortality rate from the disease.[153] The highest cancer rates occur in African American men in the United States and the lowest in men living in China.[154]

Prostate cancer cells are thought to be androgen dependent. This notion is supported by the finding that prostate cancer does not occur in eunuchs. A diet rich in saturated fat is associated with increased risk of prostate cancer. Lycopene, vitamin E, and other antioxidants may reduce the risk, and selenium may have a protective effect. Exposure within the rubber, fertilizer, and textile industries, as well as exposure to cadmium (a zinc antagonist), may be related to an increase in prostate cancer risk.

Diagnosis

AUA screening recommendations state that both PSA and digital rectal examination should be offered annually to men beginning at the age of 50 years. Younger men at risk (African Americans and those with a family history, especially in first-degree relatives) should be screened starting at the age of 40 years. Screening asymptomatic men for prostate cancer is controversial.[155–157] The reader is also referred to a summary on screening for prostate cancer by the National Cancer Institute (http://www.cancer.gov) and to the discussion of pertinent issues regarding screening guidelines in Chapter 24, Cancer Incidence, Screening, and Prevention.

Signs and Symptoms

There are often no signs or symptoms associated with early (nonmetastatic) prostate cancer. Local disease may present with irritative voiding symptoms similar to those seen in men with BPH. Hematospermia is a very rare presenting symptom of prostate cancer. In advanced disease, bony pain due to bone metastases may rarely be a presenting symptom.

Prostate-Specific Antigen

PSA is a serine protease produced by the prostatic epithelium and secreted in seminal fluid. It is specific to the prostate but not to prostate cancer. Its function is to liquefy the ejaculate,

enabling fertilization. Serum PSA can be affected by a number of factors, including serum androgen concentrations, prostate volume, race, age, BPH, prostatic inflammation or infection, prostate cancer, prostate needle biopsy, urine infection, urinary retention, and bladder catheterization. Digital rectal examination has been shown to cause a subclinical rise in PSA.

Controversy continues regarding PSA's role in the screening of asymptomatic men, but nevertheless, its utility as a tumor marker in established disease is unquestioned.[158–165] Serum PSA concentration correlates well with pathologic tumor stage and volume. Generally, a serum PSA greater than 4 ng/mL is considered to be an elevated reading. However, other criteria have been used in addition to or instead of an absolute cutoff for PSA. Serum PSA levels can be interpreted in a number of ways (e.g., PSA density, PSA velocity, age-adjusted PSA ranges, free PSA). These techniques may improve detection rates but may also tend to increase the number of unnecessary biopsies. These adjunctive assays appear to have the most utility in men with PSA levels of 4–10 ng/mL, men with prostates larger than 45 g (estimated on digital rectal examination), and men older than 70 years. No uniform standard exists for the clinical use of PSA and, if a laboratory changes its assay kit, the serial PSA assay may yield nonequivalent PSA values.

The positive predictive value of digital rectal examination is improved when combined with serum PSA. Digital rectal examination was the only screening test for prostate cancer before PSA become clinically available. Roughly 50% of suspicious lesions palpated on digital rectal examination are found to be prostate cancer on biopsy. Suspicious lesions include discrete or hard nodules, focal induration, diffusely hard gland, or asymmetry. It is important to assess the seminal vesicles for the extent of disease on digital examination. A thorough evaluation includes complete examination of the chest, abdomen, pelvis, and genitalia—especially for adenopathy, lower extremity edema, and bony tenderness because these findings may herald metastatic disease.

Further evaluation is recommended for men with normal digital rectal examination results or an abnormal elevation in PSA, although how an abnormal PSA is defined is somewhat controversial. A transrectal ultrasound (TRUS) scan is used to examine the prostate for hypoechoic areas, which are associated with but not diagnostic of prostate cancer. TRUS is very operator dependent, does not assess pelvis lymph node status, and does no better than digital rectal examination in predicting extracapsular tumor extension or seminal vesicle invasion.[166] Prostate biopsy is usually performed via the transrectal approach under ultrasound guidance using a spring-driven biopsy gun. It can also be performed transurethrally (cystoscopically) or transperineally. Typically, a total of 6–18 needle biopsy specimens are taken from the peripheral and transition zones systematically, regardless of ultrasound findings. TRUS-guided prostatic biopsies are generally recommended for men with at least 10 years of life expectancy who have abnormal digital rectal examination results and/or an elevated serum PSA level. Complications of TRUS-guided biopsy include bleeding, infection, and sepsis.[167–170]

Screening methods for the detection of prostate cancer are associated with high false-positive rates and may identify tumors that will not be clinically significant to a patient's health.[171–174] The upper limit of the normal range of PSA is not well defined, nor is the threshold for biopsy.[175] A National Cancer Institute–sponsored multicenter trial is ongoing to study the value of early detection in reducing prostate cancer–specific mortality.[176]

Tumor Histology

More than 95% of prostate cancers are adenocarcinomas that arise from prostatic acinar cells in the peripheral zone of the gland (70%), the transition zone (20%), or the central zone (10%). Conversely, BPH develops from the transition zone of the prostate (i.e., periurethral prostate tissue). Squamous cell carcinoma (0.5%) and transitional cell carcinoma (2–4%) occur more rarely. This discussion is limited to men with adenocarcinoma of the prostate.

Prostatic Intraepithelial Neoplasia

Prostatic intraepithelial neoplasia (PIN) is a dysplastic lesion consisting of benign-appearing prostate glands lined by cytologically atypical cells. PIN is considered a premalignant lesion or carcinoma in situ and is classified as either low or high grade. Twenty percent of low-grade PIN is associated with invasive prostate cancer and can be followed up without the urgent need for treatment, whereas high-grade PIN has predictive value in identifying patients at increased risk for prostate cancer, with an 80% association with invasive disease. After high-grade PIN is detected on prostate biopsy, the risk of diagnosis of prostate cancer on subsequent biopsy is 20–35%. Prostate biopsy should be repeated within 6–18 months when high-grade PIN is found.

Tumor differentiation and the degree of abnormality of histologic growth pattern correlates with the likelihood of metastases and mortality. There is marked variation in tumor histology and multifocality of tumor sites within all prostate tumors (and biopsy samples); therefore, pathologists report the range of differentiation among the malignant cells. Adenocarcinoma of the prostate is graded using the Gleason grading system, based on five grades of glandular and cellular architecture visualized microscopically under low power. The two most prominent glandular patterns are graded from 1 to 5 (although 1 is no longer used clinically or pathologically). The sum of these two patterns determines the Gleason score, ranging from 4 (well-differentiated tumor with favorable prognosis) to 10 (poorly differentiated tumor with poor prognosis). Gleason score correlates with the biologic behavior of the tumor, with decreased survival associated with higher-grade tumors.[177,178]

Prostate cancer spreads via lymphatics (e.g., external iliac, internal iliac, presacral nodes) with a higher incidence of lymphatic metastases in the larger and less-differentiated tumors. Late in the course of disease, hematogenous spread occurs to bone, lung, liver, and kidneys. Skeletal metastases are common in advanced disease. Radionuclide bone scans are the most widely used tests for detecting metastatic bony disease, the most common site of distant tumor spread. MRI is more sensitive than bone scans but is impractical for assessing the entire skeletal system. Bone scans are often reserved for high-grade, large-volume tumors with significantly elevated PSA levels ($< 20\,\mathrm{ng/mL}$) or in men with bony pain.[179,180]

Pelvic lymph node involvement generally holds worse prognosis. Pelvic lymph node dissection (PLND) is performed at the time of radical prostatectomy, and nodal status is determined as a matter of routine. However, in studies of men undergoing perineal prostatectomy with a PSA level less than $20\,\mathrm{ng/mL}$ and a low Gleason score, data suggest that PLND is unnecessary.[181,182] PLND is not generally performed for men with a PSA level less than $20\,\mathrm{ng/mL}$ and a low Gleason score who undergo brachytherapy or external-beam radiation therapy. A positive correlation between prostate biopsy Gleason score and risk of lymph node metastasis at PLND was found in a cohort study of men with clinically localized prostate cancer undergoing radical prostatectomy. The risk of nodal metastasis was 2%, 13%, and 23% for Gleason scores 5, 6, and 8, respectively.[183] CT can detect grossly enlarged lymph nodes but it not as reliable as surgical staging of lymph nodes[173,184] and is generally reserved for men with PSA levels of more than 20 ng/mL and higher Gleason scores. MRI is not useful for the assessment of nodal disease. Although there is considerable interobserver variation, MRI has been used to assess extracapsular tumor extension with a positive predictive value of about 70%. The use of an endorectal MRI coil increases the sensitivity and specificity for identification of organ-confined versus extracapsular disease.[181,185–187]

Several nomograms have been developed and validated to predict outcomes either before or after radical prostatectomy with intent to cure.[188–191] The nomograms use clinical stage, Gleason score, and PSA to predict pathologic findings (e.g., organ confinement, extracapsular disease, seminal vesicle involvement, positive lymph nodes). Other nomograms include pathologic findings (e.g., capsular invasion, surgical margins, seminal vesicle invasion, and lymph node involvement). These nomograms should not replace clinical judgment because they do not predict prognosis. Rather, they were developed in academic medical centers and may or may not be generalizable to nonacademic hospitals, where the majority of men are treated.[192,193]

Management

The management of nonmetastatic prostate cancer is controversial in many respects because it is dependent on a multitude of factors and there are few randomized clinical trials available to date. Factors to consider in management include age, life expectancy, extent of disease (e.g., tumor size, location, invasiveness, and stage), and quality of life. Two systems are used for staging prostate cancer, namely the Jewett system was described in 1975 and later modified[194] and the AJCC- and the International Union Against Cancer–adopted revised staging system designated by TNM classification that incorporates a stage for those men diagnosed through PSA screening. The AJCC TMN staging system was revised in 2002[195] and is the classification commonly used clinically.

Primary Treatment

Treatment options for nonmetastatic prostate cancer include radical prostatectomy (e.g., retropubic

open, perineal, laparoscopic, robot-assisted), interstitial brachytherapy, external-beam radiation therapy, cryotherapy, hormonal therapy, chemotherapy, and observation. Radical prostatectomy involves complete removal of the prostate, seminal vesicles, and prostatic urethra. The bladder neck is anastomosed to the distal membranous urethra. PLND is performed via a separate incision or laparoscopically when performed in conjunction with perineal prostatectomy, if indicated. Radical prostatectomy is currently the most common form of treatment for organ-confined disease. Surgery is commonly offered to men younger than 70 years of age with a better than average life expectancy.[196–198] Radical prostatectomy offers the best chance of long-term disease-free survival in organ-confined prostate cancer. Men with organ-confined disease have a 10-year disease-free survival rate of 70–85%; with focal extracapsular extension 75%; and more extensive extracapsular extension 40%.[196–198] Two RCTs of men with clinically localized prostate cancer with median follow-up of 6.2 and 23 years found no significant difference in mortality due to any cause between radical prostatectomy and watchful waiting in men with clinically detected disease.[199,200] Prostatectomy was shown to reduce the risk of treatment failure when compared with external-beam radiation in two RCTs.[199,201] After radical prostatectomy, the incidence of disease recurrence increases when there is extracapsular tumor extension or when the surgical margins are positive.[202–204] Men with extracapsular or locally advanced disease are candidates for clinical trials of postoperative radiation therapy, hormonal therapy, and cytotoxic agents.[205] Long-term outcomes for men with positive surgical margins have not been reported to date.

Complications of all types of radical prostatectomy mentioned above include the risks inherent to major abdominal surgery, cancer recurrence, erectile dysfunction (even with "nerve-sparing" techniques), and urinary incontinence. Differences in the reporting of complications involves many factors such as age differences among different patient populations; variations in surgical expertise and volume among surgeons, community hospitals, and major medical centers; selection factors; publication bias; and data-collection methods (e.g., patient report versus physician report of outcomes). Prostatectomies performed at hospitals where fewer procedures are performed have been found to have higher complication rates.[206,207] Erectile dysfunction may be avoided by performing a "nerve-sparing" prostatectomy, but this is not advisable in men with high pretreatment PSA levels or high Gleason scores (i.e., 8–10). Rates of erectile dysfunction after prostatectomy range from 10% to 75% depending on presurgical erectile function, age, history of radiation, and integrity of cavernosal nerves.[208–213] Urinary incontinence can range from posturination dribbling to urge or stress incontinence of varying severity.[208–213] The patient and treating physician must decide what the trade-offs are between the anticipated benefits and potential adverse effects of all potential treatment options for prostate cancer.

External-beam radiation therapy is recommended in the case of clinically localized prostate cancer. It typically involves a 6-week course of daily treatments. Long-term results are dependent on tumor stage. Initial PSA levels above than 15 ng/mL have been shown to be a predictor for treatment failure with conventional radiation therapy nerves.[214] Radiation achieves survival rates equivalent to radical prostatectomy at 5 years after diagnosis, but long-term recurrence and PSA failures are higher than with surgery. A retrospective review of almost 1000 men treated with radiation with intent to treat revealed their disease-specific survival by stage to be 79% for T1, 66% for T2, 55% for T3, and 22% for T4.[215] No studies directly compare radical prostatectomy and external-beam radiation therapy. Higher-grade prostate tumors (Gleason score ≥ 7) tend to respond less well to radiation, and surgery may be recommended.

Radiation offers an alternative treatment modality to men who refuse, or are not appropriate medical candidates for, surgery. To date, there have been no RCTs comparing external-beam radiation therapy to watchful waiting. Improved disease-free survival rates and fewer complications may be achievable with three-dimensional conformal radiotherapy. A systematic review found limited evidence that, in men with early-stage, low- or intermediate-risk prostate cancer, conformal radiotherapy with dose escalation reduced acute and late treatment-related morbidity compared with conventional radiotherapy. However, two RCTs found no significant survival or tumor control (at 3–5 years) between conventional and conformal radiation therapy.[216,217] External-beam radiation therapy may be combined with brachytherapy or hormonal ablation.

Complications of definitive external-beam radiation include cancer recurrence, erectile dysfunction, urinary incontinence, urinary retention, proctitis, cystitis, and enteritis.[196,211,212,218–220] Erectile function may be preserved in many cases

in the short-term but may diminish over time. A previous history of a TURP increases the risk of bladder outlet obstruction and stricture in men treated with radiation.[221–223] Men treated with radiation were less likely to report incontinence or erectile dysfunction but more likely to report bowel dysfunction, especially frequency and symptoms of proctitis.[224,225]

Interstitial brachytherapy involves ultrasound-guided implantation of radioactive seeds (iodine-125 and palladium-103) into the prostate. This therapy is an alternative to radical prostatectomy for organ-confined, early-stage prostate cancer, with PSA levels less than 10 ng/mL and Gleason score less than 6.[226] The advantage of brachytherapy over external-beam radiation therapy is that it potentially allows selective radiation to the prostate compared with surrounding structures. Patients who do not meet these criteria but opt for brachytherapy should be treated with supplemental external-beam radiation therapy or neoadjuvant hormonal therapy. There are no RCTs to date addressing the use of brachytherapy in men with prostate cancer. Relative contraindications to brachytherapy include prior TURP (associated with irritative symptoms and increased risk of urinary incontinence in up to 50% of men) and evidence for bladder outlet obstruction (greater risk of postbrachytherapy urinary retention). Complications include irritative urinary symptoms, urinary retention, urinary incontinence, proctitis, and erectile dysfunction.

Cryosurgery involves freezing the prostate by placing multiple cryoprobes into the prostate under ultrasonographic guidance. Cryotherapy can be used as primary therapy, salvage therapy after external-beam radiation therapy or brachytherapy, or palliative control of local disease.[227–229] Retreatment may be necessary. Short-term studies have shown decreases in PSA levels to undetectable levels and negative postcryotherapy biopsy results. Long-term outcomes of this treatment modality are not known. Three-year biochemical recurrence is approximately 50% after cryotherapy. There are no RCTs addressing the use of cryotherapy in men with prostate cancer. Reported complications include irritative urinary symptoms, injury to the urethra and bladder outlet, rectal injury, rectourethral fistula, urinary incontinence, and erectile dysfunction.

Watchful waiting has also been advocated for the management of clinically localized prostate cancer. Asymptomatic men, those of advanced age, or those with significant comorbid illness may be candidates for observation with no active initial treatment.[230,231] A population-based study of men with clinically localized, well- or moderately well-differentiated tumors who underwent no treatment revealed excellent survival rates, irrespective of age, with a mean observation time of 12.5 years (15 years' follow-up); these men were diagnosed before the era of PSA screening.[202] The men were followed up for a mean of 21 years after initial diagnosis and the risk of progression of disease and disease-specific death persisted throughout the follow-up period. By the end of follow-up, 16% of men in the study had prostate cancer and 91% had died of other non–prostate cancer morbidities.[232] Similar results were found in a smaller, population-based study at 4–9 years of follow-up.[233] Long-term follow-up of almost 800 men in the United States with clinically localized prostate cancer diagnosed before PSA screening managed with either observation only or androgen ablation showed a cancer-specific mortality of 6 per 1000 person-years in men with Gleason scores 2–4 after 20-year follow-up. The cancer-specific mortality for men by Gleason score was as follows: Gleason score 5, 12 deaths per 1000 person-years; Gleason score 6, 30 deaths; Gleason score 7, 65 deaths; and Gleason scores 8–10, 121 deaths.[234]

Normal and cancerous growth of the prostate is under the influence of testosterone and dihydrotestosterone. Hormonal therapy is generally reserved for men who are not appropriate surgical candidates or for those with metastatic disease. There are no RCTs addressing the use of early androgen deprivation (i.e., hormonal therapy) in asymptomatic men with clinically localized prostate cancer or in asymptomatic men with an elevated PSA level after early treatment. In men with localized or locally advanced prostate cancer, three ongoing RCTs report that, at 2–3 years, bicalutamide plus standard care reduces radiologic progression and bone metastases compared with standard care alone. Overall survival was similar in both groups.[154]

Initiation of androgen suppression at the diagnosis of prostate cancer may be beneficial. RCTs found no significant difference in overall survival rates between no androgen suppression and therapy with the adrenal androgen bicalutamide in men with localized or locally advanced prostate cancer at 2–10 years.[154,235] Bicalutamide was found to reduce objective disease progression compared with no hormonal suppression. There is evidence from RCTs that hormonal therapy is beneficial for locally advanced prostate cancer. Immediate androgen suppression after radical prostatectomy and pelvic lymphadenectomy in men with node-positive disease was found to

reduce 7-year mortality compared with radical prostatectomy and deferred androgen suppression.[236] A systematic review found early androgen suppression increased survival at 10 years compared with deferred treatment in men with locally advanced prostate cancer but not at 5 years.[237] There is limited evidence that immediate androgen suppression reduced complications compared with deferred androgen suppression.

Androgen suppression started at diagnosis in addition to external-beam radiation therapy was found to improve long-term survival compared with radiation alone or radiation with deferred androgen suppression, according to RCT data. There is RCT evidence that immediate androgen suppression reduces complications compared with deferred androgen suppression.[238,239]

Primary hormonal blockade can be accomplished with bilateral orchiectomy or the use of luteinizing hormone–releasing hormone agonists (leuprolide) alone, or in combination with antiandrogens that affect adrenal androgens (e.g., flutamide, nilutamide, bicalutamide). Adverse effects of hormonal therapy include psychological effects, hot flashes, gynecomastia, breast tenderness, decreased libido, impotence, osteoporosis, bone fractures, and a flare of symptoms and signs caused by a surge of luteinizing hormone and follicle-stimulating hormone that can occur with initial administration of hormonal therapy.[240–245] This flare phenomenon can be prevented by pretreatment with antiandrogens before beginning luteinizing hormone–releasing hormone therapy.

Neoadjuvant hormonal therapy before radical prostatectomy is not established at the present time.[246,247] It may induce a lower stage, decrease positive surgical margins, and effect a reduction in long-term cancer recurrence rates. The use of neoadjuvant hormonal therapy with radiation has been shown to reduce local progression and increase metastasis-free survival. There may also be a possible survival advantage. Neoadjuvant hormonal therapy is currently considered standard therapy when external-beam radiation therapy is administered for locally advanced prostate cancer. Androgen deprivation is currently the primary treatment for men with metastatic prostate cancer, with a 90% response rate but no improvement in survival.[235–239]

Hormonal therapy (e.g., immediate versus delayed hormonal therapy, bilateral orchiectomy, medical castration with a variety of available medications) and chemotherapy are not usually recommended for the primary treatment of organ-confined prostate cancer. Discussion of these and the other treatment modalities described above in terms of locally advanced or metastatic prostate cancer is beyond the scope of this chapter.

A systematic review of the contemporary literature was carried out to compare radical prostatectomy, radiation therapy with intent to treat, and observation as the three primary management strategies for clinically localized prostate cancer.[248] Due to poor reporting and selection factors in all 144 studies reviewed, a valid comparison of efficacy was not possible. Comparison of therapeutic modalities has been difficult in meta-analyses as well.[249] A retrospective review of patients with clinically localized prostate cancer treated expectantly revealed a 10-year disease-specific survival rate of 94% for tumors staged at Gleason scores 2–4 and 75% for tumors at Gleason scores 5–7.[250] Data from the Surveillance, Epidemiology, and End Results database reveals similar survival rates of 95% and 77%, respectively.[251] An RCT comparing prostatectomy with observation alone in men with clinically localized, early-stage disease diagnosed before the PSA era showed a statistically significant difference in overall 10-year survival.[200] After 10 years, there was a 5% (73% versus 68%) difference in survival in men younger than 65 years at the time of prostatectomy.[252] The results of an ongoing randomized trial in the United States comparing radical prostatectomy to observation using mortality as its primary end point are awaited (Prostate Intervention Versus Observation Trial).[253]

Alternative Therapy

Information about ongoing clinical trials is available from the National Cancer Institute's Web site (http://cancer.gov/clinicaltrials). An integrative medicine approach to the treatment of prostate cancer is described in Chapter 22, Integrative Medicine.

Prognosis

Survival of men with prostate cancer is related to the extent of the tumor. The prognosis for men with nonmetastatic prostate cancer is dependent on Gleason score, extent of tumor volume, time to PSA progression, PSA doubling time, and presence of prostatic capsular penetration or margin positivity at the time of prostatectomy. In addition, patient age and medical comorbidity must be taken into account when discussing management and prognosis.[158,159,230,254,255]

Biochemical recurrence or failure is defined by a rise in PSA after primary therapy. After radical prostatectomy, PSA should be undetectable and any rise in PSA to detectable levels is considered a biochemical recurrence of tumor.[163,256,257] After radiation via any modality with curative intent, persistently elevated or rising PSA may be a prognostic factor for clinical disease recurrence. In the past, many definitions of PSA failure have been used clinically and in published reports of men treated with radiation, and therefore, criteria have been developed.[258] A rise in PSA to a level greater than 0.5 ng/mL after a PSA nadir indicates biochemical recurrence. This should be confirmed by three consecutive PSA measurements, each performed 6 months apart. Data from a retrospective cohort with clinically localized prostate cancer treated with either radical prostatectomy or radiation therapy suggested that short post-treatment doubling time of less than 3 months was a useful surrogate end point for disease-specific and all-cause mortality.[259] This may or may not apply to men treated with androgen ablation and will need to be confirmed in a prospective fashion.

The reduction of PSA to undetectable levels after treatment with androgen ablation provides information on the duration of progression-free status, but decreases in PSA less than 80% may not be as useful.[158] PSA expression is under hormonal control; therefore, androgen deprivation can decrease serum PSA independent of tumor response. Clinicians and patients cannot rely solely on PSA values as response to hormonal therapy, but must also follow clinical data.[260]

In patients with late-stage disease, flow cytometry has shown that nuclear DNA ploidy is an independent prognostic indicator for progression- and disease-specific survival[261] but requires further study and standardization.[262-265] Patients with nonmetastatic prostate cancer should be monitored on a semiannual or annual basis, with digital rectal examinations to assess the prostatic fossa (after radical prostatectomy) or prostate (after radiation) for induration and nodularity and serum PSA testing to monitor that factor. Depending on the results of digital rectal examination and PSA, abdominal and pelvic CT and bone scans should be performed on what is usually a less frequent basis.

The chance that men with moderately differentiated, palpable, clinically localized prostate cancer will remain free of symptomatic progression is 70% at 5 years and 40% at 10 years.[266] Men with poorly differentiated cancer have a higher risk of symptomatic disease progression.[202] A large retrospective review[257] of men with clinically localized prostate cancer treated surgically found that the median time to development of clinical metastasis after biochemical recurrence was 8 years. After development of metastatic disease, the median time to death was an additional 5 years.[257] Morbidity from local or regional disease progression includes hematuria, bladder obstruction, and lower extremity edema. In general, median survival in excess of 5 years can be anticipated in men with clinically localized prostate cancer. The median survival in men with locally advanced disease approaches 5 years. Metastatic prostate cancer is not curable with current treatment modalities, and medical survival is usually 1–3 years. In all patients, however, indolent clinical courses spanning many years have been seen.

Conclusions

This review of several of the major clinical topics within the field of urology should provide a framework for the clinical and evidence-based general urologic care of our adult male patients. The information presented herein will continue to evolve as more evidence becomes available. We hope that this chapter will serve as a reference for general practitioners who are presented with both specific and broad urologic problems in their daily clinical practices.

References

1. Grossfeld GD, Litwin MS, Wolf JS, et al: Evaluation of asymptomatic microscopic hematuria in adults: the American Urological Association best practice policy—part I: definition, detection, prevalence, and etiology, *Urology* 57(4):599–603, 2001.
2. Woolhandler S, Pels RJ, Bor DH, et al: Dipstick urinalysis screening of asymptomatic adults for urinary tract disorders: I. hematuria and proteinuria, *JAMA* 262:1214–1219, 1989.
3. Gerber GS, Brendler CB: Evaluation of the urologic patient: history, physical examination, and urinalysis. In Walsh PC, editor: *Campbell's Urology*, ed 8, Philadelphia, 2002, Saunders, pp 83–110.
4. Lotan Y, Roehrborn CG: Sensitivity and specificity of commonly available bladder tumor markers versus cytology: results of a comprehensive literature review and meta-analyses, *Urology* 61(1): 109–118, 2003.
5. Fielding JR, Silverman SG, Samuel S, et al: Unenhanced helical CT of ureteral stones: a replacement for excretory urography in planning treatment, *AJR Am J Roentgenol* 171(4):1051–1053, 1998.
6. Caoili EM, Cohan RH, Korobkin M, et al: Urinary tract abnormalities: initial experience with multidetector row CT urography, *Radiology* 222(3): 353–360, 2002.
7. Mariani AJ, Mariani MC, Macchioni C: The significance of adult hematuria: 1,000 hematuria evaluations including a risk-benefit and cost-effectiveness analysis, *J Urol* 141(2):350–355, 1989.
8. Gasparich JP, Mason JT, Greene HL, et al: Amiodarone-associated epididymitis: drug-related epididymitis in the absence of infection, *J Urol* 133:971–972, 1985.
9. Collins MM, Stafford RS, O'Leary MP, Barry MJ: How common is prostatitis? a national survey of physician visits, *J Urol* 159:1224–1248, 1998.
10. Mittemeyer BT, Lennox KW, Borski AA: Epididymitis: a review of 610 cases, *J Urol* 95:390–392, 1966.
11. Kaver I, Matzkin H, Braf ZF: Epididymo-orchitis: a retrospective study of 121 patients, *J Fam Pract* 30:548–552, 1990.
12. Herbener TE: Ultrasound in the assessment of the acute scrotum, *J Clin Ultrasound* 24:405–421, 1996.
13. Herwig KR, Lapides J, MacLean TA: Response of acute epididymitis to oxyphenbutazone, *J Urol* 106:890–891, 1971.
14. Moore CA, Lockett BL, Lennox KW, et al: Prednisone in the treatment of acute epididymitis: a cooperative study, *J Urol* 106:578–580, 1971.
15. Eickhoff JH, Frimodt-Moller N, Walter S, Frimodt-Moller C: A double-blind, randomized, controlled multicentre study to compare the efficacy of ciprofloxacin with pivampicillin as oral therapy for epididymitis in men over 40 years of age, *BJU Int* 84:827–834, 1999.
16. Krieger JN, Nyberg LJ, Nickel JC: NIH consensus definition and classification of prostatitis, *JAMA* 282:236–237, 1999.
17. Nickel JC, Downey J, Hunter D, Clark J: Prevalence of prostatitis-like symptoms in a population-based study using the National Institutes of Health chronic prostatitis symptom index, *J Urol* 165:842–845, 2001.
18. Mehik A, Hellstrom P, Lukkarinen O, et al: Epidemiology of prostatitis in Finnish men: a population-based cross-sectional study, *Br J Urol Int* 86:443–448, 2000.
19. Schappert SM: National Ambulatory Medical Care Survey, 1991 summary, *Vital Health Stat* 13:1–110, 1994.
20. Weidner W, Schiefer HG, Krauss H, et al: Chronic prostatitis: a thorough search for etiologically involved microorganisms in 1,461 patients, *Infection* 19(Suppl 3):S119–S125, 1991.
21. Schaeffer AJ: Etiology and management of chronic pelvic pain syndrome in men, *Urology* 63:75–84, 2004.
22. Lobel B, Rodriguez A: Chronic prostatitis: what we know, what we do not know, and what we should do! *World J Urol* 21:57–63, 2003.
23. Cheah PY, Liong LM, Yuen KH, et al: Initial, long-term, and durable response to terazosin, placebo, or other therapies for chronic prostatitis/chronic pelvic pain syndrome, *Urology* 64:881–886, 2004.

24. Nickel JC, Forrest JB, Tomera K, et al: Pentosan polysulfate sodium therapy for men with chronic pelvic pain syndrome: a multicenter, randomized placebo controlled study, *J Urol* 173:1252–1255, 2005.

25. Hu TW, Wagner TH, Bentkover JD, et al: Costs of urinary incontinence and overactive bladder in the United States: a comparative study, *Urology* 63(3):461–465, 2004.

26. Thom D: Variation in estimates of urinary incontinence prevalence in the community: effects of differences in definition, population characteristics, and study type, *J Am Geriatr Soc* 46(4):473–480, 1998.

27. US Census Bureau: *National Health and Nutrition Examination Survey Data, 1999–2000*, 2001. Available at: http://www.cdc.gov/nchs/nhanes.htm.

28. Hunter KF, Moore KN, Cody DJ, et al: Conservative management for postprostatectomy urinary incontinence, *Cochrane Database Syst Rev* 2:CD001843, 2005.

29. Van Kampen M, De Weerdt W, Van Poppel H, et al: Effect of pelvic-floor re-education on duration and degree of incontinence after radical prostatectomy: a randomised controlled trial, *Lancet* 355(9198):98–102, 2000.

30. Moore KN, Griffiths D, Houghton A: Urinary incontinence after radical prostatectomy: a randomized controlled trial comparing pelvic muscle exercises with or without electrical stimulation, *Br J Urol Int* 83(1):57–65, 1999.

31. Franke JJ, Gilbert WB, Grier J, et al: Early postprostatectomy pelvic floor biofeedback, *J Urol* 163(1):191–193, 2000.

32. Burgio KL, Stutzman RE, Engel BT: Behavioral training for post-prostatectomy urinary incontinence, *J Urol* 141(2):303–306, 1989.

33. Alhasso A, Glazener CM, Pickard R, et al: Adrenergic drugs for urinary incontinence in adults, *Cochrane Database Syst Rev* 3:CD001842, 2005.

34. Ostaszkiezicz J, Johnston L, Roe B: Habit retraining for the management of urinary incontinence in adults, *Cochrane Database Syst Rev* 2:CD002801, 2004.

35. Ostaszkiezicz J, Johnston L, Roe B: Timed voiding for the management of urinary incontinence in adults, *Cochrane Database Syst Rev* 1:CD002802, 2004.

36. Wallace SA, Roe B, Williams K, et al: Bladder training for urinary incontinence in adults, *Cochrane Database Syst Rev* 1:CD001308, 2004.

37. Mourtzinos A, Smith JJ, Barrett DM: Treatments for male urinary incontinence: a review, *AUA Update Series* 24(15):122–131, 2005.

38. Imamglu MA, Tuygun C, Bakirtas H, et al: The comparison of artificial urinary sphincter implantation and endourethral macroplastique injection for the treatment of postprostatectomy incontinence, *Eur Urol* 47(2):209–213, 2005.

39. Madjar S, Jacoby K, Gilberti C, et al: Bone anchored sling for the treatment of post-prostatectomy incontinence, *J Urol* 165:72, 2001.

40. Lepor H, Lowe FC: Evaluation and nonsurgical measurement of benign prostatic hyperplasia. In Walsh PC, editor: *Campbell's Urology*, ed 8, Philadelphia, 2002, Saunders, pp 1337–1378.

41. Guess HA, Arrighi HM, Metter AJ, et al: Cumulative prevalence of prostatism matches the autopsy prevalence of benign prostatic hyperplasia, *Prostate* 17:241–246, 1990.

42. Girman CJ, Jacobsen SJ, Guess HA, et al: Natural history of prostatism: relationship among symptoms, prostate volume, and peak urinary flow, *J Urol* 153:1510–1515, 1995.

43. Roerborn CG, McConnell JD, Barry MJ, et al: *AUA Guideline on the Management of Benign Prostatic Hyperplasia (BPH)* 2003, American Urological Association Education and Research, Inc. Available at: http://www.auanet.org/guidelines.

44. McConnell JD, Roehrborn CG, Bautista OM, et al: The long-term effect of doxazosin, finasteride, and combination therapy on the clinical progression of benign prostatic hyperplasia, *N Engl J Med* 349:2387–2398, 2003.

45. Andriole GL, Guess HA, Epstein JI, et al: Treatment with finasteride preserves usefulness of prostate-specific antigen in the detection of prostate cancer: results of a randomized, double-blind, placebo-controlled clinical trial. PLESS Study Group. Proscar Long-term Efficacy and Safety Study, *Urology* 52(2):195–201, discussion 201–202, 1998.

46. Madgar I, Weissenberg R, Lunenfeld B, et al: Controlled trial of high spermatic vein ligation for varicocele in infertile men, *Fertil Steril* 63:120–124, 1995.

47. Nieschlag E, Hertle L, Fischedick A, et al: Update on treatment of varicocele: counselling as effective as occlusion of the vena spermatica, *Human Reprod* 13:101–104, 1998.

48. Hopps CV, Goldstein M: Varicocele: unified theory of pathophysiology and treatment, *AUA Update Series* 24:12, 2004.

49. Thonneau P, Marchand S, Tallec A, et al: Incidence and main causes of infertility in a resident population (1,850,000) of three French regions 1988–1989), *Hum Reprod* 6:811–816, 1991.

50. Burrows PJ, Schrepferman CG, Lipshultz LI: Comprehensive office evaluation in the new millennium, *Urol Clin North Am* 29:873–894, 2002.

51. Brugh VM, Matschke HM, Lipshultz LI: Male factor infertility, *Endo Metab Clin North Am* 32:689–707, 2003.

52. Gilbaugh JH, Lipshultz LI: Nonsurgical treatment of male infertility, *Urol Clin North Am* 21:531–548, 1994.

53. Siddiq FM, Sigman M: A new look at the medical management of infertility, *Urol Clin North Am* 29:949–963, 2002.

54. Vandekerckhove P, Lilford R, Vail A, et al: Clomiphene or tamoxifen for idiopathic oligo/asthenospermia, *Cochrane Database Syst Rev* 4:CD000151, 2005.

55. Van Peperstraten AM, Proctor ML, Phillipson G, et al: Techniques for surgical retrieval of sperm prior to ICSI for azoospermia, *Cochrane Database Syst Rev* 4:CD002807, 2005.

56. Carson C, Jordan GH, Gelbard MK: Peyronie's disease: new concepts in etiology, diagnosis, and treatment, *Contemp Urol* 11:44–64, 1999.

57. Lewis RW, Jordan GH: Surgery for erectile dysfunction. In Walsh PC editor: *Campbell's Urology*, ed 8, Philadelphia, 2002, Saunders, pp 1696–1709.

58. Hasche-Klunder R: Treatment of Peyronie's disease with para-aminobenzoacidic potassium (Potaba), *Urology* 17:224–227, 1978.

59. Teloken C, Rhoden EL, Frazziotin TM, et al: Tamoxifen versus placebo in the treatment of Peyronie's disease, *J Urol* 162:2003–2005, 1999.

60. Levine LA: Treatment of Peyronie's disease with intralesional verapamil injection, *J Urol* 158:1395–1399, 1997.

61. Winter CC, Khanna R: Peyronie's disease: results with dermo-jet injection of dexamethasone, *J Urol* 114:898–900, 1975.

62. Judge IS, Wisniewski ZS: Intralesional interferon in the treatment of Peyronie's disease: a pilot study, *Br J Urol* 79:40–42, 1997.

63. Gelbard MK, James K, Riach P, et al: Collagenase versus placebo in the treatment of Peyronie's disease: a double blind study, *J Urol* 149:56–58, 1993.

64. Wilson SK, Cleves MA, Delk JR II: Long-term followup of treatment for Peyronie's disease: modeling the penis over an inflatable penile prosthesis, *J Urol* 165:825–829, 2001.

65. Linet OI, Ogring FG: Efficacy and safety of intracavernosal alprostadil in men with erectile dysfunction, *N Engl J Med* 334:873–877, 1996.

66. El-Bahnasawy MS, Dawood A, Farouk A: Low-flow priapism: risk factors for erectile dysfunction, *Br J Urol Int* 89:285–290, 2002.

67. Montague DK, Jarow J, Broderick GA, et al: American Urological Association guideline on the management of priapism, *J Urol* 170(4 Pt 1):1318–1324, 2003.

68. Gairdner D: The fate of the foreskin: a study of circumcision, *Br Med J* 2:1433–1437, 1949.

69. Monsour MA, Rabinovitch HH, Dean GE: Medical management of phimosis in children: our experience with topical steroids, *J Urol* 162:1162–1164, 1999.

70. Litzky GM: Reduction of paraphimosis with hyaluronidase, *Urology* 50:160, 1997.

71. Cahill D, Rane A: Reduction of paraphimosis with granulated sugar, *Br J Urol Int* 83:362, 1999.

72. Stamatelou KK, Francis ME, Jones CA, et al: Time trends in reported prevalence of kidney stones in the United States: 1976–1994, *Kidney Int* 63:1817–1823, 2003.

73. Pearle MS, Calhoun EA, Curhan GC, et al: Urologic diseases in America project: urolithiasis, *J Urol* 173:848–857, 2005.

74. Pak CY: Should patients with single renal stone occurrence undergo diagnostic evaluation? *J Urol* 127(5):855–858, 1982.

75. Johnson CM, Wilson DM, O'Fallon WM, et al: Renal stone epidemiology: a 25-year study in Rochester, Minnesota, *Kidney Int* 16(5):624–631, 1979.

76. Rous SN: A review of 171 consecutive patients with urinary lithiasis, *J Urol* 126(3):376–379, 1981.

77. Sarmina I, Spirnak JP, Resnick MI: Urinary lithiasis in the black population: an epidemiological study and review of the literature, *J Urol* 138(1):14–17, 1987.

78. Maloney ME, Springhart WP, Ekeruo WO, et al: Ethnic background has minimal impact on the etiology of nephrolithiasis, *J Urol* 173(6):2001–2004, 2005.

79. Siener R, Glatz S, Nicolay C, et al: The role of overweight and obesity in calcium oxalate stone formation, *Obesity Res* 12(1):106–113, 2004.

80. Taylor EN, Stampfer MJ, Curhan GC: Obesity, weight gain, and the risk of kidney stones, *JAMA* 293(4):455–462, 2005.

81. Colistro R, Torreggiani WC, Lyburn ID: Unenhanced helical CT in the investigation of acute flank pain, *Clin Radiol* 57(6):435–441, 2002.

82. Holdgate A, Pollock T: Systematic review of the relative efficacy of non-steroidal anti-inflammatory drugs and opioids in the treatment of acute renal colic, *BMJ* 328(7453):1401–1404, 2004.

83. Autorino R, De Sio M, Damiano R, et al: The use of tamsulosin in the medical treatment of ureteral calculi: where do we stand? *Urol Res* 33(6):460–464, 2005.

84. Dellabella M, Milanese G, Muzzonigro G: Randomized trial of the efficacy of tamsulosin, nifedipine and phloroglucinol in medical expulsive therapy for distal ureteral calculi, *J Urol* 174(1):167–172, 2005.

85. Putman SS, Hamilton BD, Johnson DB: The use of shock wave lithotripsy for renal calculi, *Curr Opin Urol* 14(2):117–121, 2004.

86. Lingeman JE, Siegel YI, Steele B, et al: Management of lower pole nephrolithiasis: a critical analysis, *J Urol* 151:663–667, 1994.

87. Lee DI, Kim I, Clayman RV: Updated approach to staghorn calculi, *AUA Update Series* 24(35):306–311, 2005.

88. Socher SA: Intracorporeal lithotripsy. In Sosa RE, Albala DM, Jenkins AD, Perlmutter AD, editors: *Textbook of Endourology*, Philadelphia, 1997, WB Saunders.

89. Faerber GJ, Bloom DA: Pediatric endourology. In Gillenwater J, Grayhack J, Howards S, Duckett J, editors: *Adult and Pediatric Urology*, ed 3, New York, 1996, Mosby, pp 2739–2758.

90. Strohmaier WL: Course of calcium stone disease without treatment: what can we expect? *Eur Urol* 37(3):339–344, 2000.

91. Stoller ML: Urinary stone disease. In Tanagho EA, McAnich JW, editors: *Smith's General Urology*, ed 14, Norwalk, CT, 1995, Appleton and Lange, pp 27–34.

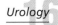
92. Esen T, Marshall VR, Rao N, Ettinger B: Medical management of urolithiasis. In Segura JW, Concort P, Hhourny S, et al, editors: *Stone Disease*, Paris, 2003, Health Publications, pp 133–149.

93. Leyva M: The role of dietary calcium in disease prevention, *J Okla State Med Assoc* 96(6):272–275, 2003.

94. Curhan GC, Willett WC, Rimm EB, et al: A prospective study of dietary calcium and other nutrients and the risk of symptomatic kidney stones, *N Engl J Med* 328(12):833–838, 1993.

95. Curhan GC, Willett WC, Knight EL, et al: Dietary factors and the risk of incident kidney stones in younger women: Nurses' Health Study II, *Arch Intern Med* 164(8):885–891, 2004.

96. Traxer O, Huet B, Poindexter J, et al: Effect of ascorbic acid consumption on urinary stone risk factors, *J Urol* 170(2 Part 1):397–401, 2003.

97. Gettman MT, Ogan K, Brinkley LJ, et al: Effect of cranberry juice consumption on urinary stone risk factors, *J Urol* 174(2):590–594, 2005.

98. Segak R, Lukka H, Klotz LH, et al: Surveillance programs for early stage non-seminomatous testicular cancer: a practice guideline, *Can J Urol* 8(1):1184–1192, 2001.

99. Blandy JP, Hope-Stone HF, Dayan A: *Tumors of the Testicle*, New York, 1970, Grune & Stratton Inc, pp 16–22.

100. Devessa SS, Blot WJ, Stone BJ, et al: Recent cancer trends in the United States, *J Natl Cancer Inst* 87:175–182, 1995.

101. American Cancer Society: Cancer facts and figures 2005. Atlanta, GA, 2005, American Cancer Society. Available at: http://www.cancer.org/docroot/STT/stt_0.asp.

102. Schmoll HJ, Souchon R, Krege S, et al: European consensus on diagnosis and treatment of germ cell cancer: a report of the European Germ Cell Cancer Consensus Group (EGCCCG), *Ann Oncol* 15(9):1377–1399, 2004.

103. Bosl GJ, Motzer RJ: Testicular germ-cell cancer, *N Engl J Med* 337:242–253, 1997.

104. Richie JR: Detection and treatment of testicular cancer, *CA Cancer J Clin* 43:151–175, 1993.

105. Garner MJ, Turner MC, Ghadirian P, et al: Epidemiology of testicular cancer: an overview, *Int J Cancer* 116(3):331–339, 2005.

106. Dieckmann KP, Pichlmeier U: Clinical epidemiology of testicular germ cell tumors, *World J Urol* 22(1):2–14, 2004.

107. Forman D, Oliver RT, Brett AR, et al: Familial testicular cancer: a report of the UK family register, estimation of risk and an HLA class I sub-pair analysis, *Br J Cancer* 65:255–262, 1992.

108. Heimdal K, Olsen H, Tretli S, et al: Familial testicular cancer in Norway and southern Sweden, *Br J Cancer* 73:964–969, 1996.

109. Westergaard T, Olsen J, Frisch M, et al: Cancer risk in father and brothers of testicular cancer patients in Denmark—a population based study, *Int J Cancer* 66:627–631, 1996.

110. Leibovitch I, Baniel J, Foster RS, et al: The clinical implications of procedural deviations during orchoectomy for nonseminomatous testis cancer, *J Urol* 154(3):935–939, 2005.

111. Capeluto CC, Clark PE, Ransil BJ, et al: A review of scrotal violation in testicular cancer: is adjuvant local therapy necessary? *J Urol* 153(3 Pt 2):981–985, 1995.

112. Testis. In Greene FL, Page DL, Fleming ID, et al, editors: American Joint Committee on Cancer: *AJCC Cancer Staging Manual*, ed 6, New York, 2002, Springer, pp 317–322.

113. Woodward PJ, Heidenreich A, Looijenga LHJ, et al: Germ cell tumours. In Eble JN, Sauter G, Epstein JI, et al: *Pathology and Genetics of Tumours of the Urinary System and Male Genital Organs*, Lyon, France, 2004, IARC Press, pp 221–249.

114. International Germ Cell Cancer Collaborative Group: International germ cell consensus classification: a prognostic factor-based staging system for metastatic germ cell cancers, *J Clin Oncol* 15(2):594–603, 1997.

115. Stephenson AJ, Sheinfeld J: The role of retroperitoneal lymph node dissection in the management of testicular cancer, *Urol Oncol* 22(3):225–233, 2004.

116. Oosterhof GO, Verlind J: Testicular tumors (nonseminomatous), *Br J Urol Int* 94(8):1196–1201, 2004.

117. Osterlind A, Berthelson JG, Abildgaard N, et al: Risk of bilateral testicular germ cell cancer in Denmark: 1960–1984, *J Natl Cancer Inst* 83(19):1391–1395, 1991.

118. Colls BM, Harvey VJ, Skelton L, et al: Bilateral germ cell testicular tumors in New Zealand: experience in Auckland and Christchurch 1978–1994, *J Clin Oncol* 14(7):2061–2065, 1996.

119. Gerl A, Clemm C, Schmeller N, et al: Late relapse of germ cell tumors after cisplatin-based chemotherapy, *Ann Oncol* 8(1):41–47, 1997.

120. Drasga RE, Einhorn LH, Williams SD, et al: Fertility after chemotherapy for testicular cancer, *J Clin Oncol* 1(3):179–183, 1983.

121. Nijman JM, Schraffordt Koops H, Kremer J, et al: Gonadal function after surgery and chemotherapy in men with stage II and III nonseminomatous testicular tumors, *J Clin Oncol* 5(4):651–656, 1987.

122. Hansen PV, Trykker H, Helkjoer PE, et al: Testicular function in patients with testicular cancer treated with orchiectomy alone or orchiectomy plus cisplatin-based chemotherapy, *J Natl Cancer Inst* 81(16):1246–1250, 1989.

123. Stephenson WT, Poirier SM, Rubin L, et al: Evaluation of reproductive capacity in germ cell tumor patients following treatment with cisplatin, etoposide, and bleomycin, *J Clin Oncol* 13(9):2278–2280, 1995.

124. Gordon W Jr, Siegmund K, Stanisic TH, et al: A study of reproductive function in patients with seminoma treated with radiotherapy and orchidectomy: (SWOG-8711). Southwest Oncology Group, *Int J Radiat Oncol Biol Phys* 38(1):83–94, 1997.

125. Schoen EJ, Oehrli M, Colby C, et al: The highly protective effect of newborn circumcision against invasive penile cancer, *Pediatrics* 105(3):E36, 2000.

126. Fetus and Newborn Committee, Canadian Paediatric Society: Neonatal circumcision revisited, *CMAJ* 154(6):769–780, 1996.

127. Christakis DA, Harvey E, Zerr DM, et al: A trade-off analysis of routine newborn circumcision, *Pediatrics* 105(1 Pt 3):246–249, 2000.

128. Del Mistro A, Chieco Bianchi L: HPV-related neoplasias in HIV-infected individuals, *Eur J Cancer* 37(10):1227–1235, 2001.

129. Griffiths TR, Mellon JK: Human papillomavirus and urological tumours: I. basic science and role in penile cancer, *Br J Urol Int* 84(5):579–586, 1999.

130. Jackson SM: The treatment of carcinoma of the penis, *Br J Urol* 53:33–35, 1966.

131. Penis. In Greene FL, Page DL, Fleming ID, et al, editors: American Joint Committee on Cancer: *AJCC Cancer Staging Manual*, ed 6, New York, Springer, pp 303–308.

132. Smith JA Jr: Lasers in clinical urologic surgery. In Dixon JA, editor: *Surgical Application of Lasers*, ed 2, Chicago, 1987, Year Book Medical Publishers, pp 218–237.

133. Horenblas S, van Tinteren H, Delemarre JF, et al: Squamous cell carcinoma of the penis: II. treatment of the primary tumor, *J Urol* 147(6):1533–1538, 1992.

134. Rosemberg SK, Fuller TA: Carbon dioxide rapid superpulsed laser treatment of erythroplasia of Queyrat, *Urology* 16(2):181–182, 1980.

135. Mohs FE, Snow SN, Messing EM, et al: Microscopically controlled surgery in the treatment of carcinoma of the penis, *J Urol* 133(6):961–966, 1985.

136. Lynch DF, Pettaway CA: Tumors of the penis. In Walsh PC, Retik AB, Vaughan ED, et al, editors: *Campbell's Urology*, ed 8, Philadelphia, 2002, Saunders, pp 2945–2947.

137. Chao KS, Perez CA: Penis and male urethra. In Perez CA, Brady LW, editors: *Principles and Practice of Radiation Oncology*, ed 3, Philadelphia, 1998, Lippincott-Raven, pp 1717–1732.

138. McLean M, Akl AM, Warde P, et al: The results of primary radiation therapy in the management of squamous cell carcinoma of the penis, *Int J Radiat Oncol Biol Phys* 25(4):623–628, 1993.

139. Harty JI, Catalona WJ: Carcinoma of the penis. In Javadpour N, editor: *Principles and Management of Urologic Cancer*, ed 2, Baltimore, 1983, Williams and Wilkins, pp 581–597.

140. Schellhammer PF, Spaulding JT: Carcinoma of the penis. In Paulson DF, editor: *Genitourinary Surgery*, vol 2, New York, 1984, Churchill Livingston, pp 629–654.

141. Johnson DE, Lo RK: Tumors of the penis, urethra, and scrotum. In deKernion JB, Paulson DF, editors: *Genitourinary Cancer Management*, Philadelphia, 1987, Lea and Febiger, pp 219–258.

142. Theodorescu D, Russo P, Zhang ZF, et al: Outcomes of initial surveillance of invasive squamous cell carcinoma of the penis and negative nodes, *J Urol* 155(5):1626–1631, 1996.

143. Lindegaard JC, Nielsen OS, Lundbeck FA, et al: A retrospective analysis of 82 cases of cancer of the penis, *Br J Urol* 77(6):883–890, 1996.

144. Ornellas AA, Seixas AL, Marota A, et al: Surgical treatment of invasive squamous cell carcinoma of the penis: retrospective analysis of 350 cases, *J Urol* 151(5):1244–1249, 1994.

145. Young MJ, Reda DJ, Waters WB: Penile carcinoma: a twenty-five-year experience, *Urology* 38(6): 529–532, 1991.

145a. Neave F, Neal AJ, Hoskin PJ, Hope-Stone HF: Carcinoma of the penis: a retrospective review of treatment with iridium mould and external beam irradiation, *Clin Oncol (R Coll Radiol)* 5(4):207–210, 1993.

146. Fisher HA, Barada JH, Horton J, et al: Neoadjuvant therapy with cisplatin and 5-fluorouracil for stage III squamous cell carcinoma of the penis (abstract), *J Urol* 143(4 Suppl):A-653, 352A, 1990.

147. Pizzocaro G, Piva L: Adjuvant and neoadjuvant vincristine, bleomycin, and methotrexate for inguinal metastases from squamous cell carcinoma of the penis, *Acta Oncol* 27(6b):823–824, 1988.

148. Gagliano RG, Blumenstein BA, Crawford ED, et al: cis-Diamminedichloroplatinum in the treatment of advanced epidermoid carcinoma of the penis: a Southwest Oncology Group Study, *J Urol* 141(1): 66–67, 1989.

149. Ahmed T, Sklaroff R, Yagoda A: Sequential trials of methotrexate, cisplatin and bleomycin for penile cancer, *J Urol* 132(3):465–468, 1984.

150. Dexeus FH, Logothetis CJ, Sella A, et al: Combination chemotherapy with methotrexate, bleomycin and cisplatin for advanced squamous cell carcinoma of the male genital tract, *J Urol* 146(5): 1284–1287, 1991.

151. Hussein AM, Benedetto P, Sridhar KS: Chemotherapy with cisplatin and 5-fluorouracil for penile and urethral squamous cell carcinomas, *Cancer* 65 (3):433–438, 1990.

152. Lu-Yao G, Albertsen PC, Stanford JL, et al: Natural experiment examining impact of aggressive screening and treatment on prostate cancer mortality in two fixed cohorts from Seattle area and Connecticut, *BMJ* 325:740, 2002.

153. Stanford JL, Stephenson RA, Coyle LM, et al: *Prostate Cancer Trends 1973–1995*, SEER Program. NIH Pub. No. 99–4543. Bethesda, MD, 1999, National Cancer Institute.

154. See WA, Wirth MP, McLeod DG, et al: Bicalutamide as immediate therapy either alone or as adjuvant to standard care of patients with localized or locally advanced prostate cancer: first analysis of the early prostate cancer program, *J Urol* 168: 429–435, 2002.

155. Garnick MB: Prostate cancer: screening, diagnosis, and management, *Ann Intern Med* 118(10):804–818, 1993.

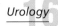
156. Krahn MD, Mahoney JE, Eckman MH, et al: Screening for prostate cancer: a decision analytic view, *JAMA* 272(10):773–780, 1994.

157. Kramer BS, Brown ML, Prorok PC, et al: Prostate cancer screening: what we know and what we need to know, *Ann Intern Med* 119(9):914–923, 1993.

158. Matzkin H, Eber P, Todd B, et al: Prognostic significance of changes in prostate-specific markers after endocrine treatment of stage D2 prostatic cancer, *Cancer* 70(9):2302–2309, 1992.

159. Pisansky TM, Cha SS, Earle JD, et al: Prostate-spécific antigen as a pretherapy prognostic factor in patients treated with radiation therapy for clinically localized prostate cancer, *J Clin Oncol* 11 (11):2158–2166, 1993.

160. Carlton JC, Zagars GK, Oswald MJ: The role of serum prostatic acid phosphatase in the management of adenocarcinoma of the prostate with radiotherapy, *Int J Radiat Oncol Biol Phys* 19 (6):1383–1388, 1990.

161. Stamey TA, Yang N, Hay AR, et al: Prostate-specific antigen as a serum marker for adenocarcinoma of the prostate, *N Engl J Med* 317(15): 909–916, 1987.

162. Stamey TA, Kabalin JN: Prostate specific antigen in the diagnosis and treatment of adenocarcinoma of the prostate: I. untreated patients, *J Urol* 141(5): 1070–1075, 1989.

163. Stamey TA, Kabalin JN, McNeal JE, et al: Prostate specific antigen in the diagnosis and treatment of adenocarcinoma of the prostate: II. radical prostatectomy treated patients, *J Urol* 141(5):1076–1083, 1989.

164. Stamey TA, Kabalin JN, Ferrari M: Prostate specific antigen in the diagnosis and treatment of adenocarcinoma of the prostate: III. radiation treated patients, *J Urol* 141(5):1084–1087, 1989.

165. Andriole GL: Serum prostate-specific antigen: the most useful tumor marker, *J Clin Oncol* 10(8): 1205–1207, 1992.

166. Smith JA Jr, Scardino PT, Resnick MI, et al: Transrectal ultrasound versus digital rectal examination for the staging of carcinoma of the prostate: results of a prospective, multi-institutional trial, *J Urol* 157 (3):902–906, 1997.

167. Ljung BM, Cherrie R, Kaufman JJ: Fine needle aspiration biopsy of the prostate gland: a study of 103 cases with histological followup, *J Urol* 135 (5):955–958, 1986.

168. Algaba F, Epstein JI, Aldape HC, et al: Assessment of prostate carcinoma in core needle biopsy—definition of minimal criteria for the diagnosis of cancer in biopsy material, *Cancer* 78 (2):376–381, 1996.

169. Webb JA, Shanmuganathan K, McLean A: Complications of ultrasound-guided transperineal prostate biopsy: a prospective study, *Br J Urol* 72(5 Pt 2):775–777, 1993.

170. Desmond PM, Clark J, Thompson IM, et al: Morbidity with contemporary prostate biopsy, *J Urol* 150(5 Pt 1):1425–1426, 1993.

171. Hinman F Jr: Screening for prostatic carcinoma, *J Urol* 145(1):126–129, discussion 129–130, 1991.

172. Gerber GS, Chodak GW: Routine screening for cancer of the prostate, *J Natl Cancer Inst* 83(5): 329–335, 1991.

173. Gerber GS, Goldberg R, Chodak GW: Local staging of prostate cancer by tumor volume, prostate-specific antigen, and transrectal ultrasound, *Urology* 40(4):311–316, 1992.

174. Catalona WJ, Smith DS, Ratliff TL, et al: Measurement of prostate-specific antigen in serum as a screening test for prostate cancer, *N Engl J Med* 324(17):1156–1161, 1991.

175. Thompson IM, Pauler DK, Goodman PJ, et al: Prevalence of prostate cancer among men with a prostate-specific antigen level < or =4.0 ng per milliliter, *N Engl J Med* 350(22):2239–2246, 2004.

176. Berg CD, NCI—Early Detection Branch: A 16-year randomized screening study for prostate, lung, colorectal, and ovarian cancer—PLCO Trial, PLCO-1, Clinical trial, Closed. Available at: http://www.nci.nih.gov/search/viewclinicaltrials. aspx?version=healthprofessional&cdrid=78532.

177. Gleason DF, Mellinger GT: Prediction of prognosis for prostatic adenocarcinoma by combined histological grading and clinical staging, *J Urol* 111(1): 58–64, 1974.

178. Gleason DF: Histologic grading and clinical staging of prostatic carcinoma. In Tannenbaum M, editor: *Urologic Pathology: The Prostate*, Philadelphia, 1977, Lea and Febiger, pp 171–197.

179. Oesterling JE, Martin SK, Bergstralh EJ, et al: The use of prostate-specific antigen in staging patients with newly diagnosed prostate cancer, *JAMA* 269 (1):57–60, 1993.

180. Huncharek M, Muscat J: Serum prostate-specific antigen as a predictor of radiographic staging studies in newly diagnosed prostate cancer, *Cancer Invest* 13(1):31–35, 1995.

181. Oesterling JE, Brendler CB, Epstein JI, et al: Correlation of clinical stage, serum prostatic acid phosphatase and preoperative Gleason grade with final pathological stage in 275 patients with clinically localized adenocarcinoma of the prostate, *J Urol* 138(1):92–98, 1987.

182. Daniels GF Jr, McNeal JE, Stamey TA: Predictive value of contralateral biopsies in unilaterally palpable prostate cancer, *J Urol* 147(3 Pt 2):870–874, 1992.

183. Fournier GR Jr, Narayan P: Re-evaluation of the need for pelvic lymphadenectomy in low grade prostate cancer, *Br J Urol* 72(4):484–488, 1993.

184. Hanks GE, Krall JM, Pilepich MV, et al: Comparison of pathologic and clinical evaluation of lymph nodes in prostate cancer: implications of RTOG data for patient management and trial design and stratification, *Int J Radiat Oncol Biol Phys* 23(2): 293–298, 1992.

185. Schiebler ML, Yankaskas BC, Tempany C, et al: MR imaging in adenocarcinoma of the prostate: interobserver variation and efficacy for

determining stage C disease, *AJR Am J Roentgenol* 158(3): 559–562, discussion 563–564 1992.

186. Consensus conference: the management of clinically localized prostate cancer, *JAMA* 258(19): 2727–2730, 1987.

187. Schiebler ML, Schnall MD, Pollack HM, et al: Current role of MR imaging in the staging of adenocarcinoma of the prostate, *Radiology* 189(2): 339–352, 1993.

188. Partin AW, Kattan MW, Subong EN, et al: Combination of prostate-specific antigen, clinical stage, and Gleason score to predict pathological stage of localized prostate cancer: a multi-institutional update, *JAMA* 277(18):1445–1451, 1997.

189. Partin AW, Mangold LA, Lamm DM, et al: Contemporary update of prostate cancer staging nomograms (Partin Tables) for the new millennium, *Urology* 58(6):843–848, 2001.

190. Kattan MW, Eastham JA, Stapleton AM, et al: A preoperative nomogram for disease recurrence following radical prostatectomy for prostate cancer, *J Natl Cancer Inst* 90(10):766–771, 1998.

191. Kattan MW, Wheeler TM, Scardino PT: Postoperative nomogram for disease recurrence after radical prostatectomy for prostate cancer, *J Clin Oncol* 17 (5):1499–1507, 1999.

192. Penson DF, Grossfeld GD, Li YP, et al: How well does the Partin nomogram predict pathological stage after radical prostatectomy in a community based population? results of the cancer of the prostate strategic urological research endeavor, *J Urol* 167(4):1653–1657, discussion 1657–1658, 2002.

193. Greene KL, Meng MV, Elkin EP, et al: Validation of the Kattan preoperative nomogram for prostate cancer recurrence using a community based cohort: results from cancer of the prostate strategic urological research endeavor (capsure), *J Urol* 171 (6 Pt 1):2255–2259, 2004.

194. Jewett HJ: The present status of radical prostatectomy for stages A and B prostatic cancer, *Urol Clin North Am* 2(1):105–124, 1975.

195. Prostate. In Greene FL, Page DL, Fleming ID, et al, editors: American Joint Committee on Cancer: *AJCC Cancer Staging Manual*, ed 6, New York, 2002, Springer, pp 309–316.

196. Catalona WJ, Bigg SW: Nerve-sparing radical prostatectomy: evaluation of results after 250 patients, *J Urol* 143(3):538–543, discussion 544, 1990.

197. Corral DA, Bahnson RR: Survival of men with clinically localized prostate cancer detected in the eighth decade of life, *J Urol* 151(5):1326–1329, 1994.

198. Zincke H, Bergstralh EJ, Blute ML, et al: Radical prostatectomy for clinically localized prostate cancer: long-term results of 1,143 patients from a single institution, *J Clin Oncol* 12(11):2254–2263, 1994.

199. Harris RP, Lohr KN, Beck R, et al: *Screening for Prostate Cancer: Systematic Evidence Review No. 16* Rockville, MD, 2001, Agency for Healthcare Research and Quality.

200. Holmberg L, Bill-Axelson A, Helgesen F, et al: A randomized trial comparing radical prostatectomy with watchful waiting in early prostate cancer, *N Engl J Med* 347:781–789, 2002.

201. Paulson DF, Lin GH, Hinshaw W, et al: Radical surgery versus radiotherapy for adenocarcinoma of the prostate, *J Urol* 128:502–504, 1982.

202. Johansson JE, Holmberg L, Johansson S, et al: Fifteen-year survival in prostate cancer: a prospective, population-based study in Sweden, *JAMA* 277 (6):467–471, 1997.

203. Adolfsson J, Rönström L, Löwhagen T, et al: Deferred treatment of clinically localized low grade prostate cancer: the experience from a prospective series at the Karolinska Hospital, *J Urol* 152(5 Pt 2):1757–1760, 1994.

204. Grossfeld GD, Chang JJ, Broering JM, et al: Impact of positive surgical margins on prostate cancer recurrence and the use of secondary cancer treatment: data from the CaPSURE database, *J Urol* 163(4):1171–1177, quiz 1295, 2000.

205. Shipley WU, Radiation Therapy Oncology Group: Phase III randomized study of radiotherapy with or without bicalutamide in patients with PSA elevation following radical prostatectomy for carcinoma of the prostate, RTOG-9601. Clinical trial, completed, 2003.

206. Lu-Yao GL, McLerran D, Wasson J, et al: An assessment of radical prostatectomy: time trends, geographic variation, and outcomes. The Prostate Patient Outcomes Research Team, *JAMA* 269 (20):2633–2636, 1993.

207. Yao SL, Lu-Yao G: Population-based study of relationships between hospital volume of prostatectomies, patient outcomes, and length of hospital stay, *J Natl Cancer Inst* 91(22):1950–1956, 1999.

208. Catalona WJ, Basler JW: Return of erections and urinary continence following nerve sparing radical retropubic prostatectomy, *J Urol* 150(3):905–907, 1993.

209. Jønler M, Messing EM, Rhodes PR, et al: Sequelae of radical prostatectomy, *Br J Urol* 74(3):352–358, 1994.

210. Geary ES, Dendinger TE, Freiha FS, et al: Nerve sparing radical prostatectomy: a different view, *J Urol* 154(1):145–149, 1995.

211. Lim AJ, Brandon AH, Fiedler J, et al: Quality of life: radical prostatectomy versus radiation therapy for prostate cancer, *J Urol* 154(4):1420–1425, 1995.

212. Litwin MS, Hays RD, Fink A, et al: Quality-of-life outcomes in men treated for localized prostate cancer, *JAMA* 273(2):129–135, 1995.

213. Potosky AL, Davis WW, Hoffman RM, et al: Five-year outcomes after prostatectomy or radiotherapy for prostate cancer: the prostate cancer outcomes study, *J Natl Cancer Inst* 96(18): 1358–1367, 2004.

214. Zietman AL, Coen JJ, Shipley WU, et al: Radical radiation therapy in the management of prostatic adenocarcinoma: the initial prostate specific

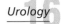

antigen value as a predictor of treatment outcome, *J Urol* 151(3):640–645, 1994.

215. Duncan W, Warde P, Catton CN, et al: Carcinoma of the prostate: results of radical radiotherapy (1970–1985), *Int J Radiat Oncol Biol Phys* 26(2): 203–210, 1993.

216. Hanks GE, Hanlon AL, Schultheiss TE, et al: Dose escalation with 3D conformal treatment: five year outcomes, treatment optimization, and future directions, *Int J Radiat Oncol Biol Phys* 41(3): 501–510, 1998.

217. Dearnaley DP, Khoo VS, Norman AR, et al: Comparison of radiation side-effects of conformal and conventional radiotherapy in prostate cancer: a randomised trial, *Lancet* 353(9149):267–272, 1999.

218. Schellhammer PF, Jordan GH, el-Mahdi AM: Pelvic complications after interstitial and external beam irradiation of urologic and gynecologic malignancy, *World J Surg* 10(2):259–268, 1986.

219. Hanlon AL, Schultheiss TE, Hunt MA, et al: Chronic rectal bleeding after high-dose conformal treatment of prostate cancer warrants modification of existing morbidity scales, *Int J Radiat Oncol Biol Phys* 38(1):59–63, 1997.

220. Hamilton AS, Stanford JL, Gilliland FD, et al: Health outcomes after external-beam radiation therapy for clinically localized prostate cancer: results from the Prostate Cancer Outcomes Study, *J Clin Oncol* 19(9):2517–2526, 2001.

221. Greskovich FJ, Zagars GK, Sherman NE, et al: Complications following external beam radiation therapy for prostate cancer: an analysis of patients treated with and without staging pelvic lymphadenectomy, *J Urol* 146(3):798–802, 1991.

222. Seymore CH, el-Mahdi AM, Schellhammer PF: The effect of prior transurethral resection of the prostate on post radiation urethral strictures and bladder neck contractures, *Int J Radiat Oncol Biol Phys* 12(9):1597–1600, 1986.

223. Green N, Treible D, Wallack H, et al: Prostate cancer—the impact of irradiation on urinary outlet obstruction, *Br J Urol* 70(3):310–313, 1992.

224. Fowler FJ Jr, Barry MJ, Lu-Yao G, et al: Outcomes of external-beam radiation therapy for prostate cancer: a study of Medicare beneficiaries in three surveillance, epidemiology, and end results areas, *J Clin Oncol* 14(8):2258–2265, 1996.

225. Potosky AL, Legler J, Albertsen PC, et al: Health outcomes after prostatectomy or radiotherapy for prostate cancer: results from the Prostate Cancer Outcomes Study, *J Natl Cancer Inst* 92(19): 1582–1592, 2000.

226. Ragde H, Blasko JC, Grimm PD, et al: Interstitial iodine-125 radiation without adjuvant therapy in the treatment of clinically localized prostate carcinoma, *Cancer* 80(3):442–453, 1997.

227. Robinson JW, Saliken JC, Donnelly BJ, et al: Quality-of-life outcomes for men treated with cryosurgery for localized prostate carcinoma, *Cancer* 86(9):1793–1801, 1999.

228. Donnelly BJ, Saliken JC, Ernst DS, et al: Prospective trial of cryosurgical ablation of the prostate: five-year results, *Urology* 60 (4):645–649, 2002.

229. Aus G, Pileblad E, Hugosson J: Cryosurgical ablation of the prostate: 5-year follow-up of a prospective study, *Eur Urol* 42(2):133–138, 2002.

230. Chodak GW, Thisted RA, Gerber GS, et al: Results of conservative management of clinically localized prostate cancer, *N Engl J Med* 330(4):242–248, 1994.

231. Whitmore WF Jr: Expectant management of clinically localized prostatic cancer, *Semin Oncol* 21 (5):560–568, 1994.

232. Johansson JE, Andrén O, Andersson SO, et al: Natural history of early, localized prostate cancer, *JAMA* 291(22):2713–2719, 2004.

233. Waaler G, Stenwig AE: Prognosis of localised prostatic cancer managed by "watch and wait" policy, *Br J Urol* 72(2):214–219, 1993.

234. Albertsen PC, Hanley JA, Fine J: 20-year outcomes following conservative management of clinically localized prostate cancer, *JAMA* 293(17): 2095–2101, 2005.

235. Byar DP, Corle DK: Hormone treatment for prostate cancer: results of the Veterans' Administration cooperative urologic research group studies, *NCI Monograph* 7:165–170, 1988.

236. Nair B, Wilt T, MacDonald R, et al: Early versus deferred androgen suppression in the treatment of advanced prostatic cancer. In *The Cochrane Library* Issue 2:CD003506, 2002.

237. The Medical Research Council Prostate Cancer Working Party Investigators Group: Immediate versus deferred treatment for advanced prostatic cancer: initial results of the Medical Research Council trial, *Br J Urol* 79:235–246, 1997.

238. Fellows GJ, Clark PB, Beynon LL, et al: Treatment of advanced localised prostatic cancer by orchiectomy, radiotherapy, or combined treatment, *Br J Urol* 70:304–309, 1992.

239. Pilepich M, Winter M, Madhu J, et al: Phase III Radiation Therapy Oncology Group (RTOG) trial 86–10 of androgen deprivation adjuvant to definitive radiotherapy in locally advanced carcinoma of the prostate, *Int J Radiat Oncol Biol Phys* 50:1243–1252, 2001.

240. Daniel HW: Osteoporosis after orchiectomy for prostate cancer, *J Urol* 157(2):439–444, 1997.

241. Soloway MS, Schellhammer PF, Smith JA, et al: Bicalutamide in the treatment of advanced prostatic carcinoma: a phase II multicenter trial, *Urology* 47(1A Suppl): 33–37, 48–53 1996.

242. Fowler FJ Jr, McNaughton Collins M, Walker Corkery E, et al: The impact of androgen deprivation on quality of life after radical prostatectomy for prostate carcinoma, *Cancer* 95(2):287–295, 2002.

243. Kirschenbaum A: Management of hormonal treatment effects, *Cancer* 75(7 Suppl):1983–1986, 1995.

244. Shahinian VB, Kuo YF, Freeman JL, et al: Risk of fracture after androgen deprivation for prostate cancer, *N Engl J Med* 352(2):154–164, 2005.

245. Smith MR, McGovern FJ, Zietman AL, et al: Pamidronate to prevent bone loss during androgen-deprivation therapy for prostate cancer, *N Engl J Med* 345(13):948–955, 2001.

246. Witjes WP, Schulman CC, Debruyne FM: Preliminary results of a prospective randomized study comparing radical prostatectomy versus radical prostatectomy associated with neoadjuvant hormonal combination therapy in T2–3 N0 M0 prostatic carcinoma. The European Study Group on Neoadjuvant Treatment of Prostate Cancer, *Urology* 49(3A Suppl):65–69, 1997.

247. Fair WR, Cookson MS, Stroumbakis N, et al: The indications, rationale, and results of neoadjuvant androgen deprivation in the treatment of prostatic cancer: Memorial Sloan-Kettering Cancer Center results, *Urology* 49(3A Suppl):46–55, 1997.

248. Wasson JH, Cushman CC, Bruskewitz RC, et al: A structured literature review of treatment for localized prostate cancer: Prostate Disease Patient Outcome Research Team, *Arch Fam Med* 2(5):487–493, 1993.

249. Austenfeld MS, Thompson IMJr, Middleton, RG: Meta-analysis of the literature: guideline development for prostate cancer treatment: American Urological Association Prostate Cancer Guideline Panel, *J Urol* 152(5 Pt 2):1866–1869, 1994.

250. Barry MJ, Albertsen PC, Bagshaw MA, et al: Outcomes for men with clinically nonmetastatic prostate carcinoma managed with radical prostatectomy, external beam radiotherapy, or expectant management: a retrospective analysis, *Cancer* 91 (12):2302–2314, 2001.

251. Lu-Yao GL, Yao SL: Population-based study of long-term survival in patients with clinically localised prostate cancer, *Lancet* 349(9056):906–910, 1997.

252. Bill-Axelson A, Holmberg L, Ruutu M, et al: Radical prostatectomy versus watchful waiting in early prostate cancer, *N Engl J Med* 352(19):1977–1984, 2005.

253. Wilt TJ, Veterans Affairs Cooperative Studies Program Coordinating Center–Perry Point: NCI high priority clinical trail-phase III randomized study of prostatectomy versus expectant management with palliative therapy in patients with clinically localized prostate cancer (PIVOT), VA-CSP-407, clinical trial, closed. *[PDQ Clinical Trial].*

254. Gittes RF: Carcinoma of the prostate, *N Engl J Med* 324(4):236–245, 1991.

255. Paulson DF, Moul JW, Walther PJ: Radical prostatectomy for clinical stage T1–2N0M0 prostatic adenocarcinoma: long-term results, *J Urol* 144(5): 1180–1184, 1990.

256. Frazier HA, Robertson JE, Humphrey PA, et al: Is prostate specific antigen of clinical importance in evaluating outcome after radical prostatectomy, *J Urol* 149(3):516–518, 1993.

257. Pound CR, Partin AW, Eisenberger MA, et al: Natural history of progression after PSA elevation following radical prostatectomy, *JAMA* 281(17): 1591–1597, 1999.

258. Consensus statement: guidelines for PSA following radiation therapy, American Society for Therapeutic Radiology and Oncology Consensus Panel, *Int J Radiat Oncol Biol Phys* 37 (5):1035–1041, 1997.

259. D'Amico AV, Moul JW, Carroll PR, et al: Surrogate end point for prostate cancer-specific mortality after radical prostatectomy or radiation therapy, *J Natl Cancer Inst* 95(18):1376–1383, 2003.

260. Ruckle HC, Klee GG, Oesterling JE: Prostate-specific antigen: concepts for staging prostate cancer and monitoring response to therapy, *Mayo Clin Proc* 69(1):69–79, 1994.

261. Pisansky TM, Kahn MJ, Rasp GM, et al: A multiple prognostic index predictive of disease outcome after irradiation for clinically localized prostate carcinoma, *Cancer* 79(2):337–344, 1997.

262. Nativ O, Winkler HZ, Raz Y, et al: Stage C prostatic adenocarcinoma: flow cytometric nuclear DNA ploidy analysis, *Mayo Clin Proc* 64(8): 911–919, 1989.

263. Lee SE, Currin SM, Paulson DF, et al: Flow cytometric determination of ploidy in prostatic adenocarcinoma: a comparison with seminal vesicle involvement and histopathological grading as a predictor of clinical recurrence, *J Urol* 140(4): 769–774, 1988.

264. Ritchie AW, Dorey F, Layfield LJ, et al: Relationship of DNA content to conventional prognostic factors in clinically localised carcinoma of the prostate, *Br J Urol* 62(3):245–260, 1988.

265. Lieber MM: Pathological stage C (pT3) prostate cancer treated by radical prostatectomy: clinical implications of DNA ploidy analysis, *Semin Urol* 8(4):219–224, 1990.

266. Adolfsson J, Steineck G, Hedund P: Deferred treatment of clinically localized low-grade prostate cancer: actual 10-year and projected 15-year follow-up of the Karolinska series, *Urology* 50: 722–726, 1997

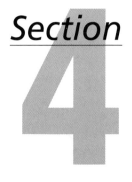

Section

Special Concerns of the Adolescent and Adult Male

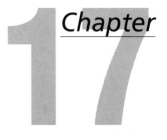

Chapter 17

Lifestyle Risks

Joel J. Heidelbaugh, MD, and Gary Yen, MD

Key Points

- Men are more likely than women to engage in various risk-taking behaviors (strength of recommendation: B).
- Smoking is the leading cause of preventable death worldwide. It has been attributed to lung cancer, coronary heart disease, chronic obstructive pulmonary disease, neonatal death resulting from smoking during pregnancy, and accidental death caused by cigarette-induced residential fires (strength of recommendation: A).
- Epidemiologic data supports that men are more likely to be binge or heavy drinkers, to drive while intoxicated, and to engage in violent altercations (strength of recommendation: B).
- Males have been found to be more likely to use marijuana, cocaine, hallucinogens, and inhalants than females; however, the rates of nonmedical use of prescription-type psychotherapeutics have been shown to be similar for both males and females (strength of recommendation: B).
- There are currently insufficient data to link tattooing and body piercing to an increased risk of hepatitis C infection (strength of recommendation: C).
- In several small epidemiologic studies, the incidence of tattoos was fairly equally distributed among men and women, yet body piercings were statistically more common in females versus males (strength of recommendation: C).
- To date, there is no consistent regulation regarding the practice of tattooing or body piercing. Future efforts to standardize these practices may limit the transmission of viral hepatitis and HIV infection (strength of recommendation: C).

Introduction

The stereotyping of males from a young age has included such typical characteristics as self-reliance, participation in dangerous activities, dominance, independence, being physically active, and aggression, among others.[1] Although this list is probably an oversimplification of the subtleties in gender difference, some of the behaviors listed above play a significant role in the challenge of caring for male patients. The image of the male as a risk taker is reflected in numerous health-related statistics. For example, in the 10–24-year-old age group, 71% of deaths can be attributed to motor vehicle crashes and other unintentional injuries, homicide, and suicide.[2] Delve deeper into the statistics and one discovers a greater male prevalence in risky behavior in the majority of categories. Fewer males wear motorcycle or bicycle helmets and seat belts and are more likely to drive while intoxicated.[2] In addition, males are more likely to carry a firearm or any form of weapon and are more likely to engage in a physically violent altercation.[2] Overall, accidents ranked as the fifth leading cause of death in the United States in 2003, with males exhibiting a disproportionate ratio of 2.2 over females.[3]

Despite these statistics, risk taking is not exclusive to the male youth demographic, and it is not solely limited to the possession of an object or substance that could lead to bodily harm to one's self or others. Risk taking is also reflected in how males choose to obtain their healthcare as well as the lifestyle choices they make as adolescents and adults. Fewer males report identifying a regular doctor and are less likely to have medical checkups and office visits for both acute and chronic medical care.[4] Males have an average life expectancy that is 5.3 years shorter than females, and of the 15 leading causes of death in the United States, males are noted to have a higher rate of death in 12 of the categories (see Chapter 4, Men and the Problem of Help Seeking).[3] The largest gender differences in mortality rates are noted in the categories of suicide, homicide, unintentional injuries, chronic liver disease and cirrhosis, Parkinson's disease, cancer, and heart disease.[3] It should come as no surprise, then, that males have a higher prevalence of obesity, smoking, and alcohol consumption.[5]

This chapter highlights statistics on four major high-risk behaviors prominent in men: smoking, alcohol consumption, illicit drug abuse, and tattoos and body piercing. Ensuring the proper and adequate health of male patients lies in the realization that, statistically, they are at a disadvantage in a number of health outcomes routinely measured. The challenge for clinicians is to empower men to invest in the importance of their health, to start addressing risk-taking behavior early in life, and to take advantage of every healthcare encounter as a counseling opportunity.

Smoking

Cigarette smoking exacts a high toll on the health of the general public and is the leading cause of preventable death globally; nearly 5 million people die each year from tobacco-related illnesses, with disproportionately higher mortality occurring in developing countries.[6] Most smokers begin the habit during their adolescent years, with the highest prevalence found in the Americas when data is examined globally (Table 17-1). Smoking has been linked to an estimated 440,000 premature deaths annually in the United States[7]; smoking-related deaths have been attributed to lung cancer, coronary heart disease, chronic obstructive pulmonary disease, neonatal death resulting from maternal smoking during pregnancy, and accidental death caused by cigarette-induced residential fires. Baseline adverse health conditions coexist with current smokers, including bronchitis in nearly one half and emphysema in nearly one quarter of all smokers, with estimates that up to 8.6 million people in the

United States have some form of a smoking-related health condition.[8]

As of 2004, the prevalence of cigarette smoking was 23.4% in adult men in the United States, down from a peak of 57% in 1955, and it was 18.5% in adult women, down from a peak of 34% in 1965 (Figure 17-1).[9] The Monitoring the Future Survey,[10] an epidemiologic study performed through the University of Michigan, found that smoking prevalence has decreased in all groups since 1996 for 8th and 10th graders and since 1997 for 12th graders (Figure 17-2). The percentage decrease since the peak year was found to be 56% in 8th graders, 47% in 10th graders, and 32% in 12th graders. These declines have coincided with an increase in tobacco-control efforts including higher excise taxes on cigarettes and other tobacco products as well as counter-advertising directed at adolescents in some states.[11] Among US high school students in 2005, the percentage of smokers was more evenly distributed between males (23.0%) and females (22.9%).[12] In 2004, the percentages of high school and middle school students who reported current use of cigarettes were 21.7% and 8.4%, respectively.[13] For comparison, the Healthy People 2010 target prevalence is 12% or below for adults who smoke and 16% or below for adolescents, specifically high school students, who smoke.[14]

Trends in smoking have been shown to differ by gender, education, and socioeconomic class. According to the American Cancer Society's Facts and Figures 2006,[15] the gender gap in smoking prevalence has narrowed over time, yet the socioeconomic gradient in tobacco smoking has widened. Smoking prevalence among adults with less than a high school degree declined from 41.7% in 1965 to 29.7% in 2004, whereas that among college graduates dropped from 35% to 10% during the same time period.[16] Trends in smoking among various ethnicities are reflected in Table 17-2. Over the past decade, surveys have consistently shown that the average daily number of cigarettes smoked by US adults is approximately 12.[17]

Annual cigar sales in the United States increased dramatically from 1993 to 1998 by almost 50% to 4.5 billion. As a result, one epidemiologic study in Massachusetts adults[18] that used a phone survey determined that cigar-smoking rates increased significantly among men aged 18–34 years between 1993 (5.8%) and 1997–1998 (18.2%) but began to decline by 2000 (13.5%). In this study, young male cigar smokers were increasingly those who had never smoked

Table 17-1. Global Youth Tobacco Survey Measure of Tobacco Use Prevalence Among Students Aged 13–15 Years, by Sex and World Health Organization Region, 1999–2005

WHO region	CURRENT USE OF ANY TOBACCO PRODUCTS						CURRENT CIGARETTE SMOKING						CURRENT OTHER TOBACCO[†] USE					
	GIRLS		BOYS		TOTAL		GIRLS		BOYS		TOTAL		GIRLS		BOYS		TOTAL	
	%	(95% CI)	%	(95% CI)	%	(95% CI)	%	(95% CI)	%	(95% CI)	%	(95% CI)	%	(95% CI)	%	(95% CI)	%	(95% CI)
Africa	13.9	(±3.1)	19.7	(±3.9)	16.8	(±2.7)	5.8	(±2.3)	13.0	(±3.6)	9.2	(±2.2)	9.9	(±2.6)	10.9	(±2.9)	10.5	(±2.2)
Americas	20.4	(±2.8)	24.0	(±3.0)	22.2	(±2.4)	17.5	(±2.6)	17.4	(±2.7)	17.5	(±2.3)	7.8	(±1.6)	14.8	(±2.2)	11.3	(±1.5)
Eastern Mediterranean	11.3	(±3.3)	18.8	(±3.6)	15.3	(±2.6)	3.2	(±2.1)	6.7	(±2.3)	5.0	(±1.7)	9.9	(±2.6)	15.6	(±3.2)	12.9	(±2.3)
Europe	17.0	(±3.2)	22.3	(±4.3)	19.8	(±3.2)	15.7	(±3.1)	19.9	(±3.8)	17.9	(±2.7)	6.0	(±2.0)	10.0	(±3.3)	8.1	(±2.3)
South-East Asia	7.1	(±2.4)	18.4	(±4.1)	12.9	(±2.7)	1.9	(±0.9)	5.8	(±1.7)	4.3	(±1.2)	8.4	(±1.6)	16.4	(±1.4)	13.3	(±1.0)
Western Pacific	7.8	(±2.0)	15.0	(±2.8)	11.4	(±1.9)	3.3	(±1.2)	8.9	(±2.8)	6.5	(±1.6)	5.4	(±1.5)	7.7	(±1.6)	6.4	(±1.2)
Total	14.3	(±2.8)	20.1	(±3.4)	17.3	(±2.5)	6.7	(±1.7)	10.5	(±2.4)	8.9	(±1.7)	7.8	(±1.8)	13.8	(±2.1)	11.2	(±1.5)

* Regional aggregations were calculated as means weighted by the population of the sampling frame. In many cases, the sampling frame was the country, but in areas where samples were drawn to be representative of a subnational population, estimates were weighted by the population of the city, state, or administrative region.

† Confidence Interval.

‡ Including chewing tobacco, snuff, dip, cigars, cigarillos, little cigars, pipes, and shisha (flavored tobacco smoked in hookah pipes).

Adapted from: Use of cigarettes and other tobacco products among students aged 13–15 years–worldwide 1999–2005, *MMWR* 55(20):553–556, 2006.

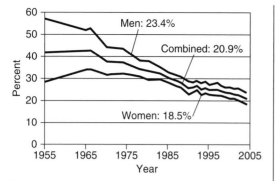

Figure 17-1. Trends in prevalence of current cigarette smoking among adults (i.e., persons 18 years and older), United States, 1955–2004. (Adapted from: Centers for Disease Control and Prevention: Cigarette smoking among adults—United States, 2004, *MMWR* 54:1121–1124, 2005.)

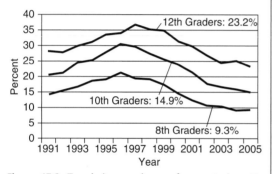

Figure 17-2. Trends in prevalence of current cigarette smoking among students, United States, 1990–2005. (Source: Monitoring the Future Survey, University of Michigan. Adapted from: Johnston L, O'Malley P, Bachman J, et al: *Monitoring the Future National Results on Adolescent Drug Use: Overview of Key Findings, 2004,* Bethesda, MD, 2005, National Institutes of Health, National Institute on Drug Abuse.)

Table 17-2. Prevalence of Cigarette Smoking by Ethnicity, United States, 2004

Ethnicity	High School Students	Adults (Age > 18 Years)
American Indian/ Alaska Natives	24.5%	33.4%
Non-Hispanic Whites	24.8%	22.2%
African Americans	11.0%	20.2%
Hispanics/Latinos	20.5%	15.0%
Asians	11.3%	11.3%

Adapted from: Centers for Disease Control and Prevention: Cigarette smoking among adults—United States, 2004, *MMWR* 54:1121–1214, 2005; and Centers for Disease Control and Prevention: National Youth Tobacco Survey, 2004. Available at: http://www.cdc.gov/tobacco/NYTS/nyts2004.htm. Accessed September 6, 2006.

cigarettes; former cigarette smokers were not found to be smoking cigars in greater numbers. Cigar smokers were three times as likely as those who did not smoke cigars to believe that cigars are a safer alternative to cigarettes.

Smokeless tobacco is also an issue that should not be overlooked in males, since they form the vast majority of users. Smokeless tobacco has been implicated in nicotine addiction, oral/pharyngeal cancers, precancerous lesions such as leukoplakia, and noncancerous damage to the gingiva and periodontium.[19,20] In 2005, the Youth Risk Behavior Surveillance System noted that 13.6% of high school males used smokeless tobacco compared with just 2.2% of females.[21] In adults, smokeless tobacco use in males was noted to be 4.5% versus 0.3% in females.[22]

The US Centers for Disease Control and Prevention (CDC) performed a surveillance of tobacco use behavior analyzing trends between 1900 and 1994. During this period, men were noted to have a greater prevalence for smoking cessation of 51.6% compared with 44.7% for women in 1991.[23] Men were also noted to have a greater prevalence for heavy smoking (defined as 25 cigarettes or more per day) of 26.4% versus 16.1% for women in 1991.[24] This latter fact was corroborated in a survey performed in the United Kingdom commissioned for the group No Smoking Day. This study also discovered that when men contemplate reducing nicotine intake, they tend to cut back on the number of cigarettes and rely on willpower rather than medical intervention to succeed. With regard to reasons for quitting, men cited more practical reasons such as improving fitness or workplace restrictions compared with more emotional reasons cited by women (e.g., family and pregnancy). The authors point out that these subtle differences should lead to different approaches when counseling men or women about smoking cessation.[25]

Physicians should discuss smoking cessation with their patients at every opportunity, discussing both health risks and benefits of quitting. Pharmacologic options include bupropion (Wellbutrin) and the newer varenicline (Chantix); nicotine patches, inhalers, and gums; acupuncture and hypnotherapy have also been used with modest success in men and women of all ages. Most insurance plans have gravitated toward increased coverage for smoking cessation aids, though Medicaid plans differ from state to state regarding coverage (Figure 17-3).

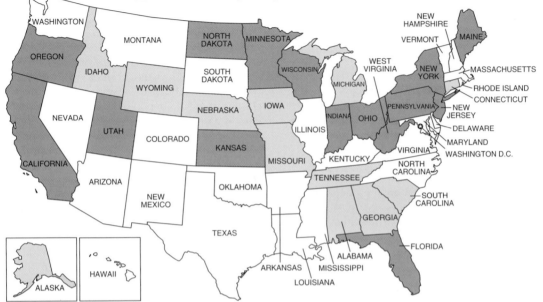

Provides full coverage for smoking cessation to all beneficiaries through Medicaid, including some form of counseling and some drug therapy.

Provides partial smoking cessation coverage through Medicaid to all or some beneficiaries, including some form of counseling or some form of drug therapy.

Provides no coverage through Medicaid to beneficiaries for smoking cessation therapies.

Figure 17-3. Insurance coverage of smoking cessation treatments for US Medicaid recipients, 2003. (Adapted from: Kaiser Family Foundation: *State Health Facts,* Provided by National Government Relations Department, American Cancer Society, 2005.)

Alcohol Abuse and Dependence

The most recent available economic data from 1998 details an estimated $185 billion in expenditures due to alcohol abuse and dependence, representing a significant public health concern in the United States.[26] The Substance Abuse and Mental Health Services Administration combined data from three consecutive National Surveys on Drug Use and Health (NSDUH) between 2002 and 2004[27] and found that 18.2 million people met the diagnostic criteria for alcohol abuse or dependence within the past year. These criteria have been best defined by the *Diagnostic and Statistical Manual of Mental Disorders*[28] (DSM-IV) as follows.

Alcohol abuse is a maladaptive pattern of alcohol use causing clinically significant distress or impairment of social or occupational functioning. Maladaptive use includes high daily consumption, regular heavy weekend drinking, and binge drinking (e.g., staying drunk for days, often after periods of abstinence). A diagnosis of abuse cannot be made when a person is dependent on alcohol. One or more of the following must have occurred as a result of recurrent alcohol use within a 12-month period:

- Failure to fulfill major role obligations (e.g., repeated absences or poor work performance related to alcohol use; suspensions or expulsion from school; neglect of the children or household)
- Exposure to physical hazards (e.g., driving an automobile or operating a machine when impaired by alcohol use)
- Legal problems (e.g., arrests for alcohol-related disorderly conduct)
- Social or interpersonal problems (e.g., arguments with partner about consequences of intoxication, physical fights while drunk)

Alcohol dependence is a maladaptive pattern of alcohol use leading to clinically significant impairment or distress, as manifested by three or more of the following occurring at any time during the same 12-month period:

- Tolerance, defined by one of the following:
  - The need for markedly increased amounts of alcohol to achieve intoxication
  - The desired effect with continued use of the same amount of alcohol with markedly diminished effect
- Withdrawal, as manifested by two or more of the following occurring after cessation or reduction after heavy prolonged alcohol use:

- Autonomic hyperactivity such as sweating or heart rate in excess of 100 beats/min
- Hand tremor
- Nausea or vomiting
- Transient visual, auditory, or tactile hallucinations
- Psychomotor agitation
- Anxiety
- Grand mal seizures
- Alcohol consumed in larger amounts over a longer period than was intended
- A persistent desire or unsuccessful efforts made to cut down or control alcohol use
- A great deal of time spent in activities necessary to obtain alcohol, consume it, or recover from its effects
- Important social, occupational, or recreational activities given up or reduced because of alcohol use
- Alcohol use is continued despite a physical or psychological problem that is likely to have been caused or exacerbated by the substance

The National Institute on Alcohol Abuse and Alcoholism sponsors the National Epidemiologic Survey on Alcohol and Related Conditions, the primary source for information and epidemiologic data on the US population for alcohol and drug use, abuse, and dependence. Data reflecting the 12-month prevalence and population estimates for alcohol abuse, as defined by the DSM-IV, are charted in Table 17-3.

The 2005 NSDUH[29] found that 51.8% of Americans aged 12 years or older reported being current drinkers of alcohol, translating to an estimated 126 million people, which is higher than the 2004 estimate of 121 million people (50.3%). More than one fifth (22.7%) of persons aged 12 years or older admitted to participating in binge drinking (defined as five or more drinks on the same occasion [e.g., at the same time or within a couple of hours of each other] on at least 1 day in the past 30 days, including heavy use) at least once in the 30 days before the survey. This equates to approximately 55 million people, comparable with the estimates reported yearly since 2002. In 2005, heavy drinking (defined as five or more drinks on the same occasion on each of 5 or more days in the past 30 days) was reported by 6.6% of the population aged 12 years or older, or 16 million people, similar to the rates of heavy drinking in 2002 (6.7%), 2003 (6.8%), and 2004 (6.9%), respectively. In 2005, roughly 10.8 million persons aged 12–20 years (28.2% of this age group) reported drinking alcohol in the past month.

Nearly 7.2 million (18.8%) were admittedly binge drinkers, and 2.3 million (6.0%) were admittedly heavy drinkers. These figures have remained essentially the same since the 2002 survey. Notably, more males than females aged 12–20 years reported current alcohol use (28.9 versus 27.5%), binge drinking (21.3 versus 16.1%), and heavy drinking (7.6 versus 4.3%) in 2005 (Figure 17-4).

In the same NSDUH report from 2005, among persons aged 12 years or older, white persons were more likely than persons of other racial/ethnic groups to report current use of alcohol (56.5%) (Figure 17-5).[29] Alcohol use rates were 47.3% for persons reporting two or more races, 42.6% for Hispanics, 42.4% for American Indians or Alaska Natives, 40.8% for African Americans, 38.1% for Asians, and 37.3% for Native Hawaiians or Other Pacific Islanders. The rate of binge alcohol use was lowest among Asians at 12.7% and was 20.3% for African Americans, 20.8% for persons reporting two or more races, 23.4% for whites, 23.7% for Hispanics, 25.7% for Native Hawaiians or Other Pacific Islanders, and 32.8% for American Indians or Alaska Natives. Among adolescents aged 12–17 years in 2005, Asians had the lowest reported rate of alcohol use within the month before the survey. Only 7.0% of Asian youths were reportedly current drinkers, whereas 11.6% of African Americans, 12.2% of American Indians or Alaska Natives, 13.0% of those reporting two or more races, 16.7% of Hispanics, and 18.5% of white youths were current drinkers.

Underage drinking continues to be a serious issue in the United States, especially on college campuses. Among adults aged 18 years or older, the NSDUH found that the rate of alcohol use in the past month increased with increasing levels of education.[29] Among adults with less than a high school education, 36.7% were current drinkers in 2005, significantly lower than the 69.4% of college graduates who were current drinkers. However, among adults aged 26 years or older, binge and heavy alcohol use rates were lower among college graduates (18.9 and 4.9%, respectively) than among adults who had not completed college (21.9 and 6.0%, respectively). Young adults aged 18 to 22 years enrolled full-time in college were more likely than their peers not enrolled full-time (e.g., part-time college students and persons not currently enrolled in college) to use alcohol in the past month, binge drink, and drink heavily.[29,30] Past-month alcohol use was reported by 64.4% of full-time college students compared with 53.2% of persons aged 18–22 years who were not enrolled full-time.

Table 17-3. Twelve-Month Prevalence and Population Estimates of DSM-IV–Defined Alcohol Abuse by Age, Sex, and Race/Ethnicity: United States, 2001–2002*

Sociodemographic Characteristic (Age in Years)	MALE %	MALE S.E.	MALE Population Estimate[†]	FEMALE %	FEMALE S.E.	FEMALE Population Estimate	TOTAL %	TOTAL S.E.	TOTAL Population Estimate
Total									
Total	6.93	0.28	6906	2.55	0.16	2762	4.65	0.18	9668
18–29	9.35	0.61	2110	4.57	0.39	1041	6.95	0.39	3151
30–44	8.69	0.49	2742	3.31	0.28	1080	5.95	0.31	3822
45–64	5.50	0.43	1719	1.70	0.20	566	3.54	0.25	2286
65+	2.36	0.32	335	0.38	0.11	75	1.21	0.15	410
White									
Total	7.45	0.33	5276	2.92	0.19	2236	5.10	0.21	7511
18–29	10.19	0.81	1405	5.56	0.54	777	7.86	0.50	2182
30–44	10.10	0.63	2166	4.13	0.38	902	7.09	0.40	3068
45–64	5.97	0.51	1425	2.02	0.26	499	3.96	0.30	1925
65+	2.38	0.35	279	0.36	0.10	58	1.21	0.16	336
Black									
Total	5.71	0.58	574	1.41	0.19	182	3.29	0.30	756
18–29	6.92	1.28	166	2.10	0.45	68	4.28	0.67	254
30–44	7.04	0.95	238	1.51	0.30	65	3.95	0.46	302
45–64	4.48	0.74	132	1.25	0.37	47	2.66	0.40	178
65+	1.79	0.59	19	0.12	0.12	2	0.78	0.25	21
Native American[‡]									
Total	7.47	1.65	157	4.18	1.25	97	5.75	1.02	253
18–29	15.25	5.68	56	6.68	3.34	33	10.35	3.11	89
30–44	7.67	3.00	54	6.52	3.01	49	7.07	2.13	102
45–64	4.85	2.12	39	0.00	0.00	0	2.57	1.14	39
65+	3.59	2.49	8	4.12	4.00	15	3.91	2.63	24
Asian[§]									
Total	3.20	0.79	140	1.13	0.41	53	2.13	0.46	193
18–29	4.77	1.81	63	3.89	1.38	47	4.35	1.25	110
30–44	4.22	1.54	64	0.23	0.22	4	2.18	0.79	68
45–64	1.13	0.78	13	0.20	0.20	3	0.61	0.32	16
65+	0.00	0.00	0	0.00	0.00	0	0.00	0.00	0
Hispanic/Latino									
Total	6.21	0.50	759	1.65	0.23	195	3.97	0.30	953
18–29	9.08	1.07	400	3.04	0.63	116	6.28	0.63	516
30–44	4.88	0.59	219	1.46	0.33	61	3.23	0.37	281
45–64	4.35	0.84	111	0.63	0.36	17	2.43	0.39	128
65+	3.69	1.62	29	0.00	0.00	0	1.56	0.66	29

DSM-IV, Diagnostic and Statistical Manual of Mental Disorders; S.E., standard error of mean.

* Data are from the NIAAA 2001–2002 National Epidemiologic Survey on Alcohol and Related Conditions (NESARC).

† Population counts are in thousands.

‡ Includes American Indians and Alaska Natives.

§ Includes Native Hawaiians and other Pacific Islanders.

Adapted from: Grant BF, Dawson DA, Stinson FS, et al: The 12-month prevalence and trends in DSM-IV alcohol abuse and dependence: United States, 1991–1992 and 2001–2002, *Drug Alcohol Depend* 74(3):223–234, 2004.

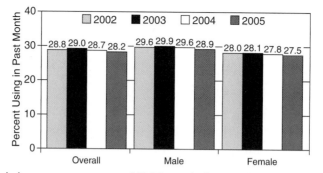

Figure 17-4. Current alcohol use among persons aged 12–20 years in the United States, by gender, 2002–2005. (Adapted from: National Survey on Drug Use and Health: Alcohol use. Available at: http://www.oas.samhsa.gov/NSDUH/2k5NSDUH/2k5results.htm#Ch3. Accessed September 8, 2006.)

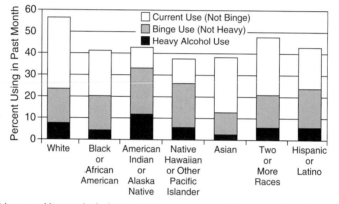

Figure 17-5. Current, binge, and heavy alcohol use among persons aged 12 years or older in the United States, by race/ethnicity, 2005. (Adapted from: National Survey on Drug Use and Health. Alcohol use. Available at: http://www.oas.samhsa.gov/NSDUH/2k5NSDUH/2k5results.htm#Ch3. Accessed September 8, 2006.)

Binge and heavy use rates for college students were 44.8 and 19.5%, respectively, compared with 38.3 and 13.0%, respectively, for 18–22-year-olds not enrolled full-time in college. The pattern of rates of current alcohol use, binge alcohol use, and heavy alcohol use among full-time college students being higher than the rates for others aged 18–22 years has remained consistent since 2002 (Figure 17-6).

In 2005, an estimated 13.0% of persons aged 12 years or older drove a motor vehicle under the influence of alcohol at least once in the past year.[29] This percentage has dropped since 2002, when it was 14.2%. The 2005 estimate corresponds to 31.7 million persons. Driving under the influence of alcohol was associated with age in 2005. An estimated 8.3% of 16- or 17-year-olds, 19.8% of 18–20-year-olds, and 27.9% of 21–25-year-olds reported driving under the influence of alcohol in the past year (Figure 17-7). Beyond the age of 25 years, these rates showed a general decline with increasing age. Among persons aged 12 years or older, males were nearly twice as

likely as females to drive under the influence of alcohol in the past year (17.1 versus 9.2%).

With sequelae from alcohol abuse leading to such long-term health consequences as liver disease, heart disease, neurologic dysfunction, and

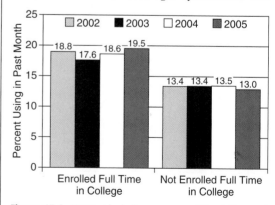

Figure 17-6. Heavy alcohol use among US adults aged 18–22 years, by college enrollment, 2002–2005. (Adapted from: National Survey on Drug Use and Health: Alcohol use. Available at: http://www.oas.samhsa.gov/NSDUH/2k5NSDUH/2k5results.htm#Ch3. Accessed September 8, 2006.)

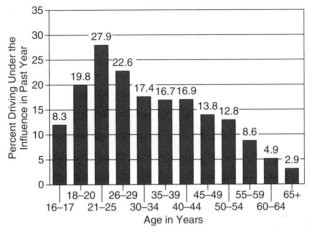

Figure 17-7. Driving under the influence of alcohol in the past year among persons aged 16 years or older in the United States, by age, 2005. (Adapted from: National Survey on Drug Use and Health: Alcohol use. Available at: http://www.oas.samhsa.gov/NSDUH/2k5NSDUH/2k5results.htm#Ch3. Accessed September 8, 2006.)

alterations to the immune system,[31] it is important to consider how likely men may be willing to seek treatment for their alcohol abuse or dependence. In analyzing trends between 1979 and 1990, men (particularly young and middle-aged men younger than 50 years) tended to seek help for an alcohol abuse problem more frequently than women, with the greatest proportion seeking help from either Alcoholics Anonymous or some other form of alcohol rehabilitation program.[32] The percentage of men who sought help increased in the 3 years that were surveyed (1979, 1984, and 1990), yet in 1990, 8.3% of the total number of men surveyed sought help versus 2.0% of the total number of women.[33]

In the Marin Institute's recent Alcohol Policy,[34] numerous statistics were highlighted based on epidemiologic data regarding the relationship between alcohol and violent assaults. Alcohol use was found to be frequently associated with violence between intimate partners; two thirds of victims of intimate partner violence reported that alcohol was involved in the incident. In one study of interpersonal violence,[35] men had been drinking in an estimated 45% of cases and women had been drinking in 20% of cases. Women whose partners abused alcohol were 3.6 times more likely than other women to be assaulted by their partners.[35] In 2002, more than 70,000 students between the ages of 18 and 24 years were victims of alcohol-related sexual assault in the United States.[34] In those violent incidents recorded by the police in which alcohol was a factor, approximately 9% of the offenders and nearly 14% of the victims were younger than 21 years.[34]

An estimated 480,000 children are mistreated each year by a caretaker with alcohol problems.[34]

Illicit Drug Use

The NSDUH, along with the National Institute on Drug Abuse, obtains information annually on the use of nine different categories of illicit drugs of abuse: marijuana, cocaine, heroin, hallucinogens, and inhalants, and the nonmedical use of prescription-type pain relievers, tranquilizers, stimulants, and sedatives.[36,37] It is widely held as the most accurate source for population data regarding the use of these substances. Methamphetamine use is thought to be significantly underestimated in this report due to its inclusion with survey questions regarding the use of prescription medications, namely prescription stimulants.

According to the NSDUH in 2005, an estimated 19.7 million Americans aged 12 years or older (8.1% of the US population) were current illicit drug users, behavior defined as use during the month before the survey interview.[36] The overall rate of current illicit drug use among persons aged 12 years or older in 2005 (8.1%) was similar to the rates in 2004 (7.9%), 2003 (8.2%), and 2002 (8.3%). Marijuana was the most commonly used illicit drug (14.6 million past-month users) and, in 2005, it was used by 74.2% of current illicit drug users. Among current illicit drug users, 54.5% admitted to using only marijuana, 19.6% used marijuana and another illicit drug, and the remaining 25.8% used only an illicit drug other than marijuana in the past month.

As in prior years, the NSDUH[36] reported that in 2005 males were more likely to report current illicit drug use than females (10.2 and 6.1%, respectively). Males were more than twice as likely to use marijuana as females (8.2 versus 4.0%); however, the rates of nonmedical use of prescription-type psychotherapeutics were similar for both males (2.8%) and females (2.5%). Among youths aged 12–17 years, the rate of current illicit drug use was similar for boys (10.1%) and girls (9.7%). Although boys aged 12–17 years had a higher rate of marijuana use than girls (7.5 versus 6.2%), the rate for nonmedical use of prescription-type psychotherapeutics was similar for boys and girls (3.1 and 3.6%, respectively). Past-month marijuana use declined from 2002 to 2005 for both male youths (9.1% to 7.5%) and female youths (7.2% to 6.2%) (Figure 17-8).

The incidence of drug abuse is often correlated with age. Among youths aged 12–17 years, the rates of current illicit drug use were found to increase with age: 3.8% at ages 12 or 13 years, 8.9% at ages 14 or 15 years, and 17.0% at ages 16 or 17 years (Figure 17-9).[36] The highest rate of illicit drug use was found to be among persons aged 18–20 years (22.3%). The rate was 18.7% among those aged 21–25 years and declined with increasing age among older adults.

According to the NSDUH in 2005, there were 2.4 million persons who were current cocaine users, greater than the reported rate of 2.0 million users in 2004.[36] However, the change in the rate of current use of cocaine between 2005 and 2004 (1.0 and 0.8%, respectively) was not statistically

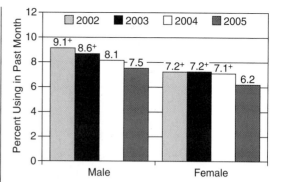

Figure 17-8. Past-month marijuana use among youths aged 12–17 years, by gender, 2002–2005. [+]Difference between estimate and the 2005 estimate is statistically significant at the .05 level. (Adapted from: National Survey on Drug Use and Health: Illicit drug use. Available at: http://www.oas.samhsa.gov/NSDUH/2k5NSDUH/2k5results.htm#Ch2. Accessed September 10, 2006.)

significant. Similarly, the number of reported current crack cocaine users increased from 467,000 in 2004 to 682,000 in 2005, yet the change in the rate of current use of crack between 2004 and 2005 (0.2 and 0.3%, respectively) was not statistically significant.

The NSDUH reports that hallucinogens were used in the past month by 1.1 million US persons (0.4%) in 2005, including 502,000 (0.2%) who had used methylenedioxymethamphetamine (MDMA; Ecstasy); these estimates are similar to the corresponding estimates for 2004.[36] There was no significant change in the number of current heroin users in 2005, (136,000) nor in the

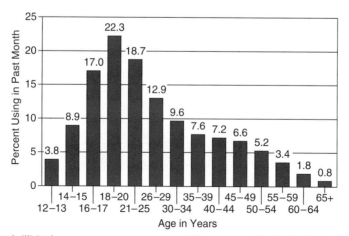

Figure 17-9. Past-month illicit drug use among persons aged 12 years or older in the United States, by age, 2005. (Adapted from: National Survey on Drug Use and Health: Illicit drug use. Available at: http://www.oas.samhsa.gov/NSDUH/2k5NSDUH/2k5results.htm#Ch2. Accessed September 10, 2006.)

rate of heroin use (0.1%), compared with estimates from 2004. There were 9.0 million people aged 12 years or older (3.7%) who were current users of illicit drugs other than marijuana in 2005 (Figure 17-10). Approximately 6.4 million (2.6%) admitted to using psychotherapeutic drugs for nonmedical purposes. Of these, 4.7 million used pain relievers, 1.8 million used tranquilizers, 1.1 million used stimulants (including 512,000 using methamphetamine), and 272,000 used sedatives. Each of these estimates is statistically similar to the respective corresponding estimates for 2004.

Studies have been performed in an attempt to explain the gender discrepancy in illicit drug use between males and females. One study postulated that the difference relates to males being more frequently exposed to the opportunity to use drugs rather than being more likely to progress from exposure to actual use.[38] In four types of illicit drugs studied (i.e., marijuana, cocaine, hallucinogens, and heroin), males were more likely than females to have the opportunity to use the substance in all cases. However, once exposure and the opportunity to use the illicit drug occurred, females were found to be just as likely as males to progress to actual use.[38] This study led the authors to propose that a way to screen for drug abuse risk, namely, to inquire about opportunities to obtain and use illicit drugs, specifically measured the frequency of exposure to illicit substances.[38,39] Studies have also been performed to address any gender differences in abuse of prescription medications. One investigation[40] concluded that, after controlling for multiple variables such as illicit drug use, alcohol use, and other factors, female gender resulted in a 43% increased odds of abusing a prescription psychotherapeutic medication compared with men, particularly narcotics and tranquilizers.

McCabe and colleagues[41] at the University of Michigan and Harvard University analyzed data from the 2001 Harvard School of Public Health College Alcohol Study, which surveyed 10,904 randomly selected students enrolled at 119 colleges across the United States. Overall, 4% of the respondents reported having taken a stimulant medication without a prescription at least once during the previous year. In this study, men were twice as likely as women (5.8% versus 2.9%) to have abused methylphenidate (Ritalin), dextroamphetamine (Dexedrine), and amphetamine/dextroamphetamine (Adderall). Stimulant medication abuse was found to be more prevalent among white persons (4.9%, versus 1.6% for African Americans and 1.3% for Asians); members of fraternities or sororities (8.6%, versus 3.5% for nonmembers); and students earning lower grades (5.2% for those with a grade point average of B or lower versus 3.3% for B+ or higher). Students who abused prescription stimulants reported higher levels of cigarette smoking, heavy consumption of alcohol, risky driving, and abuse of marijuana, MDMA, and cocaine.

Tattoos and Body Piercing

Body modification via tattooing and piercing has been an increasingly popular means of expression in today's society. With constant visual reminders from professional athletes to celebrities on television, the practice is certainly more mainstream and not relegated to any particular ethnic group, gender, or age demographic.

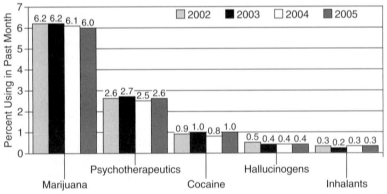

Figure 17-10. Past-month use of selected illicit drugs among persons aged 12 years or older in the United States, 2002–2005. Psychotherapeutics: prescription-type pain relievers, tranquilizers, stimulants, and sedatives; hallucinogens: LSD, PCP, peyote, mescaline, mushrooms, and Ecstasy (MDMA); inhalants, amyl nitrite, cleaning fluids, gasoline, paint, and glue. (Adapted from: National Survey on Drug Use and Health: Illicit drug use. Available at: http://www.oas.samhsa.gov/NSDUH/2k5NSDUH/2k5results.htm#Ch2. Accessed September 10, 2006.)

Mayers and colleagues[42] performed a survey study on undergraduates at an American university that used a questionnaire on a voluntary and anonymous basis to inquire about age, sex, body piercing and tattooing at various body sites, and any complications associated with these practices (women were specifically asked not to include pierced earlobes). There were 454 completed questionnaires from 218 men and 236 women, accounting for approximately 15% of the total undergraduate population, and the average age of the respondents was 21 years. Body piercing was found to be present in 42% of men and 60% of women undergraduates, with 315 piercings in 229 students, with a maximum of five piercings. In men, 31% had pierced ears, with tongue, eyebrow, nipple, genitals, and navel in 2% or fewer for each. Additionally, 7% of students had ear piercings removed, and tongue, nipple, and navel piercings had been removed in 2% or fewer. By comparison, 29% of women had pierced navels, 27% had pierced ears (excluding pierced earlobes), 12% had a pierced tongue, and 5% had a pierced nipple, with genitals, nose, or lip in 2% or fewer. Additionally, 4% of those surveyed had tongue piercings removed, 3% had navel piercings removed, and ear, eyebrow, nose, lip, nipple, and genital piercings had been removed in 2% or fewer.

Complications were reported in 17% of piercings, the most common being bacterial infections, bleeding, and local trauma. No cases of viral infection (e.g., hepatitis B or C, human immunodeficiency virus [HIV] infection) were reported. Tongue piercing was associated with subsequent oral or dental injury in 10% of students surveyed. Tattoos were found to be present in 22% of men and 26% of women undergraduates, with one to three sites per individual. Common sites of tattooing for men were hand or arm, back, and shoulder, and the back was the predominant site for women. No complications from tattooing were reported in this study.

In 2006, a dermatology group from the University of Chicago performed a national survey to obtain demographic data on the practice of tattooing and body piercing in the United States.[43] In reviewing the 500 interviews completed, the researchers were able to obtain a fairly representative sample of a cross-section of the US population. In this study, 24% of the 500 surveyed had at least one tattoo and 14% had at least one body piercing, with 8% having both. Tattoos were fairly equally distributed among men and women, but body piercings were statistically more common in females versus males. The proportion of respondents who either had received or had considered getting a tattoo and/or body piercing increased as the demographic became younger.

A study by Armstrong[44] conducted at a Midwestern military installation surveyed 1835 recruits with a questionnaire regarding tattooing experiences. Almost half (48%) of the soldiers were either serious or very serious about getting a tattoo, with 31% stating that there were "no reasons" to keep them from getting one. More than one third (36%) already had a tattoo, and 22% possess three or more. Many soldiers (64%) entered the military already having tattoos. Limited use (15%) of alcohol or illicit drugs before tattooing was reported. Overall, the study findings included a high incidence of tattooing, a strong determination to obtain tattoos, the possession of tattoos for self-identity reasons, and the supportive role of friends.

Tattoos and body piercing are not without risks. Tattooing has been implicated in the transmission of hepatitis B, hepatitis C, and syphilis[45–47]; the literature is less definitive on HIV transmission via tattooing. However, situations of increased risk can be defined. For example, tattooing in prisons is often performed with nonsterile equipment[48] in a setting where the presence of confirmed acquired immunodeficiency syndrome is 3.5 times higher in comparison with the general population.[49]

Body piercings can lead to a variety of complications depending on the site that is pierced. As piercings become more common, many persons have recommended that healthcare providers become familiar with health risks so that they can better counsel their patients. Some complications are present regardless of site, including allergic reaction (especially to nickel, often used in jewelry), local infection, swelling, pain, hematoma formation, trauma from accidental pulling of the jewelry, and keloid formation.[50] More specifically, oral piercings can lead to trauma to the teeth (e.g., chipping and fracturing) and damage to the gingival tissue.[51] Naval piercing can lead to scarring of the skin. Genital piercings can lead to significant infection, paraphimosis in men, or failure of barrier contraceptives.[50]

In addition to counseling for negative health consequences, healthcare providers should also observe for risk-taking behaviors associated with tattoos or body piercings. One survey of adolescents between the ages of 12–22 years showed that those with a tattoo and/or body piercing were significantly more likely to engage in drug abuse, sexual activity, disordered eating behavior, or suicide.[52] However, the literature is not consistent regarding this association. Another study tried to correlate healthy behavior with fewer tattoos and/or body piercings but could not find such a correlation. More significantly, a larger than expected portion of respondents in this study had not considered health risks, and those who were aware of health risks cited only localized infection as the major adverse effect, without consideration for transfusion-transmitted viral diseases associated with tattoos and body piercing.[53]

With the increasing popularity of tattoos and body piercing, some researchers have advocated the regulation of facilities that perform these services. Currently, there is little uniformity for regulation across the United States. A 1998 survey of all 50 state health departments plus that in the District of Columbia showed that the vast majority of states perform only cursory regulation at a local level. Only 13 states have regulated tattoo facilities, and only four states have regulated body piercing facilities.[48] The task of developing and enforcing a consistent and uniform policy and agreeing on the literature is challenging. For example, in the *Morbidity and Mortality Weekly Report* from 1998[54] focusing on recommendations for prevention and control of the hepatitis C virus, the CDC stated that insufficient data existed in the United States to link tattooing and body piercing to an increased risk of hepatitis C infection. A subsequent investigation argued that this report did not have the benefit of tests developed to detect subclinical hepatitis C infections at that time. With the advent of more sensitive and specific testing methodologies, a strong link between tattoos and hepatitis C seropositivity was noted, leading the authors to advocate more strict regulation and inspection of facilities and practices.[55]

Although it is not possible at the present time to predict how many persons will contract a serious viral infection from body piercing or tattooing, we do know that there may be an increased risk depending on the procedure used and the setting. In the meantime, although some fear that a significant public health problem may be surfacing, persons considering tattooing and/or body piercing should be aware that there may be risks. Both on the federal and state levels, it is believed that this industry should be carefully regulated, single-use sterile devices should be mandatory, and hepatitis B vaccination for those performing the procedures should be standard policy.

Conclusion

Men have been stereotypically cast as risk takers based on epidemiologic data supporting their higher incidence of smoking, alcohol and substance abuse, preventable accidents, and suicide. Additional studies have demonstrated the challenges in getting men to visit a physician in the first place. The next logical steps are to encourage routine health maintenance examinations for men to provide an opportunity for pertinent and comprehensible education to decrease significant morbidity and mortality associated with various lifestyle risks.

References

1. Martin CL: Stereotypes about children with traditional and nontraditional gender roles, *Sex Roles* 33 (11/12):727–752, 1995.
2. Youth Risk Behavior Surveillance—United States, 2005. Available at: http://www.cdc.gov/mmwr/PDF/SS/SS5505.pdf. Accessed September 20, 2006.
3. Hoyert DL, Heron MP, Murphy SL, et al: Deaths. final data for 2003, National Center for Health Statistics, *National Vital Stat Rep* 54(13):1–120, 2006.
4. Kandrack MA, Grant KR, Segall A, et al: Gender differences in health related behaviour: some unanswered questions, *Soc Sci Med* 32(5):579–590, 1991.
5. State-specific prevalence of selected chronic disease–related characteristics—behavioral risk factor surveillance system, 2001. Available at: http://www.cdc.gov/mmwr/PDF/ss/ss5208.pdf. Accessed September 20, 2006.
6. Peto R, Lopez AD: Future worldwide health effects of current smoking patterns. In Koop CD, Pearson C, Schwarz MR, editors: *Critical Issues in Global Health*, New York, 2001, Jossey-Bass.
7. Annual smoking-attributable mortality, years of potential life lost, and economic costs—United States, 1995–1999. *MMWR* April 11, 2002.
8. Cigarette smoking-attributable morbidity—United States, 2000. *MMWR* Sept 5, 2003.
9. Cigarette smoking among adults—United States, 2004. Available at: http://www.cdc.gov/mmwr/PDF/wk/mm5444.pdf. Accessed September 20, 2006.
10. Johnston L, O'Malley P, Bachman J, et al: *Monitoring the Future National Results on Adolescent Drug Use: Overview of Key Findings, 2004*, Bethesda, MD, 2005, National Institutes of Health, National Institute on Drug Abuse.
11. Cokkinides V, Bandi P, Ward E, et al: Progress and opportunities in tobacco control, *CA Cancer J Clin* 56:135–142, 2006.
12. Cigarette use among high school students—United States, 1991–2005. *MMWR* July 7, 2006.
13. Corrected text: tobacco use, access, and exposure to tobacco in media among middle and high school students—United States, 2004. *MMWR* April 1, 2005.

14. Healthy People 2010: Leading health indicators. Available at: http://www.healthypeople.gov/Document/html/uih/uih_bw/uih_4.htm. Accessed September 20, 2006.

15. American Cancer Society: *Cancer Prevention and Early Detection, Facts & Figures, 2006*, Atlanta, GA, 2006, American Cancer Society.

16. US Department of Health and Human Services: *Health, United States, 2005, with Chartbook on Trends in the Health of Americans*, DHHS Publication No. 205–1232, Washington, DC, 2005, Department of Health and Human Services, Centers for Disease Control and Prevention, National Center for Health Statistics.

17. Ministry of Health, New Zealand Health Information Service: Tobacco facts 2005. Available at: http://www.moh.govt.nz/moh.nsf/by+unid/8BDA2162 5203A2DDCC25708B00783A1F?Open. Accessed September 7, 2006.

18. Nyman AL, Taylor TM, Biener L: Trends in cigar smoking and perceptions of health risks among Massachusetts adults, *Tobacco Control* 11(Suppl II):1125–1129, 2002.

19. Advisory Committee of the US Surgeon General: The health consequences of using smokeless tobacco. Available at: http://profiles.nlm.nih.gov/NN/B/B/F/C/_/nnbbfc.pdf. Accessed September 20, 2006.

20. Spangler JG, Salisbury PL III: Smokeless tobacco: epidemiology, health effects and cessation strategies, *Am Fam Phys* 52(5):1421–1430,1433–1434, 1995.

21. Youth Risk Behavior Surveillance—United States, 2005. Available at: http://www.cdc.gov/mmwr/PDF/SS/SS5505.pdf. Accessed September 20, 2006.

22. Nelson DE, Mowery P, Tomar S, et al: Trends in smokeless tobacco use among adults and adolescents in the United States, *Am J Public Health* 96(5): 897–905, 2006.

23. Centers for Disease Control and Prevention: Cigarette smoking among adults—United States, 2004, *MMWR* 54:1121–1124, 2005.

24. Surveillance for selected tobacco-use behaviors—United States, 1900–1994. Available at: http://www.cdc.gov/mmwr/PDF/ss/ss4303.pdf. Accessed September 20, 2006.

25. West R, McEwen A: Sex and smoking: comparisons between male & female smokers, a report for No Smoking Day. Available at: http://www.ash.org.uk/html/health/html/nsdr99.html. Accessed September 20, 2006.

26. Tenth Special Report to Congress on Alcohol and Health from the Secretary of Human Services, June 2000, DHHS Publication No. 00–1583.

27. The NSDUH report: alcohol dependence or abuse: 2002, 2003, and 2004. Available at: http://oas.samhsa.gov/2k6/AlcDepend/AlcDepend.pdf. Accessed September 20, 2006.

28. American Psychiatric Association: *Diagnostic and Statistical Manual of Mental Disorders*, ed 4, Washington, DC, 1994, American Psychiatric Association.

29. National Survey on Drug Use and Health: Alcohol use. Available at: http://www.oas.samhsa.gov/NSDUH/2k5NSDUH/2k5results.htm#Ch3. Accessed September 8, 2006.

30. Centers for Disease Control and Prevention: Quick stats: excessive alcohol use and risks to men's health. Available at: http://www.cdc.gov/alcohol/quick-stats/mens_health.htm. Accessed September 8, 2006.

31. 10th special report to the U.S. Congress on Alcohol and Health. Available at: http://pubs.niaaa.nih.gov/publications/10report/intro.pdf#search=%22special%20report%20to%20the%20us%20congress%20on%20alcohol%22. Accessed September 20, 2006.

32. Weisner C, Greenfield T, Room R: Trends in the treatment of alcohol problems in the US general population, 1979 through 1990, *Am J Public Health* 85(1):55–60, 1995.

33. National Institute on Alcohol Abuse and Alcoholism of the National Institutes of Health. Available at: http://www.niaaa.nih.gov. Accessed September 8, 2006.

34. The Marin Institute: Alcohol policy. Available at: http://www.marininstitute.org/alcohol_policy/violence.htm. Accessed September 9, 2006.

35. Roizen J: Issues in the epidemiology of alcohol and violence. In Martin SE, editor: *Alcohol and Interpersonal Violence: Fostering Multidisciplinary Perspectives*, Bethesda, MD, 1993, National Institute on Alcohol Abuse and Alcoholism, pp 3–36. NIAAA Research Monograph No. 24.

36. National Survey on Drug Use and Health: Illicit drug use. Available at: http://www.oas.samhsa.gov/NSDUH/2k5NSDUH/2k5results.htm#Ch2. Accessed September 10, 2006.

37. National Institute on Drug Abuse. Available at: http://www.nida.nih.gov. Accessed September 8, 2006.

38. Van Etten ML, Neumark YD, Anthony JC: Male-female differences in the earliest stages of drug involvement, *Addiction* 94(9):1413–1419, 1999.

39. Van Etten ML, Anthony JC: Comparative epidemiology of initial drug opportunities and transitions to first use: marijuana, cocaine, hallucinogens and heroin, *Drug Alcohol Dependence* 54(2):117–125, 1999.

40. Simoni-Wastila L, Ritter G, Strickler G: Gender and other factors associated with the nonmedical use of abusable prescription drugs, *Substance Use Misuse* 39(1):1–23, 2004.

41. McCabe SE, Knight JR, Teter CJ, Wechsler H: Nonmedical use of prescription stimulants among US college students: prevalence and correlates from a national survey, *Addiction* 100(1):96–106, 2005.

42. Mayers LB, Judelson DA, Moriarty BW, Rundell KW: Prevalence of body art (body piercing and tattooing) in university undergraduates and incidence of medical complications, *Mayo Clin Proc* 77:29–34, 2002.

43. Laumann AE, Derick AJ: Tattoos and body piercings in the United States: a national data set, *J Am Acad Dermatol* 55:413–421, 2006.

44. Armstrong M: Tattooed army soldiers: examining the incidence, behavior and risk, *Military Med* 165 (2):135–141, 2000.

45. Hayes MO, Harkness GA: Body piercing as a risk factor for viral hepatitis: an integrative research review, *Am J Infect Contr* 29:271–274, 2001.

46. Yee LJ, Weiss HL, Langner RG, et al: Risk factors for acquisition of hepatitis C virus infection: a case series and potential implication for disease surveillance, *BMC Infect Dis* 1:8, 2001.

47. Long GE, Rickman LS: Infectious complications of tattoos, *Clin Infect Dis* 18(4):610–619, 1994.

48. Braithwaite RL, Stephens T, Sterk C, Braithwaite K: Risks associated with tattooing and body piercing, *J Public Health Policy* 20(4):459–470, 1999.

49. Maruschak LM: HIV in prisons and jails, 2002. Available at: http://www.ojp.usdoj.gov/bjs/pub/pdf/hivpj02.pdf. Accessed September 20, 2006.

50. Meltzer DI: Complications of body piercing, *Am Fam Phys* 72(10):2029–2034, 2005.

51. De Moor RJG, De Witte AM, Delme KI, et al: Dental and oral complications of lip and tongue piercings, *Br Dent J* 199(8):506–509.

52. Carroll ST, Rittenburgh RH, Roberts TA, Myhre EB: Tattoos and body piercings as indicators of adolescent risk-taking behaviors, *Pediatrics* 109(6): 1021–1027, 2002.

53. Huxley C, Grogan S: Tattooing, piercing, healthy behaviours and health value, *J Health Psychol* 10 (6):831–841, 2005.

54. Recommendations for prevention and control of hepatitis C virus (HCV) infection and HCV-related chronic disease. Available at: http://www.cdc.gov/mmwr/PDF/rr/rr4719.pdf. Accessed September 20, 2006.

55. Haley RW, Fischer RP: The tattooing paradox: are studies of acute hepatitis adequate to identify routes of transmission of subclinical hepatitis C infection? *Arch Intern Med* 163(9):1095–1098, 2003.

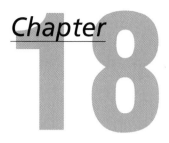

Chapter 18

Suicide

Lisa Seyfried, MD, and Joel J. Heidelbaugh, MD

Key Points

- The US Preventive Services Task Force concluded that evidence is insufficient to recommend for or against routine screening for suicide during office visits (strength of recommendation: C).
- Contracts for safety in patients who may be at an increased risk for suicide have not been proved to be effective in reducing attempts or deaths from suicide (strength of recommendation: C).
- Although a black box warning has been issued concerning increased suicidal ideation and behavior associated with antidepressant (specifically SSRI) drug treatment in children and adolescents, this is not an absolute contraindication. Consultation with a pediatric mental health professional should be considered when treating children and adolescents with major depressive disorder who may be at an increased risk of suicide (strength of recommendation: C).

Introduction

According to the National Center for Health Statistics, suicide was the eleventh leading cause of mortality in the United States in 2003, accounting for 31,484 deaths or 1.3% of total US deaths.[1] Men were 4.3 times more likely to die by suicide; the ratio of completed suicide in both of African American and Hispanic men as related to non-Hispanic white men was 0.4 in 2003.[1] Suicidology literature consistently demonstrates that, worldwide, men of all ages are at a higher risk for suicide than women, with only few exceptions.[2,3]

The act of suicide is the result of a complex interaction between risk and protective factors. Population studies have identified several factors associated with suicide completion in men; yet, at an individual level, these data do little to help the clinician determine which patients will eventually commit suicide. Given the low baseline rate of suicide in the population, even in populations at high risk, it is almost statistically impossible to reliably predict suicidality at the level of the individual. In a 2006 review, Paris[4] concluded that "given our present knowledge... it is not possible to predict suicide with any degree of accuracy."

Despite a lack of evidence-based guidelines for suicide risk assessment, clinicians must carry on in their attempts to predict and prevent suicide in their patients. Given that one half to two thirds of persons who complete suicide have visited a primary care professional within 1 month of their death,[5] we are commonly placed in a unique position to appropriately detect and intervene. The assessment of suicide and suicidal behavior is relevant to all clinicians and is not limited solely to mental health professionals.

The Gender Paradox

Although men tend to complete suicide more often than women, women attempt suicide far more often than men. This trend is often referred to as the "gender paradox" of suicidal behavior.[6] Several explanations for this paradox have been proposed. One of the most frequently posited reasons relates to gender difference in choice of suicide method. Men who commit suicide tend to choose more violent and immediately lethal means, such as firearms, at a higher rate than

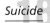

women.[7] Although a considerable number of women do use firearms, they are more likely to choose less lethal means including drug overdose and carbon monoxide poisoning.[8] One interpretation of these data is that these findings reflect a difference in level of intent; some studies[9] report that men have higher level of intent than women to actually succeed in killing themselves, whereas others[6,8] have not supported that conclusion.

Another theory related to this paradox suggests that gendered beliefs and attitudes about suicide contribute to differences in suicidal behavior. It has been suggested that, in the United States, attempting suicide tends to be thought of as a somewhat "feminine" behavior in contrast to committing suicide, which is perceived as a "masculine" behavior.[10] In research on the role of gender in attitudes toward suicidal behavior, men appear to be more accepting of suicide and tend to view it as a matter of individual right.[11] Early work by Linehan[12] discovered that males who survived a suicide attempt were viewed as less masculine and potent by their peers than those who succeeded in killing themselves. Men may be viewed as acting "powerfully" when committing suicide in response to a debilitating illness or a serious achievement failure[10]; there have been examples of this trend that have received national media attention in recent years. In lieu of attempting suicide, males are statistically more likely to engage in more "socially acceptable" self-destructive and high-risk behavior including alcohol and illicit drug abuse. In a comprehensive review of this issue, Canetto and Sakinofsky[6] concluded that "an important influence on the gender paradox may be cultural expectations about gender and suicidal behavior."

Gender, Depression, and Suicide

Depression is one of the most commonly cited risk factors for suicide. Large-scale epidemiologic studies have repeatedly demonstrated a significant gender difference in rates of major depressive disorder, with prevalence of depression twice as high in women than in men[13,14]; criteria for major depressive disorder are listed in Table 18-1. Still, despite lower identified rates of depression in males, men are successful at committing suicide far more often than women.

Gender differences in depression have been well investigated in the literature. One of the most consistent findings is the 2:1 (female to male) gender ratio in the prevalence of major

Table 18-1. Criteria for Major Depressive Disorder*

- Depressed mood most of the day, nearly every day, as indicated by either subjective report (e.g., feels sad or empty) or observation made by others (e.g., appears tearful) (In children and adolescents, this may be characterized as an "irritable" mood.)
- Markedly diminished interest or pleasure in all, or almost all, activities most of the day, nearly every day
- Significant weight loss when not dieting or weight gain (e.g., a change of more than 5% of body weight in a month) or decrease or increase in appetite nearly every day
- Insomnia or hypersomnia nearly every day
- Psychomotor agitation or retardation nearly every day
- Fatigue or loss of energy nearly every day
- Feelings of worthlessness or excessive or inappropriate guilt nearly every day
- Diminished ability to think or concentrate, or indecisiveness, nearly every day
- Recurrent thoughts of death (not just fear of dying), recurrent suicidal ideation without a specific plan, or a suicide attempt or a specific plan for committing suicide

*A person with a major depressive disorder must either have a depressed mood or a loss of interest or pleasure in daily activities consistently for at least a 2-week period. This mood must represent a change from the person's normal mood; social, occupational, educational, or other important functioning must also be negatively impaired by the change in mood. A depressed mood caused by substances (e.g., drugs, alcohol, medications) is not considered a major depressive disorder, nor is one that is caused by a general medical condition. Major depressive disorder cannot be diagnosed if a person has a history of manic, hypomanic, or mixed episodes (e.g., bipolar disorder) or if the depressed mood is better accounted for by schizoaffective disorder and is not superimposed on schizophrenia, a delusion, or psychotic disorder.

Furthermore, to qualify as a major depressive disorder, the symptoms are not better accounted for by bereavement (i.e., after the loss of a loved one), the symptoms persist for longer than 2 months or are characterized by marked functional impairment, morbid preoccupation with worthlessness, suicidal ideation, psychotic symptoms, or psychomotor retardation.

Reprinted with permission from *The Diagnostic and Statistical Manual of Mental Disorders,* Fourth Edition, Text Revision (Copyright 2000). American Psychiatric Association.

depression.[15] This difference in prevalence begins around puberty and persists through the fifth decade of life. Numerous explanations have been posited to explain this difference in prevalence, although none have been sufficiently supported by clinical evidence. Some researchers have proposed that gender differences in the course of depression might explain the lower prevalence among males. Although several studies have reported a similar course for men and women, the majority have identified lower relapse and nonremission rates among men.[16] Differences in help-seeking behavior may artificially increase the difference in prevalence (see Chapter 4, Men and the Problem of Help Seeking). Men often have longer delays and lower rates of treatment contact than women.[17,18] Some research suggests that men are less reliable historians when it comes to affective states and have difficulty recalling the frequency and duration of their depressive episodes[19]; however, there is also substantial evidence against this theory.[16,20] Another controversial explanation for the difference in prevalence suggests that men are less likely than women to experience an episode of major depression in response to stressful life events.[21]

Limited research has addressed gender-related variations in the symptoms of depression, and a significant proportion is conflicting. For example, a large community-based study of depressed outpatients found no gender differences in the severity or symptomatology of depression,[22] yet numerous additional studies have noted some differences. Several researchers have attempted to distinguish a separate "male depressive syndrome," proposing that there is an inherent gender-related bias in our current criteria.[23] Rutzt and Walinder[24] describe a male subtype of depression characterized in part by temporary lower stress tolerance, acting out, aggression, low impulse control, indecisiveness, irritability, substance abuse, and anti-social features. Other studies also report that depressed men, compared with women, tend to experience lower impulse control, increased irritability, and anger.[25] In addition, men appear more likely to complain of insomnia and agitation.[26] Many studies suggest that men are less likely to have a significant change in appetite, hypersomnia, fatigue, and psychomotor retardation.[27,28] In both sexes, major depression has been shown to lead to limitations and impairments in daily activities, yet men appear more likely to report impairments in work and leisure activities.[29,30]

Physicians are less likely to recognize depression and suicidality in male patients than in females. It appears that gender-related stereotypes on the part of clinicians play a role in the underdiagnosis of major depression in men.[31] In turn, men are much less likely to acknowledge and discuss physical and psychological distress when meeting with their physicians and find it more difficult to divulge personal information that may be at the root of such mood changes.[32] This dangerous combination presents a significant challenge to the identification of men with depression and suicidal ideation.

Identifying Men at Risk

No one can predict with certainty whether an individual will or will not attempt suicide. At present, there are no risk-assessment techniques,

no diagnostic criteria, and no screening tools available that can accurately predict suicidal behavior in any given patient. The US Preventive Services Task Force[33] 2004 review of studies on routine screening by primary care clinicians to detect suicide risk in the general population concluded that the evidence is insufficient to recommend for or against this practice. The goal of a suicide assessment is therefore not to predict suicidal behavior but rather to identify those people who may be at a greater risk and to evaluate individual factors that may influence acute risk so as to inform clinical practice.[34,35]

Table 18-2 lists several factors that have been associated with an increased suicide risk. As the table demonstrates, male-to-female predominance in suicide in the United States continues across the life span, and the largest gender difference in suicide rates occurs among older age groups. For example, men who are 65–74 years old are nearly six times more likely to commit suicide than age-matched females. It is also important to remember that suicide is the third leading cause of death in young men between the ages of 15 and 24 years.

Table 18-2. Risk Factors for Suicide

Demographic features	Male gender Widowed or divorced Age 60 years or older White race
Psychosocial features	Living alone Unemployed or with financial problems Recent stressful life event
Psychiatric diagnoses	Major depressive disorder (see Table 18-1) Alcohol/substance abuse Cluster B personality disorders
Psychological features	Feeling of hopelessness Severe or unremitting anxiety Panic attacks
Genetic and familial effects	Family history of suicide (particularly in first-degree relatives) Family history of mental illness, including substance use disorders
Additional features	History of suicide attempts or ideation Access to firearms

Adapted from: American Psychiatric Association: *Practice Guidelines for the Assessment and Treatment of Patients with Suicidal Behaviors*, Washington, DC, 2003, American Psychiatric Association.

Race may also be an important consideration because the risk of completing suicide is more than double for the white population compared with the African American population.[1] White males over the age of 85 years have the highest suicide rates compared with all age and gender groups. Data from the National Survey of American Life[36] sampled 5181 blacks aged 18 years and older who were categorized as African Americans and Caribbean Americans. The reported lifetime prevalence for suicidal ideation in this study group was 11.7% and for suicide attempts was 4.1%. Among the respondents who reported suicidal ideation, 34.6% actually transitioned to making a plan and only 21% made an unplanned attempt. This study determined that blacks at a higher risk for suicide attempts were in younger birth cohorts, less educated, and residents of the Midwestern United States and had one or more psychological disorders classified by the *Diagnostic and Statistical Manual of Mental Disorders,* Fourth Edition.

Past psychiatric history is one of the strongest predictors of suicide because approximately 90% of persons who commit suicide have a diagnosable mental illness.[37] As discussed previously, it is estimated that 50% of men who commit suicide have major depressive disorder.[38] In a meta-analysis of 249 studies, Harris and Barraclough[39] estimated the suicide risk associated with common psychiatric disorders. They demonstrated that the rate of suicide exceeded the expected rate in the general population by 20 times in major depression, 10 times in panic disorder, 7 times in personality disorder, and nearly 6 times in alcohol abuse. A history of past suicide attempts was found to be correlated with a suicide risk 38 times greater than that of the expected population. These results are consistent with those from numerous other studies; however, the vast majority of patients with psychiatric illness do not commit suicide. The challenge herein is to recognize what psychological characteristics place some patients at a higher risk than others for attempting and completing suicide. Mann and colleagues[40] found that the severity of subjective feelings of depression and suicidal ideation were both indicators of an elevated risk for future suicidal acts. This ideal is consistent with earlier work suggesting that the more severe the depression, the higher the acute risk of a suicide attempt.[41]

Alcohol abuse and dependence is an important risk factor for suicide and, like suicide, is a gendered phenomena.[42] Alcohol use disorders occur more frequently in men compared with women. In the National Comorbidity Survey in the United States, the 12-month prevalence of alcohol dependence in males was 20.1%—approximately 2.5 times the rate in females.[13] In a review of the literature, Murphy and Wetzel[43] found that the lifetime risk of suicide in patients with alcoholism was between 60 and 120 times that of the non–psychiatrically ill. They estimate that 25% of persons who commit suicide have an alcohol use disorder. Several studies have demonstrated that acute alcohol use is also associated with suicidal behavior.[44] It is possible that this notion is a direct result of alcohol's physiologic effects, which include increasing aggressiveness and decreasing inhibition. Some studies have suggested that ingestion of alcohol might predispose persons to the choice of guns for committing suicide, but current data are conflicting.[45,46]

A growing body of evidence exists that suggests that impulsive and aggressive behaviors in depressed men may play a significant role in suicide.[40] In a 2005 study of male suicide completers, impulsive-aggressive personality disorders and alcohol abuse or dependence were found to be two independent predictors of suicide in cases of major depressive disorder.[47] This finding was consistent with numerous other studies that have identified borderline and antisocial personality disorders as risk factors for suicidal behavior. The "cluster B" personality disorders (commonly referred to as the *dramatic and erratic personalities*), particularly the borderline and antisocial personality disorders, are highly correlated with impulsivity and aggression. In this study, 70% of completed suicides in patients with a known cluster B personality disorder had concomitant problems with alcohol and/or drug abuse or dependence.[47]

Numerous medical illnesses have been associated with increased risk of suicide, some independent of the effects of comorbid psychiatric disorders. Pulmonary disease (particularly chronic obstructive pulmonary disease), congestive heart failure, urinary incontinence, peptic ulcer disease, cancer, migraine with aura, epilepsy, stroke, multiple sclerosis, traumatic brain injury, Huntington's disease, and acquired immunodeficiency syndrome all carry a higher risk for suicide.[48-51] In addition, the risk is greatly increased among patients with multiple chronic illnesses.[48]

A final risk factor to consider in suicidality is the experience of hopelessness. A high degree of hopelessness is more significantly related to suicidal behavior than depressed mood alone.[40] A 1990 study of 1958 psychiatric outpatients found that those with greater levels of hopelessness were 11 times more likely to commit suicide than the rest of the outpatients.[52] Depressed patients who are "future oriented," defined as those who look to the future with a generally positive outlook and who can identify goals and reasons for living, have fewer and less intense thoughts of attempting suicide.[53]

Protective factors, specifically those associated with a reduced risk for suicide, must also be considered. Married men experience lower suicide rates than those who are divorced or separated.[54,55] Having children, particularly younger children in the home, is also associated with a reduced suicide risk.[56] Overall, persons who have a strong religious faith and believe that suicide is morally wrong or sinful also appear to have decreased risk.[57,58] Social connectedness, problem-solving confidence, and an internal locus of control are thought to be protective against suicide attempts in young adults.[59]

Acute Risk Factors: Warning Signs for Suicide

An emerging area of suicidology research concerns itself with the warning signs for suicide. As Rudd and colleagues[60] have noted, compared with the aforementioned risk factors, warning signs "suggest a more proximal rather than distal relationship to suicidal behaviors." They imply more imminent risk (i.e., days to weeks) than do risk factors, which suggest long-term risk (i.e., months to years). Using a consensus process, the American Association of Suicidology has developed a list of suicide warning signs for use by clinicians and the lay public. This list is summarized by the mnemonic "IS PATH WARM?"[60,61]:

- I: Ideation (suicidal ideation)
- S: Substance abuse (increasing alcohol or illicit drug use)
- P: Purposelessness (no reason to live, no sense of purpose in life)
- A: Anxiety
- T: Trapped (feeling like there is no way out)
- H: Hopelessness
- W: Withdrawal (withdrawing from friends, family, or society)
- A: Anger (rage, revenge seeking)
- R: Recklessness (engaging in risky behaviors)
- M: Mood changes

These various signs reflect the current state of the patient and may be useful to the clinician in the assessment of impending suicide risk. When inquiring about suicidal risk, documentation of any or all of the above signs is paramount, as well as ensuring the immediacy of patient safety.

The Psychiatric Interview

A thorough psychiatric examination is the foundation of any suicide assessment. The psychiatric interview and mental status examination are essential elements in determining risk and protective factors for suicide. In addition, the interview can help to establish a rapport between the patient and clinician. Of note, interviewer gender may influence disclosure in mental health interviews. Some research suggests that men interviewed by a woman are likely to report slightly more symptoms of depression than those interviewed by a man.[62] Collateral information should also be obtained from family members, other physicians, and the medical record when allowed by the patient. Important elements of the psychiatric interview include the following[63]:

- The patient's psychiatric history: Obtaining the patient's personal psychiatric history is critical. This can often be approached during the review of systems or while obtaining the medical history. It is also important to ask specific and directed questions about any past suicidal behavior. Prior suicide attempts are among the strongest risk factors for completed suicide and may be the best single predictor of completed suicide.[64]
- Family history: The family psychiatric history may provide important clues to understanding the patient's current mental state. It is often easiest to obtain this information while gathering the family medical history. Topics of particular importance include mood disorders and substance abuse or dependence, as these may indicate a genetic vulnerability in the patient. Men have a 60% increased risk for alcohol abuse and dependence if they report that their father has a history of heavy drinking.[65] Numerous studies have determined that a family history of suicide is associated with an increased risk of suicidal behavior.[66, 67]
- Social history: This is an opportunity for the clinician to not only gather data but also to assess the patient's overall social situation. Questions about work, home life, religion, and legal issues should be posed. Men appear to be particularly vulnerable to depression during times of marital discord and economic hardship.[68]
- Mental status examination: The mental status examination is a systematic assessment of

the patient's current mental state. The most pertinent elements include the following:

- Appearance: Patients who are very depressed often have difficulty attending to activities of daily living, including grooming. The level of psychomotor activity should be noted; in depressed patients, this can range anywhere from slowed to agitated.
- Mood and affect: The assessment of a patient's mood has two salient components, namely what the patient reports as his mood and what the clinician observes; these determinations can occasionally be incongruous. The term *affect* refers to the observable expression of emotion such that a man who appears sad and tearful may report that his *mood* is "fine."
- Hallucinations and delusions: Some patients will develop psychotic symptoms as part of their depression. This is important to assess because psychosis is an independent risk factor for suicide.
- Suicidal ideation: The specifics of suicide assessment are covered below.

Assessment of Suicidal Ideation

Forming an accurate assessment of suicidal ideation in men is particularly challenging. As noted earlier in this chapter, most men have a difficult time discussing their true feelings. In addition, the stigma surrounding mental illness and suicide often deters them from seeking treatment in the first place.[69] Very few men will spontaneously disclose suicidal ideations to their physician.[70,71] In turn, physicians are sometimes uncomfortable discussing these issues with their patients because suicide assessment in particular may provoke anxiety in some clinicians; physicians may hesitate to ask their patients about suicide in the belief that this could trigger suicidal thoughts and behavior despite the lack of any empiric evidence supporting this fear. Still others may believe that the patient will spontaneously communicate suicidal intent himself.[72] Given that suicidal patients are far more likely to anticipate difficulty in talking to their physicians about psychiatric problems than those who are not suicidal,[73] the responsibility to explore these issues falls on the primary care clinician.

A hierarchical stepwise approach to questioning has been recommended by several expert suicidologists.[74,75] This method is consistent with the American Psychiatric Association's *Practice Guidelines for the Assessment and Treatment of Patients with Suicidal Behaviors*.[34] In this type of interview, the clinician typically begins with general and open-ended questions (e.g., "How are things going in your life?") in an attempt to identify any current stressors. Then, the intensity and degree of detail in questioning is slowly increased. Questions such as "Have you ever felt that life was not worth living?" and "Did you ever wish you could go to sleep and just not wake up?" help to broach the subject of death. In addition, it can be helpful for the clinician to normalize these thoughts (e.g., "Sometimes people who are depressed/divorcing/just lost their job/etc. have thoughts that it would be better to not go on. Have you had any thoughts like that?"). It is important to then follow up with specific directed questions about thoughts of self-harm or suicide. Questions like "Is death something you've thought about recently?" and "Have things ever reached the point that you've thought about harming yourself?" can be helpful in eliciting such thoughts.

By approaching a suicide assessment in this manner, the clinician should be able to establish a better rapport with the patient, thereby allowing him to feel more comfortable about sharing difficult and potentially disturbing thoughts over time and through subsequent encounters. If the patient admits to having thoughts of death or suicide, then the clinician should continue his or her line of questioning by inquiring about detailed aspects of the suicidal thoughts. The patient should be asked about specific plans for suicide and any steps that have been taken toward enacting those plans. To assess type of method, one might simply ask, "What have you been thinking of doing?" and follow up with "Have you considered any other methods?" A highly organized and detailed plan is generally associated with a greater risk, although suicide attempts can occur impulsively with little or no planning.[34] A plan involving a violent, lethal, and easily accessible method is particularly concerning because it implies a high level of intent; the notion of intent refers to the degree of seriousness of the patient's wish to die. When assessing intent, it is important to ascertain the patient's beliefs and knowledge about the suicide method. For example, he may believe that acetaminophen is relatively safe in an overdose since it is available over the counter. Thus, he may have a low intent but may have a plan that is highly lethal. The converse of this relationship is true as well, as some people will devise a plan that they erroneously believe will be lethal in a sincere wish to die. These people should be considered at a higher risk for suicide based on their level of intent.

Management

Once it has been determined that a patient is suicidal, the clinician must devise a comprehensive treatment plan that addresses patient safety based on level of risk for suicidal behavior.[76] Immediate action must be taken when a man is judged to be at imminent risk. Rapid evaluation by a mental health professional is warranted with inpatient psychiatric hospitalization a likely and practical outcome. Often, this will involve transferring the patient by ambulance to a nearby hospital and direct communication of medical information and concerns between the clinician and mental health professional who will be evaluating and treating the suicidal patient. Regardless of the patient's level of cooperation, one-to-one constant staff observation is indicated while these arrangements are being made. The situation becomes more difficult if the patient rejects the physician's recommendations. In these cases, the clinician must explore medical-legal avenues with appropriate risk-management experts, which typically involve calling local authorities for assistance. Although this can be anxiety provoking for the physician and can strain the doctor-patient relationship, ultimately patient safety must be the first priority.

If the patient is believed to be at a moderate but not imminent risk for suicide, he often can be managed in the outpatient setting. If allowed by the patient, family or others close to him should be actively involved in the treatment plan. The patient should be made aware of the availability of any available 24-hour emergency or crisis intervention services. It is often helpful to increase the frequency and duration of outpatient visits in these cases, during which frequent reevaluation of suicide risk should be performed and documented in detail. Depending on the clinician's level of comfort with psychiatric problems, a referral to a mental health specialist may be indicated. Patients with suicidal behaviors frequently benefit from treatment involving a multidisciplinary team that may include several mental health professionals.

The use of suicide prevention contracts as a part of a clinical treatment plan is controversial at best. Contracts are often used in an attempt to ensure that a patient will inform someone if he feels unable to resist his suicidal thoughts.

No studies to date have demonstrated their effectiveness in reducing suicide. In fact, studies of competed suicides have shown that a significant number had such a contract in place at the time of their suicidal act[34]; however, some clinicians find them to be a useful tool in assessing risk and strengthening the therapeutic alliance.

Lastly, the management of any patient at risk for suicide, particularly high-risk men, must include a conversation about firearms. The presence of one or more guns in the home is associated with a four-fold increased risk of suicide.[7] Men with firearms in the home are 10 times more likely to commit suicide than men without guns in the home.[77] The clinician who is interviewing a depressed or potentially suicidal patient should recommend that the patient remove any firearms from his house. This practice can prove to be a difficult negotiation with some patients. Clinicians should also attempt to educate the patient and his family about the aforementioned risks and suggest that all firearms be made inaccessible to the patient. Patients, in an attempt to be reassuring, may state that they keep their guns unloaded and in a locked location. There is a large body of research that demonstrates a strong association between guns and risk of suicide exists regardless of storage practice, type of gun, or number of firearms in the home.[77] The removal of all firearms from the home is the safest option.

Suicide and the Potential Link to Pharmacotherapy

The controversy regarding the relationship between selective serotonin reuptake inhibitors (SSRIs) and suicidality dates back to the early 1990s. Although the first agent reported to be associated with suicidality was fluoxetine, in 2003 the British Medicines and Healthcare Products Regulatory Agency warned about a possible risk of suicidality in children and adolescents treated with paroxetine for major depressive disorder. This warning was soon extended to the SSRIs as an entire class as well as venlafaxine and mirtazapine.[78] In 2004, the US Food and Drug Administration issued a "black box warning" concerning increased suicidal ideation and behavior associated with antidepressant (specifically SSRI) drug treatment in children and adolescents. Despite numerous studies and reviews examining this topic, it is still largely unknown whether antidepressant agents, specifically the SSRIs, actually increase the risk of suicide death in children or adults, as current data are conflicting.[79]

Bostwick[80] comments that "after regulatory agencies in the United Kingdom and the US recommended severe restrictions on antidepressant use in children, many lessons were learned, although one was not that these drugs cause suicide. There has been enormous speculation that pharmaceutical companies selectively released data that reflected positively on their products and that combining suppressed and published data suggested that most of these medications had questionable efficacy. We also learned that the studies lacked uniformity both in which age groups constituted children and which behavior was considered suicidal."

A 2006 meta-analysis by Hall and Lucke[81] reviewed the evidence on the effects of SSRIs and their relationship to decreased suicide rates in the population as well as increased suicide rates in some individuals early in their treatment. They found that SSRIs increase suicidal ideation compared with placebo but that observational studies suggest that SSRIs do not increase suicide risk to a greater degree than older, non-SSRI antidepressants. If SSRIs truly increase suicide risk in some patients, then the number of additional deaths is very small, since ecologic studies have generally found that suicide mortality has declined (or at least not increased) as SSRI use has increased substantially in the United States since their breakthrough in the 1980s.[81]

Simon and colleagues[82] evaluated population-based data to evaluate the risk of suicide death and serious suicide attempt in relation to the initiation of antidepressant treatment with SSRIs. The risk of death by suicide was not found to be significantly higher in the month after starting medication compared with the subsequent months of pharmacotherapy. The risk of suicide attempt was found to be highest in the month before starting antidepressant treatment and declined progressively after starting medication.[82] Available data to date do not indicate a significant increase in risk of suicide or serious suicide attempt after starting treatment with newer antidepressant drugs.

Apter and colleagues[83] conducted a double-blinded trial of potential suicidal events by comparing incidence rates between 642 paroxetine- and 549 placebo-treated pediatric patients. They determined that suicide-related events occurred more often in paroxetine-treated (22 of 642; 3.4%) than placebo-treated groups (5 of 549; 0.9%) with an odds ratio of 3.86. All suicide-related events occurred in adolescents of at least 12 years of age, except for 1 of 156 paroxetine-treated children, and all suicide attempts occurred in patients with major depressive disorder; few suicide-related events occurred in patients with solely a primary anxiety disorder. They concluded that adolescents treated with paroxetine showed an increased risk of suicide-related events, yet suicidality rating scales used in the study did not show this risk difference.[83] The presence of uncontrolled suicide risk factors, the relatively low incidence of these events, and their predominance in adolescents with major depressive disorder make it difficult to identify a single cause for suicidality in these pediatric patients.

Olfson and colleagues[79] conducted a matched case-control study on Medicaid recipients from all 50 US states who had received inpatient treatment for major depression. In adults aged 19–64 years, antidepressant (SSRI) drug treatment was not significantly associated with suicide attempts (odds ratio, 1.10) or suicide deaths (odds ratio, 0.90). However, in children and adolescents aged 6–18 years, antidepressant drug treatment was significantly associated with suicide attempts (odds ratio, 1.52) and suicide deaths (odds ratio, 15.62). The authors concluded that, in these high-risk patients, antidepressant drug treatment does not seem to be related to suicide attempts and death in adults but might be related in children and adolescents.[79]

Juurlink and colleagues[84] explored the relationship between the initiation of therapy with SSRIs and completed suicide in older patients. In their study, during the first month of therapy, SSRIs were associated with a nearly five-fold higher risk of completed suicide compared with other antidepressants (adjusted odds ratio, 4.8). The risk was believed to be independent of a recent diagnosis of depression or the receipt of psychiatric care, and suicides of a violent nature were distinctly more common during SSRI therapy. No disproportionate suicide risk was seen during the second and subsequent months of treatment with SSRI antidepressants, and the absolute risk of suicide with all antidepressants was low.[84] The authors concluded that initiation of SSRI therapy is associated with an increased risk of suicide during the first month of therapy compared with other antidepressants, yet the absolute risk is low, suggesting that an idiosyncratic response to these agents may provoke suicide in a vulnerable subgroup of patients.[84]

Conventional wisdom has stressed that treatment of major depressive disorder with SSRIs may increase the risk of impulsive acts including suicide, whereas data from epidemiologic studies suggest that the effect of SSRIs in elderly persons may actually be beneficial. Elderly depressed patients treated with antidepressants may be at a reduced risk of attempting suicide, yet these findings need support from rigorous prospective randomized trials.[85]

Conclusions

Whether a male patient will attempt suicide is impossible to predict, even in cases of major depressive disorder and other psychiatric illnesses. Clinicians are urged to screen for high-risk behaviors and depression when indicated, then to consider asking first open-ended and then directed questions about suicidal intent whenever suspicion is present. The importance of forming a meaningful rapport with male patients to ensure a bidirectional level of comfort with communication is paramount.

References

1. Hoyert DL, Heron MP, Murphy SL, Kung HC: Deaths: final data for 2003, *Natl Vital Stat Rep* 54 (13):1–120, 2006.
2. Phillips MR, Li X, Zhang Y: Suicide rates in China, 1995–99, *Lancet* 359(9309):835–840, 2002.
3. Schmidtke A, Bille-Brahe U, DeLeo D, et al: Attempted suicide in Europe: rates, trends and socio-demographic characteristics of suicide attempters during the period 1989–1992. Results of the WHO/EURO Multicentre Study on Parasuicide, *Acta Psychiatr Scand* 93(5):327–338, 1996.
4. Paris J: Predicting and preventing suicide: do we know enough to do either? *Harv Rev Psychiatry* 14 (5):233–240, 2006.
5. Luoma JB, Martin CE, Pearson JL: Contact with mental health and primary care providers before suicide: a review of the evidence 10.1176/appi.ajp.159.6.909, *Am J Psychiatry* 159(6):909–916, 2002.
6. Canetto SS, Sakinofsky I: The gender paradox in suicide, *Suicide Life Threat Behav* 28(1):1–23, 1998.
7. Kellermann AL, Rivara FP, Somes G, et al: Suicide in the home in relation to gun ownership, *N Engl J Med* 327(7):467–472, 1992.
8. Denning DG, Conwell Y, King D, Cox C: Method choice, intent, and gender in completed suicide, *Suicide Life Threat Behav* 30(3):282–288, 2000.
9. Rich CL, Ricketts JE, Fowler RC, Young D: Some differences between men and women who commit suicide, *Am J Psychiatry* 145(6):718–722, 1988.
10. Canetto SS: Gender and suicidal behavior: theories and evidence. In Canetto SS, Maris RW, Silverman MM, editors: *Review of Suicidology*, New York, 1997, Guilford, pp 138–167.
11. Dahlen ER, Canetto SS: The role of gender and suicide precipitant in attitudes toward nonfatal suicide behavior, *Death Stud* 26(2):99–116, 2002.
12. Linehan MM: Suicide and attempted suicide: study of perceived sex differences, *Percept Mot Skills* 37 (1):31–34, 1973.
13. Kessler RC, McGonagle KA, Zhao S, et al: Lifetime and 12-month prevalence of DSM-III-R psychiatric disorders in the United States: results from the National Comorbidity Survey, *Arch Gen Psychiatry* 51(1):8–19, 1994.
14. Kessler RC, Berglund P, Demler O, et al: The epidemiology of major depressive disorder: results from the National Comorbidity Survey Replication (NCS-R), *JAMA* 289(23):3095–3105, 2003.
15. Weissman MM, Bland RC, Canino GJ, et al: Cross-national epidemiology of major depression and bipolar disorder, *JAMA* 276(4):293–299, 1996.
16. Kuehner C: Gender differences in the short-term course of unipolar depression in a follow-up sample of depressed inpatients, *J Affect Disord* 56(2–3): 127–139, 1999.
17. Wang PS, Berglund P, Olfson M, et al: Failure and delay in initial treatment contact after first onset of mental disorders in the national comorbidity survey replication, *Arch Gen Psychiatry* 62(6):603–613, 2005.
18. Kessler RC, Brown RL, Broman CL: Sex differences in psychiatric help-seeking: evidence from four large-scale surveys, *J Health Soc Behav* 22(1):49–64, 1981.
19. Angst J, Dobler-Mikola A: Do the diagnostic criteria determine the sex ratio in depression? *J Affect Disord* 7(3–4):189–198, 1984.
20. Kendler KS, Gardner CO, Prescott CA: Are there sex differences in the reliability of a lifetime history of major depression and its predictors? *Psychol Med* 31(4):617–625, 2001.
21. Maciejewski PK, Prigerson HG, Mazure CM: Sex differences in event-related risk for major depression, *Psychol Med* 31(4):593–604, 2001.
22. Hildebrandt MG, Stage KB, Kragh-Soerensen P: Gender and depression: a study of severity and symptomatology of depressive disorders (ICD-10) in general practice, *Acta Psychiatr Scand* 107 (3):197–202, 2003.
23. Rutz W, Wallinder J, Von Knorring L, et al: Prevention of depression and suicide by education and medication: impact on male suicidality. An update from the Gotland study, *Int J Psychiatry Clin Pract* 1(1):39–46, 1997.
24. Walinder J, Rutzt W: Male depression and suicide, *Int Clin Psychopharmacol* 16(Suppl 2):S21–S24, 2001.
25. Winkler D, Pjrek E, Kasper S: Anger attacks in depression—evidence for a male depressive syndrome, *Psychother Psychosom* 74(5):303–307, 2005.
26. Khan AA, Gardner CO, Prescott CA, Kendler KS: Gender differences in the symptoms of major depression in opposite-sex dizygotic twin pairs, *Am J Psychiatry* 159(8):1427–1429, 2002.
27. Silverstein B: Gender differences in the prevalence of somatic versus pure depression: a replication, *Am J Psychiatry* 159(6):1051–1052, 2002.
28. Kroenke K, Spitzer RL: Gender differences in the reporting of physical and somatoform symptoms, *Psychosom Med* 60(2):150–155, 1998.

29. Breslin FC, Gnam W, Franche RL, et al: Depression and activity limitations: examining gender differences in the general population, *Soc Psychiatry Psychiatr Epidemiol* 41(8):648–655, 2006.

30. Kornstein SG, Schatzberg AF, Thase ME, et al: Gender differences in chronic major and double depression, *J Affect Disord* 60(1):1–11, 2000.

31. Stoppe G, Sandholzer H, Huppertz C, et al: Gender differences in the recognition of depression in old age. *Maturitas* 32(3):205–212, 1999.

32. Corney RH: Sex differences in general practice attendance and help seeking for minor illness, *J Psychosom Res* 34(5):525–534, 1990.

33. US Preventive Services Task Force: Screening for suicide risk: recommendation and rationale, *Ann Intern Med* 140(10):820–821, 2004

34. American Psychiatric Association: *Practice Guidelines for the Assessment and Treatment of Patients with Suicidal Behaviors*, Washington, DC, 2003, American Psychiatric Association.

35. Simon R: Suicide risk assessment: what is the standard of care? *J Am Acad Psychiatry Law* 30(3):340–344, 2002.

36. Joe S, Baser RE, Breedon G et al: Prevalence of and risk factors for lifetime suicide attempts among blacks in the United States, *JAMA* 296:2112–2123, 2006.

37. Rich CL, Young D, Fowler RC: San Diego suicide study: I. young vs old subjects, *Arch Gen Psychiatry* 43(6):577–582, 1986.

38. Lesage AD, Boyer R, Grunberg F, et al: Suicide and mental disorders: a case-control study of young men, *Am J Psychiatry* 151(7):1063–1068, 1994.

39. Harris EC, Barraclough B: Suicide as an outcome for mental disorders: a meta-analysis, *Br J Psychiatry* 170:205–228, 1997.

40. Mann JJ, Waternaux C, Haas GL, Malone KM: Toward a clinical model of suicidal behavior in psychiatric patients, *Am J Psychiatry* 156(2):181–189, 1999.

41. Hagnell O, Rorsman B: Suicide in the Lundby study: a comparative investigation of clinical aspects, *Neuropsychobiology* 5(2):61–73, 1979.

42. Sher L: Alcoholism and suicidal behavior: a clinical overview, *Acta Psychiatr Scand* 113(1): 13–22, 2006.

43. Murphy GE, Wetzel RD: The lifetime risk of suicide in alcoholism, *Arch Gen Psychiatry* 47(4):383–392, 1990.

44. Cherpitel CJ, Borges GL, Wilcox HC: Acute alcohol use and suicidal behavior: a review of the literature, *Alcohol Clin Exp Res* 28(5 Suppl):18S–28S, 2004.

45. Brent DA, Perper JA, Allman CJ: Alcohol, firearms, and suicide among youth: temporal trends in Allegheny County, Pennsylvania, 1960 to 1983, *JAMA* 257(24):3369–3372, 1987.

46. Rich CL, Dhossche DM, Ghani S, Isacsson G: Suicide methods and presence of intoxicating abusable substances: some clinical and public health implications, *Ann Clin Psychiatry* 10(4):169–175, 1998.

47. Dumais A, Lesage AD, Alda M, et al: Risk factors for suicide completion in major depression: a case–control study of impulsive and aggressive behaviors in men, *Am J Psychiatry* 162(11):2116–2124, 2005.

48. Juurlink DN, Herrmann N, Szalai JP, et al: Medical illness and the risk of suicide in the elderly, *Arch Intern Med* 164(11):1179–1184, 2004.

49. Goodwin RD, Kroenke K, Hoven CW, Spitzer RL: Major depression, physical illness, and suicidal ideation in primary care, *Psychosom Med* 65(4):501–505, 2003.

50. Arciniegas DB, Anderson CA: Suicide in neurologic illness, *Curr Treat Options Neurol* 4(6):457–468, 2002.

51. Bjorkenstam C, Edberg A, Ayoubi S, Rosen M: Are cancer patients at higher suicide risk than the general population? *Scand J Public Health* 33(3): 208–214, 2005.

52. Beck AT, Brown G, Berchick RJ, et al: Relationship between hopelessness and ultimate suicide: a replication with psychiatric outpatients, *Am J Psychiatry* 147(2):190–195, 1990.

53. Hirsch JK, Duberstein PR, Conner KR, et al: Future orientation and suicide ideation and attempts in depressed adults ages 50 and over, *Am J Geriatr Psychiatry* 14(9):752–757, 2006.

54. Smith JC, Mercy JA, Conn JM: Marital status and the risk of suicide, *Am J Public Health* 78(1):78–80, 1988.

55. Kposowa AJ: Marital status and suicide in the National Longitudinal Mortality Study, *J Epidemiol Community Health* 54(4):254–261, 2000.

56. Qin P, Mortensen PB: The impact of parental status on the risk of completed suicide, *Arch Gen Psychiatry* 60(8):797–802, 2003.

57. Stack S, Lester D: The effect of religion on suicide ideation, *Soc Psychiatry Psychiatr Epidemiol* 26(4): 168–170, 1991.

58. Dervic K, Oquendo MA, Grunebaum MF, et al: Religious affiliation and suicide attempt, *Am J Psychiatry* 161(12):2303–2308, 2004.

59. Donald M, Dower J, Correa-Velez I, Jones M: Risk and protective factors for medically serious suicide attempts: a comparison of hospital-based with population-based samples of young adults, *Aust N Z J Psychiatry* 40(1):87–96, 2006.

60. Rudd MD, Berman AL, Joiner TE Jr, et al: Warning signs for suicide: theory, research, and clinical applications, *Suicide Life Threat Behav* 36(3):255–262, 2006.

61. American Association of Suicidology: Suicide fact sheet, Warning signs. Available at: http://www.suicidology.org/associations/1045/files/Mnemonic.pdf.

62. Pollner M: The effects of interviewer gender in mental health interviews, *J Nerv Ment Disord* 186 (6):369–373, 1998.

63. Slavney P: *Psychiatric Dimensions of Medical Practice*, Baltimore, 1998, The Johns Hopkins University Press.

64. Joiner TE Jr, Conwell Y, Fitzpatrick KK, et al: Four studies on how past and current suicidality relate even when "everything but the kitchen sink" is covaried, *J Abnorm Psychol* 114(2):291–303, 2005.

65. Crum RM, Harris EL: Risk of alcoholism and parental history: gender differences and a possible reporting bias, *Genet Epidemiol* 13(4):329–341, 1996.

66. Roy A, Rylander G, Sarchiapone M: Genetic studies of suicidal behavior, *Psychiatr Clin North Am* 20 (3):595–611, 1997.

67. Roy A: Family history of suicide, *Arch Gen Psychiatry* 40(9):971–974, 1983.

68. Kendler KS, Thornton LM, Prescott CA: Gender differences in the rates of exposure to stressful life events and sensitivity to their depressogenic effects, *Am J Psychiatry* 158(4):587–593, 2001.

69. USDHHS, Mental Health: *A Report of the Surgeon General.* Rockville, MD, 1999, U.S. Department of Health and Human Services, Substance Abuse and Mental Health Services Administration, Center for Mental Health Services, National Institutes of Health, National Institute of Mental Health.

70. Houston K, Haw C, Townsend E, Hawton K: General practitioner contacts with patients before and after deliberate self harm, *Br J Gen Pract* 53(490): 365–370, 2003.

71. Matthews K, Milne S, Ashcroft GW: Role of doctors in the prevention of suicide: the final consultation, *Br J Gen Pract* 44(385):345–348, 1994.

72. Stoppe G, Sandholzer H, Huppertz C, et al: Family physicians and the risk of suicide in the depressed elderly, *J Affect Disord* 54(1–2):193–198, 1999.

73. Zimmerman M, Lish JD, Lush DT, et al: Suicidal ideation among urban medical outpatients, *J Gen Intern Med* 10(10):573–576, 1995.

74. Bryan CJ, Rudd MD: Advances in the assessment of suicide risk, *J Clin Psychol* 62(2):185–200, 2006.

75. Jacobs D, Brewer M, Klein-Benheim M: Suicide assessment: an overview and recommended protocol. In Jacobs DG, editor: *The Harvard Medical School Guide to Suicide Assessment and Intervention*, San Francisco, 1999, Jossey-Bass, pp 3–39.

76. Hirschfeld RMA, Russell JM: Assessment and treatment of suicidal patients, *N Engl J Med* 337(13): 910–915, 1997.

77. Dahlberg LL, Ikeda RM, Kresnow MJ: Guns in the home and risk of a violent death in the home: findings from a national study, *Am J Epidemiol* 160 (10): 929–936, 2004.

78. Giner L, Nichols CM, Zalsman G, Oquendo MA: Selective serotonin reuptake inhibitors and the risk for suicidality in adolescents: an update, *Int J Adolesc Med Health* 17(3):211–220, 2005.

79. Olfson M, Marcus M, Steven C, Shaffer D: Antidepressant drug therapy and suicide in severely depressed children and adults: a case-control study, *Arch Gen Psychiatry* 63(8):865–872, 2006.

80. Bostwick JM: Do SSRIs cause suicide in children? the evidence is underwhelming, *J Clin Psychol* 62 (2):235–241, 2006.

81. Hall WD, Lucke J: How have the selective serotonin reuptake inhibitor antidepressants affected suicide mortality? *Austral N Z J Psychiatry* 40:941–950, 2006.

82. Simon GE, Savarino J, Operskalski B, Wang PS: Suicide risk during antidepressant treatment, *Am J Psychiatry* 163(1):41–47, 2006.

83. Apter A, Lipschitz A, Fong R, et al: Evaluation of suicidal thoughts and behaviors in children and adolescents taking paroxetine, *J Child Adolesc Psychopharmacol* 16(1–2):77–90, 2006.

84. Juurlink DN, Mamdani MM, Kopp A, Redelmeier DA: The risk of suicide with selective serotonin reuptake inhibitors in the elderly, *Am J Psychiatry* 163(5):813–821, 2006.

85. Barak Y, Olmer A, Aizenberg D: Antidepressants reduce the risk of suicide among elderly depressed patients, *Neuropsychopharmacology* 31(1):178–181, 2006.

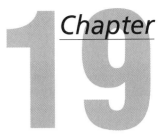

Chapter
19

Nutrition

Mark Mirabelli, MD, and Ramsey Shehab, MD

Key Points

- Foods containing carbohydrates from whole grains, fruits, vegetables, and low-fat milk are important components of and should be included in a healthy diet (strength of recommendation: A).
- With regard to the glycemic effects of carbohydrates, the total amount of carbohydrates in meals is more important than the source (i.e., starches or sugars) or type (i.e., GI) (strength of recommendation: B).
- There is no evidence to support that sodium restriction reduces morbidity or mortality in patients with hypertension, nor that modest sodium restriction is harmful (strength of recommendation: A).
- Diets that result in long-term weight loss of 5–7%, along with exercise of moderate intensity for at least 150 min/week (average of 30 minutes 5 times/week) have been shown to reduce the incidence of type 2 diabetes (strength of recommendation: A).
- Adherence to any diet with caloric restriction below the usual energy requirements will result in weight loss (strength of recommendation: B).
- Consumption of dietary fiber improves lipid profiles and may reduce cardiovascular morbidity and mortality (strength of recommendation: B).
- Consumption of omega-3 fatty acids improves lipid profiles and may reduce cardiovascular morbidity and mortality (strength of recommendation: B).
- For persons who consume alcohol, limiting consumption to 1–2 drinks daily may reduce mortality (strength of recommendation: B).
- Low-carbohydrate diets do not adversely affect and may improve lipid profiles, but evidence of their effect on long-term cardiovascular health is lacking (strength of recommendation: C).
- Low-fat diets can improve total cholesterol and may reduce cardiovascular risk factors (strength of recommendation: C).
- Low-carbohydrate diets are slightly more effective than low-fat diets for initial, short-term weight loss (3–6 months), but they are no more effective after 1 year (strength of recommendation: C).
- Because long-term data on patient-oriented outcomes are lacking for many diets, it is not possible to clearly endorse one diet over another (strength of recommendation: C).

Introduction

A healthy diet is essential to disease prevention, treatment, and perhaps longevity. Over the past few decades, mounting evidence has implicated diet not only as a cause, but also an adjunct to treatment for many chronic diseases such diabetes mellitus, stroke, cardiovascular disease, and obesity. These chronic diseases disproportionately affect developed countries and especially men, for whom these chronic diseases are leading causes of death. This chapter will provide a historical background of governmental nutritional guidelines, an overview of general nutrition, dietary assessment, and various guidelines that exist for low-fat, low-carbohydrate, and low-calorie options. In addition, we will examine the role of nutrition in the prevention and treatment of chronic diseases in men and conclude with evidence-based dietary recommendations to help foster change and promote healthy living.

Government Regulation

In the United States, Recommended Dietary Allowances (RDAs) were established by the Food and Nutrition Board of the National Academy of Sciences in 1941 and have since been updated 10 times. The first attempts at establishing dietary standards were made in 1894, and again during World War I, and were then formalized in 1933 with recommendations from the US Department of Agriculture (USDA) on consumption of calcium, iron, phosphorus, vitamin A, and vitamin C. The original goal of establishing an RDA for a particular nutrient was neither to treat or to prevent a chronic disease nor to optimize health, but rather to prevent a nutritional deficiency. RDAs constitute the levels of intake of essential nutrients that are adequate to meet the known needs of almost all healthy persons. In 1953, as a way to explain the RDAs to the public, the USDA introduced the four food groups: the meats, poultry, fish, and egg group; the dairy group; the breads and grains group; and the fruits and vegetables group.

In 1973, the USDA established its own set of RDAs based on those of the Food and Nutrition Board, designed to replace the minimum daily requirements that had previously been used for labeling. The final revision was established in 1989 when RDAs were determined for protein, 11 vitamins, and 7 minerals. These RDAs were set for different age groups, for men and women, and for pregnant and nursing mothers. Finally, the Board also established Estimated Safe and Adequate Daily Dietary Intakes for seven other nutrients for which insufficient data were available to establish a certain RDA. Also in 1989, the Food and Nutrition Board published a comprehensive volume, *Diet and Health,* which reviewed the available scientific literature and was later reduced into more usable forms for medical professionals and the lay public.[1]

Despite decades of constant revision, by the early 1990s the US RDAs were quickly becoming outdated and inadequate for determining optimal nutrition. An expanding interest in nutrition by both the scientific and lay communities led to questions on the importance of higher intakes of some nutrients to improve health, prevent or treat disease, or even improve performance. The RDAs were criticized for not acknowledging individual differences and emphasizing only population-level recommendations. Some consumer advocacy groups also criticized the USDA and the Food and Nutrition Board for adjusting RDAs in response to pressure from the meat and dairy industries. The USDA published the first Food Guide Pyramid in 1992 to replace the four food groups. Finally, food fortification and dietary supplements were subject to decreased regulation with the advent of the Dietary Supplement Health and Education Act of 1994.[2] Thus, from 1996 through 1997, the Food and Nutrition Board developed a new, more comprehensive approach to setting dietary guidelines. The current RDAs were revised and replaced with Dietary Reference Intakes (DRIs) to provide recommended nutrient intakes for use in a variety of settings.[3]

Each DRI value has specific recommendations based on age and gender. To help balance individual needs versus general recommendations, RDAs, adequate intakes (AIs), and tolerable upper intake levels are used as guidelines for individuals, whereas estimated average requirements provide guidelines for groups and populations (Table 19-1). The 1997 revisions also incorporated, for the first time, factors that might modify these guidelines, such as bioavailability of nutrients from different sources, nutrient-nutrient and nutrient-drug interactions, and intakes from food fortifiers and supplements.

RDAs and DRIs are used as the baseline in making more general recommendations regarding which foods to consume. Recommendations now focus on altering dietary components to reduce the risk of disease as well as highlighting the types and amounts of foods required to prevent deficiencies. Using the Food and Nutrition Board's new DRIs as a base, these recommendations are published jointly by the USDA and US Department of Health and Human Services as the Dietary Guidelines for Americans and have been updated every 5 years since 1980, with the most recent update in 2005.[4]

Other governmental and public and private nonprofit groups such as the American Heart Association (AHA), the American Diabetes Association (ADA), the World Health Organization, the Institute of Medicine, the National Research Council, Physicians Committee for Responsible Medicine, Oldways Preservation and Exchange Trust, and various branches within the National Institutes of Health have also published guidelines and recommendations on the role of diet in health. Private industry lobbying groups, such as the National Dairy Council, the United Fresh Fruit and Vegetable Association, the Soft Drink Association, the American Meat Institute, the Cattlemen's Beef Association, and the Wheat Foods Council, may also promote certain foods to the public and the government.[5]

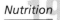

Table 19-1. US Department of Agriculture Dietary Reference Intakes

Recommended dietary allowance (RDA)	Average daily nutrient intake level that is sufficient to meet the nutrient requirements of nearly all persons (97–98%) in a given life stage and gender group, intended for assessing the diets of healthy individuals, not for assessing or planning diets for groups
Acceptable macronutrient distribution range	Range of macronutrient intakes for a particular energy source associated with reduced risk of chronic disease while providing adequate intakes of essential nutrients
Adequate intake	Recommended average daily nutrient level based on observed or experimentally determined estimates of average nutrient intakes by a group of healthy persons, used when the RDA cannot be determined and may be used to plan and evaluate diets of individuals or groups
Tolerable upper intake level	The highest daily nutrient intake that is likely to pose no risk of toxicity for almost all individuals in a given life stage and gender group
Estimated average requirement	Nutrient intake value estimated to meet the requirement defined by a specific indicator of adequacy in 50% of individuals in a given life stage and gender group and is expressed as a daily value over time (e.g., at least 1 week), including adjustments for bioavailability, and should not be used as an intake goal for an individual

Adapted from: Nutrition.gov. Available at http://www.nutrition.gov. Accessed August 4, 2006.

Nutritional Basics

From an evolutionary standpoint, human biology encourages and is well adapted to the consumption and storage of food whenever available. Humans are naturally omnivorous and have evolutionarily driven preferences for foods that contain nutrients, such as salt or fat, that were historically scarce or good sources of energy. Although there is considerable debate on the "original" or Paleolithic diets of early man, unquestionably, social changes over the millennia have made all types of nutrients more accessible, with a resultant impact on health. The relationship between diet and health is extraordinarily complex, which makes it difficult to define nutritional quality.

Clearly, nutritional quality is determined by the nutrient composition of the diet. *Nutrients* are substances in food that provide energy and contribute to the structure and function of all biologic processes that are essential to life. Food is built from essential and nonessential nutrients as well as nonnutritive compounds. More than 45 individual nutrients are classified as *essential* to human life, meaning that they must be provided regularly through the diet. *Nonessential* nutrients can be made by the body in sufficient quantity and thus are not required to be ingested. *Macronutrients* include carbohydrates, lipids, and proteins and are required in relatively large amounts (i.e., gram and kilogram quantities) by the body as they are energy containing; although it contains no energy, water is also considered to be a macronutrient. *Micronutrients* include vitamins and minerals and are required in relatively small amounts (i.e., microgram or milligram quantities). Other substances including alcohol may also be consumed in the diet but do not fit into any of these classes because they are not required by the body. Some non-nutritive substances may play important roles in promoting health and minimizing disease. Optimal nutrition results from the proper combination of nutrients from foods.

Macronutrients

Lipids

Fats (i.e., solids at room temperature) and oils (i.e., liquids at room temperature) are the major forms of lipids consumed in the diet. Lipids are the most concentrated energy source at 9 kilocalories (Calories) per gram. The USDA suggests that 20–35% of the diet consist of fat. Based on a 2200-Calorie/day diet, this allows for approximately 50–85 g of fat per day. No RDA or AI has been set for lipid intake. The acceptable macronutrient distribution range, which provides a minimum amount required for physiologic function, suggests 20–35 g/day for a 70-kg male.[6] Lipids, which may be of either animal or plant origin, include fatty acids, glycerides, phospholipids, and sterols.

Fatty acids may be saturated (containing no carbon-carbon double bonds), monounsaturated (containing one double bond), or polyunsaturated (multiple double bonds). Increasing the double bonds lowers the melting temperature, which is why mono- and polyunsaturated fatty acids are more likely to be liquid at room temperature. Common saturated fatty acids include palmitic and stearic acids and are often found in animal sources. Tropical oils such as palm, palm kernel, and coconut also contain saturated fatty acids. The DRI for saturated fats suggest an intake as low as possible because they have no physiologic requirement in the body. Monounsaturated fatty acids are most commonly obtained as oleic acid, which is prevalent in olive, peanut, and canola oils. Approximately one half of the daily fat intake should be in the form of monounsaturated fats.

Polyunsaturated fatty acids are named for the location of the first double bond in the carbon chain. The most important of these are the essential fatty acids (EFAs). These include linoleic acid and arachidonic acid, which are omega-6 (n-6) fatty acids, and alpha-linolenic acid, eicosapentaenoic acid (EPA), and docosahexaenoic acid (DHA), which are omega-3 (n-3) fatty acids. In the body, arachidonic acid can be made from linoleic acid, and EPA and DHA can be made from linolenic acid. Although these fatty acids can be manufactured by the body, they are considered essential because the rate at which they are synthesized may not be sufficient to meet the body's needs. EFAs are needed for many physiologic processes, including maintaining the integrity of the skin and the structure of cell membranes and synthesizing prostaglandins and leukotrienes. EPA and DHA are important components of the brain and retina. Alpha-linoleic acid is found vegetable oils, and EPA is primarily obtained from cold-water fish oils. Linoleic acid is the primary omega-6 fatty acid in the American diet and is obtained from corn, soybean, and safflower oils. Omega-3 fatty acids may have a protective benefit in heart disease.[7]

EFAs are damaged by processing in the manufacture of cooking oils, margarines, shortenings, partially hydrogenated vegetable oils, and *trans*-fatty acids, and are also damaged by sautéing and frying. The RDAs for an adult male are 1.6 g/day of omega-3 fatty acids and 17 g/day (decreasing to 14 g/day for men older than 50 years) of omega-6 fatty acids.[6] Deficiencies of fatty acids are rare in the US and include nonspecific dermatitis, liver abnormalities, impaired wound healing and vision.

Trans-fatty acids (also called *trans-fat*) are those unsaturated fatty acids in which the hydrogen atoms are found on opposite sides of the double-bond ("trans" configuration), which is opposite of the normal *cis* configuration usually found in nature. *Trans*-fats are formed during the hydrogenation of oils, a processing technique used in commercial foods by bubbling hydrogen gas through liquid vegetable oils. The resulting product, partially hydrogenated vegetable oil, has improved storage characteristics and an increased melting point. Diets with increased *trans*-fats have been shown to raise low-density lipoprotein (LDL) cholesterol and decrease high-density lipoprotein (HDL) cholesterol. Recent recommendations regarding the role of *trans*-fats in the diet have called for mandatory reporting of amounts in food and suggestions for elimination. The AHA 2006 Diet and Lifestyle Recommendations call for *trans*-fat to be limited to less than 1% of total caloric intake. The USDA Dietary Guidelines call for *trans*-fat to be limited to as little as possible.

Other types of lipids are also important in the diet. Most fatty acids in food are found as a component of glycerides; triglycerides are the most common form of lipid in both food and in the body. Phospholipids are those containing a phosphate group, such as phosphoglycerides. Sterols are lipids composed of multiple carbon rings; cholesterol is the most well known lipid in this class. Although cholesterol is essential to the body, it is manufactured in significant quantities by the liver and is thus not an essential lipid. Intake of cholesterol should be as low as possible, ideally below 200 mg daily.[6]

Carbohydrates

Carbohydrates are energy-containing compounds composed of carbon, hydrogen, and oxygen that supply 4 Calories/g. They are classified as either *simple* carbohydrates (i.e., simple sugars) or *complex* carbohydrates (i.e., starches). Glucose is the end product of all carbohydrate digestion and serves as the primary energy source for the body. Glucose metabolism in healthy adults is tightly regulated primarily by the endocrine pancreas, which produces both insulin and glucagon. Monosaccharides, including glucose, are the basic component of all carbohydrates. Other monosaccharides include galactose, which is rarely found in food, and fructose, which is found in honey, fruits, and vegetables. Disaccharides include maltose (found in breads), sucrose (table sugar, found in honey, cane sugar, and maple syrup), and lactose (found in milk). Lactose consumption is a common cause of diarrhea, abdominal cramping, and bloating in persons who are lactase deficient, a problem which occurs rarely in Northern Europeans but is more common in East Asians. Complex carbohydrates are termed *polysaccharides* and include glycogen in animals and starch and fiber in plants. Plant starch is found as either amylose, which consists of long chains of glucose, or amylopectin, which consists of branched chains of glucose. The RDA for carbohydrates for adult men is 130 g/day. Added sugars should be limited to no more than 25% of total caloric intake.[6]

Although simple and complex carbohydrates have different biochemical properties, their physiologic action in the body may or may not significantly differ. A recent and increasingly popular method of understanding how carbohydrates work in the body is a rating scale called the *glycemic index* (GI) (Figure 19-1). This scale is a relative ranking of a carbohydrate's ability to raise plasma glucose on a scale from 0 to 100, with low-glycemic foods rated below 55 and those rated over 70 considered to have a high GI.[8] GI is not an unalterable and intrinsic property of a food, like fat or vitamin content, but rather it is a relative property in comparison to other foods. It is determined by feeding 50 g of the food to 10 healthy people after an overnight fast. Finger-stick blood glucose samples are taken at 15–30-minute intervals over the next 2 hours. These blood samples are then averaged and used to construct a blood sugar response curve for the 2-hour period. The area under the curve (AUC) is calculated to reflect the total rise in blood glucose levels after the test food is eaten. The GI rating (%) is calculated by dividing the AUC for the test food by the AUC for the reference food (50 g of glucose) and multiplying by 100.[8] Foods with a high GI are rapidly digested and absorbed and result in a rapid increase in plasma glucose. High-GI foods include maltose, glucose, dextrose, white breads and rice, and pancakes and muffins. Watermelons, bananas, pineapple, raisins, corn, potatoes, carrots, and turnips are also high-GI foods. Low-GI foods have a slower rate of rise in plasma glucose and a smaller related increase in insulin. These include most fruits, vegetables, and whole-grain products. Pasta, due to the presence of gluten, is a low- to intermediate-GI food. Dark chocolate (over 60% cocoa) is also a low-GI food.

The term *glycemic load* builds on this concept. A GI value describes how quickly a carbohydrate increases serum glucose but does not describe the amount of carbohydrate in a particular food. The glycemic load is the GI divided by 100, multiplied by its available carbohydrate content (i.e., carbohydrates minus fiber) in grams.[9] A glycemic load of 20 or more is high, a glycemic load of 11–19 is medium, and a glycemic load of 10 or less is low. Foods that have a low glycemic load almost always have a low GI. Foods with an intermediate or high glycemic load range from very low to very high GI. High-GI foods, however, may be useful for quickly restoring glycogen stores after exercise. Low-GI carbohydrates form the basis of many of the low-carbohydrate diets.[10] Diets with low-GI foods and low overall glycemic load may result in weight loss, improvement in serum lipid levels, and improved insulin sensitivity.[11] A standard reference for GI was published as the International Tables of Glycemic Index by *The American Journal of Clinical Nutrition* in 1995 and 2002.[8,12]

Although the GI and glycemic load are useful pieces of information, they have several limitations. First, these numbers are not readily obtainable by consumers. Second, a food's GI is influenced greatly by processing, storage, and preparation. Third, the GI for a food is specific for only that food consumed individually, which is not how most people eat. Others foods and beverages consumed at the same time affect GI. Finally, the GI may confuse consumers into believing that all high-GI foods are unhealthy (including watermelons, corn, carrots, and baked potatoes) and all low-GI foods are good (including french fries), which is not necessarily the case.

Protein

Proteins are the most complex and diverse group of macronutrients in the diet. They are organic, nitrogen-containing compounds composed of amino acids. Protein is obtained from both animal sources and plant sources. Animal sources are considered to be complete because they provide all essential amino acids in the proper proportions for human use. Plant sources are incomplete protein sources because they individually cannot provide all essential amino acids. There are 20 amino acids that form the building blocks of all proteins in the diet; 9 of these are essential, and 11 are nonessential and are formed

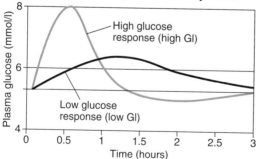

Figure 19-1. Glycemic response in health adults. GI, Glycemic index. (Adapted from: Home of the glycemic index. University of Sydney. Available at: http://www.glycemicindex.com. Accessed August 4, 2006.)

from the transamination of other amino acids. The essential amino acids include the three branched-chain amino acids valine, isoleucine, and leucine, as well as lysine, methionine, phenylalanine, threonine, tryptophan, and histidine. Alanine, arginine, asparagine, aspartic acid, cysteine, tyrosine, glutamic acid, glutamine, glycine, proline, and serine are nonessential.

Protein provides structure for the body, regulates metabolism, and provides energy. Through the digestive process, protein is denatured and absorbed in the small intestine as tripeptides and smaller structures, which are eventually completely degraded into their constituent amino acids. This digestive process is imperfect and occasionally results in disease. Food allergies are caused by abnormal foreign body immune response to normal proteins in the intestinal tract. Gluten sensitivity, or celiac disease, is an enteropathy resulting in intestinal inflammation from a reaction to gluten protein, which is found in wheat, oats, barley, and rye.

Like carbohydrates, protein contains 4 Calories/g. Protein beyond that required by the diet is used for energy or converted into fat or carbohydrate stores. The RDA for protein in adult males is 0.8 g/kg, or 56 g/day in an average-sized (70-kg) male.[6] A severe infection may increase protein needs by one third. Burns increase protein requirements by two- to four-fold. Endurance athletes and other athletes who are actively building muscle mass may require a higher amount of protein, in the range of 1.0–1.5 g of protein per kilogram of body weight.[6]

The amount of protein required by the body depends greatly on the current nitrogen balance. If more nitrogen is lost than is ingested, the body is in a negative nitrogen balance and intake should be increased. This occurs when stress is applied to the body—such as when burns, infection, or trauma occur—without a compensatory increase in the protein intake. A positive nitrogen balance occurs when less nitrogen is lost than ingested. This could occur during times of wound healing, muscle building, or growth. If a negative nitrogen balance is experienced long enough, disease will arise. Kwashiorkor is a rare yet severe type of protein-energy malnutrition that occurs with extremely low protein intake. Typically thought of as a disease of children in developing countries, kwashiorkor may also occur in hospitalized and chronically ill adult men. Marasmus is another severe type of protein-energy malnutrition in which massive chronic caloric deficits results in ketosis and eventual muscle wasting. This occurs during starvation that may be seen during famine and certain types of eating disorders. Protein and energy supplementation in the form of commercial shakes, such as Boost or Ensure, may have a beneficial effect on weight gain and mortality but lack evidence for improvement in clinical outcome, functional benefit, or reduction in length of hospitalization according to a review of 49 trials covering 4970 patients conducted by the Cochrane Database.[13]

Water

Water is essential for survival. The average adult male can survive only a few days without fluid intake. Approximately 60% of body mass in an adult male is composed of water, approximately two thirds of which is blood, interstitial fluid, and other extracellular fluids. Water serves as a universal solvent in the body, maintains homeostasis, and allows for transport of nutrients to cells and removal and excretion of waste products of metabolism. Water balance is tightly regulated by the body through interactions of the pituitary-renal axis via arginine vasopressin (antidiuretic hormone). Typical water loss for an adult male is 2 liters of urine per day, 200 mL of water lost in feces, and 1.5 liters are excreted in insensible losses. The AI for adult males is thus approximately 3.7 liters of water per day obtained through both food and beverage.[14] There is no upper limit listed for water because water intoxication is extremely rare in healthy adults.

Micronutrients

Vitamins

Vitamins are essential nutrients. An organic compound is classified as a vitamin if a lack of the compound in the diet results in symptoms that are then relieved by addition of the substance back into the diet. Vitamins promote and regulate a variety of chemical reactions in the body, act as coenzymes, and are necessary for many physiologic processes. Vitamins are named alphabetically in the order they were discovered. Some substances originally classified as vitamins were later found to be nonessential and were thus dropped, resulting in gaps in the list. Others, such as the B vitamin series, were once thought to be one compound but later found to be many different substances and were thus numbered. There are 13 recognized vitamins that are classified as either water soluble or fat soluble. Several vitamin-like compounds, including choline, carnitine, taurine, inositol, ubiquinone (coenzyme

Q 10), and lipoic acid, serve essential physiologic functions but are not known to be required in the diet because they are synthesized in the body in adequate amounts. Although choline is not a vitamin, the Food and Nutrition Board established an AI of 550 mg/day with a upper limit of 3.5 g daily.[15]

Water-Soluble Vitamins. The water-soluble vitamins include the entire B complex series and vitamin C.

Thiamine, also called *vitamin B₁* or aneurine, acts as a coenzyme in the metabolism of carbohydrates and branched-chain amino acids. Good sources of thiamine include enriched or fortified bakery products and cereals, whole grains, nuts, legumes, seeds, and pork. Deficiency results in depression, weakness, and eventual loss of coordination (Wernicke's encephalopathy) and paresthesias that constitute "dry" beriberi. Advanced or "wet" beriberi results from heart failure and weakening of the capillary walls and subsequent edema. Persons with alcoholism are particularly susceptible to thiamine deficiency because of increased need for the vitamin with alcohol metabolism and decreased absorption and intake. There is no known toxicity for thiamine. The RDA in adult males for thiamine is 1.2 mg/day with no upper limit.[15]

Riboflavin, *vitamin B₂*, forms the coenzymes flavin mononucleotide and flavin adenine dinucleotide, which work in the citric acid cycle and in the breakdown of fatty acids. These coenzymes also are active in the electron transport chain. Good sources of riboflavin include milk and other dairy products, red meat, fish, poultry, asparagus, broccoli, and mushrooms. Ariboflavinosis results from a sustained deficiency over a period of months and consists of conjunctivitis, glossitis, and dermatitis. There is no known toxicity for riboflavin, although high intakes will result in brightly yellow urine. The RDA in adult males for riboflavin is 1.3 mg/day with no upper limit.[15]

Niacin, *vitamin B₃*, acts as a coenzyme in a variety of reduction-oxidation reactions. Two forms, nicotinic acid and nicotinamide, are obtained from the diet. Either form can be converted into nicotinamide adenine dinucleotide and nicotinamide adenine dinucleotide phosphate. These coenzymes act in glycolysis, the citric acid cycle, and the electron transport chain. Good sources of niacin include meat, fish, whole grains, asparagus, peanuts, and mushrooms. Niacin can be synthesized in the body from tryptophan. Deficiency results in pellagra ("raw skin"), a disease consisting of *d*ermatitis and *d*iarrhea with eventual progression to *d*ementia and *d*eath (i.e., "the four Ds"). There is no known toxicity for niacin, although high intakes may cause flushing and elevation in liver enzyme levels. Niacin is indicated in high doses (1–2 g daily) as a pharmacologic agent in hypercholesterolemia and mixed dyslipidemia. The RDA in adult males for niacin is 35 mg/day with no upper limit.[15]

Vitamin B₆, or pyridoxine, is actually a group of closely related compounds that are converted into a coenzyme, pyridoxal phosphate. Six compounds, pyridoxamine, pyridoxine, pyridoxal, and three 5'-phosphates (PLP, PMP, PNP) are commonly consumed in the diet. Vitamin B₆ acts as a coenzyme in the metabolism of glycogen, amino acids, and sphingoid bases. Good sources include chicken, fish, pork, liver, whole grains, brown rice, soybean, peanuts, walnuts, eggs, yeast, bananas, broccoli, and spinach. Vitamin B₆ is lost quickly with processing during food preparation. Vitamin B₆ supplementation has not been helpful for the relief of carpal tunnel syndrome.[16,17] Results of the Norwegian Vitamin Trial[18] found that vitamin B₆ and folate may worsen cardiovascular disease outcome when used to treat elevated homocysteine levels. Vitamin B₆ supplementation did not improve short-term mood or cognitive functions in a trial of 76 elderly men.[19] Deficiency results in depression, headaches, confusion, and possible seizures. Important nutrient-drug interactions include hydralazine and isoniazid, which both interfere with metabolism of the vitamin. Sensory neuropathy may result from toxic overdose. The RDA in adult males for pyridoxine is 1.3 mg/day for adult men younger than 50 years and 1.7 mg for men aged 50 years and older, with an upper limit of 100 mg daily.[15]

Vitamin B₁₂, also called cobalamin or cyanocobalamin, is group of cobalt-containing coenzymes. Vitamin B₁₂ is synthesized by bacteria, fungi, and algae and accumulates in animals. Good sources include beef and poultry. Algae and fermented soy products such as miso and tempeh are some of the few available plant-based sources. Absorption of vitamin B₁₂ requires the presence of intrinsic factor, a protein secreted by parietal cells in the stomach. The presence of gastric acid, pancreatic bicarbonate, and trypsin is also required. As such, alcoholics, elderly persons, patients with pancreatic insufficiency, patients taking acid-blocking medications, and those who have undergone gastrectomy or other radical gastric surgery are at high risk for folate deficiency. Because plant sources are very poor in vitamin B_{12}, vegetarians may be at risk for developing deficiency. Deficiency of folate results in pernicious anemia, characterized by macrocytic anemia and severe irreversible peripheral and central neuropathy. Although vitamin B_{12} has a clear role in treatment of pernicious anemia, supplementation in the well-known vitamin B_{12} injections for undifferentiated fatigue have no established benefit. A Cochrane Database of Systematic Reviews[20] found insufficient evidence to support the efficacy of vitamin B_{12} in improving cognitive function in patients with dementia and low serum vitamin B_{12} levels. There is no known toxicity for vitamin B_{12}. The RDA in adult males for vitamin B_{12} is 2.4 μg/day with no upper limit.[15]

Folate or *folic acid* are general terms for a group of closely related B-complex vitamins including folacin and pteroylpolyglutamates. They serve as coenzymes in nucleic acid production and metabolism of amino acids. Good sources of folate include liver, yeast, spinach, and legumes. Folate is naturally unstable and easily degraded during food preparation. Persons with alcoholism are at high risk for folate deficiency. Deficiency of folate results in megaloblastic or macrocytic anemia. Caution should be exercised when supplementing folate empirically for macrocytic anemia because replacement may mask vitamin B_{12} deficiency. Folate supplementation is also used to prevent neural tube defects in pregnancy. There is no known toxicity for folate. The RDA in adult males for folate is 400 μg/day with a 1000-μg upper limit.[15]

Biotin is another B-complex vitamin that serves as a coenzyme in carboxylation reactions. Good sources of biotin include egg yolks, soy, cereal, and yeast. Foods containing raw egg whites contain a protein called *avidin* that binds with biotin, interfering with its absorption. Deficiency is uncommon but may be seen in persons who frequently consume raw egg whites and those with different types of malabsorption syndromes. Symptoms of deficiency include nausea, loss of hair and change in hair color, depression, and paresthesias. There is no known toxicity level for biotin. Although no RDA exists, the AI in adult males for biotin is 30 μg/day with no upper limit.[15]

Pantothenic acid is a part of coenzyme A, involved in the metabolism of protein, carbohydrates, and fat. It is also involved in cholesterol and fatty acid synthesis. Good sources of pantothenic acid include meat, eggs, whole grains, legumes, egg yolks, tomatoes, and broccoli. Deficiency is uncommon. There is no known toxicity level for pantothenic acid. Although no RDA

exists, the AI in adult males for pantothenic acid is 5 mg/day with no upper limit.[15]

Vitamin C, or ascorbic acid, serves many purposes. It acts as an electron donor in hydroxylation reactions, serving as a cofactor for reactions requiring reduced copper or iron metalloenzymes, and it also acts as an antioxidant. Vitamin C regenerates the antioxidant properties of vitamin E and improves intestinal absorption of iron. Vitamin C plays a crucial role in the formation of collagen. Good sources of vitamin C include citrus fruits, berries, melons, and members of the cabbage family. Scurvy results from deficiency, with symptoms of poor wound healing, gingival bleeding, bone and joint pains, and hemorrhage. Toxicity results in nausea, diarrhea, and abdominal cramps. Kidney stones, acid-base imbalances, and destruction of vitamin B_{12} may also occur. Vitamin C supplementation is commonly used to prevent and treat upper respiratory viruses, although research has been equivocal. Vitamin C is also used at dosages of 1 g/day for 3 weeks before competition for athletes, but no conclusive evidence of improved performance has been noted. The RDA in adult males for vitamin C is 90 mg/day with a 2000-mg upper limit; persons who smoke require an additional 35 mg of vitamin C daily.[21]

Fat-soluble Vitamins. The fat-soluble vitamins are A, D, E, and K.

Vitamin A comes in the forms of retinoids or carotenoids. Retinoids include retinal, retinol, and retinoic acid and are used in vision, growth, reproduction, and maintenance of epithelial tissue. Liver, eggs, and dairy products are particularly good sources of retinoids. At least 50 provitamin carotenoids can be converted into vitamin A, with beta-carotene as the most potent. These yellow, orange, and red pigments are found in carrots, squash, apricots, peppers, and green leafy vegetables. Vitamin A is also obtained through the use of retinoid-containing skin products. Deficiency of vitamin A may result in night blindness, xerophthalmia, and impaired immunity. Although vitamin A acts as an antioxidant, no protective role has clearly been established in preventing cancer and other diseases or slowing the aging process. Vitamin A is toxic in acute or chronic overdose and may cause hypercarotenemia, in which carotenoids deposited in body fat cause the skin to appear yellow. Toxic levels of vitamin A may worsen or predispose men to osteoporosis. The RDA in adult males for vitamin A is 900 μg with an upper limit of 3000 μg/day.[22]

Vitamin D, or calciferol, is in many aspects as much a hormone as a vitamin. It is produced in the skin from exposure to sunlight and has multiple effects on other organs. It is considered a vitamin because it becomes essential in the diet for persons who have limited sun exposure. Good sources of vitamin D include liver, fish, and fortified dairy products. Vitamin D exists in two forms: ergocalciferol (D_2) from plant sources and cholecalciferol (D_3) from animal sources. Both types are inactive until they are converted into 25-hydroxy vitamin D in the liver and then 1,25-dihydroxy vitamin D in the kidney. Vitamin D acts in the body to regulate calcium and phosphorus metabolism through interaction with parathyroid hormone and calcitonin. Deficiency results in rickets in children and osteomalacia in adults. Vitamin D may be more important than calcium in maintaining bone health.[23] Vitamin D is more likely to be deficient in homebound elderly persons and patients with end-stage kidney disease. Vitamin D is toxic in low levels of overdose, resulting in hypercalcemia. Although no RDA exists, the AI in males 19–50 years old for vitamin D is 5 µg, increasing to 10 µg daily in men aged 51–70 years and 15 µg daily for men older than 70 years, with an upper limit of 50 µg/day.[24] Vitamin D intake is also often expressed in international units (IU), where 40 IU equals 1 µg.

Vitamin E, or tocopherol, exists in several different forms. Alpha-tocopherol is the most common and most potent form. Good sources of vitamin E include plant oils, grains, nuts, and leafy green vegetables. The exact physiologic function of vitamin E has not been established but it is thought to function as an antioxidant. No conclusive studies have linked vitamin E with decreased rates of cancer or established it as an effective treatment for heart disease. Vitamin E has recently been included in a mixture of antioxidants that convincingly slowed the progression of age-related macular degeneration in the Age-Related Eye Disease Study.[25] Vitamin E deficiency is rare but may result in intravascular hemolysis and subsequent anemia; toxicity is likewise uncommon. Vitamin E interferes with vitamin K absorption and, therefore, supplementation should be cautioned for persons taking Coumadin (warfarin). The RDA in adult males for vitamin E is 15 µg with an upper limit of 1000 µg/day.[21]

Vitamin K, like all fat-soluble vitamins, exists in multiple forms: phylloquinone from plants and menaquinone from animals and intestinal microflora. Good sources of vitamin K include dark green, leafy vegetables, vegetable oils, and liver. Vitamin K is also obtained from production by intestinal microflora. Vitamin K is used in the production of prothrombin and other clotting factors. Vitamin K also interacts with vitamin D in bone metabolism. Deficiency of vitamin K results in uncontrolled hemorrhage. This fact is used by blood-thinning medications derived from coumarol and dicumarol, including Coumadin. Therefore, although patients taking warfarin should not be discouraged from eating dark, leafy vegetables and taking multivitamins containing vitamin K, caution and frequent monitoring is suggested if these are suddenly introduced or removed from the diet. Although no RDA exists, the AI in adult males is 120 µg daily with no determination on an upper limit.[22]

Minerals

Minerals are nonorganic elements that are essential for a wide array of biologic processes. They may be grouped as either major or trace minerals. Major minerals are required in amounts of 100 mg or more per day or are present in the body in greater than 0.01% of body weight and include four cations (i.e., sodium, potassium, magnesium, calcium) and three anions (i.e., phosphorus, chloride, and sulfur). Bicarbonate also serves as a major anion but is not considered a micronutrient.

Major Minerals. *Sodium* is the major electrolyte in blood and therefore a principal regulator of fluid volume in the body and a key factor in nerve transmission. It is obtained from a wide variety of dietary sources, as most processed foods contain added sodium chloride. Even softened drinking water may contain a significant amount of sodium. Serum sodium is tightly regulated by the renin-angiotensin system. Because the typical American diet is high in sodium, chronic deficiency is extremely rare. However, acute hyponatremia may occur in endurance and high-performance athletes who lose more sodium than they replace. Acute hyponatremia may present with muscle cramps and nausea and progress to confusion and coma. Persons with salt-sensitive hypertension (approximately half of those with primary hypertension) should be counseled to follow a low-sodium diet, which is discussed later in this chapter. Typical American dietary intake in men is approximately 4 g of sodium daily, which is above the recommended upper limit. Despite this, no toxic effects from high sodium intake are usually observed. A Cochrane Database review found that a low-salt diet in normotensive persons had a statistically significant but clinically insignificant effect on blood pressure but was helpful in short-term reduction of blood pressure in white persons with elevated blood pressure.[26] Although no RDA exists, the AI in adult males is 1.5 g/day in men aged 18–50 years, 1.3 g in men aged 50–70 years, and 1.2 g in men older than 70 years with an upper limit of 2.3 g.[14]

Potassium is another major electrolyte, serving as a major intracellular ion and functioning in nerve transmission. Like sodium, it is regulated by the kidney. It is obtained from fresh fruits, vegetables, and unprocessed meats. Potassium deficiency is much more common than sodium deficiency. Persons with high-salt diets and those taking most types of diuretics are likely to have lower serum potassium levels. Symptoms of deficiency may include arrhythmia, fatigue, and muscle cramps. Toxicity from hyperkalemia is common in end-stage renal failure but extremely uncommon in patients with normal renal function and may result in cardiac arrhythmias. The AI is 4.7 g/day with no upper limit.[14]

Chloride serves as the opposite, negatively charged, extracellular ion to sodium. Chloride balance is also regulated by the kidney. Chloride is usually obtained in the diet as salt with sodium. Deficiencies in chloride are uncommon, although hypochloremia may occur with prolonged vomiting and with use of diuretic medications. The AI in adult males is 2.3 g/day for men aged 18–50 years, decreasing to 2.0 g in men aged 50–70 years and 1.8 g in men older than 70 years, with an upper limit of 3.6 g daily.[14]

Calcium is the most abundant mineral in the body. Ninety-nine percent of total body calcium is bound with phosphorus in hydroxyapatite, found in bones and teeth. The remainder is found in both intravascular and extravascular fluid, where it is involved with nerve transmission, muscular contraction, and blood clotting. Calcium is commonly obtained as a salt in the diet in the forms of calcium carbonate, citrate, phosphate, gluconate, malate, and lactate. Good sources of calcium include dairy, bony fish, and leafy green vegetables. Calcium is best absorbed in the presence of vitamin D, whereas absorption is decreased in the presence of magnesium and iron. Calcium is tightly regulated and balanced with phosphorus via the actions of calcitonin and parathyroid hormone, as well as vitamin D from the kidney. A diet high in calcium—and in particular, dairy foods—may increase weight loss in patients on low-calorie diets.[27] However, diets high in calcium from dairy foods have been

linked to increased rates of prostate cancer in some studies, including a prospective trial of 2776 men.[28] Calcium supplementation is also being investigated in the prevention of adenomatous colonic polyps.[29] Calcium deficiency may result in muscle cramps and osteoporosis. Toxicity may result in a predisposition to nephrolithiasis, constipation, and inhibition of absorption of other minerals. The AI in adult males is 1 g/day for men aged 18–50 years, increasing to 1200 mg in men older than 50 years with an upper limit of 2.5 g daily.[24]

Phosphorus is bound to calcium in bones and teeth. In addition, it exists in both intravascular and extravascular fluid, where it acts as a buffer, is a major constituent of nucleic acids, and is involved intimately in energy production as adenosine diphosphate and triphosphate. Good sources of phosphorus include meat, dairy, cereals, and other baked goods. Deficiency is uncommon but may result in weakness, bone loss, and lack of appetite; toxicity may result in bone resorption. The RDA in adult males is 700 mg/day with an upper limit of 4 g daily decreasing to 3 g daily for men older than 70 years.[24]

Magnesium is involved in energy production and nerve and muscle function. It is involved in numerous enzymatic reactions including glycolysis, fat oxidation, protein synthesis, and adenosine triphosphate synthesis. The majority of magnesium in the body is in bone, with 40% found in muscle and soft tissue. A small amount is in extracellular and intravascular fluid. Concentration of magnesium is regulated by the kidney. Good sources of magnesium from the diet include nuts, leafy green vegetables, and whole grains. Magnesium absorption is enhanced by vitamin D. Although magnesium has been touted as an ergogenic aide, no studies have shown that magnesium supplementation can increase performance in athletes with normal diets. Symptoms of deficiency include nausea, vomiting, weakness, and cardiac arrhythmias. Patients with alcoholism or end-stage kidney disease are at high risk for magnesium deficiency. Magnesium toxicity may result in diarrhea, nausea, and hypotension. The RDA in adult males is 420 mg/day with an upper limit of 350 mg/day of supplement beyond any amount obtained in the diet.[24]

Sulfur, or sulfate, is an important component of the essential amino acid methionine and the nonessential amino acid cysteine. It is involved in acid–base balance. No deficiencies or toxicities are known. There is no RDA, AI, nor upper limit for sulfur.[14]

Trace Minerals. The trace minerals group includes 19 different chemical elements that serve as important nutrients to various extents in the human body. They include 14 known to be essential: arsenic, boron, copper, chromium, fluoride, iodine, iron, manganese, molybdenum, nickel, selenium, silicon, vanadium, and zinc. Five others may also play a role in health but have not been conclusively demonstrated as essential. These include cadmium, cobalt, lead, lithium, and tin. Several of these minerals, such as arsenic, cadmium, and lead are normally toxic but are safe in trace amounts. There are also trace minerals that may be found in the body but have no known biologic function. Their presence in the diet and the body likely reflects only their concentration in nature. This category is fairly loose, changing from time to time, and includes bromine, mercury, tungsten, and aluminum.

Arsenic, found in organic forms from fish and grains, is generally nontoxic. It is used in heart function and cell growth. Inorganic arsenic may be fatal in toxic doses as small as 0.6 mg/kg.[30] There is no RDA, AI, nor upper limit for arsenic, although arsenic needs are estimated at 12–15 μg daily.[22]

Boron is involved in calcium and magnesium metabolism. As such, it plays a role in bone health. Fruits, vegetables, and nuts are high in boron. There is no RDA or AI for boron, but estimated needs are about 0.5–3 mg daily; the upper limit is 20 mg daily.[22]

Chromium is used in glucose metabolism to facilitate insulin action and is obtained from brewer's yeast, nuts, whole grains, and mushrooms. Deficiency may result in diabetes-like symptoms. Despite claims for anabolic or ergogenic actions, no adequate studies have shown that chromium supplementation can increase performance in athletes with normal diets. The AI in adult males is 35 μg/day for men 18–50 years old and 30 μg daily for men older than 50 years, with no determined upper limit.[22]

Copper is important in wound healing and in the formation of ceruloplasmin. Deficiency leads to anemia and impaired antibody formation and inflammatory responses. Toxicity, as evidenced by Wilson's disease, may result in cirrhosis and chronic liver failure. The RDA for adult men is 900 μg/day with an upper limit of 10,000 μg.[22]

Fluoride is present in small amounts in all soil, water, plants, and animals. The main source in the United States is from fluoridated water supplies. Fluoride supplementation is indicated for the prevention of dental caries. Fluoride is also involved in bone health. Toxicity may result in paradoxic fractures. The RDA for adult men is 4 mg/day with an upper limit of 10 mg.[24]

Iodine is obtained mainly from seafood and iodized (dietary) salt. Iodine is an essential component of thyroid hormone. Deficiency results in cretinism in children, characterized by failure to thrive and mental retardation. In adults, iodine deficiency results in hypothyroidism and the formation of a goiter. Toxicity results in paradoxic goiter from hyperthyroidism. Although iodine supplementation clearly increases the body's iodine status, the Cochrane Database[31] found insufficient evidence for improvements in other, more patient-oriented outcomes. The RDA for adult men is 150 μg/day, with an upper limit of 1.1 mg.[22]

Iron is quickly bound to transferrin and carried throughout the body, most importantly to the bone marrow, where it is used for the production of hemoglobin. Heme iron sources such as red meat and liver are better absorbed than non-heme sources, such as dark leafy vegetables. A low gastric pH also facilitates absorption. The average adult male consumes approximately 15 mg of iron per day but absorbs only about 1–2 mg daily. Unlike women, men do not have a constant source iron loss beyond normal gastrointestinal and skin sloughing, which accounts for about 1–2 mg of iron loss daily. Also unlike women, middle-aged men are more likely to have iron deficiency anemia than younger men. Iron supplements used to correct deficiency should be taken with vitamin C to improve absorption. Low iron stores, as evidenced by ferritin levels below 50 μg/liter, may result in a wide variety of symptoms, including fatigue, paresthesias, and restless legs syndrome. Low ferritin levels, even in the absence of frank anemia, are an indication for supplementation. The RDA for adult men is 8 mg/day with an upper limit of 45 mg.[22]

Manganese is obtained from whole grains, cereal, and nuts. It is involved in carbohydrate and lipid metabolism. Deficiency is exceedingly rare but may result in nonspecific dermatitis and alterations in glucose and lipid metabolism. Toxicity may result in neuropathy. The AI for adult men is 2.3 mg/day with an upper limit of 11 mg.[22]

Molybdenum acts as a cofactor for several enzymatic reactions. It is obtained from dairy products, organ meats, cereals, and legumes. Deficiency is extremely rare, and toxicity may cause gout-like symptoms of arthritis. The RDA for adult men is 45 μg/day with a upper limit of 2000 μg daily.[22]

Nickel is found in chocolate, nuts, legumes, and grains. Nickel acts as a cofactor in a variety of enzymatic reactions and affects the distribution and function of other nutrients including zinc, iron, and calcium. Deficiency is uncommon, causing failure to thrive and decreased sexual function. There is no RDA or AI for nickel, although daily needs are estimated at 60–260 μg daily with an upper limit of 1 mg.[22]

Selenium acts as an antioxidant and is found in seafood, liver, kidney, and eggs, as well as some seeds and grains. Selenium interacts with vitamin E and other antioxidants as an essential part of glutathione peroxidase. Selenium has been studied in the prevention of a variety of cancers, including prostate cancer, without definitive results, but considerable epidemiologic promise.[32] The Randomized Study of Selenium and vitamin E for the Prevention of Prostate Cancer (SELECT Trial) has enrolled more than 32,000 men and should provide clarity on this topic when data are reported. Deficiency may result in muscle pain, weakness, and a rare cardiac condition called *Keshan disease*. Toxicity may cause fingernail changes and hair loss. The RDA for adult men is 55 μg/day with an upper limit of 400 μg daily.[21]

Silicon is involved in collagen synthesis and calcification of bone. Dietary sources include grains and root vegetables. Deficiency is uncommon, causing failure of wound healing and connective tissue and bone abnormalities. There is no RDA, AI, nor upper limit for silicon, although daily needs are estimated at 5–20 mg.[22]

The exact role of *vanadium* in health is currently unclear but it is believed to be an essential mineral; deficiency may predispose a person to bipolar disease. There is no RDA or AI for vanadium, although daily needs are estimated at 5–20 mg. The upper limit is 1.8 mg/day.[22]

Zinc is abundant in red meats, dairy products, seafood, and wheat germ. Zinc is omnipresent in the body and acts as a cofactor for numerous enzymes. The signs and symptoms of zinc deficiency include anorexia, growth retardation, delayed sexual maturation, hypogonadism and hypospermatogenesis, alopecia, immune disorders, dermatitis, night blindness, impaired taste (i.e., hypogeusia), and impaired wound healing. Zinc deficiency may result from acrodermatitis enteropathica, a recessively inherited partial defect in intestinal zinc absorption. Biochemical signs associated with zinc deficiency include decreased levels of plasma zinc (<70 μg/dL), alkaline phosphatase, and plasma testosterone. Clinical assessment of mild zinc deficiency is difficult because many of the signs and symptoms are nonspecific. Nonetheless, if a malnourished person has a borderline-low plasma zinc level, is subsisting on a high-fiber and high-phytate diet (which reduces zinc absorption), and has reduced signs and symptoms compatible with deficiency, empiric treatment with zinc supplements (15–25 mg/day) may be tried. A Cochrane Database review[33] found zinc supplementation ineffective for the treatment of leg ulcers. Zinc depletion may adversely affect strength and cardiorespiratory performance in deficient athletes through decreased activity of the zinc-dependent enzyme, carbonic anhydrase.[34] No studies have shown that zinc supplementation can increase performance in athletes with normal diets. Toxicity may result in impaired immune function and impairment of copper absorption. The RDA for adult men is 11 mg/day with an upper limit of 40 mg daily.[22]

Non-nutritive Components of Food

Alcohol

Ethyl alcohol, or ethanol, is an energy-containing compound; 1 g of alcohol yields 7 Calories. Alcohol is absorbed primarily in the stomach and duodenum. One 12-oz beer, a 1.5-oz 80-proof shot of liquor, and a 5-oz glass of wine each have approximately 15 g of alcohol. Many studies have supported benefits from low to moderate intake of alcohol with detrimental effects occurring with larger amounts. Light to moderate amounts of alcohol increase insulin sensitivity and raise HDL cholesterol levels. A systematic review of 32 studies on alcohol intake concluded that moderate amounts of alcohol (1–3 drinks/day), when compared with no alcohol use, was associated with a 33–56% lower incidence of diabetes and a 34% lower incidence of diabetes-related coronary heart disease.[35] Conversely, the study also noted that, compared with moderate intake, chronic ingestion of greater than 45 g/day can cause deterioration in glucose control and a 43% increase in incidence of diabetes. Moderate amounts of alcohol with food have no acute effect on blood glucose and insulin levels. Light to moderate alcohol intake does not increase blood pressure, but amounts greater 30–60 g/day may cause elevated blood pressure. These hypertensive effects from excess alcohol are reversed after abstinence. This systematic review and other studies suggest a J-shaped mortality curve for alcohol consumption, with lowest all-cause mortality at between 1 and 2 drinks

(15–30 g) per day for an adult male.[35] Of significance in nutrition, alcohol-containing beverages generally contain few other nutrients, may reduce nutrient intake by replacing more nutritious foods, and can decrease absorption of a number nutrients and alter their storage, metabolism, and excretion. Thiamine, niacin, folate, zinc, and vitamins B_6, B_{12}, A, D, and K are commonly deficient in alcoholics.

USDA guidelines recommend moderate intake for persons who choose to drink alcohol. If male patients choose to drink alcohol, they should limit their intake to no more than 2 drinks/day. Persons with diabetes may consume moderate amounts without concern of acute effect on glycemic control, blood pressure, or triglycerides. Men with a history of alcohol abuse, liver disease, and other high-risk conditions should be encouraged to abstain from alcohol completely.

Fiber

Fiber is a non–energy-containing carbohydrate compound. The consumption of dietary fiber is encouraged by all major health and dietary organizations. Although small amounts of fiber may be digested by intestinal microflora, fiber generally cannot be broken down by the digestive process into energy extractable products. Fiber is classified as either functional (soluble) or dietary (insoluble). Total fiber is the sum of dietary and functional fiber. Functional or soluble fibers dissolve or swell in water and include pectin, mucilage, psyllium, and gums. Sources are oat bran, legumes, fruit, and seaweed, which contain carrageenan. Soluble fibers can hold 20–30 times their weight in water. This causes the formation of more viscous chyme in the digestive tract, which slows the rate of nutrient absorption. Soluble fibers bind bile acids and interfere with enterohepatic circulation, thus sequestering and ultimately decreasing serum cholesterol. Insoluble fibers do not dissolve in water. These include cellulose, hemicellulose, and lignin (which is technically a noncarbohydrate). Sources of insoluble fiber include grain brans and cruciferous vegetables. Insoluble fibers increase the bulk of intestinal contents. This increased stool bulk combined with increased intraluminal fluid from soluble fibers stimulates peristalsis and reduces transit time. Reduced transit time may reduce the incidence of hemorrhoids and diverticuli, as noted in the US Physician's Health Study of nearly 44,000 men.[36] Fiber also has a beneficial effect on cardiovascular health. Fiber intake in quantities over 50 g daily may have a

beneficial effect on glycemia, insulinemia, and lipemia. The Framingham Offspring Study[37] found that the prevalence of both insulin resistance and the metabolic syndrome was significantly lower among persons eating the most cereal fiber from whole grains compared with those eating the least. Recent ADA guidelines suggest, however, that there is no reason to recommend greater amount of fiber intake in persons with diabetes.[38] The AI for fiber in adult males is 38 g/day, decreasing to 30 g/day in men older than 50 years of age.[6] Although large amounts of daily fiber (>50 g daily) require large amounts of water intake to ensure normal colonic transit, there is no upper limit on safe fiber intake.

Phytochemicals

This group includes a wide array of non–energy-containing and apparently nonessential chemical compounds found in plants. These compounds are the current subject of multiple investigations and may have physiologic or pharmaceutical actions in the body because many are thought to have antioxidant properties. Some, such as ephedrine, are used as the basis of current and future pharmaceuticals. Phytochemicals include carotenoids from red, yellow, and orange foods, such as carrots, yams, and tomatoes; lycopene in tomato-based products; lutein and zeaxanthin from leafy greens, such as spinach, endive, and romaine lettuce; and flavonoids in brightly colored fruits and vegetables, such as blueberries, cherries, and strawberries. Two flavonoids, rutin, and hesperidin, are referred to as vitamin P, although they have no recognized nutritional necessity. Phytosterols impair intestinal absorption of cholesterol and may significantly reduce LDL levels.[39] Plant sterols are now being used in commercial spreads, such as Benecol, for this purpose. Polyphenols in dark chocolate have been found to improve vascular function in male smokers[40] and flavonols in chocolate may also have favorable cardiovascular effects. Policosanols derived from rice are being investigated as cholesterol reducers. Phytoestrogens, such as isoflavones, may be associated with a decreased risk of lung cancer.[41] In Kuopio Ischaemic Heart Disease Risk Factor Study,[42] 1889 men were prospectively monitored for the development of cardiovascular disease in relation to intake of enterolactone, an intestinal microflora-modified phytochemical. Men with the highest quartile of intake had significantly lower rates of coronary heart disease and cardiovascular disease. Although there is no USDA recommendation on phytochemical intake, the current recommendation for 5–9 servings of fruits and vegetables daily would include a considerable amount and array of phytochemicals.

Sugar Substitutes

A variety of products are currently used in food in place of the naturally occurring sugars such as glucose, fructose, lactose, and sucrose (dextrose). Sugar alcohols are chemical derivatives of sugar that provide minimal energy. They include mannitol, sorbitol, xylitol, maltitol, and lactitol. Cyclamate was one of the earliest artificial sweeteners, provides no energy, and is 30 times sweeter than sucrose. It was banned by the US Food and Drug Administration (FDA) in 1969 because of studies that suggested an increase cancer risk in laboratory animals.[43]

Another early sugar substitute is saccharin (Sweet 'n' Low), which is about 300 times sweeter than sucrose. Findings from animal studies indicated that high does of saccharin could cause bladder cancer; however, human studies have not shown any link between bladder cancer risk and saccharin intake.[44] In 1977 and continuing through today, the FDA placed a warning on the use of saccharin while safety studies continue. Aspartame (NutraSweet, Equal) contains two amino acids: aspartic acid and phenylalanine. It is 200 times as sweet as sucrose and contains 4 Calories/g. Aspartame is metabolized to several products, including the amino acid phenylalanine, which means that persons with phenylketonuria should not consume aspartame. Neotame, an aspartame derivative that is considered safer for patients with phenylketonuria, was approved in 2002. Acesulfame potassium (Sweet and Safe, Sunett) is 200 times as sweet as sucrose and contains no energy. Sucralose (Splenda) is an increasingly popular artificial sweetener that is a chlorinated sucrose derivative. No specific cautions have been found for acesulfame potassium, sucralose, and Neotame. Persons with diabetes and patients trying to lose weight should be encouraged to use sugar substitutes when appropriate. However, artificial sweeteners may still cause an increase in insulin after consumption, thus tempering some of their usefulness for diabetics. Non-nutritive sweeteners are safe when consumed within the acceptable daily intake (ADI) established by the FDA.[45] Each non-nutritive sweetener has its own ADI. For example, aspartame has an ADI of 50 mg/kg, which translates into approximately 15 cans of diet soda daily for a 60-kg male.[46]

Nutritional Assessment

The nutritional assessment is a specialized and comprehensive evaluation of a patient's nutritional status and requirements based on data obtained from the medical history, physical exam, and laboratory values. A proper assessment is the foundation on which further recommendations on proper diet for the prevention and treatment of disease can be based. These assessments are routinely performed by registered dietitians and nutritionists and should also be used by physicians when evaluating the nutritional status of any patient. A complete assessment proceeds in three parts[47]:

1. Define the patient's nutritional status with respect to energy, protein, vitamin, and mineral intake.
2. Establish optimal levels of nutritional intake for the individual patient's needs and make dietary recommendations based on those needs.
3. Conduct assessments in a serial fashion to assess the effects of dietary recommendations on health.

A complete medical history is the first step in the assessment.[48] In the past medical history and surgical history, specific inquiry of cardiovascular disease, diabetes mellitus, gout, alcoholism, cancer, immunodeficiencies, and pulmonary, gastrointestinal, or renal diseases should be made. The disease itself or medical or surgical interventions used to treat it may affect the nutritional status of the patient. In addition to standard medications and allergies, the patient should be asked whether he takes any vitamins, minerals, or supplements and whether he has any food allergies or sensitivities, including lactose intolerance. Certain medications, such as laxatives, diuretics, and antacids may directly affect the nutritional status of a patient or, in the case of vitamin K–containing green vegetables, may present problems of drug-nutrient interactions. A family history of osteoporosis, cardiovascular disease, diabetes, hypertension, or obesity is important to note. The patient's social history should be evaluated for caffeine, alcohol, and tobacco use.

A complete understanding of the patient's social background will improve the clinician's ability to formulate a successful dietary recommendation, and a specific dietary history should be elicited at this time (Table 19-2)[49]; a daily food log may be helpful as well. A complete review of systems is useful to further elicit any other significant problems a patient may have that can

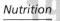

Table 19-2. Key Questions for the Dietary History

Do you have a history of "dieting"?
Do you follow a special diet? (low-salt, vegetarian, etc.)
How successful are you at following this diet?
How many meals and snacks do you eat daily?
Do you avoid any specific foods? Why?
What types of food do you frequently/infrequently eat?
Who prepares your meals? (e.g., self, spouse, restaurant, caregiver)
How much water/soft drinks/coffee/juice/tea/alcohol do you drink?
Describe your typical daily food and beverage intake, including meals and snacks (i.e., usual dietary intake history).
Describe everything you ate and drank within the past 24 hours, including the quantities consumed and methods of preparation (i.e., 24-hour recall).

Adapted from: Morrison G, Hark L: *Medical Nutrition: A Case-Based Approach,* Malden, MA, 2003, Blackwell Publishing.

herald a nutritional concern. The review of systems is subjective and organ system based and should be appropriately tailored to the age and general health of the patient. Gastrointestinal symptoms such as heartburn, dyspepsia, abdominal bloating, gas, constipation, and diarrhea may be particularly salient.

The physical examination provides more objective measurements of the nutritional status of a patient. For example, a patient who, according to his history, has no medical problems, takes no medicines, refrains from alcohol and tobacco, and claims to eat a low-fat diet rich in fruits and vegetables yet appears morbidly obese, hypertensive, and is noted to have acanthosis nigricans should immediately focus the attention of the physician on a nutritional imbalance. Malnutrition may cause a myriad of physical findings in any number of organ systems, the specifics of which are beyond the scope of this chapter. The most important baseline data to be gathered during the exam are vital signs, including blood pressure, and an accurate height and weight measurements. These numbers can be used to calculate a variety of anthropometric measurements that better quantify the size of a patient. Ideal body weight (for men more than 5 feet tall, 106 pounds + 6 pounds ± 10% for each inch over 5 feet) and percent ideal body weight (current/ideal weight) are useful rules of thumb, as is the USDA Healthy Weight for Adults table. Body mass index (BMI; kg/m^2) should be calculated and is the standard measure used in the diagnosis of obesity[50]:

- Normal BMI: 18–25
- Overweight: 25–30
- Obese: 30–40
- Morbidly obese: >40

Distribution of body fat is typically more visceral in males than in females, likely due to hormonal differences, resulting in a greater abdominal-to-waist ratio. Other measurements, such as estimated percent body fat by underwater weighing and bioelectric impedance, triceps or abdominal skin fold testing, mid-arm circumference, and mid-arm muscle circumference are not routinely needed. These measurements alone may not be accurate in establishing overnourishment or undernourishment in specific types of patients, including amputees, acutely ill patients, patients with recent trauma or burns, and athletes with significant muscle bulk. Magnetic resonance imaging, dual-energy x-ray absorptiometry, and other advanced imaging is usually unnecessary to determine body fat distribution.

The final part of a complete nutritional assessment is laboratory analysis.[49] This provides a final piece of objective data to support the clinician's diagnosis. No single laboratory test completely measures total nutritional status in a patient; therefore, laboratory tests are best used as an extension of the history and physical examination. Levels of serum electrolytes and minerals including sodium, potassium, chloride, calcium, phosphorus, and magnesium are routinely assessed. A measurement of serum iron and zinc levels may also be useful in certain patients. Testing for other types of minerals and metals is less commonly necessary and should be done with an appropriate index of suspicion. A fasting serum lipid panel including total cholesterol, HDL cholesterol, LDL cholesterol, very-low-density lipoproteins, and triglycerides serves as a useful laboratory test and should be routinely performed for a complete nutritional assessment. Measures of vitamin levels, including thiamine, folate, B_{12}, and 25-OH vitamin D are useful in appropriate patients, as are measures of liver and renal function.

Protein status should routinely be assessed via serum blood urea nitrogen and creatinine levels, yet these levels are highly dependent on hydration status and baseline renal function. Therefore, protein status can also be assessed using a variety of markers for patients for whom reduced protein and caloric intake is a concern. Each of these markers may also be affected by not only nutrition and hydration, but also diseases, surgery, and impaired liver function. Serum albumin has the longest half-life (18–21 days) and is useful for evaluating nutritional status over the past several months. Significantly depressed levels of albumin are associated with increased morbidity and mortality. Serum transferrin has a shorter half-life (8–9 days) but is also affected by iron status, in addition to protein and caloric intake. Serum prealbumin has a short half-life (2–3 days), which makes it useful for nutritional status assessment over the past week. Serum retinol-binding protein has the shortest half-life of commercially available protein markers (12 hours), which makes it the most sensitive for daily protein and caloric intake. Serum retinol-binding protein levels are also affected by vitamin A status.

Dietary Choices

One of the most common questions asked of physicians by their patients is "What should I eat to stay healthy?" Adult American men are increasingly looking for an ideal diet that maintains health, prevents disease, and provides an abundance of energy while remaining enjoyable and easy to follow. A bewildering array of choices exist, from low-fat and low-carbohydrate diets, to low-sodium and low-calorie diets, to other diets that have been promoted for prevention or treatment of specific diseases or that focus on particular types or amounts of food. A Google search performed in mid 2006 for "diet AND men" revealed an astonishing 70 million-plus references.

The earliest data collected on the association of different diets and disease were from The Seven Countries Study[51] carried out from 1958 to 1970. This study explored associations among diet, risk, and disease experience in contrasting populations (i.e., United States, Japan, Greece, England, Finland, Italy, and Yugoslavia). Men aged 40–59 years in 18 areas of seven countries were studied, and results demonstrated that levels of saturated fatty acids and mean serum cholesterol predict present and future population rates of coronary heart disease. Moreover, it served as basis for the concept of population and dietary causes in the development of obesity, hypertension, coronary disease, and stroke.

Based upon the Seven Countries Study's demonstrated risk of cardiovascular disease with increased levels of saturated fats, the focus for the last 25 years has been on decreasing fat intake. As a result, the average American's fat consumption dropped from 40% to 34% of total calories.[52] Despite these data, according to the Centers for Disease Control and Prevention, between 1971 and 2000 American men increased their caloric intake by 7%.[52] Concurrently, obesity, hypertension, diabetes, and cardiovascular disease rates have continued to increase in men.[53]

Low-Fat Diets

High-fat diets are associated with increasing rates of obesity and cardiovascular disease.[51] The Multiple Risk Factor Intervention trial[54] conducted during the 1970s was the first trial that examined the role of a low-fat diet in reducing the risk of atherosclerosis in men. More than 6000 male patients were placed on a low-fat diet, encouraged to exercise, and advised to quit smoking. The trial concluded that low-fat diets, when combined with smoking cessation and exercise, could reduce the risk of heart disease in men. The Lipid Research Clinics Coronary Primary Prevention Trial[55] was conducted in the United States from 1976 to 1983 and involved 3806 men. This trial also found evidence that a diet low in saturated fat could reduce heart disease.[55]

Currently, there are a variety of low-fat dietary plans that share similar principles but demonstrate different food choices. The USDA, Dietary Approaches to Stop Hypertension (DASH), Weight Watchers, Mediterranean, and vegetarian diets are established and well-studied low-fat diets. More recently, the Healing Foods Pyramid diet from the University of Michigan Medical School and the Healthy Eating Pyramid from the Harvard School of Public Health were introduced; these share a similar core of recommendations with other low-fat diets:

- More fruits, vegetables, and whole grains
- Less cholesterol, saturated fats, sweets, and salt
- Modest amount of alcohol
- Smaller meals

USDA/My Pyramid

The Dietary Guidelines for Americans[56] are written to "promote good dietary habits, reserve health and reduce risk for major chronic diseases" (Table 19-3). Like all low-fat diets, the emphasis in the USDA food guide diet is on fruits, vegetables, and whole grains. The Dietary Guidelines are explained in visual form as the USDA My Pyramid, an evolution from the previous USDA Food Guide Pyramid. In 2005, the USDA food guide pyramid was rebuilt with the food groups being represented by a rainbow of colored, vertical stripes and an illustration of a person climbing steps to emphasize the importance of exercise (Figure 19-2). It was also individualized for age, gender, and activity level and simplified

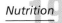
Table 19-3. Key Recommendations from the USDA Dietary Guidelines for Americans

Topic	Recommendations
Adequate nutrients within calorie needs	Consume a variety of nutrient-dense foods and beverages within and among the basic food groups while choosing foods that limit the intake of saturated and *trans*-fats, cholesterol, added sugars, salt, and alcohol.
	Meet recommended intakes within energy needs by adopting a balanced eating pattern, such as the USDA Food Guide or the DASH Eating Plan.
	Persons older than 50 years of age should consume vitamin B_{12} in its crystalline form (e.g., fortified foods or supplements).
	Older adults, persons with dark skin, and persons exposed to insufficient ultraviolet-band radiation (e.g., sunlight): Consume extra vitamin D from vitamin D–fortified foods and/or supplements.
Food groups to encourage	Consume a sufficient amount of fruits and vegetables while staying within energy needs. Two cups of fruit and 2½ cups of vegetables per day are recommended for a reference 2000-Calorie intake, with higher or lower amounts depending on the Calorie level.
	Choose a variety of fruits and vegetables each day. In particular, select from all five vegetable subgroups (dark green, orange, legumes, starchy vegetables, and other vegetables) several times a week.
	Consume 3 or more ounce-equivalents of whole-grain products per day, with the rest of the recommended grains coming from enriched or whole-grain products. In general, at least half the grains should come from whole grains.
	Consume 3 cups per day of fat-free or low-fat milk or equivalent milk products.
	Children and adolescents: Consume whole-grain products often; at least half the grains should be whole grains. Children aged 2–8 years should consume 2 cups of fat-free or low-fat milk or equivalent milk products per day. Children 9 years of age and older should consume 3 cups of fat-free or low-fat milk or equivalent milk products per day.
Fats	Consume less than 10% of calories from saturated fatty acids and less than 300 mg of cholesterol per day, and keep *trans*-fatty acid consumption as low as possible.
	Keep total fat intake to between 20% and 35% of calories, with most fats coming from sources of polyunsaturated and monounsaturated fatty acids such as fish, nuts, and vegetable oils.
	When selecting and preparing meat, poultry, dry beans, and milk or milk products, make choices that are lean, low in fat, or fat free.
	Limit intake of fats and oils high in saturated and/or *trans*-fatty acids, and choose products low in such fats and oils.
	Children and adolescents: Keep total fat intake to between 30% and 35% of Calories for children 2–3 years of age and between 25% and 35% of calories for children and adolescents 4–18 years of age, with most fats coming from sources of polyunsaturated and monounsaturated fatty acids, such as fish, nuts, and vegetable oils.
Carbohydrates	Choose fiber-rich fruits, vegetables, and whole grains often.
	Choose and prepare foods and beverages with little added sugar or caloric sweetener, such as amounts suggested by the USDA Food Guide and the DASH Eating Plan.
	Reduce the incidence of dental caries by practicing good oral hygiene and consuming sugar- and starch-containing foods and beverages less frequently.
Alcoholic beverages	Persons who choose to drink alcoholic beverages: Do so sensibly and in moderation—defined as the consumption of up to one drink per day for women and up to two drinks per day for men.
	Alcoholic beverages should not be consumed by some persons, including those who cannot restrict their alcohol intake, children and adolescents, persons taking medications that can interact with alcohol, and those with specific medical conditions.
	Alcoholic beverages should be avoided by persons engaging in activities that require attention, skill, or coordination, such as driving or operating machinery.

Table continued on following page

Table 19-3. Key Recommendations from the USDA Dietary Guidelines for Americans (Continued)

Topic	Recommendations
Sodium and potassium	Consume less than 2300 mg (approximately 1 tsp of salt) of sodium per day.
	Choose and prepare foods with little salt. At the same time, consume potassium-rich foods, such as fruits and vegetables.
	Persons with hypertension, African Americans, and middle-aged and older adults: Aim to consume no more than 1500 mg of sodium per day, and meet the potassium recommendation (4700 mg/day) with food.

USDA, US Department of Agriculture; DASH, Dietary Approaches to Stop Hypertension.
Adapted from: US Department of Agriculture: Dietary guidelines for Americans. Available at: http://www.health.gov/DietaryGuidelines/. Accessed July 22, 2006.

to make serving sizes and food choices easier to comprehend by the public. A Web site highlighting this diet (http://www.mypyramid.gov) allows individuals to receive a personal, tailored diet regimen plan. This in turn creates an individualized approach to balancing nutrition and exercise, which is promoted to lead to a better lifestyle. Unfortunately, the basic pyramid contains no text and has an abstract illustration that limits its usefulness to individuals with access to it—persons with access to the Web site or a full copy.

The Diabetes Prevention Program[57] examined the USDA diet in a 27-center, randomized, clinical trial that evaluated the effects of lifestyle intervention and pharmacotherapy on the incidence

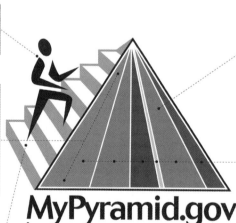

Figure 19-2. A, Anatomy of MyPyramid. (Adapted from: MyPyramid.gov. Available at: http://www.mypyramid.gov/downloads/MyPyramid_Anatomy.pdf. Accessed July 22, 2006.)

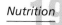

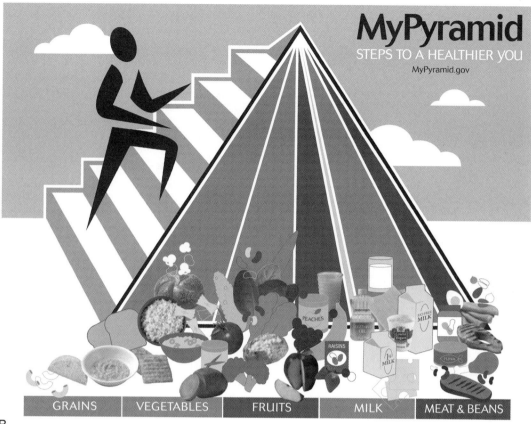

GRAINS | VEGETABLES | FRUITS | MILK | MEAT & BEANS

B

Figure 19-2. B, MyPyramid—Steps to a Healthier You. USDA, US Department of Agriculture. (Adapted from: MyPyramid. gov. Available at: http://www.mypyramid.gov/downloads/MiniPoster.pdf. Accessed July 22, 2006.)

of type 2 diabetes in persons with impaired glucose tolerance. In this study, 3234 overweight participants (32% men) were randomly assigned to one of three groups: (1) placebo plus standard lifestyle recommendations, (2) metformin plus standard lifestyle recommendations, and (3) intensive lifestyle intervention. Participants in the medication and placebo groups were provided written information on the food guide pyramid and were seen annually in individual sessions. Patients in the intensive lifestyle group also followed the food guide pyramid but received closer follow-up. Participants in the intensive lifestyle group lost significantly more weight than those in the metformin and placebo groups. The intensive lifestyle group also had a significantly lower incidence of type 2 diabetes than the placebo or metformin group at 1 year.

AHA Diet

The AHA changed its dietary recommendations for 2006 introducing the "No-Fad" Diet.[58] The

AHA acknowledges that losing weight is difficult and designed this diet based on three concepts that allow each individual to personalize a weight-loss plan (Figure 19-3).

Think Smart. According to the AHA, good planning, rather than sheer willpower, is the key to losing weight. They advocate planning day-to-day activities to support weight-loss efforts because this will make it easier to maintain weight loss. Other key recommendations include the following:

- Think about something that represents inner strength and use this image to boost the self resolve needed for successful weight loss.
- Set reasonable, realistic, and measurable short- and long-term weight-loss goals.
- Write goals in a weight-loss diary to make them real.
- Reassess progress every 6 weeks and make changes accordingly.

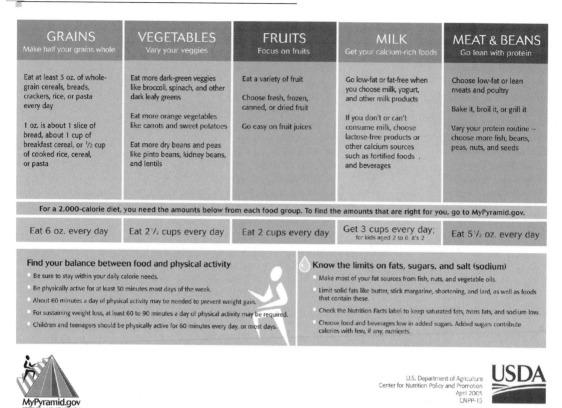

GRAINS Make half your grains whole	VEGETABLES Vary your veggies	FRUITS Focus on fruits	MILK Get your calcium-rich foods	MEAT & BEANS Go lean with protein
Eat at least 3 oz. of whole-grain cereals, breads, crackers, rice, or pasta every day 1 oz. is about 1 slice of bread, about 1 cup of breakfast cereal, or ½ cup of cooked rice, cereal, or pasta	Eat more dark-green veggies like broccoli, spinach, and other dark leafy greens Eat more orange vegetables like carrots and sweet potatoes Eat more dry beans and peas like pinto beans, kidney beans, and lentils	Eat a variety of fruit Choose fresh, frozen, canned, or dried fruit Go easy on fruit juices	Go low-fat or fat-free when you choose milk, yogurt, and other milk products If you don't or can't consume milk, choose lactose-free products or other calcium sources such as fortified foods and beverages	Choose low-fat or lean meats and poultry Bake it, broil it, or grill it Vary your protein routine — choose more fish, beans, peas, nuts, and seeds

For a 2,000-calorie diet, you need the amounts below from each food group. To find the amounts that are right for you, go to MyPyramid.gov.

| Eat 6 oz. every day | Eat 2½ cups every day | Eat 2 cups every day | Get 3 cups every day;
for kids aged 2 to 8, it's 2 | Eat 5½ oz. every day |

Find your balance between food and physical activity
- Be sure to stay within your daily calorie needs.
- Be physically active for at least 30 minutes most days of the week.
- About 60 minutes a day of physical activity may be needed to prevent weight gain.
- For sustaining weight loss, at least 60 to 90 minutes a day of physical activity may be required.
- Children and teenagers should be physically active for 60 minutes every day, or most days.

Know the limits on fats, sugars, and salt (sodium)
- Make most of your fat sources from fish, nuts, and vegetable oils.
- Limit solid fats like butter, stick margarine, shortening, and lard, as well as foods that contain these.
- Check the Nutrition Facts label to keep saturated fats, trans fats, and sodium low.
- Choose food and beverages low in added sugars. Added sugars contribute calories with few, if any, nutrients.

MyPyramid.gov
STEPS TO A HEALTHIER YOU

U.S. Department of Agriculture
Center for Nutrition Policy and Promotion
April 2005
CNPP-15

USDA

USDA is an equal opportunity provider and employer

C

Figure 19-2. C, MyPyramid—Steps to a Healthier You. USDA, US Department of Agriculture. (Adapted from: MyPyramid.gov. Available at: http://www.mypyramid.gov/downloads/MiniPoster.pdf. Accessed July 22, 2006.)

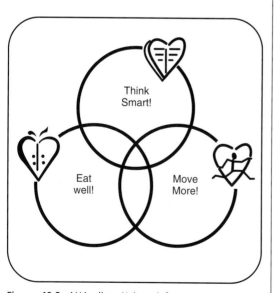

Figure 19-3. AHA diet. (Adapted from: American Heart Association. Available at: http://www.americanheart.org. Accessed July 22, 2006.)

- Be persistent and practice new behaviors until they become habit.

Eat Well. The emphasis here is on not only following a diet plan until weight is lost, but making a commitment to choose foods wisely. Other helpful tips include the following:
- Set a personal weight-loss goal and start with a goal of losing about 10% of current body weight.
- Keep a food diary.
- Watch nutrition labels.
- Include high-fiber foods, such as whole grains, fruits, and vegetables, in your diet since they take longer to digest and make you feel full longer.
- Identify the nonessential, high-calorie foods bought out of habit, and stop buying them.

Move More. The AHA agrees that diet alone is not enough. Regular physical activity is needed to help lose the weight and maintain the weight loss. Activity is an integral part of the recommendations, which include the following:

- Decide on a personal fitness goal and write it down. Start at 10 minutes each day, and progress to 30–60 min/day.
- Choose an activity that fits into your lifestyle because that increases the likelihood of maintaining it.
- Find a friend who will join in the activity.
- Set aside a 30-minute block of time each day to devote to the activity.
- Make physical fitness a priority in life.
- Monitor progress, and reassess every 6 weeks.

DASH Diet

The DASH eating plan was designed from the Dietary Approaches to Stop Hypertension clinical study funded by the National Heart, Lung, and Blood Institute in 1997.[59] This study found that populations who consume diets rich in vegetables and fruits have lower blood pressures than those whose diets are low in vegetables. In addition to fruits and vegetables, this diet is rich in dietary fiber, potassium, calcium, and magnesium, and protein (Figure 19-4).

In the original DASH trial, Appel and colleagues[59] evaluated 459 patients who had hypertension and, after a 3-week run-in period, subjects were randomly assigned to a control diet (rich in fruits and vegetables) or a DASH-type diet. At 8 weeks, there was a significant decrease in blood pressure of 5.5 mm Hg in the DASH group. More recently, the PREMIER[60] trial investigated the effects of the DASH diet combined with recommendations known to lower blood pressure (e.g., sodium and alcohol restriction, exercise, weight loss) and evaluated for reductions in weight and hypertension. A total of 810 participants were randomly assigned to a control group (including a single advice-giving session for consuming a DASH diet) or one of two intervention groups. One intervention group followed the DASH diet and exercised. The other was encouraged to participate in calorie restriction and exercise. There was significantly greater weight loss in both intervention groups at 6 months, with the greatest weight loss noted in patients who followed the DASH diet and exercise plans.

A further modification of the DASH diet was conducted in the OmniHeart Randomized Trial.[61] This three-armed trial compared a standard diet similar to the DASH diet with modified diets based on the DASH diet with either high proportions of proteins or monounsaturated fats. One hundred sixty-four patients (55% men) were enrolled and were crossed-over to each diet at 6-week intervals. Compared with the standard DASH diet, partial substitution of carbohydrates with either monounsaturated fats or proteins provided improved blood pressure control and lipid levels and reduced estimated cardiovascular risk.

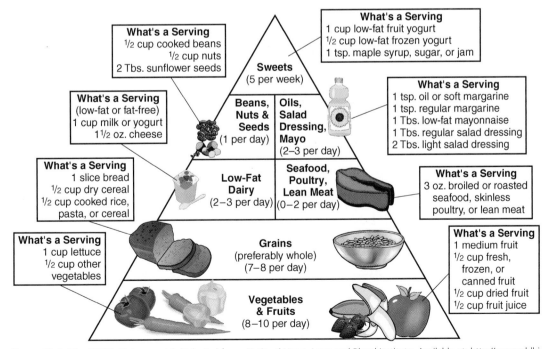

What's a Serving
1 cup low-fat fruit yogurt
1/2 cup low-fat frozen yogurt
1 tsp. maple syrup, sugar, or jam

What's a Serving
1/2 cup cooked beans
1/2 cup nuts
2 Tbs. sunflower seeds

What's a Serving
(low-fat or fat-free)
1 cup milk or yogurt
1 1/2 oz. cheese

What's a Serving
1 slice bread
1/2 cup dry cereal
1/2 cup cooked rice, pasta, or cereal

What's a Serving
1 cup lettuce
1/2 cup other vegetables

What's a Serving
1 tsp. oil or soft margarine
1 tsp. regular margarine
1 Tbs. low-fat mayonnaise
1 Tbs. regular salad dressing
2 Tbs. light salad dressing

What's a Serving
3 oz. broiled or roasted seafood, skinless poultry, or lean meat

What's a Serving
1 medium fruit
1/2 cup fresh, frozen, or canned fruit
1/2 cup dried fruit
1/2 cup fruit juice

Sweets (5 per week)

Beans, Nuts & Seeds (1 per day)

Oils, Salad Dressing, Mayo (2–3 per day)

Low-Fat Dairy (2–3 per day)

Seafood, Poultry, Lean Meat (0–2 per day)

Grains (preferably whole) (7–8 per day)

Vegetables & Fruits (8–10 per day)

Figure 19-4. The DASH diet pyramid. (Adapted from: National Heart, Lung and Blood Institute. Available at: http://www.nhlbi.nih.gov/health/public/heart/hbp/dash.)

Mediterranean Diet

There is not a universal "Mediterranean" diet. Many countries border the Mediterranean Sea, and differences in culture, ethnicity, and agriculture lead to variations in their diets. In addition to the well-known Mediterranean diet, Latin American and Asian diet pyramids have also been devised; these are based on similar principles but use traditional ethnic foods in place of those found in the Mediterranean region. These diets have been clearly illustrated and explained by the Oldways Preservation and Exchange Trust.[62] Regardless of their background, all Mediterranean-style diets have a few things in common (Figure 19-5):

- Abundant use of olive oil
- High consumption of fruits, vegetables, breads, nuts, fish
- Limited amount of red meat

The Mediterranean diet does not regard all fat as unhealthy. The emphasis is not to limit fat consumption, but rather make good choices about the types of fat to include in the diet. This diet is low in saturated and *trans*-fats, but high in omega-3 fatty acids and monounsaturated fats. Omega-3 fatty acids are found in fatty fish including salmon, trout, and sardines, whereas monounsaturated fat is abundant in olive oil, nuts, and avocados.

A popular ingredient in the Mediterranean diet is olive oil, which is predominantly monounsaturated fat. Olive oil has been shown to also decrease triglycerides and increase HDL levels.[63] In addition to improving the lipid profile, olive oil may contribute to the cardioprotective effect of the Mediterranean diet in several other ways, including lowering blood pressure, providing antithrombotic effects, and improving insulin sensitivity.[64]

Fish consumption has long been recognized as important in the prevention of coronary artery disease (CAD). In the United States Physicians' Health Study[65] of more than 20,000 men over 11 years, consumption of more than one serving of

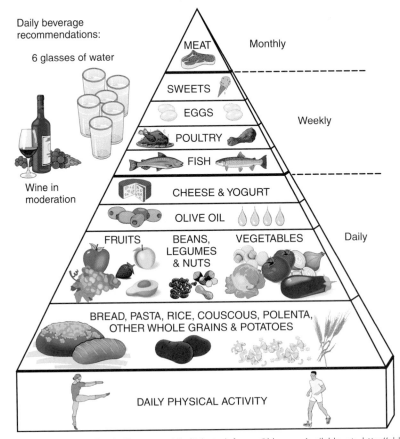

The Traditional Healthy Mediterranean Diet Pyramid

Daily beverage recommendations:

6 glasses of water

Wine in moderation

MEAT — Monthly

SWEETS
EGGS
POULTRY
FISH — Weekly

CHEESE & YOGURT

OLIVE OIL

FRUITS | BEANS, LEGUMES & NUTS | VEGETABLES — Daily

BREAD, PASTA, RICE, COUSCOUS, POLENTA, OTHER WHOLE GRAINS & POTATOES

DAILY PHYSICAL ACTIVITY

Figure 19-5. The Mediterranean food diet pyramid. (Adapted from: Oldways. Available at: http://oldwayspt.org/med_pyramid.html. Accessed July 24, 2006.)

fish per week was associated with a 52% decrease in sudden cardiac death. The Nurses Health Study[66] supported this finding and found a negative relation between fish intake and risk of coronary heart disease. This protective effect is likely the result of the cardiovascular benefits of omega-3 fatty acids, which include lowering triglyceride levels and providing anti-inflammatory effects.

In the Diet and Reinfarction Trial,[67] 2033 men with prior myocardial infarction were randomly assigned to receive different kinds of dietary advice. After 2 years, the group that was advised to increase omega-3 fatty acid intake by eating fish or taking a fish oil supplement had a 29% reduction in mortality from any cause. In the GISSI-Prevenzione study,[68] a 3½-year trial involving more than 11,000 patients, the administration of a supplement containing 850 mg of omega-3 fatty acids decreased the risk of sudden cardiac death by 45% and improved all-cause mortality by 20%, even in patients who were already receiving standard therapies (e.g., beta-blockers, statins, and aspirin).

In addition to proteins, carbohydrates, and fats, nuts contain other important nutrients including fiber, vitamin E, folic acid, potassium, and magnesium. Although nuts do contain a high proportion of fat, most of it is in the form of monounsaturated fat and omega-3 fatty acids. Several large studies have examined the relationship between the risk of heart disease and intake of omega-3 fatty acids from plant sources. In the Health Professionals Follow-up Study,[69] which involved over 43,700 male healthcare professionals, increased intake of alpha-linolenic acid (found in nuts) lowered the risk of a heart attack by 60%. The Seventh-Day Adventist Health Study,[70] which had more than 31,000 participants, found that eating nuts more than four times per week had a 50% CAD risk–lowering effect. Similar results were seen in the Nurses' Health Study,[66] which found eating nuts regularly cut CAD risk by 35%, compared with the results in those who rarely ate nuts.

Vegetarian Diet

According to a Time/CNN poll in 2002,[71] 4% of the US population identified themselves as vegetarian. People usually choose vegetarian diets for religious, ethical, or health reasons. Vegetarians do not eat meat, chicken, or fish, and their diet consists mostly of plant-based foods such as fruits, vegetables, whole grains, legumes, and nuts. This type of diet contains less total fat and cholesterol and includes more dietary fiber.

In the early 1970s, Frank Sacks,[72] through his work at the Harvard School of Public Health, demonstrated that blood pressure and plasma levels of lipids were lower in vegetarians than in persons who ate meat. The American Dietetic Association now states that vegetarian diets are associated with a reduced risk of obesity, hypertension, hyperlipidemia, type 2 diabetes mellitus, coronary heart disease, and some forms of cancer including prostate, colon, and other gastrointestinal malignancies.[73] This is thought to be due to a higher intake of fruit, vegetables, fiber, and antioxidants and a lower intake of saturated fat and cholesterol (Figure 19-6).

Some of the strongest epidemiologic evidence in support of vegetarian diets has been provided by the China-Oxford-Cornell Diet and Health Project (the China Study). The China Study was a collaboration between Cornell University, Oxford University, and the Chinese Academy of Preventive Medicine and examined the relationship between diet and the risk of developing disease.[74] The study's concept was rooted in data and hypotheses linking Western-style diets with increased risks of chronic disease summarized by the National Academy of Sciences in 1982.[75] The project collected mortality data on more than 50 diseases from 130 villages in 65 rural counties in China. Blood, urine, and food samples and dietary data were collected from 50 adults in each village from 1983 to 1984 and combined with historical mortality data from 1973 to 1975.

A follow-up study (the China II Study), resurveyed the same 6500 persons in 1989–1990, adding mortality data from 1986–1988 as well as participants from new counties in China and Taiwan. The results were published in a manuscript,[76] spawning dozens of studies, abstracts, and reviews and eventually a best-selling book for the public.[77] Although strictly an observational study, multiple papers spawned from the study reached several conclusions and generated many more hypotheses. Increased plasma cholesterol levels were associated with animal protein intake and positively associated with increased cancer mortality rates. Cardiovascular disease was also associated with increased animal protein intake (such as casein) but not plant protein (such as gluten). Western-type diseases, in aggregate, were significantly *correlated* (although not definitively caused) with increasing concentrations of plasma cholesterol, which are associated in turn with increasing intakes of animal-based foods.[78]

Vegetarians can be subdivided into groups defined by the types of animal-based foods they eat:

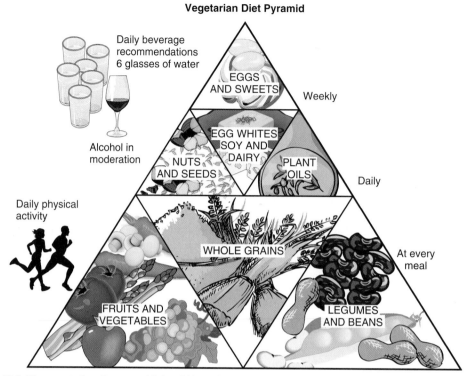

Figure 19-6. The vegetarian diet pyramid. (Available at: http://www.vpul.upenn.edu/ohe/HealthLinks/vegetarian-pyramid.jpg. Accessed July 24, 2006.)

- Lacto-ovo vegetarians: eliminate meat, slaughterhouse products, fish, and poultry, but eat/drink eggs, milk, and milk products
- Ovo-vegetarians: eat eggs but not dairy products
- Lacto-vegetarians: eliminate meat, fish, poultry, and eggs, but eat/drink milk and milk products
- Vegans: eliminate all foods from animals, including meat, slaughterhouse products, fish, poultry, milk, eggs, and dairy products
- Fruitarians: restrict vegan diet to fruits, nuts, honey, and olive oil
- Macrobiotic vegetarians: restrict vegan diet, stressing whole grains and vegetables

The greatest risks associated with inadequate nutrient intake from a vegetarian diet occur during periods of growth. The more restricted the diet, the more difficult it is to get all of the necessary nutrients. Yet, vegetarians can meet their nutritional needs with a carefully planned diet with particular attention to a few nutrients. As discussed earlier, plant proteins are incomplete. To correct this deficiency, vegetarians should be encouraged to add milk and eggs to their diet, since these items have an equivalent amount of essential amino acids to animal protein, or to eat soybean products, which have all essential amino acids with the exception of methionine.

Concerns about iron nutrition arise from the differences between heme (meat-based) and non-heme (plant-based) iron. Since heme iron is more readily absorbed than non-heme iron (15–35% and 2–20%, respectively), vegetarians should include vitamin C sources with each meal to enhance absorption of non-heme iron, and they should avoid heavy intake of tea, which inhibits iron absorption. In addition to cow's milk, other excellent vegetarian sources of calcium include dark green leafy vegetables, dried figs, blackstrap molasses, soy milk, and calcium-fortified cereals, pastas, and tofu.

Plant foods do not contain vitamin B_{12} except when they are contaminated or processed by microorganisms. Thus, vegetarians need to look to other sources to get vitamin B_{12} in their diet. Although the minimum requirement for vitamin B_{12} is quite small (1–2 µg/day), B_{12} deficiency can lead to anemia and irreversible nerve damage. Possible vitamin B_{12} sources include eggs, milk, and milk products for lacto-vegetarians and B_{12}-fortified soy milk, B_{12}-fortified meat analogs, and vitamin B_{12} supplements for vegans.

Weight Watchers

The Weight Watchers diet is a commercial diet program based on a low-calorie and low-fat philosophy.[79] The program uses a point system that encourages a sensible diet consisting of healthy, ordinary foods, exercise, and a positive attitude. The plan is flexible and allows considerable variability and choice, but it requires relatively strict caloric restriction. In addition to the actual diet, in-person group meetings and weigh-ins are important parts of the program that encourage adherence to the plan.

The Weight Watchers diet has proven effective in weight loss in multiple studies. A systematic review of the effectiveness of five commercial diet programs compared eDiets.com, Health Management Resources, Take Off Pounds Sensibly, OPTIFAST, and Weight Watchers.[80] Of three randomized, controlled trials of Weight Watchers, the largest reported a loss of 3.2% of initial weight at 2 years. Although most of the diets showed a large weight loss, most were associated with high-cost, high-attrition rates and a high probability of regaining weight. With the exception of Weight Watchers, the review found poor evidence to support other commercial weight-loss programs. A separate randomized trial compared two low-carbohydrate diets (Atkins and The Zone) with a low-fat cardiac diet (the Ornish Diet) and Weight Watchers.[81] Each diet achieved between 2 and 3 kg of weight loss at 1 year and significantly reduced the LDL/HDL cholesterol ratio by approximately 10% but had no significant effects on blood pressure or glucose levels. Adherence for all the diets was considered poor.

Healing Foods and Healthy Foods Pyramids

The Healthy Foods Pyramid was designed in 2001 and revised in 2005 as an evidence-based response to the USDA Food Pyramid. It promotes the treatment and prevention of disease through an evidence-based diet, including whole grains, eliminating refined starches, and reducing red meat and dairy intake.[82] The Healing Foods Diet is a recent addition to low-fat diets (Figure 19-7). The diet includes principles of a plant-based diet with components of food that are healthy for both the individual and the earth.[83] Alcohol, especially wine (which contains saponins, resveratrol, and tannins), dark chocolate (which contain bioflavonoids), and teas (which contain multiple antioxidants) are included as daily accompaniments because of their phytochemical content.

Monounsaturated and polyunsaturated fats from olive or canola oil, nuts, seeds, and avocado are recommended. Five tenets are emphasized:

- Healing foods: Only foods that contain high proportions of essential nutrients and those with established healing properties are included.
- Plant-based choices: Plants constitute the majority of the diet; in particular, two to four servings of fruit and essentially unlimited servings of vegetables are recommended.
- Variety and balance: Balance and variety of color, nutrients, and portion size are encouraged.
- Support of a healthful environment: Persons are encouraged to make food selections so as to be respectful of environment, emphasizing organic foods raised without or with minimum additions of pesticides, hormones, medications, or contaminants.
- Mindful eating: Dieters are reminded to eat slowly and enjoy and focus on what is consumed.

Low-Carbohydrate Diets

Currently, one of the most popular approaches to weight loss is the low-carbohydrate diet (Table 19-4). In 2003, a systematic review including over 107 studies, 24 of which were randomized controlled trials, evaluated the efficacy of these diets.[84] The analysis concluded that the diets were generally effective but that weight loss was associated with decreased caloric intake, rather than true amount of carbohydrates in the diet. Both low- and higher-carbohydrate dieters lost similar amounts of weight (2–3 kg) and had no differences in cardiovascular effects after 90 days. Proponents of these diets argue that high glycemic carbohydrates are the cause for the weight gain because they result in a rapid rise in blood sugar followed by a surge in insulin. This insulin surge decreases blood sugar levels, which in turn results in craving for more carbohydrates, which results in more food ingestion and subsequent conversion into triglycerides. It is thus hypothesized that the body then continually needs glucose and relies on food as opposed to burning its own fat. These diets focus on changing the body's fuel source from dietary carbohydrates to adipose tissue. These diets are sometimes referred to as *ketogenic diets* because the increase in fat breakdown commonly results in ketone production.

Since low-carbohydrate diets are generally high in protein content (which has been shown to be more hunger satisfying than carbohydrates

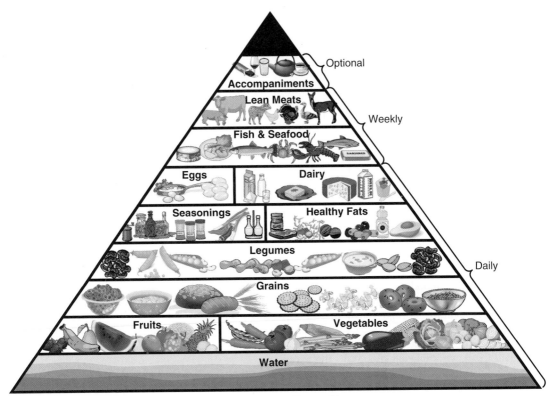

Optional
Accompaniments
Lean Meats
Weekly
Fish & Seafood
Eggs | Dairy
Seasonings | Healthy Fats
Legumes
Daily
Grains
Fruits | Vegetables
Water

Healing Foods Pyramid

Figure 19-7. The Healing Foods Pyramid. (University of Michigan Integrative Medicine: Healing Foods Pyramid. 2004. Available at: http://www.med.umich.edu/umim/clinical/pyramid/index.htm. Accessed July 24, 2006.)

or fats), dieters often consume fewer total calories, which aids in the weight loss. Finally, low-carbohydrate diets can induce significant water diuresis as a result of glycogenolysis from increased protein consumption. As glycogen stores (which are bound to water) are consumed for energy, two to four times that amount in weight-equivalent free water is diuresed through the urine. Thus, a portion of the early weight loss in these diets is simply water weight.[85]

Many versions of the low-carbohydrate diet exist, each with a unique interpretation of optimal low-carbohydrate eating.

The Atkins Diet

The Atkins Diet (Figure 19-8) was first published in the 1970s by Dr. Robert Atkins[86] but did not gain popularity until the late 1990s. The diet works by promoting a 2-week induction phase that restricts carbohydrates to 20 g/day, followed by an ongoing weight-loss phase that slowly increases carbohydrates in at a rate of 5 g/week. Finally, a maintenance phase with a goal carbohydrate level of 40–90 g/day is entered; this phase is designed to maintain weight loss.

In 2003, Foster et al[87] randomly assigned 63 obese people to follow either the Atkins diet or a conventional low-fat, low-calorie diet. Although the Atkins group had statistically significant greater weight loss at 3 months, there was no significant difference in weight loss, total cholesterol, or LDL cholesterol levels at 1 year. However, the subjects in the Atkins group did have greater HDL cholesterol and lower triglyceride levels.

South Beach Diet

The South Beach Diet was based on the 2003 best-selling book by Dr. Arthur Agatston.[88] It incorporates some of the elements of the Atkins diet but in a less restrictive form. Phase 1 of the diet limits fat to monounsaturated sources and includes only low-GI carbohydrates. As the various phases progress, the proportion of carbohydrates increases and the proportions of fat and protein decrease. In phase 2, "healthy carbohydrates" with a low GI are introduced slowly. Here, each dieter's reaction to carbohydrates is monitored by their weight to make changes necessary to continue to lose weight. Finally, lifelong maintenance (phase 3) is reached when the right balance between intake and weight

Table 19-4. Low-Carbohydrate/High-Protein Diet Summaries

	Atkins	Zone	Protein Power	Sugar Busters	Stillman	South Beach
Diet philosophy	Eating excess CHO releases insulin in large quantities, contributing to obesity and health problems. Restricting CHO intake leads to ketosis, which decreases hunger and increasing metabolism. Three phases are involved.	Eating the right combination of foods to optimize metabolic functions lowers insulin levels and desirable eicosanoid levels, thus leading to decreased hunger, weight loss, and increased energy.	Eating CHO releases insulin in large quantities, which contributes to obesity and other health problems.	Sugar is "toxic" to the body and causes release of insulin, which promotes fat storage.	High-protein foods burn body fat. If CHO are consumed, the body stores fat instead of burning it.	Eating the "right carbs" and the "right fats" results in health and weight loss. "Bad carbs" create urges to overeat and store fat. Three phases are involved.
Foods to eat	All meats, fish, poultry, eggs, cheese, low-CHO vegetables Butter, oils No alcohol Mega vitamins and mineral supplements daily (MVIs recommended)	40% CHO, 30% protein (based on lean body mass), 30% fat Mono fats, lean meats Low-GI foods Alcohol in moderation 200 IU vitamin E	15-35% CHO, 30-45% protein (based on lean body mass) 30-50% fat Meat, fish, poultry, eggs, cheese Low-CHO vegetables High fiber (25 g/day) Butter, oil, salad dressings Alcohol in moderation 8 glasses water/day MVI, vitamin C, chromium, potassium	Protein and fat Low-GI foods Olive oil, canola oil in moderation Alcohol in moderation Fruits must be eaten alone 3 meals/day	Lean meat and fish, skinless poultry Eggs No alcohol Skim milk, skim cheeses and cottage cheese	Meat, poultry, and fish, reduced-fat cheese, eggs Healthy oils and nuts Vegetables "Right carbohydrates and sweets"—low GI Three meals and two snacks Dessert after dinner
Menu analysis (based on computer analysis of 2-3 days menus provided in books)	1st 2 weeks: 1400 kcal/day; 28 g/day CHO (8%); 125 g/day protein (36%); 83 g/day fat (53%); 29 g/day saturated fat (19%); 5 g/day fiber	1430 kcal/day; 135 g/day CHO (38%); 111 g/day protein (31%); 50 g/day fat (31%); 14 g/day saturated fat (9%); 17 g/day fiber (protein requirement based on 1.6 g/kg)	1475 kcal/day; 47 g/day CHO (13%); 110 g/day protein (30%); 86 g/day fat (52%); 32 g/day sat fat (20%); 14 g/day fiber; increase CHO gradually	1000 kcal/day; 114 g/day CHO (46%); 71 g/day protein (28%); 28 g/day fat (25%); 7 g/day saturated fat (6%); 16 g/day fiber	1038 kcal/day; 7 g/day CHO (3%); 162 g/day protein (64%); 80 g/day fat (33%); 13% saturated fat	1st 2 weeks: 1409 kcal/day; 72 g/day CHO (20%); 122 g/day protein (35%); 67 g/day fat (43%); 20 g/day saturated fat

Table continued on following page

Table 19-4. Low-Carbohydrate/High-Protein Diet Summaries (Continued)

	Atkins	Zone	Protein Power	Sugar Busters	Stillman	South Beach
	Ongoing weight loss phase: 1840 kcal/day; 33 g/day CHO (7%); 161 g/day protein (35%); 118 g/day fat (58%); 39 g/day saturated fat (19%); 6 g/day fiber Maintenance phase: 1800 kcal/day; 128 g/day CHO (31%); 110 g/day protein (24%); 80 g/day fat (40%); 31 g/day saturated fat (16%); 20 g/day fiber						(13%); 15 g/day fiber Ongoing weight loss phase: 1220 kcal/day; 125 g/day CHO (41%); 70 g/day protein (23%); 53 g/day fat (38%)
Foods to limit or avoid	1st 2 weeks: CHO 20 g/day CHO Ongoing weight loss: gradual increase in CHO over 2 months Maintenance diet: 25–90 g/day CHO	CHO; specifically, bread, pasta, fruit (some types) Saturated fats and arachidonic acid	CHO limited to 30 g/day in phase 1, 55 g/day in phase 2, increase in maintenance Count CHO from alcohol	Potatoes, white rice, corn, carrots, beets, white bread, all refined white flour products	All CHO: specifically, bread, pasta, fruit (some types) Vegetables Fats, oils Dairy products	Phase 1: Fatty meats; whole milk cheese; high-GI vegetables; all fruit; fruit juices; all starchy foods; all dairy; alcohol Phase 2: bagels, white flour, potatoes, white rice; beets; carrots, corn; bananas; canned fruit, juice, pineapple

CHO, Carbohydrates; GI, glycemic index; MVI, multivitamin.

Adapted from: St. Jeor ST, Howard BV, Prewitt TE, et al: Dietary protein and weight reduction: a statement for healthcare professionals from the Nutrition Committee of the Council on Nutrition, Physical Activity, and Metabolism of the American Heart Association, *Circulation* 104:1869–1874, 2001; and from the Registered Dietitians at the University of Michigan Cardiovascular Center.

THE ATKINS LIFESTYLE FOOD GUIDE PRYAMID™

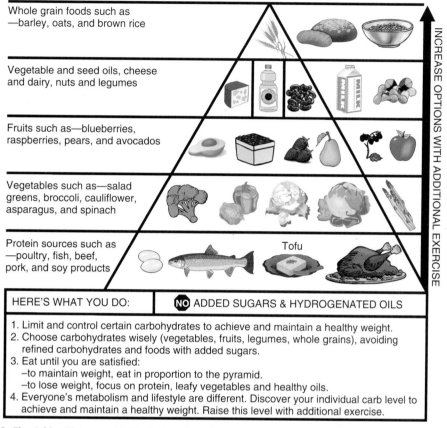

Whole grain foods such as
—barley, oats, and brown rice

Vegetable and seed oils, cheese
and dairy, nuts and legumes

Fruits such as—blueberries,
raspberries, pears, and avocados

Vegetables such as—salad
greens, broccoli, cauliflower,
asparagus, and spinach

Protein sources such as
—poultry, fish, beef,
pork, and soy products

Tofu

INCREASE OPTIONS WITH ADDITIONAL EXERCISE

HERE'S WHAT YOU DO: **NO** ADDED SUGARS & HYDROGENATED OILS

1. Limit and control certain carbohydrates to achieve and maintain a healthy weight.
2. Choose carbohydrates wisely (vegetables, fruits, legumes, whole grains), avoiding refined carbohydrates and foods with added sugars.
3. Eat until you are satisfied:
   –to maintain weight, eat in proportion to the pyramid.
   –to lose weight, focus on protein, leafy vegetables and healthy oils.
4. Everyone's metabolism and lifestyle are different. Discover your individual carb level to achieve and maintain a healthy weight. Raise this level with additional exercise.

Figure 19-8. The Atkins Diet pyramid. (Available at: http://www.atkins.com. Accessed July 24, 2006.)

is reached. In 2004, Aude and colleagues[89] randomly assigned 60 obese patients to follow either the South Beach Diet or a low cholesterol diet. At 3 months, weight loss was almost double in the South Beach group (13.6 versus 7.5 pounds) with no statistically significant differences in the lipid profiles between the two groups.

Other Low-Carbohydrate Diets

The Zone Diet[90] and the Sugar Busters Diet[91] are also modified low-carbohydrate diets that allow 40% of calories from carbohydrates. The Zone Diet recommends a balanced approach of 40% carbohydrates, 30% protein, and 30% fat and a return to the diet of our human ancestors, where meats, fruits, and vegetables were the main dietary sources. This plan theoretically achieves the correct ratio of carbohydrates to proteins and fats to control basal insulin levels. According to its author, Barry Sears, PhD,[90] this diet optimizes the body's metabolic function through the regulation of blood glucose.

The Sugar Busters Diet[91] not only promotes avoidance of high glycemic carbohydrates but also encourages the consumption of monounsaturated fats such as olive and canola oils. The authors of this diet also stress the avoidance of saturated and *trans*-fats to reach a balanced nutritional concept. A modified food pyramid is created that emphasizes moderation in portion sizes and the consumption of grains, fruits, and vegetables.

In 2002, Bouche and colleagues[92] examined whether glucose, lipids, and total fat mass could be improved in nondiabetic men by adhering to a low-GI diet similar to the Zone or Sugar Buster Diet. Participants in the low-glycemic group were instructed to consume foods with a GI less than 45 (e.g., proteins, tofu, nuts, seeds, berries, avocados, and most vegetables), whereas those in the high-GI group were asked to consume foods with a GI greater than 60 (e.g., white bread, white rice, potatoes, sweets). No significant changes in body weight were observed during the 5 weeks in either group; however, those who consumed a low-glycemic diet had lower postprandial plasma glucose, cholesterol, and triglyceride levels than their counterparts.

There are many other low-carbohydrate diets available. Some of the more popular include the Protein Power and Protein Power Lifeplan, the Scarsdale Medical Diet (Dr. Tarnower's Diet), and one of the earliest low-carbohydrate diets, The Doctor's Quick Weight Loss Diet (i.e., the Stillman Diet).

Dietary Guidelines for the Prevention and Management of Chronic Disease

Lifestyle modifications including healthier dietary choices and exercise are always recommended as first-line treatment for obesity, hypertension, diabetes mellitus, and cardiovascular disease. This next section examines the evidence for specific dietary recommendations that have been evaluated as part of this first-line treatment.

Obesity

The prevalence of obesity is rapidly increasing worldwide, with more than 64% of US adults overweight or obese by BMI according to results from the 1999–2000 National Health and Nutrition Examination Survey (NHANES).[93] This figure represents a 14% increase in the prevalence rate from NHANES III (1988–1994) and a 36% increase from NHANES II (1976–1980) (Table 19-5). Men have lower rates of obesity than women (27.7% versus 34% between the ages of 20 and 74 years), although prevalence for men has more than doubled since the first NHANES survey in 1960–1962, in which just 10.7% of males were obese.[94] Despite its prevalence, the prevention and management of obesity remains controversial.

A review of the literature reveals that many studies demonstrating that calorie restriction can achieve short-term weight loss, yet the lack of long-term, high-quality trials has led to a lack of consensus among clinicians regarding the best dietary approach to treat obesity.

In November 2004, the Cochrane Database of Systematic Reviews updated *Advice on Low-fat Diets for Obesity*.[95] This was a collection of all available randomized clinical trials of low-fat diets versus other weight-reducing diets. This review focused on adults who were overweight or clinically obese and were dieting for the purpose of weight reduction. The main outcome measure was weight loss, and the participants were followed up for at least 6 months. The results of this systematic review showed no significant difference between low-fat diets and other weight-reducing diets in terms of long-term weight loss. In most of the studies, there were small, nonsignificant differences in weight loss between low-fat diet groups and the comparison groups. The two main limitations of this review were the lack of long-term studies and large losses of participants to follow-up.

Currently, a systematic review is being collected by the Cochrane group evaluating low-GI diets for obesity.[96] Until the results of that review are revealed and more long-term clinical trials undertaken, there will continue to be much controversy about the type of weight-loss diet that can be proven to be most efficacious in the long-term treatment and management of obesity.

Hypertension

Although a variety of dietary modifications have been shown to be beneficial in treating hypertension, approximately 50 million persons in the United States are still affected. In fact, a

Table 19-5. Prevalence of Obesity from 1988 to 2000

	MEN PREVALENCE (%)		WOMEN PREVALENCE (%)	
Age (Years)	1988–1994	1999–2000	1988–1994	1999–2000
20–34	14.1	24.1	18.5	25.8
35–44	21.5	25.2	25.5	33.9
45–54	23.2	30.1	32.4	38.1
55–64	27.2	32.9	33.7	43.1
65–74	24.1	33.4	26.9	38.8
75 and older	13.2	20.4	19.2	25.1

Adapted from: National Center for Health StatisticsPrevalence of overweight and obesity among adults: United States, 1999–2002. Available at: http://www.cdc.gov/nchs/products/pubs/pubd/hestats/obese/obse99.htm.

relationship between weight loss and decreased blood pressure was first noted as early as the 1920s.[97] Since then, many trials have demonstrated that weight loss in overweight patients, salt and alcohol restriction, and incorporation of a vegetarian or DASH-type diet (see Figure 19-4) can improve blood pressure.[98]

Solid evidence for weight loss was collected by the Cochrane group in a 2005 systematic review.[99] This review sought to evaluate whether weight-loss diets are more effective than regular diets in controlling blood pressure. Eighteen randomized controlled trials involving 2611 participants concluded that weight-reducing diets in overweight hypertensive persons resulting in weight loss of an average of 3–9% of body weight are associated with a decrease of 3 mm Hg of both systolic and diastolic blood pressure.[100]

The workshop on *Sodium and Blood Pressure* was convened by the National Heart, Lung, and Blood Institute in Bethesda, MD, in January 1999. It reviewed evidence from the previous decade on the relationship between sodium intake and blood pressure. The group concluded that a higher sodium intake is associated with higher blood pressure levels and that blood pressure can be lowered with reductions in sodium intake reductions in sodium intake of 40–50 mmol in both hypertensive and nonhypertensive persons.[100]

In 2001, Sacks and colleagues[101] evaluated the effect of varying sodium intake in combination with consumption of a DASH diet. In this study, 412 participants were randomly assigned to follow either a control or a DASH diet and, within each diet, participants ate foods with three different levels of sodium content for 30 days. Their findings revealed that reducing sodium intake to levels below 100 mmol/day and the DASH diet both lower blood pressure substantially. The greatest effects were observed in the low-sodium DASH group that had decreases in blood pressure comparable to those observed with anti-hypertensive patients.

Diabetes Mellitus

Lifestyle modifications including diet and exercise have been considered to be effective first-line treatment for type 2 diabetes for many years. The US Diabetes Prevention Program Study[57] demonstrated that the onset of type 2 diabetes can be prevented—or at least delayed—with dietary effort and increased physical activity. A diet with greater low-fat dairy intake was found to lower the risk for type 2 diabetes in men in the Health Professions Follow-up Study, which examined 41,254 male patients.[102] Yet, the optimal diet for patients with diabetes remains controversial. Significant amounts of carbohydrates worsen hyperglycemia, whereas fats increase the risk of atherosclerosis, and proteins may promote diabetic nephropathy. In 2004, the ADA updated its statement on the topic[103] and provided the following top-level evidence-based recommendations based on multiple population risk strata:

- Foods containing carbohydrates from whole grains, fruits, vegetables, and low-fat milk should be included in a healthy diet.
- With regard to the glycemic effects of carbohydrates, the total amount of carbohydrates in meals or snacks is more important than the source or type.
- Less than 10% of energy intake should be derived from saturated fats.
- Dietary cholesterol intake should be less than 300 mg/day.
- In insulin-resistant persons, reduced energy intake and modest weight loss improve insulin resistance and glycemia in the short term.
- Structured programs that emphasize lifestyle changes, including education, reduced fat (< 30% of daily energy) and energy intake, regular physical activity, and regular participant contact, can produce long-term weight loss on the order of 5–7% of starting weight.
- Exercise and behavior modification are most useful as adjuncts to other weight-loss strategies. Exercise is helpful in the maintenance of weight loss.
- Standard weight-reduction diets, when used alone, are unlikely to produce long-term weight loss; structured intensive lifestyle programs are necessary.

The Cochrane Database of Systematic Reviews examined all randomized trials of 6 months' duration or longer in which dietary advice was the main intervention in adults with type 2 diabetes.[104] Data from 36 articles reporting a total of 18 trials monitoring 1467 participants were collected. Different dietary approaches, as well as the addition of exercise to each diet, were the main analyses, whereas weight and micro- and macrovascular diabetic complications were the main outcome measures. Unfortunately, there were insufficient data in the review to reach any valid conclusions regarding the type of dietary advice most suitable for patients with diabetes. However, there was solid evidence for the use of exercise as an adjunct to dietary modifications because this was associated with a statistically significant decrease in mean glycosylated hemoglobin levels of 0.9% at 6 months and 1% at 12 months.[22]

Currently, the National Institutes of Health is evaluating the long-term health effects of weight loss in adults who are overweight and have type 2 diabetes. This new study entitled "Look AHEAD" is well underway and will follow up with participants for up to 11 years, which should help clarify the role of dietary treatment in type 2 diabetes.

Metabolic Syndrome

The constellation of dyslipidemia, elevated blood pressure, impaired glucose tolerance, and central obesity defines the metabolic syndrome. The National Cholesterol Education Program–Adult Treatment Panel III (NCEP-ATP III) identified metabolic syndrome as an independent risk factor for cardiovascular disease and considered it an indication for intensive lifestyle modification.[105] The two essential components of lifestyle modification are diet and exercise. Since skeletal muscle is the most insulin-sensitive tissue in the body, it should be a primary target for affecting insulin resistance. Physical training has been shown to reduce skeletal muscle lipid levels and improve insulin resistance, regardless of BMI.[106]

Unfortunately, very few randomized controlled trials exist to specifically examine the treatment of metabolic syndrome with specific dietary interventions. Azadbakht and colleagues[107] conducted a randomized controlled outpatient trial conducted on 116 patients with the metabolic syndrome. These patients were assigned to follow one of six diets and were followed up over a period of 6 months. Relative to the control diet, the DASH diet resulted in higher HDL cholesterol (7 and 10 mg/dL), lower triglycerides (−18 and −14 mg/dL), lower systolic blood pressure (−12 and −11 mm Hg), lower diastolic blood pressure (−6 and −7 mm Hg), lower weight (−16 and −14 kg), decreased fasting blood glucose (−15 and −8 mg/dL), and decreased weight (−16 and −15 kg) among men and women, respectively (all $P < .001$).

Cochrane Database systematic reviews[108,109] support the role of dietary interventions in helping to reduce cardiovascular risk. These reviews demonstrated that a low-sodium diet was enough to maintain a lower blood pressure after withdrawal of antihypertensive medications and also showed that low-fat diets in which participants were involved for more than 2 years showed significant protection from cardiovascular events (relative risk, 0.84; 95% confidence interval, 0.72–0.99).

Coronary Artery Disease

An important emphasis of the latest AHA dietary guidelines for the secondary prevention of CAD (last updated in 2006)[110] is lipid management. The recommendations include the following:

- Dietary therapy should proceed in all patients, including a goal of less than 7% of caloric intake provided by saturated fat and an intake of less than 200 mg dietary cholesterol and *trans*-fatty acids per day.
- LDL cholesterol should be less than 100 mg/dL (at baseline or on medical treatment); levels less than 70 mg/dL are also reasonable, especially in persons with diabetes.
- Triglyceride levels should be less than 150 mg/dL and HDL cholesterol levels should be greater than 40 mg/dL (at baseline or on medical treatment).
- The goal BMI should be 18–25 kg/m^2.
- Increased intake of omega-3 fatty acids in the form of fish or capsules should be encouraged.

Early studies with conventional dietary modification (National Cholesterol Education Program Step 1 and 2 diets) yielded little benefit on established coronary disease; however, more positive results were reported in the early 1990s,[111] with aggressive dietary therapy aimed at reducing dietary saturated fat and cholesterol. The St. Thomas Atheroma Regression Study (STARS) randomly assigned men with coronary heart disease and total cholesterol levels exceeding 232 mg/dL to receive conventional care versus a low-fat diet with a target cholesterol consumption of 100–120 mg/day. At 3 years, the diet-treated group was noted to have a slower progression rate of coronary atherosclerosis, more regression of coronary atherosclerotic lesions based on angiography, and less severe angina pectoris.[111] The Lyon Diet Heart Study[112] evaluated the effects of a Mediterranean diet in 605 patients after a first myocardial infarction. At 27 months, patients following this diet had lower rates of deaths and myocardial infarctions (primary end points) as well as unstable angina, stroke, heart failure, and pulmonary embolisms (secondary end points). This benefit was also noted up to 4 years.

The Cochrane Group recently examined the AHA's advice regarding omega-3 fatty acids in the treatment of cardiovascular disease in a recent review.[113] They collected data from 48 randomized controlled trials including 36,913 participants. Pooled trial results did not show a reduction in the risk of total mortality or combined cardiovascular events in persons taking additional omega-3 fats. They concluded that there is no evidence to advise people to stop taking rich sources of omega-3 fats, but further high-quality trials are needed to confirm suggestions of a protective effect of omega-3 fats on cardiovascular health.

The Portfolio Diet is a special low-fat diet designed to reduced cholesterol.[114] A research intervention, rather than a commercial service or book, it was designed as a "portfolio" of current recommendations from the NCEP-ATP III and the AHA Step II diet for foods that are known to reduce cholesterol. This portfolio of cholesterol-reducing foods was compared with statin medications in a randomized trial. This vegetarian diet is low in saturated fat and encourages plant sterols and viscous fibers, soy protein, and almonds. Psyllium, in the form of Metamucil, barley, and oats were preferred grains; eggplants and okra were preferred vegetables. Margarine and butter were substituted with spreads containing omega-3 fatty acids and plant sterols, such as Benecol, Take Control, and Smart Balance. In this small trial, 25 men and 21 women were randomly assigned to participate in one of three interventions for 1 month: a control standard low-fat diet based on milled whole-wheat cereals and low-fat dairy foods, the same diet plus lovastatin 20 mg/day, or the dietary portfolio. Results from the diet showed a significant difference between the control diet, which reduced cholesterol by 8% and C-reactive protein (CRP) by 10%, and the other two arms.[22] The control diet plus lovastatin reduced cholesterol by 31% and CRP by 33% and was not significantly different than the dietary portfolio, which reduced cholesterol by 29% and CRP by 28%.[22]

Other Diseases

Persons with chronic gastrointestinal diseases, such as peptic ulcer disease, gastroesophageal reflux disease, malabsorptive syndromes, and inflammatory bowel disease, should adhere to specific diets that treat the symptoms of the disease or prevent problems associated with it. Persons with chronic pulmonary diseases, such as chronic obstructive pulmonary disease and cystic fibrosis, and patients with chronic renal insufficiency and renal failure also benefit from adherence to a diet specifically designed to address their medical problems. For men with these problems, specific consultation with a physician regarding nutritional issues should be encouraged.

Fostering Change

Physicians should take an active role in guiding their patients toward their nutritional goals. This should include not only educating them regarding the different dietary choices but also assisting them in setting reasonable goals that are possible to maintain. Because no one superior diet exists, the choice of an acceptable diet is not as important as its incorporation as part of an overall healthy lifestyle. The importance of regular physical activity is not to be underestimated because long-term weight loss and maintenance of optimal weight and body composition is difficult without exercise. Scheduled-interval patient follow-ups for support and tracking progress are of great importance because they will decrease the likelihood of relapse into poor dietary habits. Finally, both physicians and dieting persons need to be patient and flexible because successful weight loss is a long-term process that is both challenging and rewarding. The following basic steps provide the groundwork toward achieving dietary goals:

- Provide a thorough evaluation of a patient's nutritional status in the context of his overall health.
- Educate and devise a plan together.
- Set realistic short- and long-term goals.
- Consider early referral to a nutritionist or dietitian as well as other medical subspecialists when indicated.
- Monitor and track changes through use of a food diary, and review it at scheduled visits.
- Provide support and encouragement along the way through frequent follow-up visits.
- Be flexible and consider changing the plan if compliance is a concern.
- Be available for any questions or problems that may arise.

Conclusion

Diet plays a critical role in the etiology of chronic disease and as an adjunct to treatment. Despite growing public awareness and scientific research, the incidence of chronic diseases such cardiovascular disease and diabetes continue to increase. Various dietary options exist that can potentially minimize morbidity and mortality in both healthy patients and in those with chronic diseases. Patients should consult their physicians as to proper guidance regarding dietary recommendations, employing dietitians and nutritional counselors when available.

References

1. Woteki C, Thomas P: *Eat for Life*, Washington DC, 1992, National Academy Press.
2. Commission on Dietary Supplement Labels: Report of the Commission on Dietary Supplement Labels. 1997. Available at: http://www.health.gov/dietsupp/cover.htm.
3. Nutrition.gov. Available at: http://www.nutrition.gov.
4. US Department of Agriculture: Dietary guidelines for Americans 2005. Available at: http://www.health.gov/dietaryguidelines/dga2005/document.
5. Aboud L: Expect a food fight as U.S. sets to revise diet guidelines, *Wall Street J* August 8, 2003, B1.
6. Institute of Medicine: *Dietary Reference Intakes for Energy, Carbohydrate, Fiber, Fat, Fatty Acids, Cholesterol, Protein, and Amino Acids*, Washington DC, 2002, National Academy Press.
7. Leaf A, Kang J, Xiao YF, et al: Clinical prevention of sudden cardiac death by n-3 polyunsaturated fatty acids and mechanism of prevention of arrhythmias by n-3 fish oils, *Circulation* 107:2646–2652, 2003.
8. Foster-Powell K: International table of glycemic index and glycemic load values: 2002, *Am J Clin Nutr* 76(1):5–56, 2002.
9. Wolever TM, Vorster HH, Bjorck I, et al: Determination of the glycemic index of foods: interlaboratory study, *Eur J Clin Nutr* 57(3):475–482, 2003.
10. Brand-Miller J, Foster-Powell K, Colquir S, et al: *The New Glucose Revolution Low GI Guide to Losing Weight: The Only Authoritative Guide to Weight Loss Using the Glycemic Index*, New York, 2006, Marlowe and Company.
11. Pereira MA, Swain J, Goldfine AB, et al: Effects of a low-glycemic load diet on resting energy expenditure and heart disease risk factors during weight loss, *JAMA* 292(20):2482–2490, 2004.
12. Home of the glycemic index University of Sydney. Available at: http://www.glycemicindex.com.
13. Milne AC, Potter J, Avenell A, et al: Protein and energy supplementation in elderly people at risk from malnutrition, *Cochrane Database Syst Rev* 2:CD003288, 2006.
14. Institute of Medicine: *Dietary Reference Intakes for Water, Potassium, Sodium, Chloride and Sulfate*, Washington DC, 2004, National Academy Press.
15. Institute of Medicine: *Dietary Reference Intakes for Thiamin, Riboflavin, Niacin, Vitamin B₆, Folate, Vitamin B₁₂, Pantothenic Acid, Biotin, and Choline*, Washington DC, 1998, National Academy Press.
16. Stransky M, Rubin A, Lava NS, Lazaro RP: Treatment of carpal tunnel syndrome with vitamin B6: a double-blind study, *South Med J* 82:841–842, 1989.
17. Spooner GR, Desai HB, Angel JF, et al: Using pyridoxine to treat carpal tunnel syndrome: randomized control trial, *Can Fam Phys* 39:2122–2127, 1993.
18. Bonaa KH, et al, for NORVIT Trial Investigators: Homocysteine lowering and cardiovascular events after acute myocardial infarction, *N Engl J Med* 354 (15):1578–1588, 2006.
19. Deijen JB: Vitamin B6 supplementation in elderly men: effects on mood, memory, performance and mental effort, *Psychopharmacology (Berl)* 109(4):489–496, 1992.
20. Malouf R: Vitamin B₁₂ for cognition, *Cochrane Database Syst Rev* 2:CD004394, 2006.
21. Institute of Medicine: *Dietary Reference Intakes for Vitamin C, Vitamin E, Selenium, and Carotenoids*, Washington DC, 2000, National Academy Press.
22. Institute of Medicine: *Dietary Reference Intakes for Vitamin A, Vitamin K, Arsenic, Boron, Chromium, Copper, Iodine, Iron, Manganese, Molybdenum, Nickel, Silicon, Vanadium, and Zinc*, Washington DC, 2001, National Academy Press.
23. Steingrimsdottir L, Gunnarsson O, Indridason OS, et al: Relationship between serum parathyroid hormone levels, vitamin D sufficiency, and calcium intake, *JAMA* 294:2336–2341, 2005.
24. Institute of Medicine: *Dietary Reference Intakes for Calcium, Phosphorous, Magnesium, Vitamin D, and Fluoride*, Washington DC, 1997, National Academy Press.
25. Age-Related Eye Disease Study Research Group: A randomized, placebo-controlled, clinical trial of high-dose supplementation with vitamins C and E, beta carotene, and zinc for age-related macular degeneration and vision loss: AREDS report no. 8, *Arch Ophthalmol* 119(10):1417–1436, 2001.
26. Jurgens G, Graudal NA: Effects of low sodium diet versus high sodium diet on blood pressure, renin, aldosterone, catecholamines, cholesterols, and triglycerides, *Cochrane Database Syst Rev* 2:CD004022, 2006.
27. Zemel MB, Thompson W, Milstead A, et al: Calcium and dairy acceleration of weight and fat loss during energy restriction in obese adults, *Obes Res* 12(4):582–590, 2004.
28. Keese E, Bertrais S, Astorg P, et al: Dairy products, calcium and phosphorus intake, and the risk of prostate cancer: results of the French Prospective SU.VI.MAX (Supplementation en Vitamines et Mineraux Antioxydants) Study, *Br J Nutr* 95(3):539–545, 2006.
29. Holt PR: Modulation of abnormal colonic epithelial cell proliferation and differentiation by low-fat dairy foods: a randomized controlled trial, *JAMA* 280:1074–1079, 1998.
30. Yip L, Dart R: Arsenic, In Sullivan JB, Krieger GR, eds: *Clinical Environmental Health and Toxic Exposures*, ed 2. Philadelphia, 2001, Lippincott, William & Williams, pp 858–866.
31. Wu T, Liu GJ, Li P, Clar C: Iodised salt for preventing iodine deficiency disorders, *Cochrane Database Syst Rev* 3:CD003204, 2002.
32. Chan JM, Stampfer MJ, Giovannucci EL: What causes prostate cancer? a brief summary of the epidemiology, *Semin Cancer Biol* 8:263–273, 1998.
33. Wilkinson EAJ, Hawke CI: Oral zinc for arterial and venous leg ulcers, *Cochrane Database Syst Rev* 2:CD001273, 2000.

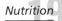
34. Lukaski HC: Low dietary zinc decreases erythrocyte carbonic anhydrase activities and impairs cardiorespiratory function in men during exercise, *Am J Clin Nutr* 81(5):1045–1051, 2005.

35. Howard AA, Arnsten JH, Gourevitch MN: Effect of alcohol consumption on diabetes mellitus: a systematic review, *Ann Intern Med* 140(3):211–219, 2004.

36. Aldoori WH, Giovannucci EL, Rockett HR, et al: A prospective study of dietary fiber types and symptomatic diverticular disease in men, *J Nutr* 128 (4):714–719, 1998.

37. McKeown NM, Meigs JB, Liu S, et al: Carbohydrate nutrition, insulin resistance, and the prevalence of the metabolic syndrome in the Framingham Offspring Cohort, *Diabetes Care* 27 (2):538–546, 2004.

38. Anderson JW, Randles KM, Kendall CW, Jenkins DJ: Carbohydrate and fiber recommendations for individuals with diabetes: a quantitative assessment and meta-analysis of the evidence, *J Am Coll Nutr* 23(1):5–17, 2004.

39. Blair SN, Capuzzi DM, Gottlieb SO, et al: Incremental reduction of serum total cholesterol and low-density lipoprotein cholesterol with the addition of plant stanol ester-containing spread to statin therapy, *Am J Cardiol* 86(1):46–52, 2000.

40. Hermann, F, Spieker, LE, Ruschitzka, F, et al: Dark chocolate improves endothelial and platelet function, *Heart* 92(1):119–120, 2006.

41. Schabath MB, Hernandez LM, Wu X, et al: Dietary phytoestrogens and lung cancer risk, *JAMA* 294 (12):1493–1504, 2005.

42. Vanharanta, M, Voutilainen, S, Rissanen, TH, et al: Risk of cardiovascular disease–related and all-cause death according to serum concentrations of enterolactone: Kuopio Ischaemic Heart Disease Risk Factor Study. *Arch Intern Med* 163(9): 1099–1104, 2003.

43. Brower LP: Sodium cyclamate and bladder carcinoma, *Science* 170(957):558, 1970.

44. Howe GR, Burch JD, Miller AB, et al: Artificial sweeteners and human bladder cancer, *Lancet* 2 (8038):578–581, 1977.

45. US Food and Drug Administration: Artificial sweeteners: no calories…sweet! *FDA Consumer Mag* 2006. Available at: http://www.fda.gov/fdac/features/2006/406_sweeteners.html.

46. US Food and Drug Administration Web site. Available at: http://www.fda.gov.

47. Smolin L: *Nutrition Science and Application*, New York, 1999, John Wiley and Sons.

48. Khalidi N, Btaiche I, Kovacevich D, et al, editors: *The University of Michigan Hospitals and Health Centers Parenteral and Enteral Nutrition Manual*, Chicago, 2003, University of Michigan Press.

49. Morrison G, Hark L: *Medical Nutrition: A Case-based Approach*, Malden, MA 2003, Blackwell Publishing.

50. Kushner RF: Risk assessment of the overweight and obese patient, *J Am Diet Assoc* 105(5 Suppl 1): S53–S62, 2005.

51. Keys A, Aravanis C, Blackburn HW, et al: Epidemiologic studies related to coronary heart disease: characteristics of men aged 40–59 in seven countries, *Acta Med Scand* 460(Suppl):1–392, 1967.

52. National Center for Health Statistics Web site. Centers for Disease Control and Prevention. Available at: http://www.cdc.gov/nchs.

53. Mokdad AH, Ford ES, Bowman BA, et al: Prevalence of obesity, diabetes and obesity-related risk factors, 2001, *JAMA* 289:76–79, 2003.

54. Multiple Risk Factor Intervention Trial Research Group: Mortality rates after 10.5 years after participants in the MRFIT, *JAMA* 263:1795–1801, 1990.

55. The LRC-CPPT Authors: The Lipid Research Clinics Coronary Primary Prevention Trial results: I. reduction in incidence of coronary heart disease, *JAMA* 251(3):351–364, 1984.

56. US Department of Agriculture: Dietary guidelines for Americans. Available at: http://www.health.gov/DietaryGuidelines.

57. Knowler WC: Reduction in the incidence of type 2 diabetes with lifestyle intervention or metformin, *N Engl J Med* 346:1829–1830, 2002.

58. American Heart Association: *No-fad Diet: A Personal Plan for Healthy Weight Loss*. 2007. Available at: http://www.americanheart.org/presenter.jhtml?identifier=3031890.

59. Appel LJ, Moore TJ, Obarzanek E, et al: A clinical trial of the effects of dietary patterns on blood pressure: DASH Collaborative Research Group, *N Engl J Med* 336:1117–1124, 1997.

60. Appel LJ: Effects of comprehensive lifestyle modification on blood pressure control, *JAMA* 2889:2083, 2003.

61. Appel LJ, Sacks FM, Carey VJ, et al: Effects of protein, monounsaturated fat, and carbohydrate intake on blood pressure and serum lipids: results of the OmniHeart randomized trial, *JAMA* 294: 2455–2464, 2005.

62. Oldways Preservation and Exchange Trust Web site. Available at: http://www.oldwayspt.org.

63. World Health Organization: *Diet, Nutrition, and the Prevention of Chronic Diseases: Report of a WHO Study Group*, Geneva, 1990, WHO Technical Report Series 797.

64. Trichopoulou A, Costacou T, Bamia C, Trichopoulos D: Adherence to a Mediterranean diet and survival in a Greek population, *N Engl J Med* 348:2599–2608, 2003.

65. Albert CM: Fish consumption and risk of sudden cardiac death, *JAMA* 279:23–28, 1998.

66. Hu FB: Fish and omega-3 fatty acid intake and risk of coronary heart disease in women, *JAMA* 287:1815–1821, 2002.

67. Burr ML: Effects of changes in fat, fish, and fibre intakes on death and reinfarction: diet and Reinfarction Trial (DART), *Lancet* 2:757–761, 1989.

68. GISSI-Prevenzione Investigators: Dietary supplementation with n-3 polyunsaturated fatty acids and vitamin E after myocardial infarction: results of the GISSI-Prevenzione trial, *Lancet* 354:447–455, 1999.

69. Ascherio A: Dietary intake of marine n-3 fatty acids, fish intake and risk of coronary heart disease among men, *N Engl J Med* 332:977–982, 1995.

70. Loma Linda University: The Adventist Health Study: findings for nuts. 2006. Available at: http://www.llu.edu/llu/health/nuts.html.

71. Corliss R: Should we all be vegetarians? *Time* July 7, 2002.

72. Sacks FM, Kass EH: Low blood pressure in vegetarians: effects of specific foods and nutrients, *Am J Clin Nutr* 48(3 Suppl):795–800, 1988.

73. Position statement of the American Dietetic Association, *J Am Diet Assoc* 103:748–765, 2003.

74. Campell TC: Diet, lifestyle, and the etiology of coronary artery disease: the China Cornell Study, *Am J Cardiol* 82(10B):18T–21T, 1998.

75. Committee on Diet Nutrition and Cancer, Commission on Life Sciences, National Research Council: *Diet, Nutrition and Cancer: Directions for Research*, Washington, DC, 1983, National Academy Press.

76. Chen J, Campbell TC, Li J, Peto R: *Diet, Life-style and Mortality in China: A Study of the Characteristics of 65 Chinese Counties*, Ithaca, NY, 1991, Cornell University Press.

77. Campbell TC: *The China Study: The Most Comprehensive Study of Nutrition Ever and the Startling Implications for Diet, Weight Loss and Long-term Health*, Dallas, 2005, Benbella Books.

78. Campbell TC, Cambell T: Diet and chronic degenerative diseases: perspectives from China, *Am J Clin Nutr* 59(5 Suppl):1153S–1161S, 1994.

79. Weight Watchers website. Available at: http://www.weightwatchers.com.

80. Tsai AG: Systematic review: an evaluation of major commercial weight loss programs in the United States, *Ann Intern Med* 142(1):56–66, 2005.

81. Dansinger ML: Comparison of the Atkins, Ornish, Weight Watchers, and Zone diets for weight loss and heart disease risk reduction: a randomized trial, *JAMA* 293(1):43–53, 2005.

82. Willet W: *Eat Drink and Be Healthy*, New York, 2005, Free Press/Simon & Schuster.

83. University of Michigan Integrative Medicine: Healing Foods Pyramid. 2004. Available at: http://www.med.umich.edu/umim/clinical/pyramid/index.htm.

84. Bravata DM, Sanders L, Huang J, et al: Efficacy and safety of low-carbohydrate diets: a systematic review, *JAMA* 289(14):1837–1850, 2003.

85. Shiles ME: *Modern Nutrition in Health and Disease*, ed 9, Baltimore, MD, 1999, Williams and Wilkins, p 904.

86. Atkins RC: *Dr. Atkins' Diet Revolution: The High Calorie Way to Stay Thin Forever*, New York, 1973, Bantam.

87. Foster GD, Wyatt HR, Hill JO, et al: A randomized trial of a low-carbohydrate diet for obesity, *N Engl J Med* 348:2082–2090, 2003.

88. Agatston A: *The South Beach Diet*, New York, 2003, Rodale.

89. Aude Y: The National Cholesterol Education Program diet vs a diet lower in carbohydrates and higher in protein and monounsaturated fat, *Arch Intern Med* 164:2141–2146, 2004.

90. Sears B: *The Zone: Revolutionary Life Plan to Put Your Body in Total Balance for Permanent Weight Loss*, New York, 1995, Regan Books.

91. Steward L: *Sugar Busters! Cut Sugar to Trim Fat*, New York, 1998, Ballantine Books.

92. Bouche C: Five-week, low glycemic index diet decreases total fat mass and improves plasma lipid profile in moderately overweight nondiabetic men, *Diabetes Care* 25:822–828, 2002.

93. National Center for Health StatisticsPrevalence of overweight and obesity among adults: United States, 1999–2002. Available at: http://www.cdc.gov/nchs/products/pubs/pubd/hestats/obese/obse99.htm.

94. Flegal KM, Carroll MD, Ogden CL, Johnson CL: Prevalence and trends in obesity among U.S. adults, 1999–2000, *JAMA* 288:1723–1727, 2002.

95. Pirozzo S: Advice on low-fat diets for obesity, *Cochrane Collaboration* 3:CD003640, 2005.

96. Thomas DE: Low glycemic index diets for overweight and obesity, *Cochrane Collaboration* 3: CD005105, 2005.

97. Terry AH: Obesity and hypertension, *JAMA* 81 (15):1283–1284, 1922.

98. Chobanian AV: The seventh report of the Joint National Committee on Prevention, Detection, Evaluation, and Treatment of High Blood Pressure, *JAMA* 289:2560–2572, 2003.

99. Mulrow CD: Dieting to reduce body weight for controlling hypertension in adults, *Cochrane Collaboration* 3:CD000484, 2005.

100. Chobanian AV, Hill M: National Heart, Lung, and Blood Institute Workshop on Sodium and Blood Pressure: a critical review of current scientific evidence, *Hypertension* 35:858–863, 2000.

101. Sacks FM, and the DASH-Sodium Collaborative Research Group: Effects on blood pressure of reduced dietary sodium and the Dietary Approaches to Stop Hypertension (DASH) diet, *N Engl J Med* 344:3–10, 2001.

102. Choi HK, Willett WC, Stampfer MJ, et al: Dietary consumption and risk of type 2 diabetes mellitus in men: a prospective study, *Arch Intern Med* 165 (9):997–1003, 2005.

103. American Diabetes Association: Evidence-based nutrition principles and recommendations for the treatment and prevention of diabetes and related complications, *Diabetes Care* 25:202–212, 2002. Available at: http://care.diabetesjournals.org/cgi/content/full/25/1/202.

104. Moore H: Dietary advice for treatment of type 2 diabetes mellitus in adults, *Cochrane Collaboration* 3:CD004097, 2005.

105. National Institutes of Health: *Third Report of the National Cholesterol Education Program Expert Panel on Detection, Evaluation, and Treatment of High Blood Cholesterol in Adults (Adult Treatment*

Panel III): Executive Summary, NIH publication no. 01–3670.Bethesda, MD, 2001, National Institutes of Health, National Heart Lung and Blood Institute.

106. Goodpaster BH, He J, Watkins S, Kelley DE: Skeletal muscle lipid content and insulin resistance: evidence for a paradox in endurance-trained athletes, *J Clin Endocrinol Metab* 86:5755–5761, 2001.

107. Azadbakht L, Mirmiran P, Esmaillzadeh A, et al: Beneficial effects of a dietary approaches to stop hypertension eating plan on features of the metabolic syndrome, *Diabetes Care* 28(12):2823–2831, 2005.

108. Hooper L, Bartlett C, Davey SG, Ebrahim S: Advice to reduce dietary salt for prevention of cardiovascular disease, *Cochrane Database Syst Rev* 2: CD003656, 2004.

109. Hooper L, Summerbell CD, Higgins JP, et al: Reduced or modified dietary fat for preventing cardiovascular disease, *Cochrane Database Syst Rev* 2:CD002137, 2004.

110. Smith SC, Allen J, Blair SN, et al: AHA/ACC guidelines for secondary prevention for patients with coronary and other atherosclerotic vascular disease: 2006 update, *Circulation* 113:2363–2372, 2006. Available at: http://circ.ahajournals.org/cgi/content/full/113/19/2363.

111. Watts GF: Effects of coronary artery disease of lipid lowering diet in the St. Tomas Atherosclerosis Regression Study (STARS), *Lancet* 339:563–569, 1992.

112. De Lorgeril M: Mediterranean diet, traditional risk factors, and the rate of cardiovascular complications after myocardial infarction: final report of the Lyon Heart Study, *Circulation* 99:770–785, 1999.

113. Hooper L: Omega 3 fatty acids for prevention and treatment of cardiovascular disease, *Cochrane Collaboration* 1:CD003177, 2006.

114. Jenkins DJ, Kendall CW, Marchie A, et al: Effects of a dietary portfolio of cholesterol-lowering foods vs lovastatin on serum lipids and C-reactive protein, *JAMA* 290:502–510, 2003.

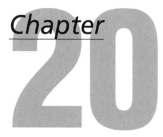

Chapter

20

Stress and the Modern Male

Denise K.C. Sur, MD, Robert Maurer, PhD, and Keyvan Hariri, MD

Key Points

- Stress in males contributes to increased rates of cardiovascular disease (strength of recommendation: B).
- Stress reduction can improve overall health (strength of recommendation: B).
- Asking male patients about their fears and stressors is an effective first step in addressing stress management (strength of recommendation: C).
- Exercise, yoga, meditation, and peer counseling are effective stress reducers (strength of recommendation: C).

Introduction

Stress remains both a challenge and an enigma to the clinician and patient alike. To the lay public, the term *stress* generally conjures up a negative connotation and is often considered in the context of a difficult job, financial problems, a challenging interpersonal relationship, or simply too much work to complete within too little time. Dr. Hans Selye was the originator of the concept of stress and the general adaptation syndrome in the early 1920s. If he were alive today, the contexts of these stressors might pain him deeply. In his writings, Selye described that a person's problems were the "stressors" and that the human body's inability to respond to them in a healthy and positive fashion constituted the "stress syndrome." He discovered that patients with a variety of ailments manifested many similar constitutional symptoms, which he ultimately attributed to their bodies' efforts to respond to the stresses of being ill. Seyle might

have been confused by the modern-day concept of a physician completing a disability form for a patient who is reportedly "too stressed to work," implying that the patient's environment has caused a medical problem. Through his hundreds of research articles and landmark textbooks *The Stress of Life*[1] and *Stress Without Distress*,[2] Selye demonstrated the role of emotional responses in causing or combating much of the "wear and tear" experienced by human beings throughout their lives that serves as a framework for our understanding of stress and its effects on the human body in today's society.

History may judge the concept of a stress disorder with confusion and disdain. Nonetheless, *stress* is, in its simplest form, another term for chronic sympathetic nervous system arousal. What science has successfully done is to outline the details of what happens to the body during this biologic phenomenon. Yet what may be overlooked with major implications for understanding male stress is perhaps a cultural abhorrence or denial of one of the body's most basic, vital, and pervasive emotions: fear. As a general rule, adult humans do not express their fear in a comfortable, natural way; any practicing physician has witnessed this phenomenon. Children will easily discuss or show their fear of the bogeyman, a vaccination, or the surgery for which someone is preparing them. By the time we have become "adulterated," fear seems to no longer be an acceptable word. You can test this theory by asking any adult, during a pause in a dinnertime conversation, "What are you afraid of?" Both your discomfort in asking this question and the peculiar look you may receive from your dinner partner will prove this point.

Fear implies a personal experience and response to an anxiety-provoking event. Stress often leads us to focus more heavily on the external event than on an individual's inability to deal with such an event, and to treat this seemingly normal emotion as a disease to be treated or avoided. Asking a male patient about his fears will likely feel awkward and may be poorly received, whereas asking about his stressors will likely inspire the patient to discuss the circumstances in his life that are anxiety provoking and disagreeable.

Sociologically, because men may have great difficulty acknowledging and accepting fear as a natural and healthy part of life, effective coping strategies for stress and fear may be limited. Often, a man's stress or fear leads to other significant problems within his life and has a negative impact on his overall health and well-being. This chapter aims to outline several of the unhealthy responses to unacknowledged and untreated stress before discussing healthy coping strategies and their inherent barriers for male patients through guidelines and advice found in both the medical and lay literature.

Common Unhealthy Responses to Stress in Males

Illicit substance abuse is one of the most common responses to stress or fear in men. In studies of gender responses to post-traumatic stress disorder, men have been shown to be more likely to respond by developing a substance abuse disorder than women. By adolescence, boys are three times more likely to use and abuse alcohol than girls and 50% more likely to use other illicit drugs such as marijuana and cocaine and to abuse prescription drugs to cope with post-traumatic stress.[3,4]

Because food is thought to be the fastest-acting tranquilizer available, overeating is also commonly seen in men as a response to stress and fear.[5] The moment that food reaches the tongue, the amygdala (i.e., the primitive portion of the brain that controls our sympathetic arousal) assumes that the proverbial "lion has gone away" and shuts off the involuntary fear or stress response immediately. The problem, of course, is that food has no true half-life, and as soon as food is swallowed, troubling thoughts trigger the amygdala again, requiring another dose of pleasurable ice cream, cookies, or potato chips!

Although violent or aggressive behavior is more likely to occur in males as a response to stress,[3] in women, depression is a far more

prevalent coping strategy for chronic stress.[6] A study to determine the relationship between the type A behavior pattern in males and angiographically documented coronary artery disease revealed that patients aged 45 years or younger were more likely to have severe coronary artery disease when age-matched to type B control subjects.[7] The verbal or physical expression of hostility in males has been a consistent finding in type A, or "coronary-prone" men.[8] Men who scored in the top quartile of the hostility subsection of the Minnesota Multiphasic Personality Inventory were seven times more likely to die of coronary disease by the age of 60 years compared with age-matched male control subjects who scored in the lowest quartile.[9]

Another unhealthy response to men ignoring stress is the potential risk of increased cardiac disease and premature death. It has been postulated that men's intense response to environmental stressors stems from their role in the hunter-gatherer era as predators of other animals and protectors of the tribe. The stereotypical male response to stress tends to be more intense and more long-lasting than that of women. Studies examining the parasympathetic response of males to common stressors found this response to be markedly slower compared with that of females. As a result, men would tend to remain upset and agitated for up to 24 hours longer than a female with the same stressor.[8,9] Coronary heart disease symptoms have traditionally appeared 10 years earlier in US men compared with women, and the onset of a coronary event is usually seen 20 years earlier. Before the age of 65 years, the rate of death from heart disease is three times higher in American men compared with women.

Of course, not all of these disparities are attributable solely to stress, but the effect of stress on the heart has been clearly demonstrated. For example, men's sympathetic arousal is more easily and intensely activated and slower to return to normal than that of females.[10–12] A compelling theory regarding these gender differences is that males have historically been biologically rewarded for their rapid response to any perceived threat. An intense fight-or-flight response would lead to a more robust response to any threat and increase their chances of survival. The female response may have historically favored the protection of offspring and the inhibition of the fight-or-flight mechanism.[13]

The association of stress with cardiovascular disease and sudden death has been studied for decades from an epidemiologic standpoint. More recently, the field of neuroimmunology has provided growing evidence suggesting that atherosclerosis is an inflammatory process that can be directly linked to proinflammatory cytokines and adhesion molecules that are released and activated in response to stress.[14] In addition, a recent study of the more immediate effects of mental stress on coronary flow velocity in men demonstrated a significant reduction in flow that lasted up to 30 minutes after mental stress testing.[10] Since cardiovascular disease is the number one cause of death in American men, there is significant cause for ongoing research to further examine these proinflammatory processes. Equally important is the need for research into effective stress-reduction strategies and their potential impact on minimizing the onset and incidence of cardiovascular disease. In a recent randomized controlled trial of 94 male and 42 female patients with stable ischemic heart disease and exercise-induced myocardial ischemia, the authors were able to demonstrate that exercise and stress management training improved markers of cardiovascular risk including left ventricular ejection fraction and wall motion abnormalities, flow-mediated dilatation, and cardiac autonomic control to a greater degree than standard medical care.[15] Currently, the five skills of self-observation, cognitive restructuring, relaxation training, time management, and problem solving form the core of almost all stress-management training. Clearly, defining the effectiveness of each of these skills and their combined use in cardiac disease prevention and management is an important next direction for clinical research in this area.

The defense mechanisms of denial and stonewalling are also common unhealthy responses to stress exhibited in males. Because males are less likely to talk about their emotions, they may be less aware of these feelings and are thus more likely to be unaware and uninterested in their fears or stressors.[16] Dramatic evidence to support this theory appears in Gottman's research[17] that has resulted in highly accurate predictors of divorce. After a single 15-minute interview, he was able to predict the likelihood that a couple would be happily married 4 years later versus reporting severe distress or divorce. One of Gottman's predictors in this study directly relates to male responses to stress. He determined that certain patterns of arguing were accurately predictive of divorce. The most serious form of arguing he dubbed "stonewalling," which referred to physical or emotional withdrawal during a conflict. Stonewalling was initially observed in his laboratory when he would have couples discuss

a topic on which they had disagreed in the past. While conversing, these couples were videotaped and were "wired" for various physiologic parameters. The videotape was used to assess affect, while two scales were used to measure the stress of the subjects. One was the Emotional Facial Action Scale, which has reliability and validity for assessing facial muscle contractions associated with specific emotions.[18] Gottman[17] created a second scale to evaluate emotional expressions other than the face including measurements of voice and language. While the couples were discussing areas of disagreement, they were monitored for interbeat intervals of heart periodicity and peripheral autonomic measures of ear pulse, ear pulse transit time, and respiration. In some of these studies, Gottman also assayed stress-related hormones in the blood and urine. Although males appeared to be more stoic to the observer, all of the physiologic measures indicated significant sympathetic arousal. The male stress response was found to be highly elevated and could remain so for several hours after the conversation ended. This pattern of hiding one's emotions, a largely male phenomenon, Gottman dubbed *stonewalling* because he believed that this defense mechanism reflects the male's ineffective and personally and socially destructive way of coping with strong and intolerable feelings.[17]

The link between ignored stress and subsequent illness has been well studied and documented throughout the medical literature, and it precedes the work of Selye. Intuitively, most physicians have recognized these links simply because most patients have described somatic distress in the setting of unpleasant or stressful events. As early as the 17th century, Dr. William Harvey was referencing the relationship between stressful life events and the onset of illness.[19] Early studies involving both animals and humans documented the immediate or short-term physiologic responses to stress involving the autonomic nervous system. Some of the well-documented physiologic responses have included elevations in blood pressure, impaired gastric motility, and fluctuations in various hormone levels.[19]

The challenge of the 20th and 21st centuries has been in demonstrating the associations between stress and specific illnesses and disease states. Current work in this area has raised many new questions and opened up new areas of research centered on the following questions:

- Does an acute stressful event cause disease, or does it uncover a subclinical condition?
- What is the role of chronic stress in medical illness?

- What is the role of stress in the modulation of the immune system and inflammatory responses?

Relevant to a discussion of stress and its implications for male patients is the study of their responses to stress relative to their perception of the stress as well as their coping strategies. With this must come an acknowledgment of a lack of studies of gender-specific links between medical illness and stress in general.

The field of psychoneuroimmunology, or the study of multidirectional interactions among the brain, one's behavior, and the immune system, has been providing increasing evidence that both acute and chronic stress contribute to decreases in the body's overall defense system. Practically, this is manifested in the increased incidence of viral infections noted in both stressed and depressed persons.[20] Of even greater interest are studies that demonstrate that measurable effects on immunity can be modulated by stress-relieving activities.[21,22] Research in this area has and will continue to provide a greater understanding of the important links between stress and specific disease states.

Additional data support the association of chronic stress with an increased susceptibility to viral diseases such as influenza, herpes simplex virus, Epstein-Barr virus, and the common cold.[23,24] The existence of this association has been supported by in vivo measures of disease-specific immunity in response to psychological stress.[25,26] Equally exciting have been the studies demonstrating that stress-reducing interventions can increase in vivo measures of disease-specific immunity. These interventions include exercise, meditation, dietary changes, yoga, and cognitive behavioral counseling.[15,27] Human immunodeficiency virus (HIV) and its relationship to stress is an active area of research in men's health. Current data support that chronic stress contributes to immune system decline and rapid HIV replication.[28,29]

Finally, the research has been undertaken from a more clinical angle in the evaluation of stress management relative to specific diseases. Some studies have demonstrated measurable responses to strategies to decrease stress for male patients with rheumatoid arthritis,[30] inflammatory bowel disease,[31] and psoriasis.[32] This area warrants greater attention if disease management is to improve.

Healthy Responses to Stress

The fight-or-flight mechanism is an involuntary response present in all mammals. It is believed that non-mammals are "hard-wired," such that their response to sympathetic nervous system arousal is preprogrammed before birth. Therefore, when animals becomes frightened, the deer runs away, the bird flies away, the mouse burrows, and the lion charges. What is the healthy human response to fear or stress? In several studies, the answer is consistent. The human response to fear is to reach to others for support. A willingness to confide in others and ask for support is correlated with lower rates of illness,[33] lower values of cholesterol,[8,34] and higher rates of creativity.[35] These studies support the common observation of what parents observe when a child is frightened by a nightmare or a barking dog. Without any training, they automatically run to the parent, and this usually calms the fear or stress response. In the human, this response may be discouraged by cultural or familial influences.

Male Obstacles to Healthy Responses to Stress

There are two major obstacles to males responding to stress in healthy ways, predominantly alexithymia and the fight-or-flight response versus "tend and befriend" concept.[13] The term *alexithymia* is derived from a Greek word that means "difficulty in identifying and communicating one's feelings." Persons with alexithymia have been described as "human robots," or "emotional illiterates" because their interpersonal relationships are frequently hampered by poor emotional communication. They typically score very low on measures of emotional intelligence and are likely to fare rather poorly in life, regardless of their intellectual capabilities.[36] Many persons with alexithymia also have chronic medical problems, particularly psychosomatic or somatoform illnesses.

Imagine for a moment that you were asked what color car is currently parked two cars to the right of yours. Aside from thinking that this is a rather foolish question, you would probably admit you did not know the answer. Yet, if each day when you came to work a colleague asked you this same question, in a matter of a week's time the hippocampus would decide that this somehow must be an important question because of the repetition, and it would begin storing this information in the brain's short-term memory. An example of the dysfunction that can occur through alexithymia would be a male growing up in a family without anyone asking him about his feelings; he would be much less likely to develop the skills required to identify his emotions. The male's body would then be reacting to emotions without any conscious awareness. If men are unaware of their fears, then they are less likely to seek healthy ways of dealing with them. Alexithymia is more common in men than in women and contributes to both physical and psychiatric difficulties.[37] The inability to read one's feelings makes it impossible to recognize fear or anger and, therefore, asking for help is unlikely. This leaves the male with chronic sympathetic arousal and the eventual cascade of physical and emotional distress. This trait may have been useful in the times of hunter-gatherers because the physical aggression necessary for hunting and for combat would not encourage awareness of feelings but rather a suppression of fear and worry because actions would be preferred over intuitive thoughts.

The second challenge for men is the tendency to use the fight-or-flight response rather than the tend-and-befriend response as a healthy coping style to manage stress. Dr. Shelley Taylor believes that women are predisposed by biology and culture to respond with nurturing—which she calls the tend-and-befriend response—when they are afraid.[35] She attributes this to the women's traditional role of tending to children and the family as well as inherent hormonal differences. In contrast, in most cultures men were expected to enter into a fight mode in response to threats. Taylor's study of modern families supports this tendency toward support for females and away from support for males. After a hard day at work, women tended to want to discuss their day and would nurture the children whereas men tended to withdraw and become irritable.[35] Many studies have found men much less likely to seek help for a wide variety of problems ranging from depression to substance abuse. In addition, epidemiologic studies report that only one third of mental health outpatient visits are with men, just as they are much less likely to visit a physician when ill.[38]

Clinical Suggestions

Ideally, the subject of a male's stress and fear would be addressed during routine medical visits, when appropriate. Asking male patients about their current stressors and how they are coping with them could raise the patient's awareness and advertise the physician's interest to the subject. It is also useful for the physician to consider stress or fear in considering the etiology and treatment of many vague and potentially psychosomatic complaints. During routine visits, a patient's strategies for stress management should be reviewed.

Men traditionally have had difficulty acknowledging emotional issues and even more difficulty seeking help (see Chapter 4, Men and the Problem of Help Seeking). If a male patient wishes to remain stoic or alexithymic and has trouble seeking the support of others, then it is advisable to recommend strategies that are likely to be acceptable. Aerobic exercise and stress-management training have been found to reduce both subjective and objective measures of stress and depression. Scores on depression inventories such as the Beck or Hamilton as well as serum cortisol levels have been used to assess the effects of treatment interventions.[14,15,34] Exercise strategies should be carefully negotiated with the patient to keep this intervention from causing harm. The amount of time spent exercising should be restricted and properly allocated so as to avoid adding additional pressure to the patient's schedule. If the patient is highly competitive, then the recommended exercise activity should be solitary, such as walking or running to avoid potential additional stress of competition. Asking patients who have many time commitments to add exercise to their day can lead to increased pressure, so it may be advisable to start with 1–5-minute increments with gradual increases in the amount over time.[39]

Stress-reduction techniques such as slowing down breathing and controlling where one's thoughts are focused can be done in classes or through readings. Books such as *The Male Stress Survival Guide*,[38] *Treating Type A Behavior and Your Heart*,[34] and *Anger Kills*[9] can be very useful for a man's self-management of stress. Alexithymic patients often prefer the cookbook-type approach that provides them with specific tools for change and improvement. Meditation techniques can be found in each of these books or in any of the majority of books on stress management. Biofeedback and yoga may appeal to some male patients as ways of improving their health and minimizing stress.[40]

For patients who are open to discussing their styles of coping with stress or fear, it is helpful to mention the studies that overwhelmingly demonstrate the protective and healing power of reaching for support and communicating one's feelings and needs. For the athletically oriented patient, Lance Armstrong's book, *It's Not About the Bike: My Journey Back to Life*[41] describes how his battle with testicular cancer helped him to learn the power of letting others help him with his fears and how this support was instrumental not only in his recovery from cancer but also in his effective use of the team in the Tour de France. After recovering from testicular cancer, Armstrong became so discouraged that he quit racing. He gives credit to a small group of friends who gently but persistently encouraged him to return. He describes in the book his realization that he needed the team to win, and that he could not win races alone. For spiritually oriented patients, Larry Dossey's book, *Healing Words*[42] can also be useful in helping men to manage their stress and address their fears.

For a male patient who is willing to discuss his alexithymia, pointing out the childhood origins of his stoicism may be insightful. Invariably, persons with alexithymia report learning early in life that they should not seek help from their parents. Sometimes, these patients have no clear recollection of their childhood experiences. In this case, it is helpful to ask the male patient whether he would take his problems to his parents today and, if not, specifically why he would not. This inquiry usually leads to the same awareness of the childhood origins of this pattern.[43] A male patient may recognize the pattern of avoiding others in his time of need if he is asked whether he would want his spouse, child, or employees to their keep problems to themselves or to bring them to the patient. An excellent book to recommend is Pennebaker's *Opening Up: The Healing Power of Confiding in Others*,[33] which provides step-by-step exercises to work on learning to seek and accept help.

Conclusion

In summary, stress is not merely a state of chronic sympathetic nervous system arousal. It is when the instinctual fight-or-flight physiologic response to fear becomes maladaptive and injurious. Although stress is not an exclusively male response, men usually react to stress in a more exaggerated and prolonged manner than women for several reasons. The male gender's historical role as the protector of the tribe has necessitated a more intense reaction to perceived threats. Moreover, men are usually expected by society to have a more stoic response to challenges and are hence more prone to have alexithymia, a difficulty in identifying and communicating their feelings and fears. This makes it harder for men to address their tension in constructive ways, thus making them much more likely than women to revert to destructive coping mechanisms such as overeating, substance abuse, or violence.

Men's tendency to internalize their negative emotions could be one explanation for their increased rate of premature death from heart disease. There is also a well-established connection between chronic stress and an increased susceptibility to viral infections such as influenza and the common cold, suggesting that stress lowers the immune response. These medical conditions are in addition to the predictable psychological conditions such as depression and anxiety that are often associated with persistent stress. In this light, the benefits of identifying and addressing stress are as indisputable as the association between stress and certain disease states. As clinicians, the most important intervention we can make for our male patients is questioning them about the fears and stressors in their lives. This may be the only chance for some patients to acknowledge previously ignored feelings and raise their awareness about the importance of stress reduction in overall well-being. This then creates an opportunity for the physician to prescribe healthful stress-relieving activities such as aerobic exercise, yoga, meditation, and peer counseling. The challenge going forward is to identify those stress-reducing interventions that produce positive health outcomes for men including reductions in obesity, alcohol abuse, and cardiovascular disease.

References

1. Selye H: *The Stress of Life,* New York, 1978, McGraw-Hill Book.
2. Selye H: *Stress Without Distress,* New York, 1974, Lippincott, Williams and Wilkins.
3. Breslau N, Davis GC, Andreski P, et al: Sex differences in posttraumatic stress disorder, *Arch Gen Psychiatry* 54(11):1044–1048, 1997.
4. Zlotnick C, Zimmerman M, Wolfsdorf BA, et al: Gender differences in patients with posttraumatic stress disorder in general psychiatric practice, *Am J Psychiatry* 158:1923–1925, 2001.
5. Kouvonen A, Kivimäki M, Cox SJ, et al: Relationship between work stress and body mass index among 45,810 female and male employees, *Psychosomatic Med* 67:577–583, 2005.
6. Nolen-Hoeksema S, Larson J, Grayson C: Explaining the gender difference in depressive symptoms, *J Pers Soc Psychol* 77(5):1061–1072, 1999.
7. Williams RB, Barefoot JC, Haney TL, et al: Type A behavior and angiographically documented coronary atherosclerosis in a sample of 2,289 patients, *Psychosom Med* 50(2):139–152, 1988.
8. Friedman M, Rosenman RH: *Type A Behavior and Your Heart,* New York, 1974, Fawcett Press.
9. Willimas R: *Anger Kills,* New York, 1998, Harper Collins.

10. Hasagawa R, Daimon M, Toyoda T: Effects of mental stress on coronary flow velocity reserve in healthy males, *Am J Cardiol* 96(1):137–140, 2005.

11. Pollack WS, Gump BH: *New Psychotherapy in Males,* New York, 1998, Wiley.

12. Witkin G: *The Male Stress Survival Guide,* New York, 2002, New Market Press.

13. Taylor S: *The Tending Instinct,* New York, 2002, HarperCollins.

14. Saddock B, Sadock VA, Kaplan HI: Stress and psychiatry, *Comp Textbook Psychiatry* (2):2180–2195, 2005.

15. Blumenthal JA, Sherwood A, Babyak M, et al: Effects of exercise and stress management training on markers of cardiovascular risk in patients with ischemic heart disease, *JAMA* 293(12):1626–1634, 2005.

16. Goleman D: *Emotional Intelligence,* New York, 1995, Bantam Books.

17. Gottman J: *Why Marriages Succeed and Fail,* New York, 1994, Simon & Schuster.

18. Eckman P, Friesen RW: *Facial Action Coding System,* Palo Alto, CA, 1978, Consulting Press.

19. Yount L: *William Harvey: Discoverer of How Blood Circulates,* New York, 1999, Enslow.

20. Cohen S, Tyrrell DA, Smith MP: Psychological stress and susceptibility to the common cold, *N Engl J Med* 325(9):606–612, 1991.

21. Schedlowski M, Tewes U, editors: *Psychoneuroimmunology: An Interdisciplinary Introduction,* New York, 1999, Springer.

22. Vedhara K, Irwin MR, editors: *Human Psychoneuroimmunology,* London, 2005, Oxford University Press.

23. Cohen S, Doyle WJ, Alper CM: Emotional style and susceptibility to the common cold, *Psychosom Med* 65:652–657, 2003.

24. Marnocha SK: Chronic stressors increased susceptibility to colds, *Evid Based Nurs* 2:54–64, 1999.

25. McEwen BS: Protective and damaging effects of stress mediators, *N Engl J Med* 338:171–179, 1998.

26. Schattner A: The emotional dimension and the biological paradigm of illness, *QJM* 96:617–621, 2003.

27. Ornish D, Scherwitz LW, Doody RS, et al: Effects of stress management training and dietary changes in treating ischemic heart disease, *JAMA* 249(1): 574–585, 1983.

28. Treisman G, Angelino A, Hutton H: Psychiatric issues in the management of patients with HIV infection, *JAMA* 286(22):2857–2864, 2001.

29. Motivala SJ, Hurwitz BE, Liabre ML, et al: Psychological distress is associated with decreased memory helper T-cell and B-cell counts in Pre-AIDS HIV seropositive men and women but only in those with low viral load, *Psychom Med* 65: 627–635, 2003.

30. Patterson RM, Craig JB, Waggoner RW: Studies of the relationship between emotional factors and rheumatoid arthritis, *Am J Psychiatry* 99:775–780, 1943.

31. Gurrera RJ: Sympathoadrenal hyperactivity and etiology of neuroleptic malignant syndrome, *Am J Psychiatry* 156:169–180, 1999.

32. Picardi A, Mazzotti E, Gaetano P: Stress, social support, emotional regulation, and exacerbation of diffuse plaque psoriasis, *Psychosomatics* 46:556–564, 2005.

33. Pennebaker JW: *Opening Up: The Healing Power of Confiding in Others,* New York, 1990, William Morrow.

34. Friedman M, Ulmer D: *Treating type A Behavior and Your Heart,* New York, 1985, Fawcett.

35. Gardner H: *Creating Minds: An Anatomy of Creativity Seen Through the Lives of Freud, Einstein, Picasso, Stravinsky, Eliot, Graham, and Gandhi,* New York, 1993, Basic Books.

36. Kooiman CG, Bolk JH, Brand R: Is alexithymia a risk factor for unexplained physical symptoms in general medical outpatients? *Psychosom Med* 62: 768–778, 2000.

37. Conrad R, Schilling G, Langenbuch M: Alexithymia in male fertility, *Human Reprod* 16:587–592, 2001.

38. Witkin G: *The Male Stress Survival Guide,* New York, 2002, New Market Press.

39. Maurer RJ: *One Small Step Can Change Your Life,* New York, 2004, Workman Press.

40. Pollack WS, Levant RF: *New Psychotherapy for Men,* New York, 1998, Wiley.

41. Armstrong L Jenkins S: *It's Not About the Bike: My Journey Back to Life,* New York, 2000, Putnam.

42. Dossey L: *Healing Words,* San Francisco, 1997, Harper Press.

43. Levant RF: The masculinity crisis, *J Men Studies* 5:56–71, 1997.

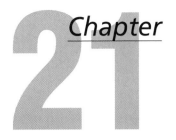

Chapter

21

Exercise and Fitness

Robert Kiningham, MD, MA, Tarannum Master-Hunter, MD, and Arno K. Kumagai, MD

Key Points

- The American Cancer Society guidelines recommended that adults should engage in at least 30 minutes of moderate to vigorous physical activity above their usual activities on 5 or more days of the week; 45–60 minutes of intentional physical activity are preferable (strength of recommendation: C).
- Vigorous exercise (>60% aerobic capacity) results in greater improvements in aerobic fitness, diastolic blood pressure, and glucose control, but not systolic blood pressure, lipid profiles, or body fat loss compared with moderate-intensity exercise when total energy expenditure is similar (strength of recommendation: C).
- Physical activity and physical fitness have been shown to decrease all-cause cardiovascular morbidity and mortality in numerous cohort studies (strength of recommendation: B).
- Strong clinical evidence supports a critical role of exercise in the prevention and management of type 2 diabetes mellitus (strength of recommendation: B).
- Before persons with diabetes engage in exercise, consideration should be given to assessment for possible underlying cardiovascular disease. Persons who are using insulin or who have proliferative retinopathy or significant neuropathy should take precautions during exercise to prevent hypoglycemia (strength of recommendation: C).
- Multiple cohort studies have reported a decreased colon cancer risk of 20–40% in men who habitually engage in moderate to vigorous physical activity. Regularly done

exercise may also decrease the risk of prostate and lung cancer, but the magnitude of the benefit is unclear (strength of recommendation: C).
- Exercise training is an effective treatment of major depression disorder equal in efficacy to medications and psychotherapy (strength of recommendation: C).
- A physically active lifestyle can reduce the risk of developing dementia; elderly adults with dementia can also improve both physical and cognitive functioning with physical and exercise training (strength of recommendation: C).
- The primary risks of physical activity in men are musculoskeletal injuries and sudden cardiac death. The risk of sudden cardiac death in healthy men aged 30–65 years is estimated as 1 death per year for every 15,240–18,000 Goggers (strength of recommendation: C).

Introduction

The rise of incommunicable diseases as the major cause of death in industrialized societies corresponds to a decrease in the population's physical activity.[1] Multiple epidemiologic studies conducted since the 1950s have concluded that this relationship is not a coincidence.[2,3] Physical inactivity is a major risk factor for the development of multiple chronic diseases and ultimately contributes to early mortality. To address this issue, the US Department of Health and Human Services published the first Surgeon General's report on physical activity and health in 1996.[4]

The report concluded that people of all ages benefit from regular physical activity and recommended a "minimum of 30 minutes of physical activity of moderate intensity (such as brisk walking) on most, if not all, days of the week." The report also stated that greater health benefits could be obtained by engaging in physical activity of more vigorous intensity or of longer duration.

These recommendations echoed the conclusions of the Centers for Disease Control and Prevention (CDC), the American College of Sports Medicine (ACSM),[5] the National Institutes of Health,[6] and the American Heart Association[7] in separate reports published between 1995 and 1996. Countless epidemiologic studies conducted since the release of these reports have reinforced the significant impact that physical activity has on health. Consistent participation in moderate to vigorous physical activity has been found to reduce overall mortality rates, cardiovascular diseases, cancer, type 2 diabetes mellitus, osteoarthritis, obesity, and dementia, as well as improving mental health and overall quality of life.[4]

Physical inactivity in men is the most prevalent of the controllable major risk factors for cardiovascular disease. The CDC estimates that 74% of US adults do not engage regularly in moderate intensity physical activity, and 22% engaging in no leisure-time physical activity at all.[8] Approximately 25% of adult US men smoke cigarettes regularly,[9] 28% are hypertensive,[10] and 44% have a low-density lipoprotein cholesterol level greater than 130 mg/dL.[11] Therefore, increasing physical activity has the greatest potential to significantly improve men's health in the United States.

This chapter will review the epidemiologic evidence regarding the health benefits of habitual physical activity. Special attention will be given to exercise and fitness recommendations for men with cardiovascular disease, diabetes mellitus, cancer, and mental health disorders. Specific recommendations regarding the type of exercise and the intensity, duration, and frequency will also be critically reviewed and summarized.

General Concepts

Physical activity, exercise, and *physical fitness* are distinct terms. *Physical activity* is a behavior consisting of bodily movement produced by skeletal muscles that requires energy expenditure. *Exercise* is a type of physical activity that is performed purposely to improve or maintain one or more of the components of physical fitness. *Physical fitness* is a set of attributes that determines the ability of a person to perform physical activity.[12]

Each of the components of physical fitness (i.e., endurance, power, and flexibility) can be measured and quantified accurately. However, physical fitness measurements are time, labor, and cost intensive, particularly over the large study populations needed for epidemiologic research. Physical activity is usually assessed by questionnaires or interviews that are much easier to obtain in a large population. Therefore, much of the epidemiologic literature examining the relationship between physical activity and health is based on subjective questionnaires. These methods are subject to a number of potential errors and are generally considered, at best, to be estimates of actual physical activity. The correlation between physical fitness and activity levels measured in the same population has ranged from 0.3 to 0.5.[13] This modest correlation may reflect a genetic component contributing to physical fitness[14] or the imprecision of the physical activity measurement.[15]

Frequency, Duration, Intensity, and Type of Exercise for Optimal Health

Although compelling research evidence exists to show that habitual physical activity is beneficial to health, the specifics regarding the optimal amount, intensity, frequency, and type of exercise for health benefits has not been established.[16] Much of the research that established a relationship between physical activity and health involved large populations using measurements of physical activity that are not very precise. Extrapolating specific exercise dose recommendations from these studies is difficult.[17] Confounding the attempt to derive a single "exercise prescription" for optimal health is the possibility that the amount and type of exercise best for one area of health may not be sufficient for benefits in another area. People also differ widely in their physiologic and psychological response to exercise.[18] In addition, chronic disease states may influence the response to exercise and the amount and type that is most beneficial.

Despite these obstacles, several large organizations have issued public health statements regarding the amount of physical activity recommended for good health.[5,6,19–21] Most of these statements reinforce the 1995 recommendations of the CDC and ACSM. This report recommended that "every US adult should accumulate

30 minutes or more of moderate-intensity physical activity on most, preferably all, days of the week."[5] Moderate-intensity physical activity is defined as requiring an absolute energy expenditure of 3–6 or metabolic equivalents of the task (METs), or 3.5–7 kcal/min, whereas vigorous activity requires an energy expenditure of greater than 6 METs, or more than 7 kcal/min (Table 21-1).[22] One MET is the estimated adult baseline metabolic oxygen consumption, estimated to be 3.5 mL of oxygen per kilogram of body weight per minute (or approximately 1.5 kcal/min).[23] Examples of moderate-intensity physical activity are walking at a pace of 3–4.5

Table 21-1. Various Intensity Levels Related to Activity

Light-Intensity Activities (<3.0 METs):
Walking slowly (1–2 miles/hour)
Golf, powered cart
Swimming, slow treading
Gardening or pruning
Bicycling, very light effort
Dusting or vacuuming
Conditioning exercise, light stretching, or warming up
Moderate-Intensity Activities (3.0–6.0 METs):
Walking briskly (3–4 miles/hour)
Golf, pulling or carrying clubs
Swimming, recreational
Mowing lawn, power motor
Tennis, doubles
Bicycling 5–9 miles/hour, level terrain, or with a few hills
Scrubbing floors or washing windows
Weight lifting, Nautilus machines, or free weights
Vigorous-Intensity Activities (>6.0 METs):
Racewalking, jogging, or running
Swimming laps
Mowing lawn, hand mower
Tennis, singles
Bicycling more than 10 miles/hour or on steep uphill terrain
Moving or pushing furniture
Circuit training

Note: Higher-intensity activities require less time spent performing exercise; lower-intensity activities require more time.

MET, Metabolic equivalent.

Adapted from: Ainsworth BE, Haskell WL, Leon AS, et al: Compendium of physical activities: classification of energy costs of human physical activities, *Med Sci Sports Exerc* 25(1):71–80, 1993.

miles/hour or bicycling at a speed of 5–9 miles/hour.[24] The Institute of Medicine panel report differed from the CDC report in that it recommended "60 minutes of daily moderate intensity physical activity."[20] However, the Institute of Medicine report focused on weight loss and has been criticized for discounting the significant health benefits (including weight control) of 30 minutes of moderate-intensity activity.[25]

One of the challenges of making public health exercise recommendations is balancing the amount and intensity of exercise that may optimize health and disease risk reduction with the minimum amount and intensity that has been shown to significantly reduce risk. The CDC/ACSM report acknowledged that more intense exercise may accrue additional health benefits.[5] Similarly, the American Cancer Society guidelines recommended that adults "engage in at least 30 minutes of moderate to vigorous physical activity, above usual activities, on 5 or more days of the week," and then added the statement, "Forty-five to 60 minutes of intentional physical activity are preferable."[21] The danger of recommending the "optimal" amount of exercise is that this amount may not be achievable by the majority of the adult population.[25] These recommendations may then be misinterpreted to mean that only this amount of exercise is beneficial, so if a person cannot devote the time and energy to this amount, they might as well remain sedentary. That is clearly not the public health message that needs to be delivered and is not supported by the literature.[25,26]

Since the CDC/ACSM report from 1995, researchers have attempted to better determine the impact of different durations, frequencies, and intensities of exercise on various health outcomes. Reports from three large epidemiologic studies of middle-aged men suggest that exercise needs to be at least of moderate intensity to be beneficial. Lee and colleagues[27] examined the physical activity patterns of 13,485 men in the Harvard Alumni Health Study (average age, 57.5 years) and found that energy expenditure was inversely related to mortality over 15 years of follow-up. Participation in vigorous activities had the greatest benefit, whereas participation in light activities was not associated with mortality, regardless of total energy expenditure.[27] A cohort of 44,452 healthy men was followed up for 10 years in the Health Professionals' Follow-up Study, which determined that intensity of exercise was related to a decreased risk of fatal coronary heart disease (CHD) and nonfatal myocardial infarction independent of total exercise volume, with a 4% reduction in risk for each 1-MET increase in intensity. Time spent walking was not significantly related to risk in analyses that controlled for walking pace, indicating that no amount of leisurely walking affected cardiac risk.[28] The Caerphilly study[29] was a prospective cohort study of 1975 middle-aged healthy, primarily sedentary men followed up for 11 years. The amount of self-reported leisure-time physical activity correlated with a decreased risk of all-cause and CHD mortality, even when adjusting for age and risk factors for CHD. However, light and moderate physical activity alone had no significant effect on mortality rates.

A recent systematic review of the literature specifically examined studies that evaluated the impact of various intensities of exercise on risk factors for CHD and CHD incidence. The authors concluded that vigorous exercise (6 METs or more) was consistently found to reduce CHD risk more than moderate-intensity exercise when controlling for total energy expenditure.[30] It is important to note, however, that almost all epidemiologic studies look at an absolute intensity of exercise, rather than a relative intensity. The studies that have found that only vigorous activity decreases CHD and total mortality risk have involved primarily middle-aged men. Studies that include older men and women consistently report a reduced risk of CHD with moderate and even lower intensities of physical activity. Thus, one can assume that it is the relative intensity of exercise that is most important rather than the absolute intensity.[26] A cohort of 7337 healthy men in the Harvard Alumni Study rated their physical activity in terms of perceived intensity. There was an inverse relationship observed between the amount of exercise performed that was perceived as moderate or greater and the risk of CHD, even among men who engaged in activities with absolute intensities of less than 3 METs.[31] Therefore, even exercise considered to be "low intensity" by most epidemiologic studies was found to be beneficial in deconditioned men.

Clinical trials have also examined the effect of different intensities and frequencies of exercise on fitness and CHD risk factors. In their review, Swain and Franklin[30] concluded that vigorous exercise (greater than 60% aerobic capacity) results in greater improvements in aerobic fitness, diastolic blood pressure, and glucose control, but not systolic blood pressure, lipid profiles, or body fat loss compared with moderate-intensity exercise when total energy expenditure is similar. A recent large randomized clinical trial

involving healthy middle-aged men and women found that moderate-intensity walking performed 5–7 days/week, but not 3–4 times/week, significantly improved aerobic fitness, similar to more vigorous walking conducted 3–4 times per week.[32] Therefore, even in healthy middle-aged men, moderate exercise may be beneficial if performed frequently.[22]

Before the 1995 CDC/ACSM report, it was commonly believed that aerobic exercise needed to be conducted continuously for at least 20 minutes to be beneficial. The CDC/ACSM report challenged this assumption and instead focused on the total volume of exercise performed per week.[5] Several clinical trials have compared the effect of continuous versus intermittent exercise. Dunn and colleagues[33] compared a traditionally structured exercise group (50–85% aerobic capacity 5 days/week) to a "lifestyle physical activity" group advised to accumulate 30 minutes of moderate-intensity physical activity on most, preferably all, days of the week. Subjects were initially sedentary middle-aged men and women. After 2 years study, results found similar, significant improvements in cardiorespiratory fitness, blood pressure, and percent body fat in the two groups.[33] A crossover study involving middle-aged (average age, 44.5 years) men and women compared 30 minutes of continuous walking to three 10-minute sessions per day, both at 70–80% maximum heart rate, performed 5 days/week for 6 weeks. Both training regimens were found to significantly improve aerobic capacity (with the greatest improvement with the short-bout program) and increased high-density lipoprotein cholesterol levels.[34] Manini and colleagues[35] took a different approach to this issue and measured total energy expenditure for 2 weeks in 302 high-functioning community-dwelling elderly adults (aged 70–82 years). After 6 years of follow-up, free-living energy expenditure (equal to total energy minus resting metabolic rate) was significantly inversely related to total mortality when controlling for potential confounders, with the lowest activity group having three times the mortality rate of the highest activity group.[35] These studies support the concept that intermittent exercise can be beneficial as long as frequency is adequate.

Most of the literature involving health benefits of exercise focuses on aerobic exercise and fitness, yet there is a growing body of research that associates muscular strength and overall health. The Canadian Fitness Survey of 1981 involved 8116 adults (3933 men) with an average age of 36.5 years who had a number of aerobic and musculoskeletal fitness measurements performed at baseline. Age-adjusted models revealed that subjects in the lowest quartile of performed sit-ups had 2.7 times the risk of mortality over 13 years of follow-up compared with the highest quartile, independent of other covariates.[36] There have been a number of studies relating low hand grip strength and mortality in both middle-aged[37–39] and elderly men.[40,41] The Honolulu Heart Program study included 6040 men with an average age of 54 years who had their baseline grip strength assessed. After 30 years of follow-up, men in the lowest and middle tertiles of grip strength at baseline had significantly increased mortality compared with men in the highest tertile that was independent of body mass index (BMI) and physical activity level.[38] Men in the lowest tertile of grip strength also had twice the risk of developing functional disability.[37] Disability with aging has been related to a general decrease in neuromuscular performance, including decreased muscular strength, impaired balance, and reduced walking speed. Studies involving resistance and balance training programs in middle-aged and elderly men indicate that these declines in neuromuscular performance with aging can be prevented, thus decreasing the development of age-associated disability.[42] The ACSM recommends that all adults engage in resistance training two to three times a week to "enhance strength, muscular endurance, and maintain fat-free mass."[43]

Physical activity in men has been shown to have a beneficial effect in a number of health areas, including decreasing all-cause mortality, cardiovascular disease, cardiovascular risk factors (including hypertension and hyperlipidemia), obesity, type 2 diabetes mellitus, colon and possibly prostate cancer, depression and anxiety, and functional disability in elderly persons.[4,7] The specific amount and intensity of physical activity that is required to induce health benefits remains unclear, but the CDC/ACSM guideline of "30 minutes of moderate-intensity physical activity done on all, or most, days of the week" appears to be a good starting point. Vigorous exercise done frequently probably incurs the greatest health benefit. However, the benefits of recommending such an exercise program to previously sedentary adult men must be weighed against the increased risk of injury and difficulties with sustaining compliance over time.[16]

Exercise intensity is best thought of in relative terms, particularly in the case of elderly men. There is solid evidence to support that even exercise that objectively is considered low intensity can incur significant health benefits in previously deconditioned men as outlined above. It is important to help younger men make the transition from thinking of exercise as a way to improve performance in competitive situations to a way of improving or maintaining overall health and well-being. Exercise is important for men throughout their lifespan. At any age, consistently done exercise improves the quality of life and decreases morbidity and mortality.

Physical Activity and Cardiovascular and All-Cause Mortality

Numerous epidemiologic studies have established an inverse relationship between physical activity and cardiovascular and all-cause mortality.[2,44,45] Four of the largest and most extensive studies evaluating the relationship of physical activity and the development of cardiovascular disease are summarized in Table 21-2. All of these studies are cohort-designed studies with follow-up periods ranging from 8 to 23 years. The Framingham study was one of the earliest studies to make the statistical association between physical activity and reduced risk of cardiovascular disease and all-cause mortality. This study was a cohort study composed of 5209 male and female residents of Framingham, MA, that began in 1948. A "physical activity index" was calculated for each subject based on a questionnaire that inquired about the number of hours spent doing various activities on "an average day" from 1956 to 1958. After 14 years of follow-up, physical activity was found to be inversely associated with cardiovascular mortality even when age and known cardiovascular disease risk factors were accounted for (relative risk of cardiovascular death was 0.77 for "active" versus "sedentary" men).[46] A second physical activity assessment was conducted from 1969 to 1973. Among 962 men free of cardiovascular disease at the second assessment, both overall and cardiovascular mortality were found to be significantly lower in the most active tertile of men in the study compared with the least active tertile, even when cardiovascular risk factors were accounted for; only the most recent physical activity index was related to cardiovascular disease development and death.[47]

The largest study of the relationship between physical activity and cardiovascular disease was the Harvard Alumni Study. This prospective cohort study sent questionnaires to 16,936 male Harvard alumni who entered college between

Table 21-2. Physical Activity and Cardiovascular and All-Cause Mortality in Men

Study	Number of Subjects	Activity Measurement	Follow-up (years)	RR CVD Mortality	RR All-Cause Mortality
Harvard Alumni (Paffenbarger et al, 1986)[50]	16,241	Leisure PA	15	0.54	0.62
British Regional (Shaper and Wannamethee, 1991)[51]	7735	Leisure PA	8	0.50*	NR
Framingham (Kannel and Sorlie, 1979)[46]	1909	Total PA	14	0.77	NS
Framingham (Sherman et al, 1999)[47]	962	Total PA	16	NR	0.58
Honolulu Heart (Rodriguez et al, 1994)[53]	7074	Total PA	23	0.85	NR

CVD, Cardiovascular disease; PA, physical activity; NR, not reported; NS, not significant.
All values are statistically significant (P ≤ .05) unless otherwise indicated.
*Relative risk (RR) for cardiovascular disease events (i.e., fatal and nonfatal myocardial infarction) of most active to least active groups, age adjusted.

Adapted from: Kannel WB, Sorlie P: Some health benefits of physical activity: the Framingham study, *Arch Intern Med* 139:857–861, 1979; Sherman SE, D'Agostino RB, Silbershatz H, Kanel WB: Comparison of past versus recent physical activity in the prevention of premature death and coronary artery disease, *Am Heart J* 138:900–907, 1999; Paffenbarger RS, Hyde RT, Wing AL, Hsieh CC: Physical activity, all-cause mortality, and longevity of college alumni, *N Engl J Med* 314:605–613, 1986; Shaper AG, Wannamethee G: Physical activity and ischaemic heart disease in middle-aged British men, *Br Heart J* 66:384–394, 1991; Rodriguez BL, Curb D, Burchfiel CM, et al: Physical activity and 23-year incidence of coronary heart disease morbidity and mortality among middle-aged men: the Honolulu heart program, *Circulation* 89:2540–2544, 1994.

1916 and 1950. Physical activity was assessed by inquiring about the number of city blocks walked, stairs climbed, and types of sporting activity played each week. A physical activity index was calculated and expressed in kilocalories per week of physical activity.[48–50] Physical activity was found to be an independent risk factor for cardiovascular disease and total mortality after 15 years of follow-up in 16,241 men free of cardiovascular disease and cancer at baseline (relative risk, 0.54 for cardiovascular mortality and 0.62 for all-cause mortality for the most active group compared with the least active group).[49] Total mortality steadily decreased from an estimated energy expenditure of 500 kcal/week to 3500 kcal/wk.[50]

The British Regional Study surveyed 7735 men between the ages of 40 and 59 years from various towns in Great Britain. Leisure-time physical activity was assessed by a questionnaire. After 8 years of follow-up, men free of cardiovascular disease at baseline who reported moderate to moderately vigorous physical activity were found to have 50% fewer myocardial infarctions than men classified as inactive. The risk of myocardial infarction was increased in men who engaged in vigorous activity.[51] Subsequent analysis revealed that this increased risk of myocardial

infarction with vigorous activity occurred only in hypertensive men.[52]

The Honolulu Heart Program[53] calculated the Framingham physical activity index for 8006 men of Japanese ancestry who were free of cardiovascular disease at the initial assessment in the period of 1965–1968. Cardiovascular disease incidence and mortality was found to be significantly reduced in the men in the highest tertile of reported physical activity compared with the lowest group after age adjustment. However, physical activity was not significantly correlated with cardiovascular disease incidence, mortality, and death after adjustment for known cardiovascular risk factors. Therefore, in this study, the impact of physical activity on cardiovascular disease appeared to occur through its effect on traditional cardiovascular disease risk factors including hypertension, diabetes mellitus, hypercholesterolemia, and obesity.[53]

The consistent association between physical activity and reduced cardiovascular disease and mortality is all the more remarkable considering the difficulty in accurately assessing physical activity across large populations. Questionnaires assessing physical activity, including the ones used in the Framingham and Harvard Alumni studies, are very rough estimates of actual physical activity.[54] However, if these assessment tools were entirely inaccurate, then it would be expected that there would not be a consistent finding of a significant relationship between physical activity and improved health outcomes, yet the opposite trend is true. Multiple studies across multiple populations have found an approximate 33% reduction in cardiovascular disease and overall mortality in physically active men compared with sedentary men.[2,44,45] This consistency suggests that the relationship between physical activity and cardiovascular disease and mortality is very strong, and that the questionnaires are able to at least distinguish physically active from inactive men.

All of the aforementioned studies have correlated a baseline measurement of physical activity with the subsequent development of cardiovascular disease and death over a period of 8–23 years. The study designs assume that physical activity is relatively constant over time or that physical activity affects health for several years; both of these assumptions are probably not true. The Harvard Alumni Study and Framingham Study cohorts both had multiple measurements of physical activity performed over several years. Physical activity at one time period was found not to be a very accurate predictor of physical activity at another time period in either study. In the Framingham Study, physical activity levels of men free of cardiovascular disease measured 11–17 years apart had a correlation of 0.16.[47] The Harvard Alumni Study had a cohort of 6092 healthy men without cancer or cardiovascular disease in 1988 that had assessments of physical activity assessed during the years 1962–1966, 1977, and 1988. The correlation of the physical activity index (a measurement of energy expenditure based on activity, represented in kilojoules per week) and collegiate sports activity was poor at all 3 measurement periods (0.16, 0.16, and 0.11, respectively). The correlation of the physical activity index from each measurement period was also very poor (0.39 between the 1962/1966 measurement and 1977 measurement and 0.27 between the 1962/1966 measurement and 1988 measurement).[55] Thus, these studies collectively conclude that physical activity levels are clearly not stable over time.

In the Framingham Study,[47,56] Harvard Alumni Study,[55,57] and British Regional Heart Study,[58] the most recent measurement of physical activity was the best predictor of future cardiovascular disease and mortality. In all three studies, becoming physically active reduced the risk of developing cardiovascular disease, whereas becoming sedentary increased risk. Coronary

events in the first 2–3 years of these studies were excluded in each analysis to minimize the possibility that occult disease present during the physical activity assessment caused decreased activity. The fact that men who altered their physical activity levels also changed their cardiovascular disease risk indicates that these studies are not simply identifying men in whom low physical activity is a marker for undetected or predetermined heart disease and early mortality. The impact of physical activity appears to be ongoing, with both the beneficial effects of becoming physically active and the detrimental effects of becoming sedentary occurring relatively quickly.

Physical Fitness and Cardiovascular and All-Cause Mortality

Physical fitness is a set of attributes that allows people to perform physical activities. Cardiovascular fitness is often quantified by measuring or estimating peak oxygen consumption during exercise testing (VO_2 max). Medical research commonly converts VO_2 max into METs (defined above). Several studies have examined the relationship between cardiovascular fitness and future morbidity and mortality; three of the larger studies are summarized in Table 21-3.

The largest and most extensively analyzed study of the health effects of cardiovascular fitness is from the Cooper Clinic in Dallas, TX.[59] The original cohort in the Aerobics Center Longitudinal Study included 13,344 healthy subjects (10,224 men) who underwent treadmill exercise testing and then were followed up for an average of 8 years. The subjects ranged in age from 40 to 56 years; most subjects were well-educated and white. The least fit quintile of men was found to have more than a three-fold greater risk of death than the most-fit quintile. This increased risk remained statistically significant even when adjusted for known cardiovascular risk factors, with a relative risk of 1.82. This relationship was not weakened by eliminating the first 3 years of follow-up in the study, which was done to avoid the possibility of occult disease causing decreased physical fitness. Cardiovascular disease and cancer death rates showed a strong gradient from least to most fit groups, but no such relationship existed for other causes of death. Higher fitness levels than a peak exercise capacity of 10 METs were not associated with any further reduction in mortality.[59]

Table 21-3. Physical Fitness and Cardiovascular and All-Cause Mortality in Men

Study	Number of Subjects	Follow-up (Years)	Fitness Measure	Outcome Measure	Relative Risk
Aerobics Center Longitudinal Study/ Cooper Clinic (Blair et al, 1989)[59]	10,224 (Healthy)	8	Maximal aerobic capacity	All-cause mortality, CVD mortality	3.4* 8.0*
Palo Alto (Myers et al, 2002)[61]	3679 (CVD)	6.3	Maximal aerobic capacity	All-cause mortality	4.1*
Palo Alto (Myers et al, 2002)[61]	2534 (Healthy)	6.3	Maximal aerobic capacity	All-cause mortality	4.5*
Mayo Clinic (Roger et al, 1998)[62]	1452 (Healthy)	6.3	Maximal aerobic capacity	Cardiac events, all-cause mortality	1.20† 1.25†

CVD, Cardiovascular disease.

*Compares least fit quintile to most fit quintile, age adjusted unless otherwise indicated. All values are statistically significant ($P \leq .05$) unless otherwise indicated.

†Multivariate analysis including risk factors, age, symptoms, and electrocardiogram, all values were statistically significant ($P < .001$).

Adapted from: Blair SN, Kohl HW, Paffenbarger RS, et al: Physical fitness and all-cause mortality. prospective study of healthy men and women, *JAMA* 262:2395–2401, 1989; Myers J, Prakash M, Froelicher V, et al: Exercise capacity and mortality among men referred for exercise testing, *N Engl J Med* 346:793–801, 2002; Roger VL, Jacobsen SJ, Pellikka PA: Prognostic value of treadmill exercise testing: a population-based study in Olmstead County, Minnesota, *Circulation* 98:2836–2841, 1998.

A subsequent study from the Cooper Clinic involving an even larger cohort of 25,341 men with an average age of 45 years compared the impact of fitness level to other traditional risk factors for cardiovascular disease on all-cause and cardiovascular mortality.[60] Table 21-4 compares the relative risk of the various cardiovascular risk factors examined in this study. Low fitness, defined as the lowest 20% of total group, was an independent risk factor comparable in impact to cigarette smoking on overall and cardiovascular disease mortality.[60]

Myers and colleagues[61] from Palo Alto, CA, studied 6213 men (average age, 59 years) who were referred for exercise treadmill testing for various reasons. The group was divided into two subgroups: (1) 3679 men with a history of cardiovascular disease, pulmonary disease, and/or an abnormal exercise test result, and (2) 2534 men without disease and with normal exercise test results. Both subgroups were followed up for 6.5 years. Peak exercise capacity was found to be the best predictor of death in both groups, significantly stronger than hypertension, cigarette smoking, hypercholesterolemia, obesity, or diabetes. Men in the least-fit quintile had a 4.5 times greater mortality rate compared with men in the most-fit quintile among initially healthy subjects, and 4.1 times greater mortality among subjects with disease or an abnormal exercise test result. Every 1-MET increase in exercise capacity corresponded to a 12% improvement in survival.[61]

A Mayo Clinic study of 1452 men who underwent exercise treadmill testing for various clinical reasons reported similar findings to the Palo Alto study. Exercise capacity was found to be a significant predictor of all-cause mortality. After adjustment for age and other cardiovascular disease risk factors, an increase of 1 MET in workload was associated with a 17% decrease in cardiac events and a 20% decrease in total mortality, even when early deaths were excluded.[62]

Table 21-4. Risk Factors for Mortality in Men, Aerobics Center Longitudinal Study

Mortality Predictor	Relative Risk* (95% confidence interval)
Smoking	1.65 (1.39–1.97)
Abnormal ECG	1.64 (1.34–2.01)
Chronic illness	1.63 (1.37–1.95)
Low fitness	1.52 (1.28–1.82)
Serum cholesterol $\geq$ 240 mg/dL	1.34 (1.13–1.59)
Elevated systolic blood pressure ($\geq$ 140 mm Hg)	1.30 (1.08–1.58)
Body mass index $\geq$ 27 kg/m³	1.02 (0.86–1.22)

ECG, Electrocardiogram.

*All comparisons are high-risk group to low-risk group, adjusted for age, examination year, and other potential risk factors.

Adapted from: Blair SN, Kampert JB, Kohl HW, et al: Influences of cardiorespiratory fitness and other precursors on cardiovascular disease and all-cause mortality in men and women. *JAMA* 276:205–210, 1996.

Physical fitness has a significant modifying effect on other risk factors for cardiovascular disease. Studies from the Cooper Clinic have found that men in the lowest quintile of physical fitness have a 62% increased risk of developing hypertension compared with men in the highest quintile fit. Unfit men who became fit had a 56% decreased risk of developing hypertension than men who remained unfit.[63] Increased fitness level has been shown to improve survival among men with hypertension, hypercholesterolemia, obesity, and a family history of CHD.[59–61]

When the Palo Alto cohort was classified by other risk factors for cardiovascular disease, all-cause mortality was almost double in subjects with exercise capacity less than 5 METs compared with men with an exercise capacity higher than 8 METs in each subgroup.[61] Lee and colleagues[64] examined a cohort of 21,925 healthy men (average age, 43.8 years) who had percent body fat measured at baseline in addition to an exercise treadmill test; these subjects were monitored for 8 years. Although there was a significant direct relationship between body fat composition and all-cause and cardiovascular mortality, the relationship was significantly affected by fitness level. Unfit (defined as the lowest 20%, with an average maximal MET level of 9.0), lean (i.e., less than 16.7% body fat) men were found to have twice the mortality rate of fit lean men and fit obese (i.e., greater than 25% body fat) men. The total mortality of fit obese men was not found to be significantly higher than that of fit lean men.[64] It appears that aerobic fitness has a greater impact on mortality than leanness and can somewhat modify the negative impact of obesity.

Changes in physical fitness have been associated with changes in cardiovascular risk and mortality. Within the Cooper clinic cohort, 9777 men completed two exercise tests, with an average interval between tests of 4.9 ± 4.1 years. The average follow-up was 5 years after the second exercise test. Men in the lowest quintile of aerobic fitness were classified as "unfit." This finding corresponded to less than 10 METs for men aged 20–39 years, less than 9.2 METs for men aged 40–49 years, less than 8.4 METs for men aged 50–59 years, and less than 7.0 METs for men aged 60 years and older. Men with findings greater than these cut-offs were considered "fit." Men who went from unfit on the first test to fit on the second test had a relative risk of all-cause mortality of 0.56 and a relative risk of cardiovascular mortality of 0.48 compared with men who were unfit on both tests. After adjustment for potential confounders, each minute

increase in treadmill time from the first to the second test was associated with a decrease in cardiovascular death by 8.6% and total mortality by 7.9%. A 1-MET increase in exercise capacity decreased mortality by 15%.[65] A group of 1756 healthy Norwegian men performed maximal bicycle exercise tests an average of 7 years apart. After 13 years of follow-up, an increase in physical fitness significantly reduced all-cause mortality irrespective of initial fitness level and other cardiovascular risk factors.[66]

Three prospective cohort studies of men have simultaneously measured physical fitness by exercise testing and physical activity by questionnaire.[67–69] In all three studies, physical fitness was a significant predictor of cardiovascular disease and mortality, with physical activity also a significant factor in two of the studies. A recent study by Myers and colleagues[70] measured physical activity by the Harvard Alumni questionnaire in 842 men who also underwent exercise treadmill testing. Although physical fitness correlated poorly with adulthood physical activity, in a multivariate analysis, only exercise capacity and physical activity energy expenditure were found to be significant predictors of mortality. Physical fitness was shown to be a stronger predictor of mortality than was physical activity, and both were significantly stronger than other risk factors for cardiovascular disease. Both a 1000-kcal/week increase in activity and a 1-MET increase of physical fitness were associated with a decrease in mortality by 20%.[70] In their review, Lee and Paffenbarger[44] estimated that a middle-aged person gains approximately 2 years of life from being physically active. Physical activity does not appear to extend the life span, but it is thought to decrease the risk of premature death.

Overall, physical fitness appears to have an even stronger impact on cardiovascular disease and mortality than physical activity. Habitual physical activity increases physical fitness, but there is also a large genetic component to physical fitness. Genetic factors are estimated to contribute 30–50% of VO_2 max.[14] Correlations between physical activity and physical fitness measured at the same time range from 0.09 to 0.60.[13,70,71] These relatively poor correlations could reflect the genetic component of physical fitness, as well as the imprecision of assessing physical activity by questionnaire. However, the fact that changes in physical fitness result in changes in health outcomes indicates that the impact of physical fitness on health is alterable by changes in physical activity.

Physical Activity and Fitness in Men with Coronary Heart Disease

Physical activity and physical fitness have also been shown to reduce mortality in men with known CHD. Among the subset of men in the British Regional Heart Study who had established CHD, those who engaged in light (i.e., regular walking plus some recreational activity) to moderately vigorous (i.e., sporting activity at least once a week plus frequent recreational activities or walking, or frequent sporting activities only) physical activity had significantly reduced mortality rates over the 5 years of follow-up compared with inactive men with CHD.[72] In the Cooper Clinic studies, men with low levels of fitness who had cardiovascular disease had a relative risk of 2.5 for cardiovascular mortality and 1.6 for all-cause mortality compared with more-fit men with cardiovascular disease over 8.4 years of follow-up.[60] Myers and colleagues[70] reported that increased fitness was associated with decreased mortality in both healthy men and men with cardiovascular disease. After an average follow-up of 5.5 years, every 1 MET of improved fitness was related to a 12% reduction in mortality.

A 2004 systematic review and meta-analysis of exercise-based rehabilitation for patients with CHD reported a 20% decrease in total mortality and a 26% decrease in cardiac mortality for patients with CHD who engaged in exercise training compared with CHD patients receiving usual care.[73] In this study, there were no significant differences noted in rates of nonfatal myocardial infarctions and revascularization. Iestra

and colleagues[74] conducted a systematic review examining the impact of lifestyle and dietary changes in men with established CHD. Table 21-5 summarizes their estimates of the impact of various lifestyle changes compared with the impact of pharmacologic therapy after myocardial infarction. In men with CHD, increasing physical activity has a comparable impact on mortality reduction as pharmacologic therapy with beta-adrenergic blockers, statins, and angiotensin- converting enzyme inhibitors.[74]

As in healthy men, exercise training in men with CHD must be done consistently to be effective. The National Exercise and Heart Disease Project[75] was a multicenter randomized clinical trial that examined the impact of a 3-year supervised exercise training program on long-term survival in 651 men with recent myocardial infarctions. Men were randomly assigned to either an exercise training or a non-exercise standard care group; both groups underwent exercise tests to determine cardiovascular fitness every 6 months. Total and cardiovascular disease-related mortality was found to be nonsignificantly reduced in the exercise group at 3 and 5 years of follow-up when analyzed on an "intent to treat" basis. By the 10th year of follow-up, mortality rates were essentially the same in both groups without any statistically significant difference. However, when analyzed by fitness level, each 1-MET increase in work capacity from baseline to the third year resulted in a significant 8–14% reduction in total and cardiovascular mortality at each follow-up period for up to 19 years. The authors concluded that men who maintained or improved their fitness over time

Table 21-5. Comparison of Lifestyle and Pharmacologic Interventions for Prevention and Treatment of CAD in Men

Intervention	CAD Patients Mortality Risk Reduction	General Population Mortality Risk Reduction
Smoking cessation	36%	50%
Increased physical activity	24%	25%
Moderate alcohol intake	20%	15%
Combination of dietary changes*	44%	15–40%
Low-dose aspirin	18%	NR
Statins (HMG CoA reductase inhibitors)	21%	NR
Beta-adrenergic blockers	23%	NR
ACE inhibitors	26%	NR

CAD, Coronary artery disease; NR, not reported; HMG CoA, 3-hydroxy-3-methylglutaryl coenzyme A; ACE, angiotensin-converting enzyme.
*Primarily, decreased saturated fat and increased fish oil consumption.

Adapted from: Iestra JA, Kromhout D, van der Schouw YT, et al: effect size estimates of lifestyle and dietary changes on all-cause mortality in coronary artery disease patients: a systematic review, *Circulation* 112:924–934, 2005.

had reduced mortality rates regardless of initial group assignment.[75]

Exercise and Prevention of Type 2 Diabetes Mellitus

The various ways in which muscle contraction and exercise enhance skeletal muscle glucose transport are the focus of current intense research investigation. Of major clinical relevance, however, is whether exercise is an affective approach to the prevention or management of type 2 diabetes mellitus.

With regard to prevention, almost all of the major long-term clinical trials investigating this issue have failed to address the impact of exercise alone on development of diabetes, but rather, they have focused on a broader lifestyle intervention approach (e.g., exercise, diet, and weight loss) to determine whether modifiable conditions and behaviors may be effective in preventing disease onset. Numerous epidemiologic studies, including the Malmo Study, Nurses Health Study, and Physicians Health Study, have documented the association between sedentary lifestyles and type 2 diabetes in both men and women.[76–80] Over the past two decades, several large clinical trials have prospectively investigated the effects of lifestyle modification, including exercise, on the incidence of type 2 diabetes in various population groups at risk for the disease.

One of the first major prospective intervention trials was Da Qing IGT (impaired glucose tolerance) and Diabetes Study,[81] in which 577 men and women with documented impaired glucose tolerance from community clinics in Da Qing, China, were assigned to either one of four cohorts: dietary intervention alone, diet and exercise intervention, exercise alone, or no intervention (control). A proportional hazards analysis of data (adjusted for BMI and fasting glucose) gathered in 2-year intervals over the 6-year trial demonstrated that diet, exercise, and diet and exercise interventions resulted in 31%, 46%, and 42% reductions in the risk of developing type 2 diabetes, respectively.[81] Interestingly, although both diet and exercise lowered the risk of development of diabetes, there was no statistically significant difference between the two interventions, and the effects were not found to be additive in the combined diet-exercise group.[81]

The Finnish Diabetes Prevention Study (DPS) was a prospective, randomized, controlled trial in which 522 overweight men and women with impaired glucose tolerance were assigned to either a control or intervention group and underwent follow-up for an average of 3.5 years to determine whether lifestyle changes (e.g., exercise, dietary changes, and weight loss) resulted in a lower risk for the development of type 2 diabetes.[82] The intervention consisted of intensive individualized instruction and counseling sessions aimed at lowering intake of dietary fat and increasing weight loss, exercise, and intake of fiber. Subjects in the intervention group were specifically counseled on increasing endurance-type (i.e., "cardiovascular") physical activities, including walking, jogging, swimming, skiing, or aerobic ball games, and in addition, circuit-type resistance training sessions were offered. In contrast, subjects in the control group received oral and brief written instructions at baseline and at yearly intervals. At the end of 4 years, the cumulative incidence of diabetes was 11% in the intervention group, compared with 23% in the control group, a total reduction of 58% among those in the intervention group. Among the male subjects in the intervention group, the decrease in the incidence of diabetes at 4 years was 63%, and among the female subjects there was a 54% lower incidence. The results also demonstrated a strong inverse correlation between the degree to which the recommended goals of dietary and exercise interventions were met and the incidence of diabetes.[82]

Both the Da Qing and DPS trials demonstrated the effectiveness of lifestyle changes on the prevention of type 2 diabetes, but with respect to application to the US population, there were limitations. The Da Qing study was not randomized, and the BMI of the majority of the Chinese subjects was less than 25 kg/m^2, which reflects the lower association between obesity and diabetes in Asian populations. In the Finnish DPS, the study group was ethnically homogenous, and therefore, generalization to an ethnically diverse society, such as that in the United States, is problematic.

To address this question in a diverse population, the Diabetes Prevention Program (DPP) was initiated in the United States.[83,84] The DPP was a prospective, randomized control trial involving 3234 persons with impaired glucose tolerance followed up at 27 study centers. Participants had a mean age of 51 years, a mean BMI of approximately 31 kg/m^2, and impaired glucose tolerance, determined by elevated serum glucose concentrations either after an overnight fast or 2 hours after a 75-g glucose load. Sixty-eight percent of the participants were women, and 45% were ethnic minorities (20% African American, 16% Hispanic/Latino, 5% Native American, 4%

Asian American).[83] Subjects were randomly assigned into one of three groups: a metformin-treated group (850 mg twice daily), a placebo control group, and a lifestyle intervention group. The goals of the latter group included weight loss and maintenance of 7% of initial body weight as well as at least 150 minutes of moderate physical activity per week equal or similar in intensity to brisk walking, including bicycle riding, aerobic dance, and swimming.[83] Participants were asked to perform these activities a minimum of three times weekly, with a minimum of 10 min/session. Attainment and maintenance of goals were assisted by case managers or "lifestyle coaches" who frequently met individually with each participant and developed personal dietary and exercise plans. The standardization of instruction of the lifestyle intervention group was achieved through a required "core curriculum" of 16 individual didactic sessions spread over the first 24 weeks of the trial that case managers covered with the subjects; additional (and post-core curriculum) contacts between case managers and individual subjects allowed for "customization" of the approaches to account for ethnic, educational, and linguistic diversity. In contrast, participants in the metformin or placebo groups received written standard lifestyle recommendations and an annual 20–30-minute individual didactic session that emphasized the importance of a healthy lifestyle.[83]

Participants in this trial received follow-up for an average of 2.8 years (range, 1.8–4.6 years). The DPP was terminated 1 year early on the advice of the data-monitoring board. At the end of the core curriculum (24 weeks), 58% of the participants in the lifestyle-intervention group had met the target weight loss goal of at least 7% of their initial body weight, and 38% met the target at their final follow-up visit. The average weight loss of the placebo, metformin, and lifestyle-intervention groups were 0.1, 2.1, and 5.6 kg, respectively, and were statistically different for each comparison ($P < .001$).[84] Based on individual exercise logs, the percentage of subjects in the lifestyle intervention group that performed more than 150 minutes of exercise per week was 74% and 58% at the 24-week and final visits, respectively. The incidence of diabetes at the end of the trial was 11.0, 7.8, and 4.8 per 100 patient-years in the placebo, metformin, and lifestyle intervention groups, respectively. At the end of 3 years, the estimated cumulative incidence of diabetes was 28.9%, 21.7%, and 14.4%, respectively, among the placebo, metformin, and lifestyle-intervention groups, and these figures were found to be statistically significant for all comparisons. These differences therefore translated into a 58% lower incidence of diabetes in the lifestyle-intervention group than in the placebo group and a 39% lower incidence in the metformin group versus placebo.

Taken together, the Da Qing, Finnish DPS, and the DPP trials provide convincing evidence that exercise, incorporated as part of a lifestyle intervention plan that also includes weight loss and a healthy diet, is effective in preventing the development of type 2 diabetes in persons at risk for the disease.

Exercise and Management of Type 2 Diabetes Mellitus

Numerous clinical trials have studied the effects of exercise on metabolic control in persons with type 2 diabetes; however, the numbers of study participants have been small, and the results are often conflicting.[85–95] To clarify this issue, Boule and coworkers[96] screened approximately 1500 clinical trials and selected 14 (11 randomized control trials and 3 clinical control trials) for meta-analysis based on specific inclusion and exclusion criteria, which included randomized or nonrandomized controlled clinical trials in subjects with type 2 diabetes of at least 8 weeks in duration and the use of specific exercise interventions with verification of adherence to the regimen based on exercise diaries or direct supervision. The majority of the 11 randomized trials used forms of aerobic activity for exercise; two trials used resistance-type exercises; and one used aerobic exercise with the addition of resistance exercises.[96] Based on the analysis of the 14 trials, Boule and coworkers reported that, in subjects with type 2 diabetes, exercise was associated with a statistically significant 0.66% reduction in glycosylated hemoglobin values without a reduction in body mass.[96] Possible explanations for the lack of effect of exercise on body mass in these trials include the relatively short duration of the activities, the possibility that study subjects reduced their other daily physical activities in proportion to an increase in exercise, and the possibility of an increase in lean body mass in relatively inactive persons who initiate an exercise program.[96] Nonetheless, the results of this meta-analysis emphasize the important clinical observation that improvement in glycemic control may be achieved independent of significant weight loss and provide a clinical corollary to the basic science observations that enhanced skeletal muscle glucose transport may occur through intracellular signal transduction pathways, independent of insulin's actions on glucose metabolism and homeostasis.

The effects of sustained exercise on glycemic control in persons with type 2 diabetes may be explained on a cellular level. In experimental models of type 2 diabetes in rats, sustained exercise (either through cardiovascular or resistance-type exercises) results in increased insulin-sensitive glucose transport and GLUT4 glucose transporter expression in the affected skeletal muscles.[97–99] Therefore, not only does exercise enhance glucose transport and lower blood glucose concentrations in an insulin-independent manner during the immediate exercise period (thus overcoming skeletal muscle insulin resistance), but in addition, sustained or regular exercise may result in longer-term cellular adaptations that lead to increased insulin sensitivity in skeletal muscle and improved metabolic control. Furthermore, although no prospective randomized controlled trials of the effects of exercise on cardiovascular mortality have been performed, a large observational study has documented an inverse association between cardiorespiratory fitness and mortality from cardiovascular events in men with type 2 diabetes.[100,101]

The *Handbook of Exercise in Diabetes* from the American Diabetes Association (ADA)[102] proposes several recommendations regarding exercise in persons at risk for, or affected by, type 2 diabetes. These recommendations, along with the levels of evidence supporting the recommendation, are listed in Table 21-6.

Additional Issues Regarding Exercise and Diabetes

Cardiovascular Evaluation of Patients with Diabetes Before an Exercise Program Is Begun

Because of the likelihood that persons with diabetes of long duration also have some degree of underlying cardiovascular disease, it is critical to screen for cardiovascular disease before the initiation of any exercise program. A recent ADA position statement[103] recommends that a graded exercise stress test may be helpful in persons with the following characteristics:

- Age older than 35 years
- Age younger than 25 years and type 2 diabetes of less than 10 years' duration or type 1 diabetes of less than 15 years' duration
- Any additional risk factor for cardiovascular disease
- Microvascular complications (e.g., retinopathy, neuropathy, nephropathy)
- Peripheral vascular disease
- Autonomic neuropathy

In particular, the presence of microalbuminuria, like peripheral vascular disease, is an independent risk factor for the presence and severity of coronary artery disease,[104,105] and therefore,

Table 21-6. Recommendations for Prevention and Management of Type 2 Diabetes Mellitus

	Recommendation	Level of Evidence*
Prevention of type 2 diabetes in persons with impaired glucose tolerance	Program of weight control, including at least 150 min/week of moderate to vigorous physical activity and a healthful diet with modest energy restriction	A
Exercise in persons with type 2 diabetes	For metabolic control, reduction of CVD risk, and weight loss: at least 150 min/week over at least 3 days/week of moderate aerobic physical activity (40–60% of VO₂ max or 50–70% of maximum heart rate) For CVD risk reduction: at least 4 hours/week or moderate-vigorous aerobic or resistance exercise For long-term maintenance of major weight loss (greater than 13.6 kg or 30 pounds), larger amounts (e.g., 7 hours/week) of moderate to vigorous aerobic exercise may be helpful	Metabolic control: A; Reduction of CVD risk: B; Long-term maintenance of weight loss: B

CVD, Cardiovascular disease; VO₂ max, peak oxygen consumption during exercise testing.

*The levels of evidence are from the American Diabetes Association's Evidence Grading System and are paraphrased as follows: *A*, clear or supportive evidence from well-designed, randomized, controlled, multicenter trials or meta-analyses with quality ratings in the analysis; *B*, supporting evidence from well-conducted prospective cohort or registry studies or case-controlled studies; *C*, supporting evidence from poorly controlled or uncontrolled studies or conflicting studies where the weight of evidence supports the recommendation; *E*, expert consensus or clinical experience.

Adapted from: Ruderman N, Devlin JT, Schneider SH, et al: *Handbook of Exercise in Diabetes: Exercise in Diabetes,* Alexandria, VA, American Diabetes Association, 2002.

persons with evidence of even early diabetic nephropathy should be screened for underlying cardiovascular disease.

Retinopathy

Persons who have active proliferative retinopathy are said to be at a higher risk for vitreous hemorrhage or retinal detachment during activities that involve straining or Valsalva maneuvers (e.g., heavy weight lifting) or contact sports. The ADA therefore recommends that these activities be avoided in persons with advanced retinopathy.[103]

Peripheral Neuropathy/Diabetic Foot Problems

Persons with peripheral neuropathy may be at a higher risk of ulceration or damage to joints with weight-bearing exercises, and the ADA recommends limiting these types of activities in the presence of significant diabetic neuropathy.[103] A reasonable alternative, however, is an activity such as swimming or water aerobics that does not place unusual pressure or strain on the joints or feet.

Exercise and Insulin Therapy

Since contracting muscle increases glucose uptake independently of insulin action, and since regular exercise enhances peripheral insulin sensitivity, the adjustment of insulin regimens must be taken into account when starting an exercise program to avoid exercise-associated hypoglycemia. The adjustment of insulin regimens must be individualized; for persons with type 1 or type 2 diabetes who are following a multiple-daily insulin regimen, lowering the dose of rapid-acting insulin or the meal before the activity by 1–2 units for every 30 minutes of moderate activity is often a good starting point. Extended periods of increased activity (e.g., vacations that involve hiking, extensive walking, or other physical activities) may require adjustment of the basal (long-acting) insulin regimen as well. For many persons with diabetes, adjustments in insulin dosing before exercise is often easier to accept than recommendations to consume large amounts of carbohydrates; since a common goal of exercise (particularly in type 2 diabetes) is weight loss, intake of additional calories is frequently viewed as "defeating the purpose" of the exercise.

In persons with type 1 diabetes, particular care must be taken to avoid hypoglycemia during and after exercise. In the period after intensive exercise, glucose uptake into skeletal muscle persists due to the increased need for glucose to replete skeletal muscle glycogen stores[106] and, as a consequence, children and adults with type 1 diabetes are at particularly high risk of nocturnal hypoglycemia in the post-exercise period.[107,108] Intensive control of type 1 diabetes is frequently associated with defects in the hormonal counter-regulatory responses to hypoglycemia,[109] and although controversial,[110] prior exercise may impair these responses as well.[111] Therefore, attention should be paid to avoid nocturnal hypoglycemia after exercise or vigorous physical activity (e.g., yard work, heavy lifting), either through a bedtime snack of complex carbohydrates or avoidance of bedtime injections of short-acting insulin.

Exercise and Cancer

For several decades, researchers have hypothesized that regular exercise reduces the risk of cancer.[112,113] However, the limitations of epidemiologic research and the multifactorial nature of cancer development have made establishing a beneficial effect of exercise difficult. Different cancers have different etiologies and risk factors, so it has been postulated that the impact of physical activity depends on the specific type of cancer. Also, many cancers go through a prolonged preclinical prodromal phase before being clinically detected. Physical activity or exercise could be most effective at an early stage of cancer development or at more advanced stages. Therefore, assessments of physical activity should ideally be very specific about when physical activity has occurred in the person's life. Most physical activity questionnaires inquire about "average" physical activity or recent physical activity. Given the limitations of the assessment tools of physical activity and the uncertainty regarding the early natural history of different cancers, any relationship between physical activity and cancer risk would have to be very strong to be detected.[113] Despite the difficulties in research, the American Cancer Society has estimated that one third of annual cancer deaths that occur in the United States can be attributed to dietary factors and insufficient physical activity.[114]

Several prospective cohort studies have examined the relationship between physical activity or fitness and all-cancer mortality.[3] Many of these studies have severe methodologic flaws, particularly with the measurement of physical activity or fitness. Despite these difficulties, some of the larger and higher-quality studies report a significant reduction in cancer death among more active subjects. The Harvard Alumni Study found that men who exerted less than 500 kcal/week in physical activity had 1.5 times the rate of cancer death than men who exerted more than 2000 kcal/week.[115] The British Regional Heart study reported a 1.7 times greater risk of cancer death for inactive men compared with active men during 9.5 years of follow-up.[116] In the Cooper Clinic trial, men in the least fit quintile had 4.3 times the risk of cancer death compared with men in the most fit quintile.[59]

Prostate, lung, and colon cancer are the leading causes of site-specific cancer in men.[114] Colon cancer has been the most extensively studied in relation to physical activity. Several extensive systematic reviews and meta-analyses examining the relationship between physical activity and colon cancer incidence have been published.[3,112,113,117–120] Physical activity has repeatedly been found to reduce colon cancer risk in men by approximately 20–50%. This reduced risk has been found to be independent of known or suspected risk factors for colon cancer such as dietary habit and body weight. The consistency of this finding is remarkable considering that these studies used different measurements of physical activity in different populations of men. Friedenreich and Orenstein[118] found that 43 of 51 studies reported a significant effect of physical activity on colon cancer risk, with an average risk reduction of 40–50% in the most active groups compared with the least active. A significant dose-response between physical activity and decreased colon cancer risk was found in 25 of the 29 studies in which it could be calculated.[118] Lee[112] surveyed 50 studies and calculated a median risk reduction of 30% in colon cancer in physically active men. Slattery[119] estimated that 13–14% of colon cancer in the population can be attributed to physical inactivity, yet physical activity has not been found to decrease the risk of rectal cancer.[3,112,118,119]

Several mechanisms have been proposed by which physical activity decreases the risk of colon cancer. Exercise helps reduce total body fat, which has been associated with increased colon cancer risk.[119] However, physical activity reduces colon cancer risk even when statistically controlling for body weight change.[121] Regularly performed exercise decreases bowel transit time[122,123] and thereby could reduce the duration of contact between fecal carcinogens and colonic mucosa.[118,121,124,125] Acute exercise increases the F-series prostaglandins, which increase gut motility and inhibit colonic cell proliferation. Exercise training decreases prostaglandin E_2 (PGE_2), which decreases gut motility and increases colonic cell proliferation. This change in prostaglandin ratio between PGF and PGE_2 could result in reducing the potential for colon cancer.[113,119,125]

Men with type 2 diabetes mellitus and hypertriglyceridemia have an increased risk of colon cancer.[126] This observation has led to research into the impact of insulin and insulin-like growth factors (IGF) on colon cancer development. Both insulin and IGF promote colonic cell growth and proliferation. High levels of circulating insulin and IGF-1 and low levels of IGF binding proteins have been associated with increased risk of colon cancer.[126,127] Exercise training increases insulin sensitivity and decreases insulin levels. Acute exercise may raise IGF-1 initially, but exercise training increases IGF binding proteins and thus decreases IGF activity.[121] Consistently performed physical activity may thereby lower colon cancer risk by decreasing insulin and physiologically active IGF-1 levels.[121,126]

The epidemiologic evidence linking exercise and a decreased risk of prostate cancer is not as strong as it is for colon cancer. Friedenreich and Orenstein[118] reviewed 30 studies examining an association between physical activity and prostate cancer and found that 17 studies reported a decreased risk for more active men, with a 10–30% average risk reduction. Torti and Matheson[128] found in their review that 16 of 27 studies showed a decreased risk of prostate cancer, but only 9 studies reported a statistically significant risk reduction in physically active men. Lee[112] reviewed 36 studies and calculated a non–statistically significant median risk reduction of 10% for physically active men versus sedentary men. Overall, it appears that exercise may reduce prostate cancer risk, yet the magnitude of the effect is relatively small compared with the impact that exercise has on decreasing colon cancer risk.

Exercise may reduce prostate cancer risk by lowering testosterone levels.[128] Endurance-trained men have been found to have lower testosterone levels than untrained men.[129,130] Exercise also increases the production of sex hormone–binding globulin, which results in lower levels of free testosterone.[131] Whether or not these changes are sufficient to alter prostate cancer development or progression is unknown. Other proposed mechanisms whereby regular exercise could lower prostate cancer risk include enhancement of the immune system (particularly natural killer cells), an improved antioxidant defense system, and a decrease in percent body fat.[118,128,131] At this point, the relationship between these potential exercise-induced changes and prostate cancer remains purely theoretical.

Relatively few studies to date have evaluated the impact of physical exercise on lung cancer development. It appears that increased physical activity may decrease lung cancer risk in men by 20–30%.[112,118] However, the magnitude of the impact of cigarette smoking on lung cancer risk is so great that it is difficult to completely account for in epidemiologic studies.[112] Most reviewers consider physical activity as possibly associated with decreased lung cancer risk.

Exercise training has also been studied in men with diagnosed cancer and has been shown to improve physical well-being and endurance, decrease fatigue, and improve psychological functioning both during and after treatment for cancer.[132–134] It is currently unknown whether exercise training will reduce the recurrence of cancer or extend the survival after cancer is diagnosed.[135] The specific duration, intensity, and frequency of exercise that is effective in decreasing cancer risk is unclear. The studies that have examined colon cancer risk suggest that exercise needs to be at least of moderate intensity to have a favorable impact.[112,119] It is also unknown when during the life cycle of possible cancer development exercise is effective. Studies have not found a decreased risk of cancer in college athletes,[119,136] indicating that more recent exercise has a more favorable effect on reducing cancer risk than remote exercise.

In summary, men who habitually participate in moderate to vigorous physical activity reduce their risk of colon cancer by 20–40%.[112,119,120] There is some evidence that exercise can reduce the risk of prostate and lung cancer, but the magnitude of the benefit is unclear.[112] Exercise training has been shown to improve immune function, decrease body fat, and improve antioxidant defense, all of which could potentially decrease the risk of developing cancer.[118] The reduction of insulin and IGF with exercise training also has the potential to reduce cancer risk.[127] The American Cancer Society recommends that adults engage in 30 minutes or more of moderate to vigorous exercise on 5 or more days of the week to reduce cancer risk.[137] In men with diagnosed cancer, exercise training can improve physical and mental functioning.[134]

Exercise and Mental Health

Multiple studies have been conducted on men from teenagers to the elderly that report mental health improvements with exercise.[138] A recent review of the epidemiologic literature reported a strong, consistent dose-response relationship between chronic exercise and energy level.[139] Men who are physically active in their leisure time have an approximate 40% reduced risk of experiencing low energy and fatigue and a 50% reduced risk of depression compared with sedentary men.[139] The Cooper Institute reported data from 5451 men enrolled in the Aerobic Center Longitudinal Study who had depressive symptoms and emotional well-being measured by self-report scales, in addition to physical fitness and physical activity assessments. There was an inverse, graded dose-response relationship between both cardiorespiratory fitness and physical activity levels and depressive symptoms. Emotional well-being was found to be positively associated with physical fitness and physical activity.[140]

Epidemiologic associations do not prove causation, and it is possible that men with less energy and more depressive feelings are less physically active because they feel poorly. Three major meta-analyses and a systematic review have been published regarding the effect of exercise training on clinical depression.[141–143] All three reviews concluded that exercise training is as effective as psychotherapy and antidepressant medication, and more effective than no treatment, in decreasing depressive symptoms in men diagnosed with major depressive disorder. However, all three reviews also comment on the significant methodologic shortcomings of most of the studies.

The Standard Medical Intervention and Long-term Exercise study by Blumenthal and colleagues[144,145] is a methodologically rigorous study that examined the impact of exercise training on clinical depression. Subjects were 156 adults (43 males) older than 50 years diagnosed with major depressive disorder who were not being treated for depression at the beginning of the study. Subjects were randomly assigned to one of three groups: aerobic exercise training (40-minute sessions three times a week for 16 weeks), medication (sertraline, 50–200 mg/day), or exercise training and medication. Depression symptoms were measured quantitatively by the Hamilton Rating Scale for Depression and the Beck Depression Inventory. At 16 weeks, members of all three groups exhibited statistically and clinically significant reductions in depression on both scales. More than 60% of subjects in all three groups no longer met criteria for major depression. The authors estimated that only 20–30% of subjects would be expected to recover from depression based on the placebo effect alone over the course of 16 weeks.[144]

Follow-up of the subjects 6 months after conclusion of the initial study found that participants in the exercise group had significantly lower rates of depression (30%) than participants in the original medication (52%) and combination (55%) groups. At that time, 64% of the participants in the exercise group were exercising regularly, compared with 66% in the combination group and 48% in the medication group. The study revealed that antidepressant medication was being taken by 40% of the combination group, 26% of the medication group, and 7% of the exercise group. Multiple logistic regression analyses revealed that patients who reported engaging in habitual aerobic exercise during the follow-up period were less likely to be classified as depressed, even when adjusting for age, gender, depression level at entry, and medication use. Each 50-minute increase in exercise per week was associated with a 50% decrease in the chances of being classified as depressed 6 months after the conclusion of the active portion of the study.[145] This study gives compelling evidence for the effectiveness of exercise in the treatment of major depression in older patients.

The current literature provides a more mixed opinion with regard to the impact of exercise training on depressive symptoms in healthy persons. Several studies have demonstrated a decrease in depressive symptoms in conjunction with exercise training, whereas several others do not report any effect.[146–148] These varying results may be due to a paucity of depressive symptoms among the subjects in some studies, thereby not providing an opportunity for improvement.[147]

Exercise training has been found to be effective in decreasing depressive symptoms in patients with chronic medical conditions.[146,147] Cardiac rehabilitation studies have consistently reported a decrease in depressive symptoms in patients with CHD who undergo exercise training.[147,149] Many of these studies are small with brief trial periods, and all have problems controlling for self-selection bias.[147] Despite the inherent limitations in the literature, exercise training should be strongly considered for stable patients with CHD, particularly if they manifest signs or symptoms of depression. Exercise has proven benefits in reducing CHD risk and may improve depression as well.[149]

Acute exercise bouts have been reported to reduce state anxiety.[138,150] In an extensive literature review, Yeung[150] concluded that "exercise may be a useful short-term strategy for alleviating psychological distress." Both aerobic and resistance exercise have been found to decrease anxiety[138,150,151] and appear to be as effective as other anxiety-reducing treatments such as relaxation and meditation.[138] The improved mood after an acute bout of exercise generally lasts 3–4 hours but can persist up to 24 hours.[150] Exercise training has been less consistently found to decrease trait anxiety.[138] In patients with panic disorder, exercise has been found to raise anxiety in some cases.[152,153] Aerobic exercise training has been reported to significantly decrease panic and depressive symptoms in agoraphobic patients over placebo, but has less of an effect than psychotropic medications.[154]

Dementia is a major public health problem, with Alzheimer disease affecting approximately 4.5 million people in the United States.[155] Exercise may help delay or reduce cognitive deterioration with aging. Aerobic exercise training has been consistently found to improve the performance of cognitive tasks in elderly adults.[156,157] A meta-analysis conducted in 2003 combined the results of 18 randomized controlled trials involving aerobic exercise training and cognitive function and concluded that aerobic fitness training improved cognitive performance by an average of 50% regardless of the type of cognitive task, training method, or participant characteristics. Exercise bouts within the training program were required to be at least 30 minutes in duration to be effective.[157] Several studies have examined the association of physical activity and the development of dementia. A literature review from 2004 reported that 6 of 9 studies found a significant inverse relationship between physical activity and the development of dementia in older adults based on cohort studies, with an average follow-up of 4.7 years. A review of the methods of these studies reveals considerable diversity and imprecision in the assessment of physical activity, which may account for the mixed results.[158–161]

Two more recent studies report a strong inverse association between exercise and the onset of dementia. In the Honolulu Heart Program cohort, elderly men (average age, 77 years) who walked more than 2 miles/day on average had an incidence of dementia 1.8 times less than men who walked less than a quarter of a mile a day at 4–6 years of follow-up.[162] Adults older than 65 years who exercised for 15 minutes at least three times a week were found to have a 32% reduced risk of developing dementia over an average follow-up of 6.2 years compared with more sedentary adults in the Group Health Cooperative cohort. Interestingly, the greatest dementia risk reduction with exercise was observed in elderly adults who had relatively poor physical function at baseline.[163]

Exercise training in mid-life has also been found to decrease the risk of developing dementia later in life. A prospective study of 1449 healthy Finnish adults assessed physical activity at baseline (average age, 50.6 years) and followed up with them for an average of 21 years. Physical activity was measured by inquiring about the frequency of physical activity that lasts at least 20–30 minutes and causes breathlessness and sweating. This definition includes only relatively intense exercise compared with the criteria used to determine physical activity in other studies. Forty-one percent of the cohort engaged in this intensity and duration of physical activity at least twice a week. This "active" group was found to have a 60% lower rate of developing Alzheimer disease and a 52% lower rate of all-cause dementia than adults who engaged in physical activity less than twice a week, even when controlling for age, sex, education, vascular disorders, smoking, alcohol intake, locomotor disorders, follow-up time, and *APOE* genotype.[164]

The previously cited studies examining physical activity and dementia involved adults who were fully intact at baseline from a cognitive standpoint. Exercise training can also improve cognitive function in elderly adults who have already developed cognitive impairment and dementia. Heyn and colleagues[165] conducted a meta-analysis of exercise-training studies that involved adults older than 65 years with cognitive impairment. Thirty trials involving 2020 subjects met the appropriate criteria for inclusion in the meta-analysis. The average age of the subjects was 80 years (range, 66–91 years), and the average length of the training programs was 23 weeks (range, 2–112 weeks). Walking was the most common exercise treatment, with some studies using other aerobic activities, and two studies using weight training. Overall, subjects who engaged in exercise training significantly improved cardiovascular fitness, muscular strength, physical function, cognitive function, and "positive behavior" compared with non-exercising control subjects.[165]

In summary, exercise training has been shown to have a beneficial impact on mental health in men from teenagers[166] to the elderly. Exercise training is an effective treatment of major depression disorder equal in efficacy to medications and psychotherapy. There is accumulating evidence that a physically active lifestyle can reduce the risk of developing dementia. Elderly adults with dementia can also improve both physical and cognitive functioning with exercise training. Moderate-intensity aerobic exercise has been the most studied, but mental health benefits from resistance exercise have also been reported. The specific mode, intensity, and duration of exercise that is most beneficial to mental health has not been identified and may vary depending on a man's age, baseline mood state, and cognitive and physical characteristics.

Risks of Exercise

Most forms of exercise are considered to be a safe activity for the vast majority of men.[167] In men with chronic diseases including diabetes mellitus, cardiovascular disease, asthma, and chronic obstructive pulmonary disease, precautions must be taken to ensure that exercise does not exacerbate the underlying condition. Other chronic diseases such as neuromuscular diseases, obesity, and osteoporosis may predispose men to musculoskeletal injury with exercise. However, even in men with these conditions, exercise can be performed safely and can be of great benefit for overall health and well-being.

The primary hazards of physical activity in healthy men are predominantly musculoskeletal injuries and sudden cardiac death. The risk of sudden cardiac death in healthy men aged 30–65 years is estimated as 1 death per year for every 15,240–18,000 joggers.[168] The sudden death rate observed with jogging is approximately seven times the rate reported during more sedentary activities.[168] The increased risk of sudden cardiac death during vigorous exercise compared with rest is actually higher in younger men than in older men, due to the exceedingly low rate of sudden cardiac death at rest in younger men. The absolute risk of sudden cardiac death during either rest or exercise is much higher in older men. Men aged 30–39 years have an estimated relative risk for sudden cardiac death during jogging that is 99 times greater than the risk during less vigorous activities. By the ages of 40–49 years, the relative risk for sudden cardiac death during jogging is only 13 times greater than the risk during less vigorous activities.[168] The rate of myocardial infarction during heavy physical activity, and up to 1 hour after activity, is approximately 2–17 times greater than the rate during less strenuous activity.[169–172] The relative risk of sudden death during and up to 30 minutes after vigorous exertion was 16.9 among men in the Physicians' Health Study (average age, 54 years). However, to put things in perspective, the absolute risk of sudden cardiac death for any particular bout of vigorous activity has been reported to be 1 sudden death per 1.51 million episodes of exertion in this population of previously healthy men.[172]

The major cause of exertional sudden cardiac death and myocardial infarction in men older than 35 years is underlying coronary artery disease.[168–173] Atherosclerotic plaque rupture with acute coronary artery thrombosis induces myocardial ischemia,[168] which leads to hypoperfusion and sudden cardiac death.[173] Acute strenuous exercise can facilitate plaque disruption by increasing platelet aggregation.[168] Acute exercise can also be associated with a number of other prothrombotic effects that can contribute to acute coronary artery thrombosis, especially in chronically sedentary men.[168] The sympathetic nervous system is activated during exercise, which may cause an acute increase in susceptibility to ventricular fibrillation, particularly in the setting of myocardial ischemia.[172] In men younger than 35 years of age, structural heart disease is the primary cause of sudden cardiac death with exercise. Hypertrophic cardiomyopathy is the most common finding at autopsy, followed by congenital aberrant coronary arteries.[174–175]

Habitually physically active men have a much lower risk for exercise-induced myocardial infarction and sudden cardiac death compared with sedentary men.[169–171] Mittleman and colleagues[170] reported progressively lower relative risks of myocardial infarction during exertion with increasing levels of habitual physical activity. Sedentary men were 100 times more likely to experience sudden cardiac death during exertion than at rest, whereas men who exercised five or more times a week had only a 2.4 increased risk of sudden cardiac death during exertion compared with a resting state.[170] Among men in the Physicians' Health Study, the relative risk of sudden cardiac death during and within 30 minutes after vigorous exercise ranged from 74 in men exercising less than once a week to 11 in men exercising five or more times a week.[172]

Although acute physical activity increases the risk of sudden cardiac death and acute myocardial infarction, sedentary men are at much greater risk for sudden cardiac death during exercise and at rest than habitually active men. These observations make it even more important that men remain physically active throughout their lives. In previously sedentary men, exercise should be conducted moderately and increased gradually to minimize the acute inherent risks of exercise. When performed sensibly, the overall cardiovascular health benefits of exercise for men far outweigh the acute risks of sudden cardiac death and myocardial infarction.[176]

Only a few studies have examined the risks of musculoskeletal injury from exercise in adults who are not performance athletes. Hootman and colleagues[177] from the Cooper Clinic administered an injury survey to 5028 men in the Aerobics Center Longitudinal Study. This group of men underwent exercise stress tests to determine their maximal aerobic capacity and was then followed over several years for health outcomes. They also had their physical activity habits assessed by a self-reported questionnaire. At the time of the injury survey, 67% of the men reported being physically active at least twice a week in the previous 12 months. One quarter of all men reported at least one musculoskeletal injury in the preceding 12 months, of which 82% were attributed to physical activity. Lower extremity injuries accounted for 68% of the injuries, with the knee being the most common site (23% of total injuries). Men who were found to be the most fit had significantly higher rates of all-cause (30.5%) and activity-related (24.9%) injuries than the least fit men (18.7% for all-cause and 13.4% for activity related injuries) during the preceding year. Sedentary men had significantly lower injury rates than the physically active men. Men who participated in sports but did not walk or jog regularly for exercise had the highest injury rates at 31% for all-cause injuries and 27.6% for activity-related injuries.[177]

The largest randomized trial that included an exercise component and reported injury data was conducted by the Diabetes Prevention Program Research Group.[178] Participants were 3234 nondiabetic persons (1043 men) with elevated fasting and post-load plasma glucose levels who were randomly assigned to one of three groups: placebo, treatment with metformin, or intensive lifestyle intervention, which included moderate-intensity exercise for at least 150 min/week. Injuries and "musculoskeletal symptoms" were not found to be significantly different between groups, ranging from 20 to 24 per 100 persons per year.[178]

Osteoarthritis of the back, hips, and knees are common problems, particularly as people age. Traditionally, osteoarthritis has been attributed to "wearing out the joint" due to overuse. A concern has been that increased physical activity will put more stress on the joint and result in more frequent and severe osteoarthritis.[179] However, several studies have reported no increased rate of knee, hip, or back osteoarthritis in habitual runners compared with sedentary men.[180-183] High-level competitive athletes, in contrast to recreational athletes, may have more osteoarthritis later in life than the nonathletic population. Former Finnish elite competitive endurance athletes had a 1.7-2.17 times greater rate of hospital admission for lower extremity osteoarthritis than healthy nonathletic control subjects. However, the first admission to the hospital occurred at the highest age in endurance athletes (70.6 years) compared with power athletes (61.9 years) and nonathletic control subjects (61.2 years).[184] The rate of back pain in this study was reported to be lower among the athletes than the control group.[185]

Several studies have demonstrated that exercise actually decreases the progression of knee and hip osteoarthritis and disability in older adults.[186-188] The Fitness Arthritis and Seniors Trial randomly assigned 439 adults older than 60 years of age with radiographically evident knee osteoarthritis, subjective pain, and self-reported physical disability to follow one of three regimens: aerobic exercise, resistance exercise, or a health education program. Exercise was conducted three times a week as a group at a facility for 3 months, and then was home based for 15 subsequent months. After 18 months, both the aerobic- and resistance-trained subjects reported significant improvements in measures of disability, physical performance, and knee pain compared with the health education group.[186] Fries and colleagues[182] compared a cohort of recreational runners (average age, 58 years) to community control subjects for 8 years; disability was assessed by the Health Assessment Questionnaire. They determined that men initially in the running club had significantly less progression of disability compared with the sedentary group over 8 years of follow-up, even when controlling for age, body weight, comorbid conditions, radiologic evidence of knee osteoarthritis, and several other possible confounders.[182] Therefore, rather than avoid exercise to minimize "stress" on the joints, the literature suggests that even men with established osteoarthritis should embark on a moderate exercise program to improve symptoms and forestall the development of significant disability.

Conclusion

Several major health organizations have endorsed the importance of habitual exercise and maintenance of physical fitness to prevent the onset, progression, and severity of chronic disease. Scores of studies with significant proportions of male subjects have demonstrated a relationship between regular exercise and reduced risk of cardiovascular disease, diabetes mellitus, cancer, and Alzheimer disease–related dementia. Primary care clinicians are strategically poised to discuss the relationship between exercise and improved health and well-being during both routine visits and health maintenance examinations.

References

1. McTiernan A: Physical activity, exercise, and cancer: prevention to treatment—symposium overview, *Med Sci Sports Exerc* 35:1821–1822, 2003.
2. Kiningham RB: Exercise and the primary prevention of cardiovascular disease, *Clin Fam Pract* 3: 707–732, 2001.
3. Kiningham RB: Physical activity and the primary prevention of cancer, *Prim Care* 25:515–536, 1998.
4. Department of Health and Human Services: *Physical Activity and Health: A Report of the Surgeon General*, Atlanta, GA, 1996, U.S. Department of Health and Human Services, Centers for Disease Control and Prevention, National Center for Chronic Disease Prevention and Health Promotion.
5. Pate RR, Pratt M, Blair SN, et al: Physical activity and health: a recommendation from the Centers for Disease Control and Prevention and the American College of Sports Medicine, *JAMA* 273: 402–407, 1995.
6. National Institutes of Health Consensus Conference: Physical activity and cardiovascular health, *JAMA* 276:241–246, 1996.
7. Fletcher GF, Balady G, Blair SN, et al: Statement on exercise: benefits and recommendations for physical activity programs for all Americans. A statement for health professionals by the committee on exercise and cardiac rehabilitation of the council on clinical cardiology, American Heart Association, *Circulation* 94:857–862, 1996.
8. Centers for Disease Control and Prevention: Trends in leisure-time physical inactivity by age, sex and race/ethnicity—United States, 1994–2004, *MMWR Weekly* 54:991–994, 2005.
9. Centers for Disease Control and Prevention: State-specific prevalence of current cigarette smoking among adults—United States, 2003, *MMWR Weekly* 53:1035–1037, 2004.

10. Wolf-Maier K, Cooper RS, Banegas JR: Hypertension prevalence and blood pressure levels in 6 European countries, Canada, and the United States, *JAMA* 289:2363–2369, 2003.
11. Centers for Disease Control/National Center for Health Statistics: *National Health and Nutrition Examination Survey III (NHANES III)* 1999–2002.
12. Caspersen CJ, Powell KE, Christensen GM: Physical activity, exercise, and physical fitness: definitions and distinctions for health-related research, *Public Health Rep* 100:126–131, 1985.
13. Eaton CB: Relation of physical activity and cardiovascular fitness to coronary heart disease: part II. cardiovascular fitness and the safety and efficacy of physical activity prescription, *J Am Board Fam Pract* 5:157–166, 1992.
14. Bouchard C, Daw EW, Rice T, et al: Familial resemblance for VO2 max in the sedentary state: the HERITAGE family study, *Med Sci Sports Exerc* 30:252–258, 1998.
15. LaPorte RE, Montoye HJ, Casperson CJ: Assessment of physical activity in epidemiological research: problems and prospects, *Public Health Rep* 100:131–146, 1985.
16. Kesaniemi YA, Danforth E, Jensen MD, et al: Dose-response issues concerning physical activity and health: an evidence-based symposium, *Med Sci Sports Exerc* 33:S351–S358, 2001.
17. Schriger DL: Analyzing the relationship of exercise and health: methods, assumptions, and limitations, *Med Sci Sports Exerc* 33:S359–S363, 2001.
18. Bouchard C, Rankinen T: Individual differences in response to regular physical activity, *Med Sci Sports Exerc* 33:S446–S451, 2001.
19. Thompson PD, Buchner D, Pina IL, et al: Exercise and physical activity in the prevention and treatment of atherosclerotic cardiovascular disease: a statement from the Council on Clinical Cardiology (subcommittee on exercise, rehabilitation, and prevention) and the Council on Nutrition, Physical Activity, and Metabolism (subcommittee on physical activity), *Circulation* 107:3109–3116, 2003.
20. Institute of Medicine of the National Academies of Science: *Dietary Reference Intakes for Energy, Carbohydrate, Fiber, Fat, Fatty Acids, Cholesterol, Protein, and Amino acids (Macronutrients)*, Washington, DC, National Academy Press, 2002.
21. Kushi LH, Byers T, Doyle C, et al: American Cancer Society guidelines on nutrition and physical activity for cancer prevention: reducing the risk of cancer with healthy food choices and physical activity, *CA Cancer J Clin* 56:254–281, 2006.
22. Blair SN, LaMonte MJ: How much and what type of physical activity is enough? What physicians should tell their patients, *Arch Intern Med* 165:2324–2325, 2005.
23. American College of Sports Medicine: *Resource Manual for Guidelines for Exercise Testing and Prescription*, ed 2, Philadelphia, Lea & Febiger, 1993, p 64.
24. Ainsworth BE, Haskell WL, Leon AS, et al: Compendium of physical activities: classification of energy costs of human physical activities, *Med Sci Sports Exerc* 25:71–80, 1993.
25. Blair SN, LaMonte MJ, Nichaman MZ: The evolution of physical activity recommendations: how much is enough? *Am J Clin Nutr* 79:913S–920S, 2004.
26. Lee IM: No pain, no gain? Thoughts on the Caerphilly study, *Br J Sports Med* 38:4–5, 2004.
27. Lee IM, Paffenbarger RS: Associations of light, moderate, and vigorous intensity physical activity with longevity: the Harvard Alumni Health Study, *Am J Epidemiol* 151:293–299, 2000.
28. Tanasescu M, Leitzmann MF, Rimm EB, et al: Exercise type and intensity in relation to coronary heart disease in men, *JAMA* 288:1994–2000, 2002.
29. Yu S, Yarnell JWG, Sweetnam PM, Murray L: What level of physical activity protects against premature cardiovascular death? The Caerphilly study, *Heart* 89:502–506, 2003.
30. Swain DP, Franklin BA: Comparison of cardioprotective benefits of vigorous versus moderate intensity aerobic exercise, *Am J Cardiol* 97:141–147, 2006.
31. Lee IM, Sesko HD, Oguma Y, et al: Relative intensity of physical activity and risk of coronary heart disease, *Circulation* 107:1110–1116, 2003.
32. Duncan GE, Anton SD, Sydeman SJ, et al: Prescribing exercise at varied levels of intensity and frequency: a randomized trial, *Arch Intern Med* 165:2362–2369, 2005.
33. Dunn AL, Marcus BH, Kampert JB, et al: Comparison of lifestyle and structured interventions to increase physical activity and cardiorespiratory fitness, *JAMA* 281:327–334, 1999.
34. Murphy M, Nevill A, Neville C, et al: Accumulating brisk walking for fitness, cardiovascular risk, and psychological health, *Med Sci Sports Exerc* 34:1468–1474, 2002.
35. Manini TM, Everhart JE, Patel KV, et al: Daily activity energy expenditure and mortality among older adults, *JAMA* 296:171–179, 2006.
36. Katzmarzyk PT, Craig CL: Musculoskeletal fitness and risk of mortality, *Med Sci Sports Exerc* 34:740–744, 2002.
37. Rantanen T, Masaki K, Foley D, et al: Grip strength changes over 27 yr in Japanese-American men, *J Appl Physiol* 85:2047–2053, 1998.
38. Rantanen T, Harris T, Leveille SG, et al: Muscle strength and body mass index as long-term predictors of mortality in initially healthy men, *J Gerontol Med Sci* 55A:M168–M173, 2000.
39. Fujita Y, Nakamura Y, Hiraoka J, et al: Physical-strength tests and mortality among visitors to health-promotion centers in Japan, *J Clin Epidemiol* 48:1349–1359, 1995.
40. Newman AB, Kupelian V, Visser M, et al: Strength, but not muscle mass, is associated with mortality in the health, aging and body composition study cohort, *J Gerontol Med Sci* 61A:72–77, 2006.
41. Metter EJ, Talbot LA, Schrager M, Conwit R: Skeletal muscle strength as a predictor of all-cause mortality in healthy men, *J Gerontol Biol Sci* 57A:B359–B365, 2002.

42. Warburton D, Gledhill N, Quinney A: Musculoskeletal fitness and health, *Can J Appl Physiol* 26:217–237, 2001.

43. American College of Sports Medicine: ACSM position stand on the recommended quantity and quality of exercise for developing and maintaining cardiorespiratory and muscular fitness, and flexibility in adults, *Med Sci Sports Exerc* 30:975–991, 1998.

44. Lee IM, Paffenbarger RS: Do physical activity and physical fitness avert premature mortality? *Exerc Sports Sci Rev* 24:135–171, 1996.

45. Warburton D, Nicol CW, Bredin S: Health benefits of physical activity: the evidence, *CMAJ* 174: 801–809, 2006.

46. Kannel WB, Sorlie P: Some health benefits of physical activity: the Framingham study, *Arch Intern Med* 139:857–861, 1979.

47. Sherman SE, D'Agostino RB, Silbershatz H, Kanel WB: Comparison of past versus recent physical activity in the prevention of premature death and coronary artery disease, *Am Heart J* 138:900–907, 1999.

48. Paffenbarger RS, Wing AL, Hyde RT: Physical activity as an index of heart attack risk in college alumni, *Am J Epidemiol* 108:161–175, 1978.

49. Paffenbarger RS, Hyde RT, Wing AL, Steinmetz CH: A natural history of athleticism and cardiovascular health, *JAMA* 252:491–495, 1984.

50. Paffenbarger RS, Hyde RT, Wing AL, Hsieh CC: Physical activity, all-cause mortality, and longevity of college alumni, *N Engl J Med* 314:605–613, 1986.

51. Shaper AG, Wannamethee G: Physical activity and ischaemic heart disease in middle-aged British men, *Br Heart J* 66:384–394, 1991.

52. Shaper AG, Wannamethee G, Walker M: Physical activity, hypertension and risk of heart attack in men without evidence of ischaemic heart disease, *J Human Hypertension* 8:3–10, 1994.

53. Rodriguez BL, Curb D, Burchfiel CM, et al: Physical activity and 23-year incidence of coronary heart disease morbidity and mortality among middle-aged men: the Honolulu heart program, *Circulation* 89:2540–2544, 1994.

54. Ainsworth BE, Leon AS, Richardson MT, et al: Accuracy of the College Alumnus Physical Activity Questionnaire, *J Clin Epidemiol* 46:1403–1411, 1993.

55. Lee IM, Paffenbarger RS, Hsieh CC: Time trends in physical activity among college alumni, 1962–1988, *Am J Epidemiol* 135:915–925, 1992.

56. Franco OH, de Laet C, Peeters A, et al: effects of physical activity on life expectancy with cardiovascular disease, *Arch Intern Med* 165:2355–2360, 2005.

57. Paffenbarger RS, Hyde RT, Wing AL, et al: The association of changes in physical activity level and other lifestyle characteristics with mortality among men, *N Engl J Med* 328:538–545, 1993.

58. Wannamethee GS, Shaper AG, Walker M: Changes in physical activity, mortality, and incidence of coronary heart disease in older men, *Lancet* 351: 1603–1608, 1998.

59. Blair SN, Kohl HW, Paffenbarger RS, et al: Physical fitness and all-cause mortality. prospective study of healthy men and women, *JAMA* 262:2395–2401, 1989.

60. Blair SN, Kampert JB, Kohl HW, et al: Influences of cardiorespiratory fitness and other precursors on cardiovascular disease and all-cause mortality in men and women, *JAMA* 276:205–210, 1996.

61. Myers J, Prakash M, Froelicher V, et al: Exercise capacity and mortality among men referred for exercise testing, *N Engl J Med* 346:793–801, 2002.

62. Roger VL, Jacobsen SJ, Pellikka PA: Prognostic value of treadmill exercise testing: a population-based study in Olmstead County, Minnesota, *Circulation* 98:2836–2841, 1998.

63. Blair SN, Goodyear NN, Gibbons LW, et al: Physical fitness and the incidence of hypertension in healthy normotensive men, *JAMA* 252:487–490, 1984.

64. Lee CD, Blair SN, Jackson AS: Cardiorespiratory fitness, body composition, and all-cause and cardiovascular disease mortality in men, *Am J Clin Nutr* 69:373–380, 1999.

65. Blair SN, Kohl HW, Barlow CE, et al: Changes in physical fitness and all-cause mortality, *JAMA* 273:1093–1098, 1995.

66. Erikssen G, Liestol K, Bjornholt J, et al: Changes in physical fitness and changes in mortality, *Lancet* 352:759–762, 1998.

67. Sobolski J, Kornitzer M, DeBacker G, et al: Protection against ischemic heart disease in the Belgian physical fitness study: physical fitness rather than physical activity? *Am J Epidemiol* 125:601–610, 1987.

68. Hein HO, Suadicani P, Gyntelberg F: Physical fitness or physical activity as a predictor of ischaemic heart disease? a 17-year follow-up in the Copenhagen Male Study, *J Intern Med* 232:471–479, 1992.

69. Lakka TA, Venalainen JM, Rauramaa R, et al: Relation of leisure-time physical activity and cardiorespiratory fitness to the risk of acute myocardial infarction in men, *N Engl J Med* 330:1549–1554, 1994.

70. Myers J, Kaykha A, George S, et al: Fitness versus physical activity patterns in predicting mortality in men, *Am J Med* 117:912–918, 2004.

71. Siconolfi SF, Garber CE, Lasater TM, Carleton RA: Simple, valid step-test for estimating maximal oxygen uptake in epidemiologic studies, *Am J Epidemiol* 121:382–390, 1985.

72. Wannamethee SG, Shaper A, Walker M: Physical activity and mortality in older men with diagnosed coronary heart disease, *Circulation* 102: 1358–1363, 2000.

73. Taylor RS, Brown A, Ebrahim S, et al: Exercise-based rehabilitation for patients with coronary heart disease: systematic review and meta-analysis of randomized controlled trials, *Am J Med* 116: 682–692, 2004.

74. Iestra JA, Kromhout D, van der Schouw YT, et al: Effect size estimates of lifestyle and dietary changes on all-cause mortality in coronary artery

disease patients: a systematic review, *Circulation* 112:924–934, 2005.

75. Dorn J, Naughton J, Imamura D, et al: Results of a multicenter randomized clinical trial of exercise and long-term survival in myocardial infarction patients: the National Exercise and Heart Disease Project (NEHDP), *Circulation* 100:1764–1769, 1999.

76. Eriksson KF, Lindgarde F: No excess 12-year mortality in men with impaired glucose tolerance who participated in the Malmo Preventive Trial with diet and exercise, *Diabetologia* 41(9):1010–1016, 1998.

77. Hu FB, Leitzmann MF, Stampfer MJ, et al: Physical activity and television watching in relation to risk for type 2 diabetes mellitus in men, *Arch Intern Med* 161(12):1542–1548, 2001.

78. Hu FB, Li TY, Colditz GA, et al: Television watching and other sedentary behaviors in relation to risk of obesity and type 2 diabetes mellitus in women, *JAMA* 289(14):1785–1791, 2003.

79. Hu FB, Manson JE, Stampfer MJ, et al: Diet, lifestyle, and the risk of type 2 diabetes mellitus in women, *N Engl J Med* 345(11):790–797, 2001.

80. Tanasescu M, Lietzmann MF, Rimm EB, Hu FB: Physical activity in relation to cardiovascular disease and total mortality among men with type 2 diabetes [see comment], *Circulation* 107(19): 2435–2439, 2003.

81. Pan XR, Li GW, Hu YH, et al: Effects of diet and exercise in preventing NIDDM in people with impaired glucose tolerance: the Da Qing IGT and Diabetes Study, *Diabetes Care* 20(4):537–544, 1997.

82. Tuomilehto J, Lindstrom J, Eriksson JG, et al: Prevention of type 2 diabetes mellitus by changes in lifestyle among subjects with impaired glucose tolerance, *N Engl J Med* 344(18):1343–1350, 2001.

83. The Diabetes Prevention Program Research Group: The Diabetes Prevention Program (DPP): description of lifestyle intervention, *Diabetes Care* 25 (12):2165–2171, 2002.

84. The Diabetes Prevention Program Research Group: Reduction in the incidence of type 2 diabetes with lifestyle intervention or metformin, *N Engl J Med* 346(6):393–403, 2002.

85. Dunstan DW, Puddey IB, Beilin LJ, et al: Effects of a short-term circuit weight training program on glycaemic control in NIDDM, *Diabetes Res Clin Pract* 40(1):53–61, 1998.

86. Raz I, Hauser E, Bursztyn M: Moderate exercise improves glucose metabolism in uncontrolled elderly patients with non–insulin-dependent diabetes mellitus, *Isr J Med Sci* 30(10):766–770, 1994.

87. Kaplan RM, Hartwell SL, Wilson DK, Wallace JP, et al: Effects of diet and exercise interventions on control and quality of life in non–insulin-dependent diabetes mellitus, *J Gen Intern Med* 2 (4):220–228, 1987.

88. Lehmann R, Vokac A, Neidermann K, et al: Loss of abdominal fat and improvement of the cardiovascular risk profile by regular moderate exercise training in patients with NIDDM, *Diabetologia* 38 (11):1313–1319, 1995.

89. Mourier A, Gautier JF, De Kerviler E, et al: Mobilization of visceral adipose tissue related to the improvement in insulin sensitivity in response to physical training in NIDDM: effects of branched-chain amino acid supplements, *Diabetes Care* 20 (3):385–391, 1997.

90. Wing RR, Epstein LH, Paternostro-Bayles M, et al: Exercise in a behavioural weight control programme for obese patients with type 2 (non–insulin-dependent) diabetes, *Diabetologia* 31(12): 902–909, 1988.

91. Tessier D, Menard J, Fulop T, et al: Effects of aerobic physical exercise in the elderly with type 2 diabetes mellitus, *Arch Gerontol Geriatr* 31(2):121–132, 2000.

92. Dunstan DW, Mori TA, Puddey IB, et al: The independent and combined effects of aerobic exercise and dietary fish intake on serum lipids and glycemic control in NIDDM: a randomized controlled study, *Diabetes Care* 20(6):913–921, 1997.

93. Honkola A, Forsen T, Eriksson J: Resistance training improves the metabolic profile in individuals with type 2 diabetes, *Acta Diabetol* 34(4):245–248, 1997.

94. Agurs-Collins TD, Kumanyika SK, Ten Have TR, Adams-Campbell LL: A randomized controlled trial of weight reduction and exercise for diabetes management in older African-American subjects, *Diabetes Care* 20(10):1503–1511, 1997.

95. Vanninen E, Uusitupa M, Siitonen O, et al: Habitual physical activity, aerobic capacity and metabolic control in patients with newly-diagnosed type 2 (non–insulin-dependent) diabetes mellitus: effect of 1-year diet and exercise intervention, *Diabetologia* 35(4):340–346, 1992.

96. Boule NG, Haddad E, Kenny GP, et al: Effects of exercise on glycemic control and body mass in type 2 diabetes mellitus: a meta-analysis of controlled clinical trials [see comment], *JAMA* 286 (10):1218–1227, 2001.

97. Lee JS, Bruce CR, Tunstall RJ, et al: Interaction of exercise and diet on GLUT-4 protein and gene expression in Type I and Type II rat skeletal muscle, *Acta Physiol Scand* 175(1):37–44, 2002.

98. Terada S, Yokozeki T, Kawanaka K, et al: Effects of high-intensity swimming training on GLUT-4 and glucose transport activity in rat skeletal muscle, *J Appl Physiol* 90(6):2019–2024, 2001.

99. Becker-Zimmermann K, Berger M, Berchtold P, et al: Treadmill training improves intravenous glucose tolerance and insulin sensitivity in fatty Zucker rats, *Diabetologia* 22(6):468–474, 1982.

100. Wei M, Gibbons LW, Kampert JB, et al: Low cardiorespiratory fitness and physical inactivity as predictors of mortality in men with type 2 diabetes, *Ann Intern Med* 132(8):605–611, 2000.

101. Church TS, Cheng YJ, Earnest CP, et al: Exercise capacity and body composition as predictors of mortality among men with diabetes, *Diabetes Care* 27(1):83–88, 2004.

102. Ruderman N, Devlin JT, Schneider SH, et al: *Handbook of Exercise in Diabetes: Exercise in Diabetes*, Alexandria, VA, American Diabetes Association, 2002.

103. American Diabetes Association: Position Statement: Physical activity/exercise and diabetes, *Diabetes Care* 27(Suppl 1):58S–62S, 2004.

104. Tillin T, Forouhi N, McKeigue P, Chaturvedi N: Microalbuminuria and coronary heart disease risk in an ethnically diverse UK population: a prospective cohort study [see comment], *J Am Soc Nephrol* 16(12):3702–3710, 2005.

105. Lekatsas I, Kranidis A, Ioannidis G, et al: Comparison of the extent and severity of coronary artery disease in patients with acute myocardial infarction with and without microalbuminuria, *Am J Cardiol* 94(3):334–337, 2004.

106. Richter EA: Glucose utilization, In Rowell LB, Shepherd JT, editors: *Handbook of Physiology*, New York, 1996, Oxford University Press, pp 912–951.

107. Tsalikian E, Mauras N, Beck RW, et al: Impact of exercise on overnight glycemic control in children with type 1 diabetes mellitus, *J Pediatr* 147(4): 528–534, 2005.

108. Epidemiology of severe hypoglycemia in the diabetes control and complications trial. The DCCT Research Group [see comment], *Am J Med,* 90(4): 450–459, 1991.

109. Cryer PE: Banting lecture. Hypoglycemia: the limiting factor in the management of IDDM, *Diabetes* 43(11):1378–1389, 1994.

110. McGregor VP, Greiwe JS, Banarer S, Cryer PE: Limited impact of vigorous exercise on defenses against hypoglycemia: relevance to hypoglycemia-associated autonomic failure, *Diabetes* 51(5): 1485–1492, 2002.

111. Sandoval DA, Guy DL, Richardson MA, et al: Effects of low and moderate antecedent exercise on counterregulatory responses to subsequent hypoglycemia in type 1 diabetes, *Diabetes* 53(7): 1798–1806, 2004.

112. Lee IM: Physical activity and cancer prevention—data from epidemiologic studies, *Med Sci Sports Exerc* 35:1823–1827, 2003.

113. McTiernan A, Ulrich C, Slate S, Potter J: Physical activity and cancer etiology: association and mechanisms, *Cancer Causes Control* 9:487–509, 1998.

114. *American Cancer Society Facts and Figures 2005,* Atlanta, GA, 2005, American Cancer Society, p 45.

115. Paffenbarger RS, Hyde RT, Wery AL: Physical activity and incidence of cancer in diverse populations: a preliminary report, *Am J Clin Nutr* 45: 312–317, 1987.

116. Wannamethee G, Shaper AG, Macfarlane PW: Heart rate, physical activity, and mortality from cancer and other noncardiovascular disease, *Am J Epidemiol* 137:735–748, 1993.

117. Colditz GA, Cannuscio CC, Frazier AL: Physical activity and reduced risk of colon cancer: implications for prevention, *Cancer Causes Control* 8: 649–667, 1997.

118. Friedenreich CM, Orenstein MR: Physical activity and cancer prevention: etiologic evidence and biological mechanisms, *J Nutr* 132:3456S–3464S, 2002.

119. Slattery ML: Physical activity and colorectal cancer, *Sports Med* 34:239–252, 2004.

120. Samad AK, Taylor RS, Marshall T, Chapman MA: A meta-analysis of the association of physical activity with reduced risk of colorectal cancer, *Colorectal Dis* 7:204–213, 2005.

121. Westerlind KC: Physical activity and cancer prevention—mechanisms, *Med Sci Sports Exerc* 35: 1834–1840, 2003.

122. Cordain L, Latin R, et al: The effects of an aerobic training program on bowel transit time, *J Sports Med* 26:101–104, 1986.

123. Oettle GJ: Effect of moderate exercise on bowel habit, *Gut* 32:941–944, 1991.

124. Batty D, Thune I: Does physical activity prevent cancer? *Br Med J* 321:1424–1425, 2003.

125. Quadrilatero J, Hoffman-Goetz L: Physical activity and colon cancer: a systematic review of potential mechanisms, *J Sports Med Phys Fitness* 43:121–138, 2003.

126. Giovannucci E: Insulin, insulin-like growth factors and colon cancer: a review of the evidence, *J Nutr* 131:3109S–3120S, 2001.

127. Yu H, Rohan T: Role of insulin-like growth factor family in cancer development and progression, *J Natl Cancer Inst* 92:1472–1489, 2000.

128. Torti DC, Matheson GO: Exercise and prostate cancer, *Sports Med* 34:363–369, 2004.

129. Hackney AC, Sinning WE, Bruot BC: Reproductive hormonal profiles of endurance-trained and untrained males, *Med Sci Sports Exerc* 20:60–65, 1988.

130. Wheeler GD, Wall SR, Belcastro AN, et al: Reduced serum testosterone and prolactin levels in male distance runners, *JAMA* 252:514–516, 1984.

131. Friedenreich CM, Thune I: A review of physical activity and prostate cancer risk, *Cancer Causes Control* 12:461–475, 2001.

132. Fairey AS, Courneya KS, Field CJ, Mackey JR: Physical exercise and immune system function in cancer survivors: a comprehensive review and future directions, *Cancer* 94:539–551, 2002.

133. Courneya KS, Friedenreich CM: Physical exercise and quality of life following cancer diagnosis: a literature review, *Ann Behav Med* 21:171–179, 1999.

134. Courneya KS: Exercise in cancer survivors: an overview of research, *Med Sci Sports Exerc* 35:1846–1852, 2003.

135. Meyerhardt JA, Heseltine D, Niedzwiecki D, et al: Impact of physical activity on cancer recurrence and survival in patients with stage III colon cancer: findings from CALGB 89803, *J Clin Oncol* 24:3535–3541, 2006.

136. Polednak AP: College athletics, body size, and cancer mortality, *Cancer* 38:382–387, 1976.

137. American Cancer Society: *Guidelines for Eating Well and Being Active* Atlanta, GA, 2002, American Cancer Society.

138. Paluska SA, Schwenk TL: Physical activity and mental health, *Sports Med* 29:167–180, 2000.

416

139. Puetz TW: Physical activity and feelings of energy and fatigue: epidemiologic evidence, *Sport Med* 36: 767–780, 2006.

140. Galper DI, Trivedi MH, Barlow CE, et al: Inverse association between physical inactivity and mental health in men and women, *Med Sci Sports Exerc* 38:173–178, 2006.

141. Craft LL, Landers DM: The effect of exercise on clinical depression and depression resulting from mental illness: a meta-analysis, *J Sport Exerc Psychol* 20:339–357, 1998.

142. Lawlor DA, Hopker SW: The effectiveness of exercise as an intervention in the management of depression: systematic review and meta-regression analysis of randomized controlled trials, *BMJ* 322:763–767, 2001.

143. North TC, McCullagh P, Tran ZV: Effect of exercise on depression, *Exerc Sport Sci Rev* 18:379–415, 1990.

144. Blumenthal JA, Babyak MA, Moore KA, et al: Effects of exercise training on older patients with major depression, *Arch Intern Med* 159:2349–2356, 1999.

145. Babyak M, Blumenthal JA, Herman S, et al: Exercise treatment for major depression: maintenance of therapeutic benefit at 10 months, *Psychosom Med* 62:633–638, 2000.

146. Barbour KA, Blumenthal JA: Exercise training and depression in older adults, *Neurobiol Aging* 26S: S119–S123, 2005.

147. Brosse AL, Sheets ES, Lett HS, Blumenthal JA: Exercise and the treatment of clinical depression in adults: recent findings and future directions, *Sports Med* 32:741–760, 2002.

148. Ernst C, Olson AK, Pinel JPJ, et al: Antidepressant effects of exercise: evidence for an adult-neurogenesis hypothesis? *J Psychiatry Neurosci* 31: 84–92, 2006.

149. Lett HS, Davidson J, Blumenthal JA: Nonpharmacologic treatments for depression in patients with coronary heart disease, *Psychosom Med* 67(Suppl 1):S58–S62, 2005.

150. Yeung RR: The acute effects of exercise on mood state, *J Psychosomatic Res* 40:123–141, 1996.

151. Martinsen EW, Hoffart A, Solberg O: Aerobic and non-aerobic forms of exercise in the treatment of anxiety disorders, *Stress Med* 5:115–120, 1989.

152. Broocks A, Meyer T, Bandelow B, et al: Exercise avoidance and impaired endurance capacity in patients with panic disorder, *Neuropsychobiology* 36:182–187, 1997.

153. Rief W, Hermanutz M: Responses to activation and rest in patients with panic disorder and major depression, *Br J Clin Psychol* 35:605–616, 1996.

154. Broocks A, Bandelow B, Pekrun G, et al: Comparison of aerobic exercise, clomipramine, and placebo in the treatment of panic disorder, *Am J Psychiatry* 155:603–609, 1998.

155. Hebert LE, Scherr PA, Bienias JL, et al: Alzheimer disease in the US population: prevalence estimates using the 2000 census, *Arch Neurol* 60:1119–1122, 2003.

156. Fratiglioni L, Paillard-Borg S: An activity and socially integrated lifestyle in late life might protect against dementia, *Lancet Neurol* 3:343–353, 2004.

157. Colcombe S, Kramer AF: Fitness effects on the cognitive function of older adults: a meta-analytic study, *Psychol Sci* 14:125–130, 2003.

158. Lindsay J, Laurin D, Verreault R, et al: Risk factors for Alzheimer's disease: a prospective analysis from the Canadian Study of Health on Aging, *Am J Epidemiol* 156:445–453, 2002.

159. Yoshitake T, Kiyihara Y, Kato I, et al: Incidence and risk factors of vascular dementia and Alzheimer's disease in a defined elderly Japanese population: the Hisayama Study, *Neurology* 45: 1161–1168, 1995.

160. Wilson RS, Mendes de Leon CF, Barnes LL, et al: Participation in cognitively stimulating activities and risk of incident Alzheimer disease, *JAMA* 287:742–748, 2002.

161. Verghese J, Lipton RB, Katz MJ, et al: Leisure activities and the risk of dementia in the elderly, *N Engl J Med* 348:2508–2516, 2003.

162. Abbott RD, White LR, Webster Ross G, et al: Walking and dementia in physically capable elderly men, *JAMA* 292:1447–1453, 2004.

163. Larson EB, Wang L, Bowen JD, et al: Exercise is associated with reduced risk for incident dementia among persons 65 years of age and older, *Ann Intern Med* 144:73–81, 2006.

164. Rovio S, Kareholt I, Helkala E, et al: Leisure-time physical activity at midlife and the risk of dementia and Alzheimer's disease, *Lancet Neurol* 4: 705–711, 2005.

165. Heyn P, Abreu C, Ottenbacher KJ: The effects of exercise training on elderly persons with cognitive impairment and dementia: a meta-analysis, *Arch Phys Med Rehabil* 85:1694–1704, 2004.

166. Steptoe A, Butler N: Sports participation and emotional wellbeing in adolescents, *Lancet* 347: 1789–1792, 1996.

167. American College of Sports Medicine: The recommended quantity and quality of exercise for developing and maintaining cardiorespiratory and muscular fitness, and flexibility in healthy adults, *Med Sci Sports Exerc* 30:975–991, 1998.

168. Thompson PD: Cardiovascular risks of exercise, *Phys Sportsmed* 29:33–47, 2001.

169. Giri S, Thompson PD, Kiernan FS, et al: Clinical and angiographic characteristics exertion-related acute myocardial infarction, *JAMA* 282:1731–1736, 1999.

170. Mittleman MA, MaClure M, Tofler GH, et al: Triggering of acute myocardial infarction by heavy physical exertion: protection against triggering by regular exertion, *N Engl J Med* 329:1677–1683, 1993.

171. Willich SN, Lewis M, Lowell H, et al: Physical exertion as a trigger of acute myocardial infarction, *N Engl J Med* 329:1684–1690, 1993.

172. Albert CM, Mittleman MA, Chae CU, et al: Triggering of sudden death from cardiac causes by vigorous exertion, *N Engl J Med* 343:1355–1361, 2000.

173. Kohl HW, Powell KE, Gordon NF, et al: Physical activity, physical fitness and sudden cardiac death, *Epidemiol Rev* 14:37–58, 1992.

174. Maron BJ, Shirani J, Poliac LC, et al: Sudden death in young competitive athletes, *JAMA* 276:199–204, 1996.

175. Liberthson RR: Sudden death from cardiac causes in children and young adults, *N Engl J Med* 334:1039–1044, 1996.

176. Maron BJ: The paradox of exercise, *N Engl J Med* 343:1409–1411, 2000.

177. Hootman JM, Macera CA, Ainsworth BE, et al: Epidemiology of musculoskeletal injuries among sedentary and physically active adults, *Med Sci Sports Exerc* 34:838–844, 2002.

178. Diabetes Prevention Program Research Group: Reduction in the incidence of type 2 diabetes with lifestyle intervention or metformin, *N Engl J Med* 346:393–403, 2002.

179. Buckwalter JA, Lane NE: Athletics and osteoarthritis, *Am J Sports Med* 25:873–881, 1997.

180. Lane NE, Michel B, Bjorkengren A, et al: The risk of osteoarthritis with running and aging: a 5-year longitudinal study, *J Rheumatol* 20:461–468, 1993.

181. Lane NE, Bloch DA, Jones HH, et al: Long-distance running, bone density, and osteoarthritis, *JAMA* 255:1147–1151, 1986.

182. Fries JF, Singh G, Morfeld D, et al: Running and the development of disability with age, *Ann Intern Med* 121:502–509, 1994.

183. Panush RS, Schmidt C, Caldwell JR, et al: Is running associated with degenerative joint disease? *JAMA* 255:1152–1154, 1986.

184. Kujala U, Kaprio J, Sarna S: Osteoarthritis of weight bearing joints of lower limbs in former elite male athletes, *Br Med J* 308:231–234, 1994.

185. Videman T, Sarna S, Battie MC, et al: The long-term effects of physical loading and exercise lifestyles on back-related symptoms, disability, and spinal pathology among men, *Spine* 20:699–709, 1995.

186. Ettinger WH, Burns R, Messier SP, et al: A randomized trial comparing aerobic exercise and resistance exercise with a health education program in older adults with knee osteoarthritis, *JAMA* 277:25–31, 1997.

187. Thomas KS, Muir KR, Doherty M, et al: Home-based exercise programme for knee pain and knee osteoarthritis: randomized controlled trial, *BMJ* 325:752–756, 2002.

188. Kovar PA, Allegrante JP, MacKenzie R, et al: Supervised fitness walking in patients with osteoarthritis of the knee, *Ann Intern Med* 116:529–534, 1992.

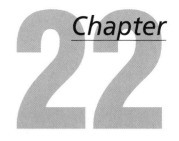

Integrative Medicine

David Rakel, MD

Key Points

Integrative Medicine Treatment Plan for Prostate Cancer

Lifestyle (strength of recommendation for all: C)

- Encourage the patient to strive to maintain an ideal weight and BMI.
- Recommend the incorporation of a regular movement and exercise routine into a daily lifestyle.
- Counsel the patient to avoid exposure to substances that may have a hormonal influence on the body:
  - Xenobiotics (e.g., pesticides, herbicides, rBGH)
  - Drugs and supplements (e.g., DHEA, androstenedione, testosterone, human growth hormone)
- Encourage consumption of organic foods and filtered drinking water, and cooking/storing food and drink in glass (non-plastic) containers.

Mind–Body Connection (strength of recommendation for all: C)

- Create a plan that empowers the patient to be an active participant in treating his prostate cancer. This will enhance a sense of control that will improve quality of life and may, in itself, positively affect prostate cancer.
- Consider recommending a mindfulness class to help the patient learn to live in the moment and not in memories of the past or desires of the future. This will help reduce emotions that can stimulate anxiety.
- *"I am an old man and have known a great many troubles, but most of them never happened."*—Mark Twain

Spirituality (strength of recommendation for all: C)

- Ask the patient, "Has being diagnosed with prostate cancer helped you reconnect with those things that give you the most meaning in your life?"
- Ask the patient, "What has helped you get through this difficult time?"
- Ask, "Do you have a spiritual practice and a community that helps this connection grow?"

Nutrition

- Recommend a reduction in intake of saturated fat, particularly in the form of dairy products and red meat (strength of recommendation: B).
- The patient should avoid intake of hormone-containing foods such as cow's milk that may contain bovine growth hormone (strength of recommendation: C).
- Soy products can be substituted for dairy products (strength of recommendation: B).
- Intake of lycopene-rich foods (strength of recommendation: C) and cruciferous vegetables (strength of recommendation: C) should be increased.
- Recommend that the patient substitute green tea for coffee and soda (strength of recommendation: C).
- Suggest that the patient consider drinking 8 oz of pomegranate juice daily (strength of recommendation: C).

Supplements (strength of recommendation for all: C)

- Vitamin E supplementation can take the form of mixed tocopherols that include alpha, beta, and gamma forms. No more than 400 IU daily should be ingested.

- Consider recommending 100–200 µg of selenium daily along with vitamin E, since they work synergistically.
- Monitor 25-hydroxy vitamin D levels and supplement with vitamin D₃ to keep levels between 30 and 100 ng/dL (general dose is 800 IU daily).
- Counsel the patient to avoid taking zinc at high doses (>100 mg) for prolonged periods of time since it can reduce the body's ability to absorb minerals such as copper, iron, and calcium.

Botanicals (strength of recommendation for all: C)

- Herbs that are commonly used for inflammation and benign prostatic hypertrophy (BPH) (such as saw palmetto, pygeum, stinging nettle root, and pumpkin seed extract) are also rich in beta-sitosterol, which reduces the absorption of cholesterol and may reduce the hormonal influences on prostate cancer.
- The recommended dose of beta-sitosterol is 60 mg twice daily, yet it is recommended to avoid supplementation with this isolated ingredient and to encourage consumption of the plants and vegetables that contain it so that it can be used synergistically with other plant nutrients.

Introduction

Integrative medicine is defined as healing-oriented medicine that takes into account the concept of "the whole person" (i.e., encompassing body, mind, and spirit), including all aspects of one's lifestyle. It emphasizes the therapeutic relationship and makes use of all appropriate therapies, both conventional and alternative.[1] This philosophy is not a new concept; in fact, it dates back to the time of Aristotle. With the growth of technology and the advent of pharmaceutical sciences, the "holistic" understanding of the multiple influences on health has been overshadowed by our successes in treating the body's parts. This reductionistic model has served acute healthcare needs well, but it has limitations in treating the growing problem of chronic disease.

In the mid 1990s, the public became frustrated by this traditional model and started to look elsewhere for health-related care beyond pharmaceuticals and surgical options. In fact, there were more visits to complementary and alternative medicine (CAM) providers in the early 1990s than to all primary care medical physicians, and patients paid for these visits out of pocket with

an estimated expenditure of $13 billion.[2] This trend continued throughout the 1990s, with 42% of the public using alternative therapies, increasing expenditures to $27 billion between 1990 and 1997.[3] The public also started reading headlines announcing that adverse effects from pharmaceutical agents were the sixth leading cause of hospital deaths in the United States,[4] and they viewed complementary approaches to be more aligned with "their own values, beliefs, and philosophical orientations toward health and life."[5]

Data collected from National Health Interview Survey, which was conducted by the Centers for Disease Control and Prevention's National Center for Health Statistics, showed that 62% of US adults used CAM within 12 months of being interviewed (Figure 22-1). The 10 most commonly used CAM therapies included the following:

- Use of prayer specifically for one's own health (43.0%)
- Prayer by others for one's own health (24.4%)
- Natural products (18.9%)
- Deep-breathing exercises (11.6%)
- Participation in prayer group for one's own health (9.6%)
- Meditation (7.6%)
- Chiropractic care (7.5%)
- Yoga (5.1%)
- Massage (5.0%)
- Diet-based therapies (3.5%)

CAM was most often used to treat back pain, colds, neck pain, joint stiffness, and depression. Almost 55% of patients believed that combining CAM with conventional care would provide an added benefit.[6]

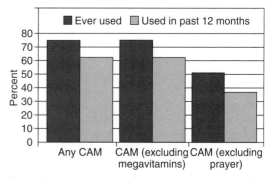

Figure 22-1. Percentage of Americans using complementary and alternative medicine (CAM). (Adapted from: Rakel DP, Weil A: Philosophy of integrative medicine. In Rakel DP, editor: *Integrative Medicine*, ed 2, Philadelphia, 2007, Saunders, pp 1–13. Data source: National Health Interview Survey, 2002.)

Tools Versus Process

In the mid 1990s, there was an increase in the use of tools that fell under the label of CAM. In fact, in 1994 botanicals were the largest growth area in retail pharmacy,[7] and at the same time, the cost of healthcare in the United States began spiraling out of control. The amount of money allocated to healthcare over the past 10 years has almost doubled, from $391 to $668 billion. The healthcare market grows when more attention is focused on diseases that can be treated with drugs, botanicals, and/or procedures. In 2003, spending allocated to pharmaceutical products in the United States rose 11% to $180 billion and is now 15% higher than any other health-related expenditure.[8] If our healthcare system continues to focus simply on the tools and not the process, then healthcare costs will continue to rise significantly. The underlying philosophy of integrative medicine focuses on the process of first understanding what is needed for the body to heal so that fewer, not more, external influences are required to maintain health, be they drugs or acupuncture needles (Table 22-1). Unfortunately, this philosophy is neither supported nor rewarded by our current economic healthcare model.

The process of integrative medicine involves exploring how the nonphysical influences the physical (Figure 22-2) and how lifestyle choices and the motivation to practice them will result in a decreased need for expensive interventions. If someone in a high-stress profession does not recognize how stress can be directly related to increased blood pressure, headaches, and dysfunctional bowel syndromes, then they will

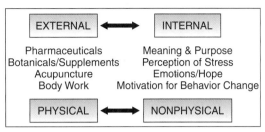

Figure 22-2. Importance of recognizing both the external, physical and the internal, nonphysical aspects on health. (Adapted from: Rakel DP, Weil A: Philosophy of integrative medicine. In Rakel DP, editor: *Integrative Medicine,* ed 2, Philadelphia, 2007, Saunders, pp 1–13.)

require more medications and procedures to treat their diseases. Healing-oriented medicine uses relationship-centered care to allow time to hear the patient's story to bring insight and understanding regarding how lifestyle, nutrition, mind–body connection, and spiritual influences can be used to "stack the deck" in favor of self-healing. This type of approach will not be successful until we help facilitate the internal dialogue of how nonphysical emotions influence the external physical process. In conventional medicine, healing occurs *outside* of the body-mind construct and is viewed as something "done to the patient." In integrative medicine, healing occurs *within* the body-mind construct and requires active participation of the patient.

An Integrative Medicine Approach to a Patient with Prostate Cancer

JD is a 72-year-old man who was found to have an elevated prostate-specific antigen (PSA) level on routine screening. He was referred to a urologist for an ultrasound-guided biopsy of the prostate, which revealed adenocarcinoma with a Gleason score of 4. JD was told that this was not an aggressive form of prostate cancer and that it was recommended that he simply have this monitored over time with PSA testing every 6 months.

There are few diseases that warrant an integrative approach more than prostate cancer. For a low-grade prostate tumor that does not warrant aggressive therapy, a trial of "watchful waiting" is often prescribed. When physicians tell a patient that they have "The Big C" (i.e., cancer), and that we are going to watch and see what it does over short intervals of time, watchful waiting quickly becomes watchful anxiety! The primary care

Table 22-1. Defining Integrative Medicine

Grounded in relationship-centered care
Integrates conventional and complementary methods for treatment and prevention
Involves removing barriers that may activate the body's innate healing response
Uses natural, less invasive interventions before costly, invasive ones whenever possible
Engages mind, body, spirit, and community to facilitate healing
Healing is always possible, even when curing is not

Adapted from: Rakel DP, Weil A: Philosophy of integrative medicine. In Rakel DP, editor: *Integrative Medicine,* ed 2, Philadelphia, 2007, Saunders, pp 1–13.

provider can take this opportunity to educate the patient on how nutrition, supplements, and the mind-body and spiritual connections can be used to empower him to be an active participant in his healthcare. This approach helps to take a situation in which a patient has anxiety with a loss of a sense of control and helps him to learn how men can be active participants in their care, creating a mind-body shift that facilitates hope.

Mind–Body Influences on Health

The mind–body/body–mind connection is present in every symptom and illness. Dividing the human condition into separate entities of mind and body is misleading because, in reality, they are one and cannot be separated. The main challenge for healthcare providers is to encourage our patients to appreciate this intricate connection and to use this insight to improve health and quality of life.

Control

Men, by nature, like to be in control of their surroundings. Studies have shown that acute, sudden loss of control typically leads to anxiety, whereas long-term perceived loss of control results in learned helplessness. One particular study exposed male subjects to loud noises. One half of the subjects had no control over the disturbing noise, and the other half was able to control the loud noise by using a button. The group without control showed an increase in self-ratings of helplessness, tension, stress, unhappiness, anxiety, and depression. Physiologic studies also demonstrated increased stimulation of the sympathetic nervous system, hypothalamic-pituitary-adrenal axis, and adrenocorticotropic hormone secretion.[9]

In another study, researchers arranged for nursing home residents to receive one of two interventions depending on the floor they lived on. On one floor, residents were given responsibility for deciding how to arrange their rooms and spend their time, and they were given plants to care for. The other group was reminded of all the options available to them provided by the home. In short, in one group the emphasis was on the participants' control and responsibility over their lives, and in the other, the emphasis was on the home's control and responsibility. Eighteen months later, the

residents with the increased control were not only more active and happier, but also more likely to be alive. Only 15% of those residents with more control had died versus 30% in the group who had less control.[10]

Addressing a man's psychological well-being can have a significant influence on his survival and can improve quality of life in patients with prostate cancer. One study revealed that men who were taught new coping skills (e.g., mental relaxation and imagery techniques, stress management, ways to develop self-esteem and spirituality, receptive imagery/intuition and problem solving, and how to create a personal health plan/goal) lived twice as long as men in the control group.[11] When a man is diagnosed with cancer, it is imperative that we give him an opportunity to be actively involved in his treatment plan, whether it involves watchful waiting or surgery.

Mindfulness

Learning to train the mind how to recognize how our thoughts can influence anxiety may affect serum PSA levels. Mindfulness-based stress reduction coupled with a plant-based diet has been shown to slow PSA doubling time in men with biochemical recurrence after radical prostatectomy and prolong survival in men with metastatic prostate cancer.[12,13] Mindfulness is the practice of being aware of the present moment and involves the following philosophical foundations:[14]

- Humans are largely unaware of their moment-to-moment experiences, often operating on "auto-pilot."
- Humans are capable of developing the ability to sustain attention to mental content.
- Developing this ability is gradual, progressive, and requires regular practice.
- Moment-to-moment awareness replaces unconscious reactivity and will provide a richer and more vital sense of life.
- Persistent, non-evaluative observation of mental content will gradually give rise to more accurate perceptions.
- As a more accurate perception of one's own mental response to external stimuli is achieved, additional information is gathered that will enhance effective action and lead to a greater sense of control, peace, and a sense of well-being.

Mindfulness classes are offered throughout the United States and are generally 8 weeks in length. A systematic review of the effects of mindfulness on persons with cancer supported its benefit in improving mood, sleep quality, and stress reduction, with a dose-response effect.[15] One of the studies reviewed showed a prolonged doubling time of PSA from 6.5 to 17.7 months when mindfulness-based stress reduction was combined with a diet and exercise program. This study was limited by its small size and lack of a control group.[12]

Spirituality

When defined appropriately, spirituality is one of the most important aspects of health and healing. It is often not until our sense of control is threatened by serious disease that there is motivation to explore our spiritual connection and define it. Spirituality is not something that we give to our patients, it is something that we help them find. Defining its meaning is a personal exploration and a question to which we should encourage patients to find their own answers. In doing so, it is important to understand the differences between religion and spirituality, initially through definitions:

- *Religion:* A body of beliefs and practices defined by a community or society to which its adherents mutually prescribe
- *Spirituality:* An inherent aspect of every human being that relates to the Absolute—that domain where values and meaning exist

Although not everyone may practice a certain religion, everyone has a spiritual meaning. An analogy that helps prepare us in approaching this aspect of healthcare with patients is to view religion as a poem that describes the flower (i.e., spirit). There are many different poems that describe the flower. Our job is not to project our own belief as to which poem a patient should choose, but rather to learn which poem may resonate the most with him or her so that his or her connection to the flower results in a stronger sense of meaning and purpose. It is *connection, meaning,* and *purpose* that help physicians understand how to communicate about spirituality with patients to help foster hope in the setting of disease. More specifically, it is often the life-threatening disease that encourages this exploration.

There are a number of mnemonics that can be used to guide a physician in conducting patient assessments regarding spirituality. These include FICA,[16] HOPE,[17] and SPIRIT[18] (Table 22-2).

Helpful questions that can aid the clinician in starting this rewarding conversation include the following:

- In a time of need, to whom do you turn for help?
- What gives you a sense of meaning and purpose in life?
- Sometimes being diagnosed with prostate cancer can bring new meaning to life. What meaning does this experience have for you?
- What helps you get through tough times?
- Sometimes having cancer can leave a person feeling empty. With what are you filling this emptiness?

It is through these ideas that patients can find meaning and purpose in their lives, and in this way they are best able to understand what is needed to self-heal. It is through spiritual exploration that we may gain insight into those relationships that result in peace, joy, and happiness, even if physical disease persists.

Pain and Suffering

A good example of the mind-body-spiritual influences on health is the difference between pain and suffering. Pain is our physical body's response to an external stimulus, whereas suffering is our perception of pain. The more suffering a human being is experiencing, the more pain is perceived (Figure 22-3). If clinicians treat pain without addressing a person's suffering, then more narcotics, epidural blocks, manipulations, and acupuncture treatments will be required. If healthcare providers first address the patient's suffering, however, then we are best able to reduce the pain to the most physiologic reason for its existence. In addressing suffering, clinicians need to address a patient's spiritual connection that results in their meaning and purpose. In helping this grow, pain severity decreases.

Nutrition

Education and research regarding how nutrition influences health is a key aspect of integrative medicine. It resonates with the philosophy of using natural and less invasive interventions before costly and invasive ones whenever possible. If more attention was given to proper nutrition, then there would be less disease and fewer medications needed to treat it. Prostate cancer

Table 22-2. Spiritual Assessment Tools

FICA—Pulchaski, 1999
F: Faith or belief—What is your faith or belief?
I: Importance and influence—Is it important in your life? How?
C: Community—Are you part of a religious community?
A: Awareness and addressing—What would you want me as your physician to be aware of? How would you like me to address these issues in your care?
HOPE—Anandarajah and Hight, 2001
H: Hope—What are your sources of hope, meaning, strength, peace, love, and connectedness?
O: Organized—Do you consider yourself part of an organized religion?
P: Personal spirituality and practices—What aspects of your spirituality or spiritual practices do you find most helpful?
E: Effects—How do your beliefs affect the kind of medical care you would like me to provide?
SPIRIT—Maugans, 1996
S: Spiritual belief system—What is your formal religious affiliation?
P: Personal spirituality—Describe the beliefs and practices of your religion or spiritual system that you personally accept/do not accept.
I: Integration with a spiritual community—Do you belong to a spiritual or religious group or community? What importance does this group have for you?
R: Ritualized practices and restrictions—Are there specific practices that you carry out as part of your religion/spirituality (e.g., prayer and meditation)? What significance do these practices or restrictions have to you?
I: Implications for medical care—What aspects of your religion/spirituality would you like me to keep in mind as I care for you?
T: Terminal events planning—As we plan for your care near the end of life, how does your faith impact on your decisions?

Adapted from: Puchalski CM: Taking a spiritual history: FICA, *Spirituality Med Connect* 3:1, 1999; Anandarajah G, Hight E: Spirituality and medical practice: using the HOPE questions as a practical tool for spiritual assessment, *Am Fam Phys* 63:81–88, 2001; Maugans TA: The SPIRITual history, *Arch Fam Med* 5:11–16, 1996.

offers a good example of how appropriate nutrition can be used to potentially prevent this common condition.

Saturated Fat and Obesity

Conditions of the prostate such as benign prostatic hypertrophy (BPH) and cancer are hormonally dependent. With the epidemic of obesity in the Western hemisphere, we will continue to see how stored subcutaneous fat becomes an active endocrine gland, creating a disruption in the balance of hormones in the body. Men who are obese and have the highest body mass index (BMI) levels have a higher overall incidence of prostate cancer.[19] Intake of foods rich in saturated fat increase hormones such as estrogen that play a role in the health of the prostate. Men who consume significant amounts of red meat have double the risk of developing prostate cancer.[20] Epidemiologic

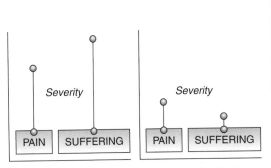

Suffering's effect on the same source of pain. Treating suffering will help reduce the severity of pain and improve quality of life and should be at the core of our work in integrative medicine.

Figure 22-3. Suffering's effect on a source of pain. (Adapted from: Rakel DP, Weil A: Philosophy of integrative medicine. In Rakel DP, editor: *Integrative Medicine*, ed 2, Philadelphia, 2007, Saunders, pp 1–13.)

studies show that the incidence of prostate cancer is lower in countries such as Japan where less red meat is consumed, but when Japanese men immigrate to America and adopt a "Western" diet, their incidence of prostate cancer has been shown to increase seven-fold.[21,22] The incidence of prostate cancer, particularly advanced forms of disease, is greatest in countries with the highest calorie and saturated fat consumption.[20,23,24]

Saturated fat is also a rich source of the main inflammatory precursor arachidonic acid, a molecular building block of prostaglandins, leukotrienes, and thromboxanes that stimulates hypertrophy and cancer cell growth in the prostate. Prostate cancer cells have been found to produce up to 10 times as much prostaglandin E_2 compared with normal prostate cells.[25] A class of series four leukotrienes, *5-HETE*, has been shown to stimulate prostate cancer growth and to prevent prostate cell apoptosis (programmed cell death).[26] Meat-based diets and most saturated cooking oils (with the exception of monounsaturated oils such as canola and olive oils) increase arachidonic acid formation. In contrast, following a vegan diet can lower arachidonic acid production by 30%.[27]

Saturated fat is a rich source of cholesterol. High serum cholesterol levels have been associated with an increased incidence of BPH and prostate cancer. Its metabolites (epoxycholesterols) have been found to accumulate in hyperplastic and cancerous prostate glands. Cholesterol is also a precursor for the production of estrogen and testosterone. Treatment of hypercholesterolemia with pharmaceutical agents that lower cholesterol (i.e., 3-hydroxy-3-methylglutaryl coenzyme A [HMG-CoA] reductase inhibitors) has been associated with a lower risk of BPH and prostate cancer.[28]

The consumption of cow's milk and other dairy products has been a controversial topic with regard to prostate cancer. There are three components of dairy products that may influence prostate health—namely saturated fat, calcium, and various hormones. Surprisingly, Veierod and colleagues[19] found that Norwegian men who drank skim milk were more likely to have prostate cancer than men who drank whole milk. Although there is good evidence to support the negative influence of saturated fat on the prostate, this study helped to trigger a search for other harmful nutrients found within dairy products, one of which was calcium.

Calcium

Vitamin D is an important cofactor required for calcium absorption, and thus the intake of excessive calcium can reduce the levels of the body's most active form of vitamin D, *1,25 dihydroxy vitamin D*. It is thought that vitamin D may help protect against prostate cancer and that the calcium found in milk may help explain why drinking cow's milk has been associated with an increased incidence of prostate cancer. The Health Professionals Follow-up Study found a 70% increase in prostate cancer in men who consumed large amounts of cow's milk and a threefold increased risk in men who took calcium supplements.[20] The Physician's Health Study[29] found that men who drank more than 2.5 servings/day of cow's milk had lower levels of 1,25 dihydroxy vitamin D than those who drank less than 0.5 servings/day. Men who consumed the most milk in this study had a 32% higher risk of prostate cancer than those in the lowest intake group. These data were not supported by a recent randomized controlled trial that found no increased risk in men who supplemented their diets with calcium for up to a period of 3 years.[30] Even if saturated fat and calcium are found to play a minor role in the development of prostate cancer, it appears that more substantive evidence is mounting regarding the hormonal influences associated with consuming cow's milk.

Insulin-Like Growth Factor-1

Insulin-like growth factor-1 (IGF-1) is a hormone produced in the liver and other tissues that acquired its name because of its insulin-like activity in adipose tissue and chemical structure, which is very similar to that of pro-insulin. Production of IGF-1 is stimulated by human growth hormone, and it acts to promote cell growth of both normal and malignant cells.[31] Serum levels of IGF-1 generally peak during puberty and gradually decrease with age. At the age of 70 years, serum levels are half the normal expected adult value of 200 ng/mL. IGF-1 has been found to play a role not only in prostate cancer but also in childhood cancers, breast cancer, small cell lung cancer, melanoma, and pancreatic cancer.[32] Harvard researchers found that men with elevated levels of IGF-1 between 300 and 500 ng/mL had four times the risk of the development of prostate cancer than persons with levels of 100–185 ng/mL.[33]

Many US dairy cows are injected in 2-week intervals with synthetic recombinant bovine growth hormone (rBGH) to increase their milk production by 14%.[34] Levels of IGF-1 in the milk of cows that are injected can range from 2 to 10 times greater than levels in cows that are not injected.[35,36] The US Food and Drug Administration (FDA) does not require identification of dairy products that come from rBGH-treated cows, so it is difficult for consumers to know the IGF-1 concentration in the products they purchase. Other countries such as Australia, New Zealand, and Japan have banned rBGH, whereas Europe and Canada have taken strides to limit its use. The company that produces rBGH actually supplied most of the data and evidence that the FDA used to approve the use of this hormone. The counter-argument for the safety of rBGH is that the level of IGF-1 is no different than that found in human breast milk and that digestive enzymes break down the hormone in the gut after it is ingested.[37] Few would argue that humans require IGF-1 for development as an infant, but we do not continue to drink breast milk into adulthood. In fact, humans are the only mammals that continue to drink milk into adulthood. IGF-1 is not destroyed by pasteurization, and there is evidence that demonstrates that it is absorbed systemically after oral ingestion.[34] An animal study of male rats showed that serum levels of IGF-1 increased after oral ingestion.[38]

In summary, saturated fat and stored adipose tissue increase the incidence of prostate cancer by promoting hormones, cholesterol, and arachidonic acid, which promote inflammation and prostate cancer cell growth. This influence on endocrine function helps us to understand why men with insulin resistance and the metabolic syndrome have twice the risk of prostate cancer.[39] It would appear that saturated fat, excess calcium, and IGF-1 render cow's milk and dairy products foods that men would want to avoid in excessive amounts. Some men may find it advantageous to switch to soy-based products.

Soy Protein

Soy protein is derived from soybeans and contains the isoflavones *genistein* and *daidzein*, which have been found to be beneficial in preventing BPH and prostate cancer. In Japanese men, the incidence of prostate cancer is much lower compared with men in the Western world, probably related to their high intake of soy products as well as their lower intake of saturated fat. In one study, Japanese men were found to have urinary isoflavone concentrations 30 times higher and serum concentrations 100 times higher than

Western males.[40] These isoflavones have been found to inhibit prostate cancer cell growth via a number of different beneficial mechanisms.[41] Genistein has been shown to inhibit prostate cancer cell growth both in vitro and in vivo by promoting apoptosis, blocking beta-estrogen receptor activity, inhibiting angiogenesis and endothelial cell proliferation, and blocking 5-alpha reductase, aromatase, and tyrosine-specific protein kinase activity.[21,42,43] A prospective study of 12,395 Seventh-day Adventist men revealed 225 cases of prostate cancer. Men who drank at least one glass of soymilk daily had a 70% reduction in the risk of developing this disease.[44] Researchers found that men taking 100 mg of soy isoflavones twice daily slowed the growth of an aggressive form androgen-insensitive prostate cancer by 35% and slowed overall cancer growth by 84%.[45]

There is some concern that genetically modified soy may not provide the same health benefits as non–genetically modified soy; for prostate cancer prevention, the equivalent of 80 mg of genistein daily (approximately 4 oz of soy milk) should be recommended. High-fiber cereal with soy milk each morning instead of cow's milk would help men incorporate this amount on a daily basis. For active treatment, 200 mg daily has been suggested. Commercially available soy protein bars and either sweetened or unsweetened soy powder can also supplement dietary soy intake to provide this recommended dosage.

Lycopene

Lycopene is a carotenoid that gives many fruits and vegetables its rosy red color. Foods rich in lycopene include tomatoes, strawberries, watermelon, apricots, pink grapefruit, and guava juice. There have been a number of prospective studies showing the benefits of lycopene in the prevention of prostate cancer.[46–48] A prospective cohort study showed that men who consumed tomato products four times weekly reduced their prostate cancer risk by 20%, and those that ate 10 or more helpings weekly reduced their risk by 45%. Men who ate a half cup of strawberries daily significantly lowered their risk of developing prostate cancer.[49]

Some evidence exists to suggest that lycopene also appears to be beneficial in treating established prostate cancer. One study demonstrated that men with prostate cancer had significantly lower serum levels of lycopene, but levels of other carotenoids such as beta-carotene did not differ between men with and without the disease.[50] To determine whether ingesting a lycopene-rich food would have an effect on prostate cancer, a study of African American men with either prostate cancer or an elevated PSA level consumed tomato sauce–based pasta dishes that were equivalent to 30 mg/day of lycopene for 3 weeks. Men with established prostate cancer had a 28.3% reduction in DNA damage to cancer cells, and men with an elevated PSA level but no definable prostate cancer were shown to have a reduction of PSA levels by approximately 17.5%.[51] Due to the promising evidence and the limited harm of eating lycopene-rich foods, encouraging their consumption should be a part of routine dietary education for patients.

Cruciferous Vegetables

Eating fruits and vegetables is important for promoting good health in general. In the case of prostate cancer, eating a plant-based diet can slow PSA doubling time in men with recurrent prostate cancer[12]; cruciferous vegetables appear to be particularly protective.[52] The term *cruciferous* is derived from the Latin word *cruc*, (translates to *cross*), which describes the four main leaves that cross on the plant of these vegetables. Cruciferous vegetables come from the *Brassica* genus and include broccoli, brussels sprouts, cabbage, collards, cauliflower, kale, kohlrabi, mustard greens, rapeseed, and root vegetables such as turnips and rutabagas. Their benefit may be partly related to a common substance they contain called *sulforaphane*.[53] They are also a rich source of *indole-3 carbinol*, a popular cancer-related nutritional supplement. There is some promising human research in its use for hormone-sensitive cancers (e.g., cervical cancer), but to date no valid human research has been performed related to prostate cancer treatment or prevention. The recommended daily dietary intake of indole-3-carbinol is typically 20–120 mg, whereas the recommended supplementing dose is 200 mg daily (one head of cabbage contains approximately 1200 mg of indole-3-carbinol). It is recommended to consume the foods from which these products are naturally found since much of the positive benefit likely occurs on account of synergy between a variety of different chemicals within the plant, which is not gained by taking a supplement that consists of only one chemical found within the plant.

Green Tea (*Camellia sinensis*)

Tea is the most commonly consumed beverage on the planet. Its common use in Asian countries may help explain the lower incidence of prostate cancer in these cultures.[54] Men who drink tea regularly in England and China have a lower incidence of prostate cancer.[55,56] The difference between green, oolong, and dark tea is the amount of fermentation that has occurred. Green tea appears to be most beneficial due to its rich source of polyphenols called *catechins* that have been found to have cancer-protecting properties. More human studies need to be performed on tea's role in prostate cancer, but animal research is encouraging, as green tea was found to inhibit the growth of prostate cancer cells and reduce the size of existing tumors in rodents.[57] Another rodent study using a population with an aggressive prostate cancer cell line were given a green tea extract oral liquid, equivalent to the human consumption of 6 cups of green tea a day. The group that received the extract resulted in almost complete inhibition of metastasis of the prostate cancer, and it stimulated significant apoptosis in the prostate cancer cells compared with those mice that were given plain water.[58] The effects of green tea appear to be dose dependent, and they also appear to be synergistic with soy protein, enhancing its effect.[59] Encouraging tea consumption in place of coffee would likely have a significant health benefit.

Pomegranate Juice

Like green tea, pomegranate is also rich in polyphenolic flavonoids. The phenol *punicalagin* is responsible for more than 50% of the juice's potent antioxidant activity. It appears that pomegranate juice has higher levels of punicalagin because the rind is used in its production. In fact, there is actually more antioxidant activity from the tannins in the juice than there is in the fruit itself.[60] A 2-year, single-center clinical trial was completed for 48 men with prostate cancer and a rising PSA level after either surgery or radiotherapy for the treatment of prostate cancer. Men in this study consumed 8 oz of pomegranate juice daily. Their mean PSA doubling time (a favorable result) significantly increased with pomegranate juice supplementation, from a mean of 14–26 months.[61]

There is currently less incentive for investigators to perform high-quality, expensive research on naturally occurring substances found in foods and their effects on disease due to the limited potential for economic gain compared with that possible in the pharmaceutical field. When research teaches us the health benefits of whole food nutrients, and we combine this with their low potential harm, clinicians can feel confident about making recommendations that honor the Hippocratic oath of "First do no harm."

Supplements

Nutritional supplements are compounds that include vitamins, antioxidants, and isolated nutrients that are thought to have positive health benefits. They differ from botanicals in that the latter consists of whole plants, whereas a supplement is often an isolated compound found in nature. Examples of supplements thought to potentially influence prostate cancer include selenium, tocopherols (e.g., vitamin E), zinc, and vitamin D.

Selenium

Selenium is a trace mineral ingested by consuming food that incorporates it into its structure from the soil in which it grows. In the United States, the Eastern Coastal Plains and the Pacific Northwest have the lowest soil selenium levels. Selenium is primarily found in grains, meats, and fish. Foods with the highest concentration include brewer's yeast, wheat germ, grains, garlic, sunflower seeds, Brazil nuts, and shellfish. Eating two Brazil nuts (the most neglected nut in the mixed nut bowl) a day provides the equivalent of 200 μg of selenium. A potent antioxidant, selenium regulates the activity of *glutathione peroxidase* enzymes, which convert hydrogen peroxide to water instead of toxic free oxygen (hydroxyl) radicals that hamper the immune system and stimulate prostate cancer cell growth.[62]

The popularity regarding selenium and its effects on prostate cancer arose from a double blind, placebo-controlled trial of selenium and skin cancer prevention. Although a protective effect of selenium was not seen for the development of skin cancer, taking 200 μg/day for 4.5 years resulted in a two-thirds reduced risk of prostate cancer compared with control subjects.[63] A follow-up study revealed that men with the highest serum levels of selenium had a 65% lower risk of prostate cancer.[64] When baseline serum selenium levels were measured in men enrolled in the Baltimore Longitudinal Study of

Aging, the men found to have the lowest levels 3.8 years before diagnosis were four to five times more likely to develop prostate cancer than men with higher levels.[65] Due to the potential positive health benefits, the country of Finland began fortifying agricultural fertilizers with selenium in 1984 in an attempt to increase soil levels. Although this practice increased dietary selenium intake two- to three-fold, the national incidence of prostate cancer did not significantly decrease during the first decade studied.[66]

Serum selenium levels significantly decrease as we age, and supplementation may be particularly beneficial in older men, yet there appears to be a therapeutic window. Selenium can be toxic if taken for prolonged periods at a dose greater than 400 μg/day. Signs and symptoms that suggest selenium toxicity include brittle hair and fingernails and a breath odor that resembles garlic.[67] Whether persons with nutritionally adequate selenium intake may benefit from selenium supplementation still remains to be proven. Three large studies are currently underway to help clarify the role of selenium in prostate health, namely Selenium and Vitamin E Cancer Prevention Trial (SELECT), Australian Prostate Cancer Prevention Trial Using Selenium, and the Progression of High Grade PIN [prostatic intraepithelial neoplasia] to Cancer (Southwest Oncology Group study 9916).[68]

Vitamin E

Vitamin E is the most common supplement used by men with prostate cancer.[69] Confidence regarding the use of this supplement has been shaken due to the potential increased risk of cardiovascular events with doses greater than 400 IU/day in men younger than 65 years of age.[70] The popularity of using vitamin E to prevent prostate cancer was derived from research showing that it decreased prostate cancer incidence and mortality in one particular study.[71] The exact mechanism of action for this trend is unknown, but it is theorized that vitamin E prevents prostate cancer by inhibiting the accumulation of toxic hydrogen peroxide and nitric oxide products within the prostate.[72] One study demonstrated that supplementing diet with as little as 50 IU of vitamin E daily reduced the incidence of prostate cancer by one third and the mortality rate by 40%.[71] Vitamin E appears to work synergistically with selenium; this was demonstrated in in vitro experiments where the two supplements together achieved greater cell growth inhibition than either alone.[73]

Mixed tocopherols (i.e., alpha-, beta-, and gamma-tocopherol) may confer additional protection than using alpha-tocopherol in isolation.[74] Unfortunately, the SELECT trial is only using alpha-tocopherol in its synthetic (*dL*-alpha tocopherol) form, which is not as well absorbed as the tocopherol in its natural state (*d*-alpha tocopherol). If vitamin E supplements are to be recommended, a mixed formulation of tocopherols should be encouraged, and they should be used in conjunction with selenium.

Vitamin D

There is a growing body of evidence regarding the beneficial relationship between vitamin D and prostate cancer. A few interesting observations include the fact that there are lower rates of prostate cancer in men who spend more time outdoors,[75] and a higher incidence exists among African American men, whose darker skin color may be associated with less vitamin D conversion in the skin.[76] An association between low vitamin D levels and an increased incidence of prostate cancer has also been determined.[77] In a Harvard study involving 1029 men with prostate cancer and more than 1300 healthy men, researchers analyzed the men's blood, looking for several factors including levels of vitamin D. They concluded that men with the highest levels of vitamin D had a significantly lower overall risk of prostate cancer (45%), including aggressive forms of prostate cancer.[78]

When evaluating serum vitamin D levels, a 25-hydroxy vitamin D level should be assayed, not a 1,25 dihydroxy vitamin D level. A normal value of the former molecule is greater than 16 ng/dL, but clinicians should consider supplementing if levels are below 30 ng/dL, not to exceed 100 ng/dL. A commonly used therapeutic goal is 50 ng/dL. The kidney normally produces more of this active hormone to compensate for low 25-hydroxy vitamin D stores in the liver. A normal or even high value of 1,25 dihydroxy vitamin D may give a false sense of security regarding adequacy. Replacement dosing for subtherapeutic values is 50,000 IU of vitamin D_2 (ergocalciferol; prescription strength) weekly for 8 weeks, then maintenance dosing twice monthly. Vitamin D_3 (cholecalciferol, over the counter) appears to be better absorbed than other forms.

Most white men require only 15 minutes of direct sunlight to produce enough vitamin D for 1 week, whereas darker-skinned men require up to 45 minutes. Men who live at more northern latitudes (e.g., Minnesota, Canada) may require vitamin D supplementation during the winter months since the sun is lower on the horizon and even ultraviolet exposure at midday may not be strong enough to convert vitamin D in the skin.

Zinc

The prostate gland has the highest levels of zinc of any human organ. This notion may be inherent to the natural antibacterial properties of zinc in the protection against ascending infection. It has been shown that there is an 80% reduction of prostatic zinc concentration in men with chronic prostatitis, as well as in those with prostate cancer.[79] Despite these variations, it is unknown whether this is a causative effect or a result of the disease. An in vitro study showed that zinc inhibits carcinoma cell growth by inducing cell cycle arrest and apoptosis.[80] Zinc inhibits 5-alpha reductase as well as the binding of androgens to their receptors in the prostate.[81,82] This latter effect is thought to occur due to zinc's ability to inhibit prolactin that, like estrogen, increases the receptors for dihydrotestosterone (DHT) in the prostate. Therefore, zinc not only decreases the production of DHT, but it also inhibits DHT binding to its receptors, which hypothetically may have a positive effect on prostate cancer. Unfortunately, oral zinc supplementation does not appear to influence tissue levels within the prostate gland,[83] although it has been shown to normalize seminal fluid zinc levels and reverse prostatitis-induced infertility.[84] Zinc supplementation should be used with caution since it interferes with the absorption of certain minerals, particularly copper, iron, and calcium.

Botanicals

In 2002, 10–19% of the US population used herbs to treat various health conditions, and the annual expenditures for herbs and dietary supplements exceeded $4 billion annually.[6] There are some challenges in prescribing herbs due to the limited FDA oversight. In 1994, the Dietary Supplements Health Education Act was passed, allowing products to be sold without the prior approval for efficacy and safety by the FDA. Manufacturers are permitted to claim that the product affects the structure or function of the body, as long as there is no claim of "effectiveness for the prevention or treatment of a specific disease." For example, a label for St. John's Wort can claim that it "has a positive effect on mood," but it cannot say that it "treats depression." The manufacturer is ultimately responsible for the quality, safety, and truthfulness of claims placed on the label of any botanical product and must have the evidence to support these claims. If there is a concern regarding safety of a botanical preparation, then the FDA is responsible for reviewing the product and evaluating its risk of harm. For example, the past removal of ephedra-containing products provides a good example of this trend.

The FDA is now proposing good manufacturing practices for herbal products, which set standards for strength and potency of the supplements to reflect what is actually stated on the product label. Facilities where botanicals and supplements are manufactured will need to meet certain standards for cleanliness, equipment maintenance, staff training, and record keeping of raw materials. This change will provide greater consumer confidence that the product reflects what is stated on the label.[85] A guide to effectively reading labels for botanical supplements can be found in Figure 22-4.

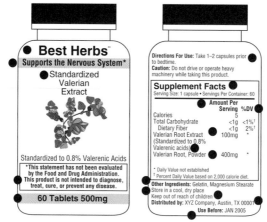

Figure 22-4. How to effectively read a label on a botanical product.

Items 1–6: Interpreting Product Labels

1. Brand name
2. Product/herb name
3. Herbal products and other "dietary supplements" may make "statements of nutritional support," often referred to as "structure/function claims," as long as they are truthful and not misleading, are documentable by scientific data, do not claim to diagnose, cure, treat, or prevent any disease, and carry a disclaimer on the product label to this effect. The disclaimer must also note that the FDA has not evaluated the claim. The product manufacturer must also notify the FDA of the structure/function claim within 30 days of bringing the product to market. According to current FDA regulations, examples of acceptable structure/function claims include "supports the immune system" and "supports a healthy heart," while claims such as "helps treat the common cold" and "helps prevent heart disease" are considered unacceptable, as these are considered drug claims. Thus, "helps maintain urinary tract health" is acceptable while "helps prevent urinary tract infections" is not.
4. A structure/function claim requires this disclaimer when it appears on the label of a dietary supplement, as well as in any brochures or advertising. The disclaimer must be in bold type and in a box.
5. Number of tablets or capsules, and net weight of each in package
6. Directions for use and cautions

Items 7–10: Supplement Facts Panel

7. "Serving Size" is the suggested number of tablets, capsules, softgels, tea bags, liquid extract, or tincture to take at one time.
8. "Amount per Serving" first indicates the nutrients present in the herb and then specifies the quantity. The following items must be declared if in excess of what can legally be declared as zero: calories, fat, carbohydrates, sodium, and protein. In addition, the following nutrients must also be declared if present in quantities exceeding what can legally be declared as zero: vitamins A, C, D, E, K, B_1, B_2, B_3, B_6, B_{12}, folic acid, biotin, calcium, iron, phosphorus, iodine, magnesium, zinc, selenium, copper, manganese, chromium, molybdenum, chloride, and potassium. Most herbal products contain negligible amounts of these nutrients.
9. "Percent Daily Value" (%DV) indicates the percentage of daily intake provided by the herb. An asterisk under the "Percent Daily Value" heading indicates that a Daily Value is not established for that dietary ingredient.
10. Herbs should be designated by their standardized common names as listed in the book *Herbs of Commerce*, published in 1992 by the American Herbal Products Association. If the common name is not listed in *Herbs of*

Commerce, then the common name must be followed by the herb's Latin name. The plant part must be listed for each herb. The amount in milligrams of each herb must be listed unless the herbs are grouped as a proprietary blend, then only the total amount of the blend need be listed. For herbal extracts, the following information must be disclosed:

A. The ratio of the weight of the starting material to the volume of the solvent (even for dried extracts where the solvent has been removed, the solvent used to extract the herb must be listed)

B. Whether the starting material is fresh or dry

C. The concentration of the botanical in the solvent

11. Standardization: If a product is chemically standardized, then the product label may list the component used to measure standardization (e.g., ginsenosides in Asian ginseng, valerenic acids in valerian, etc.) and the level to which the product is standardized (e.g., 4% ginsenosides). Therefore, if a product contained 100 mg of Asian ginseng extract per capsule and the extract was standardized to 4% ginsenosides, one capsule would contain 4 mg of ginsenosides. In most but not all cases, the component used to measure standardization is bioactive, although the standardization component may not be responsible for the intended primary activity of the herbal supplement, other active compounds may be responsible. Products can also be standardized to "marker compounds" for purposes of quality control. Those markers may or may not be active.

12. A list of all other ingredients, in decreasing order by weight, must appear outside the Supplement Facts box. In herb formulas containing multiple herbal ingredients, the herbs must be listed in descending order of predominance.

13. The proper location for storage of herbal products is typically labeled as "a cool, dry place."

14. All herbal products and other dietary supplements should be kept out of the reach of children.

15. The herb should be used before the expiration date for maximum potency and effectiveness. Expiration dates are often arbitrarily established by the manufacturer, regardless of the ingredients and their relative stability. Such dates are routinely set at 2 years from the date of manufacture of the finished dietary supplement, although this period may be longer or shorter depending on the manufacturer's policies, stability testing, dosage form, and other variables.

16. The product must list the manufacturer or distributor's name, city, state, and zip code.Go to http://www.herbalgram.org for more information on the American Botanical Council's additional resources and continuing medical education for healthcare providers.

Adapted with permission from: Interpreting product labels. In *Blumenthal M, Brickmann J, Wellschlaeger B (eds): The ABC Clinical Guide to Herbs*, 2003, American Botanical Council, New York, 2003, Thieme, pp xxiv; and Gardiner P, Lowdog T: Prescribing botanicals. In Rakel DP, editor: *Integrative Medicine*, ed 2, Philadelphia, 2007, Saunders, pp. 1110–1111.

Plant Sterols

Many of the botanical products that have been found to be beneficial for the treatment of BPH contain plant sterols at high doses. Botanicals such as saw palmetto, soy products, pygeum bark, stinging nettle root, and pumpkin seed extract are rich in plant sterols. Sterols are the plant equivalent of cholesterol. Beta-sitosterol is the most common sterol and can often be found in supplement form over the counter. The exact mechanism of its action is unknown, but it is believed to work through inhibition of cholesterol and hormonal influences that trigger inflammation. Sterols block the absorption of cholesterol from the intestinal tract and are the active ingredient in cholesterol-lowering margarine such as Take Control (beta-sitosterol) and Benecol (sitostanol). Sterols may also have benefit because they cannot be converted to testosterone in the body. A Cochrane review examined the benefit of beta-sitosterol on BPH and found it to improve urinary symptoms and urinary flow measures. As with the case of saw palmetto, beta-sitosterol did not reduce the size of the prostate, and its effect on prostate cancer has not been established.[86] The recommended dose of beta-sitosterol is 20–30 mg three times a day, and it should not be taken with fatty foods since the two inhibit absorption of each other. As with any supplement, it is always best to obtain these recommended nutrients through whole food nutrition. Eating virtually any vegetable or plant is going to provide adequate levels of plant sterols to help reduce cholesterol as well as inflammation of the prostate.

PC-SPES

Since both BPH and prostate cancer have a common hormonal influence, it would make sense that herbal products that have been found useful in treating BPH may also have benefit in treating prostate cancer. For instance, saw palmetto has been found to induce cell death and apoptosis of prostate cancer cells in vitro.[87] PC-SPES is a combination of botanical products that has been used for the treatment of prostate cancer and includes eight different herbs: *Isatis indigotica* (da qing ye), *Glycyrrhiza glabra* and *Glycyrrhiza uralensis* (gan cao), *Panax pseudoginseng* (san qi), *Ganoderma lucidum* (ling zhi, reishi), *Scutellaria baicalensis* (huang qin), *Dendranthema* (*Chrysanthemum*) *morifolium*, *Rabdosia rubescens*, and *Serenoa repens* (saw palmetto).[88] The name *PC-SPES* is derived from *p*rostate *c*ancer and the Latin word *spes*, which means "hope." Its formula was developed in 1990 by a chemist named Dr. Sophie Chen, who tailored it on the basis of an herbal recipe that was handed down from court physicians to the emperor of China. It is theorized that, by working synergistically, the herbs within PC-SPES inhibit angiogenesis and cell proliferation, down-regulate androgen receptors, stimulate the immune system, induce apoptosis, and inhibit 5-alpha reductase.[89,90] Original trials using PC-SPES were promising, showing a reduction of PSA values from an average of 7.9 ng/mL to undetectable levels in 81.3% of men after taking the supplement for a mean of 23 weeks. No patients in this study showed progression of prostate cancer up to 74 weeks after treatment commenced.[91] Unfortunately, the supplement also resulted in hormone-related adverse effects including nausea, impotence, breast tenderness, fluid retention, skin rash, blood clots, and pulmonary embolus. Due to pharmaceutical contamination, it has since been taken off the market in the United States.

Conclusion

Integrative medicine recognizes all of the potential influences on one's health. It is the study of the human ecology that includes the physical and nonphysical factors of how humans interact with their environment. Care is applied through relationships that provide insight into each individual's unique situation and needs. Evidence and research will continue to help us understand which therapies (e.g., pharmaceuticals, botanicals, acupuncture, meditation) will help the body heal. For patients with prostate cancer, this treatment involves much more than a surgical and pharmaceutical intervention. Our partnership with our male patients will help empower them to seek an understanding of how they can be active participants in their care, resulting in a more successful treatment outcome and quality of life for all involved.

References

1. Rakel DP, Weil A: Philosophy of integrative medicine. In Rakel DP editor, *Integrative Medicine*, ed 2, Philadelphia, 2007, Saunders, pp 1–13.
2. Eisenberg DM, Kessler RC, Foster C, et al: Unconventional medicine in the United States: prevalence, costs and patterns of use, *N Engl J Med* 328(4): 246–252, 1993.
3. Eisenberg DM, Davis RB, Ettner SL, et al: Trends in alternative medicine use in the United States, 1990–1997: results of a follow-up national survey, *JAMA* 280(18):1569–1575, 1998.
4. Lazarou J, Pomeranz BH, Corey PN: Incidence of adverse drug reactions in hospitalized patients, *JAMA* 279(15):1200–1205, 1998.
5. Astin JA: Why patients use alternative medicine: results of a national study, *JAMA* 279(19): 1548–1553, 1998.
6. Barnes PM, Powell-Griner E, McFann K, et al: Complementary and alternative medicine use among adults: United States, 2002, *Adv Data Vital Health Stat* 343:1–20, 2004.
7. Brevoort P: The United States botanical market—an overview, *Herbal Gram* 36:49–57, 1996.
8. National Center for Health Statistics: Trends in the health of Americans Hyattsville, MD 2004. Available at: http://www.cdc.gov/nchs. Accessed June 9, 2006.
9. Brier A, Albus M, Pickar D, et al: Controllable and uncontrollable stress in humans: alterations in mood and neuroendocrine and psychophysiological function, *Am J Psychiatry* 144(11):1419–1425, 1987.
10. Langer EJ: *The Psychology of Control,* Beverly Hills, CA, 1983, Sage.
11. Shrock D, Palmer RF, Taylor B: Effects of a psychosocial intervention on survival among patients with stage 1 breast and prostate cancer: a matched case-control study, *Altern Ther Health Med* 5:49–55, 1999.
12. Saxe GA, Hebert JR, Carmody JF, et al: Can diet in conjunction with stress reduction affect the rate of increase in prostate specific antigen after biochemical recurrence of prostate cancer? *J Urol* 166 (6): 2202–2207, 2001.
13. Schacht MJ, Saxe GA, Bauer-Wu S, et al: Integrative Tumor Board: recently diagnosed prostate cancer, *Integr Cancer Ther* 2(1):63–90, 2003.
14. Grossman P, Neimann L, Schmidt S, et al: Mindfullness-based stress reduction and health benefits: a meta-analysis, *J Psychosom Res* 57(1):35–43, 2004.
15. Smith JE, Richardson J, Hoffman C, et al: Mindfulness-based stress reduction as supportive therapy in cancer care: systematic review, *J Adv Nurs* 53(5): 618, 2006.
16. Puchalski CM: Taking a spiritual history: FICA, *Spirituality Med Connect* 3:1, 1999.
17. Anandarajah G, Hight E: Spirituality and medical practice: using the HOPE questions as a practical tool for spiritual assessment, *Am Fam Phys* 63: 81–88, 2001.
18. Maugans TA: The SPIRITual history, *Arch Fam Med* 5:11–16, 1996.
19. Veierod MB, Laake P, Thelle DS: Dietary fat intake and risk of prostate cancer: a prospective study of 25,708 Norwegian men, *Int J Cancer* 73(5):634–638, 1997.
20. Giovannucci E, Rimm EB, Colditz GA, et al: A prospective study of dietary fat and risk of prostate cancer, *J Natl Cancer Inst* 85(19):1571–1579, 1993.

21. Reiter RE, deKernion JB: Epidemiology, etiology, and prevention of prostate cancer. In Walsh PC, Retik AB, Vaughan ED, Jr, et al, editors: *Campbell's Urology*, ed 8, Philadelphia, 2002, Saunders, pp 3003–3024.

22. Muir CS, Nextoux J, Staszewski J: The epidemiology of prostate cancer: geographical distribution and time-trends, *Acta Oncol* 30(2):133–140, 1991.

23. Kolonel LN, Nomura MY, Cooney RV: Dietary fat and prostate cancer: current status, *J Natl Cancer Inst* 91(5):414–428, 1999.

24. Hayes RB, Ziegler RG, Gridley G, et al: Dietary factors and risks for prostate cancer among blacks and whites in the United States, *Cancer Epidemiol Biomarkers Prev* 8(1):25–34, 1999.

25. Myers CE, Steck SS, Myers RS: *Eating Your Way to Better Health: The Prostate Forum Nutrition Guide*, Charlottesville, VA, 2000, Rivanna Health Publications, pp 15–16.

26. Ghosh J, Myers CE: Arachidonic acid metabolism and cancer of the prostate, *Nutrition* 14(1):48–49, 1998.

27. Myers CE: Differentiating agents and nontoxic therapies, *Urol Clin North Am* 26(2):341–351, 1999.

28. Padayatty SJ, Marcelli M, Shao TC, et al: Lovastatin-induced apoptosis in prostate stromal cells, *J Clin Endocrinol Metab* 82(5):1434–1439, 1997.

29. Chan JM, Stampfer MJ, Ma J, et al: Dairy products, calcium and prostate cancer risk in the Physician's Health Study, *Am J Clin Nutr* 74:549–554, 2001.

30. Baron JA, Beach M, Wallace K, et al: Risk of prostate cancer in a randomized clinical trial of calcium supplementation, *Cancer Epidemiol Biomarkers Prev* 14(3):586–589, 2005.

31. Cohen P, Peehl DM, Lamsom G, et al: Insulin-like growth factors (IGFs), IGF receptors, and IGF-binding proteins in primary cultures of prostate epithelial cells, *J Clin Endocrinol Metab* 73(2):401–407, 1991.

32. LeRoith D, Werner H, Neuenschwander S, et al: The role of the insulin-like growth factor-I receptor in cancer, *Ann N Y Acad Sci* 766:402–408, 1995.

33. Chan JM, Stampfer MJ, Giovannucci E, et al: Plasma insulin-like growth factor-I and prostate cancer risk: a prospective study, *Science* 279(5350):563–566, 1998.

34. Epstein SS: Unlabeled milk from cows treated with biosynthetic growth hormones: a case of regulatory abdication, *Int J Health Serv* 26(1):173–185, 1996.

35. Epstein SS: Potential public health hazards of biosynthetic milk hormones, *Int J Health Serv* 20(1):73–84, 1990.

36. Mepham TB, Schofield PN, Zumkeller W, et al: Safety of milk from cows treated with bovine somatotrophin, *Lancet* 344(8916):197–198, 1994.

37. Daughaday WH, Barbano DM: Bovine somatotropin supplementation of dairy cows—is the milk safe? *JAMA* 264(8):1003–1005, 1990.

38. Juskevich JC, Guyer CG: Bovine growth hormone: human food safety evaluation, *Science* 249:875–884, 1990.

39. Laukkanen JA, Laaksonen DE, Niskanen L, et al: Metabolic syndrome and the risk of prostate cancer in Finnish men: a population-based study, *Cancer Epidemiol Biomarkers Prev* 13(10):1646–1650, 2004.

40. Adlercreutz H, Markkanen H, Watanabe S: Plasma concentration of phytoestrogens in Japanese men, *Lancet* 342:1209–1210, 1993.

41. Fair WR, Fleshner NE, Heston W: Cancer of the prostate: a nutritional disease? *Urology* 50(6):840–846, 1997.

42. Gruber CJ, Tschugguel W, Schneeberger C, et al: Production and actions of estrogens, *N Engl J Med* 346(5):340–352, 2002.

43. Castle EP, Thrasher JB: The role of soy phytoestrogens in prostate cancer, *Urol Clin North Am* 29(1):71–81, 2002.

44. Jacobsen BK, Knutsen SF, Fraser GE: Does high soy milk intake reduce prostate cancer incidence? the Adventist Health Study (United States), *Cancer Causes Control* 9(6):541–543, 1998.

45. Hussain M, Banerjee M, Sarkar FH, et al: Soy isoflavones in the treatment of prostate cancer, *Nutr Cancer* 47(2):111–117, 2003.

46. Miller EC, Giovannucci E, Erdman JW, et al: Tomato products, lycopene, and prostate cancer risk, *Urol Clin North Am* 29(1):83–93, 2002.

47. Ansari MS, Gupta NP: Lycopene: a novel drug therapy in hormone refractory metastatic prostate cancer, *Urol Oncol* 22(5):415–420, 2004.

48. Hwang E-S, Bowen PE: Can the consumption of tomatoes or lycopene reduce cancer risk? *Integr Cancer Ther* 1(2):121–132, 2002.

49. Giovannucci E, Ascherio A, Rimm EB, et al: Intake of carotenoids and retinol in relation to risk of prostate cancer, *J Natl Cancer Inst* 87(23):1767–1776, 1995.

50. Rao AV, Fleshner N, Agarwal S: Serum and tissue lycopene and biomarkers of oxidation in prostate cancer patients: a case-control study, *Nutr Cancer* 33(2):159–164, 1999.

51. Chen L, Stacewicz-Sapuntzakis M, Duncan C, et al: Oxidative DNA damage in prostate cancer patients consuming tomato sauce–based entrees as a whole-food intervention, *J Natl Cancer Inst* 93(24):1872–1879, 2001.

52. Fahey JW, Talalay P: The role of crucifers in cancer chemoprotection. In Gustine DL, Flores HE, editors: *Phytochemicals and Health*, Rockville, MD, 1995, American Society of Plant Physiologists, p 88.

53. Heber D, Fair WR, Ornish D: *Nutrition and Cancer Prostate: A Monograph from the CaP CURE Nutrition Project*, ed 2, Santa Monica, CA, 1998. The Association for the Cure of Prostate Cancer, p 11.

54. Gupta S, Mukhtar H: Green tea and prostate cancer, *Urol Clin North Am* 29:49–57, 2002.

55. Heilbrum LK, Nomura A, Stemmerman GN: Black tea consumption and cancer risk: a prospective study, *Br J Cancer* 54:677–683, 1986.

56. Jian L, Xie LP, Lee AH, et al: Protective effect of green tea against prostate cancer: a case-controlled study in southeast China, *Int J Cancer* 108(1):130–135, 2004.

57. Liao S, Umekita Y, Guo J, et al: Growth inhibition and regression of human prostate and breast

tumors in athymic mice by tea epigallocatechin gallate, *Cancer Lett* 96(2):239–243, 1995.

58. Gupta S, Hastak K, Ahmad N, et al: Inhibition of prostate carcinogenesis in TRAMP mice by oral infusion of green tea polyphenols, *Proc Natl Acad Sci USA* 98(18):10350–10355, 2001.

59. Zhou JR, Yu L, Zhong Y, et al: Soy phytochemicals and tea bioactive components synergistically inhibit androgen-sensitive human prostate tumors in mice, *J Nutr* 133(2):516–521, 2003.

60. Gil MI, Tomas-Barberan FA, Hess-Pierce B, et al: Antioxidant activity of pomegranate juice and its relationship with phenolic composition and processing, *J Agric Food Chem* 48(10):4581–4589, 2000.

61. Pantuck AJ, Leppert JT, Zomorodian N, et al: Phase II study of pomegranate juice for men with rising PSA following surgery or radiation for prostate cancer, *J Urol* 173(Suppl 4):225–226, 2005, Abstract 831.

62. Baker AM, Oberley LW, Cohen MB: Expression of antioxidant enzymes in human prostatic adenocarcinoma, *Prostate* 32(4):229–233, 1997.

63. Clark LC, Combs GF Jr, Turnbull BW, et al: Effects of selenium supplementation for cancer prevention in patients with carcinoma of the skin: a randomized controlled trial. Nutritional Prevention of Cancer Study Group, *JAMA* 276(24):1957–1963, 1996.

64. Yoshizawa K, Willett WZ, Morris SJ, et al: Study of the pre-diagnostic selenium levels in toenails and the risk of advanced prostate cancer, *J Natl Cancer Inst* 90(16):1219–1224, 1998.

65. Brooks JD, Metter EJ, Chan D, et al: Plasma selenium level before diagnosis and the risk of prostate cancer development, *J Urol* 166(6):2034–2038, 2001.

66. Aro A, Alfthan G, Varo P: Effects of supplementation of fertilizers on human selenium status in Finland, *Analyst* 120(3):841–843, 1995.

67. Institute of Medicine, National Academy of Sciences, Food and Nutrition Board, Panel on Dietary Antioxidants and Related Compounds: *Dietary Reference Intakes for Vitamin C, Vitamin E, Selenium, and Carotenoids*, Washington, DC, 2000, National Academy Press.

68. Klein EA: Selenium: epidemiology and basic science, *J Urol* 171(2 Pt 2):S50–S53, 2004.

69. Woo WW, Quinn M, Figg W: The use of complementary and alternative medicine in prostate cancer patients, *Oncol Issues* 15(6):23–27, 2000.

70. Miller ER 3rd, Pastor-Barriuso R, Dalal D, et al: Meta-analysis: high-dosage vitamin E supplementation may increase all-cause mortality, *Ann Intern Med* 142(1):37–46, 2005.

71. Heinonen OP, Albanes D, Virtamo J, et al: Prostate cancer and supplementation with alpha-tocopherol and beta-carotene: incidence and mortality in a controlled trial, *J Natl Cancer Inst* 90(6):440–446, 1998.

72. Myers CE: *Prostate Forum Newsletter* 3(6):3–4, 1998.

73. Zu K, Ip C: Synergy between selenium and vitamin E in apoptosis induction is associated with activation of distinctive initiator caspases in human prostate cancer cells, *Cancer Res* 63(20):6988–6995, 2003.

74. Helzlsouer KJ, Huang HY, Alberg AJ, et al: Association between alpha-tocopherol, gamma-tocopherol, selenium and subsequent prostate cancer, *J Natl Cancer Inst* 92(24):2018–2023, 2000.

75. John EM, Schwartz GG, Koo J, et al: Sun exposure, vitamin D receptor gene polymorphisms, and risk of advanced prostate cancer, *Cancer Res* 65(12):5470–5479, 2005.

76. Luscombe CJ, French ME, Liu S, et al: Outcome in prostate cancer associations with skin type and polymorphism in pigmentation-related genes, *Carcinogenesis* 22(9):1343–1347, 2001.

77. Kibel AS, Isaacs SD, Isaacs WB, et al: Vitamin D receptor polymorphisms and lethal prostate cancer, *J Urol* 160(4):1405–1409, 1998.

78. Brigham and Women's Hospital and Harvard University School of Public Health: News release Orlando, Florida, February 17–19, 2005, Multidisciplinary Prostate Cancer Symposium, cosponsored by the American Society of Clinical Oncology, the Prostate Cancer Foundation, the American Society for Therapeutic Radiology and Oncology, and the Society of Urologic Oncology.

79. Partin AW, Rodriguez R: The molecular biology, endocrinology and physiology of the prostate and seminal vesicles. In Walsh PC, Retik AB, Vaughan ED Jr, et al, editors: *Campbell's Urology*, ed 8, Philadelphia, 2002, Saunders, p 1279.

80. Liang JY, Liu YY, Zou J, et al: Inhibitory effect of zinc on human prostatic carcinoma cell growth, *Prostate* 40(3):200–207, 1999.

81. Leake A, Chisholm GD, Habib FK: The effect of zinc on the 5-α-reduction of testosterone by the hyperplastic human prostate gland, *J Steroid Biochem* 20:651–655, 1984.

82. Leake A, Chisholm GD, Busuttil A, et al: Subcellular distribution of zinc in the benign and malignant human prostate: evidence for a direct zinc androgen interaction, *Acta Endocrinol* 105:281–288, 1984.

83. Fair WR, Couch J, Wehner N: Prostatic antibacterial factor: identity and significance, *Urology* 7(2):168–177, 1976.

84. Marmar Jl, Katz S, Praiss DE, et al: Semen zinc levels in infertile and postvasectomy patients and patients with prostatitis, *Fert Steril* 26(11):1057–1063, 1975.

85. Federal Register: Dietary Supplements; Current Good Manufacturing Practice Regulations; Public Meetings. Available at: http://ww.cfsan.fda.gov/~lrd/fr030328.html. Accessed June 9, 2006.

86. Wilt T, Ishani A, MacDonald R, et al: Beta-sitosterols for benign prostatic hyperplasia, *Cochrane Database Syst Rev* 2:CD001043, 2000.

87. Iguchi K, Okumura N, Usui S, et al: Myristoleic acid, a cytotoxic component in the extract from *Serona repens*, induces apoptosis and necrosis in human prostatic LNCaP cells, *Prostate* 47(1):59–65, 2001.

88. Lewis J: *The Herbal Remedy for Prostate Cancer*, Westbury, NY, 1999, Health Education Literary Publisher, pp 34–37.

89. Halicka HD, Ardelt B, Juan G, et al: Apoptosis and cell cycle effects induced by extracts of the Chinese herbal preparation PC SPES, *Int J Oncol* 11:437–448, 1997.

90. Chen S: In vitro mechanism of PC SPES, *Urology* 58(2 Suppl 1):S28–S35, discussion S38, 2001.

91. Small EJ, Frohlich MW, Bok R, et al: Prospective trial of the herbal supplement PC-SPES in patients with progressive prostate cancer, *J Clin Oncol* 18(2):3595–3603, 2000.

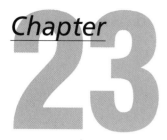

Cosmetic Plastic Surgery

*Douglas Sammer, MD, PhD, M. Haskell Newman, MD, and
William M. Kuzon, Jr, MD*

Key Points

- Males are opting for cosmetic surgery in increasing numbers, with the 1.2 million procedures performed on male patients in 2005 representing a 44% increase compared with data from 2000 (strength of recommendation: C).
- The available literature demonstrates a higher rate of personality disorders in patients undergoing aesthetic surgery than in the general population, including an increased baseline incidence of anxiety disorders, neuroticism, depression, and dysmorphic disorders (strength of recommendation: B); males presenting for aesthetic surgery may have a higher incidence of these diagnoses than in female patients (strength of recommendation: C).
- Because of the highly personal nature of cosmetic surgery, there is no 1:1 relationship between a physical finding and a surgical procedure, and there is no "ideal" result for any given operation (strength of recommendation: C).
- There is no evidence that autoimmune or other systemic diseases result from the use of silicone prostheses (strength of recommendation: C).

Introduction

The official definition of *cosmetic surgery*, as stated by the American Society of Plastic Surgeons (ASPS) and the American Medical Association,[1] is a surgical procedure "performed to reshape *normal* structures of the body in order to improve the patient's appearance and self-esteem." The most comprehensive source for demographic and statistical data on cosmetic surgery is the American Society of Plastic Surgeons.[2] These data are compiled for ASPS members only, but they clearly indicate that cosmetic surgery has become a growth industry in the United States; the number of cosmetic surgical procedures performed annually has grown dramatically in the past 10 years. In 2005, an estimated 10.2 million cosmetic procedures were performed in the United States alone, which is an 11% increase over 2004. The target market is no longer only the "rich and famous," but all socioeconomic groups. In addition, males are opting for cosmetic surgery in increasing numbers; 1.2 million procedures were performed on male patients in 2005, representing a 44% increase compared with 2000. Table 23-1 summarizes statistical data on the prevalence of cosmetic surgery in the United States.

The news and entertainment media have sensationalized cosmetic surgery, often providing misleading or incorrect information. Our goals in this chapter are to provide accurate and practical information for primary care and other referring physicians to assist patients considering cosmetic surgery and to give a brief overview of the most common aesthetic surgery procedures for men. Although this book focuses exclusively on male patients, the major considerations for a prospective aesthetic surgery patient are the same for men and women. Preeminent among these considerations are the choice of a cosmetic surgeon and what comprises a good candidate for cosmetic surgery.

Table 23-1. Top Cosmetic Surgical Procedures for Males in 2005

Surgical Procedure	Number
Nose reshaping	99,680
Hair transplantation	39,244
Liposuction	35,673
Eyelid surgery	32,988
Breast reduction	16,275
Minimally Invasive Procedure	
Botox injections	313,519
Microdermabrasion	201,051
Laser hair removal	173,387
Chemical peels	108,998
Laser skin resurfacing	37,998

Adapted from: American Society of Plastic Surgeons: Procedural statistics. 2006.

Choosing a Cosmetic Surgeon

Plastic surgeons were the first to develop and use the majority of cosmetic surgical procedures performed today, yet it is important for a prospective cosmetic surgery patient to know that the terms *plastic surgery* and *cosmetic surgery* are not synonymous. Plastic surgery is a broad surgical specialty that treats a wide range of congenital and acquired deformities, and plastic surgeons are broadly trained in both reconstructive and aesthetic surgery of all parts of the body. An increasing trend is for non–plastic surgeons to perform cosmetic surgical procedures. How can a prospective patient choose an aesthetic surgeon who is both well trained and competent?

Although there is considerable controversy over who is "qualified" to perform aesthetic surgical procedures, with some acrimony between specialties, we believe that the best advice in this regard is to rely on the American Board of Medical Specialties (ABMS) as the organization with the highest standards for the certification of medical specialists in the United States. In our opinion, patients should look for a specialist who holds certification in their specialty from an ABMS member board *and* who has specific training for the procedures that are being contemplated. For example, an otolaryngologist has specific training in rhinoplasty and facial aesthetic procedures but not in body contouring or breast surgery. An oculoplastic surgeon has training in blepharoplasty but not in rhinoplasty. For plastic surgeons, the signature of their broad training in *all* areas of aesthetic surgery is membership in the ASPS, which has as a membership requirement certification by the American Board of Plastic Surgery, an ABMS board. Although a surgeon who has credentials from a non-ABMS board may be good a cosmetic surgeon, there is no way for a prospective patient to be assured of rigorous and uniform training if a given specialist is not certified by an ABMS board.

The Cosmetic Surgery Patient

By definition, because cosmetic surgical procedures are elective and are not deemed "medically necessary," there are a number of considerations that come into play that do not apply for other types of surgical treatments. Several of these considerations are quite obvious: (1) almost all health insurance carriers do not cover cosmetic surgical services; (2) the patient is exposed to the risk of surgical complications for the sake of their appearance only; and (3) patients must be in good health to be considered candidates for aesthetic surgery, given that various medical conditions that impair wound healing or tissue circulation will disqualify patients from these elective procedures. In terms of outcomes, the measurement of the results of cosmetic surgery is imprecise and highly individual. The critically important determinant of the success of aesthetic surgery is for the patient to have appropriate expectations.

The optimal candidate for cosmetic surgery is a healthy patient who simply wants to look better, who has realistic expectations about what can be accomplished, and who understands that surgical procedures have inherent risks. It is most important to recognize that surgical complications, however uncommon they may be for a given procedure, can occur and can result in morbidity, increased expense, and suboptimal results. The same principal applies to expectations regarding surgical outcomes. The changes resulting from many aesthetic procedures are subtle, and the procedures have limitations that must be accepted. Because the issue of patient expectation is more critical than for other types of medical treatment, many, if not most, aesthetic surgeons will require two or sometimes more preoperative consultations to provide education and to ensure that the patient has a reasonable understanding of realistic expectations. In aesthetic surgery, the desired outcomes are patient satisfaction, an improved appearance, and the attendant improvement in self-confidence and self-esteem. As such, a majority of poor outcomes in aesthetic surgery do not stem from complications or from what the surgeon might consider a suboptimal result, but from a failure to meet patient expectations.

The Aesthetic Surgery Consultation

The preoperative consultation for cosmetic surgery is unlike most other doctor-patient interactions. Rather than trying to make a medical diagnosis and to effect treatment, the goals are to determine what the patient desires, to judge his or her suitability as a candidate for aesthetic surgery, and to provide education about risks and realistic outcomes. The "diagnosis" is often complex and is a combination of a physical evaluation of anatomy and an assessment of the patient's motivations, personality, and psychology. Although it was once believed that the majority of cosmetic surgery candidates manifested personality or psychiatric disorders, more recent data indicate that the majority of patients undergoing cosmetic surgery are free of such issues.[3] Nevertheless, the available literature demonstrates a higher rate of personality disorders in patients undergoing aesthetic surgery than in the general population, including an increased baseline incidence of anxiety disorders, neurosis, depression, and body dysmorphic disorders; males presenting for aesthetic surgery may have a higher incidence of these diagnoses than that seen in female cosmetic surgery patients.[4,5] Body dysmorphic disorder is a well-publicized, and fortunately rare condition in which attempts to improve appearance through surgery become a pathological obsession.[6] Personality and psychiatric factors are primary reasons that a given patient may not be considered as optimal candidates for aesthetic surgery.

Once a patient is deemed a suitable candidate for a given plastic surgery procedure, the preoperative consultation focuses on planning the procedure and reducing complications. Preoperative photographs are routine for all aesthetic procedures. Most aesthetic surgeons will decline to perform facelifts, abdominoplasties, and other procedures where tissue blood supply may be compromised if the patient is a current smoker. Use of medications, including herbal preparations, many of which reduce platelet function or impair clotting, must be discontinued.[7] For some procedures, pretreatments may be prescribed before an aesthetic procedure; an example would be the use of isotretinoin (Retin-A) for patients undergoing facial rejuvenation procedures.[8]

Many cosmetic treatments are staged, and "touch-up" operations are very common after gynecomastia procedures, liposuction, and body-contouring operations. Patients must be prepared to accept the potential for multiple interventions to obtain optimal results.

A necessary part of the aesthetic surgery consultation involves a discussion of the costs of surgery, including whether the management of complications or "touch-up" procedures would incur additional cost. Most aesthetic surgeons require cash in advance before performing any procedure; many have financing available through their offices or through a multitude of companies that specialize in loans for cosmetic surgery. National data on the average cost of the most commonly performed aesthetic procedures in men is summarized in Table 23-2.

Clearly, the aesthetic surgery consultation involves a significant level of complexity and subtlety that has a major effect on subsequent outcome. Managing this interaction is, even more than technically virtuosity, what distinguishes a successful aesthetic surgeon.

Common Cosmetic Surgery Procedures

In the paragraphs that follow, a brief description of the most commonly performed aesthetic surgical procedures in men is presented. The goal of these summaries is to give the non–plastic surgeon a basic understanding of these procedures to provide accurate and appropriate advice to their patients (and friends and relatives!). For each procedure the general indications, basic evaluation, general nature of the procedure, and possible complications are discussed. For some procedures, examples of results that could be considered "average" are presented. Because of the highly personal nature of cosmetic surgery, there is no 1:1 relationship between a physical finding and a surgical procedure, and there is no "ideal" result for any given operation.

Body Contouring

Gynecomastia Correction

Gynecomastia, or male breast enlargement, is a common condition resulting from a relative hyperestrinism, which can be due to multiple factors including liver disease, aging (with increased adrenal estrogen production), drugs (especially alcohol, antiviral agents, marijuana, steroids, and anabolic agents), genetic conditions such as

Table 23-2. Cosmetic Surgery Procedural Statistics

Procedure	Number of Procedures 2004	Number of Procedures 2005	% Change 2004 vs. 2005	National Average Surgeon's Fee*
Breast reduction in men (for gynecomastia)	13,963	16,275	17%	$2981
Calf augmentation	N/A	337	—	$2221
Ear surgery/otoplasty	25,915	27,993	8%	$2437
Eyelid surgery/ blepharoplasty	233,334	230,697	−1%	$2534
Facelift/rhytidectomy	114,279	108,955	−5%	$4484
Forehead lift	54,993	55,518	1%	$2420
Hair transportation	48,925	47,462	−3%	$4755
Liposuction	324,891	323,605	0%	$2323
Nose reshaping/ rhinoplasty	305,475	298,413	−2%	$3511
Pectoral implants	N/A	206	—	$3642
Thigh lift	8123	9533	17%	$4181
Upper arm lift	9955	11,873	19%	$3261

*Surgeon's fee does not include anesthesia and facility charges.
Adapted from: American Society of Plastic Surgeons: Procedural statistics. 2006.

Klinefelter syndrome, and testicular neoplasms. Preoperative evaluation for the patient with gynecomastia should include a thorough history and physical examination and, if indicated, a referral to an endocrinologist or other specialist for proper medical evaluation. Obviously, any underlying treatable causes of gynecomastia should be managed appropriately, and only after all other possible causes have been excluded should the most common diagnosis of idiopathic gynecomastia be assigned.

The choice of a surgical procedure for gynecomastia will depend on the patient's age, the degree of excess breast parenchyma, the amount of excess skin, and the size of the nipple/areolar complex. In young patients with good skin tone, a small amount of breast parenchyma, and normal areolae, liposuction can often achieve a very reasonable correction with an acceptable male chest profile (Figure 23-1). For patients with moderate degrees of excess skin and parenchyma and moderate areolar enlargement, a combination of liposuction with a circumareolar skin excision and direct parenchymal excision works well. This leaves a scar at the periphery of the areola only, and the surgeon has reasonable control over the resection of the parenchyma. For patients with significant breast enlargement, especially older patients with poor skin tone, a circumareolar approach is inadequate to allow the degree of

parenchymal resection, and areolar reduction is necessary to provide an adequate correction. For these patients, a formal skin excision must be combined with areolar reduction and repositioning. There are many variations of this procedure (Figure 23-2).

In addition to complications that are generic for any surgical procedure (e.g., infection, skin loss, scars), the feared complication of a gynecomastia excision is over-resection, creating a "saucer" chest.[9] This deformity is difficult, if not impossible, to correct. For this reason, the prudent surgeon will be conservative at the time of a primary gynecomastia excision, and touch-up procedures are exceedingly common. Gynecomastia excision, regardless of the technique used, is generally performed on an outpatient basis, usually with the patient under general anesthesia. Recovery time for patients undergoing liposuction only is 3–6 weeks; patients requiring direct excision of skin and parenchyma will not be able to fully return to normal activities for 2–3 months.

Liposuction

Liposuction is the most commonly performed invasive aesthetic surgical procedure and is used as an adjunctive technique in virtually all body-contouring procedures. Developed in the 1970s, this technique involves making small, 1-cm-long

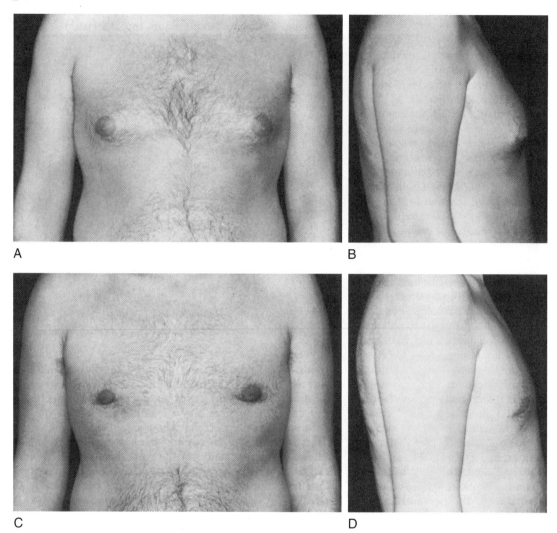

Figure 23-1. Mild gynecomastia treated with liposuction alone. Anterior (A) and lateral (B) views before surgery; anterior (C) and lateral (D) views after breast reduction. (From Mladick RA: Gynecomastia, _Clin Plast Surg_ 18:797–822, 1991.)

incisions and introducing hollow metal cannulae with side holes near the tip. By applying negative pressure to the lumen, small fragments of fat tissue are drawn into the cannula when it is moved in a reciprocating fashion, and the fragments of fat in the lumen are transected and removed into a suction reservoir. This simple concept has wide application in aesthetic surgery and has spawned a large body of literature on variations of this basic technique.[10] The most commonly used technique today is that of "tumescent" liposuction, in which a dilute solution of Xylocaine and epinephrine is infused into the target area before liposuction is performed. This has the advantage of more efficient removal of subcutaneous fat and excellent anesthesia and hemostasis.

The ideal candidate for liposuction is a patient who is at or near their ideal body weight and who has localized deposits of subcutaneous fat that are recalcitrant to reduction via diet or exercise. In males, liposuction is most commonly used in the abdomen, suprapubic area, and submental area. There are also patients who may be candidates for "large-volume" liposuction, in which the aspirated volume is greater than 1000 mL during a single procedure. This technique can be applied to more generalized subcutaneous fat deposition, with reports of 8000–10,000 mL being aspirated during a single procedure.[11]

The preoperative evaluation of a patient for liposuction includes the "pinch test," in which

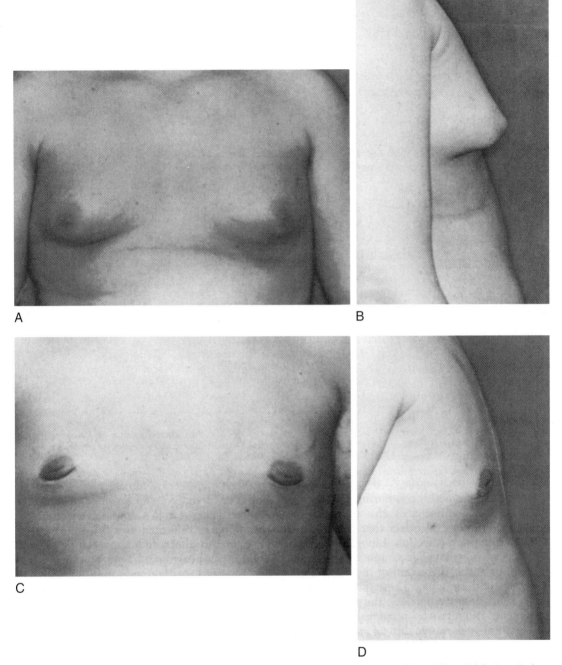

Figure 23-2. Moderate gynecomastia treated with parenchyma resection. Anterior (A) and lateral (B) views before surgery; anterior (C) and lateral (D) views after breast reduction. (From Mladick RA: Gynecomastia, *Clin Plast Surg* 18:797–822, 1991.)

the amount of subcutaneous fat is estimated. This is especially important in the abdomen since some male patients deposit the majority of their abdominal fat in the omentum and intestinal mesentery, and not in the subcutaneous space. These patients are generally not good candidates for liposuction and should focus on weight reduction over surgical removal of fat.

The most common complication of liposuction is local contour irregularities, and it is common for patients to require "touch-up" procedures to improve aesthetic appearance. For patients undergoing lower extremity liposuction, and especially in the case of large-volume liposuction, deep venous thrombosis and pulmonary emboli can occur.[10–12] Liposuction, when performed in isolation, is an outpatient surgical procedure. Patients typically have minimal pain, yet bruising is common and often persists for 1–2 weeks. A compression garment is often prescribed to minimize swelling and to help with tissue remodeling. Depending on the number of areas treated and the aspirated volume, most patients can return to work within 3 weeks.

Dermolipectomy

Dermolipectomy, or the resection of skin and underlying subcutaneous tissue, is a broad category of body-contouring procedures that includes "tummy tucks," thigh reductions, and brachioplasty. These procedures have in common an elliptical excision of skin and underlying subcutaneous fat, with closure along a straight or curved line once the excess tissue is removed. Individual procedures differ mainly in the design of the skin excision patterns. There have been both speculation and case-report data asserting that liposuction or dermolipectomy procedures may ameliorate the severity of diabetes and possibly improve risk profile for cardiac and peripheral vascular disease.[13] Subsequent studies, however, have put this speculation in question,[14] and at the present time patients should be advised that removal of subcutaneous fat does not significantly alter their obesity-related risk factors. In these patients, weight loss to reduce visceral fat should be a primary therapeutic objective.

Abdominal Procedures

Abdominal dermolipectomies or tummy tucks are designed to remove excess abdominal skin and fat, commonly referred to as a "spare tire." This procedure has a number of variations. A mini-abdominoplasty is appropriate for patients who have only a small amount of excess abdominal skin and fat that is confined to the infra-umbilical abdomen. In this procedure, a transverse ellipse of skin and fat is removed from the lower abdomen, leaving a curvilinear scar in the lower abdomen, where it is commonly covered by clothing. Liposuction is used to help remove excess fat from the upper abdomen and flanks ("love handles"). Candidates for this procedure must have good skin tone and should not require a transverse reduction of skin to achieve a good contour.

A full abdominoplasty is a more complex and invasive procedure and is indicated for patients with substantial excess skin and subcutaneous tissue and who have laxity of the abdominal myofascial structures. This procedure begins with a transverse lower abdominal incision. Then, a flap of abdominal skin and subcutaneous tissue is elevated as far cranial as the costal margin; the umbilicus is incised and left on its stalk. The abdominal skin is then re-draped, and the excess is excised. A vertically oriented excision to address transverse skin excess can be incorporated, leaving a midline abdominal scar. The abdominal musculofascial laxity can be addressed by placating the midline with a running suture from the xiphoid to the pubis. The umbilicus is brought through a new incision in the re-draped flap (Figure 23-3).

The most extensive version of the abdominal dermolipectomy is the circumferential abdominoplasty or belt lipectomy. In this procedure, a circumferential excision of skin and subcutaneous tissue is performed (Figure 23-4). For patients who are morbidly obese, an abdominal panniculectomy may be appropriate. This procedure is generally reserved for patients who experience health-limiting ulcerations, intertrigo, folliculitis, and panniculitis caused by the pannus, as well as limitations in physical mobility. The procedure consists of a straightforward elliptical wedge excision of lower abdominal skin and fat without undermining. This procedure is limited by infection, seroma, and wound dehiscence rates ranging from 30% to 70% in published series.[15] Although this procedure is functional (or reconstructive) and is not considered cosmetic in nature, it is mentioned as part of the continuum of dermolipectomy procedures for the abdomen.

The most common and problematic complications after abdominal dermolipectomy include wound dehiscence and seroma formation. The more extensive the skin resection, the more likely these complications are to occur. Full and circumferential abdominoplasties are usually performed as inpatient procedures.

Thigh Contouring

Thighplasty refers to the resection of excess skin and fat from the medial thigh via horizontal or vertical ellipse excisions. Because the resection is performed from the lower extremity and overlying the course of the saphenous vein, the risk of deep venous thrombosis is of greater concern than for other dermolipectomy procedures, and patients should receive appropriate prophylaxis (e.g., subcutaneous heparin). The major downside of this procedure is the risk of significant medial thigh scars.

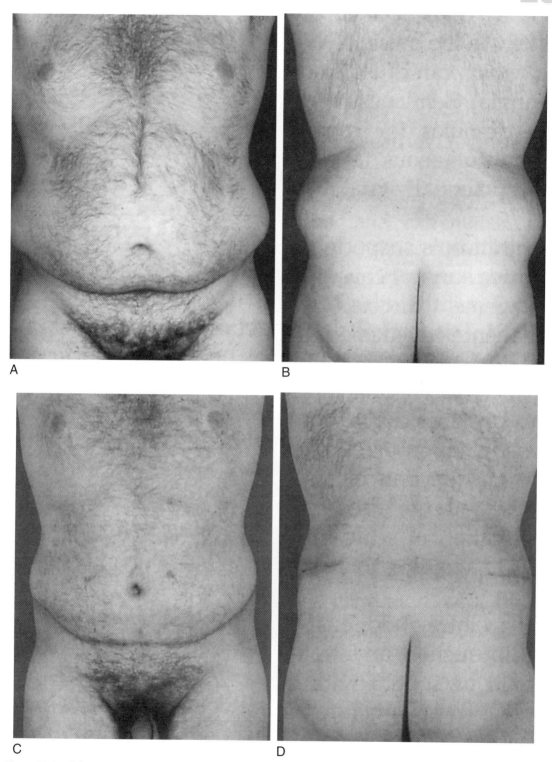

Figure 23-3. Abdominal lipodystrophy treated with full abdominoplasty. Anterior (A) and posterior (B) views prior to surgery; anterior (C) and posterior (D) views after abdominoplasty. (From Pitman G: Abdominal contouring. In Marchac D, Granick MS, Solomon MP, Robbins LB, editors: *Male Aesthetic Surgery,* Boston, 1996, Butterworth-Heinemann, pp 301–311.)

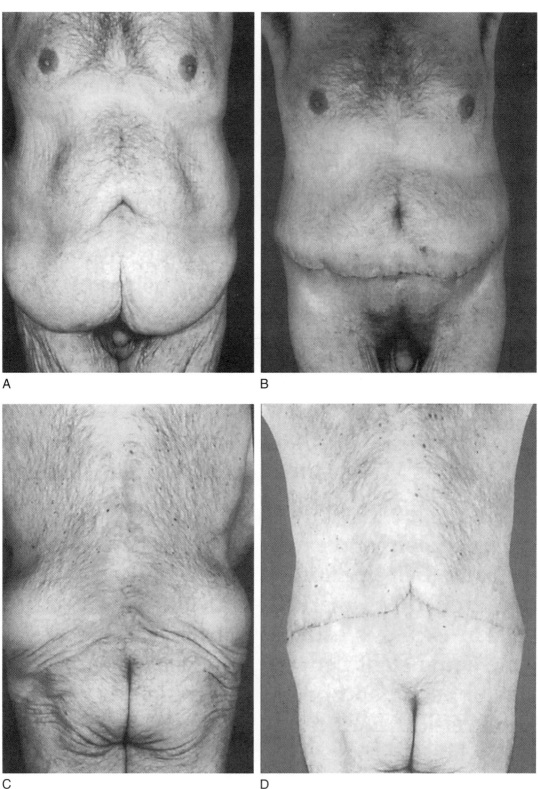

Figure 23-4. Circumferential abdominoplasty or "belt" dermolipectomy. Anterior view before (A) and after (B) surgery; posterior view before (C) and after (D) surgery; lateral view before (E) and after (F) surgery. (From Pitman G: Abdominal contouring. In Marchac D, Granick MS, Solomon MP, Robbins LB, editors: *Male Aesthetic Surgery,* Boston 1996, Butterworth-Heinemann, pp 301–311.)

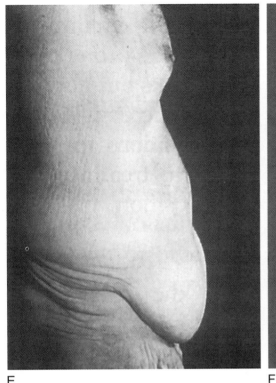

E

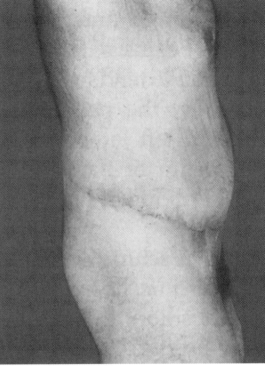

F

Figure 23-4—cont'd.

Arm Contouring

The corollary of thighplasty in the upper extremity is the *brachioplasty*. Excision of longitudinal and/or transverse ellipses of skin from the inner arm can eliminate redundancy at the expense of significant medial arm scars that are not easily covered by clothing. Because of this, this operation has been reserved chiefly for patients who have lost massive amounts of weight.

Post–Weight Loss Procedures

The obesity epidemic in the United States has been well documented and has spawned an enormous increment in bariatric surgical procedures.[16] These procedures have resulted in a large population of patients who have lost significant amounts of weight, often in excess of 100 pounds. These patients are typically left with significant excess skin in the arms, breasts, abdomen, buttocks, and thighs after such a significant weight loss (Figure 23-5). With minor modifications, the procedures described for abdominal, thigh, and arm dermolipectomy are applied to this population, and the procedure to address excess skin in the breast region is similar to procedures used in the treatment of gynecomastia.

Special considerations in this patient population include how to appropriately stage these operations if multiple body areas must be addressed and the high incidence of concomitant incisional hernias in patients who have undergone an open gastric bypass procedure. Often, these patients have unrealistic expectations of what can be accomplished with body-contouring procedures, and their cases must be managed appropriately to avoid significant postoperative patient dissatisfaction. In this population, skin-reduction procedures are in a "grey zone" between reconstructive and aesthetic surgery. For an abdominal dermolipectomy in a patient whose weight loss exceeds 100 pounds, a pannus overhanging the pubis and a health condition requiring treatment (usually recurrent intertrigo) are typical prerequisites for insurance companies to consider these procedures as medically necessary, and thus for coverage under a patient's benefits. Dermolipectomies in other areas of the body

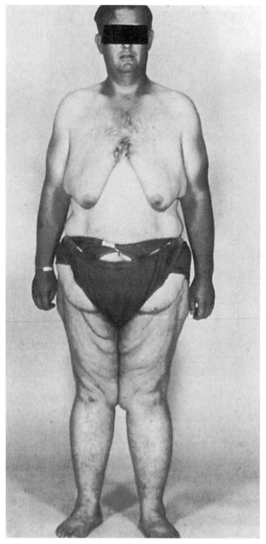

Figure 23-5. Resultant deformity after massive weight loss. (From Mladick RA: Gynecomastia, *Clin Plast Surg* 18: 797–822, 1991.)

are rarely covered by health insurance plans and are generally considered to be cosmetic, even when a significant deformity exists.

Implants

The term *implant* refers to any artificial material that is surgically implanted into the body. In plastic surgery, implants are used to improve the size and shape of various areas of the body for either cosmetic or reconstructive purposes. Although implants have been used for many years for breast reconstruction and augmentation in women, the use of implants for cosmetic body contouring in men has only recently become widely accepted. Today, plastic surgeons

routinely use implants in men to improve the appearance of the chest and calves. Implants are also used in other locations such as the buttocks or biceps, although augmentation of these areas is much less common. Although contour changes can be effected using implants, prospective patients should be advised that any medical implant may need to be revised or removed in the future. That is, implants are designed for long-term use, but cannot be considered "maintenance free."

Complications can occur with any implant operation. Some of the more common complications include contour irregularity or asymmetry, shifting of the implant out of the desired position, bleeding into the wound (hematoma), or infection of the implant. If severe enough, any of these complications can require a return to the operating room for treatment. Periprosthetic infections generally require removal of the device to control the process. Under most circumstances, the implant could be reinserted once the infection has been cleared for 6–12 months. It should be noted that, unlike the breast implants used in women, which consist of a silicone shell filled with a liquid or gel, the implants used for body contouring in men consist of solid yet soft silicone. Because of this, many of the complications associated with breast implants, such as a rupture or a leakage of fluid, do not occur with the implants used in men.

Pectoral

Pectoral implants are used to increase the size and improve the shape of the male chest for either cosmetic reasons (Figure 23-6) or for reconstruction of congenital or acquired deformities such as Poland's syndrome (a deficiency of subcutaneous fat and muscles on one side of the body, often affecting the pectoralis major and minor).[17] The implants commonly used are made of solid yet soft silicone and must be custom manufactured for each patient. In the weeks before surgery, a mold of the patient's chest is taken in clinic, and a temporary wax version of the implant is created. The patient may need to return to clinic several times for sculpting and fine-tuning of the temporary implant before the final customized implant is ordered and manufactured.

Implant placement is an outpatient operation requiring general anesthesia and usually takes 1–3 hours. An incision is made in the axilla, allowing the surgeon to create a pocket under the pectoralis major muscle. Creation of the pocket can be performed either endoscopically or via an open operation. Using an endoscope makes it

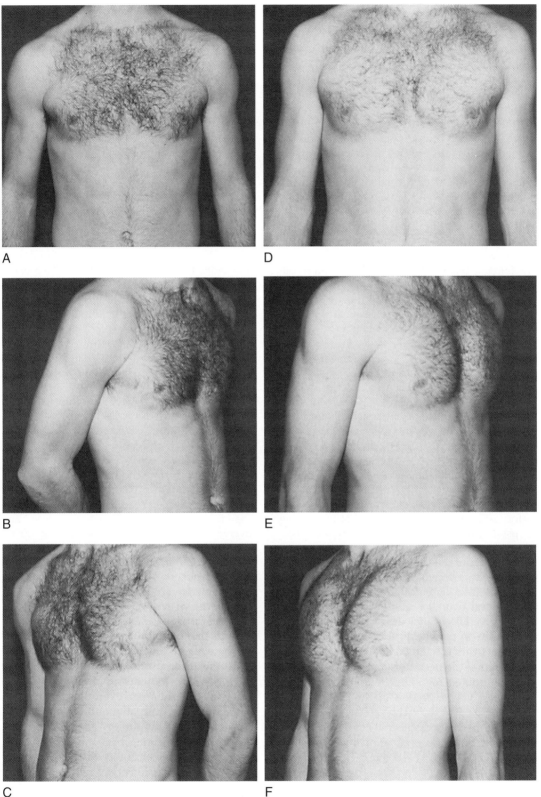

Figure 23-6. Cosmetic chest augmentation with pectoral implants. Anterior (A) and oblique (B and C) views before surgery; anterior (D) and oblique (E and F) views after augmentation. (From Novack BH: Alloplastic implants for men, *Clin Plast Surg* 18:829–855, 1991.)

possible to perform the surgery through a smaller incision but is technically more difficult. Once the pocket is developed, the implant is passed through the incision into the pocket and lies deep to the pectoralis major muscle. A small drain may be placed to reduce fluid buildup around the implant (seroma). The patient is taught to care for the drain and to measure the output at home. Once the drain output has decreased to an amount that can be absorbed by the body (usually less than 30 mL/day), the drain is removed in clinic. The patient can usually return to work within 2–3 weeks with limited upper extremity use; full recovery takes approximately 6 weeks.

Common complications of pectoral implants include hematoma and seroma formation, infection of the implant, asymmetry, displacement of the implant, and changes in nipple or skin sensation. Some complications including hematoma, infection, or displacement may require a return to the operating room for readjustment and appropriate treatment as described above.

Calf

Calf implants are used to increase the size and improve the shape of the posterior leg and are generally used for cosmetic enhancement (Figure 23-7). Like pectoral implants, calf implants are made of solid yet soft silicone. One or two implants may be used for each calf, depending on the size and shape of the patient's legs. Although it is possible to use "stock" implants, the surgeon may prefer to create custom implants. This process takes place in the weeks before surgery and is similar to that of creating a custom pectoral implant. A mold of the posterior leg is taken in the clinic, and a temporary wax version of the implant(s) is created. Sculpting and fine-tuning of the temporary model before the final implants are manufactured may be necessary.

The operation takes 2–3 hours and is performed on an outpatient basis. A general anesthetic is usually required, although a local or spinal anesthetic combined with intravenous sedation may be used. A transverse incision is made in a natural crease behind the knee. A pocket is created deep to the skin and fat of the posterior superior leg, superficial to the gastrocnemius muscle. The implants are then inserted into the pocket and the skin is closed. A drain may be placed to help reduce seroma formation, and it is removed in the clinic once the output has decreased sufficiently. The patient should plan to stay off work for 3–6 weeks after this operation, depending on how much activity

is required. Physical activity is strictly limited immediately after surgery but is gradually advanced over the next 6–8 weeks, until the patient can resume full activity.

Potential complications of calf implants include hematoma, seroma, infection, displacement, asymmetry, and visibility of the implant. Injury to major nerves or blood vessels can occur during dissection in the popliteal fossa, although this is quite rare.

Otoplasty

Cosmetic ear surgery or *otoplasty* is most commonly performed to reposition prominent ears close to the head or to reduce large ears. The operation, for the most part, is performed in children older than 4 years of age when the ear is almost fully developed; the earlier the surgery is performed, the less ridicule the child will need to endure. Congenital ear deformities are gender equal, but because of the difficulties of hair camouflage, otoplasty is more commonly performed on male patients. Ear surgery in an adult patient is also possible, and there are no additional risks associated with the advancing age of the patient. Children and adults generally return to normal activity within 1 week.

During an otoplasty, the ear cartilage is exposed through an incision on the back of the ear. The cartilage framework is repositioned and secured with permanent sutures, reduced with cartilage incision or expanded by cartilage grafting. The skin is re-draped over the modified cartilage framework, then the incision is closed and covered with an occlusive dressing. The operative procedure usually takes 2–3 hours and is performed on an outpatient basis. In young patients general anesthesia is required, but in older children and adults local anesthesia with sedation may be preferred.

Postoperative complications are uncommon but include infection of the cartilage, wound disruption, excessive scarring, and hematoma formation that may require evacuation. Recurrence of protrusion, contour distortion, or mismatch may require repeat surgery.

Rhinoplasty

Rhinoplasty, or surgery to reshape the nose, is the most common of all aesthetic procedures performed in males.[2] Rhinoplasty can reduce or increase the size of the nose, change the shape of the tip or dorsum of the nose, change the shape of the nostrils, enhance or reduce nasal

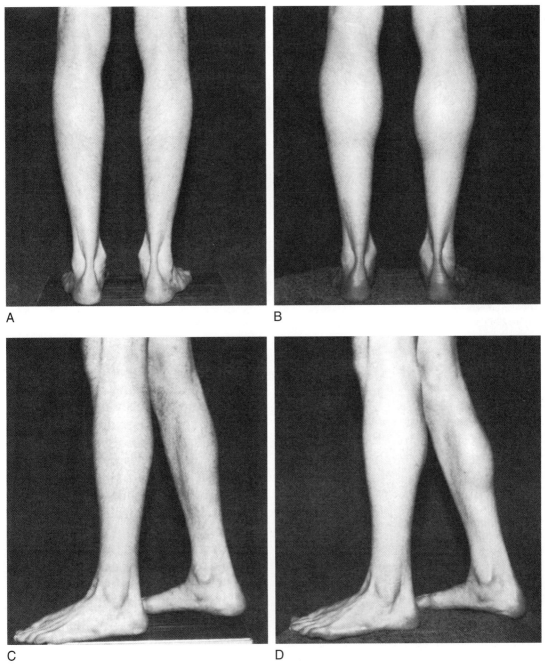

A   B

C   D

Figure 23-7. Cosmetic calf augmentation with calf implants. Anterior views before (A) and after (B) surgery. Oblique views before (C and E) and after (D and F) surgery. (From Novack BH: Alloplastic implants for men, *Clin Plast Surg* 18:829–855, 1991.)

projection, change the angle between the nose and lip, relieve nasal obstruction, or correct a deviated septum or crooked nose.

The best candidates for rhinoplasty are physically healthy, psychologically stable patients with realistic expectations. Most surgeons prefer not to perform elective rhinoplasty in teenage males until they are emotionally mature and have obtained full nasal growth, generally between 16 and 18 years of age. Rhinoplasty can be performed either with the patient under general anesthesia or with local anesthesia and intravenous sedation. Depending on the extent of the procedure and patient/surgeon preference, rhinoplasty is

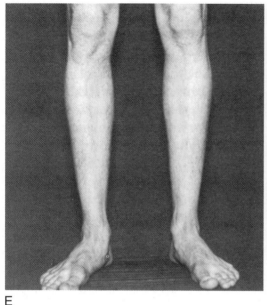 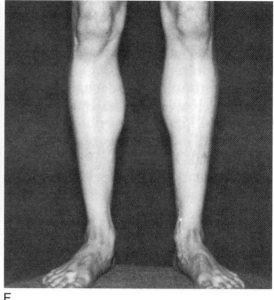

E   F

Figure 23-7—cont'd.

generally performed as an outpatient procedure and takes between 1 and 3 hours, although complicated procedures may take longer.

During surgery, the skin of the nose is separated from the supporting framework of cartilage and bone. The skeletal support is modified to the desired shape by reduction, augmentation, or suture repositioning. The skin is re-draped over the modified framework and supported for 1 or occasionally 2 weeks with a combination of external splinting and intranasal plastic splints or nasal packing to stabilize the septum and reduce postoperative bleeding.

When rhinoplasty is performed by a qualified surgeon, complications are usually minor and infrequent. When they do occur, they can include hemorrhage, infection, nasal obstruction, or a residual deformity, which may necessitate corrective surgery. Healing is a gradual process and subtle swelling may be present for months, especially in the nasal tip. The final result of a rhinoplasty may not be apparent for a year or more. A second procedure to correct a residual deformity is indicated in 10–15% of primary rhinoplasty procedures; an additional cost may be incurred.

Hair Restoration

Scalp hair loss in men is an extremely common problem and may occur for multiple reasons. For certain types of hair loss, effective nonsu-

rgical treatments exist that include various medical therapies. These options should be explored with a dermatologist before surgical intervention is considered. If medical management is not recommended or is ineffective, then surgery should be considered. All surgical techniques involve moving existing hair from one part of the patient's scalp to another to restore a more normal hair pattern. For small areas of baldness, transplantation of small grafts of hair-bearing tissue from one part of the scalp to the bald area can be effective. When hair loss is extensive, large rotation flaps, excision of bald areas, or even tissue-expansion techniques may be required. A combination of techniques is often necessary to achieve the best result. In all cases, the results that can be achieved surgically are limited by the amount of hair-bearing scalp that patient still has. A patient who has little hair left on the scalp may not be a candidate for hair-restoration surgery. It is best to perform hair-restoration surgery once hair loss has stabilized because ongoing hair loss after surgery can adversely affect the results of the operation.

Hair transplantation involves harvesting many small grafts of hair-bearing scalp and transplanting them to the bald area to restore a more youthful hair pattern. Hair transplants are classified according to the size of the grafts. Punch grafts contain approximately 10–15 hairs/graft, mini-grafts contain approximately

2–4 hairs/graft, and micro-grafts contain only 1–2 hairs each. A combination of punch, mini-, and micro-grafts is usually necessary to obtain the best cosmetic result. Smaller grafts are best used near the visible hair-line, whereas larger grafts can be used to fill in less visible areas. Slit grafts and strip grafts are long, narrow grafts containing 5–10 and 40–50 hairs/graft, respectively, and these can be used as well.

Hair transplantation is an outpatient surgery that can be performed in the office using a local anesthetic with or without sedation. If an extensive area is to be treated, the surgeon may harvest a sufficiently large strip of hair-bearing scalp, usually from the back of the head. The donor site is sutured closed, and grafts of varying sizes are taken from the harvested strip of scalp. If less extensive transplanting is planned, the surgeon can harvest grafts individually from the hair-bearing scalp without taking a large strip of tissue. The grafts are then transplanted into small incisions in the bald area. Depending on the size of the bald spot, anywhere from 50 to well over 500 grafts can be transplanted in one session. Approximately 1 month after surgery, the transplanted hairs will shed, followed by regrowth within 4–6 weeks. This normal process may be discouraging to the patient if he is not prepared for it to occur before the initial procedure. Once hair growth has stabilized, it is almost always necessary to perform repeat grafting to achieve the best final result (Figure 23-8).

Other hair restoration procedures include scalp reduction surgery (excision of bald areas), flap surgery, and tissue expansion. These techniques are more invasive than hair transplantation but may be necessary to achieve an optimal result. These operations, although usually performed on an outpatient basis, sometimes require general anesthesia.

Scalp-reduction surgery is the simplest of these techniques and can be used alone to treat small areas of baldness or may be combined with other techniques to treat larger areas. Here, an ellipse of bald scalp is excised, the surrounding scalp is undermined and stretched, and the elliptical defect is sutured closed in a straight or gently curved line. Because the scalp does not stretch like other areas of skin may, the results of a single scalp-reduction operation are usually modest. Scalp reduction can be performed serially, allowing the surrounding scalp to relax and stretch between operations, which ultimately allows for a larger area to be excised.

Flap surgery involves making large incisions in the patient's remaining hair-bearing scalp and elevating a flap of hair-bearing tissue. The flap remains attached to the surrounding scalp at its base, such that blood flow to the flap is preserved. The area of bald scalp to be replaced by the hair-bearing flap is excised, and the flap is rotated on its base into the recipient site and sutured in place. The flap donor site is closed with stitches.

Tissue expansion may be necessary when there is a very large bald area and little remaining hair-bearing scalp. Tissue expansion involves the placement of a plastic tissue expander (similar to a deflated balloon) underneath the area of hair-bearing scalp. Once the incision has healed sufficiently, expansion is initiated. This process involves injecting sterile saline into the expander

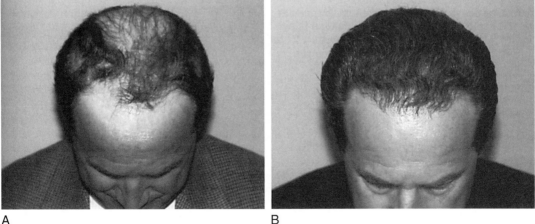

A   B

Figure 23-8. Frontal hair loss treated with hair transplantation. Before hair transplantation (A) and after transplantation (B). (From Barrera A: Hair restoration. In McCarthy JG, Galiano RD, Boutros SG, editors: *Current Therapy in Plastic Surgery*, Philadelphia, 2006, Saunders, pp 333–337.)

using a needle and syringe. A small amount of saline is injected once or twice a week for a number of weeks. As the tissue expander fills with fluid, the overlying hair-bearing scalp stretches and undergoes new tissue growth. The bulging area of scalp may be quite unsightly during the expansion process, which is one of the main reasons patients do not like this operation. Once the hair-bearing scalp has been expanded, the patient is taken back to the operating room for the second operation. The tissue expander is removed, and the expanded area of hair-bearing scalp is used to cover the bald areas.

Potential complications of hair restoration surgery include infection, bleeding, extrusion of the tissue expander (if used), and unsightly scarring. With hair-transplantation techniques, the donor sites in the hair-bearing scalp are usually well camouflaged by the remaining hair. However, if hair loss continues after surgery, the donor site scars may become more visible. The other techniques described require larger incisions and may result in more extensive scarring. Scars on the scalp from flap surgery, scalp-reduction surgery, and tissue expansion may become widened because of tension across the wounds as they heal.

Surgery of the Aging Face

Dynamics of Facial Aging

With aging, generalized facial and cervical laxity with sagging are progressive and objectionable to many persons. Smoking and sun exposure are believed to significantly exacerbate skin changes with age.[18] Forehead and glabellar wrinkling, brow ptosis, lateral hooding and drooping of upper eyelid skin, and lower lid puffiness appear in the upper face. Deepening of the nasolabial folds, jowling, and cervical laxity affect the lower face and neck.[19] The major forces contributing to facial aging include skeletal remodeling, subcutaneous fat redistribution, hormonal imbalance, and gravity.

Aging of the craniofacial skeleton is a result of focal bone atrophy and bone expansion.[20] There is a reduction in facial height and a small increase in facial width due to changes in the maxilla and mandible. The orbits increase in size, whereas the maxilla decreases, accentuating the descent of the malar fat pad and deepening of the nasolabial fold. Alveolar bone resorption enhances perioral wrinkling and reduces lip fullness.

Facial aging is associated with loss of soft tissue fullness in the periorbital forehead, malar, temporal, mandibular, and mental sites and persistence or hypertrophy of fat in others (e.g., submental, lateral nasolabial fold, infraorbital fat pouches, and malar fat pad). Skin wrinkling appears in the periorbital and perioral areas due to repeated underlying muscle action and volume loss. Jowl and submental sagging occurs due to a relative excess of skin or lack of elastic recoil as well as fat accumulation. Volume changes with the loss of temporal support, coupled with a reduction of upper eyelid fullness, creates the impression of brow ptosis with the eyebrow descending to a position at or below the supraorbital rim. In addition, there is a relative excess of upper eyelid skin accentuated by a reduction in periorbital volume. The loss of subcutaneous fullness and a downward displacement of intraorbital fat over a weakened orbital septum create a deeper and wider orbit and convex deformity of the lower eyelid. Additionally, subcutaneous thinning of the lower eyelid confers a dark coloration to the thin infraorbital skin, enhancing the "tired eye" appearance. Consequent to these structural changes, the facial convexities of youth are altered. From the front, the jawline appears scalloped; the suborbital, buccal, and temporal areas are hollow; and the forehead and brow lose their anterior projection.

Most conventional face, neck, and brow lift procedures incorporate elevation and tightening to reverse soft tissue descent that results from atrophy and loss of skin elasticity. Current trends in facial rejuvenation focus on deep aponeurotic and muscular manipulation plus volume restoration.[21–23]

Blepharoplasty

Cosmetic surgery of the eyelids (i.e., *blepharoplasty*) includes a variety of operative procedures designed to remove or reposition herniated orbital fat or skin and muscle from the upper and lower eyelids (Figure 23-9). The surgical objectives are to correct drooping upper eyelids, puffy lower eyelids, and eyelid malposition. Upper lid blepharoplasty, performed for the correction of visual obstruction, may be considered reconstructive, and the costs are often partially covered by certain insurance policies. Upper and lower eyelid surgery may be combined with browlift and cervicofacial lift procedures, when indicated. Blepharoplasty after rhinoplasty is the second most commonly performed cosmetic procedure in men.[2]

Upper and lower lid incisions follow the natural lines of the lids to conceal resultant scars. Typically, the scars lie in the natural crease of the upper lid and below the lashes of the lower

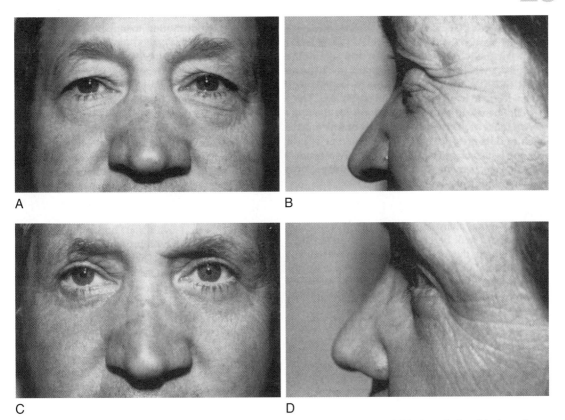

Figure 23-9. Bilateral upper and lower lid blepharoplasty. Anterior (A) and lateral (B) views before blepharoplasty; anterior (C) and lateral (D) views after blepharoplasty. (From Ellis DS: Blepharoplasty. In Marchac D, Granick MS, Solomon MP, Robbins LB, editors: *Male Aesthetic Surgery*, Boston, 1996, Butterworth-Heinemann, pp 157–170.)

eyelid, extending into the furrow at the outer can-thus. In younger patients with more elastic skin, transconjunctival blepharoplasty is performed through an incision inside the lower eyelid, leaving no visible scar. Depending on the rate of healing, most bruising and swelling are resolved by the second operative week, but the scars will remain pink for 6 months or more after surgery.

Browlift

A forehead lift or browlift is a surgical procedure designed to correct drooping brows and hooding of the upper eyelids and to improve horizontal furrows and glabellar frown lines (Figure 23-10). A forehead lift is often performed in combination with facelift to provide a more harmonious result. Blepharoplasty may also be performed in combination with a forehead lift if the patient has brow ptosis with significant overhang of the upper lids.

The operative approach may be through an incision at or just behind the hairline. Alternatively, the procedure may be performed endos-copically through small hairline incisions. Patients with male pattern baldness are not ideal candidates for browlift procedures, but incisions can be modified to accomplish the necessary brow elevation and reduce forehead creases. Working through the incisions, the surgeon lifts the skin of the forehead to expose the underlying muscles for modification, then releases, elevates, and secures the forehead soft tissue to maintain the desired forehead and eyebrow position.

Postoperative adverse effects may include temporary swelling, forehead or scalp numbness, itching, or hair loss. Injury to the temporal branch of the facial nerve is rare and usually transient. Permanent injury can result in an ipsilateral loss of forehead motion.

Facelift (Rhytidectomy)

Face and neck lifting procedures are designed to tighten the aponeurotic structures underlying the skin, reposition the skin, and remove skin sufficient to correct tissue laxity. The best candidate is a patient whose face and neck have begun to

453

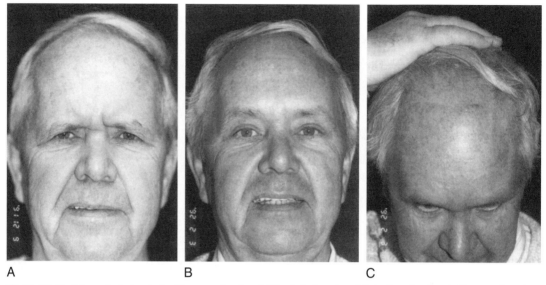

Figure 23-10. Brow ptosis treated with open forehead lift. Anterior view (A) before forehead lift; anterior view (B) after forehead lift; frontal view (C) after forehead lift. (From Camirand A: Browlift. In Marchac D, Granick MS, Solomon MP, Robbins LB, editors: *Male Aesthetic Surgery,* Boston, 1996, Butterworth-Heinemann, pp 135–156.)

sag, but whose bone structure is properly defined and whose skin has retained some elasticity. Most facelift candidates are aged between their 40s and 60s, but face and neck lifts can be performed on persons in their 70s and 80s as well.

Face and neck lift procedures usually take 2–4 hours or longer if combined with other procedures such as blepharoplasty or browlift. Depending on the recommendation of the surgeon or the preference of the patient, local anesthesia with sedation or general anesthesia may be most appropriate.

Incisions usually begin above the ear in the temporal scalp or the lower border of the temporal hairline, extend in the natural preauricular crease or free margin of the tragus, and continue around the earlobe, crossing the postauricular skin and scalp. When healed, incision lines are usually well concealed but visible on close inspection. In cases of advanced neck laxity, a small submental incision may be added.

Postoperatively, facial features are distorted by swelling and bruising with improvement over several weeks. Generally by the third week, patients achieve a socially acceptable appearance and can resume normal activity. During the early stages of recovery, it is not uncommon for patients to feel disappointment or depression.

Transient numbness and facial asymmetry are common symptoms, but these generally resolve within weeks. Hematoma, infection, partial skin loss, wound disruption, and the development of objectionable scars may require adjunctive

treatment and result in delayed recovery. Transient facial weakness may complicate recovery, but permanent facial nerve damage is rare.

Additional risks are attendant in male facelift surgery. Men may need to shave behind the ears and the lateral neck where areas of bearded skin are transferred. During the healing phase, scars may be problematic unless camouflaged by hairstyle or makeup. Many men are reluctant to accept such grooming modifications.

Ancillary Procedures

When indicated, adjunctive liposuction may be used to reduce excess facial or cervical fat deposits. In contrast, autologous fat injection or soft tissue fillers are appropriate to plump deeper facial furrows or areas of facial atrophy or for lip augmentation. Facial lifting improves tissue laxity but does not correct fine facial or perioral wrinkling. Ancillary procedures such as laser resurfacing, chemical peel, or dermabrasion remove the superficial dermis and accomplish varying degrees of improved skin texture and luster. Because many of the ancillary procedures to assist with facial rejuvenation are less invasive than open surgery, many non-surgeon physicians are beginning to perform botulinum toxin (Botox) injections, placement of fillers, and other "minor" cosmetic procedures. There are now weekend courses for primary care physicians who want to learn to do Botox injections and to use fillers. Prospective patients should be cautioned to insist on appropriate training before selecting a physician to perform even minor procedures. Again, ABMS certification in a relevant specialty is a good signature of a well-trained cosmetic surgeon.

Botox

The injection of botulinum toxin for wrinkle reduction is an extremely common procedure, with over 2 million injections performed each year.[2] Botox is the brand name of the only botulinum toxin preparation that has been approved by the US Food and Drug Administration (FDA) for cosmetic use. Botulinum toxin is a naturally occurring substance produced by *Clostridium botulinum*, a common anaerobic bacterium found in soil and other locations. The toxin binds to motor nerve endings at the neuromuscular junction and prevents release of the neurotransmitter acetylcholine, resulting in muscle paralysis. It is the same toxin that is responsible for botulism food poisoning, and it can be lethal. However, the toxin can be purified and used safely in small doses for medical purposes.

The FDA has approved Botox for cosmetic use in the glabellar region between the eyebrows, although it is commonly used "off-label" in other areas of the face. By paralyzing specific facial muscles that cause the overlying skin to wrinkle, botulinum toxin causes wrinkles and fine lines to smooth out. Botox begins to work within a week after injection, and maximum results are seen within 2 weeks. The results can last up to 4 months, and repeat injections are often requested. With repeat treatments, the paralysis effect lasts longer.

When performed by an experienced surgeon, Botox injections are safe and effective; however, potential complications do exist. If injected incorrectly, temporary numbness, drooping of the eyelids, or unwanted paralysis of other facial muscles can occur. Rare allergic reactions to the preparation can occur and could be life-threatening. In addition, some people develop antibodies to the botulinum toxin after repeated treatments and are no longer able to benefit from injections.

Soft Tissue Fillers

Soft tissue fillers are injectable substances that are used to smooth out facial wrinkles, furrows, and creases. They are also used to fill out focally depressed areas in the face or to add fullness to the lips. Many types of fillers already exist, and the number of fillers entering the market is increasing dramatically. However, not every filler that one may read or hear about is available for use in the United States. Some of the more commonly used fillers are discussed below, although the list is certainly not comprehensive.

Injection with soft tissue fillers is usually performed in the office or clinic setting and can take anywhere from a few minutes to an hour to perform. Although a topical anesthetic is applied to the skin before the procedure, these injections can be quite painful. An injected local anesthetic is much more effective for controlling pain, but its use in this situation is often limited because the injected anesthetic distorts the skin and soft tissue in the area of interest. If the patient cannot tolerate the filler injections, sedation or even a brief general anesthetic may be necessary. The results are often immediate, and the duration depends on the type of filler used.

Fillers may be derived from naturally occurring substances such as bovine collagen, or they may be completely synthetic, like silicone. Other fillers are a combination of natural and synthetic materials. For example, Artecoll is a filler composed of microspheres of polymethylmethacrylate imbedded in collagen. In addition, autogenous tissue may be injected as a filler. Most commonly, this is the patient's own fat, harvested by liposuction from another area of the body.

Fillers can be classified as temporary, semipermanent, or permanent. Temporary fillers usually last between 1 and 6 months and occasionally up to a year. Semipermanent or permanent fillers may last 5 years or longer. At first glance, it may seem that permanent fillers would be preferable to temporary fillers because of the longer duration of results. However, one of the complications that can occur with any filler is the creation of new and unsightly contour irregularities. Although temporary fillers lose their effect over time, they are more forgiving. When a bad result occurs with a permanent filler, it is extremely difficult to correct.

Fat is the most commonly used autologous filler, with more than 50,000 fat injections performed each year in the United States.[2] Fat works well to treat larger depressions or deep creases, but it does not work as well for fine wrinkles. The fat to be injected is generally harvested from a remote location on the patient's body, often the abdomen, using a liposuction cannula inserted through a small incision hidden in the umbilicus. It is then prepared for injection by centrifugation, which separates the liquid and other tissues from the fat cells. The fat is then injected into the area of soft tissue deficit. The area is initially overfilled because reabsorption of approximately 70% of the injected volume is expected. The best results are obtained with repeat treatments over a 6–12-month period. Occasionally there is some degree of permanent improvement, but the results are usually temporary, lasting from months to a year. Because the fat is derived from the patient's own body, the allergic reactions that can be seen with other fillers do not occur.

Collagen has long been the most popular soft tissue filler. Over 500,000 people undergo collagen injections each year in the United States,[2] and the number is growing. Collagen fillers are used to treat many types of facial wrinkles and creases but are especially effective for lip augmentation and for treating perioral wrinkles and the nasolabial folds. Collagen fillers are usually derived from bovine tissue (e.g., Zyderm), although human-derived collagen preparations are available. Collagen is a temporary filler, and the results generally last up to 6 months. The major drawback of bovine collagen is that it can cause a local or systemic allergic reaction. Because of this, a skin test is performed a month before the actual procedure is undertaken. The human-derived preparations have a decreased risk of allergic reaction but are more expensive and may be more quickly reabsorbed than bovine collagen, depending on the preparation. It is also possible to harvest the patient's own skin and have the collagen processed for injection, which does eliminate the risk of allergic reaction. However, since this process is time consuming and expensive and requires the excision of skin, this option is very rarely chosen.

Hyaluronic acid is a chemical that is naturally found in human skin and soft tissue, as well as in the skin and soft tissue of other animals. There are multiple hyaluronic acid filler preparations on the market, which vary significantly in terms of cost, permanence, and ease of use. Restylane and Captique are the most commonly used products and are approved by the FDA. Both of these hyaluronic acid preparations are produced without the use of human or animal tissue. The preparations available in the United States are temporary fillers, and results may last up to a year. Allergic reactions to hyaluronic acid fillers can occur but are much less common than with collagen.

There are many other permanent and semipermanent fillers used outside the United States that are currently in various stages of FDA study or approval.[24] Artecoll and Radiesse are preparations commonly used in Canada and Europe. Artecoll is a semipermanent to permanent filler made of polymethylmethacrylate microspheres embedded in bovine-derived collagen. Radiesse is a semipermanent filler made of hydroxyapatite—a chemical found in bone—suspended in a gel. These products give long-lasting results but may become lumpy over time and can result in granuloma formation.

Silicone is sometimes used as a permanent injectable filler and deserves special mention. Silicone is easy to use, is long lasting, and can give very acceptable cosmetic results initially. However, the complications associated with free silicone injection can be disastrous and disfiguring. Contour irregularities and severe granulomatous reactions can occur, and these are often impossible to correct. Even though these problems do not occur in every patient who undergoes a silicone injection, we strongly recommend against its use. It should be noted, however, that there is no evidence to date that autoimmune or other systemic diseases occur as a result of silicone injection.[25]

Peels

Chemical facial peels involve the treatment of the facial skin with a solution that "peels" away the outer surface. As the injured skin heals after the treatment, it becomes tighter, smoother, and more evenly pigmented, resulting in a healthier, more youthful appearance. In general, chemical peels are most effective and have fewest complications in fair-skinned persons. The two most common types of chemical peel are the phenol peel and the trichloroacetic acid (TCA) peel. In addition, lighter peels can be performed with alpha-hydroxy acids (AHAs) or beta-hydroxy acids (BHAs).

Phenol peels result in a deep chemical injury that extends into the dermis. As the facial skin heals, it becomes tighter, smoother, more evenly pigmented, and lighter in color. The procedure itself is usually performed in the office under light sedation and may take up to 2 hours. The facial skin is first cleaned, followed by careful application of the phenol solution. After treatment, petroleum jelly is applied to the injured skin to protect it and keep it from drying out. The skin takes up to 3 weeks to heal after a phenol peel. Crusting often occurs and can last up to 2 weeks after the peel. It is also common to have facial redness that may take up to 6 months to resolve. The final results of phenol peels are permanent, although as the body continues to age, new wrinkles and pigment changes will develop.

TCA peels are medium-depth peels and do not injure the skin as deeply as the phenol peels. Like the phenol peel, TCA peels are performed in the office but usually only take 20–30 minutes to complete. Recovery is quicker than from a phenol peel, and the skin usually heals within 7–10 days. There may be crusting, irritation, and redness for a few weeks after a TCA peel. Like phenol peels, TCA peels result in smoothing and tightening of skin, although the results are not as dramatic as those seen with phenol peels. To maximize the results of a TCA peel, the surgeon may prescribe AHAs or hydroquinone treatments (a bleaching agent) in the weeks before the TCA peel. Unlike phenol peels, the results of TCA peels are usually temporary. The duration of results varies depending on the skin type and the depth of the peel, but it is common to need one or two repeat treatments to achieve maximum results. Because the TCA peel is not as deep as the phenol peel, it results in less pigment change and is better suited to patients with darker skin.

Light chemical peels can be performed with topical AHAs or BHAs. AHAs include glycolic acid, lactic acid, and various fruit acids. Salicylic acid is a BHA that is commonly used in light peels. Light peels with AHAs or BHAs take 10–20 minutes to perform, and recovery time is minimal. The results are much less dramatic than those seen with phenol or TCA peels. Therefore, patients usually undergo scheduled treatments every few weeks or months. When treatment is started, patients often experience skin irritation, flaking, and redness. These are usually mild and resolves quickly.

Chemical peels are not without complication. All peels, especially phenol and TCA peels, cause some degree of erythema during the healing process. During this period, which can last up to 6 months with phenol peels, it is extremely important to protect the skin from the sun through minimization of exposure and judicious use of sunscreen. Failure to do so can result in scarring or permanent pigment changes. In addition, because phenol peels result in permanent lightening of the skin, patients who have had a phenol peel must be vigilant about sun protection for the rest of their lives. Although lightening of the skin may be acceptable or desirable in fair-skinned persons, lines of demarcation between treated and untreated skin may develop, requiring coverage with makeup. In darkly pigmented persons, patchy depigmentation can occur, and thus phenol peels are contraindicated. More rarely, TCA or phenol peels may result in skin injury deep enough to cause permanent scarring. Again, this is more likely to occur with a phenol peel, which naturally penetrates the skin more deeply. In addition, patients should be aware that any peel can cause a reactivation of herpes virus infections, including cold sores or shingles. This can be prevented or minimized by pretreatment with oral antiviral medications. Finally, a complication unique to phenol peels is cardiac arrhythmia, which can occur if too much phenol is absorbed systemically during the peel. Cardiac monitoring is therefore necessary phenol peels are performed, and phenol peels are avoided in patients with cardiac disease.

Lasers

Laser stands for light amplification by the stimulated emission of radiation. A laser is a very intense coherent beam of light that can deliver focused energy in a precise fashion. As such, it is a useful tool for facial resurfacing. The histologic changes in skin after laser resurfacing are similar to those seen after chemical peels. However, unlike chemical peels, the laser allows the surgeon to more precisely control the depth of treatment.

Laser resurfacing or "laser peel" is usually performed with a carbon dioxide (CO_2) laser. The CO_2 laser can be used to improve fine wrinkles and is especially useful around the eyes and mouth. It can also be used to treat uneven or patchy pigmentation and may be used in conjunction with a facelift or blepharoplasty. The CO_2 laser is used to direct brief bursts of high-energy light, vaporizing the outer layers of facial skin to a precisely controlled depth. During the 1–2 weeks after treatment, the facial skin heals, resulting in smoother, tighter, more evenly pigmented skin.

The erbium:yttrium aluminum garnet (erbium:YAG) laser, has recently become a popular tool for facial resurfacing, although it has not replaced the CO_2 laser. The energy of the erbium laser is absorbed by water in superficial skin cells, resulting in their destruction and removal. As the skin heals after treatment, it becomes tighter, smoother, and more evenly pigmented. The erbium laser is less destructive than the CO_2 laser. Because of this, it does not tighten skin as well as the CO_2 laser does, and the results of erbium laser resurfacing are less long-lasting. However, patients experience significantly less redness after treatment with the erbium laser and have a shorter recovery time. Because there are fewer pigment changes with the erbium laser, it is better suited than the CO_2 laser for use in darkly pigmented patients.

Laser resurfacing is an outpatient operation and is usually performed in the office or in an outpatient surgery center. Treatment duration ranges from a few minutes to 2 hours, with variations based on the surface area treated. Depending on the duration of the treatment, light sedation may be required. Afterward, patients experience mild swelling and discomfort for a few days. If the CO_2 laser is used, the skin will crust for 7–10 days and will be erythematous for 3–4 weeks. If the erbium laser is used, there is minimal crusting, and the facial redness resolves more quickly. With both lasers, the skin reaches its final post-treatment appearance within 3–4 months. The results of CO_2 laser resurfacing are long-lasting (up to years) but not permanent. The results of the erbium laser last for months, and repeat treatments may be required.

Laser resurfacing has potential complications. Burns and scarring are uncommon, but they can occur. Permanent darkening or lightening of the treated area can also occur, a problem more common in darkly pigmented patients. Pigment changes occur more often with the CO_2 laser, making the erbium laser better suited for use in patients with darker skin. As with chemical peels, herpes virus infections including cold sores and shingles can be reactivated, and this risk can be decreased by appropriate antiviral treatment preoperatively.[26]

Finally, there are many non-ablative lasers on the market that, unlike the CO_2 and erbium: YAG lasers, do not remove the top layer of skin but rather deliver energy beneath the surface. These lasers are believed to stimulate collagen formation, resulting in skin tightening and smoothing of wrinkles. These lasers certainly have fewer adverse effects and require less downtime after treatment. Their main disadvantage, however, is the slight degree of improvement that can be obtained, and the need for multiple repeat treatments to achieve results.

Conclusion

Cosmetic surgery has the potential to significantly improve the sense of well-being and quality of life for male patients. A wide array of major and minor procedures are now available to alter (and hopefully improve) virtually every part of the human anatomy. For referring physicians and prospective patients, the preeminent considerations when considering cosmetic surgery are the appropriate choice of a qualified surgeon, having realistic expectations of the outcomes of cosmetic surgery, understanding and accepting the risks involved, and choosing the best procedure for each patient from the myriad of options now available. Despite the fact that there is a meager supportive evidence base for most aesthetic procedures, there is every indication that the recent surge in the popularity of cosmetic surgery will continue and will increasingly involve the activities of physicians from many specialties.

References

1. American Society of Plastic Surgeons: Physician's guide to cosmetic surgery: overview of cosmetic surgery 2006. Available at: http://www.plasticsurgery.org/medical_professionals/publications/Physicians-Guide-to-Cosmetic-Surgery-Overview.cfm.
2. American Society of Plastic Surgeons: *Procedural statistics* 2006.
3. Hasan JS: Psychological issues in cosmetic surgery: a functional overview, *Ann Plast Surg* 44(1):89–96, 2000.
4. Kisely S, Morkell D, Allbrook B, et al: Factors associated with dysmorphic concern and psychiatric morbidity in plastic surgery outpatients, *Austr N Z J Psychiatry* 36(1):121–126, 2002.
5. Wright MR: The male aesthetic patient, *Arch Otolaryngol Head Neck Surg* 113(7):724–727, 1987.
6. Castle DJ, Rossell S, Kyrios M: Body dysmorphic disorder, *Psychiatric Clin North Amer* 29(2):521–538, 2006.
7. Heller J, Gabbay JS, Ghadjar K, et al: Top-10 list of herbal and supplemental medicines used by cosmetic patients: what the plastic surgeon needs to know, *Plast Reconstr Surg* 117(2):436–445, 2006.
8. Graf RM, Bernardes A, Auerswald A, Noronha L: Full-face laser resurfacing and rhytidectomy, *Aesthet Plast Surg* 23(2):101–106, 1999.
9. Letterman G, Schurter M: Gynecomastia. In Goldwyn R, editor, *The Unfavorable Result in Plastic Surgery: Avoidance and Treatment*, ed 2, Boston, 1984, Little Brown, pp 779–787.
10. Kenkel J: Practice advisory on liposuction, *Plast Reconstr Surg* 113(5):1494–1496, 2004.
11. Commons GW, Halperin B, Chang CC: Large-volume liposuction: a review of 631 consecutive cases over 12 years, *Plast Reconstr Surg* 108(6):1753–1756, 2001.
12. Trott SA, Beran SJ, Rohrich RJ, et al: Safety considerations and fluid resuscitation in liposuction: an analysis of 53 consecutive patients, *Plast Reconstr Surg* 102(6):2220–2229, 1998.
13. Giese SY, Bulan EJ, Commons GW, et al: Improvements in cardiovascular risk profile with large-volume liposuction: a pilot study, *Plast Reconstr Surg* 108(2):510–511, 2001.
14. Klein S, Fontana L, Young VL, et al: Absence of an effect of liposuction on insulin action and risk factors for coronary heart disease, *N Engl J Med* 350(25):2549–2557, 2004.
15. Shermak M, Manahan M: Massive panniculectomy after massive weight loss, *Plast Reconstr Surg* 117(7):2191–2197, 2006.
16. Buchwald H, Williams SE: Bariatric surgery worldwide 2003, *Obesity Surg* 14(9):1157–1164, 2004.

17. Borschel GH, Izenberg PH, Cederna PS: Endoscopically assisted reconstruction of male and female poland syndrome, *Plast Reconstr Surg* 109(5): 1536–1543, 2002.
18. Ernster VL, Grady D, Miike R, et al: Facial wrinkling in men and women by smoking status, *Am J Public Health* 85:78–82, 1995.
19. Zimbler MS, Kokoska MS, Thomas JR: Anatomy and pathophysiology of facial aging, *Fac Plast Surg Clin North Amer* 9:179–187, 2001.
20. Bartlet SP, Grossman R, Whitaker LA: Age related changes of the craniofacial skeleton: and anthropomorphic and histologic analysis, *Plast Reconstr Surg* 90:592–600, 1992.
21. Ramirez OM: Endoscopic full facelift, *Aesthet Plast Surg* 18:363–374, 1994.
22. Coleman SR: *Structural Fat Grafting,* St Louis, 2004, Quality Medical Publishing.
23. Little JW: Volumetric perceptions in midfacial aging with altered priorities for rejuvenation, *Plast Reconstr Surg* 5:252–266, 2000.
24. Rohrich RJ, Rios JL, Fagien S: A role of new fillers in facial rejuvenation: a cautious outlook, *Plast Reconstr Surg* 112:1899–1902, 2003.
25. Narins RS, Beer K: Liquid injectable silicone: a review of its history, immunology, technical considerations, complications, and potential, *Plast Reconstr Surg* 118(3 Suppl):77S–84S, 2006.
26. Nestor MS: Prophylaxis for and treatment of uncomplicated skin and skin structure infections in laser and cosmetic surgery, *J Drugs Dermatol* 4(6 Suppl): S20–S25, 2005.

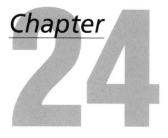

Chapter 24

Cancer Incidence, Screening, and Prevention

Joel J. Heidelbaugh, MD

Key Points

- For patients at low risk for testicular cancer, the US Preventive Services Task Force (USPSTF) and Canadian Task Force on Preventive Health Care (CTFPHC) state that there is insufficient evidence to indicate that screening—either via testicular self-examination or by a primary care physician—would result in a decrease in mortality (strength of recommendation: B).
- For patients at high risk for testicular cancer, the USPSTF and CTFPHC state that they should be informed of their increased risk and counseled regarding screening options (strength of recommendation: C).
- The American Cancer Society (ACS), USPSTF, and American Urological Association recommend that the DRE and PSA tests should be offered annually beginning at the age of 50 years for men who have a life expectancy of at least 10 more years, and that a discussion between male patients and their physicians should occur regarding the potential benefits, limitations, and harms associated with testing (strength of recommendation: C).
- The USPSTF concludes that the evidence is insufficient to recommend for or against screening asymptomatic persons for lung cancer with low-dose computerized tomography (LDCT), chest radiograph (CXR), sputum cytology, or a combination of these tests (strength of recommendation: B).
- The USPSTF strongly recommends that clinicians screen men 50 years of age or older for colorectal cancer (CRC); colonoscopy is the current gold-standard screening modality (strength of recommendation: A).
- The USPSTF has concluded that current evidence is insufficient to recommend either for or against routine screening for skin cancer using a total body skin examination (TBSE) for the early detection of cutaneous melanoma, basal cell cancer, or squamous cell skin cancer (strength of recommendation: C).

Introduction

For 2006, it was estimated that there would be 720,280 new cases of cancer in men leading to 291,270 resultant deaths (Figures 24-1 and 24-2).[1] Cancer is the second leading cause of mortality in the United States, accounting for more than 500,000 deaths in 2002, with an age-adjusted male-to-female death rate of 1.5 (Table 24-1).[2] Since 1999, when deaths are aggregated by age, cancer has surpassed heart disease as the leading cause of death for patients younger than 85 years of age.[3] The US death rate from all cancers combined has decreased by 1.5% per year since 1993.[3] Nonetheless, the lifetime probability of a man developing cancer for all sites remains a staggering 1 in 2 (Table 24-2).[2] Cancer incidence rates in African American men exceed those in white men for all anatomic sites (Table 24-3).[2]

The American Cancer Society (ACS) stresses that periodic encounters with primary care clinicians for health maintenance examinations offer the potential for discussion regarding cancer screening. These encounters should include the performance of or referral for conventional cancer screening tests

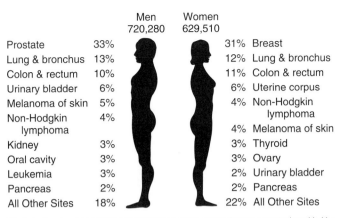

Men 720,280		Women 629,510	
Prostate	33%	31%	Breast
Lung & bronchus	13%	12%	Lung & bronchus
Colon & rectum	10%	11%	Colon & rectum
Urinary bladder	6%	6%	Uterine corpus
Melanoma of skin	5%	4%	Non-Hodgkin lymphoma
Non-Hodgkin lymphoma	4%	4%	Melanoma of skin
Kidney	3%	3%	Thyroid
Oral cavity	3%	3%	Ovary
Leukemia	3%	2%	Urinary bladder
Pancreas	2%	2%	Pancreas
All Other Sites	18%	22%	All Other Sites

*Excludes basal and squamous cell skin cancers and in situ carcinomas except urinary bladder
Source: American Cancer Society, 2006.

Figure 24-1. Estimated cancer cases, United States, 2006. (From American Cancer Society: Cancer statistics 2006: a presentation from the American Cancer Society. Available at: http://www.cancer.org/downloads/STT/Cancer_Statistics_2006_Presentation.ppt. Accessed August 28, 2006.)

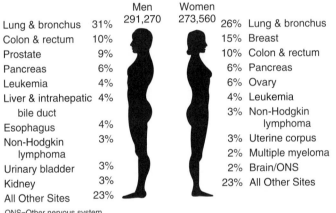

Men 291,270		Women 273,560	
Lung & bronchus	31%	26%	Lung & bronchus
Colon & rectum	10%	15%	Breast
Prostate	9%	10%	Colon & rectum
Pancreas	6%	6%	Pancreas
Leukemia	4%	6%	Ovary
Liver & intrahepatic bile duct	4%	4%	Leukemia
Esophagus	4%	3%	Non-Hodgkin lymphoma
Non-Hodgkin lymphoma	3%	3%	Uterine corpus
Urinary bladder	3%	2%	Multiple myeloma
Kidney	3%	2%	Brain/ONS
All Other Sites	23%	23%	All Other Sites

ONS=Other nervous system
Source: American Cancer Society, 2006.

Figure 24-2. Estimated cancer deaths, United States, 2006. (From American Cancer Society: Cancer statistics 2006: a presentation from the American Cancer Society. Available at: http://www.cancer.org/downloads/STT/Cancer_Statistics_2006_Presentation.ppt. Accessed August 28, 2006.)

as appropriate by age and gender, as well as instruction on self-examination techniques and increased awareness about signs and symptoms that may herald the early detection of cancer.[4] This chapter highlights data reflecting the incidence of some of the more commonly occurring cancers in men and summarizes the most current guidelines for cancer screening and prevention.

Testicular Cancer

Testicular cancer is the most commonly occurring cancer in American males between the ages of 15 and 34 years, and the incidence is increasing.[5] There will be an estimated 8250 cases in the United States in 2006 and, as a result, an estimated 370 deaths.[1] The lifetime probability of developing testicular cancer is 0.30%, whereas the mortality rate approaches 0.03%, representing approximately 1.1% of cancers among men.[5] Denial and embarrassment regarding the testicles and their examination is thought to contribute to testicular cancer being one of the least mentioned and appreciated cancers. Although the exact cause of testicular cancer is unknown, risk factors include an undescended testicle, young age, white race, and HIV infection. Cancer risk remains elevated even if the testicle has been surgically relocated to the scrotum; the majority of men who develop testicular cancer do not have a history of an undescended testicle. Signs and symptoms of testicular cancer can include any of the following[6]:

Table 24-1. Number of US Deaths by Leading Cause, 2002

Cause of Death	Number	% Total Deaths	Male:Female
Heart diseases	696,947	28.5	1.4
Malignant neoplasms	557,271	22.8	1.5
Cerebrovascular diseases	162,672	6.7	1.5
Chronic lower respiratory diseases	124,816	5.1	1.0
Accidents (unintentional injuries)	106,742	4.4	1.4
Diabetes mellitus	73,249	3.0	2.2
Influenza/pneumonia	65,681	2.7	1.4
Alzheimer's disease	58,866	2.4	0.8
Nephritis, nephrotic syndrome and nephrosis	40,974	1.7	1.5
Septicemia	33,865	1.4	1.2
Intentional self-harm/suicide	31,655	1.3	4.4
Chronic liver disease/cirrhosis	27,257	1.1	2.0
Essential hypertension/hypertensive renal disease	20,261	0.8	1.0
Assault/homicide	17,638	0.7	5.7
Pneumonitis due to solids and liquids	17,593	0.7	1.1
All other causes	407,900	—	—

Adapted from: Kochanek KD, Murphy SL, Anderson RN, Scott C. Deaths: Final Data for 2002. National Vital Statistics Reports. Volume 53, Number 5. Retrieved August 22, 2006, from: http://www.cdc.gov/nchs/data/nvsr/nvsr53/nvsr53_05acc.pdf.

Table 24-2. Lifetime Probability of a Male Developing Cancer, United States, 2000–2002[*]

Site	Risk
All sites[†]	1 in 2
Prostate	1 in 6
Lung and bronchus	1 in 13
Colon and rectum	1 in 17
Urinary bladder[‡]	1 in 28
Non-Hodgkin lymphoma	1 in 46
Melanoma	1 in 52
Kidney	1 in 64
Leukemia	1 in 67
Oral cavity	1 in 73
Stomach	1 in 82

[*]For those free of cancer at beginning of age interval. Based on cancer cases diagnosed during 2000 to 2002.
[†]All sites exclude basal and squamous cell skin cancers and in situ cancers except urinary bladder.
[‡]Includes invasive and in situ cancer cases.

From: American Cancer Society: Cancer statistics 2006. Available at: http://www.cancer.org/downloads/STT/Cancer_Statistics_2006 _Presentation.ppt. Accessed August 28, 2006. Source: DevCan: Probability of Developing or Dying of Cancer Software, Version 6.0 Statistical Research and Applications Branch, NCI, 2005. http:// srab.cancer.gov/devcan.

- A usually nonpainful lump or enlargement in either testicle
- A feeling of heaviness or fullness in the scrotum
- A dull ache in the abdomen or groin
- A sudden collection of fluid in the scrotum
- Pain or discomfort in a testicle or the scrotum
- Breast enlargement or tenderness
- Unexplained fatigue

Clinical examination of the testicles and scrotum by a physician and self-examination are the potential screening options for testicular cancer. Little evidence exists to assess the accuracy, yield, or benefits of such screening. Most testicular cancers are discovered either by patients themselves or by their partners, either unintentionally or via self-examination. There is no current evidence to suggest that instructing young men on how to examine themselves for testicular cancer would improve health outcomes, even among men at high risk, including men with a history of undescended testes or testicular atrophy.[7]

In patients believed to be at a low risk for testicular cancer, the Canadian Task Force on Preventive Health Care[5] (CTFPHC) and the US Preventive Services Task Force[7] (USPSTF) state that there is insufficient evidence to indicate that screening, either via testicular self-examination or by a primary care physician, would result in a decrease in mortality.

Table 24-3. Male Cancer Deaths in Which Death Rates for African Americans* Exceeds Death Rates for White Persons,* United States, 1998–2002

Site	African American	White	Ratio of African American/White
All sites	339.4	242.5	1.4
Prostate	68.1	27.7	2.5
Larynx	5.2	2.3	2.3
Stomach	12.8	5.6	2.3
Myeloma	8.8	4.4	2.0
Oral cavity and pharynx	7.1	3.9	1.8
Esophagus	11.2	7.5	1.5
Liver and intrahepatic bile duct	9.5	6.2	1.5
Small intestine	0.7	0.5	1.4
Colon and rectum	34.0	24.3	1.4
Lung and bronchus	101.3	75.2	1.3
Pancreas	15.8	12.0	1.3

*Per 100,000, age-adjusted to the 2000 US standard population.
From: American Cancer Society: Cancer statistics 2006. Available at: http://www.cancer.org/downloads/STT/ Cancer_Statistics_2006_Presentation.ppt. Accessed August 28, 2006. Source: Surveillance, Epidemiology, and End Results Program, 1975–2002, Division of Cancer Control and Population Sciences, National Cancer Institute, 2005.

In contrast, the ACS[8] advises a testicular examination as part of a routine cancer-related checkup. Even in the absence of screening, the current treatment interventions provide very favorable health outcomes.

In patients who are believed to be at a high risk for the development of testicular cancer, the CTFPHC[5] and the ACS[8] recommend that patients with a history of testicular atrophy, ambiguous genitalia, or cryptorchidism be informed of their increased risk and counseled regarding screening options. Although the ACS suggests monthly examinations in high-risk patients, the CTFPHC indicates that the optimal frequency of such examinations has not been determined and should be left to clinician discretion. The American Academy of Family Physicians formerly recommended a testicular examination for all males aged 13–39 years with a history of cryptorchidism, orchiopexy, or testicular atrophy, yet currently it does not provide any recommendations for testicular cancer screening in the general population.[9]

Clinicians should be aware of testicular cancer as a possible diagnosis when young men present to them with suggestive signs and symptoms. Some evidence exists to support that patients who present initially with symptoms of testicular cancer are frequently diagnosed as having epididymitis, testicular trauma, hydrocele, or other benign disorders. Efforts to promote prompt assessment and better evaluation of testicular problems may be more effective than widespread screening as a means of promoting early detection.[7] A more detailed discussion of diagnosis and treatment options for testicular cancer can be found in Chapter 16, Urology.

Prostate Cancer

Prostate cancer is currently the most commonly diagnosed cancer in men and is the third leading cause of male cancer death in the United States. For 2006, it was estimated that prostate cancer will account for 33% of all cancers in men and 9% of cancer deaths in men, accounting for an overall 1 in 6 lifetime risk (see Figures 24-1 and 24-2 and Table 24-2).[1] African American males have the highest age-standardized incidence and death rates for prostate cancer (272.0 and 68.1, respectively) compared with white males (169.0 and 27.7, respectively), Hispanic males (141.9 and 23.0, respectively), Asian males (101.4 and 12.1, respectively), and American Indian/Alaskan Native males (50.3 and 18.3, respectively).[1] A detailed discussion on the various forms of prostate cancer, treatment, and prognosis is provided in Chapter 16, Urology.

The ACS and USPSTF agree insufficient evidence currently exists to recommend that average-risk men undergo regular screening for prostate cancer via either digital rectal examination (DRE) or the prostate-specific antigen (PSA) serologic test.[10,11] The USPSTF found good evidence to support that PSA screening can detect early-stage prostate cancer, yet found mixed and inconclusive evidence that would support early detection improving health outcomes.[11] Prostate cancer screening may be associated with certain important harms, including frequent false-positive results and unnecessary anxiety, biopsies, and potential complications of treatment that may never have affected a patient's health. The USPSTF concludes that evidence is insufficient to determine whether benefits outweigh harms for a screened population.[11]

Nonetheless, the ACS, USPSTF, and the American Urological Association recommend that the DRE and PSA should be offered annually beginning at the age of 50 years for men who have a life expectancy of at least 10 more years, and that a discussion between male patients and their physicians should occur regarding the potential benefits, limitations, and harms associated with testing.[10–12] The ACS Advisory Committee strongly recommends shared decision making between clinicians and patients regarding prostate cancer screening, stressing that a clinical policy of not offering testing or discouraging testing in men who request early prostate cancer detection tests is inappropriate.[13] Likewise, the ACS Advisory Committee also concluded that if a man asks his healthcare provider to make the testing decision on his behalf after a discussion about benefits, limitations, and risks associated with prostate cancer testing, then he should be tested.[13]

The most current ACS recommendations from a systematic review in 2006[14] state that men who are at a high risk of development of prostate cancer, including men of sub-Saharan African descent and those men with a first-degree relative diagnosed before the age of 65 years, should begin prostate cancer screening at the age of 45 years. Men at an even higher risk of developing prostate cancer due to more than one first-degree relative diagnosed before the age of 65 years could begin testing at the age of 40 years, and if the PSA measurement is less than 1.0 ng/mL, then no additional testing is needed until the age of 45 years. In this population, if the PSA value is between 1.0 and 2.5 ng/mL, then annual testing is recommended. If the PSA measurement is greater than 2.5 ng/mL, then further evaluation including urology referral for a transrectal ultrasound (TRUS)-directed biopsy should be considered.[14]

The PSA is a biologic serum marker specific for prostatic tissue, not for prostate cancer itself. Elevated PSA values can be caused by any or all of the following[15]:

- Benign prostatic hypertrophy (BPH)
- Prostatitis
- Normal aging, even in the absence of prostate abnormality
- Ejaculation (physicians may suggest that men abstain from ejaculation for several days before PSA testing)
- Manipulation of the prostate during DRE
- Medicines (e.g., finasteride and dutasteride may falsely *lower* PSA levels)
- Some herbal preparations may also affect blood PSA levels, especially those marketed as being "for prostate health." (Saw palmetto, an herb used by some men to treat BPH, does not seem to interfere with the measurement of PSA.)

Conventionally, the normal range of PSA levels has been between 0 and 4.0 ng/dL. Although PSA levels less than 4.0 ng/dL have an increased sensitivity as a screening test for prostate cancer, there is no specific cutoff level at which prostate cancer is not present. In most cases of prostate cancer, the PSA level usually rises above 4.0 ng/mL. If the PSA level falls in the borderline range between 4.0 and 10.0 ng/mL, then there is an approximated 25% chance of having prostate cancer. If the PSA value is greater than 10.0 ng/mL, then the odds of having prostate cancer are greater than 50%, and the odds increase further as the PSA level increases. Approximately 15% of men with a PSA level below 4.0 ng/mL will have prostate cancer on TRUS-directed biopsy of the prostate.[15]

The PSA occurs in two major forms in the serum: either bound to albumin or unbound (free). The percent-free PSA assay indicates the amount of PSA that circulates free compared with the total serum PSA level. The percentage-free PSA level is lower in men with prostate cancer. For men with total serum PSA results that fall between 4.0 and 10.0 ng/mL, restricting the TRUS-directed biopsy to men with less than 20% free-PSA improves testing accuracy; a free PSA value less than 10% means that the likelihood of having prostate cancer is approximately 50%.[12] Applying this strategy to men with PSA levels between 2.5 and 10.0 ng/mL may lead to the detection of early disease in a larger number of men and may result in a lower TRUS biopsy rate compared with older strategies. A recent study found that if men with borderline PSA results underwent prostate biopsies only when their percent-free PSA was 25% or less, approximately 20% of unnecessary prostate biopsies could be avoided, and almost 95% of cancers would still be detected.[15]

The PSA velocity indicates how fast the PSA value rises over time. If the PSA rises faster than 0.75 ng/mL/year over a period of 18 months, then a TRUS-directed biopsy should be considered, even if the total PSA value is less than 4 ng/mL.[12] A PSA result that falls within the borderline range of 4.0–10.0 ng/mL might be very worrisome in a 50-year-old man but is less so in an 80-year-old man, and carries a lower likelihood of malignancy.[15] Although is it widely held that PSA values increase as males age, even in the absence of prostate cancer, the usefulness of age-specific PSA ranges is not well proven, and thus most physicians and professional organizations do not recommend their use at this time.

Due to the various uncertainties and controversy surrounding prostate cancer screening, clinicians should order the PSA test only after a detailed discussion with the patient regarding the potential but uncertain benefits and the potential harms of such screening. Potential benefits include a possible reduction of morbidity and mortality from prostate cancer; potential harms include anxiety associated with false-positive results that may lead to unnecessary biopsies and the inherent possible complications of treatment. Men should be informed of the current evidence and should be assisted in considering their personal preferences and risk profile before consenting for screening.[14,16]

If the early detection of prostate cancer can be shown to improve morbidity and mortality outcomes, then the population most likely to benefit from screening will be those men of average risk aged 50–70 years and men older than the age of 45 years who are at increased risk.[16] Such benefits may be smaller in Asian Americans, Hispanics, and other racial and ethnic groups who carry a lower risk of prostate cancer development. Older men and men with other significant medical problems who have a life expectancy of less than 10 more years are unlikely to benefit from prostate cancer screening but should still be offered screening after informed consent.[10]

The worldwide difference in prostate cancer incidence has been attributed to varying dietary patterns across the globe. Specific dietary factors and the roles they play in prostate cancer prevention are explained in more detail in Chapter 22, Integrative Medicine via a case discussion. For example, the higher consumption of soy protein in Asian countries compared with that of North Americans may explain a lower prostate cancer incidence and mortality. Several studies have demonstrated that the isoflavones genistein and daidzein (which may act as weak estrogens) found in soy proteins have been shown to inhibit prostate cancer cell growth by blocking estrogen receptor activity.[17,18] The lower incidence rates of prostate cancer in Asian countries may also be explained by the high intake of green tea in the Eastern world. Consumption of foods rich in lycopenes, selenium, zinc, and vitamins D and E are all thought to potentially lower prostate cancer risk. Considerable evidence suggests that prostate cancer is more common in obese men and those with a high intake of saturated fat in their diets.

The correlation of prostate cancer risk and vasectomy remains controversial. It has been postulated that a biologic mechanism whereby vasectomy influences the rate of prostate cancer may be related to a diminished secretory rate of prostatic fluid after vasectomy, or alternatively, to the post-vasectomy immune response to sperm antigens, which may cross-react with tumor-associated antigens and suppress tumor immunosurveillance mechanisms.[19] Two studies from *The Journal of the American Medical Association* in 1993[19,20] (one prospective, one retrospective) supported an increased risk of prostate cancer after vasectomy, yet it was noted in both studies that the association may be purely causal. In the first (prospective) study, the men who had undergone a vasectomy were slightly greater than 1.5 times as likely as those who did not have a vasectomy to develop prostate cancer.[20] In the second (retrospective) study, the results were virtually the same when compared with the first study.[19] If the result of these large studies are accurate, then the risk of developing prostate cancer after vasectomy increases from 7 to 11 per 1000 men per year, or just over a 60% increase.[19,20] A study published in 1999 examined men with prostate cancer and looked retrospectively to determine the likelihood that any of these men had a vasectomy before the development of prostate cancer. Sixteen percent of men with prostate cancer had had a vasectomy, whereas 15% who were healthy had had a vasectomy. In this study, men who had prostate cancer who were younger than 55 years of age were almost twice as likely to have had a vasectomy.[21] However, it is widely held that there is a significant lack of data to support any direct link between prostate cancer and vasectomy.

Lung and Bronchus Cancer

Cancer of the lung and bronchus is currently the second most commonly diagnosed cancer and the leading cause of cancer death in the United States. It was estimated that, in 2006, cancer of the lung and bronchus would account for 13% of all cancers in men, as well as 31% of cancer deaths in men, accounting for an overall 1 in 13 lifetime risk (see Figures 24-1 and 24-2 and Table 24-2).[1] The overall incidence of lung cancer has slightly decreased in recent decades (Figure 24-3), and there has been a decline in mortality since the peak around 1990 (see Table 24-3). African American males have the highest age-standardized incidence and death rates for lung cancer (113.9 and 101.3, respectively) compared with white males (76.7 and 75.2, respectively), Asian males (59.4 and 39.4, respectively), Hispanic males (44.6 and 38.7, respectively), and American Indian/Alaskan Native males (42.6 and 47.0, respectively).[1]

The main risk factor for the development of lung and bronchus cancer is cigarette smoking, which accounts for approximately 87% of cases and is, obviously, preventable. Radon gas exposure accounts for between 15,000 and 22,000 lung cancer deaths (approximately 12%) each year in the United States.[22] Home test kits to determine radon concentration in subterranean basements can be purchased inexpensively, and one's risk of radon exposure can be determined. Other major risk factors for the development of lung and bronchus cancer include cigar and pipe smoking and secondhand smoke exposure.

The benefit of screening for lung cancer has not been established in any group, including asymptomatic high-risk populations such as older smokers. The balance of harms and benefits becomes increasingly unfavorable for persons at lower risk, such as nonsmokers. Through systematic reviews of the literature, the USPSTF, CTFPHC, and American College of Chest Physicians found insufficient evidence to recommend either for or against lung cancer screening via low-dose computerized tomography (LDCT), chest radiographs (CXR), or single or serial sputum cytology evaluations.[23–25] None of these methodologies have been proved effective to detect lung cancer at an earlier stage than would be detected in an unscreened population. These groups also concluded that there is poor evidence to suggest that any screening strategy for lung cancer decreases mortality.[23–25] Due to the invasive nature of diagnostic testing and the possibility of a high number of false-positive test results in certain populations, there may be potential for significant harms from screening for lung cancer. The sensitivity of LDCT for detecting lung cancer is four times greater than the sensitivity of CXR, but it is also associated with a greater number of false-positive results, more radiation exposure, and increased costs compared with CXR.[23]

Due to the high rate of false-positive results, many patients will undergo invasive diagnostic procedures including transbronchial biopsy and lobar resections as a result of lung cancer screening. Although the morbidity and mortality rates from these procedures in asymptomatic persons are not available, mortality rates due to complications from surgical interventions in symptomatic patients reportedly range from 1.3% to 11.6%; morbidity rates range from 8.8% to 44%, with

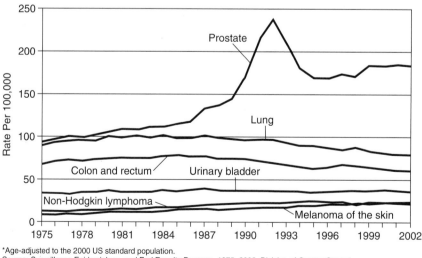

*Age-adjusted to the 2000 US standard population.
Source: Surveillance Epidemiology, and End Results Program, 1975–2002, Division of Cancer Control and Population Sciences, National Cancer Institute, 2005.

Figure 24-3. Cancer incidence rates for men, United States, 1975–2002. (From American Cancer Society: Cancer statistics 2006: a presentation from the American Cancer Society. Available at: http://www.cancer.org/downloads/STT/Cancer_Statistics _2006_Presentation.ppt. Accessed August 28, 2006.).

higher rates associated with larger resections.[23] Other potential harms of screening include potential anxiety and concern as a result of false-positive test results, as well as possible false reassurance because of false-negative results. Despite the insufficient evidence to date regarding lung cancer screening, smoking cessation should be emphasized for all patients as the preferred modality for reducing lung cancer mortality. The ACS emphasizes the importance of informed decision making for persons who elect to be tested for early lung cancer detection and recommend that testing should be performed only in experienced centers characterized by multispecialty groups with experience in testing, diagnosis, and appropriate follow-up.[4]

Colon and Rectum Cancer

Colorectal cancer (CRC) is currently the third most commonly diagnosed cancer and the second leading cause of cancer death in the United States. It was estimated that, in 2006, CRC would account for 10% of all cancers in men, accounting for an overall 1 in 17 lifetime risk (see Figures 24-1 and 24-2 and Table 24-2).[1] Risk factors for the development of CRC include increasing age, a family history of CRC, obesity, a sedentary lifestyle, a diet high in red meat and low in vegetables, and excessive alcohol or tobacco use. Several case-controlled and cohort studies have found an inverse association between physical activity and risk in men of all ages, as well as in various racial and ethnic groups in diverse geographic areas around the world.[26,27] African Americans have a higher likelihood of dying from CRC than do white persons (odds ratio, 1.4), as it has been postulated that they may have a more proximal distribution of colonic adenomas and carcinomas than the general population that may be more commonly missed on suboptimal screening (see Table 24-3).[28] Overall, deaths due to CRC have been decreasing since 1980 due to increased surveillance and screening (Table 24-4).

Approximately 75% of CRCs are diagnosed in persons who have no risk factors other than advanced age; 90% of cases occur in persons older than 50 years of age. Additional risk factors include prior or family history of CRC or adenomatous polyps, chronic inflammatory bowel disease (e.g., ulcerative colitis, Crohn's disease), and various genetic syndromes, as up to 30% of CRCs are believed to arise as the result of a

Table 24-4. Summary Comparison of Screening Modalities for Colorectal Cancer

	Fecal Occult Testing	Flexible Sigmoidoscopy	Colonoscopy	Air Contrast Barium Enema
Purpose	Chemically tests for blood in stool	Directly looks in last third of colon	Directly looks in all of colon	Uses radiograph to look in the colon
How to do it	Patient collects stool on a stick and touches the stool to a special card	Doctor inserts a 2-foot flexible instrument into the colon	Doctor inserts a 3-foot flexible instrument into the colon	Radiologist inserts air and barium into the colon, then radiographs are taken
Preparation	Small	Moderate	Intense	Intense
	Diet low in lightly-cooked meats and certain vegetables	Take a medication that stimulates a bowel movement and clear liquid diet for a day	Take a medication that stimulates a bowel movement and use an enema to clean out the stool	Take a medication that stimulates a bowel movement and use an enema to clean out the stool
Pain	None	Mild to moderate	Moderate to severe Requires anesthesia	Mild to moderate
Test accuracy	Fair	Good-limited; only 1/3 of colon seen. Limited if stool still in bowel	Excellent-limited only if bowel still has stool inside	Excellent-limited only if bowel still has stool inside
How often?	Annually	Every 5 years	Every 10 years	Every 5–7 years
Other testing involved?	If blood found, need colonoscopy	Biopsy done at time of test. If abnormal, need colonoscopy	Biopsy done at time of test	If abnormal, need colonoscopy

Adapted from: Nease DE, Stoffel E, Turgeon DK, Ruffin MT: Colorectal cancer screening, *Clin Fam Pract* 6(3):693–707, 2004.

genetic predisposition. Approximately 20% of cases occur among patients who have a history of CRC in a first-degree relative. Approximately 6% of cases are attributable to identifiable, inherited genetic mutations known as hereditary CRC syndromes (e.g., familial adenomatous polyposis and hereditary nonpolyposis CRC). Although these syndromes are relatively uncommon, they confer a lifetime risk of CRC ranging from 80% to 100%.[29]

Currently accepted screening options for CRC include fecal occult blood testing (FOBT) via the DRE or home test, flexible sigmoidoscopy, the combination of FOBT and flexible sigmoidoscopy, colonoscopy, and the double-contrast barium enema (DCBE) (see Table 24-4). Each screening option has advantages and disadvantages that vary for individuals and practice settings. Choosing a specific screening strategy should be based on patient preferences after targeted education about the various methodologies, medical contraindications, and available resources for testing and follow-up with appropriate attention to the patient's insurance coverage. According to the American Gastroenterological Association, "[T]he relative virtues of each screening test can be debated, but the best test is that one that gets done."[30] Studies reviewed by the USPSTF indicate that CRC screening is likely to be cost-effective (less than $30,000 per additional year of life gained) regardless of the specific screening strategy chosen.[31]

The FOBT is a simple, inexpensive, and minimally invasive test that can be routinely performed in the office during yearly health maintenance examinations via DRE. The DRE allows for palpation of the internal anal canal, examination of the prostate, and sampling of stool within the rectoanal vault. Whenever a DRE is performed, a stool guaiac test should be performed to assess for occult blood. The DRE itself has a very low diagnostic yield because very few colorectal tumors are discovered via this approach. Proven methods of FOBT screening use guaiac-based test cards prepared at home by patients from three consecutive stool samples that are then brought to the physician. Neither the DRE nor the testing of a single stool specimen obtained during DRE is recommended as an adequate screening strategy for CRC. A retrospective study of patients who had a colonoscopy for the evaluation of a positive FOBT result obtained by DRE and no definable gastrointestinal symptoms revealed that adding a single FOBT discovered adenomas or carcinomas in 28% of patients.[32]

Several large randomized controlled clinical trials have demonstrated that screening for CRC with FOBT reduces mortality from CRC.[33,34] The reduction found ranged from 33% using annual screening to 15% with biannual screening. The specificity and sensitivity of FOBT for CRC detection vary considerably, depending on the technique that is used for testing. FOBT screening has an advantage in that it is convenient, and compliance rates in the general population are likely to be higher than those for invasive methods. The sensitivity of a single office FOBT is likely to be substantially lower than the screening strategy of using multiple sample cards, defined as samples from three consecutive bowel movements. Recent evidence has shown concern over the quality of FOBT, finding that the one-time FOBT testing using the take-home method was only 13% sensitive for cancer, with poorer performance attributable to in-office processing of test results.[35] Patients should not take aspirin, iron, or vitamin C or consume red meat several days before undergoing FOBT to minimize the risk of false-positive results.

Flexible sigmoidoscopy has been shown to be an efficient screening tool for persons who are at an average risk for CRC, allowing for direct visualization and biopsy of the colonic mucosa in the rectosigmoid, descending, and distal transverse colon. To date, there are no randomized controlled trials or case-controlled studies that have demonstrated that screening via this method decreases CRC mortality for tumors within the reach of the standard 60-cm sigmoidoscope.[36] The limitation of this method is that advanced lesions may be missed in the ascending and proximal transverse colon in persons who do not have distal polyps. Flexible sigmoidoscopy is advocated as being more convenient than colonoscopy because the procedure is generally performed in the office without the need for conscious sedation, yet it is estimated that only 30% of eligible patients undergo screening with flexible sigmoidoscopy.[36] The combination of FOBT and flexible sigmoidoscopy may detect more cancers and more large polyps than either test alone, but the additional benefits and potential harms of combining the two tests are uncertain. In a study of US veterans that combined flexible sigmoidoscopy and FOBT, the combination strategy failed to detect 24% of advanced neoplastic lesions.[37] In general, FOBT should precede sigmoidoscopy because a positive test result is an indication for colonoscopy, obviating the need for a sigmoidoscopy.[31]

Colonoscopy provides the most complete visualization of the entire colon and is considered to be the gold standard test for CRC screening. Since more than half of all persons who have advanced proximal adenomas may not have distal polyps, many investigators advocate the use of colonoscopy as the primary modality for CRC screening.[31] The presence of neoplasms in the distal colon increases the risk of advanced neoplasia in the proximal colon. In a large Veterans Affairs study,[38] approximately 50% of patients with proximal advanced neoplasms were found to have no distal polyps; this study also found that using colonoscopy as a screening tool allowed for the discovery of advanced villous adenomas in 10.5% of subjects. The removal of precancerous adenomas decreases CRC incidence by as much as 76–90% compared with no screening methodology. Colonoscopy carries a higher risk of adverse events attributed to therapeutic interventions such as biopsy and polyp removal compared with FOBT, DCBE, and flexible sigmoidoscopy, specifically bowel perforation and postpolypectomy hemorrhage.

The sensitivities for DCBE vary widely, ranging from 50% to 80% for polyps less than 1 cm, 70–90% for polyps greater than 1 cm, and 55–85% for Dukes stage A and B colon cancers.[39] A comparison study between colonoscopy and DCBE revealed that the sensitivity of barium enema for neoplasia was significantly lower than that for colonoscopy, with a sensitivity of 32% for polyps less than or equal to 5 mm, 53% for polyps measuring 0.6–10 mm, and 48% for polyps greater than 1 cm.[40] DCBE has been combined with flexible sigmoidoscopy to improve sensitivity of the barium enema up to 99% by better visualization of the rectosigmoid area. Overall, there is no direct evidence that DCBE is effective in reducing mortality rates from CRC.[31] Any suspected lesions that are identified by DCBE need to be confirmed, biopsied, and removed by colonoscopy. Rarely, the classic "apple core" hallmark sign of a colonic mass may be visualized on DCBE.

Several novel modalities for CRC screening are currently being investigated. Virtual colonoscopy (i.e., computed tomographic [CT] colonography) uses ultra-thin-section helical-CT scans to generate high-resolution two-dimensional images that are reconstructed into three-dimensional images of the colon to evaluate for the presence of polyps. Direct comparison of CT colonography to colonoscopy in asymptomatic adults has shown sensitivity and specificity for polyp detection to be comparable to that of colonoscopy for polyps greater than 6 mm in diameter.[41] As with conventional colonoscopy, CT colonography is limited by the quality of the bowel preparation, procedural cost, lack of insurance coverage, variability in physician training, and procedural time.[36] Capsule endoscopy involves an overnight fast and the ingestion of a disposable capsule, which is usually expelled within 48 hours of ingestion. The recorded information from the capsule is then downloaded and reviewed for abnormal pathology. Molecular and biochemical stool markers are also being studied as adjunct methodologies for CRC screening. Before the advent of virtual colonoscopy, capsule endoscopy, and stool-based biomarkers as options for routine CRC screening, rigorous trials examining cost-effectiveness and long-term follow-up compared with conventional colonoscopy need to be performed. The USPSTF found insufficient evidence that these newer screening technologies are effective in improving health outcomes.[31]

Current recommendations for CRC screening for are based on the USPSTF and the American Gastroenterological Association consortium panel updated review, both of which have been reviewed and endorsed by the ACS.[4,31,42] The current recommendations state that men of average risk for CRC should be offered options for CRC screening at the age of 50 years. Surveillance screening for high-risk populations is summarized in Table 24-5. The advantages and disadvantages for each screening option should be discussed and patients should be given a choice regarding the screening modality that is best suited for them with respect to insurance coverage.

Trials studying the prevention of CRC are being largely aimed at chemoprevention and nutrition. The long-term use of aspirin may be associated with a decreased risk of CRC, yet the risk/benefit profile for chemoprevention cannot justify broad recommendations for its use in the general population.[43] Diets high in fiber, fruits, vegetables, and calcium may offer some protective benefit, yet to date these data have been inconclusive. The potential benefits of dietary fiber in the prevention of colorectal adenomas and carcinomas are not evident in randomized controlled trials with 2–4-year follow-up.[44] The daily intake of 1 g of dietary calcium may have a moderate protective effect on development of colorectal adenomatous polyps, but the evidence is insufficient to recommend general use of calcium supplements to prevent CRC.[45] Antioxidant and selenium supplementation has not been

Table 24-5. Surveillance for Colorectal Cancer in Patients at Increased Risk

Risk	When to Start Screening	Screening Intervals
Personal History		
Single, small (1 cm) adenoma	3–6 years after polypectomy	Colonoscopy every 3–5 years
Large (> 1 cm) adenoma, multiple adenomas, adenoma with high-grade dysplasia, or villous changes	3 years after initial polypectomy	Colonoscopy every 3–5 years
Curative-intent resection of colorectal cancer	1 year after cancer resection	Colonoscopy repeated at 3 years, then every 5 years
Inflammatory bowel disease Ulcerative colitis Crohn's disease	Cancer risk significantly increases 8 years after pancolitis or 12–15 years after left-sided colitis	Colonoscopy every 1–2 years with biopsies for dysplasia
Family History		
Colorectal cancer or adenomatous polyp in any first-degree relative before the age of 60	Age 40 or ten years before the youngest case in the family	Colonoscopy every 5 years
Colorectal cancer or adenomatous polyp in any first-degree relative over age of 60, or two second-degree relatives	Age 40 or ten years before the youngest case in the family	Colonoscopy every 10 years
Colorectal cancer or adenomatous polyp in two or more first-degree relatives at any age (if not hereditary syndrome)	Age 40 or ten years before the youngest case in the family	Colonoscopy every 5 years
Family history of FAP	Puberty	Colonoscopy every year, genetic counseling
Family history of HNPCC	Age 20–25	Colonoscopy every 1–2 years genetic counseling

FAP, Familial adenomatous polyposis; HNPCC, hereditary nonpolyposis colorectal cancer.
Adapted from: Nease DE, Stoffel E, Turgeon DK, Ruffin MT: Colorectal cancer screening, *Clin Fam Pract* 6(3):693–707, 2004.

recommended for gastrointestinal cancer prevention and requires further in-depth study.[45]

Skin Cancer/Malignant Melanoma

The ACS estimated that there would be 34,260 new cases of malignant melanoma in 2006, accounting for 5% of all male cancers, as well as 6990 deaths, accounting for just less than 3% of all male cancer deaths.[1] Overall, the incidence of melanoma has been increasing since the 1970s (see Table 24-3). Approximately 83% of malignant melanomas are diagnosed at a localized stage (83% in white persons, 64% in African Americans), 11% at a regional stage (11% in whites, 20% in African Americans), and 3% at a distant stage (3% whites, 12% in African Americans).[1] Five-year survival statistics have increased since 1974, most likely due to increased awareness and education, attempts at prevention, and early detection. For all races, the 5-year

survival rate from 1995 to 2001 was 92%, whereas that for white persons was 92% and that for African Americans was 76%.[1]

Risk factors for both melanoma and nonmelanoma skin cancers include the following[46]:

- Unprotected and/or excessive exposure to ultraviolet (UV) radiation
- Fair complexion
- Occupational exposures to coal tar, pitch, creosote, arsenic compounds, or radium
- Family history
- Multiple or atypical moles
- Severe sunburns as a child

The best ways to lower the risk of skin cancer are to avoid intense sunlight for long periods of time and to practice sun safety. The ACS recommends the following[46]:

- Avoid the sun between 10 AM and 4 PM.
- Look for shade, especially in the middle of the day when the sun's rays are strongest.
- Cover up with protective clothing to guard as much skin as possible when you are out in the sun.

- Choose comfortable clothes made of tightly woven fabrics that cannot be seen through when held up to a light.
- Use sunscreen with a sun protection factor (SPF) of 15 or higher, applying a generous amount and reapplying after swimming, toweling dry, or perspiring.
- Cover your head with a wide-brimmed hat, shading your face, ears, and neck.
- If you choose a baseball cap, remember to protect your ears and neck with sunscreen.
- Wear sunglasses with 99–100% UV absorption to provide optimal protection for the eyes and the surrounding skin.
- Follow these practices to protect your skin even on cloudy or overcast days because UV rays travel through clouds.

The USPSTF and the CTFPHC state that for patients at a low risk for the development of cutaneous melanoma, basal cell carcinoma, or squamous cell skin carcinoma, there is insufficient evidence to determine whether a decrease in mortality occurs with a total body skin examination (TBSE) by either primary care physicians or via self-examination (Table 24-6).[47,48] Several studies have shown that patients who have TBSEs are 6.4 times more likely to have a melanoma detected compared with patients who undergo partial skin examinations, yet no outcome data were reported.[49] The ACS recommends a cancer-related checkup, including a TBSE, at least once every 3 years in patients between 20 and 40 years of age and yearly in patients older than 40 years.[46] The American Medical Association advises patients to discuss the frequency of skin cancer screening with their physicians and perform skin self-examinations monthly, and annual skin examinations are recommended in patients at moderately increased risk.[50] The American Academy of Dermatology recommends that persons adopt a comprehensive sun protection program and

Table 24-6. Evidence-Based Approach to Skin Cancer Screening and Prevention

Practice Intervention	Effectiveness	Study Design	Evidence Recommendation
Total body skin examination (TBSE)	Not proved to be effective for normal-risk persons	Comparison of times and places	Poor evidence exists to include or exclude a TBSE in the general population.*
	For persons at increased risk (e.g., family melanoma syndrome [MM] or first-degree relative with melanoma), it is prudent to undertake regular skin examinations.	Comparison of times and places	Fair evidence exists for the inclusion of a TBSE for a select sub-group of persons.*
Self-examination	No evidence to suggest that patient ability to detect lesions or of physician ability to alter patient screening skills or behavior improves clinical outcomes.	Comparison of times and places	Poor evidence exists to include or exclude TBSE in the periodic health examination.†
Avoidance of sun exposure and use of protective clothing	Supported by evidence focusing on etiology, prudence, and low cost vs. adverse effects.	Epidemiologic and case-control studies	On the basis of data and prudence, there is fair evidence to include recommendations in the periodic health examination.*
Use of sunscreens	Studies have indicated no effect or raised concerns of increased risk among sunscreen users.	Cohort and case-control studies	Poor evidence exists for the inclusion or exclusion of advice on sunscreen use for skin cancer prevention.†

*The Canadian Task Force (CTF) concludes that there is fair evidence to recommend the clinical preventive action.
†The CTF concludes that the existing evidence is conflicting and does not allow making a recommendation for or against use of the clinical preventive action; however, other factors may influence decision making.
  Adapted from: Canadian Task Force on Preventive Health Care: CTFPHC Systematic reviews and recommendations. Available at: http://www.ctfphc.org. Accessed September 1, 2006.

perform regular self-examinations of the skin, and that any conspicuous skin changes should be evaluated.[49] The USPSTF and CTFPHC recommend that patients at a high risk of development of melanoma (e.g., patients with familial melanoma syndrome or a first-degree relative with melanoma) should be referred to a dermatologist for TBSEs and subsequent monitoring.[47,48] However, the USPSTF did not examine the outcomes related to the surveillance of these patients who are at higher risk.[51]

Expert opinion states that clinicians should remain alert for skin lesions with malignant features noted in the context of physical examinations performed for other purposes.[52] The ABCDE classification system—asymmetry, border irregularity, color variability, diameter greater than 6 mm, and/or elevation or enlargement—should alert patients and physicians to consider either biopsy or excision of concerning lesions to evaluate for potential malignancy.

Pancreatic Cancer

Pancreatic cancer is currently the tenth most commonly diagnosed cancer in men and the fourth leading cause of male cancer deaths in the United States. It was estimated that, in 2006, pancreatic cancer would account for 2% of all cancers in men, as well as 6% of cancer deaths in men (see Figures 24-1 and 24-2).[1] Due to the often late presentation, almost all patients with pancreatic cancer are expected to die from their disease. Major risk factors include advancing age, a history of tobacco or alcohol use, and chronic pancreatitis; diabetes mellitus, peptic ulcer disease, high-fat and -carbohydrate diets, and familial cancer syndromes may also play roles in the development of pancreatic cancer. Given the generally poor prognosis of patients diagnosed with pancreatic cancer, there is a significant interest in primary prevention, yet the evidence for diet-based prevention of pancreatic cancer is limited and conflicting. Some experts recommend lifestyle changes to help prevent pancreatic cancer, including the cessation of using tobacco products, moderation of alcohol intake, and adoption of a balanced diet with sufficient fruits and vegetables.[53] Persons with hereditary pancreatitis may have a higher lifetime risk for developing pancreatic cancer, yet there is no current evidence to support the routine screening of these patients.

The diagnosis of pancreatic cancer is rarely made early in the course of the disease due to the presence of vague presenting symptoms of nonspecific abdominal pain, weight loss, cachexia, and painless obstructive jaundice. Approximately 85% of patients present with either locally, advanced, or metastatic disease and have a median survival of between 3 and 12 months.[54] Pancreatic cancer may be detected via ultrasound, CT, magnetic resonance imaging, endoscopic ultrasound, endoscopic retrograde cholangiopancreatography, laparoscopy, or surgical biopsy. For patients diagnosed with pancreatic cancer, conventional treatments including surgery (e.g., Whipple procedure, pancreaticoduodenectomy) may be offered. This procedure consists of the removal of the gallbladder, common bile duct, part of the duodenum, and head of the pancreas. Radiation and chemotherapy have not been shown to have a substantially positive impact on survival. Endoscopic ultrasound and newer generation high-resolution CT allow for better preoperative selection for patients likely to benefit from exploration for resection. Only 15% of patients present with resectable disease and go to surgery. Unfortunately, the prognosis remains poor due to high local and metastatic recurrence rates, with a 5-year survival rate of less than 10%.[54]

Currently under investigation is vaccine therapy for the treatment of pancreatic cancer. Panvac VF (Therion, Cambridge, MA) is an injection with a benign virus loaded with genes culled from pancreatic cancer cells, which triggers the immune system to produce cancer-killing cells.[55] Gvax (Cell Genesys, San Francisco, CA) is another vaccine currently in phase II trials that uses an injection of pancreatic cancer cells along with a molecule designed to attract immune cells and sensitize them to deadly growth.[56] Before vaccine therapy becomes a viable standard of care in the treatment of pancreatic cancer, rigorous trials will be required.

Conclusion

Cancer continues to be a leading cause of morbidity and mortality in males in the United States and worldwide (Figure 24-4). Numerous screening strategies exist for some of the most common cancers that we encounter in primary care. Options for screening, as well as risks and benefits of various modalities, should be discussed with patients on regular intervals in an educative format, allowing patients to choose tests based on evidence-based recommendations. Every attempt to discuss cancer prevention should be taken during office visits when appropriate screening is offered.

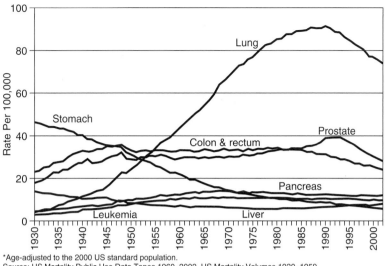

*Age-adjusted to the 2000 US standard population.
Source: US Mortality Public Use Data Tapes 1960–2002, US Mortality Volumes 1930–1959,
National Center for Health Statistics, Centers for Disease Control and Prevention, 2005.

Figure 24-4. Cancer death rates for men, United States, 1930–2002. (From American Cancer Society: Cancer statistics 2006: a presentation from the American Cancer Society. Available at: http://www.cancer.org/downloads/STT/Cancer_Statistics_2006_Presentation.ppt. Accessed August 28, 2006.)

References

1. Jemal A, Siegel R, Ward E, et al: Cancer statistics, 2006, *CA Cancer J Clin* 56(2):106–130, 2006.
2. Kochanek KD, Murphy SL, Anderson RN, Scott C: Deaths: final data for 2002, *Natl Vital Stat Rep* 53 (5):1–115, 2004. Available at: http://www.cdc.gov/nchs/data/nvsr/nvsr53/nvsr53_05acc.pdf. Accessed April 22, 2006.
3. Jemal A, Murray T, Ward E, et al: Cancer statistics, 2005, *CA Cancer J Clin* 55(1):10–30, 2005.
4. Smith RA, Cokkinides V, Eyre HJ: American Cancer Society Guidelines for the early detection of cancer, 2006, *CA Cancer J Clin* 56:11–25, 2006.
5. Canadian Task Force on Preventive Health Care: CTFPHC Systematic reviews and recommendations. Available at: http://www.ctfphc.org. Accessed April 22, 2006.
6. Mayo Foundation for Medical Education and Research: Testicular cancer. Available at: http://www.mayoclinic.com/health/testicular-cancer/DS00046. Accessed April 22, 2006.
7. US Preventive Services Task Force: *Screening for Testicular Cancer: Recommendation Statement*, Rockville, MD, 2004, Agency for Healthcare Research and Quality.
8. American Cancer Society: Testicular cancer. Available at: http://www.cancer.org/downloads/PRO/TesticularCancer.pdf. Accessed April 22, 2006.
9. Zoorob R, Anderson R, Cefalu C, et al: Cancer screening guidelines, *Am Fam Phys* 63:1101–1112, 2001.
10. Recommendations from the American Cancer Society Workshop on Early Prostate Cancer Detection, May 4–6, 2000 and ACS guideline on testing for early prostate cancer detection: update 2001, *CA Cancer J Clin* 51(1):39–44, 2001.
11. US Preventive Services Task Force: Screening for prostate cancer: recommendations and rationale, *Ann Intern Med* 137(11):915–916, 2002.
12. American Urological Association: Urology Health. org. Adult conditions: prostate. Available at: http://www.urologyhealth.org/adult/index.cfm?cat=09&topic=39. Accessed May 28, 2006.
13. Smith RA, von Eschenbach AC, Wender R, et al: American Cancer Society guidelines for the early detection of cancer: update of early detection guidelines for prostate, colorectal, and endometrial cancers, *CA Cancer J Clin* 51:38–75, 2001.
14. Smith RA, Cokkinides V, Eyre HJ: American Cancer Society Guidelines for the early detection of cancer, 2006, *CA Cancer J Clin* 56:11–25, 2006.
15. American Cancer Society: Detailed guide: can prostate cancer be found early? Available at: http://www.cancer.org/docroot/CRI/content/CRI_2_4_3X_Can_prostate_cancer_be_found_early_36.asp. Accessed May 28, 2006.
16. Berg AO: Screening for prostate cancer: recommendations and rationale, *Am J Nurs* 103(3):107–110, 2003.
17. Castle EP, Thrasher JB: The role of soy phytoestrogens in prostate cancer, *Urol Clin North Am* 29(1):71–81, 2002.
18. Fair WR, Fleshner NE, Heston W: Cancer of the prostate: a nutritional disease? *Urology* 50(6): 840–846, 1997.

19. Giovannucci E, Tosteson TD, Speizer FE, et al: A retrospective cohort study of vasectomy and prostate cancer in US men, *JAMA* 269(7):878–882, 1993.

20. Giovannucci E, Ascherio A, Rimm EB, et al: A prospective cohort study of vasectomy and prostate cancer in US men, *JAMA* 269(7):873–877, 1993.

21. Stanford JL, Wicklund KG, McKnight B, et al: Vasectomy and risk of prostate cancer, *Cancer Epidemiol Biomarkers Prev* 8(10):881–886, 1999.

22. American Lung Association: What causes lung cancer? Available at: http://www.lungusa.org/site/pp.asp?c=dvLUK9O0E&b=35427#what. Accessed May 23, 2006.

23. US Preventive Services Task Force. Lung cancer screening: recommendation statement, *Ann Intern Med* 140(9):738–739, 2004.

24. Palda VA, Van Spall HGC: *Screening for Lung Cancer: Updated Recommendations from the Canadian Task Force on Preventive Health Care,* London, Ontario, Canada, 2003, Canadian Task Force on Preventive Health Care.

25. Bach PB, Niewoehner DE, Black WC: Screening for lung cancer: the guidelines. American College of Chest Physicians, *Chest* 123(1 Suppl):83S–88S, 2003.

26. Batty D, Thune I: Does physical activity prevent cancer? Evidence suggests protection against colon cancer and probably breast cancer, *BMJ* 321(7274):1424–1425, 2000.

27. Boutron-Ruault MC, Senesse P, Meance S, et al: Energy intake, body mass index, physical activity, and the colorectal adenoma-carcinoma sequence, *Nutr Cancer* 39(1):50–57, 2001.

28. Pignone M, Rich M, Teutsch SM, et al: Screening for colorectal cancer in adults at average risk: a summary of the evidence for the US Preventive Services Task Force, *Ann Intern Med* 137(2):132–141, 2002.

29. Giardello FM, Petersen GM, Piantadosi S, et al: APC gene mutations and extraintestinal phenotype of familial adenomatous polyposis, *Gut* 40(4):521–525, 1997.

30. Burt RW, Winawer SJ, Bond JH, et al: Preventing colorectal cancer: a clinician's guide. *American Gastroenterological Association Monograph* 2004. Available at: http://www.gastro.org/edu/CRCpreventionMonograph.pdf. Accessed May 15, 2005.

31. US Preventive Services Task Force: Screening for colorectal cancer: recommendations and rationale, *Ann Intern Med* 137(2):129–131, 2002.

32. Brint SL, DiPalms JA, Herrera JL: Is a hemoccult-positive rectal examination clinically significant? *South Med J* 86(6):601–603, 1993.

33. Mandel JS, Bond JH, Church TR, et al: Reducing mortality from colorectal cancer by screening for fecal occult blood. Minnesota Colon Cancer Control Study, *N Engl J Med* 328(19):1365–1371, 1993.

34. Robinson MH, Marks CG, Farrands PA, et al: Screening for colorectal cancer with an immunological faecal occult blood test: 2-year follow-up, *Br J Surg* 83(4):500–501, 1996.

35. Imperiale TF, Ransohoff DF, Itzkowitz SH, et al: Fecal DNA versus fecal occult blood for colorectal-cancer screening in an average-risk population, *N Engl J Med* 351:2704–2714, 2004.

36. Nease DE, Stoffel E, Turgeon DK, Ruffin MT: Colorectal cancer screening, *Clin Fam Pract* 6(3):693–707, 2004.

37. Lieberman DA: the Veterans Affairs Cooperative Study Group: One-time screening for colorectal cancer with combined fecal-occult blood testing and examination of the distal colon, *N Engl J Med* 345(8):555–560, 2001.

38. Lieberman DA, Weiss DG, Bond JH, et al: Use of colonoscopy to screen asymptomatic adults for colorectal cancer. Veterans Affairs Cooperative Study Group 380, *N Engl J Med* 343(3):162–168, 2000.

39. Winawer SJ, Fletcher RH, Miller L, et al: Colorectal cancer screening: clinical guidelines and rationale, *Gastroenterology* 112(2):594–642, 1997.

40. Winawer SJ, Stewart ET, Zauber AG: A comparison of colonoscopy and double-contrast barium enema for surveillance after polypectomy. National Polyp Study Work Group, *N Engl J Med* 342(24):1766–1772, 2000.

41. Fenlon H, Nunes D, Schroy P, et al: A comparison of virtual and conventional colonoscopy for the detection of colorectal polyps, *N Engl J Med* 341:1496–1503, 1999.

42. Winawer S, Fletcher R, Rex D, et al: Colorectal cancer screening and surveillance: clinical guidelines and rationale. Update based on new evidence, *Gastroenterology* 124(2):544–560, 2003.

43. Baron JA, Cole BF, Sandler RS, et al: A randomized trial of aspirin to prevent colorectal adenomas, *N Engl J Med* 348(10):891–899, 2003.

44. Asano TK, McLeod RS: Dietary fibre for the prevention of colorectal adenomas and carcinomas, *Cochrane Database Syst Rev* 1:CD003430, 2002. DOI: 10.1002/14651858.CD003430.

45. Finnish Medical Society Duodecim: Prevention and screening of colorectal cancer. *In: EBM Guidelines: Evidence-Based Medicine* [CD-ROM]. Helsinki, Finland, 2005, Duodecim Medical Publications Ltd.

46. American Cancer Society: Skin cancer facts. Available at: http://www.cancer.org/docroot/PED/content/ped_7_1_What_You_Need_To_Know_About_Skin_Cancer.asp. Accessed May 22, 2006.

47. US Preventive Services Task Force: *Guide to Clinical Preventive Services,* ed 2, Baltimore, MD, 1996, Williams & Wilkins. Available at: http://text.nlm.nih.gov. Accessed April 30, 2006.

48. Canadian Task Force on Preventive Health Care: CTFPHC Systematic reviews and recommendations. Available at: http://www.ctfphc.org. Accessed April 30, 2006.

49. Rigel DS, Friedman RJ, Kopf AW, et al: Importance of complete cutaneous examination for the detection of malignant melanoma, *J Am Acad Dermatol* 14(5 pt 1):857–860, 1986.

50. American Medical Association: Cancer screening guidelines [searched under "skin cancer"]. Available at: http://www.ama-assn.org. Accessed May 20, 2006.

51. Berg AO: Screening for skin cancer: recommendations and rationale, *Am J Prev Med* 20(3 Suppl): 44–46, 2001.

52. Scottish Intercollegiate Guidelines Network: *Cutaneous Melanoma: A National Clinical Guideline,* Edinburgh, Scotland, 2003, Scottish Intercollegiate Guidelines Network.

53. US Preventive Services Task Force (USPSTF): *Screening for Pancreatic Cancer: Recommendation Statement,* Rockville, MD, 2004, Agency for Healthcare Research and Quality.

54. Jafari M, Abbruzzese JL: Pancreatic cancer: future outlook, promising trials, newer systemic agents, and strategies from the Gastrointestinal Intergroup Pancreatic Cancer Task Force, *Surg Oncol Clin N Am* 13:751–760, 2004.

55. Therion Biologics: Pancreatic cancer program. Available at: http://www.therionbio.com/studies/pancreatic_cancer.asp. Accessed April 22, 2006.

56. Cell Genesys: New treatment strategies. Available at: http://www.cellgenesys.com/clinicaltrials-pancreatic-cancer.shtml. Accessed April 22, 2006.

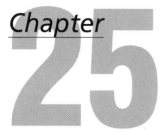
The Aging Male/End-of-Life Issues

Lourdes Velez, MD

Key Points

- Men experience more difficulties in discussing their health issues, are less inclined to seek help, and postpone healthcare until they reach more advanced stages of disease (strength of recommendation: C).
- Ethnogeriatrics allows clinicians to focus on sociologic and cultural differences, fostering a better understanding of how to provide adequate services for aging populations across various racial groups (strength of recommendation: C).
- Compared with men of other racial and ethnic populations, African American men are more likely to live alone and are less likely to live with a spouse, with recent studies showing an increase in older adults living in nursing homes (strength of recommendation: C).
- Primary care of the homebound elderly requires a seamless integration of a variety of disciplines including medical, nursing, and social work, along with the assistance of family, friends, and neighbors to prevent illness and injury and to ensure a safe home environment (strength of recommendation: C).
- Effective communication is essential to providing high-quality end-of-life care to discuss the patient's illness and prognosis, to develop a care team to include family and friends, and to provide ongoing support, especially during the last hours of living (strength of recommendation: C).

"Old age; it isn't bad when you consider the alternative."

—Maurice Chevalier, 1888–1972

Introduction

Aging is a statistical inevitability that provides challenges for healthcare providers of male patients regarding numerous biopsychosocial issues. Simply stated, the average male worldwide is living longer, will die with more chronic diseases and taking more medications, and will require more resources as he ages, through the end of his life. This chapter examines the epidemiology of the aging US population with an emphasis on the aging male and the inherent gender differences. Statistics on aging are examined from the multicultural angle of ethnogeriatrics, analyzing future population trends and how they will transcend society. Options for end-of-life care will be examined from home care to nursing home care, highlighting principles of specialized palliative and hospice care.

Epidemiology

According to data from *A Profile of Older Americans: 2004* compiled by the US Department of Health and Human Services,[1] older adults aged

65 years and older numbered 35.9 million, or 12.4% of the US population (about one in every eight Americans), in 2003. Since 1900, the percentage of older Americans has tripled from 4.1% to 12.4%, and this population has increased 11-fold, from 3.1 million to 35.9 million. The older population itself is aging, with the 65–74-year age group (18.3 million) being eight times larger than in 1900, the 75–84-year age group (12.9 million) 17 times larger, and the 85-years-and-older age group (4.7 million) an astonishing 38.5 times larger. The older population will expand even greater between the years 2010 and 2030 when the "baby boom" generation reaches age 65. By the year 2030, the population older than 65 years will be more than twice their respective number in 2000, approaching 71.5 million people. In 2002, persons reaching the age of 65 years had an average life expectancy of an additional 18.2 years; life expectancy in the United States was 74.5 years for men and 79.9 years for women (Table 25-1). Older women outnumber older men at 21.0 million to 14.9 million (approximately 140 women for every 100 men). A child born in 2002 can expect to live approximately 77.3 years or almost 30 years longer than a child born in 1900.

Many theories have been proposed to explain the gender differential in longevity. Some theories are derived from studies of the animal kingdom, whereas others stem from the study of people aged 100 years and older. From the role of testosterone in the immune system of male mammals to the role of age at childbirth, sex hormones, the Y chromosome, and menopause, this predilection

for longevity in women is multifactorial with significant implications for the prevention, diagnosis, and treatment of disease.

Urinary incontinence, with a 2:1 female-to-male ratio, is an example of how gender affects disease. In men, urinary incontinence is often caused by bladder outlet obstruction, whereas in women it is associated with risk factors related to the female pelvic anatomy and physiology. How men and women differ in their responses to pain and various pain therapies is not well understood. Women tend to have a lower pain threshold and tolerance for pain and are more likely to be inadequately treated for their pain. Physiologically, women respond differently to the effects of medication for treatment of heart disease. In general, women have higher rates of nonfatal illnesses and chronic conditions, allowing them to remain sicker yet live longer than men. Women are at a higher risk of developing diseases including irritable bowel syndrome, diabetes mellitus, osteoporosis, and autoimmune diseases; major depression, anxiety, anorexia nervosa, and bulimia are also more common in women. Men are less likely than women to report symptoms of depression, making the impact of this condition greater and the likelihood that they (men) will complete suicide more frequently.[2]

Gender, the socially constructed roles and learned behaviors associated with femininity and masculinity, has significant implications for health and well-being. Lifestyle behaviors such as smoking and drinking, occupational hazards, and other risk-taking behaviors contribute to the early onset of cardiovascular disease, cancer, emphysema, liver and kidney disease, and injury in men. In addition, older men face special challenges as they grow older and retire. Once autonomous, independent, and self-reliant, they soon find themselves dependent on others for care. As a group, they are less often prepared to face the challenges that come with the end of a working career because their identities are intimately connected to their work. Research suggests that men experience more difficulties in discussing their health issues, are less inclined to seek help, and postpone healthcare until they reach more advanced stages of disease.[3]

Chronic diseases have replaced acute infections as the major causes of death in older adults. Heart disease, cancer, stroke, and chronic lower respiratory diseases (e.g., chronic bronchitis, emphysema and asthma) are the top four leading causes of death in the United States.[4] In 2003, Alzheimer disease surpassed diabetes, influenza, and pneumonia as a leading cause of death; other

Table 25-1. Top Ten Countries With the Highest Life Expectancy in Years, 2002

Men	Women
Japan, 77.8	Japan, 85.0
Iceland, 77.6	Hong Kong, China, 82.7
Sweden, 77.5	France, 82.7
Hong Kong, China, 77.2	Spain, 82.7
Israel, 77	Sweden, 82.5
Canada, 76.6	Switzerland, 82.3
Australia, 76.4	Australia, 82.0
Norway, 75.9	Italy, 81.9
Cyprus, 75.9	Iceland, 81.9
Switzerland, 75.9	Canada, 81.9
United States, 74.5	United States, 79.9

Adapted from: Gorina Y, Hoyert D, Lentzner H, Goulding M: Trends in causes of death among older persons in the United States. Aging Trends, No. 6. Hyattsville, MD, 2006, National Center for Health Statistics.

leading causes include kidney disease, accidents, and septicemia. Pneumonia remains a leading cause of mortality among men and women aged 85 years and older.[4]

Between 1990 and 2002, all-cause mortality declined for most groups of older adults. Death rates decreased by 12% among persons in the 65–74-year age group and by 7% for those in the 75–84-year age group. Declines were higher for men than for women. For those people aged 85 years and older, the all-cause mortality rate increased 1% for women and declined approximately 9% in men. Heart disease and stroke experienced the most significant decline, and cancer death rates decreased more among men than women.[4]

Accidents remain an important cause of death for older adults, with falls (with rates increasing since 1993), motor vehicle crashes, suffocation, and burns accounting for the majority of unintentional injury deaths. Old age has been identified as one of the highest factors of suicide in the elderly. Although suicide rates have declined for persons aged 65 years and older, they remain higher for older white men than for any other group, including teenagers; the major mechanism for suicide is firearms.[4]

Aging

"Will you still need me, will you still feed me, when I'm sixty-four."

—Paul McCartney

People are living longer today thanks to successful public health policies and advances in medical science. Medicine has been extremely successful in prolonging life expectancy but not in addressing the social and cultural problems of old age. Aging is defined as an inescapable attribute of life that we cannot change or manipulate because it carries social meaning affecting attitudes, behaviors, and the way people relate to one another. To reach a certain age in life implies a certain level of maturity, accomplishment, and status. To be 21 years old is to reach adulthood, in contrast to the age of 65 years often being defined as reaching old age.

The aging process carries a unique set of physical, economic, and social challenges. *Ageism* is a term coined by Butler in 1968 to describe prejudice against the elderly, a form of bigotry defined as prejudice by one group toward another age group. This is especially prevalent in America where youth, action, and power are valued over

contemplation, reflection, experience, and the wisdom of age. Aging is often viewed as a negative attribute carrying a multitude of myths and stereotypes. Older adults are usually lumped into a category reflected by the use of expressions such as "little old ladies" and "grumpy old men." Whether this is the result of health, economic issues, or cultural expectations is an ongoing debate.

In contrast to this perception, research demonstrates that older adults are a diverse group of mostly active and independent people. There has been an upward trend in labor force participation for both women (since the mid 1980s) and men (since the mid 1990s), including persons aged 70 years and older. In 2003, 5.0 million (14.4%) Americans aged 65 years and older were in the labor force working or actively seeking work, including 3.3 million men (18.3%) and 2.1 million women (10.7%).[1]

Only 31% (10.5 million) of community-dwelling older adults live alone (7.8 million women and 2.7 men). Approximately 643,000 grandparents aged 65 years and older maintained households in which grandchildren were present, with approximately 416,000 grandparents having the primary responsibility for the grandchildren who lived with them.[1]

Successful aging is to reach extreme old age with little disability, a new paradigm focusing on primary and secondary prevention of functional morbidity and premature mortality. Oral health, vision, and hearing impairments are often overlooked components of an older person's overall health, well-being, and quality of life. Although more older people are keeping their natural teeth, there are currently no federal or state dental insurance programs to cover routine dental care; in 1995, only 22% of older persons were covered by private dental insurance.[7] Common problems associated with poor oral health include oral pain; difficulty eating because of missing teeth, ill-fitting dentures, cavities, gum disease, or infection; and the obvious negative aesthetic and functional (e.g., speech, chewing, eating) consequences of total tooth loss.[7] *Visual impairment,* defined as vision loss that cannot be corrected by glasses or by contact lenses alone, increases the risk of falls and subsequent fractures in the elderly. Most common causes of visual impairment and blindness are due to cataracts (more prevalent among women), age-related macular degeneration (the leading cause of irreversible visual impairment in the elderly), glaucoma, and diabetic retinopathy. For persons aged 70 years and older, macular degeneration is more common in women than in men. Older men are at the highest risk of developing a hearing impairment. Risk factors for age-related hearing loss include exposure to loud noises over long periods of time, smoking, history of middle ear infections, and long duration of exposure to certain chemicals including trichloroethylene, a colorless liquid commonly used as a solvent in cleaning metal parts.[8]

In general, men should be screened for hypertension, dyslipidemia, prostate and colorectal cancer, obesity and malnutrition, alcoholism, depression, memory loss, and vision and hearing deficits. All men should be counseled at least annually regarding diet, physical activity, safety and injury prevention, smoking cessation, and routine optometry and dental care; evidence-based guidelines are lacking to support recommendations regarding the frequency of routine optometry and dental care in the elderly. Counseling regarding physical activity should emphasize the advantages of promoting motility and decreasing rates of coronary artery disease and osteoporosis. A balanced exercise program includes exercises for flexibility (e.g., stretching), endurance (e.g., walking and cycling), strength (e.g., weight training), and balance (e.g., tai chi and dance). Immunizations should be an integral part of the preventive healthcare of all older adults and should include influenza, pneumonia, and tetanus vaccinations when appropriate according to standard guidelines (see Chapter 1, Organizing Preventive Healthcare in Men).

Ethnogeriatrics

"If the United States is a melting pot, the cultural stew still has a lot of lumps."

—Geri-Ann Galanti

Minority populations are projected to represent 26.4% of the elderly population in 2030, an increase from 17.6% in 2003. Between 2000 and 2030, the white population aged 65 years and older is projected to increase by 77% compared with 223% for older minorities. Persons of Hispanic origin are projected to increase by 324%; African Americans 164%; American Indians, Eskimos, and Aleuts 207%; and Asians and Pacific Islanders 302% of the older adult population over this time period.[1]

The term *Hispanic* reflects an ethnic category used by the US Census that is defined as "a person of Cuban, Mexican, Puerto Rican, South or Central American or other Spanish Culture or origin regardless of race." There is regional variation in the use of the terms *Hispanic* and *Latino*,

with the word *Hispanic* being used more frequently in the Eastern regions and *Latino* in the Western regions of the United States. Hispanic/Latino elderly persons are a significantly diverse group, each one with a unique historical and sociopolitical reality; it is dangerous and mistaken to assume that they are all alike. Spanish language is the most commonly shared characteristic and is often a significant barrier to acquiring adequate medical and social services in the United States. There is a difference between native and foreign-born elderly Hispanic/Latino persons, with the native group generally having more education, personal income, and fewer difficulties with mobility and instrumental activities of daily living. Like non-Hispanic elderly groups, this group includes more women than men older than 65 years of age. According to 2000 Census figures (www.census.gov), they are only second to Asian/Pacific Islanders in living with their relatives. Whether this is the result of healthcare issues or economic inevitability is an ongoing debate.

Hispanic/Latino elderly persons are less likely to live in nursing homes, and studies have suggested that family members care for older adults with significant disease for as long as they can before they are placed in nursing facilities.[9] Data from the Hispanic Health and Nutrition Examination Survey[9] determined that the most common causes of death in this population include coronary artery disease, cerebrovascular disease, cancer, and chronic obstructive pulmonary disease (similar to national data for all racial groups), as well as an increased prevalence of diabetes in all Hispanic groups. The use of healers and complementary and alternative medicine is often mentioned but poorly studied in the older populations. Healing systems include *curanderismo* (Mexican folk healing), *espiritismo* (Puerto Rican faith healers), and *santeria* (Cuban faith healers). Hispanic/Latino persons generally believe that there is little or no control over natural forces and tend to have a present-time orientation, making them less likely to engage in preventive care and concentrating their efforts and thoughts on surviving today.[10]

According to the 2000 Census (www.census.gov), a significant number of black persons identified themselves as "Black, African American or Negro." This category includes persons born in the United States as well as immigrants from Haiti and other islands in the Caribbean, South and Central America, and Africa. Compared with men of other racial and ethnic populations, African American men are more likely to live alone and less likely to live with a spouse, with recent studies showing an increase in older adults living in nursing homes.[11] Prostate cancer is common among African American men, and both glaucoma and dementia have higher rates in older African Americans. Heart disease, cancer, and cerebrovascular disease are all more common causes of mortality than in age-matched white persons, Asian/Pacific Islanders and Hispanic/Latino persons; diabetes is a common cause of morbidity and mortality in African Americans, with only the incidence in American Indians exceeding this racial group.[11]

American healthcare culture values autonomy and independence, often leading to conflict in the care of older adults. Cultures that value family over the individual usually prefer to make decisions as a group, emphasizing interdependence over independence. The way in which patients and families react and express emotions at the time of illness and death can often trigger antagonism with the medical staff. To avoid miscommunication, professional interpreters should be used in place of family members to translate dialogue between patients and clinicians, medical jargon should be avoided, and healthcare staff must be sensitive to communication styles, demeanor, eye contact, gesturing, touching, and health beliefs and complementary practices.[12]

Home Care

Number of centenarians that the US Census counted in 2000: 50,740

Projected number it will count in 2050: 1,149,500

—*Harper's Index,* February 2006

More than one half of community-dwelling older adults live with their spouses. Of the 21.6 million households headed by older adults, 80% are owners and 20% renters. Independence and the ability to stay in control of their lives and homes are fundamental to older adults. Primary care of a homebound elderly person requires seamless integration of a variety of disciplines including medical, nursing, and social work along with assistance of family, friends, and neighbors to prevent illness and injury and to ensure a safe home environment. Whether home care is ultimately cheaper than nursing home placement is a matter of much heated debate; although it is often highly dependent on the patient's degree of disability, it nonetheless decreases nosocomial infections, enhances human dignity, and ensures psychological well-being.

In addition to the usual health maintenance recommendations, home care providers need to remain alert to changes in cognitive status within the older population, signs of physical abuse and neglect, depression, suicide risk factors, abnormal bereavement, and the ways the use of both prescription and nonprescription medications may increase the risk of falling.

A recent study investigated sense of belonging as a predictor of reasons for living in community-dwelling adults aged 61–95 years. The study found that a higher sense of belonging predicted more reasons to live overall, in addition to more child-related concerns, greater responsibility to family, and more survival and coping beliefs, specifically.[13]

Nursing Home Care

The care of aged persons has been historically intertwined with the care of the poor and destitute. During colonial times, almshouses were public poor houses caring for parentless children, mentally retarded and insane patients, the infirm aged, and any stranger in the community who lacked family. With the passage of the Social Security Act of 1935, residents of public institutions were prohibited from receiving payments under the Old Age Assistance of the Social Security Act, leading to the development of a private, largely for-profit nursing home industry. Today, a relatively small number (1.56 million) of persons aged 65 years and older live in nursing homes. This percentage (4.5%) increases dramatically with age, ranging from 1.1% for persons 65–74 years to 4.7% for persons 75–84 years, and 18.2% for those older than 85 years. In addition, approximately 5% of older adults live in senior housing of various types, many of which have supportive services for their residents.[1]

Data analysis from the National Mortality Followback Survey[14] indicates that, over a lifetime, the risk of entering a nursing home and spending a long time there is substantial. It is projected that for persons who turned 65 years old in 1990, 43% will enter a nursing home at some time before they die with 55% spending at least 1 year and 21% 5 years or more. More women than men will enter nursing homes and will have a total lifetime nursing home use of 5 years or more.[15] The average age at the time of admission to a nursing home has increased from 81.1 years in 1985 to 82.6 years in 1997, with an increase in the number of African American residents from 6% to 10%.[16]

Although cardiovascular disease remains the most common diagnosis listed at the time of admission, moderate to severe cognitive impairment with behavioral problems (e.g., hitting,

wandering, being unable to keep oneself safe), incontinence, and functional decline remaining strong predictors for nursing home placement. Other common disorders listed on admission include Alzheimer disease, cerebrovascular disease, mood and anxiety disorders, type 2 diabetes mellitus, and hypothyroidism.

Over the years, the passage of several congressional bills has provided public funds for the construction of nursing facilities, requiring the development of laws to regulate and monitor those institutions financed by public programs. Faced with reports of substandard care and pressure from organized consumer groups, US Congress passed the Nursing Home Reform Amendments of the Consolidated Omnibus Budget Reconciliation Act (COBRA) of 1987, creating an oversight system for the nursing home industry and significantly affecting medical practice within such nursing facilities. Major areas of COBRA provide regulations concerning resident assessment and care planning, the use of physical restraints, pharmacotherapy with special attention to the use of psychotropic medications, resident's rights, and overall quality-of-care standards. In addition, changes in Medicare payments to hospitals under diagnosis-related groups provided substantial financial incentives for shorter hospital stays that in turn increase the transfer of patients to skilled nursing facilities to complete rehabilitation programs.

There are two main categories of medical care in the nursing home: skilled nursing care or rehabilitation and long-term nursing care. Additionally, hospice care is offered in many facilities through working collaboration and affiliation with community hospice agencies.

Skilled nursing care provides an option after an acute inpatient stay for those patients with significant complex medical illnesses and functional deficits that impair their ability to return home in an independent and safe manner. Common services provided include intravenous therapy, extensive wound care, and physical, occupational, and speech therapy. Typically, patients spend several days or weeks up to 6 months in this type of setting. Long-term nursing care is offered to patients who are unable to live independently in the community due to the need for 24-hour supervision and assistance with activities of daily living (e.g., bathing, dressing, eating, walking, transferring from a bed to a chair, and toileting, including the ability to get to the bathroom). Since 1985, more nursing home residents require assistance with activities of daily living than was previously documented.

Federal regulations require nursing homes to hire the services of a physician medical director to oversee the medical care of the residents and of a consultant pharmacist to review the medications administered to patients to avoid harmful drug interactions or potentially inappropriate drug prescription. Other requirements include the creation of quality assurance and infection control committees and the development of written policies and procedures covering a broad variety of issues from food handling to the evacuation of residents and how and when to notify a physician of changes in the resident's condition. Routine nursing home visit notes should begin by addressing both the resident and staff concerns, reviewing any changes in care given since the last visit, and updating the patient's medical problem list. Medication review and how each drug relates to each problem and diagnosis are essential to avoid inappropriate drug use. Indications for psychotropic use and physical restraints need to be documented carefully, including regular reassessments to discontinue their use.

Care at the End of Life

"Loveliest of what I leave behind is the sunlight, and loveliest after that the shining stars, and the moon's face, but also cucumbers that are ripe, and pears and apples."

—Praxilla, early to mid fifth century B.C.

Before the era of antibiotics, Americans died quickly, predominantly due to accidents and infectious diseases. Medicine focused on caring and support and, depending on cultural variations, the sick were generally cared for at home. Improved sanitation, antibiotics, and other therapies have allowed us to fight illness and death aggressively, leading to prolongation of life at all cost. Culturally, there has been a shift in values where death is seen mostly as an enemy to defeat; there is a sense of failure when a patient is not saved.

Although modern medicine has afforded us a cure for only a few select illnesses, Americans are generally healthier and live longer with more chronic diseases than decades ago. Older adults living in 1900 usually died at home, most medical expenses were paid by the family, and little disability was present before death. Today, the usual place of death is the hospital, although research has demonstrated that most people want to die at home when death is the expected outcome of care.[17] Most medical expenses are paid by Medicare, and most healthcare expenditures are concentrated in the years just before death with an

Table 25-2. Medications Used During the Last Hours of Life

Drug	Dosage	Notes
Lorazepam	1–2 mg buccal mucosal, PR, SL, SQ, IV, q1h to titrate, then q4–6h to maintain	If paradoxical agitation is observed, choose a non-benzodiazepine for sedation
Haloperidol	2–5 mg PR, SQ, IV q1h to titrate, then q6h to maintain	Relatively non-sedating at low doses; may require 10–30 mg daily to sedate
Chlorpromazine	10–25 mg PR, IV q4–6h	Parenteral route may require special exemptions from standard nursing policy in some settings
Scopolamine (hyoscine hydrobromide)	10–100 µg/h SQ, IV continuous infusion or 0.1–0.4 mg SQ q6h or 1–10 patches q72h	Transdermal preparation only; delivers approximately 10 µg/h and takes many hours to reach therapeutic levels
Glycopyrrolate	0.2–0.4 mg SQ q2–4h and titrate	Does not cross blood-brain barrier

PR, Per rectum; SL, sublingual; SQ, subcutaneous; IV, intravenous.
Adapted from: Ferris FD: Last hours of living, *Clin Geriatr Med* 20:641–667, 2004.

average of 2 years of disability before death.[18] A recent cross-sectional analysis of data regarding place of death for centenarians in England and Wales between 1995 and 1999 showed that for women home was the most frequent place of death, whereas for men it was the hospital.[19]

What we know of how people die in the hospital is based on a controlled trial from 1995 to improve the care of seriously ill hospitalized patients at five tertiary care teaching hospitals.[20] The study examined data from 9000 patients with life-threatening illnesses, of whom 50% died within 6 months of admission. Physical suffering at the end of life, communication about goals of medical care, concordance of care with patient and family preferences, and family and caregiver financial, physical, and emotional burden were studied. Forty percent of do-not-resuscitate (DNR) orders were written within 2 days of death, and of those patients preferring a DNR status, fewer than 50% made their doctors aware of their wishes. Three hundred and eighty-five of those patients who died spent more than 10 days in an intensive care unit. One half of the patients in this study had moderate to severe pain at the end of life. Patients required large amounts of family caregiving while family caregivers lost most of their family savings.

Other studies have documented pain and discomfort ratings for common hospital life.[21] Nasogastric tubes, mechanical ventilation, central line placement, and arterial blood gases are rated as causing moderate to severe pain in hospitalized patients. Burdensome, nonpalliative interventions such as laboratory testing, therapeutic interventions, artificial nutrition, and hydration are still received by dying patients with cancer and end-stage dementia.

Palliative and hospice care are part of the continuum-of-care model that begins at the time of

diagnosis of a chronic terminal disease and ends long after the patient's death with family support and education throughout their mourning process. Palliative medicine focuses on adequate pain and symptom management (Table 25-2), promoting function and avoiding inappropriate prolongation of the dying process. Care focuses on providing the best possible quality of life as determined by the patient, helping him or her to achieve a sense of control over his or her death, clarifying goals of care, relieving decision-making burden for the family, and strengthening relationships with loved ones (Table 25-3). Effective communication is

Table 25-3. Principles of a Good Death

To know when death is coming and to understand what can be expected
To be able to retain control of what happens
To be afforded dignity and privacy
To have control over pain relief and other symptom control
To have choice and control over where death occurs (at home or elsewhere)
To have access to information and expertise of whatever kind is necessary
To have access to any spiritual or emotional support required
To have access to hospice care in any location, not only in the hospital
To have control over who is present and shares the end
To be able to issue advance directives which ensure wishes are respected
To have time to say goodbye, and control over other aspects of timing
To be able to leave when it is time to go, and not to have life prolonged pointlessly

Adapted from: Smith R: A good death, *BMJ* 320:129–130, 2000.

essential to the provision of high-quality end-of-life care requiring family meetings to discuss the patient's illness and prognosis; the development of a care team to include family and friends; discussing rites, rituals, and funeral and memorial services; and providing ongoing support, especially during the last hours of living. How people die and how well end-of-life signs and symptoms are managed remain a vivid memory for most family members and friends left behind (Table 25-4).

Table 25-4. Physiologic Changes During the Dying Process

Physiologic Changes	Signs and Symptoms
Fatigue, weakness	Decreased function and hygiene Inability to move around in bed Inability to lift head off of pillow
Cutaneous ischemia	Erythema over bony prominences Skin breakdown Decubitus wounds and ulcers
Pain	Facial grimacing Tension in forehead and between eyebrows
Decreased food intake, wasting	Anorexia Aspiration, asphyxiation Weight loss, muscle and fat wasting (e.g., notable in facial temples)
Loss of ability to close eyes	Eyelids not completely closed White of eyes showing (with or without pupils visible)
Decreased fluid intake, dehydration	Poor intake Aspiration Peripheral edema due to hypoalbuminemia Dehydration, dry mucous membranes/conjunctiva
Cardiac dysfunction, renal failure	Tachycardia Hypertension followed by hypotension Peripheral cooling Peripheral and central cyanosis (bluing of extremities) Mottling of skin (livedo reticularis) Venous pooling along dependent skin surfaces Dark urine Oliguria, anuria
Neurologic dysfunction, including decreasing level of consciousness	Increasing drowsiness Difficulty awakening Nonresponse to verbal tactile stimuli
Decreased ability to communicate	Difficulty finding words Monosyllabic words, short sentences Delayed or inappropriate responses Lack of verbal response
Respiratory dysfunction	Change in ventilatory rate—increasing first, then slowing down Decreased tidal volume Abnormal breathing patterns—apnea, Cheyne-Stokes respirations, agonal breaths
Loss of ability to swallow	Dysphagia Coughing, choking Loss of gag reflex Buildup of oral and tracheal secretions Gurgling
Loss of sphincter control	Incontinence of urine or bowels Maceration of skin Perineal candidiasis
Terminal delirium	Early signs of cognitive failure (e.g., day-night reversal) Agitation, restlessness Purposeless, repetitious movements Moaning, groaning
Rare, unexpected events	Bursts of energy just before death occurs (e.g., the "golden glow") Aspiration, asphyxiation

Adapted from: Ferris FD: Last hours of living, *Clin Geriatr Med* 20:641–667, 2004.

Four simple phrases have been suggested to help facilitate life-closure conversations and the last good-bye: "Please forgive me," "I forgive you," "Thank you," and "I love you." In the end, these are the four things that matter most.[22]

Conclusions

As the worldwide male population lives longer, clinicians will be challenged with managing more complex medical and psychosocial issues for their patients and families. Clinicians must strive for cultural competency when caring for various ethnic groups, understanding and respecting key variations in cultures; this will serve to enhance communication and the overall care provided. The economic burden of end-of-life care appears to be staggering, with overall poor federal and state provisions at the present time. Discussions regarding end-of-life issues between the primary care clinician and the patient and their families, including long-term placement for rehabilitation and chronic care, as well as in-home care and palliative and hospice care, are of paramount importance.

References

1. Administration on Aging: *A Profile of Older Americans: 2004*, US Department of Health and Human Services, 2004. Available at: www.aoa.gov/PROF/Statistics/profile/2004/2004profile.pdf
2. Pinn VW: Sex and gender factors in medical studies, *JAMA* 289:397–400, 2003.
3. Kalache A: Gender and ageing, *Aging Male* 7(1):13, 2004.
4. Gorina Y, Hoyert D, Lentzner H, Goulding M: Trends in causes of death among older persons in the United States, *Aging Trends*, No 6, Hyattsville, MD, 2006, National Center for Health Statistics.
5. Butler RN: Age-ism: another form of bigotry, *Gerontologist* 9:243–246, 1969.
6. Butler RN: *Why survive? Being Old in America*, Baltimore, MD, 1985, Johns Hopkins University Press.
7. Vargas CM, Kramarow EA, Yellowitz JA: The oral health of older Americans, *Aging Trends*, No. 3, Hyattsville, MD, 2001, National Center for Health Statistics.
8. Desai M, Pratt LA, Lentzner H, Robinson KN: Trends in vision and hearing among older adults, *Aging Trends*, No. 2, Hyattsville, MD, 2001, National Center for Health Statistics.
9. National Center for Health Statistics: Hispanic Health and Nutrition Examination Survey, HHANES. Available at: http://www.cdc.gov/nchs/about/major/nhanes/hhanesrrm.htm. Accessed October 9, 2006.
10. Yeo G, editor, *Core Curriculum in Ethnogeriatrics: Health and Health Care of Hispanic/Latino American Elders*, ed 2, October 2000. Available at: www.stanford.edu/group/ethnoger.
11. Yeo G, editor, *Core Curriculum in Ethnogeriatrics: Health and Health Care of African American Elders*, ed 2, October 2000. Available at: www.stanford.edu/group/ethnoger.
12. Galanti GA: *Caring for Patients from Different Cultures*, ed 2, Philadelphia, 1997, University of Pennsylvania Press.
13. Kissane M, McLaren S: Sense of belonging as a predictor of reasons for living in older adults, *Death Studies* 30:243–258, 2006.
14. National Center for Health Statistics: National Mortality Followback Survey. Available at: http://www.cdc.gov/nchs/about/major/nmfs/nmfs.htm. Accessed October 9, 2006.
15. Kemper P, Murtaugh CM: Lifetime use of nursing home care, *N Engl J Med* 324:595–600, 1991.
16. Sahyoun NR, Pratt LA, Lentzner H, et al: The changing profile of nursing home residents: 1985–1997, *Aging Trends*, No. 4. Hyattsville, MD, 2001, National Center for Health Statistics.
17. The Gallup Organization: *Knowledge and Attitudes Related to Hospice Care: Survey Conducted for the National Hospice Organization*, Princeton, NJ, 1996, The Gallup Organization.
18. Lynn J, Adamson DM: *Living Well at the End of Life*, Washington, DC, 2003, RAND Health.
19. Lock A, Higginson I: Patterns and predictors of place of cancer death for the oldest old, *BMC Palliative Care* 4:6, 2005.
20. The SUPPORT Investigators: A controlled trial to improve care for seriously ill hospitalized patients, *JAMA* 274:1591–1598, 1995.
21. Morrison RS, Ahronheim JC, Morrison GR, et al: Pain and discomfort associated with common hospital procedures and experiences, *J Pain Symptom Manage* 15:91–1001, 1998.
22. Byock I: *The Four Things That Matter Most*, New York, 2004, Free Press.

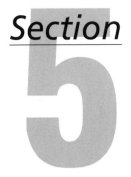
Special Populations of the Adolescent and Adult Male

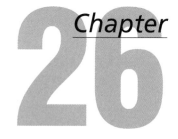
The Collegiate/Professional Male Athlete

Michael Kernan, MD, Bhuvana Raja, MD, and Jason Matuszak, MD

Key Points

- The American Heart Association (AHA) suggests that a complete cardiac evaluation should be performed in competitive athletes at a minimum of once every 2 years; the National Collegiate Athletic Association (NCAA) requires participants to undergo an initial, comprehensive preparticipation physical evaluation (PPE) upon entrance to their respective academic institutions, including a comprehensive health history, relevant physical examination, and orthopedic evaluation (strength of recommendation: C).
- PPEs are poorly predictive of which athletes are at an increased risk of orthopedic injuries (strength of recommendation: B).
- An athlete should appropriately warm up and stretch before exercise and should use cushioned insoles and appropriate footwear when training to prevent musculoskeletal injury (strength of recommendation: C).
- Any athlete who demonstrates symptoms of airway hyper-reactivity during practice or competition, whether previously diagnosed with EIA/EIB or not, must be removed from activity, promptly evaluated, and provided with emergency treatment (strength of recommendation: B).
- CT scans, MRI scans, and EEGs, although invaluable in identifying more severe intracranial pathology, are typically insensitive to measuring the subtle neuronal aspects of MTBI; their false-negative results often provide an errant basis on which return-to-play decisions are made (strength of recommendation: B).

- The use of ergogenic aids in competitive athletes should be discouraged by physicians (strength of recommendation: C).
- Creatine can be an effective ergogenic supplement maximized when used for simple, short-duration, maximal-effort anaerobic events (strength of recommendation: C).

Introduction

Collegiate and professional male athletes deserve special attention in a textbook dedicated to men's health. Many primary care physicians have a working relationship with athletics at some level. Although most will not be caring for a large population of elite athletes, more often than not primary care physicians will have some competitive athletes in their practice. This chapter highlights some of the key concepts and common medical problems encountered by collegiate and professional athletes.

Preparticipation Evaluation

More than three decades ago, in an effort to decrease the number of catastrophic events in athletes, the preparticipation physical evaluation (PPE) was born. At that time the "exam" consisted of a brief interview, a quick cardiac examination, and an awkward hernia check in males. Since then the PPE has evolved, but the desire remains the same: to effectively screen athletes to maximize their ability to participate and compete in sports safely. The latest version of the PPE is the combined work of the American Academy of Family Physicians, the American Academy of Pediatrics, the American Medical Society for Sports Medicine, the American Orthopaedic Society for Sports Medicine, and the American Osteopathic Academy of Sports Medicine, with contributions from the American Heart Association (AHA).[1,2]

Although still not universally required for participation,[3] expert opinion states that a PPE should be conducted to serve several functions. First, it should screen for conditions that would preclude or modify an athlete's ability to participate because the athlete would be placed at an elevated risk for potential life-threatening or disabling conditions. Additionally, this examination should detect any injuries incompletely or improperly rehabilitated, assess for general health and fitness, serve as an opportunity to practice preventive medicine, screen for performance-enhancing substance use and abuse, and satisfy legal and liability concerns.[1,4–8] This interchange between the athlete and physician also allows the physician to discuss proper diet and conditioning, maintenance of proper hydration, injury prevention, and education regarding the use of ergogenic aids.[9]

No current recommendations exist dictating who should perform PPEs. A survey by Pfister and colleagues[10] found that at the National Collegiate Athletic Association (NCAA) level, 75% of examinations are performed by orthopedic surgeons. The pitfall that can arise in this atmosphere is that orthopedic surgeons may be less familiar with the non-musculoskeletal portions of the PPE.

Timing and Frequency

Several authors and the recommendations made by the AHA suggest that a complete cardiac evaluation should be performed in competitive athletes at a minimum of once every 2 years. Many still prefer, or are required by state law, to have annual examinations.[3,10] The NCAA requires participants to undergo an initial, comprehensive PPE upon entrance to their respective academic institutions, including a comprehensive health history, relevant physical examination, and orthopedic evaluation. Each year thereafter, they are to submit to an interim history, and limited additional examinations may be performed if necessitated by new problems. There are not, however, standardized forms for NCAA member institutions to complete during PPEs.[11]

Most sports medicine professionals believe that the PPE should be performed approximately 6 weeks before participation in a competitive sport. This time frame will generally allow for proper investigation of any abnormalities discovered, without being constrained by the timing of the athletic season.[1,6,7,12] Difficulty may arise for collegiate athletes who live a great distance from their school and participate in fall sports. Although an examination performed before a student leaves school in the spring may often be substituted, it is important to address problems that arise over the summer. Several schools use Web-based forms to allow student-athletes to complete the interval history portion of the evaluation while still at home.[13,14]

Professional athletes may have more extensive and frequent evaluations with more diagnostic tests performed as a direct result of the economics of professional sports and inherent investment in its players. The unique situation of professional athletes also raises several ethical issues including who medical information really belongs to and who should have access to it. One National Football League (NFL) director of player personnel was quoted as saying, "The most important part of the [pre-draft] combine is the medical information. The physical exams are thorough."[15] At the NFL combine, for example, radiographs are taken of all of players' previous injuries, knee strength is tested, a urinalysis is performed, and a detailed physical examination with a particular emphasis on the orthopedic aspects is administered.[16] There is also a new question regarding which tests an athlete can be subjected to. For example, Eddy Curry, a center in the National Basketball Association (NBA), was traded after refusing genetic testing.[17] Frequency of examinations is variable, with boxers having to undergo a thorough evaluation before each fight.

Format

The two most common types of PPEs are the station-based mass screening and the office-based individual examination. The station-based format offers distinct advantages in that it is more cost and time efficient, allowing a provider to focus on one particular portion of the examination (e.g., cardiac exam only) for each of the many athletes screened. It offers the opportunity to use particular skills of examiners and allows for better communication among coaches, athletes, and the medical team. A study conducted by DuRant and colleagues[18] revealed that multiple examiners in a station-based format were more likely to find an abnormality than an individual performing the entire physical examination and were more likely to refer the athlete for more testing. The advantages of an office-based assessment include better continuity of care and having the potential for a long-standing patient-physician relationship.

The disadvantages of station-based examinations include lack of time and privacy, an uncomfortable environment, and the possibility of loss to follow-up if there are pertinent findings. Office-based physical examinations can be problematic if the athlete lacks a primary care physician or has limited financial means. In addition, there can be a lack of communication between the physician and the coaches; primary care physicians also have different levels of comfort in determining clearance for athletes.[1]

Medical History

An accurate and complete medical history is of paramount importance to uncovering reasons why an athlete may not be able to participate. Studies have demonstrated that up to 75% of all disqualifying conditions are revealed during the medical history.[9] The history places a particular emphasis on cardiac and musculoskeletal concerns[8,19] but should also include prior head injuries or other neurologic problems[9,20,21]; recent significant illnesses[9,20]; ongoing or chronic illnesses[9,21,22]; pulmonary complaints[9,21,22]; the use of prescription and nonprescription medications[1,9]; the use of supplements, vitamins, or other performance enhancers[1,9]; and allergies, skin problems, and psychosocial issues.[9,20] A history of heat illness is an emerging area of interest in the preparticipation history.[21]

Cardiovascular History

There is considerable and ongoing debate regarding the best method used to screen for the possibility of sudden cardiac death in athletes. Many authors have widely encouraged the use of universal electrocardiography (ECG) for athletes, whereas others desire two-dimensional echocardiography.[19] The proponents of such measures point to data including the demonstration that up to 90% of people with hypertrophic obstructive cardiomyopathy (HOCM) have an abnormal ECG result.[19]

A multitude of studies have investigated the effectiveness of various cardiovascular screening tests. The evidence-based review by Wingfield and colleagues[23] found that of the 12 original studies that looked at specific cardiovascular screening techniques, there was a division on the effectiveness of history, physical examination, ECG, and echocardiography for detecting risk of sudden death. Seto[19] has devised a battery of questions that providers can use when taking a thorough cardiac history (Table 26-1). The AHA has recommended that the screening of athletes at all ages be performed with a cardiovascular history that addresses the following points[24]:

- Sudden death in a family member younger than 50 years of age
- Prior heart disease in the family
- Exertional dyspnea or chest pain
- Syncope
- Excessive fatigability
- Heart murmur
- Systemic hypertension
- Parental verification of history

It is imperative for the clinician performing the PPE to remember that athletes want to compete and that they may not fully divulge all pertinent medical information if they believe it will keep them from competition. For younger participants, possibly even college student-athletes, recommendations suggest asking the athlete's parents to complete the questionnaire.[19,25]

Table 26-1. Screening Questions for Cardiovascular History in the Preparticipation Examination

1. Have you ever become dizzy or passed out during or after exercise?
2. Have you ever had chest pain during or after exercise?
3. Do you get tired more quickly than your friends do during exercise?
4. Have you ever had racing of your heart or skipped heartbeats?
5. Have you had high blood pressure or high cholesterol?
6. Have you ever been told that you had a heart murmur?
7. Has any family member or relative died of heart problems or sudden death before age 50?
8. Have you had a severe viral infection such as mononucleosis or myocarditis within the last month?
9. Has a physician ever denied or restricted your participation in sports for any heart problems?
10. Have any of your relatives ever had any of the following conditions? a. Hypertrophic cardiomyopathy b. Dilated cardiomyopathy c. Marfan syndrome d. Long QT syndrome e. Significant heart arrhythmia

Adapted from: Seto CK: Preparticipation cardiovascular screening, *Clin Sports Med* 22:23–35, 2003.

Because diseases such as HOCM, long QT syndrome, premature coronary artery disease, and Marfan syndrome can all be inherited, any family history of these diseases should result in a further workup through specialist evaluation. Thirty percent of people with HOCM have a positive family history of sudden cardiac death at age younger than 50 years.[19,21]

Athletes who already have a specific cardiovascular condition may determine their eligibility for various sports by consulting with their physician, in conjunction with the 36th annual Bethesda Conference recommendations, *Eligibility Recommendations for Competitive Athletes with Cardiovascular Abnormalities,* which are the most current eligibility recommendations for competi-

tive athletes with cardiovascular abnormalities[24] (Table 26-2).

Musculoskeletal History

Although cardiovascular problems in competitive athletes are exceedingly rare but nevertheless potentially devastating, musculoskeletal injuries are common, especially in contact and collision sports. A thorough musculoskeletal history should elicit information regarding all previous injuries, particularly those involving ligaments. Documentation should be made regarding whether surgery was required, the type and duration of rehabilitation, and return-to-play time. The NCAA Injury Surveillance System collects injury data from a representative sample of

Table 26-2. Cardiac Abnormalities and Bethesda Conference Recommendations

Abnormality	Recommendation
Hypertrophic obstructive cardiomyopathy	**No competitive sports;** possible exception of low-static, low-dynamic, low-intensity (class 1A) sports
Congenital coronary anomalies	**No competitive sports;** 6 months after corrective surgery, athlete may participate if maximal stress test is passed
Marfan syndrome	**No collision sports;** echocardiogram every 6 months to assess for aortic root dilatation or mitral regurgitation
Coarctation of aorta	Untreated: If mild (< 20 mm Hg difference, maximum SBP during exercise < 230) **allow all sports,** otherwise class IA only
	Treated: First 6 months, **no competitive sports;** at 6–12 months, mild, all but class III (A, B, and C) and high-collision sports
Aortic stenosis (AS)	Mild AS: **All sports;** yearly evaluations of severity
	Moderate AS: **Class IA sports** (select athletes—class IA, IB, IIA)
Arrhythmogenic right ventricular dysplasia	**No competitive sports,** possible exception of class IA
Brugada syndrome	**Class IA sports only**
Mitral valve prolapse (MVP)	**Allow all sports** unless prior syncope, sustained or repetitive SVT, severe mitral regurgitation, LVEF <50%, prior embolic event, or family history of MVP-related sudden death. If any of these, then **Class IA sports only.**

		INCREASING STATIC COMPONENT		
		I	II	III
INCREASING DYNAMIC COMPONENT	A	Billiards, bowling, cricket, curling, golf, riflery	Archery, auto racing, diving, equestrian, motorcycling	Bobsledding/luge, gymnastics, martial arts, sailing, climbing, water skiing, weight lifting, windsurfing
	B	Baseball, fencing, table tennis, volleyball	Football, figure skating, rodeo, rugby, sprinting, surfing	Body building, downhill skiing, snowboarding, wrestling
	C	Badminton, cross-country skiing, field hockey, race walking, racquet sports, long-distance running, soccer	Basketball, ice hockey, lacrosse, swimming	Boxing, cycling, canoeing, decathlon, rowing, triathlon

SBP, Systolic blood pressure; SVT, supraventricular tachycardia; LVEF, left ventricular ejection fraction.
Both adapted from: Maron BJ, Zipes DP, editors: Eligibility recommendations for competitive athletes with cardiovascular abnormalities: general considerations, 36th Bethesda Conference, *J Am Coll Cardiol* 45(8):1318–1321, 2005.

member institutions every year. Practice and game injuries are analyzed to determine incidence and trends of injuries. A reportable injury is any injury that "occurs as a result of participation in an organized intercollegiate practice or game; requires medical attention by a team athletic trainer or physician; and results in a restriction of the student-athlete's participation or performance for one or more days beyond the day of injury."[11]

The epidemiology of sports injuries has already helped to reduce catastrophic injuries. For example, football rules have been changed to disallow helmet collisions such as "spearing" and "butt blocking" (despite the name, it refers to blocking a player with the helmet) and to prevent "chop blocks."[6] These actions are now 15-yard penalties in football at all levels, which is a considerable penalty. Players can also be disqualified at the official's discretion and, at the professional level, even fined.

Remainder of the History

The neurologic history should focus on whether the athlete has experienced any concussions, episodes of unconsciousness on the field, head or neck injuries, stingers or burners, or seizure disorders. The pulmonary history must include screening questions for exercise-induced asthma (EIA) and primary spontaneous pneumothorax.[9,26] History of heat illness including heat cramps, exhaustion, and stroke needs to be documented because this may place the athlete at higher risk for having further difficulties, particularly if there is documented history of heat stroke or more than two episodes of heat exhaustion[27]; the guidelines for evaluation and management of heat-related illness appear in Table 26-3.[28] Medications the athlete is taking may place him

at an increased risk for suffering illnesses or injuries.

The history is a time to focus on psychosocial issues facing the athlete including stress, anxiety, depression, and the use of performance enhancers and other risky behaviors as mentioned above. Also, a thorough immunization history should be obtained and prophylactic vaccinations (e.g., combined tetanus, diphtheria, pertussis vaccine; Menactra) administered, if necessary.

Physical Examination

Cardiovascular Examination

According to the AHA, an examination of the cardiovascular system in athletes needs to include the following[29]:

- Precordial auscultation with the patient in both standing and supine positions to assess for rate, rhythm, and murmurs
- Assessment of presence of femoral pulses to exclude coarctation of the aorta
- Brachial blood pressure measured with the patient in a seated position in the standard manner
- Evaluation for the physical stigmata of Marfan syndrome (e.g., long arms, arachnodactyly, hyperextensible joints, kyphoscoliosis, pectus excavatum)

Musculoskeletal Examination

The 90-second orthopedic screening examination in conjunction with a negative history for musculoskeletal symptoms is a good screening tool for an asymptomatic athlete.[30] It consists of observing the athlete performing a series of maneuvers

Table 26-3. Evaluation and Treatment of Heat-Related Illnesses

Heat Cramps	Heat Exhaustion	Heat Stroke
- Any muscle group	- Occurs when the body is no longer able to continue to exercise in the heat	- **Medical emergency**
- Frequent in lower extremities, abdomen, and intercostals	- Weakness, fatigue, sweating, nausea, vomiting, thirst, headache	- Extreme hyperthermia—core temp $\geq 104°F$ (often 107–108°F)
- Painful tightening or spasm from long and intense exercise	- Mild mental status changes—confusion, agitation, incoordination	- Thermoregulatory failure
- No change in mental status	- Body temperature	- CNS dysfunction
- Easily treated	- **No long-term harmful effects reported**	- Hot, flushed, dry skin with failed sweat mechanism Progressive moderate to severe mental status changes (e.g., delirium, seizures, coma)

CNS, Central nervous system.
Adapted from: Wexler RK: Evaluation and treatment of heat-related illnesses, *Am Fam Phys* 65(11):2307–2314, 2002.

and assessing overall musculoskeletal health. The athlete is asked to do the following:

- Look up, side to side, and down, touch ears to shoulders (cervical spine range of motion)
- Shrug shoulders against resistance, adduct shoulders to 90 degrees (i.e., hold against resistance), followed by internal and external rotation of shoulders at 90 degrees (trapezius and deltoid strength, shoulder range of motion)
- Flex and extend elbows, pronate and supinate, with elbows flexed to 90 degrees with arms at side (elbow and wrist range of motion)
- Spread fingers apart, make a fist (hand function, any rotational deformities)
- Contract and relax quadriceps muscles (knee symmetry, patellar function, quadriceps mechanism)
- Duck-walk away from and toward examiner (hip, knee, and ankle function)
- Touch toes with legs straight (scoliosis evaluation, hamstring flexibility)
- Stand on toes; stand on heels (leg and foot strength, calf symmetry)

In an evaluation of NCAA division IA athletes, a 2-minute (12-step) orthopedic screening examination, similar to the 90-second screening described above, was found to have a sensitivity of 50.8% and a specificity of 97.5% in identifying orthopedic problems, with a sensitivity of 91.6% in identifying problems through history.[1,31]

Other Aspects of the Physical Examination

A targeted physical examination in a competitive athlete should include attention to the following:[20]

- Height/weight (body mass index if indicated for a particular sport, e.g., wrestling)
- Eyes (visual acuity, anisocoria)
- Oral cavity (assessing dentition), ears, nose
- Lungs
- Abdomen (masses, tenderness, organomegaly, single kidney)
- Genitalia (single or undescended testicle, mass, hernia)
- Skin (rashes, infectious lesions)

Outcomes of the Preparticipation Examination

Experts from various medical fields and associations recommend a thorough PPE for all athletes, yet there is some debate regarding whether this examination in fact decreases morbidity and

mortality or improves outcomes at all. A systematic review of 310 studies on PPE in athletes younger than 36 years of age that appeared in *The Journal of Family Practice* in 2005[32] revealed some surprising results: to date, there were no prospective cohort studies or randomized trials addressing the effectiveness of the PPE, nor was there any medium- or better-quality evidence that demonstrated that it reduces mortality or morbidity. A *British Medical Journal* article[33] found that PPEs were not good screening tests because the accuracy of the PPE could not be determined. One case series reviewed 158 sudden deaths of trained athletes from 1985 to 1995 and determined that 115 had undergone a standard PPE. Of those 115, only 4 were suspected of having a cardiovascular abnormality, with 1 athlete identified prospectively with the cardiovascular abnormality ultimately responsible for the patient's death.[32,34]

Also in this review, PPEs were evaluated on their ability to determine exercise-induced bronchospasm (EIB) in athletes. One prospective cross-sectional study of 352 adolescents in suburban Washington State demonstrated EIB in 9.4% of athletes tested with a 7-minute exercise challenge spirometry, whereas none were identified by physical examination alone. A questionnaire used to screen for EIB showed a sensitivity of 71% and a specificity of 47%.[32,35]

A cross-sectional study revealed that PPEs were poorly predictive of which athletes were at an increased risk of orthopedic injuries. This study determined that a history of knee or ankle injury and an abnormal finding on examination in male athletes slightly increased the likelihood of repeated injury of the same joint. A previous knee injury or knee surgery was significantly associated with further knee injuries during the subsequent sports season when compared with persons who did not report previous knee injury or surgery (30.6% versus 7.2%; $P = .0001$). However, the sensitivities of history or physical examination for ankle or knee injuries were all less than 25%.[32,33,36] This study suggests a more effective and standardized screening tool than the PPE as it is currently formatted may be necessary.

Cardiovascular Diseases
Sudden Death in Athletes

According to legend, Pheidippides was a Greek soldier who ran from the town of Marathon to Athens to announce that the Persians had been defeated in the Battle of Marathon. Upon proclaiming, "Rejoice. We conquer!" he fell dead.[37] This is one of the earliest documented stories of sudden death in an athlete, but it is probably a mixture of historical events.

Sudden death in young athletes is a rare occurrence, with an incidence of approximately 1 in 100,000–300,000.[19,23] According to the NCAA, more than 360,000 collegiate athletes compete annually, and one study[38] found nine cases of sudden cardiac arrest in intercollegiate athletes occurring between 1999 and 2005. There have also been several professional athletes who have died suddenly either on the field or immediately afterward within the past few years.[19,32,34,37] Mortality rates from sudden death in athletes are approximately five to nine times higher in males than in females.[1,9]

Sudden cardiac death is defined as a nontraumatic, nonviolent, unexpected event resulting from sudden cardiac arrest within 6 hours of a previously witnessed state of normal health.[32] When sudden death has a cardiovascular etiology, it is most often due to congenital anomalies including HOCM, coronary artery abnormalities, and increased cardiac mass. Other reported causes include myocarditis, arrhythmogenic right ventricle, acute heart failure, coronary artery disease, mitral valve prolapse, idiopathic dilated cardiomyopathy, and prolonged QT syndrome[23] (Table 26-4). HOCM is the most common cause of sudden death in young athletes younger than 30 years of age,[24] and 95% of all sudden deaths in athletes younger than the age of 30 years are the result of a structural cardiac abnormality.[19,23,32,34,37] Most congenital anomalies that can predispose an athlete to sudden cardiac death have long been disqualifying conditions[24]; however, researchers are currently examining the potential for athletes to participate in many sports using implantable cardiac defibrillators.[39] As mentioned previously, the 36th Bethesda Conference guidelines make standard recommendations for athletes attempting to compete with known cardiac diseases or congenital anomalies[24] (see Table 26-2).

Athletic Heart Syndrome

For the last few decades, it has been well noted that intense regular training leads to changes in heart structure in athletes. It becomes important for physicians dealing with competitive athletes to be familiar and comfortable assessing athletic heart syndrome (AHS). Different sports place a

Table 26-4. Common Cardiovascular Causes of Sudden Death in Athletes

1. Cardiomyopathies
   a. Hypertrophic cardiomyopathy
   b. Arrhythmogenic right-ventricular dysplasia or cardiomyopathy
   c. Dilated cardiomyopathy
   d. Idiopathic left ventricular hypertrophy

2. Commotio cordis

3. Congenital malformation of coronary arteries
   a. Coronary artery aberrancies and anomalies
   b. Intramural coronary artery (myocardial bridging)

4. Coronary artery disease

5. Myocarditis

6. Aortic rupture
   a. Marfan syndrome
   b. Coarctation of aorta

7. Valvular heart disease
   a. Aortic stenosis
   b. Mitral valve prolapse

8. Arrhythmias and conduction system abnormalities
   a. Long QT syndrome
   b. Wolff-Parkinson-White syndrome
   c. Idiopathic ventricular tachycardia

9. Use of illicit drugs

Adapted from: Maron BJ, Pelliccia A, Spirito P: Cardiac disease in young trained athletes: insights into methods for distinguishing athlete's heart from structural heart disease, with particular emphasis on hypertrophic cardiomyopathy, *Circulation* 91(5): 1596–1601, 1995; and Vasamreddy CR, Ahmed D, Gluckman TJ, Blumenthal RS: Cardiovascular disease in athletes, *Clin Sports Med* 23:455–471, 2004.

range of stresses on the cardiovascular system, resulting in the various changes seen.[24,40–43]

According to Maron and colleagues,[24] dynamic exercise is isotonic in nature and is the type of exercise performed by endurance-trained athletes. It leads to a substantial increase in oxygen demand by the large muscle mass performing predominately aerobic metabolism. A resultant increase in cardiac output, heart rate, stroke volume, and systolic blood pressure occurs, with a moderate increase in mean arterial pressure and a decrease in diastolic blood pressure. In addition, total peripheral resistance drops considerably. These changes cause a volume load on the left ventricle and eventually lead to left ventricular chamber enlargement with a smaller increase in left ventricular wall thickness, or a resultant eccentric hypertrophy. There are several sports that are dynamic in nature but have high resistance components such as cycling, rowing sports, cross-country skiing, and swimming. These sports cause large increases in both chamber size and wall thickness. It has been widely touted that Lance Armstrong (seven-time winner of the Tour de France) has a heart that is a full 30% larger than average for his height.[44]

Static exercise is isometric in nature and is the type of exercise performed by athletes who are strength trained. It leads to a relatively small increase in oxygen consumption because most high-intensity static exercise is performed anaerobically. Small increases in cardiac output and heart rate are seen because stroke volume remains relatively unchanged. The largest differences are seen in pressure load on the heart, as there are great increases in systolic, diastolic, and mean arterial pressure, without any change in total peripheral resistance. This leads to increases in left wall thickness with a relatively modest left ventricular chamber enlargement. These changes are similar to what would be expected in patients with hypertension and is a concentric hypertrophy.

The physician's responsibility to the athlete is to determine whether an enlarged heart is due to the physiologic response to intense exercise or a pathologic condition that may hasten morbidity and mortality. The results of a physical examination may help give the clinician clues regarding the diagnosis, but they are by no means definitive. A low body-fat percentage with increased muscle mass, a slow pulse rate with or without sinus arrhythmias, lateral displacement of point of maximal impulse, and low diastolic blood pressure are common findings in athletes with AHS. Also important to note is that this syndrome is commonly a reversible condition, with an athlete's heart returning to its normal size after a period of inactivity (for some this takes longer than others). Multiple studies have demonstrated the decrease in ventricular septal thickness and in cavity dimensions through deconditioning.[45,46]

A two-dimensional echocardiogram is a good first test useful for distinguishing between AHS and HOCM. Important features that can help in differentiating these two syndromes include the following[47,48]:

1. HOCM generally shows normal left ventricular chamber size (less than 45 mm) but abnormal wall thickness (greater than 14 mm).
2. Left atrial enlargement may be seen in HOCM but not usually in AHS.
3. Left ventricular diastolic internal dimensions are generally less than less than

60 mm in AHS (although up to 10–15% can be greater).
4. Normal diastolic function is noted on blood flow velocity examination in AHS.
5. Left ventricular wall thickness, while enlarged in AHS, is generally less than 12 mm, with 2% of highly trained athletes having thicknesses of 12–14 mm and very few having less than 15 mm.
6. Preservation of systolic function or left ventricular ejection fraction (LVEF) is present in HOCM less than 50% without segmental wall motion abnormalities is characteristic of AHS.
7. Changes associated with deconditioning occur in AHS; generally several months of deconditioning will result in reduced wall thickness.

Exercise stress testing may further distinguish athletes who can safely compete from those who cannot. It has been demonstrated that persons with borderline left ventricular wall thickness who were able to perform greater than 50 mL/kg/min maximum oxygen consumption (greater than 14 metabolic equivalents of the task [METs]) during stress testing were unlikely to exhibit genetic alterations compatible with HOCM.[49] Some genetic tests are available to aid in the diagnosis of HOCM and are useful in patients with a family history of HOCM, although there is debate as to whether carrying the genetic marker alone is reason for disqualification in the absence of phenotype.[50] The recent 36th Bethesda guidelines suggest that persons with preclinical HOCM (i.e., genotype-positive, phenotype-negative) not be restricted from activity.[24] However, these persons require frequent and continued observation including, on a 12–18-month basis, serial two-dimensional echocardiography, 12-lead ECG, and ambulatory Holter ECG. Less frequently, cardiac magnetic resonance imaging (MRI) and exercise stress testing to a level similar to that expected in the sport under consideration should also be performed. Without question, a cardiologist should follow-up with these persons.[24] Also, it should be noted that a freestanding automated external defibrillator should not be considered as absolute protection against sudden death and should by no means be used as a prospectively designed treatment strategy for known cardiovascular disease.[24]

Cardiac Rhythms and Dysrhythmias

Athletes may, at baseline, have a significant number of ECG abnormalities that are not pathologic (Table 26-5).[24,47] This likely results as a product

Table 26-5. Electrocardiogram Abnormalities Commonly Seen in Athletes*

Sinus bradycardia (as low as 30–40 beats/min)
Atrioventricular block - First-degree block - Mobitz type I - Mobitz type II (Wenckebach)
Increased voltage of R or S waves (25–29 mm)
U waves and early repolarization changes with up-sloping ST segments with normal T waves
Incomplete right bundle branch block
Inverted T waves

*All of these arrhythmias commonly normalize with exercise in athletes.

Adapted from: Maron BJ, Zipes DP, editors: Eligibility recommendations for competitive athletes with cardiovascular abnormalities: general considerations, 36th Bethesda Conference, *J Am Coll Cardiol* 45(8):1318–1321, 2005; and Vasamreddy CR, Ahmed D, Gluckman TJ, Blumenthal RS: Cardiovascular disease in athletes, *Clin Sports Med* 23:455–471, 2004.

of high resting vagal tone and bradycardia in combination with increased cardiac mass.[43] For a clinician unfamiliar with these normal irregularities, it can lead to an unnecessary workup in athletes. These alterations usually revert with exercise. For example, a marathon runner with a resting heart rate of 42 beats/min may have ECG evidence for Mobitz type IIA heart block. When placed on an exercise treadmill test, the ECG will revert to normal sinus rhythm. Dysrhythmias, including atrial fibrillation and supraventricular tachycardia, are common in the athletic population (Table 26-6).[24] Many do not

preclude participation according to recommendations set forth by the Bethesda Conference.[24]

Myocarditis

Inflammation of the myocardium resulting from viral illness (predominately Coxsackie virus and, secondarily, parvovirus and adenovirus) has been linked to the sudden death of some athletes. Myocarditis involves a lymphocytic infiltration of the myocardium leading to interstitial edema, focal myocyte necrosis, and replacement fibrosis. If an athlete experiences a flu-like prodrome with a new onset of chest pain, exertional dyspnea, fatigue, syncope, or palpitations, it should raise the clinical suspicion of myocarditis. Some patients may present with overt acute heart failure.

The following laboratory tests may show abnormal results in an athlete with myocarditis: a complete blood count may demonstrate leukocytosis and eosinophilia; erythrocyte sedimentation rate will be elevated; serum myocardial enzyme levels, including creatine kinase (CK, plus CKMB), troponin I, and troponin T, may be elevated. An ECG will often demonstrate diffuse, low-voltage ST-T wave changes and also has been shown to demonstrate heart block and ventricular arrhythmias. Echocardiography can show a dilated left ventricle, global hypokinesis or segmental wall abnormalities, or decreased LVEF. When there is doubt regarding the diagnosis, endocardial biopsy, often with polymerase chain reaction of viral genomes, can be performed.[24]

Current recommendations state that the athlete should withdraw from all competition for 6

Table 26-6. Common Dysrhythmias in Athletes and Recommendations for Participation

Arrhythmia	Recommendation
Sinus node disturbances (e.g., bradycardia, sick sinus syndrome)	If symptoms require pacemaker, then **no collision sports**, otherwise no treatment needed.
Premature atrial contractions	**No restrictions to activity.**
Atrial fibrillation/flutter	If no structural disease is present and athlete is rate controlled, then **low-intensity sports** are permitted. If athlete is free of arrhythmia for 6 months, then **full participation is permitted.**
Supraventricular tachycardia	If no structural disease is present, no syncope or pre-syncope is present, and events are prevented with medication, then **no restrictions.**
Wolff-Parkinson-White syndrome (pre-excitation)	If no structural disease is present and athlete is asymptomatic, **no restrictions.** If premature ventricular contractions worsen with exercise, **restrict activity.** If pre-excitation and long QT interval are present, **restrict activity.**
Heart block	If no structural disease is present and athlete is asymptomatic, **no restrictions.** If symptoms require pacemaker, **no collision sports permitted.**
Congenital long QT syndrome	**Restricted from all competitive sports.**

Adapted from: Maron BJ, Zipes DP, editors: Eligibility recommendations for competitive athletes with cardiovascular abnormalities: general considerations, 36th Bethesda Conference, *J Am Coll Cardiol* 45(8):1318–1321, 2005.

months upon probable or definitive diagnosis of myocarditis because of the danger of sudden death. After the 6-month period, the athlete may return to activity if he meets the following criteria[24]:

1. Left ventricular function, wall motion, and cardiac dimensions return to normal both at rest and with exercise.
2. Clinically relevant arrhythmias are absent on ambulatory Holter monitoring and graded exercise testing.
3. Serum markers of inflammation and heart failure have normalized.
4. The 12-lead ECG has normalized. (Some ST-T wave changes may persist, but they are not alone a reason for continued restriction.)

Musculoskeletal Disorders

Musculoskeletal injuries are divided into those that are chronic/overuse injuries and those that are acute. This section focuses on common orthopedic problems of collegiate and professional athletes that would be seen or managed in the primary care setting.

Stress Fractures

Stress fractures are exceedingly common injuries that often are managed by primary care physicians. They should be suspected anytime an athlete presents with localized bone or periosteal pain, especially if the athlete has begun a new or more demanding exercise regimen. Other risk factors include participation in running and jumping sports (lower extremity stress fractures) or throwing sports (upper extremity), rapid increase in a physical training program, poor preparticipation physical condition, low bone turnover rate, decreased bone density, decreased cortical thickness, nutritional deficiencies, extremes of body size and composition, running on irregular or angled surfaces, inappropriate footwear, inadequate muscle strength, poor flexibility, and "type A" behavior.[51]

The diagnosis of a stress fracture can often be made clinically by identifying localized bone pain that increases with weight bearing or repetitive use. Confirmation is made via nucleotide bone scan or MRI, which may better characterize the stress fracture with superiority over conventional bone scans. Plain film radiographs are often unrevealing but are typically performed initially to rule out more severe injury. Common sites for stress fractures with their associated sports are listed in Table 26-7.[51]

Table 26-7. Common Sites of Stress Fractures and Associated Sports

Location	Associated Sports
Upper extremity	
Humerus	Throwing and racquet sports
Coracoid process of scapula	Trapshooting
Olecranon	Throwing/pitching
Ulna	Racquet sports, gymnastics, swimming
Torso	
First rib	Throwing/pitching
Second to tenth ribs	Rowing/kayaking
Pars interarticularis	Gymnastics, ballet, volleyball, diving
Pubic ramus	Distance running, ballet
Lower Extremity	
Femoral neck	Distance running, jumping, ballet
Femoral shaft	Distance running
Patella	Running, hurdling
Tibial plateau	Running
Tibial shaft	Running, ballet
Fibula	Running, aerobics, ballet
Medial malleolus	Basketball, running
Calcaneus	Marching (military)
Talus	Pole vaulting
Navicular	Sprinting and middle-distance running, hurdling, jumping, football
Metatarsal	Running, ballet, marching, tennis
Sesamoids	Running, ballet, basketball, skating

Adapted from: Bruckner P, Khan K: Sports related injuries and stress fractures. In *Clinical Sports Medicine,* ed 3. 2005. Available at: http://www.clinicalsportsmedicine.com/chapters/2.htm.

Prevention

The old adage, "An ounce of prevention is worth a pound of cure" is quite illustrative when discussing stress fractures. Prevention is best accomplished by gradually increasing exercise slowly, approximately 10% of effort and intensity per week, often with the athlete starting his conditioning before the start of the season. A recent Cochrane review concluded through a review of meta-analyses and randomized controlled trials that an athlete should appropriately warm up and stretch before exercise and use cushioned insoles and appropriate footwear when training.[51]

Treatment

Conservative therapy for stress fractures generally involves resting the affected area until the athlete is pain free, often requiring up to 6–8 weeks; the athlete should be pain free for 2–3 weeks before restarting his usual workout regimen. Other conservative management options include non-steroidal anti-inflammatory drugs (NSAIDs), cryotherapy, stretching, and flexibility exercises. To maintain proper conditioning, the athlete can participate in cross-training (non–weight-bearing) exercise.

Several stress fractures require more aggressive or alternative management. For example, femoral neck fractures, if displaced, require surgical fixation, and if non-displaced require bed rest for 1 week followed by gradual return to weight bearing. If a tension-type femoral fracture is diagnosed, then internal fixation is necessary. Other stress fractures requiring special attention include the following[51,52]:

- Navicular
  - Six weeks of short leg (non–weight-bearing) cast, followed by 4–6 weeks of transitional weight-bearing cast
  - Gradual return to full weight-bearing with a semi-rigid shoe
  - Intramedullary nailing if nonunion or delayed union
  - Return to sport after 16–20 weeks (often a season-ending injury)
- Fifth metatarsal
  - Case immobilization or percutaneous screw recommended due to high incidence of nonunion
- Tibial
  - Aircast splinting*
  - Casting for mid-shaft fractures until patient is pain free
  - Intramedullary nailing and/or grafting if anterior tibial cortex shows no improvement after 6 months
- Metatarsal, base of the second and sesamoid bone of the foot
  - 4 weeks, non–weight-bearing cast
- Talus (lateral process)
  - 6 weeks of non–weight-bearing cast
  - Immobilization/surgical excision of fragment

---

* According to a recent Cochrane Review, there is a likely benefit to using an Aircast splint for tibial and fibular stress fractures with a faster return to sports participation.[51]

Common Orthopedic Injuries by Tissue Type

Bone

Acute, traumatic injury to bone often results in a fracture. Various types of fractures include open, closed, comminuted, avulsion, greenstick, torus, and epiphyseal fractures. Depending on the bone involved, the management varies from open reduction and internal fixation to simple casting. Chronic or overuse injury of bone can result in stress fractures as discussed above and can also lead to apophysitis in skeletally immature athletes.

Joints

Dislocation and subluxation can result when there is direct trauma to a joint or its supporting structures. A *dislocation* is defined as a complete displacement of joint surfaces so that they no longer make normal contact at all.[53] A *subluxation* is a partial displacement of joint surfaces, usually transient in nature.[53] Whenever a dislocation or subluxation occurs, there can be significant damage to any of the ligaments of the joint. Chronic or overuse injury of joints often results in synovitis that can be either generalized to the entire joint or localized to a particular compartment. Often, it produces a swelling of the joint that is associated with warmth, pain, and erythema that may be confused with a joint infection.

Ligaments

Acute injuries to ligamentous structures are referred to as *sprains* or *tears* and are commonly classified by the degree of fiber tear within the ligament. A first-degree sprain results in the disruption of only a few muscle fibers, and there is typically only mild swelling, pain, and disability without any instability of the joint.[53] Second-degree sprains usually indicate that there are a moderate number of fibers that have been torn, resulting in an increased amount of swelling, pain, and disability with some joint instability noted on physical examination.[53] Third-degree sprains are the result of a complete tear of the ligament[53] in which severe swelling and pain are present and there is definitive joint instability evidenced on examination. The instability can further be characterized by the distance of separation, with 1+ displaced 3–5 mm, 2+ displaced 6–10 mm, and 3+ displaced greater than 10 mm.[53] Overuse injuries to ligaments are rare but include plantar fasciitis, breaststroker's knee, and medial elbow injury. These injuries commonly occur when there is a repeated stress to a ligament, rather than one defining traumatic incident.

Muscle-Tendon Unit

Muscle-tendon unit injuries, referred to as *strains*, are usually the result of an indirect force on the unit as opposed to a direct trauma.[52] Many times, this results from the contraction of the muscle itself, as is often the case with Achilles tendon ruptures. Like sprains, strains are graded from first to third degree, with a first-degree strain being characterized as a tear of only a few muscle or tendon fibers and a third-degree sprain defined as a complete rupture of the unit. With a first-degree strain, the athlete is often able to produce a strong muscle contraction but has pain associated with the action. A second-degree strain reduces the athlete's ability to make a strong contraction and is associated with more severe pain. A third-degree strain, or rupture of the muscle-tendon unit, allows only an extremely weak or no voluntary contraction. It is often painless, although there is potential for the associated muscle to enter spasm, which can be exceedingly painful.

Direct trauma can result in a deep muscle contusion, particularly involving the quadriceps and brachialis muscles. There is potential for a deep muscle contusion to lead to myositis ossificans, a process whereby bone formation occurs at the site of the contusion, particularly after hematoma formation.

A very common site for overuse injuries, the muscle-tendon unit can result in myositis, tendonitis, and tenosynovitis. Myositis causes many distinct common syndromes that occur at the origin or insertion of the muscle. Medial and lateral epicondylitis and shin splints are frequent complaints. Tendonitis occurs when there is an inflammatory reaction within the tendon tissue itself. Three common sites of tendonitis are the Achilles tendon, the rotator cuff, and the biceps tendon. Tenosynovitis results if the inflammatory changes encompass the tissue surrounding the tendon in question. This condition classically produces a crepitation as the tendon moves through its sheath.

Common Orthopedic Injuries by Joint

Shoulder, elbow, wrist, hand, knee, ankle, and foot injuries are exceedingly common in competitive athletes. Tables 26-8 through 26-11[54–61] highlight the most common orthopedic injuries for athletes often seen and evaluated by primary care physicians.

Steroid Injections

Corticosteroid injections are widely used in sports medicine practice as a palliative measure for many different musculoskeletal injuries, although to date their role is not clearly supported by objective evidence-based data.[62] Table 26-12[53,58,62] highlights a list of common joints, conditions, and sites of injection which may be clinically encountered.

Possible complications of steroid injections include the following[62]:

- Achilles and patellar tendon injections have significant potential for tendon rupture
- Fat pad atrophy
- Postinjection steroid flare
- Crystal steroid arthropathy
- Infection/sterile abscess
- Hypopigmentation
- Necrosis of cartilage, nerve, bone, and tendon

Exercise-Induced Asthma

EIA is a common yet often unrecognized condition occurring in both known asthmatics and otherwise healthy persons. To make an accurate diagnosis, a bronchoprovocation challenge test must be performed; the current recommended test is a eucapnic voluntary hyperventilation (EVH) challenge test. Although there are a number of treatment options available, both pharmacologic and nonpharmacologic, in most cases medications are required. A range of medications are currently available to either treat or prevent EIA. It is important that the medications used are individualized to the patient's needs and monitored to ensure efficacy.

Chronic inflammation of the airways leading to airway hyper-responsiveness and airway narrowing is characteristic of asthma.[63–66] A variety of stimuli are known to trigger a bronchospastic response in patients with asthma including allergens, environmental irritants, bacterial or viral upper respiratory infection, cold air, and exercise.[63] Inhaled corticosteroids remain the cornerstone of therapy for persistent asthma.

Exercise-Induced Bronchoconstriction

More than 40 years ago, reports began to appear in the literature describing a separate and distinct group of patients in whom asthmatic symptoms occurred only after cessation of strenuous exercise.[67–70] Most of these patients had no prior history of asthma and those few who did had been

Table 26-8. Diagnosis and Treatment of Common Shoulder Injuries

Diagnosis	Anatomy/Grades	Clinical Diagnosis	Radiologic Diagnosis	Treatment, Initial
Acromioclavicular injuries	Acromioclavicular (AC) Coracoclavicular (CC) ligaments		AP and axial views Alexander view (posterior dislocation)	Initially: RICE, NSAIDs, sling immobilizer
	I: AC ligament and capsular stretching	Swelling, tender over AC without instability	Normal	Wean out of sling as tolerated; early PT with ROM and PREs for several weeks
	II: AC ligament disruption with slight upward migration of the clavicle and tearing of the CC ligaments	Snapping of AC joint on ROM, slight instability with downward pressure; crossover test painful	1.3 cm coracoacromial separation	
	III: AC and CC ligaments and intraarticular joint dislocation with the clavicle displaced upward relative to the acromion	Grades III–VI: Swelling and marked tenderness, marked asymmetry with high-riding clavicle; unable to perform crossover test	Greater then 1.3 cm separation or > 50% increase in the distance	As above, with PT for 6–8 weeks. If athlete performs throwing sport(s), surgery may benefit
	IV: A grade III with the clavicle anatomically displaced upward and posterior into or through the trapezius			Clavicle must be removed from trapezius, which is usually accomplished with closed reduction; occasionally surgery required.
	V: Severe upward dislocation of the distal clavicle relative to the acromion with complete destruction of the AC and CC and disruption of muscle attachments to clavicle			Surgical repair
	VI: Inferior dislocation of the clavicle under the coracoid; injury to underlying neurovascular structures likely			
Impingement syndrome	Bursitis, tendonitis, supraspinatus syndrome	Pain worse at night and overhead ROM, + straight-arm raising	MRI demonstrates partial and full cuff tears, bursitis, tendonitis and capsular tears	RICE, NSAIDs, injection therapy; PT improves ROM, strength; electric stimulation and US improve symptoms but not healing; consider surgery if conservative measures fail

Table continued on following page

Table 26-8. Diagnosis and Treatment of Common Shoulder Injuries (Continued)

Diagnosis	Anatomy/Grades	Clinical Diagnosis	Radiologic Diagnosis	Treatment, Initial
Rotator cuff strain	Acute or chronic tearing of rotator cuff muscle-tendon unit	Pain and weakness, especially with 70–120 degrees of arm abduction and external rotation; palpable crepitus during abduction, + impingement sign	MRI sensitive and specific for tears and may reveal evidence of wear; US sensitive and specific for 85–95% of complete tears	Initial: RICE, NSAID, sling long term: PT for ROM and PRE, emphasis on abduction and external rotation; surgery if conservative measures fail
Biceps injuries				
Biceps tendonitis	Chronic microtrauma	Crepitus and tenderness over bicipital groove; pain and snapping over proximal humerus and tendon	Tunnel views on plain radiographs, US, MRI, arthrography	RICE, NSAIDs
Biceps tendon dislocation	Acute injury after sudden forceful contraction against resistance or a direct blow	Snapping/popping sensation with external rotation		Counter-force bracing proximal to biceps belly; steroid injection therapy of biceps sheath; possibly tenodesis
Biceps tendon rupture		Ecchymoses; palpable visible gap; supination and flexion weakness; "Popeye" deformity		Surgical repair of the transverse humeral ligament
				Surgical repair for all ruptures in the elite athlete

AP, Anteroposterior; RICE, rest, ice, compression, elevation; NSAIDs, nonsteroidal anti-inflammatory drugs; ROM, range of motion; PT, physical therapy; PREs, progressive resistance exercise; US, ultrasound; MRI, magnetic resonance imaging.

Adapted from: Wexler RK: Evaluation and treatment of heat-related illnesses, *Am Fam Phys* 65(11):2307–2314, 2002.

Table 26-9. Diagnosis and Treatment of Common Elbow, Wrist, and Hand Injuries

Diagnosis	Anatomy/Grades	Clinical Diagnosis	Radiologic Diagnosis	Treatment: Initial Long-term
Lateral epicondylitis	Degenerative tendinosis of extensor carpi radialis brevis/extensor communis	Tender around lateral epicondyle, over the extensor brevis, pain with resisted wrist extension	Radiographs usually normal; rule out other conditions	RICE, NSAIDs, and activity modification Rehab to restore ROM, strengthening exercises, elbow counterforce bracing may be used, but a Cochrane Review found no benefit to bracing Steroid injections infrequently to reduce pain for optimal rehab, short-term benefit of injection vs. NSAIDs
Medial epicondylitis	Flexor/pronator group at its insertion on medial epicondyle	Pain/tender over medial epicondyle, along pronator teres and flexor carpi radialis; pain with resisted palmar flexion and pronation, and flexion of the elbow	Radiographs normal	Rehab-flexibility, strengthening, endurance Surgical decompression if no improvement with 3–6 months' conservative treatment For type I, sling, elbow immobilizer, posterior splint for 1–2 weeks with early ROM; type II/III may require surgery—orthopedic evaluation needed PRICEMM (RICE + prevention/protection, modalities, and medications) Injection therapy after NSAID trial, counter-force bracing, technique improvement; flexibility, strengthening Modify technique, counter-force elbow sleeve, rehab Ligament rupture/chronic MCL insufficiency requires surgical repair/reconstruction
Olecranon bursitis	Olecranon bursa inflammation	Fluctuant, non-tender swelling (if painful or signs of inflammation present, infection must be ruled out)	Radiographs normal	If asymptomatic, then usually self-limiting RICE, NSAIDs, elbow protective pad Aspiration; steroid injections rarely needed or useful
Scaphoid fracture	Fall on outstretched hand	"Snuff box" tenderness; ROM limited; tender over scaphoid tubercle	Radiograph with scaphoid series, if results are negative, may cast in thumb spica and repeat films in 10–14 days; MRI, CT may show immediate diagnosis	RICE, thumb spica splint Non-displaced: Long-arm spica cast for 6 weeks, followed by short-arm spica case until there is radiographic evidence of healing; protect from impact loading an additional 3 months If fracture of proximal third, displaced, or presentation > 2 weeks, orthopedic referral

Table continued on following page

Table 26-9. Diagnosis and Treatment of Common Elbow, Wrist, and Hand Injuries (Continued)

Diagnosis	Anatomy/Grades	Clinical Diagnosis	Radiologic Diagnosis	Treatment: Initial	Treatment: Long-term
De Quervain's tenosynovitis	First dorsal compartment of the wrist, repetitive injury	Finkelstein's test	Radiographs normal, used to rule out other causes		Splint with thumb spica; avoidance, rehab. Steroid injections may benefit. Surgery for resistant cases
Gamekeeper's thumb	Hyperabduction of the thumb MCP joint: Ulnar collateral ligament sprain Type 1 avulsion fracture, no displacement Type 2 avulsion fracture, displaced Type 3 torn ligament, stable in flexion Type 4 torn ligament, unstable in flexion	Stress testing as follows: 1. Anesthetize with local block or median and radial nerve blocks 2. Stabilize the thumb metacarpal with one hand and place a valgus stress on the MCP while in full flexion 3. Complete rupture if angulation > 15 degrees then normal or > 35 degrees absolute 4. Angulation less than that is considered type 3 and stable	Radiographs should be performed before stress testing of joint to reveal any avulsion fragment. If avulsion is evident, do not perform stress testing Displaced fracture > 2 mm, or rotated fracture indicates type 4 MRI may be useful	RICE	Type 1: Thumb spica cast with MCP in full extension for 4 weeks Type 2: ORIF Type 3: Thumb spica cast with IP joint free and MCP flexed 20 degrees for 3 weeks Type 4: ORIF

RICE, Rest, ice, compression, elevation; NSAIDs, nonsteroidal anti-inflammatory drugs; ROM, range of motion; MCL, medial collateral ligament; MRI, magnetic resonance imaging; CT, computed tomography; MCP, metacarpophalangeal joint; ORIF, open-reduction internal fixation; IP, interphalangeal joint.

Adapted from: Shaw J, O'Connor FG, Nirschl RP: Elbow. In Birrer RB, O'Connor FG, editors: *Sports Medicine for the Primary Care Physician*, ed 3, New York, 2004, CRC Press, pp 523–538; Brennan F, Howard T, Lillegard W: Hand and wrist injuries. In Birrer RB, O'Connor FG, editors: *Sports Medicine for the Primary Care Physician*, ed 3, New York, 2004, CRC Press, pp 551–585; and Tiedeman JJ, Ferlic TP: Hand and wrist injuries. In Mellion MB, Walsh WM, Madden CM, et al: *Team Physician's Handbook*, ed 3, Hanley & Belfus, 2002, Philadelphia, pp 427–440.

Table 26-10. Diagnosis and Treatment of Common Knee Injuries

Diagnosis	ANATOMY/GRADES Mechanism	Clinical Diagnosis	Radiologic Diagnosis	TREATMENT: INITIAL Long-term
Ligamentous Injuries				
Medial collateral ligament (MCL)	Tearing of MCL: Grades 1–3	Edema, tender, positive abduction stress test	Routine radiographs negative; MRI can distinguish grade 1 and 2 from grade 3	RICE, NSAIDs, posterior splint, crutches with weight-bearing
	Contact or non-contact in fixed-foot rotational injuries; valgus force with external tibial rotation			Grades 1 and 2, symptomatic treatment; grade 3, (isolated only) brace that prevents valgus stress
Lateral collateral ligament (LCL)	Tearing of LCL: Grades 1–3 Varus force with internal tibial rotation	Adduction stress test at 30 degrees of flexion; + posterolateral drawer; chronic cases; + reverse pivot shift and external rotation recurvatum tests	Routine radiographs negative (may see avulsion of lateral capsular ligament) MRI can distinguish grades 1 and 2 from grade 3	Initial: RICE, NSAIDs, immobilization Grades 1 and 2, bracing, crutches with weight bearing and PT (ROM and PREs); grade 3, surgical repair
Anterior cruciate ligament (ACL)	Tearing of ACL: may be torn from femur, tibia, or mid portion	Large hemarthrosis; + Lachman's test; functional instability	Routine radiographs may show lateral capsular sign MRI	RICE, NSAIDs, crutches with limited motion brace or splint
	Hyperextension, varus/internal rotation, extremes of valgus and external rotation, deceleration, or force that drives the tibia anteriorly with knee flexed			Grades 1 and 2, bracing to prevent full extension, PT for (ROM and PREs) quads and hamstrings; grade 3, surgery may be necessary, especially in the elite athlete population
Posterior cruciate ligament (PCL)	Tear of part or all of two major bundles of PCL	Abduction or adduction with full extension if valgus or varus cause + posterior drawer if traumatic functional instability	AP and lateral radiographs may show sag in tibia and bony avulsion; stress films CT good for bony structures; MRI excellent	RICE, NSAIDs
	Valgus/varus stress in full extensions, rotation, rapid deceleration; hyperextension, direct blow, or a fall on a flexed knee			Grades 1 and 2, bracing and PT; grade 3 (isolated), under debate—some prefer conservative treatment, others surgery
Meniscal Injuries				
Medial/lateral	Disruption of medial or lateral (semilunar) cartilage of the knee	McMurray, Apley tests; joint-line tenderness, quadriceps atrophy, "clunk" during anterior drawer test; inability to squat and duck walk	Routine radiographs negative; MRI the procedure of choice	RICE, NSAIDs
	Fixed-foot rotation injury while weight bearing with the knee flexed			PT for a stable tear; surgery if persistent symptoms, especially in athletes
Unhappy triad	Tear of the MCL, ACL, and medial meniscus	As above	As above	As above, operative repair

Table continued on following page

Table 26-10. Diagnosis and Treatment of Common Knee Injuries (Continued)

Diagnosis	ANATOMY/GRADES Mechanism	Clinical Diagnosis	Radiologic Diagnosis	TREATMENT: INITIAL Long-term
Patellar Injuries				
Patellofemoral syndrome	Inflammation and degeneration of patellar cartilage, also a shallow femoral groove	Malalignment with increased Q angle + patellofemoral compression and inhibition tests; patellar apprehension test	Radiographs usually negative (may demonstrate patella alta); sunrise view may demonstrate lateral tilt/subluxation; arthroscopy is gold standard	RICE, NSAIDs, patella cutout brace with inferior horseshoe / PT, functional patellar bracing, orthotics, or arch supports
Patellar subluxation/dislocation	Partial or complete lateral displacement of patella from femoral trochlea / Valgus and/or twisting action with strong quadriceps contraction	Deformity over lateral femoral condyle	AP and lateral usually normal because spontaneous relocation is typical	RICE, NSAIDs, Relocation: knee flexion knee extension gentle pressure along lateral patellar edge / Immobilize in extension with foam pad over vastus medialis obliquus and lateral buttress for 4 weeks; PT and bracing.
Tendonitis/Bursitis				
Quadriceps	Inflammation of quadriceps tendon at superior pole attachment of patella	Swelling/tenderness at superior patellar pole	Radiographs usually negative; MRI may demonstrate degenerative changes in tendon	RICE, NSAIDs
Infrapatellar	Inflammation of patellar tendon, usually at the attachment to the inferior patellar pole	Swelling/tenderness at inferior patellar pole		PT, counterforce bracing; steroid injections risky as it may promote tendon rupture
Iliotibial band syndrome	Inflammation with excessive flexion and extension of the knee as the band rubs back and forth over the lateral femoral epicondyle	Tender over lateral femoral epicondyle; Malacrea's test for pain; Renne's creak sign	Radiographs not beneficial	RICE, NSAIDs, transverse friction and ice massage / Cross-training, modalities, PT, orthotics in shoes; steroid injections beneficial

MRI, Magnetic resonance imaging; RICE, rest, ice, compression, elevation; NSAIDs, nonsteroidal anti-inflammatory drugs; PT, physical therapy; ROM, range of motion; PREs, progressive resistance exercise; AP, anteroposterior; CT, computed tomography.

Adapted from: Levandowski R, Cohen P: Knee injuries. In Birrer RB, O'Connor FG, editors: *Sports Medicine for the Primary Care Physician*, ed 3, New York, 2004, CRC Press, pp 617-645.

Table 26-11. Diagnosis and Treatment of Common Ankle and Foot Injuries

Diagnosis	ANATOMY/GRADES Mechanism	Clinical Diagnosis	Radiologic Diagnosis	Treatment
Lateral sprain	Tearing of anterior talofibular (ATF), calcaneofibular (CF), and posterior talofibular (PTF) ligaments	Tender, swelling, hemarthrosis, ecchymoses anterior drawer test: 4–14-mm, grade 2; >15-mm, grade 3; talar tilt test: 5–10 degrees, grade 2; >10 degrees, grade 3	AP, lateral, mortise views; stress films using mechanical stress device; arthroscopy, MRI	RICE, NSAIDs, posterior or air splint, no weight bearing
	Inversion, plantar flexion, and adduction, especially when landing from a jump			Grade 1, weight-bearing brace or strapping for 2–3 weeks; grade 2, walking boot, cast for 2–4 weeks, then strap at 90 degrees for 2–4 weeks; grade 3, dorsiflexion cast or weight-bearing brace for 3–6 weeks, strapping 3–6 weeks; surgical repair favored by some especially in athletes
Medial sprain	Tearing of superficial deltoid (tibionavicular), anteromedial capsule, anterior deep deltoid component, anterior tibiofibular, interosseous membrane			Grade 1, weight-bearing cast for 2–3 weeks; grade 2–3, weight-bearing cast for 5–6 weeks; follow cast with strapping for all grades; operative repair if necessary
	Eversion, dorsiflexion, and abduction			
Achilles tendonitis	Tears of collagen fibers in tendon, pseudosheath thickening	Tenderness, crepitus, dorsiflexion weak secondary to pain	None indicated	RICE, NSAIDs
	Repetitive stress, inflexibility of gastrocsoleus complex			PT (ROM + PRE), cross-training; surgical tenolysis and debridement
Achilles rupture	Rupture of tendon 2–6 cm proximal to insertion	Thompson-Doherty squeeze test; heel resistance test; gap sign	US, CT, MRI	Dependent on severity, age, and caliber of athlete
	Sudden dorsiflexion of a plantarflexed foot; pushing off the weight-bearing foot with knee locked and extended, direct blow			Nonoperative: RICE, NSAIDs, non–weight bearing, long-leg, gravity equines cast for 6 weeks; short-leg equines cast for 2 weeks; short-leg walking cast for 2 weeks (recreational athletes)
				Operative: improved strength and endurance and decreased risk of re-rupture (elite/professional athletes)

Table continued on following page

Table 26-11. Diagnosis and Treatment of Common Ankle and Foot Injuries (Continued)

Diagnosis	ANATOMY/GRADES Mechanism	Clinical Diagnosis	Radiologic Diagnosis	Treatment
Flexor hallucis longus (FHL) tendonitis	Irritation of the FHL tendon in the fibro-osseous tunnel behind medial malleolus or between sesamoids	Tender, swollen, crepitus; triggering and clawing of the hallux	None indicated	RICE, NSAIDs
	Repetitive push-offs			Surgical tenolysis for severe cases; steroids not recommended
Syndesmotic injury	Tearing of syndesmosis	Kleiger test; Squeeze test	AP, lateral, mortise; > 6 mm tibiofibular clear space and widening of the mortise	Grade 1, aggressive functional rehab; grade 2, cast immobilization with progressive weight bearing for 3–6 weeks; grade 3, ORIF with syndesmotic screw; prolonged recovery
	Forced external rotation or hyperdorsiflexion and eversion with internal tibial rotation			
Ankle fractures	Fracture of one or both malleoli, depending on the mechanism; spiral fibular fractures usually involve ankle	Tender, ecchymoses, inability to bear weight; crepitus	AP, lateral, mortise views	Splint, RICE, NSAIDs
	External rotation, eversion, abduction, or adduction with pronation or supination			Non-displaced: cast immobilization for 4–6 weeks Displaced: ORIF Open: irrigation, debridement, antibiotics
Retroachilles and retrocalcaneal bursitis	Bursa between Achilles tendon and skin; bursa between Achilles and calcaneus	Tender anterior or posterior (depending on bursa involved) without bony or Achilles tenderness	None indicated	RICE, NSAIDs
	Repetitive stress			Padded heel counter; steroid injection therapy; return to play after pain subsides

Table continued on following page

Table 26-11. Diagnosis and Treatment of Common Ankle and Foot Injuries (Continued)

Diagnosis	ANATOMY/GRADES		Clinical Diagnosis	Radiologic Diagnosis	Treatment
	Mechanism				
Plantar fasciitis	Microtears and inflammation of plantar fascia		Tender at plantar fascia insertion and calcaneus pain increases with passive dorsiflexion of hallux	Radiographs may show heel spur, but not pathognomonic; bone scan results often negative	RICE, NSAIDs
	Excessive torsion and hyperpronation; poor shock dissipation, especially with cavus foot				Soft orthotic device to create varus heel tilt; tension night splints; steroid injections; rolling pin exercises; return to play with absence of pain
Fifth metatarsal fracture— avulsion	Avulsion of the styloid process		Point tenderness at base of metatarsal	Avulsed fragment of tuberosity	RICE, NSAIDs
	Inversion with or without plantar flexion in association with contraction of the peroneus brevis muscle				Short leg cast for 4–6 weeks; eversion strapping or wooden shoe for hairline fracture; return to play after pain free and rehabilitation
Fifth metatarsal fracture— Jones	Fracture of shaft within 1.5 cm of tuberosity		Tender over base of metatarsal + tuning fork test	Radiolucent fracture line with periosteal reaction; technetium-99m bone scan	Non–weight bearing with crutches
	Repetitive microtrauma without inversion				Non–weight-bearing leg cast for 6–8 weeks; additional 2–4 months for delayed union (avascular area); operative management for competitive athletes; return to play after evidence of radiographic healing (6–8 weeks) and appropriate PT (7–14 weeks)

AP, Anteroposterior; MRI, magnetic resonance imaging; RICE, rest, ice, compression, elevation; NSAIDs, nonsteroidal anti-inflammatory drugs; PT, physical therapy; ROM, range of motion; PRE, progressive resistance exercise; US, ultrasound; CT, computed tomography; ORIF, open reduction internal fixation.

Adapted from: Birrer R: The ankle. In Birrer RB, O'Connor FG, editors: *Sports Medicine for the Primary Care Physician*, ed 3, New York, 2004, CRC Press, pp 665–685; Petrizzi MJ, Richardson DG: Foot injuries. In Birrer RB, O'Connor FG, editors: *Sports Medicine for the Primary Care Physician*, ed 3, New York, 2004, CRC Press, pp 687–710; and Brown DE: Ankle and leg injuries. In Mellion MB, Walsh WM, Madden CM, et al: *Team Physician's Handbook*, ed 3, Hanley & Belfus, 2002, Philadelphia, pp 509–520.

Table 26-12. Common Joint Diagnoses and Respective Sites of Injection of Steroid Therapy

Joint	Diagnosis	Site of Injection	Needle Size (gauge/length)	Dose of Methylprednisolone Acetate (mg)	Dose of 1% Lidocaine (mL)
Shoulder	Impingement syndrome	Subacromial bursa	22/1–1.5 in	10–20	1–2
	AC arthrosis	AC joint	22/1–1.5 in	20–40	1–2
	Bicipital tendonitis	Biceps tendon	22/1–1.5 in	5–10	1–2
	Rotator cuff tendonitis	Rotator cuff tendons	22/1–1.5 in	20–40	2–4
Elbow	Epicondylitis	Extensor muscle origin	25/1–1.5 in	15–30	2–4
Wrist	De Quervain's tenosynovitis	First extensor compartment	25–30/0.5–1 in	5–10	1–2
Hand	Flexor tenosynovitis (trigger finger)	Tendon sheath	25–30/0.5–1 in	5–10	1–2
	Ganglia		25–30/0.5–1 in	5–15	1–2
Knee	Iliotibial band tendonitis	Iliotibial band/insertion fibula head	22/1–1.5 in	10–20	2–4
Foot	Plantar fasciitis	Calcaneal origin of plantar fascia	25–30/1–1.5 in	15–30	2–4
Hip	Trochanteric bursitis	Trochanteric bursa	20–22/1–1.5 in	10–20	1–2

AC, Acromioclavicular.

Adapted from: O'Connor FG, Birrer RB: Sports injuries: a general guide for the treatment and rehabilitation of sports injuries. In Birrer RB, O'Connor FG, editors: *Sports Medicine for the Primary Care Physician*, ed 3, New York, 2004, CRC Press, pp 281–290; and Walsh WM, Hald RD, Peter LE, Mellion MB: Musculoskeletal injuries in sports. In Mellion MB, Walsh WM, Madden CM, et al: *Team Physician's Handbook*, ed 3, Hanley & Belfus, 2002, Philadelphia.

asymptomatic for years. Typically, these athletes exhibit no pulmonary symptoms while exercising vigorously because airway caliber is maintained during exercise. However, within approximately 5 minutes of cessation of exercise, symptoms of airflow obstruction develop and may persist for 30–60 minutes without bronchodilator administration.

Airflow limitation in EIB is related to thermal changes in the airways.[63,66,71,72] Exercise hyperventilation with cool inspired air leads to cooling of the airway mucosa. This ultimately causes hyperemia of the airway surface and subsequent release of fluid into the submucosal cells, stimulating the release of bronchospastic chemical mediators causing airway smooth muscle to contract with resultant airways narrowing. Minimal or no demonstrable inflammation has been reported in this group of patients compared with those with persistent asthma. Because athletes with EIB have no demonstrable inflammation, treatment with inhaled steroids (although appropriate for EIA) is unwarranted.[73]

Diagnosis

EIA/EIB must be considered when a history of respiratory symptoms including cough, wheezing, chest tightness or pain, dizziness, fatigue, or unusual or unexpected shortness of breath during or after exercise is reported. Routine pre- and post-exercise screening of all athletes during the initial PPE is recommended.

A peak expiratory flow rate (PEFR) screening test for all athletes with suspected or known EIA/EIB is recommended. An exercise challenge in the form of a 6–8-minute run at an intensity of 80% of maximum is followed by PEFR readings at 5-minute intervals for 30 minutes. A fall in PEFR of 15% from baseline (at rest) is diagnostic. A return to normal levels 30–60 minutes after exercise is confirmatory of EIB. Several other confirmatory tests are available, should the situation be less than clear, including a standard exercise study, a methacholine challenge, and an EVH study[74]; the EVH test is recommended for Olympic athletes.

Treatment

Preventive Measures

Sideline management of EIA/EIB begins with measures to prevent or attenuate exercise-associated respiratory events.[75] Athletes with chronic asthma should achieve optimum anti-inflammatory and bronchodilator regimens. Consideration of the previously mentioned environmental triggers is appropriate. Recent reports have described several dietary modifications that may attenuate the severity of EIA, such as fish oil and omega-3 fatty acids.[76]

McKenzie and colleagues[77] found that a short warm up at 80–90% of a maximum workload 15–20 minutes before practice or competition will attenuate the EIB response. Others found that pre-game calisthenics or short, repeated warm-up runs reduced the decrease in PEF in asthmatic children.[78,79]

Refractory Period

The refractory period represents the period, usually of 1–2 hours' duration, after spontaneous recovery from an episode of EIA, in which more than 50% of athletes do not experience another episode of bronchoconstriction with further exercise. Such a refractory period can be used by those athletes who experience them to lessen the severity of EIA for their "real competition."[80] The exact mechanism whereby a person becomes refractory is not known, but it may be secondary to an improved delivery of water to the airways during the second episode of exercise. This effect is short-lived, generally lasting a few hours, and can be inhibited by the use of NSAIDs, as has been well-described following the use of indomethacin for 3 days.[81–83]

Pre-Exercise Medicines

An albuterol metered-dose inhaler used 15 minutes before exercise or competition is the most commonly used pre-exercise medication to prevent EIA/EIB.[84] Longer-acting beta-2 agonists such as salmeterol and formoterol, because of their delayed onset of activity, are not effective in treating in EIA/EIB. Cromolyn sodium and nedocromil sodium are mast cell stabilizers that can be used as prophylactic medication for EIA/EIB, but these have fallen out of favor in recent years. These medications are not bronchodilators and are not effective to treat acute symptoms, but they are indicated for athletes who cannot tolerate beta-2 agonists or for whom beta-2 agonists are not completely protective.[84] Leukotriene antagonists have been demonstrated to protect against EIA in some patients but have not been shown to be as effective in the treatment of acute bronchospasm because they are given orally and have a delayed onset of action.[84]

Sideline Management

Any athlete who demonstrates symptoms of airway hyper-reactivity during practice or competition, whether previously diagnosed with EIA/EIB or not, must be removed from activity, promptly evaluated, and provided emergency treatment (Figure 26-1).[85] Comparing a sideline PEFR with the athlete's baseline measurements (obtained during the PPE) is the first step in the sideline evaluation. Occasionally, the respiratory difficulty resolves spontaneously when the athlete is removed from exercise or competition, but the usual scenario is that symptoms resolve shortly (5–10 minutes) after the inhalation of a beta-2 agonist. If the PEF is diminished 15–20%, then a short-acting beta-2 agonist should be administered.

If the symptoms do not resolve completely with sideline treatment, then the athlete must be returned to the athletic training room for further evaluation and therapy because the possibility that the episode may progress to status asthmaticus is real. The most common scenario in which an incomplete response to initial sideline bronchodilator administration occurs is in an athlete whose respiratory symptoms are due to EIA and in whom chronic persistent asthma is either previously unrecognized or inadequately treated.[86]

Concussion

The American Academy of Neurology defines *mild traumatic brain injury* (MTBI), or *concussion*, as "a trauma-induced alteration in mental status that may or may not be accompanied by a loss of consciousness."[87] Athletes with concussion may present with a wide variety of signs and symptoms (Table 26-13),[87] many of which are subtle and may go unrecognized by an untrained professional, or even the athletes themselves. A second concern is that many athletes may be reluctant to report concussive symptoms, due to the fear that they will be removed from the game, jeopardizing their status on the team, the outcome of the game, or their careers. Attempting to "play through" a concussion, however, could have long-term or even catastrophic consequences.

Clinical Concerns

Three primary issues exist in the clinical management of a head-injured athlete. First, more serious intracranial pathology in the form of skull fracture, epidural hematoma, subdural hematoma, and parenchymal hematoma must be ruled out. Clinicians should be aware that a major head injury may present with an initial lucid interval, followed by delayed neurologic deterioration.[88] A rapid progression of headache, personality change, or mental status deterioration should alert the clinician to this possibility and facilitate an emergent evaluation. A second management concern is the prevention of catastrophic outcome from *second impact syndrome* (SIS). This occurs

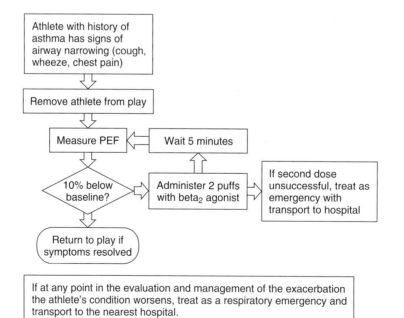

Figure 26-1. Sideline management of exercise-induced asthma. PEF, Peak expiratory flow. (Adapted from: Allen TW: Sideline management of asthma, *Curr Sports Med Rep* 4:301–304, 2005.)

Table 26-13. Frequently Observed Signs and Symptoms of Concussion

Signs observed by medical staff:
Athlete appears dazed
Vacant facial expression
Confusion about assignment
Athlete forgets plays
Disorientation to game, score, opposing team
Inappropriate emotional reaction (e.g., laughing, crying)
Athlete displays incoordination or clumsiness
Athlete is slow to answer questions
Loss of consciousness (even for seconds)
Any change in typical behavior or personality
Symptoms reported by athlete:
Headache
Nausea
Balance problems or dizziness
Double or fuzzy vision
Sensitivity to light or noise
Feeling slowed down
Feeling "foggy" or "not sharp"
Change in sleep pattern
Concentration or memory problems
Irritability
Sadness
Feeling more emotional

Note: Symptoms may worsen with exertion. Athlete should not return to play until symptom-free.

Adapted from: Collins MW, Hawn KL: The clinical management of sports concussion, *Curr Sports Med Rep* 1:12–22, 2002.

when an athlete experiences a second concussive insult soon after a first. Both the initial as well as the second insult may be considered mild, with the second impact occurring up to 10 days after the first trauma. Most athletes who have succumbed to SIS have reported discernible symptoms (e.g., headache, nausea, feeling slow) after the first insult and before the second.[89] The majority of documented cases have occurred in high school athletes, that may be secondary to specific neurodevelopmental issues or possible selection bias, as the largest athletic population is teenaged or younger.[87]

A final and much more prevalent management concern in the concussed athlete is the salient possibility of cumulative brain injury related to repeated traumas. Several neuropsychological studies have identified the possibility of cognitive

and neurobehavioral sequelae associated with two or more concussive events.[90–92] This has led to speculation that successive concussive impacts may lead to mild yet significant impairment of cognitive processes (e.g., attention, memory), personality changes, and somatic disturbances (e.g., sensitivity to light, dizziness). This collection of symptoms has been termed *postconcussion syndrome* and can be quite incapacitating. It should be noted that discernible cognitive deficits have been identified in particular athletes from a single concussive event.[93]

Evaluation

In assessing traumatic brain injury, all clinicians should be aware that neurodiagnostic techniques such as computed tomography (CT) scans, MRI scans, and the electroencephalogram (EEG), although invaluable in identifying more severe intracranial pathology, are typically insensitive to measuring the subtle neuronal aspects of MTBI.[94] Their high rate of false-negative results often provides an errant basis on which return-to-play decisions are made. However, the advent of magnetization transfer imaging[95] and the monitoring of brain electrophysiologic activity through event-related potentials,[96,97] as well as the constant evolution of positron emission tomography scanning and functional MRI[98] technology, may be able to offer the future establishment of neurodiagnostic norms with the ability to accurately assess concussion severity.

Management

Appropriate acute care of the concussed athlete begins with an accurate assessment of the gravity of the situation. As with any serious injury assessment, the first priority is always to evaluate the athlete's level of consciousness and ABCs (i.e., airway, breathing, and circulation). Next, a thorough mental status assessment should be performed (Table 26-14).[87] Once the diagnosis of concussion is delineated, making the postinjury decision to return an athlete to participation in sports is one of the major challenges of concussion management. The initial step is to assign a grade to the concussion based on symptom severity. Most guidelines were primarily developed by panels of experts in the field and are based on popular belief or practice rather than empiric evidence.[94,99] The 2001 Cantu Grading System,[100] the 1991 Colorado Medical Society Guidelines,[101] and the 1997 American Academy of Neurology Guidelines[102] collectively provide the most

Table 26-14. Mental Status Testing in a Concussed Athlete*

Cognitive testing
Orientation
Ask the athlete the following questions: - What stadium is this? - What city is this? - Who is the opposing team? - What month is it? - What day is it?
Anterograde amnesia
Ask the athlete to repeat the following words: - Girl, dog, green
Retrograde amnesia
Ask the athlete the following questions: - What happened in the prior quarter/period? - What do you remember just prior to the hit? - What was the score of the game prior to the hit? - Do you remember the hit?
Concentration
Ask the athlete to do the following: - Repeat these numbers backward: 63, 419
Word list memory

*Any failure should be considered abnormal. A physician should be consulted if the athlete exhibits any signs or symptoms of concussion.

The University of Pittsburgh Medical Center Concussion Card is a brief mental status evaluation and symptom inventory intended for sideline and athletic training room use immediately following injury. Its intended purpose is to assist the clinician in determining the presence of concussive injury, and is not for use in making decisions regarding safe return to competition.

Adapted from: Collins MW, Hawn KL: The clinical management of sports concussion, *Curr Sports Med Rep* 1:12–22, 2002.

detailed and widely used criteria for both grading concussions and providing guidelines for when a concussed athlete can return to play (Tables 26-15 and 26-16).[100–102]

Neuropsychological Testing

Traditional sports-specific neuropsychological test batteries have been proved to be both valid and reliable measures to delineate the subtle effects of concussive injury.[87] Ideally, a neuropsychological testing approach in athletic populations will involve pre- and post-concussion evaluations. The preseason test, or baseline, provides a basis for comparison if the athlete is later concussed. This is important for several reasons. First, each athlete's level of performance will likely vary considerably on the test battery. Without assessing preinjury levels, it is difficult to determine whether postinjury deficits are truly attributable to concussion. In addition, some athletes may perform more poorly due to individual discrepancies in cognitive functioning, learning disabilities, or related concerns. Lastly, prior concussions may mediate the effects of cognitive function and cloud the assessment of post-concussive test results if a baseline test has not been obtained.

Once a concussion has occurred, follow-up testing should ideally be conducted within 24–48 hours of injury and again at approximately 5–7 days postinjury (or subsequently in more severely injured athletes). Unlike the previously discussed neurodiagnostic measures that provide information on brain structure, neuropsychological testing is able to provide clinicians with a measure of functional status. In combination with an individual preseason baseline, or when compared with a database of matched control subjects, postinjury neuropsychological assessment may offer a tangible evidenced-based determination of when an athlete is able to return to participation.[87]

A major recent advancement in concussion diagnosis and management has been the development and implementation of computerized neuropsychological assessment. At the forefront of this technology is the advent of Immediate Postconcussion Assessment and Cognitive Testing (ImPACT),[103,104] a 25-minute computerized battery of neuropsychological tests prepared specifically for use in athletic concussion. This technology has made neuropsychological evaluation a practical option for athletes at all levels. Although neuropsychological testing currently appears to be the gold standard in concussion management, there are other ancillary measures that can be beneficial in the diagnosis and evaluation of concussion. Guskiewicz and colleagues[105] used the SMART Balance Master (NeuroCom International, Clackamas, OR) to test for postural instability after mild head injury, in an attempt to set the precedence for establishing recovery curves based on objective data. Their study revealed that concussed athletes exhibited increased postural instability for the first 3 days after injury. They concluded that this was due to a sensory interaction problem that caused injured athletes to fail to use their visual systems correctly. Balance testing or postural stability has recently been a popular topic among some clinicians, but current research in this area has been conducted with small sample sizes and has yet to be confirmed with larger groups of athletes.[105–107]

Table 26-15. Concussion Grading Criteria

Concussion Grade	Cantu Grading System (2001 Revision)	1991 Colorado Medical Society Guidelines	1997 American Academy of Neurology Guidelines
Grade 1 (mild)	No LOC Either PTA or post-concussion signs and symptoms that clear in less than 30 minutes	Transient mental confusion No PTA No LOC	No LOC Transient confusion Symptoms or abnormalities clear in less than 15 minutes
Grade 2 (moderate)	LOC lasting less than 1 minute and PTA *or* Post-concussion signs or symptoms lasting longer than 30 minutes but less than 24 hours	No LOC Confusion with PTA	No LOC Symptoms or abnormalities last more than 15 minutes
Grade 3 (severe)	LOC lasting more than 1 minute *or* PTA lasting longer than 24 hours *or* post-concussion signs or symptoms lasting longer than 7 days	Any LOC, however brief	Any LOC, either brief (seconds) or prolonged (minutes)

LOC, Loss of consciousness; PTA, post-trauma amnesia.

From: Cantu RC: Posttraumatic retrograde and anterograde amnesia: pathophysiology and implications in grading and safe return to play, *J Athl Train* 36(3):244–248, 2001. This grading system modifies the original Cantu grading system proposed in Cantu RC: Guidelines for return to contact sports after a cerebral concussion, *Phys Sportsmed* 14(10):75–83, 1986; Report of the Sports Medicine Committee: *Guidelines for the Management of Concussion in Sports,* Denver, CO, 1990, revised May 1991, Colorado Medical Society; American Academy of Neurology: Practice parameter: the management of concussion in sports (summary statement). Report of the Quality Standards Subcommittee, *Neurology* 48:581–585, 1997.

The study of sports concussion and management is rapidly evolving. The realization that the same seemingly minor mechanism of injury may result in one athlete being out for 2 days and another for 2 or more months underscores the importance of an individualized, evidence-based approach to concussion management. In light of these issues, use of the outlined neuropsychological testing approach can provide the clinician with an individual basis for comparison and produce evidence of an athlete's level of cognitive functioning. This is currently the clearest verification for when an athlete can safely resume participation.

Ergogenic Aids

Since the earliest days of competitive sport, athletes have been searching for a way, fair or unfair, to gain an advantage over their opponents. During the Greek and Roman games, history revealed that athletes used mushrooms and opioids as performance-enhancing supplements. Testosterone was used as early as 1940 to gain additional strength in competition, amphetamines were used extensively by some speed skaters in the 1952 Olympics in Oslo, Norway, and the 1964 Olympics in Tokyo, Japan, saw the first abuse of anabolic steroids. In 1967, a top British cyclist died ascending a mountain in the Tour de France from extensive amphetamine use. Despite a lack of strong evidence that many of the commonly used supplements are beneficial to performance, many athletes risk personal harm for the mere hope that they will gain an advantage in competition.

Recent scandal across several sports, in particular track and baseball athletes' involvement in the Bay Area Laboratory Co-Operative scandal, has caused the US Congress to investigate the use of ergogenic aids in professional sports. The 2006 Tour de France was beset by allegations of cheating, with several tour favorites disqualified before the start of the race. The term *ergogenic aids* refers to substances or devices that enhance energy production, use or recovery, and provide athletes with a competitive advantage[108] (Table 26-17). The age of "designer drugs" created specifically to circumvent existing drug tests has come about. Chemists produced tetrahydrogestrinone (THG), known as "the clear," liquid drops that could be placed under the tongue, specifically to circumvent known testing methods.

In an article published in *Sports Illustrated* in 1997,[109] a poll was conducted of 198 Olympic-level power-lifting athletes. They were all given the same scenario in which they were offered a banned substance with two guarantees: they would absolutely not be caught using the substance, and they were guaranteed to win their event. Of the 198 athletes polled, only 3 said they would not take the substance. The scenario was

Table 26-16. Guidelines for Returning to Play Post-Concussion

Concussion Grade	Number of Concussion Sustained	Cantu Guidelines (Revised)	Colorado Medical Society Guidelines	American Academy of Neurology Guidelines
Grade 1 (mild)	First	Return to play after 1 symptom-free week End season if CT or MRI abnormal	Remove from contest May return to same contest or practice if symptom free for at least 20 minutes	Remove from contest May return to play if symptom free within 15 minutes. May return to play if symptom free within 15 minutes
Grade 1 (mild)	Second	Return to play in 2 weeks after 1 symptom free week	May not return to contest or practice May return after 1 symptom-free week	May not return to contest or practice May return to play after 1 symptom-free week
Grade 1 (mild)	Third	End season May return to play next season if no symptoms	End season May return to play in 3 months if without symptoms	
Grade 2 (moderate)	First	Return to play after 1 symptom-free week	May not return to contest or practice May return to play after 1 symptom-free week	May not return to contest or practice May return to play after 1 full symptom-free week CT or MRI recommended if symptoms or signs persist
Grade 2 (moderate)	Second	May not return for minimum of 1 month May return to play then if symptom-free for 1 week Consider ending season	Consider ending season May return in 1 month if symptom-free	May not return to contest or practice May return to play after at least 2 symptom-free weeks End season if any CT or MRI abnormality
Grade 2 (moderate)	Third	End season May return to play next season if without symptoms	End season May return to play next season if without symptoms	
Grade 3 (severe)	First	May not return to play for minimum of 1 month May then return to play then after 1 symptom-free week	May not return to contest or practice Transport to hospital for evaluation May return to play in 1 month, after 2 symptom-free weeks	May not return to contest or practice Transport to hospital if unconscious or neurologic abnormality CT or MRI recommended if post-traumatic symptoms or signs persist If LOC brief (seconds). May return to play in 1 week if no symptoms or signs If LOC is prolonged (minutes), return after 2 symptom-free weeks
Grade 3 (severe)	Second	End season May return to play next season if no symptoms	End season May return to play next season if no symptoms	May not return to contest or practice May return to play after minimum of 1 symptom-free month End season if any CT or MRI abnormality

Table continued on following page

Table 26-16. Guidelines for Returning to Play Post-Concussion (Continued)

Concussion Grade	Number of Concussion Sustained	Cantu Guidelines (Revised)	Colorado Medical Society Guidelines	American Academy of Neurology Guidelines
Grade 3 (severe)	Third		End season Strongly discourage any return to contact or collision sports	

From: Cantu RC: Posttraumatic retrograde and anterograde amnesia: pathophysiology and implications in grading and safe return to play, *J Athl Train* 36(3):244–248, 2001. This grading system modifies the original Cantu grading system proposed in Cantu RC: Guidelines for return to contact sports after a cerebral concussion, *Phys Sportsmed* 14(10):75–83, 1986; Report of the Sports Medicine Committee: *Guidelines for the Management of Concussion in Sports,* Denver, CO, 1990, revised May 1991, Colorado Medical Society; American Academy of Neurology: Practice parameter: the management of concussion in sports (summary statement). Report of the Quality Standards Subcommittee, *Neurology* 48:581–585, 1997.

Table 26-17. Common Ergogenic Aids

Ergogenic Aid	Percentage of NCAA Respondents Using in Last 12 Months (2001)	Action/Desired Effect	Supporting Data*	Adverse Effects	Banned by:
Anabolic steroids	1.4%	Increase strength, lean muscle mass, and motivation	Supports use	Many (see Table 26-18)	All sports
Androstenedione	1%	Steroid precursor, may lead to increased testosterone	No benefit of use	Unknown, may pose cardiovascular risk	IOC, NCAA, NFL
Human growth hormone	3.5%	May stimulate body growth to increase muscle mass	Limited ergogenic benefits	Resistance to long-term use, myopathic muscles, carpal tunnel	IOC
Erythropoietin (EPO)	0.9%	Increases endurance, increases oxygen-carrying capacity of the blood	Supports use	Increases blood viscosity, myocardial infarction, PE	All sports
Creatine	7%	May enhance anaerobic training, increased strength and performance	Supports use	May lead to dehydration, long-term data lacking	None
Amphetamines	3.3%	Increased reaction time and endurance	Mixed, some benefits of use	Anxiety, ventricular dysrhythmias, hypertension, hallucinations, addiction, death	IOC
Ephedrine	1.2%	Boosts metabolism, burns fat, increases alertness, increases endurance	Mixed	Same as amphetamines	IOC, NCAA, NFL

*Supporting data reflect studies that have demonstrated a positive performance-enhancing result when using these substances.
NCAA, National Collegiate Athletic Association; IOC, International Olympic Committee; NFL, National Football League; PE, pulmonary embolism.
Adapted from: Tokish JM, Kocher MS, Hawkins RJ: Ergogenic aids: a review of basic science, performance, side effects, and status in sports, *Am J Sport Med* 32(6):1543–1553, 2004; Ahrendt DM: Ergogenic aids: counseling the athlete, *Am Fam Phys* 63(5):842–843, 2001; NCAA Research Staff: NCAA study of substance use habits of college student-athletes. 2001. Available at: http://www.ncaa.org/library/research/substance_use_habits/2001/substance_use_habits.pdf.

then altered to say that the athlete, if taking the substance, would win every event for 5 years but would then die from using the substance. More than half of the athletes indicated that they would still take the substance.

The use of ergogenic aids is rampant, with some studies showing as much as 40–60% of the general population taking some supplementation that they believe will augment their performance. The NCAA recently started a program of surveying college athletes to determine the use and abuse of such substances. According to survey information from 2001, more than 50% of college athletes admit to taking a dietary supplement on a regular basis; 52% of surveyed college athletes believed vitamins and minerals were beneficial to their performance, with nearly 38% finding benefit from nutritional supplements.[11]

Anabolic/Anabolic-Androgenic Steroids

Drugs that are classified as anabolic or anabolic/androgenic steroids (AAS) are chemically related to testosterone. Discovered in 1935, testosterone (and its relatives) was routinely used as a sport supplement starting in 1940 and continuing until this family of chemicals was banned from the 1976 Olympics in Montreal, Quebec, Canada. Nearly 5% of respondents reported anabolic steroid use in the 2001 NCAA survey (1.4% reported use in the previous 12 months), and more than 20% indicated use by other members on their team.[110] Only 0.4% of athletes surveyed believed that more than half of their teammates had used AAS in the previous 12 months. Twenty percent of the users of steroids felt certain their coaching staff new about their use, with 8% actually receiving the AAS from their coaches; yet most often, athletes that choose to take AAS obtain them from a physician (21%). In this survey, water polo and rifle shooting showed surprisingly high use

of AAS, along with, less surprisingly, football, baseball, and lacrosse[110] (Figures 26-2 and 26-3). It is believed that between 1 and 3 million athletes in the US alone have used anabolic steroids, with annual sales over $100 million.[111]

The effects athletes are looking to achieve when using anabolic steroids are to increase lean body mass, strength, and aggressiveness. Although the data behind early studies are skewed because of the low doses used, more recent studies have demonstrated significant gains in muscle mass, muscle size, and overall strength. One randomized double-blinded controlled 10-week trial of 40 men showed a 9% increase in muscle mass and a 23% increase in bench-press strength, compared with 3% and 9%, respectively, in placebo group.[111] The adverse effects of anabolic steroids are numerous (Table 26-18),[108] with some severe and others irreversible. In 2004, this class of compounds became listed as schedule III controlled substances.

A series of compounds classified as steroid-like substances that have similar ergogenic effects. These include dehydroepiandrosterone, androstenedione, human growth hormone, insulin-like growth factor-1, gamma-hydroxybutyrate, and clenbuterol.

Amphetamines

Amphetamines and ephedrine are chemically related to the catecholamines and indirectly affect their metabolism, leading to a release of norepinephrine from sympathetic nerves and resulting in peripheral vasoconstriction and subsequent

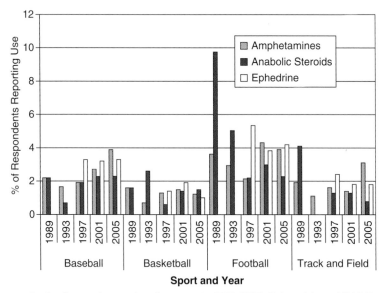

Figure 26-2. Drug use in the four major men's college sports, 1989–2005. (Adapted from: NCAA Research Staff: NCAA study of substance use habits of college student-athletes. 2001. Available at: http://www.ncaa.org/library/research/substance_use_habits/2001/substance_use_habits.pdf.)

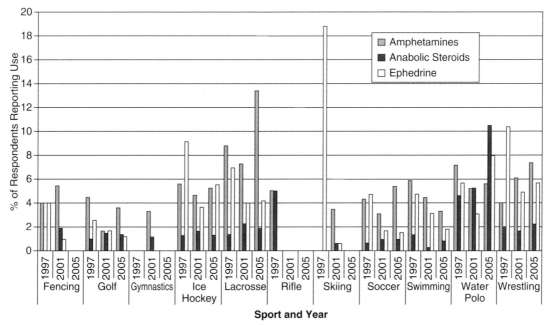

Figure 26-3. Substance use habits in men's collegiate sports, 1997–2005. (Adapted from: NCAA Research Staff: NCAA study of substance use habits of college student-athletes. 2001. Available at: http://www.ncaa.org/library/research/substance_use_habits/2001/substance_use_habits.pdf.)

Table 26-18. Potential Adverse Effects From Anabolic Steroid Use

Sexual	Gastrointestinal/Liver
Decrease in sperm production	Gastric ulcers
Decreased testicular size	Increase in transaminases
Increased/decreased libido	Cholestasis
Gynecomastia	Hepatitis
Prostatic enlargement	Liver failure
Physical/musculoskeletal	Liver neoplasm
Acne	**Psychological**
Alopecia	Aggressiveness
Edema	Irritability
Premature closure of growth plates	Depression
Increase in tendon tears	Psychosis
Metabolic	
Hyperglycemia	
Hypertension	
Hypercholesterolemia	

Adapted from: Ahrendt DM: Ergogenic aids: counseling the athlete, *Am Fam Phys* 63(5):842–843, 2001.

increased blood pressure. The action by amphetamines along the dopaminergic pathways leads to mood elevation, a boost in energy, and a decrease in response time. Amphetamines and stimulants are popular owing to the ease with which they are obtained, as well as their low cost. Many, like pseudoephedrine, are readily available over the counter, whereas others are prescribed for conditions like attention-deficit/hyperactivity disorder. The overall use of amphetamines in NCAA athletes is just over 3%, with nine sports over the mean. Rifle shooting topped the list with a reported 8.3% use rate, and lacrosse was close behind with a 7% reported use rate. When the rates of ephedrine use were combined with that of amphetamines, several sports approached 10% use, with lacrosse over 12%[110] (see Figures 26-2 and 26-3).

According to Tokish,[111] several studies have shown beneficial effects to using stimulants or amphetamines on performance. One study showed increases in time to exhaustion, quadriceps strength, and anaerobic capacity with the administration of Dexedrine (dextroamphetamine).[112] Another study showed improvements in maximum torque, peak power during cycling, and lung function after pseudoephedrine was taken.[113] Medium-distance run times have been reportedly decreased when using these drugs as well.[114,115] Although sudden death has been rarely reported in persons taking these products, it is still the most noteworthy side effect. More common adverse effects include nervousness or anxiety, ventricular dysrhythmias, hypertension, and hallucinations.

Creatine

Creatine is an amino acid that does not function in protein synthesis, but rather generates adenosine triphosphate (ATP) from adenosine diphosphate. It is synthesized by the body in the kidneys, liver, and pancreas but can also be obtained from the diet to some extent. Found predominantly in meat and fish, the daily requirement of creatine is 2 g.[111] Approximately 95% of creatine in the body is stored in skeletal muscle, especially type II muscle cells. Two thirds of the creatine stored in muscle is phosphorylated as phosphocreatine, which serves the function of rapidly producing ATP without the need for glycolysis, especially in short-term anaerobic activity. Cells typically have enough stores of ATP to endure approximately 10 seconds of high-intensity activity. Some hypothesize that high phosphocreatine levels may postpone or decrease lactate and hydrogen ion buildup from the breakdown of glucose and increase the time of maximal exercise.[6,111,116]

Creatine supplementation as a tasteless, crystalline powder that can be dissolved in liquids came to the forefront in the late 1990s. It was first noted in track athletes at the 1992 Olympics in Barcelona, Spain, and by 2000 approximately $300 million were spent in America alone on creatine supplements; there was a three-fold increase in use between 1997 and 2000. It is widely considered the most popular nutritional supplement on the market with some estimates of up to 48% of all male college athletes using the supplement.[111] An NCAA survey on habitual use among collegiate athletes found creatine supplement use second only to protein supplements.[111] A study with unpublished data by Tokish in 2002 of NFL trainers and physicians showed all teams had someone taking the supplement, with the average 33% and reports as high as 90%. Creatine is currently legal in the United States at all levels of competition.[6,110,111,116]

The data relating sports performance with creatine supplementation have been summarized by many authors. In 2004, Tokish,[111] after a review of the literature, wrote "A summary statement on these studies would be that creatine can be an effective ergogenic supplement maximized when used for simple, short-duration, maximal-effort anaerobic events." It should be added that

the benefit has only been seen in younger athletes (a study of 60–87-year-old athletes found no benefit).[111]

The most common regimen for creatine supplementation is for the athlete to take a loading dose of 20 g/day for 5–7 days, followed with 2–5 g/day for maintenance. Some studies have shown that alternative regimens may be equally effective. One such alternative was simply taking 3 g/day, without loading first.[116] Serious adverse effects have not been frequently associated with creatine, yet a few isolated cases of kidney dysfunction associated with its use have been reported. Although many believe creatine may lead to dehydration, no data on this point have been conclusive. Since creatine is sold over the counter as a nutritional supplement, there is no FDA regulation of the product.[6,111,116]

Erythropoietin and Blood Doping

From basic biochemistry, aerobic metabolism is much more effective at producing ATP than anaerobic metabolism. Keeping this in mind, athletes have known for some time that increasing the blood's ability to carry oxygen results in increased aerobic capacity, increased endurance, and the potential for enhanced performance. First noted after the 1968 Olympics in Mexico City, training at high altitudes or using altitude tents for sleeping are two practices used by athletes to increase the oxygen-carrying capacity of their blood.[111,117]

Blood doping refers to the practice of administering extra red blood cells to the athlete via intravenous transfusion. This can be accomplished via an autologous transfusion or via homologous transfusion using cross-matched blood. Erythropoietin is a hormone synthesized and released by the kidney in response to low circulating levels of oxygen that stimulates the bone marrow to produce more erythrocytes. As the level of oxygen rises, serum erythropoietin levels decrease. Recombinant erythropoietin (Epogen/EPO) was initially used for medical purposes, but its value as an ergogenic aid was quickly discovered.

Endurance athletes including cyclists and long-distance runners are more likely to abuse methods that artificially increase hematocrit because of the importance of aerobic capacity in their respective sports.[111,117] According to Shaskey and Green,[117] there is evidence that increases in hematocrit, either by blood doping or by using recombinant erythropoietin, can result in improvements in athletic performance and decreasing time to exhaustion in endurance athletes.

The potential adverse effects of using methods to artificially increase hematocrit include increasing blood viscosity, thrombogenic potential, myocardial infarction, and the inherent risks of blood transfusions (unless they are autologous). Homologous blood transfusion increases the risk of acquiring a blood-borne pathogen such as human immunodeficiency virus or viral hepatitis or of having a transfusion reaction.[111,117] From 1997 to 2000, 18 cyclists have died from stroke, myocardial infarction, or pulmonary embolism as a result of blood doping.[111,117]

Conclusion

The primary care of elite athletes can be a challenging undertaking and continues to become more complex. There is a great demand for providers who are interested in the medical management of the unique, as well as the routine, problems faced by these athletes. Today's collegiate and professional athletes depend on their health for their livelihood; the college athlete uses his investment to help him obtain an education and potentially become a professional. A primary care physician's chief role will be to continue to allow the athletes to compete in a manner that is safe and healthy.

References

1. Lombardo JA, Badolato SK: The preparticipation physical examination, *Sports Med* 3(5):10–22, 2001.
2. Glover DW, Maron BJ, Matheson GO: The preparticipation physical examination: steps toward consensus and uniformity, *Phys Sportsmed* 27:29–34, 1999.
3. Glover DW, Maron BJ: Profile of preparticipation cardiovascular screening for high school athletes, *JAMA* 279:1817–1819, 1998.
4. Loud KJ, Field AE, Micheli LJ: The adolescent male: primary care of the elite or elite-emulating adolescent male athlete, *Adolesc Med* 14(3):647–661, 2003.
5. Cavanaugh RM, Jr, Miller ML, Heneberger PK: The preparticipation athletic examination of adolescents: a missed opportunity? *Curr Probl Pediatr* 27:109–120, 1997.
6. Armsey TD, Hosey RG: Medical aspects of sports: epidemiology of injuries, preparticipation physical examination, and drugs in sports, *Clin Sports Med* 23:255–279, 2004.
7. Grafe MW, Paul GR, Foster TE: The preparticipation sports examination for high school and college athletes, *Clin Sports Med* 16(4):569, 1997.
8. Joy E, Paisley T, Price R, et al: Optimizing the collegiate preparticipation physical evaluation, *Clin J Sport Med* 14(3):183–187, 2004.
9. Patel DR, Greydanus DE, Luckstead EF: The college athlete, *Pediatr Clin North Am* 52:25–60, 2005.
10. Pfister GC, Puffer JC, Maron BJ: Preparticipation cardiovascular screening for US collegiate student-athletes, *JAMA* 283:1597–1599, 2000.
11. Klossner D: 2006–07 *NCAA Sports Medicine Handbook*, ed 18. Indianapolis, IN, 2006, National Collegiate Athletic Association Available at: http://www.ncaa.org/health-safety.
12. McKeag DB: Preseason physical examination for the prevention of sports injuries, *Sports Med* 2:413–431, 1985.
13. Peltz JE, Haskell WL, Matheson GO: A comprehensive and cost-effective preparticipation exam implemented on the World Wide Web, *Med Sci Sports Exerc* 31(12):1727–1740, 1999.
14. Flore RD: The development and implementation of a Web-based participation athletics health questionnaire, *J Athl Train NATA News* 9:49–58, 2003.
15. Goheen K: NFL teams rely on combine for draft guidance, *The Cincinnati Post* March 1, 2002. Available at: http://www.cincypost.com/bengals/2002/beng030102.html.
16. Kiper M: Sizing up the combine's pros and cons, *ESPN.com* February 23, 2007. Available at: http://espn.go.com/melkiper/s/2001/0221/1099442.html.
17. Associated Press: Bulls deal Curry after DNA test refusal, *ESPN.com* October 4, 2005. Available at: http://sports.espn.go.com/nba/news/story?id=2180298.
18. DuRant RH, Seymore C, Linder CW, Jay S: The preparticipation examination of athletes: comparison of single and multiple examiners, *Am J Dis Child* 139(7):657–661, 1985.
19. Seto CK: Preparticipation cardiovascular screening, *Clin Sports Med* 22:23–35, 2003.
20. Smith DM, Kovan JR, Rich BS, Tanner SM: *Preparticipation Physical Examination*, ed 2, Minneapolis, MN, 1997, American Academy of Family Physicians, American Academy of Pediatrics, American Medical Society for Sports Medicine, American Orthopaedic Society for Sports Medicine, and American Osteopathic Academy of Sports Medicine.
21. Kurowski K, Chandran S: The preparticipation athletic evaluation, *Am Fam Phys* 61:2683–2698, 2000.
22. Rifat SF, Ruffin MT, Gorenflo DW: Disqualifying criteria in preparticipation sports evaluation, *J Fam Pract* 41:42–50, 1995.
23. Wingfield K, Matheson G, Meeuwisse W: Preparticipation evaluation, *Clin J Sport Med* 14(3): 109–122, 2004.
24. Maron BJ, Zipes DP, editors: Eligibility recommendations for competitive athletes with cardiovascular abnormalities: general considerations, 36th Bethesda Conference, *J Am Coll Cardiol* 45(8): 1318–1321, 2005.
25. Carek PJ, Turell M, Heuston WJ: The preparticipation physical examination history: who has the correct answers? *Clin J Sport Med* 9(3):124–128, 1999.

26. Walker K, Tucker JB: *The Preparticipation Physical Examination* In Birrer RB, O'Connor FG (eds): *Sports Medicine for the Primary Care Physician*, ed 3, Boca Raton, FL, 2004, CRC Press.

27. Khosla R, Guntupalli KK: Heat-related illnesses, *Crit Care Clin* 15:251–263, 1999.

28. Wexler RK: Evaluation and treatment of heat-related illnesses, *Am Fam Phys* 65(11):2307–2314, 2002.

29. Maron BJ, Thompson PD, Puffer JC: Cardiovascular preparticipation screening of competitive athletes addendum: an addendum to a statement for health professionals from the Sudden Death Committee (Council on Clinical Cardiology) and the Congenital Cardiac Defects Committee (Council on Cardiovascular Disease in the Young), American Heart Association, *Circulation* 97:2294, 1998.

30. Carek PJ, Mainous AG 3rd: A thorough yet efficient exam identifies most problems in school athletes, *J Fam Pract* 52(2):127–134, 2003.

31. Gomez JE, Landry GL, Bernhardt DT: Critical evaluation of the 2-minute orthopedic screening examination, *Am J Dis Child* 147:1109–1113, 1993.

32. Hulkower S, Fagan B, Watts J, Ketterman E: Do preparticipation clinical exams reduce morbidity and mortality for athletes? *J Fam Pract* 54(7): 628–632, 2005.

33. Carek PJ, Mainous A: The preparticipation examination for athletics: a systematic review of current recommendations, *BMJ* 327:170–173, 2003.

34. Maron BJ, Shirani J, Pliac LC, et al: Sudden death in young competitive athletes, clinical demographic, and pathological profiles, *JAMA* 276: 199–204, 1996.

35. Hallstrand TS, Curtis JR, Koepsell TD, et al: Effectiveness of screening examinations to detect unrecognized exercise-induced bronchoconstriction, *J Pediatr* 141:343–348, 2002.

36. DuRant RH, Pendergrast RA, Seymore C, et al: Findings from the preparticipation athletic examination and athletic injuries, *Am J Dis Child* 146:85, 1992.

37. Van Camp SP, Bloor CM, Mueller FO, et al: Nontraumatic sports death in high school and college athletes, *Med Sci Sports Exerc* 27:641–647, 1995.

38. Drezner JA, Rogers KJ: Sudden cardiac arrest in intercollegiate athletes: detailed analysis and outcomes of resuscitation in nine cases, *Heart Rhythm* 3(7):755–759, 2006.

39. Kranhold K, Helliker K: Why heart trouble doesn't sideline some athletes, *Wall Street J* July 25, 2006. Available at: http://www.wsj.com.

40. Murkerji B, Albert MA, Mukerji V: Cardiovascular changes in athletes, *Am Fam Phys* 40:169–175, 1989.

41. Pluim BM, Zwinderman AH, van der Laarse A, et al: The athlete's heart: a meta-analysis of cardiac structure and function, *Circulation* 101: 336–344, 2001.

42. Pelliccia A, Maron BJ, Spataro A, et al: The upper limit of physiologic cardiac hypertrophy in highly trained elite athletes, *N Engl J Med* 324(5):295–301, 1991.

43. Holly RG, Shaffrath JD, Amsterdam EA: Electrocardiographic alterations associated with the hearts of athletes, *Sports Med* 25(3):139–148, 1998.

44. Robertson L: Inside is the heart of a champion—literally, *Miami Herald* July 21, 2005. Available at: http://www.edb.utexas.edu/coyle/content/armstrong%20media/LA-miami%20herald%207-21-05.pdf.

45. Pelliccia A, Maron BJ, De Luca R, et al: Remodeling of left ventricular hypertrophy in elite athletes after long-term deconditioning, *Circulation* 105:944–949, 2002.

46. Maron BJ, Pelliccia A, Spataro A, et al: Reduction in left ventricular wall thickness after deconditioning in highly trained Olympic athletes, *Br Heart J* 69:125–128, 1993.

47. Vasamreddy CR, Ahmed D, Gluckman TJ, Blumenthal RS: Cardiovascular disease in athletes, *Clin Sports Med* 23:455–471, 2004.

48. Maron BJ, Pelliccia A, Spirito P: Cardiac disease in young trained athletes: insights into methods for distinguishing athlete's heart from structural heart disease, with particular emphasis on hypertrophic cardiomyopathy, *Circulation* 91(5): 1596–1601, 1995.

49. Sharma S, Elliott PM, Whyte G, et al: Utility of metabolic exercise testing in distinguishing hypertrophic cardiomyopathy from physiologic left ventricular hypertrophy in athletes, *J Am Coll Cardiol* 36:864–870, 2000.

50. Maron BJ, Moller JH, Seidman CE, et al: Impact of laboratory molecular diagnosis on contemporary diagnostic criteria for genetically transmitted cardiovascular diseases: hypertrophic cardiomyopathy, long QT syndrome, and Marfan syndrome—a statement for health care professionals from the councils on clinical cardiology, cardiovascular disease in the young, and basic science, American Heart Association, *Circulation* 98(14):1460–1471, 1998.

51. Sanderlin BW, Raspa RF: Common stress fractures, *Am Fam Phys* 68(8):1527, 2003.

52. Bruckner P, Khan K: Sports related injuries and stress fractures. In *Clinical Sports Medicine*, ed 3, 2005. Available at: http://www.clinicalsportsmedicine.com/chapters/2.htm.

53. Walsh WM, Hald RD, Peter LE, Mellion MB: Musculoskeletal injuries in sports. In Mellion MB, Walsh WM, Madden CM, et al, editors: *Team Physician's Handbook*, ed 3, Hanley & Belfus, 2002, Philadelphia.

54. Halpern BC, King OS: Shoulder injuries, In Birrer RB, O'Connor FG, editors: *Sports Medicine for the Primary Care Physician*, ed 3, New York, 2004, CRC Press, pp 493–521.

55. Shaw J, O'Connor FG, Nirschl RP: Elbow. In Birrer RB, O'Connor FG, editors: *Sports Medicine for the Primary Care Physician*, ed 3, New York, 2004, CRC Press, pp 523–538.

56. Brennan F, Howard T, Lillegard W: Hand and wrist injuries. In Birrer RB, O'Connor FG, editors:

Sports Medicine for the Primary Care Physician, ed 3, New York, 2004, CRC Press, pp 551–585.

57. Levandowski R, Cohen P: Knee injuries, In Birrer RB, O'Connor FG, editors: *Sports Medicine for the Primary Care Physician*, ed 3, New York, 2004, CRC Press, pp 617–645.

58. Birrer R: The ankle. In Birrer RB, O'Connor FG, editors: *Sports Medicine for the Primary Care Physician*, ed 3, New York, 2004, CRC Press, pp 665–685.

59. Petrizzi MJ, Richardson DG: Foot injuries. In Birrer RB, O'Connor FG, editors: *Sports Medicine for the Primary Care Physician*, ed 3, New York, 2004, CRC Press, pp 687–710.

60. Tiedeman JJ, Ferlic TP: Hand and wrist injuries. In Mellion MB, Walsh WM, Madden CM, et al: *Team Physician's Handbook*, ed 3, Hanley & Belfus, 2002, Philadelphia, pp 427–440.

61. Brown DE: Ankle and leg injuries. In Mellion MB, Walsh WM, Madden CM, et al: *Team Physician's Handbook*, ed 3, Hanley & Belfus, 2002, Philadelphia, pp 509–520.

62. O'Connor FG, Birrer RB: Sports injuries: a general guide for the treatment and rehabilitation of sports injuries. In Birrer RB, O'Connor FG, editors: *Sports Medicine for the Primary Care Physician*, ed 3, New York, 2004, CRC Press, pp 281–290.

63. National Asthma Education and Prevention Program: *Highlights of the Expert Panel Report 2: Guidelines for the Diagnosis and Management of Asthma*, publication no. 97–4051. Bethesda, MD, 1997, US Department of Health and Human Services, Public Health Service, National Institutes of Health, National Heart, Lung and Blood Institute.

64. Barnes PJ: Mechanisms in COPD: differences from asthma, *Chest* 117:10–14, 2000.

65. Neven AS: Alternate treatments in asthma, *Chest* 123:1254–1265, 2003.

66. McFadden ER Jr: Exercise-induced asthma, *Chest* 91:151–157, 1987.

67. Allen TW, Cugell DW, Addington WW, et al: Post-exercise bronchospasm, *Chest* 59:157–160, 1971.

68. Allen TW, Addington W, Rosendal T, Cugell DW: Airway carbon dioxide and airway resistance in patients with postexercise bronchospasm, *Am Rev Resp Dis* 107:816–821, 1973.

69. Ferguson A: Dyspnea and bronchospasm from inappropriate post-exercise hyperventilation, *Ann Intern Med* 71:1063, 1969.

70. McNeill RS, Nairin JR, Millar JS, et al: Exercise-induced asthma, *QJ Med* 35:55, 1966.

71. Eggleston PA: Pathophysiology of exercise-induced asthma, *Med Sci Sports Exerc* 18:318–321, 1986.

72. Anderson SD: The mechanism of exercise-induced asthma is... *J Allergy Clin Immunol* 106:453–459, 2000.

73. Hermansen CL: Exercise-induced bronchospasm versus exercise-induced asthma, *Am Fam Phys* 67(4):769–774, 2003.

74. Holzer K: Screening of athletes for exercise-induced bronchoconstriction, *Clin J Sports Med* 14:134–138, 2004.

75. Brugman SM, Simons SM: Vocal cord dysfunction: don't mistake it for asthma, *Phys Sportsmed* 26:63–74, 1998.

76. Mickleborough TD, Lindley MR, Ionescu AA, Fly AD: Protective effect of fish oil supplementation on exercise-induced bronchoconstriction in asthma, *Chest* 129(1):39–49, 2006.

77. McKenzie DC, McLuckie SL, Stirling DR: The protective effect of continuous and interval exercise in athletes with exercise-induced asthma, *Med Sci Sports Exerc* 26:951–956, 1994.

78. Perez Lopez J, Rosas Vargas MA, del Rio Navarro BE, et al: Calisthenics as a preventive measure against the decrease in maximum expiratory flow in asthmatic patients before and after a soccer game, *Revista Alergia Mexico* 50:37–42, 2003.

79. De Bisschop C, Guenard H, Desnot P, Vergeret J: Reduction of exercise-induced asthma in children by short, repeated warm ups, *Br J Sports Med* 33:100–104, 1999.

80. Edmunds A: The refractory period after exercise-induced asthma: its duration and relation to the severity of exercise, *Am Rev Respir Dis* 117:247–254, 1978.

81. O'Byrne PM: The effect of indomethacin on exercise-induced bronchoconstriction and refractoriness after exercise, *Am Rev Respir Dis* 134:69–72, 1986.

82. Margolskee DJ: Indomethacin blocks airway tolerance to repetitive exercise but not to eucapnic hyperpnoea in asthmatic subjects, *Am Rev Respir Dis* 137:842–846, 1988.

83. Wilson BA: The effects of indomethacin on refractoriness following exercise both with and without bronchoconstriction, *Eur Respir J* 12:2174–2178, 1994.

84. Storms W: Exercise-induced asthma: diagnosis and treatment for the recreational or elite athlete, *Med Sci Sports Exerc* 31:S33–S38, 1999.

85. Allen TW: Sideline management of asthma, *Curr Sports Med Rep* 4:301–304, 2005.

86. Allen TW: Return to play following exercise-induced bronchoconstriction, *Clin J Sport Med* 15(6): 421–425, 2005.

87. Collins MW, Hawn KL: The clinical management of sports concussion, *Curr Sports Med Rep* 1: 12–22, 2002.

88. Bailes JE: Head injury in athletes, *Neurosurgery* 48:26–46, 2001.

89. Cantu R: Second impact syndrome: a risk in any sport, *Phys Sportsmed* 23:27–36, 1995.

90. Collins MW, Grindel SH, Lovell MR, et al: Relationship between concussion and neuropsychological performance in college football players, *JAMA* 282:964–970, 1999.

91. Gronwall D: Cumulative effects of concussion, *Lancet* 2:995–997, 1975.

92. Matser EJ, Kessels AG, Lezak MD, et al: Neuropsychological impairment in amateur soccer players, *JAMA* 282:971–973, 1999.

93. Collins MW: Concussion assessment in high school and college athletes: the ImPACT System, *Proceedings from New Developments in Sports-Related Concussion*, Pittsburgh, PA, July 27–29, 2001.

94. Echemendia RJ, Putukian M, Mackin RS, et al: Neuropsychological test performance prior to and following sports-related mild traumatic brain injury, *Clin J Sport Med* 11:23–31, 2001.

95. McGowan JC, Yang JH, Plotkin RC, et al: Magnetization transfer imaging in the detection of injury associated with mild head trauma, *Am J Neuroradiol* 21:875–880, 2000.

96. Johnston KM: A contemporary neurosurgical approach to sport-related head injury: the McGill Concussion Protocol, *J Am Coll Surg* 192:515–524, 2001.

97. Dupuis F, Johnston KM, Lavoie M, et al: Concussions in athletes produce brain dysfunction as revealed by event-related potentials, *Neuroreport* 11:4087–4092, 2000.

98. McAllister TW, Saykin AJ, Flashman LA, et al: Brain activation during working memory 1 month after mild traumatic brain injury: a functional MRI study, *Neurology* 53:1300–1308, 1999.

99. Collins M: Current issues in managing sports-related concussion, *JAMA* 282:2283–2285, 1999.

100. Cantu RC: Posttraumatic retrograde and anterograde amnesia: pathophysiology and implications in grading and safe return to play, *J Athl Train* 36(3):244–248, 2001. This grading system modifies the original Cantu grading system proposed in Cantu RC: Guidelines for return to contact sports after a cerebral concussion, *Phys Sportsmed* 14(10):75–83, 1986.

101. Report of the Sports Medicine Committee: *Guidelines for the Management of Concussion in Sports*, Denver, CO, 1990, revised May 1991, Colorado Medical Society.

102. American Academy of Neurology: Practice parameter: the management of concussion in sports (summary statement). Report of the Quality Standards Subcommittee, *Neurology* 48: 581–585, 1997.

103. Maroon JC, Lovell MR, Norwiq J, et al: Cerebral concussions in athletes: evaluation and neuropsychological testing, *Neurosurgery* 47:659–671, 2000.

104. Lovell M: The comparison of computerized versus traditional neuropsychological testing in developing objective criteria for return to play following concussion in high school athletes, Presented at the 27th Annual Meeting of the National Academy of Neuropsychology. Orlando, FL October 15–18, 2000.

105. Guskiewicz KM, Riemann BL, Perrin DH, Nashner LM: Alternative approaches to the assessment of mild head injury in athletes, *Med Sci Sports Exerc* 29:S213–S221, 1997.

106. Mrazik M, Ferrara MS, Peterson CL, et al: Injury severity and neuropsychological and balance outcomes of four college athletes, *Brain Inj* 14: 921–931, 2000.

107. Guskiewicz KM: Effect of mild head injury on postural stability in athletes, *J Athl Train* 31: 300–306, 1996.

108. Ahrendt DM: Ergogenic aids: counseling the athlete, *Am Fam Phys* 63(5):842–843, 2001.

109. Bamberger M, Yaeger D: Over the edge: special report, *Sports Illustrated* 86:64, 1997.

110. NCAA Research Staff: *NCAA study of substance use habits of college student-athletes 2001*. Available at: http://www.ncaa.org/library/research/substance_use_habits/2001/substance_use_habits.pdf.

111. Tokish JM, Kocher MS, Hawkins RJ: Ergogenic aids: a review of basic science, performance, side effects, and status in sports, *Am J Sport Med* 32 (6):1543–1553, 2004.

112. Chandler JV, Blair SN: The effect of amphetamines on selected physiological components related to athletic success, *Med Sci Sports Exerc* 12:65–69, 1980.

113. Gill ND, Shield A, Blazevich AJ, et al: Muscular and cardiorespiratory effects of pseudoephedrine in human athletes, *Br J Clin Pharmacol* 50:205–213, 2000.

114. Bell DG, Jacobs I: Combined caffeine and ephedrine ingestion improves run times of Canadian Forces Warrior Test, *Aviat Space Environ Med* 70:325–329, 1999.

115. Bell DG, McLellan TM, Sabiston CM: Effect of ingesting caffeine and ephedrine on 10–km run performance, *Med Sci Sports Exerc* 34:344–349, 2002.

116. Greydanus DE, Patel DR: Sports doping in the adolescent athlete: the hope, hype, and hyperbole, *Pediatr Clin North Am* 49:829–855, 2002.

117. Shaskey DJ, Green GA: Sports haematology, *Sports Med* 29(1):27–38, 2000.

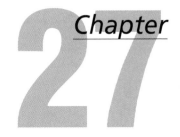

Chapter 27

The Executive Male

Sean Kesterson, MD, and Joel J. Heidelbaugh, MD

Key Points

- Executive Health Programs (EHPs) provide comprehensive evaluation and testing that is commonly not fully covered by traditional insurances and not always clearly evidence based (strength of recommendation: C).
- Companies and individuals can enjoy substantial financial benefit from EHPs (strength of recommendation: C).
- EHPs can be profitable for practices and affordable for patients with the increasing use of health savings accounts and the increasing demand for patient autonomy (strength of recommendation: C).
- Modern technology provides the opportunity for better access for executives to their EHPs to improve follow-up outcomes (strength of recommendation: C).

Introduction

"An ounce of prevention is worth a pound of cure."

—Henry de Bracton, English jurist, 13th century[1]

Although Henry de Bracton was probably not referring to health and wellness in this statement, the words obviously ring true to proponents of periodic preventive health maintenance examinations. Indeed, there is ample proof that evidence-based examinations and targeted disease screening can reduce morbidity and mortality. This concept applies when considering executive-level healthcare, except that the ripple effect of individual male business executive wellness and illness can mean the difference between brighter and darker days for not only businessmen but also for the companies, stockholders, and customers they serve. The executive/company incentive duality sustains an industrious effort to reach out to executives, encouraging them to undergo regular preventive healthcare examinations at an unprecedented rate, and executive health programs (EHPs) are now becoming ubiquitous. There is precious little evidence in the medical literature regarding the specific benefit of EHPs, despite their currently blossoming popularity. Although few cost-effectiveness analyses have been published, morbidity and mortality data comparing EHPs to standard evidence-based health maintenance examinations does not exist.

One might say that the term *executive health* is an oxymoron. When we think of the life of today's typical male executive, the picture appears somewhat contrary to a healthy lifestyle. From a biopsychosocial standpoint, the executive's world virtually mirrors the image of a hectic life. These men are psychosocially complex and plagued with work and life stressors that lead to feelings of uncertainty, chaos, and questioning—their lives are full of urgency and pressure. Calendars are commonly overbooked, with availability by meeting, telephone, pager, and e-mail filling up days and time with more work and less attention to their own personal healthcare needs. This trend is compounded by the "Superman" complex that so many high-powered male executives seem to have. Their success in life and business gives them a feeling of invincibility, as if no setback could derail their drive toward success. Literally fueled by stress, these persons push their bodies and minds to extraordinary limits. The level of intense functioning that male executives seek and attempt to maintain is unfathomable and unfamiliar to most "average mortals."

Today, men wield the command in Fortune 500 companies at a 3-to-1 ratio. But although they outnumber women in the boardroom, they do not outnumber women in the doctor's office. In modern healthcare, we accept that women seek both routine and acute healthcare, prevention, diagnosis, and treatment of disease more frequently than men. This holds especially true in the executive suite, as there is always a better reason to miss the yearly checkup: a customer to meet, a deal to make, a transaction to oversee. This denial is rationalized as looking after the needs of the company, its employees and their families, its stockholders, and specifically *not* the executive himself. This tendency toward self-neglect is commonly driven by noble, altruistic, honorable causes, but it is also driven by a passion for work and success, ambition, ego, and monetary incentives that can be gargantuan.

Principles of Executive Healthcare

EHPs are very common and relatively easy to find in the United States. They exist within both academic and nonacademic centers and health systems and are sometimes free-standing and independent agencies. These programs can be found at hospitals, outpatient clinics, and even in luxurious spa resorts. What these clinics have in common is a cash-paying clientele—namely, patients who are interested in a periodic health examination that is extensive and efficient. As with most anyone seeking preventive healthcare in today's society, male executives tend to want personal information on identifiable risk factors for diseases and early detection of disease that requires treatment. Virtually none of these programs provide services that would be fully covered by traditional medical insurance; in fact, most EHPs clearly state that their services are *not* covered by traditional medical insurance. The menu of services available in EHPs typically ranges from evidence-based testing and examinations, to batteries of tests that are exhaustive (and probably excessive), to constructive coaching about promoting a healthy lifestyle.

The executive physical is a periodic health examination for a business executive that serves two purposes. The first goal is to deliver what a periodic examination should for any man seeking preventive healthcare. The second purpose is a more financially driven goal, seemingly the business case for investing in the executive workforce. A powerful driver of the demand and market for EHPs is that businesses are extremely dependent on the output of their high-level executives. Sick days or disabling illness in the boardroom constitutes the potential for opportunity cost, loss in market share, and spiraling stock values. The executive himself benefits from the preventive examination by obtaining information on how to stay healthy, as well as how to stay available to earn the coming year's bonus, stock options, and future promotion. Therefore, there is a sizable financial incentive and motivation for a given company and its executives to participate regularly in a thorough periodic health maintenance examination. Furthermore, the higher the salary and responsibility of the executive, the higher the premium for executive-level preventive care and advice. At the highest executive levels, no expense for testing and treatment need be spared to ensure health for the individual, and ultimately, the company that this executive leads. This incentive for business is addressed more fully in the section on economic rationale below.

Changes in healthcare benefits and financing are likely to make executive physicals and preventive examinations for nonexecutives more accessible to the average male. Increasingly, companies across America appear to be converting to benefit plans that are more conducive to consumer-directed healthcare. Attractive features of these plans include more latitude on healthcare expenditures that are simultaneously tax-free and portable. Although the US Internal Revenue Service (IRS) currently regulates allowable expenses, almost all testing and preventive services provided in an EHP would be permitted.

Historical Perspective

Models of disease, health, and wellness have evolved over centuries. Developing knowledge of normal anatomy, disease and its causes, then disease and its treatment has taken a substantial amount of time. Interestingly, rigorous focus on effective means of prevention of disease for individuals is a much more modern phenomenon. In 1964, Dr. Luther Terry, the US Surgeon General, issued a landmark report linking cigarette smoking with lung cancer, throat cancer, and chronic bronchitis, drawing on evidence in thousands of medical studies and reports.[2] He then called for immediate remedial action. In 1976, Canada formed a preventive healthcare task force, followed by the United States in 1984 under the guise of the Public Health Service. Similarly, the post–World War II era marks the beginning of explosive development of effective vaccines to prevent contagious disease. This timeline closely mirrors the growth in emphasis on public preventive health and, secondarily, EHPs.

The best known EHPs are relatively new. Examples include EHPs at the Cooper Clinic in Texas, the Mayo Clinic in Minnesota, the Cleveland Clinic in Ohio, Duke University in North Carolina, and the University of California at Los Angeles (UCLA; Table 27-1). All of these programs have been in existence for less than 40 years.

Economic Rationale

The negative reverberation of a major health problem for a male executive has unfortunately been common and very high profile. Recently, illness at the executive level affected major companies such as McDonald's and Coca-Cola severely, clearly demonstrating the sizable impact of the unexpected and untimely death of world-renowned businessmen.

In April 2004, Jim Cantalupo, serving at the time as Chief Executive Officer (CEO) of the McDonald's Corporation, died suddenly of a myocardial infarction. Ironically, this came shortly after he directed the company toward the development of healthier menu items at McDonald's

Table 27-1. Features of Common Executive Health Programs

Program	Highlights*	Cost and Features†
Cooper Aerobics Clinic http://www.cooperaerobics.com Dallas, TX 1-800-444-5764	Cardiovascular prevention programs FAA certifications Lung CT Electron beam tomography Private, preventive care Ranch setting	$2600—Standard battery plus: Stress assessment Exercise assessment Nutrition consultation Body fat composition Vision and hearing screening
Duke Executive Health http://www.dukeexechealth.org Durham, NC 1-919-660-6823	Academic hospital affiliation Cardiovascular assessment including arterial stiffness, endothelial function test Affiliated with Duke School of Business Electronic patient portal for test results and reports	$2765—Standard battery plus: Stress assessment Exercise assessment Nutrition consultation Body fat composition Endoscopy *not* included
Mayo Clinic Executive Health http://www.mayoclinic.org/executive-health Jacksonville, FL Rochester, MN Scottsdale, AZ 1-800-851-9022	Standard Bearer of Executive Health Programs 3 locations in US Affiliation with premier hospital in Rochester, MN	$5714—Standard battery plus: Coronary CT scanning for CACS Hearing screening Colonoscopy replaces flexible sigmoidoscopy
UCLA Executive Health http://www.exechealth.ucla.edu Los Angeles, CA 1-866-330-EXEC	Academic hospital affiliation Premier West Coast EHP provider PET scanning for cancer detection Menu for cardiovascular preventive tests	$2400—Standard battery plus: Cardiovascular test menu‡ Pulmonary function test Body fat composition Vision and hearing screening Urologic consultation Personalized nutritional counseling (extra charge) Colonoscopy replaces flexible sigmoidoscopy Does *not* include chest radiograph

FAA, Federal Aviation Administration; CT, computed tomography; CACS, coronary artery calcium score; PET, positron emission tomography.
*Not all items are included in a standard examination.
†Charge quoted is based on standard charge, or that reported for new patient male executive examination for a man older than 50 years, August 2006. EHP listed includes all of the following as standard items unless otherwise noted: complete history and physical examination, flexible sigmoidoscopy or colonoscopy, prostate-specific antigen (PSA) test and/or free PSA test, C-reactive protein level measurement, fasting lipid profile, serum chemistry profile, electrocardiogram and cardiac stress test, chest radiograph.
‡Stress echocardiogram, coronary CT scanning for determination of CACS, serum chemistry and lipid panel, carotid intima-medial thickness testing.
Adapted from materials from the various executive programs listed above via faxed personal communication, August 2006.

restaurants, with great financial success. Loss of human life is not only difficult for close family and friends, but it can also be devastating to businesses. Urgently and eagerly, the McDonald's Corporation moved to replace their lost leader and maintain an image of control by quickly announcing Charles Bell as the new CEO. Mr. Bell, who was enormously qualified for the job, would in short time unfortunately discover his own health misfortune. Within 2 weeks of his promotion he was diagnosed with colorectal cancer, and the economic impact of poor executive healthcare hit the books and the press. Shares of the Illinois-based McDonald's Corporation fell 2.6%, or approximately 78 cents per share, immediately. The day after Mr. Cantalupo's death, more than 15 million shares exchanged hands, which was three times the average daily volume, reflecting billions of dollars. This record loss—directly related to executive illness—was one of the most significant in business history.[3,4]

Surprisingly, Coca-Cola experienced even more dramatic and persistent declines in performance upon the unfortunate death of its CEO. In 1997, after a long, steady, and successful run, Coca-Cola lost its CEO, Roberto C. Goizueta. Mr. Goizueta died in October of that year, a month after being diagnosed with lung cancer. During his 16-year leadership, the stock value of Coca-Cola increased by approximately 7100%, with campaigns such as "Coke is it," "The New Coke," and "Classic Coke." Simply stated, an investment of $1000 in 1981 was worth $71,000 in 1997. Since his death, Coca-Cola has been in a long and slow decline, and now the company has the lowest stock value and poorest stock performance of any in its relative category. The stock value that reached $87 per share at the time of Goizueta's death has fallen to $42 per share in mid 2006. With 475 million shares outstanding, the change in value reflects a loss of $21 billion.[5,6]

Whether measures aimed at targeted disease prevention and screening would have averted these scenarios may not seem perfectly clear. Yet, it is known that a key for businesses in managing leadership change is an appearance of gradual, careful, and deliberate hiring or promotion that eases the potential anxiety of the market and its stockholders and customers. Such anxiety can lead to great stockholder desertion, a slide in market value, and a drop in market share. Sudden changes that occur with health catastrophes like these garner enormous skepticism in the press and could potentially be avoided if there is earlier detection or very deliberate preventive healthcare delivered. Early detection and prevention of

disease dampens the need for urgent leadership change that can send companies into a tailspin. Fortunately, there is some rigorous evidence that preventive examinations at management levels have positive impacts on decreasing absenteeism and improve the bottom line financially, but little evidence exists to support the direct link between executive health and market value as clearly as it is made in the two cases above.

In 2002, Burton published a report analyzing outcomes of an EHP for bank executives, along with a brief review of published work on EHPs.[7] Burton's literature review concurs that the evidence is scarce on any useful information of cost benefits and outcomes of EHPs. The retrospective study of nearly 1800 persons compared executive participants and nonparticipants in the company's EHP. Participation was offered to all executives and therefore was voluntary. Sixty-nine percent of participants and 60% of nonparticipants were male ($P < .01$). The executive periodic examination for participants included the following[7]:

- Complete history and physical examination
- Fasting laboratory tests including multiphasic chemistries (e.g., complete blood count, blood chemistries, thyroid function tests)
- Serum lipid profile including triglycerides, total cholesterol, high-density lipoprotein cholesterol, and calculated low-density lipoprotein cholesterol
- Urinalysis
- Resting 12-lead electrocardiogram
- Spirometry
- Vision and glaucoma screening
- Prostate-specific antigen (PSA) screening for men older than 50 years and when clinically indicated
- Additional testing including chest radiograph, flexible sigmoidoscopy, and hemoglobin A_{1c} performed either as recommended by the American Cancer Society or when clinically indicated (see Chapter 1, Organizing Preventive Healthcare in Men)

The chief outcomes in Burton's review were reduced short-term disability days (2.78 days versus 4.08 days) and medical claims ($5361 versus $6246) over a 3-year period between participants and nonparticipants, respectively.[7] The author estimated overall direct and indirect cost benefits to the company to be $1661 per executive over the 3-year period when secondarily using the cost of lost productivity. Multiplying by the total number in the study equals a total potential cost savings of over $2.9 million.[7] This information extends and generalizes the benefits for businesses to their managers and executives well below the CEO level on an organizational chart. The preventive examination conducted in this study did not involve extraordinary or exhaustive evaluation and testing. Instead, a fairly traditional and individualized approach based on standard recommendations for prevention and symptom-based diagnosis and treatment was used.

The economic impact for the business of executive healthcare and wellness has been demonstrated, both in the medical literature and on Wall Street. From the highest executive levels to middle management, it appears to be "good business" to direct male executives to regular and periodic health examinations. Furthermore, it provides an opportunity for executives to benefit individually from such an examination. As programs and emphasis grow in this sector of healthcare delivery, there will certainly be recognition that disease prevention is just as valuable to the health of companies as it is to the health of individuals. After all, the strength of the chain is only as great as its weakest link.

Health Concerns of Male Executives

Stress

Although it seems obvious and certainly explainable that executives are subjected to enormous stress, it is very ironic that this stress and its sequelae are rarely addressed directly by EHPs. An informal and unreported survey of male executives at the University of Michigan Ross School of Business conducted during their attendance of weekend training sessions in Ann Arbor in 2006 indicates that their greatest health concern not routinely addressed in their periodic health maintenance examinations is stress. *Crain's Detroit Business*[8] reports stress management as a common request at a Southeast Michigan EHP, typically manifested by fatigue, chest pain, and insomnia in the male executive.

Although the exact direct cause of an executive's stress may or may not be clear, it is commonly apparent that they may not possess the necessary coping skills to balance inherent stress along with the demands of their careers. Divorce, alcoholism, substance abuse, depression, and suicide are probably at least as common in executives as in average populations, although accurate epidemiologic data in this demographic are somewhat lacking. Furthermore, it appears to be uncommon for executives to seek help and to counsel for stress management,[7] perhaps

because of a sense of time urgency, and perhaps because of the associated stigma.

Many EHPs, on average, unfortunately fail to screen for depression, alcoholism, anxiety disorders, and most of the aforementioned sequelae of inherent stress. Their general focus tends to be on the prevention and treatment of medical illness, though they often lack the support and expertise of mental health professionals or even personal or executive coaches. Certainly, it seems that a strong case could be made for folding in a structure of mental preventive health and treatment for executives under such great pressure.

Cardiovascular Health

The connection between catecholamines and cardiovascular events is now a generally accepted principle in medicine. The adrenaline-filled executive life gives one the sense that these men are a "heart attack waiting to happen." An executive's apparent predisposition is supported by observational outcome data from the 1950s on personality types. Business executives are almost exclusively type A personalities, and they commonly exhibit the following characteristics:

- An insatiable desire to achieve one's goals
- A strong willingness to compete in all situations
- A strong desire for recognition and advancement
- A strong desire to multitask under time constraints
- Always being in a rush to finish activities
- Above average physical and mental alertness

Further research on the type A personality and its behavior indicates that components of anger and hostility subcategorize the classification of the type A personality into the type H personality. Both type A and type H personalities have demonstrated increase risk for unfavorable lipid profiles and double the age-adjusted risk for cardiovascular events.[9] Personalities and behaviors resist change most resiliently, thus the focus for prevention in these driven persons tends to be identification of treatable lipid abnormalities and asymptomatic or minimally symptomatic coronary artery disease.[10] As demonstrated in Table 27-1, EHPs seem to emphasize this angle of preventive strategy with their clientele.

Cancer

The fourth, fifth, and sixth decades of a man's life are important times in which the focus of healthcare should be on the early detection and prevention of cancer. The most common types of cancer in men include lung, colon, prostate, and skin, all of which are amenable to preventive efforts and screening interventions for early detection. Fortunately, with the improvement in public awareness of cancer-prevention strategies, virtually all business executives should be curious about recommendations for cancer detection and prevention. Although screening for lung cancer is still difficult at best, EHPs that provide focus on smoking cessation are doing what is minimally necessary to address this continued executive-level and public health threat. Endoscopic screening for colorectal cancer is virtually standard in EHPs to date, with colonoscopy being the preferred modality. Screening for prostate cancer is also standard in EHPs, and it appears that the EHPs reviewed are recommending PSA testing for all of their male executive patients (see Table 27-1).

Erectile Dysfunction

Addressing erectile dysfunction is increasingly common in practice when men attend clinics for non–acute illness-related visits. Direct inquiry about sexual health and wellness is a desirable and timely endeavor when caring for executives because their demographic is commonly affected by sexual dysfunction. Sexual health is a major driver of a man's sense of overall health and wellness, and addressing this can significantly improve the executive's self-reported sense of well-being. Poor sexual performance may also be a sign of disease or increased risk of disease, including atherosclerosis, alcoholism, or depression. Unfortunately, most EHPs do not both diagnose and treat the executives that they evaluate, so an efficient means of addressing erectile dysfunction is uncommonly available to them. Modern EHPs should seek to rectify this shortfall and devise a systematic manner in which to treat disorders they uncover.

Service Expectations and Standards

Male executives run tight schedules and have demanding timelines to complete tasks, assignments, and goals. They are a focused and determined group with high expectations of themselves and others. Largely, they have experienced high levels of service and tend to appreciate and demand attention and efficiency not normally offered in traditional medical

settings. Therefore, successful EHPs, without exception, will go to great lengths to promise and deliver extraordinary levels of service to businessmen.

A typical EHP offers a comprehensive medical examination that can be completed within 1–2 days. These examinations often include tests performed and results interpreted by specialists including colonoscopy, coronary computed tomography scans, and echocardiography. The networks serving these EHPs must give priority to the performance, interpretation, and reporting of such testing if these programs are to meet the high standard of EHPs in the United States.

Geographic location is important to the overall success of EHPs. Although individuals may be willing to travel by airplane great distances to receive care from high-quality EHPs, the distance from the airport to EHP is usually a short one. Some EHPs are located near business centers such as Detroit, New York, Houston, or Los Angeles, making access even more ideal for the home office of major corporations. Others are located outside of business centers with easy access to airports and highways.

Academic affiliation is another important component of EHPs. Businessmen are sensitive to the notion of branding, and affiliation with centers owning an excellent clinical and academic affiliation satisfies the desire to associate with a top-quality brand. The Mayo Clinic, Duke University, and UCLA are great examples of executive programs that own excellent brand security. Although such an affiliation provides more than brand security for the EHP, larger networks that prioritize their executive healthcare work can prioritize access to testing and specialists beyond the influence of an individual practice.

Lastly, the comfort, privacy, and environment of the EHP clinic are of paramount importance. Many EHP clients will be high-profile persons who struggle to keep their lives private and will be desirous of short wait times in private waiting rooms. Some executives may wish to use assumed names during their visits to prevent curious inquiries into their personal and medical affairs. The physicians and staff of an EHP must be very deliberate in individualizing the reception and in handling the privacy of their executives who may be more instantly recognizable than average patients. Examples of EHPs with high standards of privacy and environment include the Cooper Clinic in Texas, the Mayo

Clinic in Minnesota, and the Wellmax Program (http://www.wellmax.com) at the La Quinta Resort in California.

Elements of the Executive Physical

The reality of the executive-level preventive health examination is that it is not a pure example of a purely evidence-based practice. It usually provides a standard evidence-based exam *plus* a way to determine the likelihood of disease that may affect the male executive or his business, regardless of whether it would affect the individual's morbidity or mortality. For this reason, one sees many tests offered in the executive physical examination that would not normally be recommended in a traditional male health maintenance exam. This, of course, makes good business sense because the company that pays for the examination is interested in predicting the longevity of its workforce while shoring up their health and individual productivity, regardless of whether it has been proven to make a significant difference in the length or quality of life of the individual.

Table 27-1 illustrates four of the best known EHPs in the United States along with individual program highlights, elements of the standard evaluation, optional examinations, and current fees. As noted previously, the cost of these examinations to the business is negligible in comparison to the potential benefit of early detection of disease, particularly at the highest executive levels. Coronary artery calcium (CAC) scores may provide additional information that is presumed to be useful in motivating persons toward preventive strategies when the value correlates with a potentially high risk of a cardiac event. High values have been shown to modify predicted risk obtained from Framingham risk scores alone, especially among patients in the intermediate-risk category in whom clinical decision making is most uncertain.[11] The cost/benefit analysis of these studies for businesses is probably often taken into account more so than the cost-effectiveness to the individual undergoing such testing.

Two articles that appeared in *Circulation* in 2006 under the section *Controversies in Cardiovascular Medicine* attempted to address the utility of electron-beam computed tomography (EBCT) for the noninvasive screening of coronary artery disease, and they presented quite opposing viewpoints. The first article by Clause[12] posits that CAC scores should be used as an additional predictor for future coronary events, given that the scientific basis for such a test has been validated. He concluded that CAC scores should be integrated with Framingham risk scores in intermediate- and high-risk groups and should be used as a guide for therapy in addition to correction of other cardiovascular risk factors including changes in lifestyle, diet, weight reduction, and exercise. In addition, Clause also concluded that CAC scores should be monitored sequentially over time to evaluate their significance as a predictor for future cardiac events as they relate to progression, regression, or stabilization of coronary artery disease. The second article by Chen and Krumholz[13] concluded that there has been no study to date to definitively demonstrate that screening with EBCT improves clinical outcomes by reducing morbidity or mortality from CAD, and that widespread and routine screening is unlikely to benefit either low-risk or high-risk patients. Moreover, they concluded that no study has demonstrated that EBCT reduces healthcare costs; of the few studies that have been conducted, none have highlighted male executives as research subjects.

After an executive-level health maintenance examination, a report is generated that outlines the pertinent findings and test results. This report is usually given to the executive, his primary care physician, and sometimes to the company's human resources department. Risk stratification and recommendations for further testing, as well as recommendations for lifestyle changes are commonly included in the report. Generally, the follow-up and treatment of conditions that are discovered are left up to the executive and his personal primary care physician. An EHP connected with a health system or network is very useful when positive test results are discovered in the event that the executive requests a referral for specialty care. Commonly, the executive may bring the examination report and test results to his private physician to discuss any issues and decide on further testing, treatment, or referral. Although these examinations are often extremely useful in that they are quite comprehensive, the risk of incidental false-positive results may burden practices and traditional insurances charged with determining whether the incidental findings are significant, as well as raise potential anxiety in the executive. This notion begins to make the case that some private physician practices should consider developing EHPs for their own patients, so that diagnosis, treatment, and follow-up can be more tightly connected. Present and future models of healthcare financing may make this option more feasible for such practices.

Frontiers and Opportunities in Executive Healthcare

Changes in healthcare financing, telecommunication, service orientation, and office efficiency are simultaneously creating a more conducive environment for EHPs to run well and thrive. A major stimulus in favor of EHPs is the movement toward consumer-driven healthcare. This will be a more common orientation as the financial transaction between physicians and patients becomes more direct. Patients will begin to have more choice and authority in spending for healthcare as rules for use common in managed care settings apply less and less, and restrictions are loosened as a result. The public will more actively participate in decision making with regard to the tests, treatment, medications, and other services they will have available to them. This trend has become even more prevalent and impending with changes in how businesses pay for their executive and employee healthcare.

The extreme burden for US businesses in financing healthcare has created a pressing need to create new ways for employees to obtain reasonable healthcare at a lower overall cost to their respective businesses. Simply stated, employee health benefits that require lower employer contributions drive down the cost of doing business. Before 2003, alternatives such as flexible spending accounts existed but were undesirable because of their inherent "use it or lose it" rules: tax-free dollars saved for allowable healthcare expenses had to be used within a 12–18-month period or be forfeited. When the Medicare Prescription Drug Improvement and Modernization Act was signed into law on December 8, 2003, the ability to create healthcare savings accounts (HSAs) became law. These accounts are effectively managed in a manner similar to individual retirement accounts.[14]

A number of rules apply to the creation of HSAs. Maximum liabilities and contributions are set for individuals and families, contributions must be made while enrolled in a qualified high-deductible health insurance policy (but does not have to be in effect for a withdrawal from the HSA), and only certain types of medical expenses qualify for fund withdrawal and application. HSAs are quite different from flexible healthcare savings accounts in that the funds do not have to be used during a specific time period, and they can be kept in reserve for use in future years. Thus, the "use it or lose it" rule does not apply to HSAs. These funds can be used for Consolidated Omnibus Budget Reconciliation Act (COBRA) premiums, healthcare coverage while receiving unemployment compensation, and long-term care insurance premiums.[15] Thus, HSAs seem to be a very positive and attainable option for many patients and their employers. In this scenario, the employer ultimately pays lower premiums for higher-deductible catastrophic medical insurance, and the patient has a means to use tax-exempt dollars to directly purchase healthcare services, evaluations, tests, and treatment. Although lists of eligible expenses have been drafted, none are currently definitive. According to the IRS, "the expense has to be primarily for the prevention or alleviation of a physical or mental defect or illness." Virtually everything that is commonly provided in an EHP would therefore meet the definition of an allowable expense.

Although employers traditionally cover the costs for higher level executives to have executive physicals, HSAs make executive examinations more accessible to executives, managers, directors, and employees who are not generally eligible for a company-funded executive-level physical. EHP practices can take advantage of this by creating programs that emphasize patient choice and freedom created by HSAs, encouraging them to pursue this with their employer, and creating EHPs that efficiently address their needs and preferences. Competitive pricing of office visits and evaluations can be created in a way that permits additional time for the physician to spend consulting with patients, the limits of which are a major frustration in managed care and third-party fee-for-service insurance-financed healthcare.

The facile use of modern communication equipment also provides new opportunities to improve health outcomes with executives. As previously noted, the importance of efficiency and time savings are enormously important to executives. The use of cellular phones, wireless technology, the Internet, e-mail, text pagers, and video phones makes it possible for patients and their physicians to communicate with each other, virtually face to face, anywhere, at anytime. EHPs can therefore provide additional services and prompt follow-up that is not traditionally possible. Office-initiated contact can influence outcomes by ensuring adequate follow-up on important test abnormalities, behavior and lifestyle changes, exercise and stress management, medication options and management, and guidance on specialist referral, tests, and treatment. The array of information exchange seems almost limitless. It is almost certain that access to physician-patient communication of this sort is an untapped opportunity to revolutionize ideal preventive healthcare for everyone.

Conclusion

The increasing trend toward patient preference, patient satisfaction, and consumer-driven healthcare aligns with executive healthcare and demands for high levels of service. Traditional financing has been a major driver in limiting physician time spent in direct contact with patients and results in significant lost time spent in waiting rooms and ultimately short visits with the physician. EHPs ultimately pay for more time with the physician, something that is not fundable with a traditional insurance model and standard office practices. Physician satisfaction and patient satisfaction should fit hand in glove, creating a win-win situation for both parties in their encounters. Paradigms that create more time and space to consult with patients would be a good start. As practices become more financially accountable for outcomes of disease prevention and treatment, as well as satisfaction with pay-for-performance initiatives, programs within practices like EHPs align extraordinarily well.

References

1. Wikipedia contributors: Luther Leonidas Terry. *Wikipedia: The Free Encyclopedia*, July 26, 2006, 19:43 UTC. Available at: http://en.wikipedia.org/w/index.php?title=Luther_Leonidas_Terry&oldid=66018585. Accessed August 16, 2006.
2. US Department of Health, Education and Welfare. Smoking and Health: Report of the Advisory Committee to the Surgeon General of the Public Health Service. Public Health Service Publication No. 1103 Publisher: United States. Public Health Service. Office of the Surgeon General, 1964.
3. Sad day at McDonald's. Available at: http://www.cnnmoney.com. Accessed April 19, 2004.
4. Morningstar: McDonald's stock/financial performance. Available at: http://quote.morningstar.com/Quote/Quote.aspx?ticker=MCD.
5. CNN Interactive: Coke CEO Robert C. Goizueta Dies at 65, October 18, 1997. Available at: http://www.cnn.com/US/9710/18/goizueta.obit.9am.
6. Available at: http://tools.morningstar.com/charts/Mcharts.aspx?Country=USA&Security=KO&sLevel=Acoke stock/financial performance.
7. Burton WN: The value of the periodic executive health examination: experience at Bank One and summary of the literature, *J Occup Environ Med* 44 (8):737–744, 2002.
8. Bendetti M: Heart disease, cholesterol, stress are top health issues, *Crain's Detroit Business Detroit* 16(6): 13, 2000.
9. Friedman M, Rosenman RH: Association of specific overt behavior pattern with blood and cardiovascular findings, *JAMA* 169:1286–1296, 1959.
10. Rosenman RH, Brand R, Sholtz R, Friedman M: Multivariate prediction of CHD during 8.5-year follow-up in the Western Collaborative Group Study, *Am J Cardiol* 37:903–910, 1976.
11. Greenland P, LaBree L, Azen SP, et al: Coronary artery calcium score combined with Framingham score for risk prediction in asymptomatic individuals, *JAMA* 291:210–215, 2004.
12. Clouse ME, Chen J, Krumbolz HM, et al: Noninvasive screening for coronary artery disease with computed tomography is useful, *Circulation* 113:125–146, 2006.
13. Chen J, Krumholz HM: How useful is computed tomography for screening for coronary artery disease? Screening for coronary artery disease with electron-beam computed tomography is not useful, *Circulation* 113:135–145, 2006.
14. Feldman A, Carbonara P: Are you ready to own your health care? *Money New York* 33(11):135–140, 2004.
15. Wilson PL: Health savings accounts: save now and save for later, *Agency Sales Irvine* 34(7):48–51, 2004.

28

The Incarcerated Male

R. Scott Chavez, PhD, MPA, PA

Key Points

- The NCCHC recommends screening all inmates in correction facilities for chlamydia and gonorrhea regardless of their behavioral risk for STDs or their symptomatology (strength of recommendation: C).
- Facilities that house long-term inmates (i.e., persons who will be incarcerated for 14 days or longer) should skin-test inmates using the intradermal Mantoux skin-test; facilities housing short-term inmates should consider using chest radiography to screen all inmates for TB disease upon entry into the facility. All inmates with HIV infection should undergo chest radiography, regardless of their skin-test results (strength of recommendation: C).
- See Box 28-2. Among its recommendations, the NCCHC urges the promotion of communicable disease, chronic disease, and mental illness surveillance among inmates in all correctional jurisdictions; creation of a national reporting system for prevalence data; and addressing the medical, housing, and postrelease needs of inmates in prerelease planning and making use of appropriate resources and new technologies. Each recommendation was developed by an expert consensus panel established by the NCCHC for its congressional report, *The Health Status of Soon-to-be-released Inmates*[5] (strength of recommendation: C).

Introduction

Evidence-based medicine (EBM) research involving US incarcerated men remains an elusive goal. Randomized controlled trials (RCTs), the best level of evidence for medical decision making, are profoundly lacking relative to understanding healthcare needs and practices of incarcerated men. Similarly, prospective cohort and case-controlled studies are limited at best. Federal regulations and corrections policies tightly control research practices on inmates and, as a result, the environment to propose and conduct any RCTs in this population is limited. Voluntary participation by incarcerated men in RCTs has raised ethical and procedural concerns since the inclusion of inmates in studies is never fully voluntary. In addition, prison and jail incarceration strategies to move inmates from facility to facility, or to release them back to the community, have created an additional barrier for researchers to mount EBM controlled studies.

With more than 1.4 million prisoners in federal and state adult correctional facilities, and 500,000 in city and county jails,[1] there is a great need to manage complex healthcare "behind the walls" using evidence-based practices. Three distinct case examples highlight this problem:

1. Thirteen days after his arrest, a 68-year-old male who had a medical history significant for heart disease and diabetes mellitus was found dead, naked, and lying on his back on a mat in his cell next to a half-eaten orange and a sandwich. He was on a self-medication program and was expected to administer his own insulin. The medical examiners' office reported that "the inmate died of diabetes and that heart disease may have contributed to his death."[2]

2. In an effort to maintain costs and expensive treatment, critics of the California prison system claim that officials often avoid

screening prisoners for some medical conditions, thus having inadequate information about serious diagnoses such as hepatitis C or tuberculosis (TB).[3]

3. A 37-year-old neuroleptic prisoner's medical record was found to be incomplete, with his medical condition not listed in the master problem list and no indication when he was last seen in the seizure disorder clinic. The patient was housed in the prison infirmary to enforce his compliance with anticonvulsant medications, yet there was no recent anticonvulsant blood level measurement obtained or other reason clarifying why there was such concern regarding his medication noncompliance.[4]

The failure to provide consistent and adequate healthcare services to incarcerated men has an onerous effect on the overall health of our communities.[5] High rates of communicable disease, including TB, human immunodeficiency virus (HIV) infection, and various sexually transmitted diseases (STDs), among untreated incarcerated men who are released into the community may be transmitted to the public at large. In addition, releasing inmates with untreated chronic disease likely creates a financial burden on the local community's healthcare system. Correctional institutions have a unique opportunity to improve disease control and treatment and thus reduce the community burden of providing adequate and appropriate healthcare to inmates with significant comorbid conditions after they have been released.

This chapter describes the current status of and barriers to EBM decision making and research involving US incarcerated men. It concludes with a discussion of what is needed to improve correctional health service delivery and care.

Evidence-Based Medicine at the Point of Incarceration

Incarcerated male populations arise from a mixture of various microcosms in our society including the homeless, minorities, impoverished, substance abusers, and mentally ill. Can EBM findings from these populations at large be extrapolated to medical care for incarcerated men? Are incarcerated men truly representative of patients studied in other populations? Before accepting evidence from EBM-inspired databases or from other external sources of knowledge, we must first ask how robust the conclusions are and whether those conclusions are based on long-term results relevant for the eventual fate of the patient.[6]

Incarcerated environments are truly unique and affect the clinical outcome of chronic disease in a multitude of ways. Inmates have limited options for freedom of movement, diet, exercise, and access to medical or trained operational staff. As a result, opportunities for patient self-management of chronic disease are difficult to implement in jails and prisons. Preincarceration behavior and experience mixed with a correctional institution's practices influence whether an individual will engage in risky behavior while incarcerated[7] will take action to improve treatment regimens and clinical outcomes. To understand how preincarceration behavior affects clinical care, studies on male inmates' health prior to incarceration have focused largely on drug abuse, STDs, TB, and mental illness.

Alcohol and Other Drug Abuse

A history of illegal substance use before incarceration is well documented in the literature.[8] Although this research is not exclusive to men, the majority of studies have demonstrated the response to and needs of AOD-abusing men who become incarcerated. Approximately 80% of inmates have some form of alcohol or drug abuse problem, with 25% of state and federal inmates having histories of injection drug use.[9] EBM research on alcohol practices of men before incarceration is limited and focuses mainly on mentally ill inmates.[10]

The Arrestee Drug Abuse Monitoring (ADAM) Program sponsored by the National Institute of Justice (NIJ) assesses drug use among arrestees in selected US cities on a voluntary and anonymous basis. During the time of arrest, an assessment is calculated as a percentage of arrestees with urine assays yielding results that are positive for illicit drug use. This figure provides an estimate of the percentage of inmates who test positive for any illicit substance. Jail reception centers collect the urine tests from arrestees on a voluntarily and anonymous basis and then report these data to ADAM. In 2000, ADAM data reported that 64% of male arrestees tested positive for at least one of five illicit drugs (i.e., cocaine, opioids, marijuana, methamphetamines, and phencyclidine [PCP]).[11]

Dependence on heroin and other opiates has long been associated with criminality. Jails are faced with an ever growing number of persons who have an opiate addiction, yet few receive methadone maintenance or detoxification.[12] Although EBM in the treatment and management of opiate dependence is clearly established, political, social, and judicial opposition to opioid replacement therapy in jails has thwarted EBM decision making among incarcerated males.

The Substance Abuse and Mental Health Services Administration's Center for Substance Abuse Treatment (CSAT)[13] has produced an EBM guide for the screening and treatment of alcohol and other drug (AOD) abuse in the criminal justice system. The best-practice guidelines for the treatment of AOD abuse are based on experience and knowledge of clinical, research, and administrative experts and are thus expert opinion-based recommendations. The CSAT recommends that jail and prison staff use the following evidence-based tools to screen incoming inmates for AOD abuse[12] (Box 28-1):

- Receiving screening: National Commission on Correctional Health Care (NCCHC) standards[14,15] require that an arriving inmate be immediately screened by health-trained personnel or qualified healthcare professionals for infectious diseases (e.g., TB, hepatitis, STDs, HIV status); pregnancy; acute conditions; substance use history; detoxification needs; acute intoxication; suicidality; acute mental health symptoms and past hospitalizations; history of abuse; dental problems; and allergies. In addition, correctional facility staff members are instructed to indicate their observations of appearance, behavior, state of consciousness, ease of movement, breathing, and skin manifestations (e.g., jaundice, rashes, bruises, scars, needle marks).

- Alcohol Dependence Scale (ADS): This 25-item instrument was developed to screen for symptoms of alcohol dependence. The scale performs well in community and institutional settings.

- Addiction Severity Index (ASI)-Drug Use Subscale (ASI-Drug): A 25-item instrument designed for alcohol dependence symptom screening, this tool is especially effective in community and institutional settings. Combined with the ADS, the ASI-Drug identifies AOD use problems among offenders.

- Drug Abuse Screening Test (DAST-20): The DAST-20 is another screening tool that identifies drug abuse. Questions asked include the following:
  - Have you used drugs other than those required for medical reasons?
  - Have you abused prescription drugs?
  - Can you get through the week without using drugs (other than those required for medical reasons)?

- Texas Christian University Drug Screen: This 15-item substance abuse diagnostic screen is completed by the offender and is able to quickly identify persons who report heavy drug use or dependency.

- Michigan Alcoholism Screening Test (MAST, short version): This 25-item questionnaire rapidly screens for lifetime alcohol-related problems. It is effective among adults and can be administered and scored in 15 minutes.

BOX 28-1
CSAT–Recommended Tools to Screen Inmates for Abuse of Alcohol and Other Drugs

ASI–Drug Use Subscale (ASI-Drug) is available in Center for Substance Abuse Treatment: *Screening and Assessment for Alcohol and Other Drug Abuse Among Adults in the Criminal Justice System,* Treatment Improvement Protocol (TIP) Series 7, DHHS Publication No. (SMA) 00–3477. Rockville, MD, 1994, Substance Abuse and Mental Health Services Administration.

Addiction Severity Index (ASI) developed in 1980 by A. Thomas McLellan, Lester Luborsky, George E. Woody, Charles P. O'Brien is available from the developers at Building 7, PVAMC, University Ave, Philadelphia, PA 19104; (214) 399–0890.

The Michigan Alcoholism Screening Test (MAST), developed in 1971 by Melvin L. Selzer, is free and available in the public domain. Selzer M: *Am J Psychiatry* 127(12): 1653–1658, 1971.

The Texas Christian University (TCU) Drug Screen (TCUDS) is available from the TCU Institute of

Behavioral Research (IBR) at http://www.ibr.tcu. edu.

Substance Abuse Subtle Screening Inventory-2 (SASSI-2) is available at http://www.sassi.com/sassi/index.shtml.

Simple Screening Instrument for Substance Abuse (SSI-SA) is reproduced along with instructions in Center for Substance Abuse Treatment: *Substance Abuse Treatment for Persons with Co-occurring Disorders,* Treatment Improvement Protocol (TIP) Series 42. DHHS Publication No. (SMA) 05–3992. Rockville, MD, 2005 Substance Abuse and Mental Health Services Administration.

Addiction Severity Index (ASI)/Alcohol Use Subscale (ASI-Alcohol), developed in 1980 by A. Thomas McLellan, Lester Luborsky, George E. Woody, Charles P. O'Brien is available from the authors at Building 7, PVAMC, University Ave, Philadelphia, PA 19104; (214) 399–0890.

- Substance Abuse Subtle Screening Inventory-2 (SASSI-2): The SASSI-2 has been found to effectively and quickly screen inmates for substance abuse.[16]
- Simple Screening Instrument for Substance Abuse: This screening instrument includes 16 items related to alcohol and drug use, preoccupation and loss of control, adverse consequences of use, problem recognition, and tolerance and withdrawal effects. It identifies both alcohol and drug dependence.
- ASI/Alcohol Use Subscale (ASI-Alcohol): This comprehensive drug evaluation assessment tool has been standardized to match offenders' drug problems with treatment approaches.

In light of the CSAT's recommendation, the question remains: What is the status of substance abuse screening and treatment in jails and prisons? In the spring of 2006, the NCCHC surveyed 1300 US jails and prisons on their substance abuse and mental health screening and treatment practices and resources with the goal of assessing specifically which CSAT recommendations are implemented.[17] With 226 (17.4%) facilities responding, a picture of what EBM screening and treatment tools are being used by correctional staff to assess AOD use was obtained (Table 28-1).

The survey data revealed that there is a heavy reliance on the receiving screening tool to gather information relative to AOD abuse (81.9%).[17] Unfortunately, this does not ensure that accurate AOD screening occurs. Although the NCCHC recommends standard language for receiving screening forms, there is no universal screening form that ensures consistency because correctional institutions vary in the forms that they use. Accuracy of the information is also dependent on staff training to ensure that observations and questions are obtained without bias; there is no assurance that staff training or practice is consistent. In addition, receiving screening is largely dependent on self-report from poor historians. As a result, clinicians cannot rely on receiving screening as the sole tool on which to base their EBM decision making for AOD abuse.

Fewer than half of the facilities surveyed use an evidence-based scale to screen for AOD abuse, and surprisingly, 16.4% do not use any of the CSAT recommended tools.[17] Since these screening tools were neither developed nor validated in a criminal justice setting, there may be a reluctance to use such scales. Staffing and the length of time to administer these scales may also affect the decision to use them. Studies have demonstrated that effective AOD treatment programming includes early

Table 28-1. Common Intake Screening Instruments Used to Screen for Drug Abuse (n = 226)

	Number	(%)
None of the above	94	41.6
Mental Health Screening Form-III (MHSF-III)	62	27.4
Beck Depression Inventory II (BDI-II)	52	23.0
Personality Assessment Inventory (PAI)	39	17.3
Milon Clinical Multiaxial Inventory (MCMI-III)	19	8.4
Minnesota Multiphasic Personality Inventory (MMPI-2)	15	6.6
Brief Symptom Inventory (BSI)	14	6.2
Hamilton Depression Scale (HAM-D)	10	4.4
Symptom Checklist 90, Revised (SCL-90-R)	3	1.3
General Behavior Inventory (GBI)	3	1.3
Referral Decision Scale (RDS)	0	0.0
Total = 226		

TCU, Texas Christian University.
Adapted from: National Commission on Correctional Health Care: Unpublished survey of accredited facilities on screening, treatment, and management of AOD among inmates, 2006.

(forced if necessary) treatment, continuity (some treatment is better than no treatment), extensive aftercare (found to reduce recidivism by 90%), cognitive and behavioral therapy (reduces recidivism by 35%), and anger and interpersonal control.[18] Although this EBM approach is well established, the lack of resources, well-trained staff, and use of common evidence-based screening tools remain barriers to its consistent implementation and use.

Sexually Transmitted Diseases

Studies on detecting *Chlamydia trachomatis* and *Neisseria gonorrhoeae* infections in men entering county jails have found that screening for asymptomatic men needs to improve.[19-22] Specifically, the timeliness of the screen needs to be addressed. Unfortunately, risky sexual behavior, transient lifestyles, and limited access to healthcare have all increased the risk for STDs among men who enter correctional facilities. Asymptomatic males with chlamydia have increased risks for urethral infections and complications associated with epididymitis. The Chlamydia Prevalence Monitoring

Project, an effort to collect data on screening test results from correctional facilities in 34 states, found that 5.4% of the incarcerated juvenile male population was infected with chlamydia.[23] Men entering correctional institutions have high rates of chlamydia, reportedly at a median positive rate of 6.4%, which often reflects the local community prevalence.[20,23,24]

Chlamydia screening is among the top 10 provisions for cost-effective care in the general public,[25] as it has been demonstrated that every dollar spent on screening and treatment saves approximately $12 from the cost of complications associated with an untreated infection.[20] Too often, however, jails do not have the resources to adequately screen and conduct appropriate testing; therefore, persons who are asymptomatic can be missed entirely.[21] Another reason why it is important to screen and treat asymptomatic persons with chlamydia is that the majority of jail arrestees are released within 48 hours of being detained. It is therefore especially important to screen for and treat chlamydia to prevent transmission in the community upon release.[26] Since many persons do not have continuous access to healthcare, the NCCHC recommends screening all inmates in correctional facilities for chlamydia and gonorrhea regardless of their behavioral risk for STDs or their symptomatology.[14,15]

Human Immunodeficiency Virus

A review by Wohl and colleagues[27] provides an in-depth examination of a "dual epidemic" phenomenon—namely, HIV infection and incarceration. The potential for incarceration to directly and indirectly facilitate the spread of HIV infection has been underappreciated as well as understudied from an evidence-based perspective. As a result of changes in the epidemiology of the HIV epidemic and in criminal justice policies during the past 2 decades, HIV infection in the United States has become largely concentrated in prisons and jails.[27] The prevalence of HIV infection and acquired immunodeficiency syndrome (AIDS) is significantly higher among inmates than in the total US population (Figure 28-1). Incarceration of large numbers of men can, in fact, facilitate the spread of HIV. Interventions to enhance the identification of infected inmates, to conduct prevention counseling, and to direct treatment of inmates who have HIV infection and AIDS are required to minimize the spread of HIV within the prison system and the population at large.

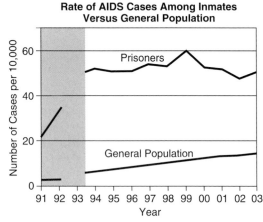

Figure 28-1. Rate of AIDS cases among inmates versus general population. (Adapted from: Wohl, DA, Rosen D, Kaplan AH: HIV and incarceration: dual epidemics, *Drug Benefit Trends* 18:392–402, 2006.)

Tuberculosis

Jails and prisons present one of the greatest reservoirs conducive for the spread of TB. Scores of incidences have been reported in which correctional institutions have had TB outbreaks, infecting inmates, staff, and visitors. The Centers for Disease Control and Prevention (CDC) and the NCCHC have EBM guidelines for the screening and treatment of TB in jails and prisons;[28] both guidelines call for aggressive screening of staff and residents. Initial and annual TB screening for facility staff should be a mandatory condition of employment; however, based on the prevalence of TB in the institution, an increase in the frequency of TB screening may be warranted. It is recommended that in "facilities which house long-term inmates [persons who will be incarcerated for 14 days or longer] should skin-test inmates using the intradermal Mantoux skin-test. Facilities housing short-term inmates should consider using chest radiography to screen all inmates for TB disease upon entry into the facility. All inmates who are HIV-positive should receive a chest radiograph, regardless of the status of their skin-test results."[28] Housing considerations for single-unit medical isolation is required, along with appropriate medical treatment.

Many institutions have a desperate shortage of medical and health staff as well as major physical limitations that prevent them from implementing EBM and effective TB screening programs.[29] As a result, current analytical research is lacking on EBM implementation of TB screening programs within US correctional institutions.

Mental Illness

The CSAT[13] recommends that one or more of the following screening instruments be used to assess the mental status of persons arriving at the jail or prison:

- Beck Depression Inventory II
- Brief Symptom Inventory
- Mental Health Screening Form-III
- Referral Decision Scale (RDS)
- Symptom Checklist 90–Revised
- General Behavior Inventory
- Millon Clinical Multiaxial Inventory III
- Hamilton Depression Scale
- Minnesota Multiphasic Personality Inventory-2
- Personality Assessment Inventory

As part of its survey to better understand the status of drug use and mental illness screening among correctional institutions, the NCCHC surveyed 1300 jails and prisons on their mental health screening practices. Table 28-2 reports data on 226 respondent facilities regarding the most commonly used evidence-based screening instruments. Surprisingly, 41.6% of the responding correctional institutions reported that none of the CSAT recommended tools are used to screen for mental health among its incoming inmates.[17] Other mental health evaluative tools may have been used by these institutions; however, CSAT-recommended tools are simple, quick, and efficient to use, and it is highly unlikely that time-consuming and difficult evidence-based tools would be used during initial screening of inmates.

Table 28-2. Common Intake Screening Instruments Used to Assess Mental Illness

	Number	(%)
Receiving Screening	185.0	81.9
Addiction Severity Index (ASI) – Alcohol Use subscale (ASI-Alcohol)	73	32.3
ASI-Drug Use subscale (ASI-Drug)	66	29.2
Substance Abuse Subtle Screening Inventory-2 (SASSI-2)	58	25.7
None of the above	37	16.4
Alcohol Dependence Scale (ADS)	35	15.5
Simple Screening Instrument for substance Abuse (SSI-SA)	31	13.7
TCU Drug Screen (TCUDS)	26	11.5

Adapted from: National Commission on Correctional Health Care: Unpublished survey of accredited facilities on screening, treatment, and management of AOD among inmates, 2006.

The RDS[30] is a 14-item measure of mental disorder symptoms developed to identify depression, bipolar disorder, and schizophrenia. The tool was developed and validated in a criminal justice setting and has been in use for more than 15 years. This screening tool is useful to detect the presence of major mental illness among jail inmates and requires no training to administer. None of the 226 responding facilities reported using this evidence-based screening tool designed for jails. Additional research is needed to understand why correctional staff members do not use the RDS.

Evidence-Based Medicine Use During Incarceration

There have been few studies to date that adequately assess the unmet needs of incarcerated men with specific chronic medical conditions such as diabetes mellitus or hypertension. Although the cumulative rate of incarcerated men with a chronic disease is unknown, it is estimated that 30% of the population has some form of a chronic disease. Estimates based on the National Health and Nutrition Examination Survey data prepared for the NCCHC suggest that asthma is more prevalent among inmates than in the overall population (9% versus 8%), whereas diabetes (4.8% versus 7%) and hypertension (18.3% versus 25%) are less prevalent among male inmates.[5]

EBM is designed to involve the patient in the medical decision-making process because patient involvement in determining the best course of action has been shown to improve clinical outcomes. A few studies have attempted to demonstrate how incarcerated populations can be invested in their healthcare, yet imprisoned males are commonly recalcitrant patients who are uninvolved in the promotion of healthy lifestyles.[5,31,32] After all, the same socioeconomic factors that lead to poor health (e.g., poverty, low educational achievement, minority populations) are the same factors that have been shown to lead to criminal activity and incarceration, and these remain a significant barrier to the application of EBM principles in correctional institutions.

NCCHC Clinical Guidelines

The NCCHC, a not-for-profit agency with a mission to improve healthcare services in correctional institutions, published a report in 2002 titled *The Health Status of Soon-To-Be-Released Inmates*. This study, conducted at the request of the US Congress and in cooperation with the NIJ, documented the prevalence of chronic and communicable diseases found in prisons. Although the report did not separate out the issues by gender, the study found diabetes and hypertension prevalence among incarcerated populations to be lower than the overall population.[5] Included in this study was the NCCHC's examination of correctional institutions' use of evidence-based guidelines in the management of chronic disease, which discovered that fewer than 63% of reporting state departments of corrections (n = 46) used any form of clinical guidelines. However, a content analysis found that many such guidelines were in fact nursing protocols for care, and many systems did not have a organized system to monitor chronic diseases.[5] Concern over these problems has led to a number of recommendations relative to healthcare services for incarcerated persons[5] (Box 28-2).

Many correctional care clinicians are focused on episodic care and do not take the time to learn the totality of the inmate's needs, lacking a professional aggressiveness to control serious conditions even for long-term patients. This is in part due to the structure of correctional healthcare systems that are based on a "sick call model" that serves the management of acute disease which is largely episodic, curable, and short-lived. Obviously, chronic care does not fit into this construct of healthcare delivery, which is a grave disadvantage to the inmate.

To remedy this situation, the NCCHC recommended that nationally accepted evidenced-based clinical guidelines for correctional institutions be developed. Subsequently, in 2002, the NCCHC published a set of evidence-based clinical guidelines for the management of incarcerated patients with hypertension, diabetes, asthma, seizure disorder, and HIV infection. The NCCHC based its correctional guidelines on the scientific evidence promulgated by the Joint National Committee on Prevention, Detection, Evaluation, and Treatment of High Blood Pressure Report (JNC 7)[33]; the American Diabetes Association[34]; the National Asthma Education Program[35]; the International Classification of Epileptic Seizures[36]; the Third Report of the National Cholesterol Education Program of the National Heart, Lung, and Blood Institute[37]; and the "Guidelines for the use of antiretroviral agents in HIV-infected adults and adolescents" published by the Department of Health and Human Services.[38]

The NCCHC guidelines address issues unique to correctional institutions, including basic intake evaluation, requirements for initial and interval follow-up, common barriers to adequate disease management in corrections, and a list of valuable quality-improvement monitors for each chronic disease. Each NCCHC guideline includes an introductory section explaining how to implement a chronic care program in a correctional setting. Within this chronic care program, a unique conceptual model is presented in which definitions of disease control are described for each chronic condition.

As often occurs in a correctional setting, clinicians subjectively form an opinion regarding how well a chronic disease is being controlled. The NCCHC approach directs clinicians to define "good control" on evidence-based targets that scientists have identified as being correlated to decreasing excess morbidity. For example, regarding the management of diabetes mellitus, *good control* is defined as the upper limit of normal on an hemoglobin A_{1c} (HbA_{1C}) assay, or less than 7.0%.[39] The American Diabetes Association recommends tight control of HbA_{1C} among incarcerated populations, owing to the fact that African Americans and Hispanic populations (predominately represented in correctional institutions) are at a higher risk for obesity and diabetes.[39] However, in a jail setting, where there is a rapid turnover of incarcerated patients, the NCCHC consensus panel recommends that definitions of control may have to be adjusted and based on random finger-stick glucose tests, where "good control" is considered to be readings of 80–120 mg/dL.[40]

The NCCHC clinical guidelines also benchmark "fair" and "poor" control indicators that are based on scientific indicators associated with long-term increases in morbidity and mortality. *Fair diabetic control* is defined as being within 2 percentage points above the upper limit of an HbA_{1C} laboratory normal, and *poor diabetic control* is defined as any range beyond the 2 percentage points above the upper limit of an HbA_{1C} laboratory normal.[40] The NCCHC chose the classification of degree of control for simplicity and clarity. Ultimately, these definitions of control help the clinician to monitor patients and guide them in achieving treatment goals.

As a result of its study and clinical guideline benchmarks, the NCCHC developed a performance-improvement measurement program to improve chronic disease management in prisons.[41] This performance-improvement measurement program seeks to redefine how clinicians monitor and reduce disease-manifested morbidity and mortality in their patients.

BOX 28-2
National Commission on Correctional Health Care: *Health Status of the Soon-to-Be-Released Inmate,* 2002.

Surveillance

The principal use of disease surveillance in correctional facilities is to monitor disease incidence, prevalence, and outcomes in the inmate population. Surveillance includes collecting health data and evaluating the data collection system to assist correctional health officials in characterizing the health status of the inmate population. The information obtained from the surveillance system is used to plan, implement, and evaluate health needs of the inmate population and their anticipated health needs upon release.

I. Congress should promote surveillance of selected communicable diseases, chronic diseases, and mental illnesses among inmates in all correctional jurisdictions. Appropriate Federal agencies in partnership with national health-related organizations should:

A. Develop surveillance guidelines to promote uniform national reporting of selected conditions to enhance epidemiologic research of these conditions and assist with accurate healthcare planning. Ensure that data collected in prisons and jails as part of the surveillance program are collected in the same manner as they are collected in the community. Surveillance guidelines should incorporate processes for protecting confidentiality of data.

B. Create a national correctional healthcare database.
 1. Develop standardized definitions and measures for reporting to assess the prevalence of selected communicable diseases, chronic diseases, and mental illnesses.
 2. Mandate national reporting of these prevalence data.
 3. Design an information system and make it available for use by local, state, and federal correctional authorities to measure and report the data with the ability to categorize the data by age, race, and gender.

C. Produce statistical reports of local, state, and national rates of selected communicable diseases, chronic diseases, and mental illnesses in prisons and jails to aid planning correctional and public health programs and allocate local resources.

D. Evaluate the utility of surveillance activities and implement improvements as appropriate.

Clinical Guidelines

Clinical guidelines provide definitions and abbreviated decision trees for the diagnosis and management of various diseases and conditions.

They guide the clinician in areas where scientific evidence of the value of selected interventions exists to improve survival and clinical outcomes and to reduce morbidity and the cost of care. Clinical guidelines are widely used outside corrections.

II. Congress should promote the use of nationally accepted evidenced-based clinical guidelines for prisons and jails. This will help ensure appropriate use of resources to prevent, diagnose, and treat selected communicable diseases, common chronic diseases, and mental illnesses that are prevalent among inmates. Appropriate federal agencies in partnership with national health-related organizations should:

A. Ensure that the clinical guidelines are consistent with nationally accepted disease definitions and evidence-based guidelines used for the non-incarcerated population.[40]

B. Disseminate the clinical guidelines to correctional healthcare professionals, public health agencies, and public policymakers.

C. Update the clinical guidelines as often as needed.

D. Develop standardized performance measures for state and local correctional authorities to determine adherence to nationally accepted clinical guidelines.

E. Train correctional health and public health professionals in the use of these clinical guidelines and performance measures.

F. Develop tools for correctional systems to assess overprescribing and underprescribing of psychotropic medications.

Immunizations

Immunizations prevent the development of a variety of communicable diseases in individuals. In the case of diseases such as hepatitis B, poliomyelitis, measles, mumps, or rubella, immunizations prevent the transmission of disease to susceptible individuals in the general population. Such immunizations are nationally accepted and promoted by the Centers for Disease Control and Prevention (CDC). Some immunizations are directly cost saving and others are highly cost effective.

III. Congress should establish and fund a national vaccine program for inmates to protect them and the public from selected vaccine-preventable communicable diseases.

A. The vaccination program should be similar to the National Vaccine Program for Children.

B. The program should conform to the recommendations of the CDC's Advisory Committee on Immunization Practices (ACIP).

Continued on following page

BOX 28-2
National Commission on Correctional Health Care: *Health Status of the Soon-to-Be-Released Inmate,* **2002. (Continued)**

National Correctional Healthcare Literature Database

To function competently, correctional healthcare clinicians require access to the medical literature, especially as it relates to correctional healthcare issues. Existing resources do not provide this level of specificity.

IV. Congress, through appropriate federal agencies and health-related national organizations, should develop and maintain a national literature database for correctional healthcare professionals, including a compendium of policies, standards, guidelines, and peer-reviewed literature.

Ethical Decision Making

Correctional healthcare professionals function in a uniquely restrictive environment with limited opportunity for peer review of medical policies and administrative actions. A national forum is needed to discuss issues, such as confidentiality, informed consent, clinical management of hepatitis C and HIV, and the availability of biomedical research.

V. Congress should establish a national advisory panel on ethical decision making among correctional and health authorities to assist those authorities in addressing ethical dilemmas encountered in correctional healthcare.

Eliminate Barriers to Inmate Healthcare

In correctional facilities, healthcare professionals face unique barriers to the delivery of health services. These include constraints on policy, budgets, priorities, and staffing. Correctional institutions are positioned to provide individual care to inmates and protect the public health through aggressive health promotion and disease-prevention efforts. At all levels of government, public policymakers should recognize that eliminating barriers to healthcare for inmates provides long-term public health benefits.

VI. Congress, through appropriate federal and state agencies and health-related national organizations, should identify and eliminate barriers to the successful implementation of public health policy.
A. Reduce obstructions to effective public health programs within correctional facilities and in the community.
B. Promote continuity of inmate healthcare by maintaining Medicaid benefits for eligible inmates throughout their incarceration.

C. Promote continuity of ex-offender healthcare by mandating immediate Medicaid eligibility upon release.
D. Provide incentives to jails and prisons to expand their alcohol and other drug treatment programs. These services should be gender specific and made available to inmates from admission through release, with special attention paid to inmates with both mental illness and substance abuse problems.

Correctional Healthcare Research

Too little is known about the epidemiology of disease in correctional populations, and too little has been done to evaluate programs designed to improve inmate health.

VII. Congress, through appropriate federal agencies and health-related national organizations, should support research in correctional healthcare to identify and address problems unique to correctional settings.
A. Fund projects to evaluate models that emphasize creative, cost-effective options for continuity of care following release.
B. Fund research programs to define effective health education and risk reduction strategies for inmates. These strategies need to deal with relevant differences between inmate and non-inmate populations. The research programs should work through public, private, and community-based healthcare agencies.
C. Fund research programs to identify correctional system barriers that prevent correctional healthcare staff from implementing prudent medical care and public health recommendations.

Improve Delivery of Healthcare

For a variety of reasons, the scope and content of correctional healthcare services vary. The quality of care is not as high as it might be, resulting in unnecessary morbidity, premature mortality, and increased costs.

VIII. Congress, through appropriate federal agencies and medically based accrediting organizations, should promote improvements to the delivery of inmate healthcare.
A. Require federal, state, and local correctional systems to adhere to nationally recognized standards for the delivery of healthcare services in corrections. These standards should include access to care, quality of care, quality

Continued on following page

BOX 28-2
National Commission on Correctional Health Care: *Health Status of the*
Soon-to-Be-Released Inmate, **2002. (Continued)**

of service, and appropriate credentialing of healthcare professionals.

B. Provide sufficient resources for correctional systems to adhere to national standards.

C. Weigh the correctional system's adherence to national standards for healthcare delivery whenever determining funding levels for the system.

Disease Prevention

Primary prevention is designed to keep disease from occurring. Examples include lifestyle choices and vaccination against selected communicable diseases. Primary prevention is widely believed to be the best and most cost-effective use of healthcare dollars. In some cases, it is also a cost saving—that is, the prevention program saves more money than it costs to implement. Secondary prevention (screening) is the early detection of disease that already exists but may not be apparent to the patient.

IX. Congress, through appropriate federal agencies and national organizations, should encourage primary and secondary disease-prevention efforts.

A. Promote primary disease-prevention measures by requiring federal, state, and local correctional agencies to:

1. Provide all inmates with a smoke-free correctional environment. Offer tobacco cessation programs for all staff and inmates as a method of achieving tobacco-free facilities.

2. Offer heart-healthy choices on institutional menus and in commissaries.

3. Make daily aerobic exercise available to all inmates.

4. Consistent with the recommendations of the ACIP, make hepatitis B vaccines available to all inmates, even when their length of incarceration is short or indeterminate.

5. Screen all female inmates for pregnancy. Test women found to be pregnant for hepatitis, HIV infection, syphilis, gonorrhea, and chlamydia. Provide HIV treatment to HIV-infected mothers to prevent transmission of the disease to the newborn.

6. Although not a correctional system responsibility, administrators should seek to collaborate with community healthcare providers to ensure the timely immunization of all infants born to mothers who test positive for hepatitis B.

7. Offer scientifically based risk-reduction education on HIV infection and sexually transmitted diseases (STDs) to all inmates.

B. Promote secondary disease-prevention measures by using nationally accepted evidence-based clinical guidelines, as appropriate.

1. Provide hypertension, obesity, asthma, and seizure disorder screening for all prison inmates.

2. Provide diabetes and hyperlipidemia screening for jail and prison inmates at high risk.

3. Provide suicide-prevention programs, including timely screening for inmates at high risk for suicide.

4. Prevent the spread of tuberculosis (TB).

   a. Consistent with nationally accepted guidelines, routinely screen inmates for TB disease and infection, and provide preventive treatment for inmates with latent TB infection.

   b. Promote the use of short-course preventive therapy (delivered over 2 months) in correctional settings.

   c. Strengthen the link of TB control efforts between correctional facilities and public health departments.

   d. On employment and annually thereafter, screen all correctional staff who have inmate contact for latent TB infection.

5. Prevent the spread of HIV infection.

   a. Encourage voluntary HIV counseling and testing of inmates.

   b. Provide appropriate treatment for HIV-positive, pregnant inmates to prevent HIV transmission to their babies.

6. Screen inmates for syphilis, gonorrhea, and chlamydia routinely upon reception at prisons and jails, and treat inmates who test positive for these infections.

Prerelease Planning

Many inmates are released into the community while still being treated for communicable and chronic diseases or mental illness. Ensuring continuity of care upon release can reduce health risks to the public, such as in cases of TB and STDs. Continuity of care upon release for inmates with co-occurring mental illness and substance abuse disorders can reduce the risk of illicit drug use in the community. It is cost-effective to the community to provide continuity of care on release for inmates with chronic disease.

X. Congress, through appropriate federal agencies and national organizations, should encourage federal, state, and local correctional

Continued on following page

BOX 28-2
National Commission on Correctional Health Care: *Health Status of the Soon-to-Be-Released Inmate,* 2002. (Continued)

---

facilities to provide prerelease planning for healthcare for all soon-to-be-released inmates.

A. Address the medical, housing, and postrelease needs of inmates in prerelease planning and make use of appropriate resources and new technologies.

B. Coordinate discharge planning efforts between appropriate public agencies—such as correctional, parole, mental health, substance abuse, and public health agencies—to prevent disease transmission and to reduce society's costs from untreated and undertreated illness.

Recommended Actions by Government Agencies

The steering committee and expert panels recognized that many federal agencies have a role in affecting the health status of soon-to-be-released inmates. Within the US Department of Health and Human Services (DHHS), for example, agencies such as the CDC, the Health Resources and Services Administration (HRSA), the Substance Abuse and Mental Health Services Administration (SAMHSA), the National Institute on Drug Abuse (NIDA), the Office of Women's Health (OWH), the Public Health Service (PHS), the Indian Health Service (IHS), and the Office of Minority Health (OMH) are actively engaged in health services programs that have an impact on inmates. In addition, within the US Department of Justice (DOJ), agencies such as the National Institute of Justice (NIJ), the Immigration and Naturalization Service (INS), the Bureau of Prisons (BOP) including the National Institute of Corrections (NIC), the Corrections Program Office (CPO), and the Office of Justice Programs (OJP) conduct programs and activities that ultimately influence inmate health. Finally, the Office of the Surgeon General (OSG) and the White House Executive Office of National Drug Control Policy (ONDCP) also impact the healthcare of inmates.

The steering committee and expert panels recommend that Congress provide the necessary authorization, funding, and other assistance to the appropriate agencies to implement the following recommendations:

I. The Secretary of the DHHS should direct appropriate agencies to collaborate with other agencies in analyzing the potential economic benefits to the community of early diagnosis and treatment of communicable diseases, chronic diseases, and mental illnesses.

II. The Secretary should direct the CDC to collaborate with NIJ, NIC, CPO, and other DOJ divisions in developing tools to assist state and local agencies in deciding when and whom to screen for communicable diseases in correctional settings.

III. The Secretary should direct all appropriate agencies within the department to work toward reducing interagency regulatory and bureaucratic barriers to testing and counseling for HIV, TB, and STDs among inmates.

IV. The Secretary and the Attorney General should involve correctional health professionals in public health planning and the evaluation of correctional healthcare programs.

V. The Secretary and the Attorney General should direct appropriate agencies to support field tests of innovative medical information systems to improve the continuity of care for inmates transferred between correctional facilities or released into the community. These efforts should concentrate on removing barriers that impede the transfer of appropriate medical information.

VI. The Secretary and the Attorney General should direct appropriate agencies to develop educational programs to inform policymakers and the public about the public health and social benefits of investing in healthcare for inmates.

VII. A federal interagency task force, currently established and co-chaired by the CDC and NIJ, should report annually to the Secretary and the Attorney General on the status of correctional healthcare in the nation and on progress made toward implementing the recommendations included in this report.

Adapted from: National Commission on Correctional Health Care: Executive summary. In *Health Status of the Soon-to-Be-Released Inmate,* Chicago, IL, 2002, National Commission on Correctional Health Care, pp xv–xix. Retrieved March, 30, 2006 from http://www.ncchc.org/stbr/Volume1/ExecutiveSummary.pdf. Used with permission from the author.

Chronic Disease Management Standards

The NCCHC maintains national standards, first promulgated by the American Medical Association, for the provision of healthcare services in correctional institutions. The NCCHC revises its standards for jails, prisons, and juvenile detention and confinement facilities every 5 years. As an extension of its landmark study to Congress, the NCCHC incorporated new language in its 2003 revision of the standards to improve patient motivation, decision support, and clinical information systems. In addition, a new standard on the management of chronic disease[14,15] was developed to promote EBM in correctional institutions. The national standard requires that:

"A chronic disease program identifies patients with chronic diseases with the goal of decreasing the frequency and severity of symptoms, including preventing disease progression and fostering improvement in function."

This standard is monitored for compliance through assessing the health services policy and defined procedures, ensuring that the responsible physician establishes and annually approves clinical protocols consistent with national clinical practice guidelines promulgated by experts in the field and that the correctional institution has clinical protocols for the management of chronic diseases, including but not limited to asthma, diabetes, hypercholesterolemia, HIV/AIDS, hypertension, seizure disorder, and TB.[14,15] Finally, the responsible physician practicing correctional medicine should implement a system to ensure continuity of medications for chronic diseases.

In addition, the NCCHC physician surveyors ascertain that documentation in the medical record confirms that clinicians are following chronic disease protocols and that, when clinically indicated, deviations from the protocols are explained. The NCCHC physician surveyors undergo medical chart review training to ensure consistency in reviews and analysis. The training is conducted by experts in the field of correctional medicine and is part of the NCCHC's ongoing quality assurance program that ensures consistency in the evaluation and quality of the accreditation program. The NCCHC's accreditation program is voluntary, and although there are no penalties associated with this medical audit, correctional physicians who undergo an audit of their medical charts benefit by having national expert physicians provide feedback on the substance of care provided to the inmate population. This audit is similar to a National Committee for Quality Assurance medical chart audit.

Evidence-Based Medicine Practice in NCCHC Facilities

Although there has been an improvement in the implementation of EBM in correctional institutions, there remains a need for practitioners to improve their evidenced-based practice parameters. In its 2005 accreditation review, the NCCHC assessed 122 facilities for their compliance to Standard G-02, the Management of Chronic Disease.[42]

A majority (86.8%; n = 106) of facilities were found to be compliant, using nationally based clinical guidelines adopted by the institutional medical director for asthma, diabetes, hyperlipidemia, HIV, hypertension, seizure disorder, and TB.

These data are encouraging, given that these standards had been in existence for 2 years, and practitioners in accredited facilities had ample time to adopt and use clinical guidelines. In four of the surveyed facilities, however, the NCCHC auditing physicians found no evidence in the medical record to support that healthcare providers were consistently following their own approved clinical guidelines in the management of chronically ill patients.[38] One facility, in fact, was using outdated protocols to guide their EBM decision making.[38] This trend indicates that correctional healthcare practitioners require additional training in the use and maintenance of current EBM guidelines.

This trend in data raises the question as to which guidelines correctional healthcare providers utilize in their EBM efforts. Many correctional institutions have outsourced their healthcare services to national, regional, or local vendors. We discovered during our 2005 accreditation review that 48 of the 106 facilities surveyed use clinical guidelines that were created by its specific healthcare contractor.[42] These guidelines, while based on national clinical guidelines, contain additional EBM directives to providers, thus ensuring consistency in their managed care approach. There were 24 institutions that used the NCCHC-approved guidelines in combination with other national EBM guidelines. We found eight prisons that were using state department of corrections–generated clinical guidelines based on national clinical guidelines standards; there were two facilities using clinical guidelines generated by the Federal Bureau of Prisons.

Six facilities were found to base their EBM decision making on national clinical guidelines from the American Diabetics Association; the National Heart, Lung, and Blood Institute; the CDC; Blue Cross/Blue Shield; the American Heart Association; the US Preventive Services Task Force; the National Institutes of Health; or their relative state health department. Sixteen facilities (13.2%) had no national- or physician-approved clinical practice guidelines in place, and many did not have a tracking system that monitored patients with chronic disease.[38] Since many facilities with smaller inmate populations do not have full-time medical or nursing staff, it stands to reason that these were the facilities that were most likely to have no physician-approved clinical practice guidelines in place. Through our survey we found that the range of average daily inmate populations for these noncompliant facilities ranged from 50 to 1519, with a median population of 561.[42] Although failure to implement EBM clinical guidelines is not solely dependent on the size of the institution, additional research is needed to fully understand the barriers to implementing EBM guidelines in correctional institutions.

Barriers to Providing Evidence-Based Medicine in Correctional Institutions

Claim: The question of whether basic healthcare should be provided to incarcerated people was settled by the US Supreme Court,[43] who in 1976 determined that prisoners are entitled, under protection of the Eighth Amendment, to healthcare for their serious medical needs. Thirty years after that seminal decision, we are still grappling with the problem of how to organize and provide acute and chronic healthcare in jails and prisons. There are a number of system barriers that prevent EBM from being practiced in correctional institutions. Although we have made considerable progress in the development of national standards, professional societies, and correctional healthcare organizations, there are still many correctional institutions that remain elusive with regard to system design, decision support, patient motivation and adherence, and clinical information systems.

From a large-scale perspective, the design and delivery of a health system greatly affects the ability of its clinicians to implement EBM in their daily practice. Correctional healthcare systems fail to provide comprehensive integrated healthcare services, lacking a continuum of care that can improve the quality of life for incarcerated men. Too often, hospital services, primary care, social services, specialty care, mental health, public health, and ancillary services are fragmented, uncoordinated, or even non-existent.

Having chronically ill patients attend regularly scheduled disease management programs or chronic care management clinics has been found to improve care and quality of life.[44] Despite this notion, most jails and prisons have not organized the management of their chronically ill patients due to either (1) a lack of sufficient personnel, (2) instability of the patient population, (3) insufficient allocation of physician time, (4) a focus on sick call and primary care complaints, and (5) appeasement of custody's demands to maintain order and deal with the most pressing problem of the day.

When correctional facilities are located in areas with a shortage of nursing personnel, decisions regarding staff assignments are both difficult and highly selective. Nurses are assigned key duties of triage of sick call requests, handling of emergencies, distribution of medication, and managing routine requests from custody and inmates regarding health services. Organizing chronic disease in a manner that permits effective monitoring of the status and condition of disease progression is a secondary effort when there is insufficient nursing and clerical personnel to track and monitor patients.

Instituting effective chronic disease management programs for incarcerated men is a challenge because the majority of inmates reside in city and county jails, where short stays and rapid turnover is the norm. In addition, more than 7 million persons are released from jails and prisons each year in the United States—the vast majority leaving city and county jails—with little or no healthcare transitional planning.

Among these inmates who are released is a startlingly disproportionate share of the total population living with communicable infectious diseases in the United States. Many institutions do not have sufficient physician time and resources to provide the necessary chronic disease services. Many correctional settings contract physicians for part-time medical services, creating situations where they may be charged with the responsibility of providing care to the incarcerated population. As a result, physicians are focused on inmate episodic care and needs but do no provide the administrative leadership for an effective or efficient healthcare delivery system.

The ability to change a delivery system assumes that one has direct control to make change; however, this is often not the case for many correctional medicine healthcare providers. There are many models of healthcare delivery in correctional settings that effect the empowerment to change delivery systems. One common model is composed of a nursing staff that reports to wardens while the physicians are under the aegis of a separate authority. Another common model is to subcontract health services out to a vendor who has no authority over correctional staff. These models make delivery system change difficult to access and implement since changes in the healthcare system may conflict with custody routines and schedules. For example, chronic care management often requires complex changes of the organization, provider, and patient[45]; a change in the chronic disease clinic schedule to accommodate a newly contracted HIV specialist could conflict with meal, court, work, school, or other programming schedules. With custody functions taking priority, such a change to the system design may not be easy to accommodate. Shortell[46] observes:

> "It appears that there may be a disconnect between evidence-based medicine (i.e., the use of diagnostic and treatment practices based on the best available biomedical and clinical research) and evidence-based management (i.e., use of management and organizational practices based on the best available managerial, organizational, and health services delivery research)."

These issues raise the following questions:

- What might account for the large amount of unwarranted variation in quality and outcomes of care?
- Why aren't evidence-based medicine and evidence-based management more widely applied in practice?
- Why are there no healthcare organizations today that can provide evidence documenting uniformly high quality of care across the board?
- Why does it take so long to incorporate advances in medical technology and treatment?

If a fundamental EBM principle is to systematically examine contemporaneous research findings to support clinical decisions, then prisons and jails create an environment that is the antithesis to an EBM practice because many correctional health systems lack sufficient resources (e.g., Internet access, medical libraries) to support a thorough literature search for acute and chronic diseases that are encountered. Although system failure to support EBM practice does not necessarily prevent it from occurring (since clinicians are forced to take extraordinary steps to ensure that they have access to the available clinical evidence), the lack of support is a major reason why EBM decision making and research lag in correctional institutions.

By following four EBM steps: "formulate a clear clinical question from a patient's problem; search the literature for relevant clinical articles; evaluate (critically appraise) the evidence for its validity and usefulness; implement useful findings in clinical practice,"[47] clinicians can make optimal decisions regarding the care and treatment of their patients. However, correctional healthcare providers ask themselves, "Are inmate-patients involved in decisions regarding their healthcare?"

Studies on decision support have found that providing patients with individualized decision support service aids improves decision outcomes.[48,49] When there is no single "best" option, individualized decision support service aids improve comprehension of the options, ease of making a choice, and clinician-patient communication. Although individualized decision support aids are a new concept, a thorough review failed to find any mention of this concept in the correctional healthcare literature. There seem to be limited options for incarcerated populations, healthcare staff have limited resources, the concept of shared decision making is not widely supported in correctional health, and correctional healthcare emphasizes "crisis management." That is to say, rather than taking an EBM approach toward planning and preparing patients to make reasonable choices, healthcare staff are more focused on the acute problems.

Conclusions

Chinnock and colleagues[50] raise the specter that EBM may not be relevant to developing countries, citing reasons that the "typical healthcare experience of a patient living in the less developed world" does not support the use of EBM. For example, patients often present to the clinic very late in the course of their disease, they have self-medicated with legend drugs or traditional treatments, the health facilities are so "poor" that they may delay diagnosis, referrals (if needed) are not easily arranged, there are problems with shortages of trained staff, there is poor infection control and a lack of follow-up care, and the "patient may be unable (e.g., because of financial hardship) to fully adhere to treatment."

Although it is certainly not suggested that correctional healthcare clinicians in the United States reject evidence-based practice, we are collectively making the argument that evidence-based studies are much harder to implement in settings where many patients are illiterate and non-adherent, and healthcare facilities are painfully inadequate. Many correctional institutions in the United States do not have access to the Internet, thus creating a barrier for clinicians to access the latest medical information while treating their patients. This environment is not conducive to EBM practice and places correctional medicine clinicians at a huge disadvantage. What needs to change is our thinking about the infrastructure of correctional institutions, providing sufficient support and staffing to augment evidence-based practice. The NCCHC has identified recommendations to improve healthcare services in correctional institutions that will ultimately create environments for EBM opportunity and improved healthcare provisions for inmates (see Box 28-1).

References

1. Harrison PM, Beck AJ: *Prisoners in 2001,* Bulletin NCJ 195189, Washington, DC, 2002, US Department of Justice, Bureau of Justice Statistics.
2. Dias M: (1998). Grim questions haunt jail death. *The Post* October 1, 1998. Available at: http://www.kypost.com/news/1998/frank100198.html. Accessed July 30, 2005.
3. California Prison Focus: Fight for the rights of prisoners with HIV/AIDS and hepatitis C. Available at: http://www.prisons.org/hivin.htm. Accessed August 14, 2006.
4. Personal analysis of a state department of corrections medical record, January 2005.
5. National Commission on Correctional Health Care: *The Health Status of Soon-to-Be-Released Inmates,* vol 1 and 2, Chicago, IL, 2002, National Commission on Correctional Health Care.
6. Rasmussen K: Evidence-based medicine and clinical practice: does it work? In Kristiansen IS, Mooney G, editors: *Evidence Based Medicine: In Whose Interests?* New York, 2004, Routledge, pp 151–159.
7. Krebs CP: High risk transmission behavior in prison and the prison subculture, *Prison J* 82(1): 19–49, 2002.
8. Peters RH, Greenbaum PE, Steinberg ML, et al: Effectiveness of screening instruments in detecting substance use disorders among prisoners, *J Subst Abuse Treat* 18:349–358, 2000.
9. The National Center on Addiction and Substance Abuse at Columbia University: *Behind Bars: Substance Abuse and America's Prison Population,* January 1998. Available at: http://www.casacolumbia.org/supportcasa/item.asp?cID=12&PID=108. Accessed November 11, 2000.
10. Stephens TT, Braithwaite R, Sprauve NE, Reeves Louis TT: Predictors of prior incarceration and alcohol use among soon-to-be-released adult male inmates, *J Correctional Health Care* 12:4–11, 2006.
11. National Institute of Justice: *2000 Arrestee Drug Abuse Monitoring: Annual Report,* April 2003. Available at: http://www.ncjrs.gov/pdffiles1/nij/193013. pdf. Accessed August 15, 2006.
12. Fiscella K, Moore A, Engerman J, Meldrum S: Management of opiate detoxification in jails, *J Addict Dis* 24(1):61–71, 2005.
13. Center for Substance Abuse Treatment: *Substance Abuse Treatment for Adults in the Criminal Justice System,* Treatment Improvement Protocol (TIP) Series 44, DHHS Publication No. (SMA) 05–4056, Rockville, MD, 2005, Substance Abuse and Mental Health Services Administration.
14. National Commission on Correctional Health Care: *Standards for Health Care in Prisons,* Chicago, IL, 2003, National Commission on Correctional Health Care.
15. National Commission on Correctional Health Care: *Standards for Health Care in Jails,* Chicago, IL, 2003, National Commission on Correctional Health Care.
16. Swartz JA: Adapting and using the substance abuse subtle screening inventory–2 with criminal justice offenders: preliminary results, *Criminal Just Behav* 25(3):344–365, 1998.
17. National Commission on Correctional Health Care: Unpublished survey of accredited facilities on screening, treatment, and management of AOD among inmates 2006.
18. Rich JD, McKenzie M, Shield DC, et al: Linkage with methadone treatment upon release from incarceration: a promising opportunity, *J Addict Dis* 24 (3):49–59, 2005.
19. Kinlock TW, Battjes RJ, Schwartz RP, and the MTC Project Team: A novel opioid maintenance program for prisoners: report of post-release outcomes, *Am J Drug Alcohol Abuse* 31(3):433–454, 2005.
20. Kraut-Becher JR, Gift TL, Haddix AC, et al: Cost-effectiveness of universal screening for chlamydia and gonorrhea in U.S jails, *J Urban Health* 81 (3):453–471, 2004.
21. Ratelle S, Nguyen MS, Tang Y, et al: Low sensitivity of the leukocyte esterase test (LET) in detecting *Chlamydia trachomatis* infections in asymptomatic men entering a county jail, *J Correctional Health Care* 10(2):217–226, 2004.
22. Nguyen MS, Ratelle S, Tang Y, et al: Prevalence and indicators of *Chlamydia trachomatis* among men entering Massachusetts correctional facilities: policy implications, *J Correctional Health Care* 10(4):543–554, 2004.
23. Centers for Disease Control and Prevention: *Sexually Transmitted Disease Surveillance, 2003,* Atlanta, GA, 2004, US Department of Health and Human Services.
24. Hammett TM, Harmon P, Rhodes W: The burden of infectious disease among inmates and releasees from correctional facilities. In *The Health Status of Soon-to-Be-Released Inmates,* vol 2, Chicago, IL, 2002, National Commission on Correctional Health Care. Available at: http://www.ncchc.org/stbr/Volume2/Report2_Hammett.pdf. Accessed March 10, 2006.
25. Centers for Disease Control and Prevention: Diseases characterized by urethritis and cervicitis: sexually transmitted diseases treatment guidelines, *MMWR Recomm Rep* 51(RR-6):30–42, 2002.
26. Mertz KJ, Voigt RA, Hutchins K, Levine WC, and the Jail STD Prevalence Monitoring Group: Findings from STD screening of adolescents and adults entering corrections facilities: implications for STD control strategies, *Sex Transm Dis* 29(12):834–839, 2002.
27. Wohl DA, Rosen D, Kaplan AH: HIV and incarceration: dual epidemics, *Drug Benefit Trends* 18: 392–402, 2006.
28. National Commission on Correctional Health Care (1996): Management of tuberculosis in correctional

facilities. Available at: http://www.ncchc.org/resources/statements/tb.html. Accessed August 15, 2006.

29. O'Neill JM: 5 hires sought for TB testing at jail, *Dallas Morning News* April 8, 2005.

30. Teplin LA, Swartz J: Referral decision scale, *Law Human Behav* 13(1):1–18, 1989.

31. Suls J, Gaes G, Philo V: Stress and illness behavior in prison: effects of life events, self-care attitudes, and race, *J Prison Jail Health* 10:117–132, 1991.

32. Anno J: Health behavior in prisons and correctional facilities. In Gochman DS editor, *Handbook of Health Behavior Research*, vol 3, Demography, development, and diversity, New York, 1997, Plenum, pp 289–303.

33. National High Blood Pressure Education Program: The seventh report of the Joint National Committee on Prevention, Detection, Evaluation, and Treatment of High Blood Pressure Reports (JNC 7). Available at: http://www.nhlbi.nih.gov/guidelines/hypertension. Accessed August 14, 2006.

34. American Diabetes Association: Diabetes management in correctional institutions, *Diabetes Care* 29 (Suppl 1):S59–S66, 2006.

35. The National Asthma Education and Prevention Program: Guidelines for the diagnosis and management of asthma—update on selected topics 2002. Available at:http://www.nhlbi.nih.gov/guidelines/asthma/index.htm. Accessed August 14, 2006.

36. The International League Against Epilepsy: *International Classification of Epileptic Seizures*. Available at: http://www.ilae-epilepsy.org. Accessed August 14, 2006.

37. The National Cholesterol Education Program (NCEP): The third report of the expert panel on detection, evaluation, and treatment of high blood cholesterol in adults (Adult Treatment Panel III). Available at: http://www.nhlbi.nih.gov/guidelines/cholesterol/index.htm. Accessed August 14, 2006.

38. Department of Health and Human Services: Guidelines for the use of antiretroviral agents in HIV-infected adults and adolescents. Available at: http://www.hivatis.org. Accessed August 14, 2006.

39. Puisis M, Appel H: Chronic disease management. In Michael Puisis, editor: *Clinical Practice in Correctional Medicine*, ed 2, Philadelphia, 2006, Mosby, pp 66–88.

40. National Commission on Correctional Health Care: Clinical guideline for correctional facilities diabetes chronic care. 2001. Available at: http://www.ncchc.org/resources/clinicalguides/adult_diabetes.pdf. Accessed June 17, 2007.

41. Kim S, Shansky R, Schiff GD: Using performance improvement measurement to improve chronic disease management in prisons. In Michael Pusis, editor: *Clinical Practice in Correctional Medicine*, ed 2, Philadelphia, 2006, Mosby, pp 503–509.

42. National Commission on Correctional Health Care: Unpublished survey of accredited facilities on compliance to standard G-02, the Management of Chronic Disease, 2006.

43. US Supreme Court: *Estelle v. Gamble*, 429 U.S. 97 (1976).

44. Gohler A, Dietz R, Osterziel K, Seibert U: Clinical effectiveness and cost-effectiveness of disease management programs for patients with heart failure. Abstracts from the 26th Annual Meeting of the Society for Medical Decision Making, Atlanta, GA, October 17–20, 2004.

45. Cretin S, Shortell, SM, Keeler EB: An evaluation of collaborative interventions to improve chronic illness care: framework and study design, *Eval Rev* 28(1):28–51, 2004.

46. Shortell SM: Increasing value: a research agenda for addressing the managerial and organizational challenges facing health care delivery in the United States, *Med Care Res Rev* 61(3):12–30, 2004.

47. Rosenberg W, Donald A: (1995). Evidence based medicine: an approach to clinical problem solving, *Br Med J* 310(6987):1122–1126, 1995.

48. Dorr DA, Wilcox A, Burns L, et al: Implementing a multidisease chronic care model in primary care using people and technology, *Dis Manage* 9(1):1–15, 2006.

49. Glasgow RE, Davis CL, Funnell MM, Beck A: Implementing practical interventions to support chronic illness self-management, *Jt Comm J Qual Saf* 29(11):563–574, 2003.

50. Chinnock P, Siegfried N, Clarke M: Is evidence-based medicine relevant to the developing world? *PLoS Med* 2(5):e107, 2005. Available at: http://www.pubmedcentral.nih.gov/articlerender.fcgi?artid=1140939. Accessed March 11, 2006.

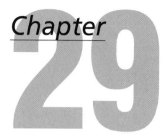

The Homosexual Male

Daniel A. Knight, MD

Key Points

- Refer to text and Table 29-5 regarding disease screening and prevention.
- Homosexual men may be at higher risk of depression, anxiety, and other mood disorders (strength of recommendation: C).
- Homosexual men, especially adolescent males, may be at higher risk for suicidal ideation and suicidal attempts than the heterosexual male population (strength of recommendation: C).
- Consider performing anal Pap smears if there is a history of anal warts and/or high-risk types of HPV infection (strength of recommendation: C).

Introduction

Homosexuality is a subject that is not commonly discussed in most healthcare settings and, frequently, the healthcare provider knows little about a patient's sexual orientation. Minimal time is spent in medical school curricula on formal healthcare for homosexuals.[1] Even less time and money is spent nationally and internationally on studies of healthcare for homosexuals.[2] Therefore, by extrapolation of existing data, healthcare for homosexual males is in many ways the same as healthcare for heterosexual males. Nonetheless, there are many additional factors that must be considered in caring for a man who identifies as homosexual or who participates in sexual activities with other males. Determining a man's sexual identity or sexual practices is often difficult. Fear of stigmatization prevents many people from identifying themselves as homosexual, as

bisexual, or as having had sex with other persons of the same gender.[3] Furthermore, prior negative experiences with healthcare workers may often limit an open discussion of sexuality.

Many physicians are unaware of the special healthcare needs of homosexuals and may, unfortunately, be openly hostile to homosexual and bisexual patients. And though some healthcare providers do not have negative attitudes toward homosexual patients, they frequently lack the specialized training and skills to appropriately care for homosexual men. In fact, two thirds of physicians never ask patients about their sexual orientation when obtaining a social history.[4] The goal of this chapter is to examine common issues in the primary care of homosexual males, specifically related to infectious diseases, psychological disorders, substance abuse, and preventive healthcare screening and counseling.

Definitions and Epidemiology

Homosexual is a term that is often defined in various ways. Some authors describe any same-sex sexual behavior as homosexuality, whereas others define a homosexual person as someone who is attracted both sexually and by affectation to someone of the same gender. Others have described a homosexual as someone who self-identifies as being attracted to the same sex, yet many men who have sex with other men describe themselves as being heterosexual. Some men have sex exclusively with other men, whereas some have sex with men and women and define themselves as *bisexual*.[5]

As it is clearly difficult to define the term *homosexual male,* it is even more difficult to determine who is homosexual or who has sex with persons of the same gender. Healthcare for homosexual males may include risks for men who have sex with men even though not all of these men may self-identify as homosexual. In the balance of this chapter, the terms *homosexual* and *homosexuality* will be used to refer generally to all men who have sex with other men unless otherwise stated.

The prevalence of homosexuality has been debated for decades. In 1953, the Kinsey Report[6] stated the prevalence of homosexuality in males was at 10% in persons who were more or less exclusively homosexual, and at 8% in persons who were exclusively homosexual for at least 3 years between the ages of 16 and 55 years. More recent data from the Kinsey Institute range from a high of 15.8% of males who have had sex with males since puberty to a low of 2.8% who self-identified as homosexual. Binson and colleagues combined data from the General Social Survey and the National AIDS Behavioral Survey (NABS) that demonstrated that 5.3% of men reported sexual activity with a same-gender partner since the age of 18 years.[6] Data from the NABS showed that 6.5% of men reported having sex with men during the previous 5 years, and the highest prevalence of 14.4% was found in central locations of the 12 largest US cities.[6] This may result from a higher concentration of homosexual men in larger cities where they may find more acceptance and anonymity. Although these figures are somewhat dated, there is a paucity of newer studies to accurately depict the current prevalence of homosexuality.

Although sexual behavior typically defines risk, other factors may contribute to problems in the homosexual male population. Society's acceptance or rejection of this behavior may be related to higher rates of depression, anxiety, and suicidal ideation in homosexual and bisexual men. Adolescents are more vulnerable to society's pressures in general and have higher rates of suicidal ideation and attempts, as well as depression.

Sexually Transmitted Diseases

Homosexual men are at risk for various medical problems including the contraction of human immunodeficiency virus (HIV) and other sexually transmitted diseases (STDs), anal cancer, and certain types of viral hepatitis (Table 29-1). Many homosexual men may not receive routine

Table 29-1. Common Sexually Transmitted Diseases in Homosexual Males

HIV (human immunodeficiency virus) infection
Gonorrhea
Chlamydia
Syphilis
Herpes simplex type 2
HPV (human papilloma virus)
Hepatitis A
Hepatitis B

primary healthcare screening as is customarily provided to the general population due to fears of self-disclosure and lack of acceptance from their physician, causing them to refrain from seeking preventive healthcare in the first place.[7] This ultimately results in a lack of counseling regarding safer-sex practices and earlier screening for STDs.

STDs disproportionately affect people with high-risk sexual behavior and those whose access to preventive care or health-seeking behavior is compromised.[8] The historical marginalization of the homosexual population places many homosexual men at a disproportionate risk for contracting STDs. Obtaining valid and precise prevalence rates of HIV and other STDs in homosexual men is difficult due to the stigma of STDs and of homosexuality in general, thus leading to the lack of disclosure of patients to healthcare providers and other survey methods.

Human Immunodeficiency Virus

HIV infection disproportionately continues to affect homosexual men at an alarming rate. For several years, the rate of newly diagnosed HIV infections by male-to-male contact was declining. Recently, many new HIV infections have occurred in men who have sex with other men, especially young, Latino, and African American men. As of 2004, 18,203 (46.9%) of newly diagnosed cases of HIV infection resulted from male-to-male sexual contact. If intravenous drug use and male-to-male sexual contact are added to these numbers, the new cases of HIV infection in this population increases to 19,575 (50.5%).[9] Adolescents and young adults account for a substantial portion of new cases of HIV infection. Approximately 25% of new cases of HIV in 2004 were in patients younger than 30 years old. In a sample of young men who have sex with men (aged 15–22 years) in six urban US counties, between 5% and 9% were found to be infected with HIV, with a significantly higher percentage of African American and Latino youth being infected than white youths.[7]

Among homosexual males who are already infected with HIV, the risk of contracting multiple-drug–resistant HIV is highest in those who have unprotected sex. There is some evidence that persons with an undetectable HIV viral load may not be as infectious as those with a higher viral load, yet there continues to be a significantly elevated risk in the spread of HIV in this population.[10]

Other Sexually Transmitted Diseases

STDs for which homosexually active men are at a high risk include hepatitis A, hepatitis B, syphilis, gonorrhea, chlamydia, non-gonococcal urethritis, herpes, and genital warts, resulting in urethritis, proctitis, pharyngitis, and/or prostatitis. From 1970 through 1997, the rates of STDs in homosexual males declined. However, in recent years, the rates of gonorrhea, chlamydia, and syphilis have been increasing.[11] According to a report of the Stop AIDS Project, a San Francisco–based community organization, that appeared in the *Morbidity and Mortality Weekly Report (MMWR)* in 1999, trends have shown increases in unprotected anal intercourse, from 57.6% in 1994 to 61.2% in 1997, and in other high-risk behaviors such as unprotected oral sex, resulting in higher rates of STDs in homosexually active males.[12] A study by The National HIV Behavioral Surveillance System from 2003 to 2005 found that 76% of 10,030 respondents reported having more than one sexual partner during the preceding 12 months. Forty-seven percent reported having unprotected anal intercourse with a male partner during the preceding 12 months. Of the HIV-negative respondents, 47% did not know the HIV status of their male sexual partner.[13]

Gonorrhea

Gonorrhea, chlamydia, and non-gonococcal urethritis rates are higher in the homosexually active male population. The incidence of *Neisseria gonorrhoeae* and other STDs among homosexual and bisexual men has increased in recent years.[11] The Gonococcal Isolate Surveillance Project sponsored by the Centers for Disease Control and Prevention (CDC)[14] reported that positive isolates of *N. gonorrhoeae* obtained from men who have sex with men increased from 4% in 1988 to 20%

in 2004, with most of the increase occurring after 1993 (Figure 29-1). STD clinics in Seattle, San Francisco, and Portland, OR, reported an increase in gonorrhea among men who have sex with men between 1993 and 1996. Seattle experienced an increase of 125% from 51 to 115 cases, whereas San Francisco had an increase of 24% from 271 to 336 cases.[14]

This trend in increased incidence of gonorrhea infection is believed to be caused by increases in unsafe sexual practices and inconsistent condom use. Gonorrhea in the homosexual male population can be pharyngeal, urethral, or anal. Most homosexual male patients with gonococcal urethritis will report symptoms such as a penile discharge or dysuria, yet a few patients may remain asymptomatic with a urethral infection. Less than half of male patients with rectal gonorrhea report anal discharge, anal pruritus, or other symptoms of proctitis. Only 16% of male patients with throat culture results positive for gonorrhea may have signs or symptoms of pharyngitis.[12] Urethral gonococcal infection has been independently associated with anal insertive intercourse and with oral insertive sex. In fact, the independent risk was found to be higher for fellatio than for anal insertive sex. This trend was postulated to be due to more consistent use of condoms during anal sex than for fellatio.[15]

Chlamydia

Chlamydia trachomatis can be detected in the male homosexual population as either a urethral or rectal infection. Although most urethral infections may be symptomatic with penile discharge or dysuria, up to one quarter may be asymptomatic.[12] For rectal chlamydia infections, approximately 67% of homosexual men are asymptomatic at the time of diagnosis. Urethral chlamydia infection is significantly associated

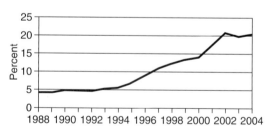

Figure 29-1. Percent of urethral *Neisseria gonorrhoeae* isolates obtained from men who have sex with men attending STD clinics, 1988–2004. (Adapted from: The Gonococcal Isolate Surveillance Project [GISP]. Available at: http://www.cdc.gov/std/stats/msm.htm. Accessed July 13, 2006.)

with young age and with anal insertive sex. Overall, the infection rate for chlamydia in the high-risk homosexual population is low at 3.5%.[15]

Non-Gonococcal Urethritis

Non-gonococcal urethritis is the most common cause of urethritis in homosexual males. It was previously believed that this condition was caused by an exposure to coliform bacteria (e.g., *Escherichia coli*) through anal sex, but studies have not substantiated this notion. It appears that up to one half of all non-chlamydial, non-gonococcal urethritis in homosexual men is acquired by oral intercourse.[12]

In the studies cited above, a history of consistent condom use offered no apparent protection from either rectal or urethral STDs.[15] In this study and a previous study by Zenilman and colleagues,[16] the authors postulated that the accuracy of patients' claims of consistent condom use was not factual and the likelihood is that patients provided socially acceptable answers concerning condom use rather than admitting to infrequent or inconsistent condom use with all partners. In both of these studies, patients who reported consistent condom use had the same frequency of STDs as those that reported no condom use. Therefore, reports of consistent condom use cannot be used as an indicator of a possible exposure to an STD.

Herpes Simplex Type 2

Infection with herpes simplex virus type 2 (HSV-2) is very common in homosexual men. Studies performed in the late 1980s through the mid 1990s, as well as more recent epidemiologic studies, have indicated that the prevalence of HSV-2 infection among HIV-negative homosexual men ranged from 26% to 40%.[17] HSV-2 seroprevalence is considerably higher according to these studies, approaching up to 70% among HIV-infected men. Some authors speculate that coinfection with HSV-2 may lead to a higher risk of acquiring HIV.[18] Studies indicate that HIV-negative homosexual men shed HSV-2 subclinically, primarily from the perianal area; most of this shedding is not accompanied by prodromal symptoms.[17] Subclinical shedding of HSV-2 may increase the period of exposure to the partners of patients that may have few or no symptoms of HSV-2 recurrence.

Syphilis

Syphilis infection seems to be having a resurgence in homosexual men. The number of primary and secondary cases of syphilis more than doubled in New York City in 2001, chiefly in men who have sex with men according to a publication in the *MMWR*.[19] Syphilis outbreaks have occurred in other major US cities including Seattle, Chicago, San Francisco, Los Angeles, and Miami. In each of these outbreaks, high rates of HIV coinfection were documented.[19] Possible contributions to these outbreaks may be increased high-risk sexual practices due to the availability of highly active antiretroviral therapy, resulting in the perception that HIV is a "treatable disease," and to "AIDS burnout," which is associated with years of exposure to prevention messages and safer-sex messages (Table 29-2). Other factors for increased sexual risk-taking among homosexual men include increased alcohol and drug abuse (especially methamphetamine use), unrecognized HIV infection, and misperception of risk-taking behaviors.[11]

Human Papilloma Virus

Human papilloma virus (HPV), the virus that causes condyloma acuminatum, has been found through serologic assays in 61–78% of HIV-negative homosexual men.[20] It is believed that certain strains of HPV (e.g., types 16 and 18 most commonly) are a causative agent for the development of anal cancer, which is at least 20-fold more

Table 29-2. Common Reasons for Increased Sexual Risk-Taking Behaviors in Homosexual Men

AIDS burnout: Fatigue of continued worry for the long AIDS epidemic
Outdated or overly simplistic safer sex messages for homosexual men
Beliefs that HAART will be effective and easy to take
Media portrayals of HAART
New HIV infection treatments and the potential for a vaccine
Lack of exposure to friends and acquaintances living with or who have died from HIV infection
Belief that STDs "won't happen to me"
Low self-esteem, depression, or lack of peer support
Lack of access to preventive services and counseling that are available to men who are more open about their homosexuality

AIDS, Acquired immunodeficiency syndrome; HAART, highly active antiretroviral therapy; HIV, human immunodeficiency virus; STDs, sexually transmitted diseases.

Adapted from: The Gay and Lesbian Medical Association Web site. Available at: http://www.glma.org. Accessed January 26, 2006.

common in homosexual men than in heterosexual men.[21] Anal cancer may progress from a lesion called *anal intraepithelial neoplasia* (AIN), which is caused by HPV, and can be diagnosed via an anal Papanicolaou (Pap) test. The potential for progression from AIN to anal cancer has yet to be determined,[22] although it is believed that AIN may mirror the progression of cervical dysplasia in women. Therefore, 30% of high-grade AIN lesions may progress to anal cancer if left untreated.

In the EXPLORE study,[23] a nationwide HIV-prevention behavioral trial involving nearly 4300 men who have sex with men, 1218 HIV-negative men in six urban populations were found to have a 57% overall prevalence of anal HPV, whereas 26% of that population were found to be infected with a type of HPV considered to be high risk for anal cancer. The genotypes particularly associated with anogenital infection, dysplasia, and malignancy include HPV genotypes 16, 18, 31, 33, and 35.[24] The main risk factors for developing anal HPV infection in HIV-negative homosexual men were found to be a history of anal intercourse and the greater number of male sex partners during the preceding 6 months. In HIV-positive homosexual men, the incidence of anal HPV rose from 85% to 93%.[25]

Hepatitis A and B

Despite a vigorous immunization program in American children, as well as updated immunization guidelines by the CDC in August 2006, many adults remain nonimmunized against hepatitis A and B. As a result, they continue to be very prevalent infections in the homosexual male population. A 2001 study by MacKellar and colleagues[26] found that 11% of homosexually active males aged 15–22 years were found to be seropositive for hepatitis B virus (HBV) infection, whereas only 9% had been immunized against HBV. Other studies have shown seroprevalence rates in homosexual and bisexual men to range from 23% to 61.5%.[27] Anal contact was strongly related to the risk of acquiring HBV infection with anal-genital intercourse as a major route for HBV transmission. Hepatitis A virus infection rates among homosexual men were found to be several times higher than heterosexual men in three studies in several countries including the United States, Canada, Australia, and Sweden.[28] The main risk factors for contracting hepatitis A include anal-oral contact, history of STDs and higher numbers of sex partners.

Sexually Transmitted Gastrointestinal Syndromes

Sexually transmitted gastrointestinal syndromes can be grouped into four broad categories: perianal disease, proctitis, proctocolitis, and enteritis. Perianal lesions are frequently caused by HPV, which causes venereal warts and, with infection via certain serotypes, carries the risk of malignant transformation. Other causes of perianal disease include infection with HSV and syphilis. *Proctitis*, an inflammation of the rectum, causes symptoms of anal discharge, bleeding, and anorectal pain or tenesmus. The most common causes of proctitis are HSV, gonorrhea, syphilis, and chlamydia; multiple pathogens may be found within the same person. Proctitis and other STD pathogens of the colon occur more frequently in homosexual men.[29] At the San Francisco municipal STD clinic, the number of cases of proctitis has increased by 26% from 159 cases in 1997 to 200 cases in 2001. On average, approximately 15 cases are diagnosed each month among approximately 600 men regularly seen at this clinic who have sex with men.[30]

Proctocolitis refers to inflammation of the colonic mucosa extending proximally from 15 cm above the anus. It is associated with symptoms of proctitis plus watery or bloody diarrhea, abdominal cramps, left lower quadrant abdominal pain, and fever. Enteric pathogens are the most likely cause, specifically *Entamoeba histolytica*, *Shigella* species, and *Campylobacter* species. Other pathogens include *C. trachomatis*, *E. coli*, *Salmonella* species, and *Yersinia* species. *Enteritis* usually results in diarrhea and abdominal cramping without signs of proctitis or proctocolitis and usually occurs among persons whose sexual practices include oral-fecal contact. In healthy persons, *Giardia lamblia* is the pathogen most frequently implicated.

Common Psychological Problems

It is unclear whether homosexual behavior or homosexual sexual orientation results in a greater prevalence of psychiatric disorders in homosexual male patients, yet many are prevalent (Table 29-3). Many believe that the historic stigmatization and marginalization of homosexuals in American society increase the likelihood of psychiatric, behavioral, and substance abuse disorders. A heightened risk of mental disorders may be related to the occurrence of victimization and abuse sustained by homosexuals, especially during adolescence. Psychosocial factors such as

Table 29-3. Behavioral Disorders Prevalent in Homosexual Men

Mood Disorders
Major depressive disorder
Adjustment disorder
Suicidal ideation and suicide attempts
Anxiety Disorders
Generalized anxiety disorder
Panic disorder
Obsessive-compulsive disorder

a sense of isolation, low levels of social support, and frequent stressful life events may contribute to elevated risk of psychiatric disorders in homosexual men.[31]

The theory of stigmatization and exposure to discriminatory behavior is consistent with the finding that homosexual men experience discrimination in multiple domains of life and that such discrimination is related to elevated levels of psychological distress. One study revealed that perceived discrimination against homosexuals may be associated with harmful effects on the quality of life and indicators of psychiatric morbidity, leading to anxiety, depression, and suicidal thoughts and behaviors.[31] The Midlife Development in the United States Study showed that homosexual and bisexual men in the study were more likely than heterosexual males to have one of the following five psychiatric disorders: major depression, generalized anxiety disorders, panic disorders, and alcohol and drug dependence. Yet, no statistically significant difference was found between the two groups in the prevalence of high levels of current psychological distress.[31]

Several studies have found that homosexuality leads to higher levels of depression, anxiety, and other psychiatric disorders than that found in the general population.[32] Data from the National Comorbidity Study (NCS), a nationally representative household survey of people aged 15–54 years carried out from 1990 through 1992, were analyzed for evidence of prevalence of a lifetime psychiatric disorder, specifically anxiety disorders and depression. Although this study had a very small subsample of homosexual males, it did demonstrate a higher risk of depression and panic in men with same-sex partners than in men with opposite-sex partners.

Based on data from the National Health and Nutrition Examination Survey III,[33] the correlation between having same-sex sexual partners and lifetime or recent major depression actually showed a trend toward the positive, but this was less clear. The Netherlands Mental Health Survey and Incidence Study (NEMESIS),[34] a large, population-based Dutch study involving face-to-face interviews, found a higher rate of mood and anxiety disorders but a lower rate of alcohol abuse in homosexual men than in heterosexual men. Homosexual men had an occurrence rate of 17.1% for mood disorders compared with 4% for heterosexual men and a 19.5% rate of anxiety disorders versus 7.6% for heterosexual men.[34] Despite an appearance of generalized elevation of risk for anxiety, mood, and substance use disorders, the low power of the studies makes it impossible to confirm the hypothesis that men with same-sex partners have a higher incidence of major depression and other affective disorders such as anxiety and panic disorder. However, it does appear reasonable to conclude that homosexual men may exhibit elevated levels of mood disorders such as depression and anxiety disorders, including generalized anxiety disorder, panic, and obsessive-compulsive disorders when compared with the general male population.

Suicidal Ideation and Suicidal Attempts

The incidence of suicidal ideation and suicidal attempts appears to be higher among homosexual men and is correlated to the large percentages of such thoughts and attempts in the adolescent male population. A comparison of 10 peer-reviewed studies found unusually high rates of suicide attempts, in the range of 20–40%, among young bisexual and homosexual research volunteers.[35] Additional studies, including a twin study in veterans[36] have shown higher rates of suicidal behaviors in adult male veterans, but the study assessed lifetime thoughts and events, not recent suicidal thoughts and attempts. As homosexual men get older, the proportion of suicidal thoughts and attempts appears to approach that of heterosexual males.

A study of adolescents in Massachusetts found elevated levels of suicidal ideation and attempts among homosexual youths, but when other factors that contribute to rates of suicidal thoughts and behaviors such as depression, victimization and recent suicide of a family member or a friend are taken into account, there remained a significant but substantially mediated elevation.[37] Similarly, a Minnesota Public School survey found that suicide attempts were associated with particular risk factors, such as

Table 29-4. Risk Factors for Adolescent Homosexual Male Suicidal Ideation and Behaviors

Depression
Victimization
Recent suicide of a family member or a friend
Self-identification as homosexual at a younger age
Substance abuse
Female gender role
Family dysfunction
Interpersonal conflict regarding sexual orientation
Nondisclosure of sexual orientation to others

Adapted from: Russell ST, Joyner K: Adolescent sexual orientation and suicide risk: evidence from a national study, *Am J Public Health* 91:1276–1281, 2001.

self-identification as homosexual at younger ages, substance abuse, female gender role, family dysfunction, interpersonal conflict regarding sexual orientation, and nondisclosure of sexual orientation to others.[37]

In the National Longitudinal Study of Adolescent Health, the greater risk of adolescent suicidal thoughts and suicide attempts was compared for homosexual youths and their peers.[38] Although this study found that the risk of suicide among youths with same-sex sexual attraction is greater than for heterosexual youths, when controlled for other factors, it may not be as great as is often cited. Other studies have shown higher rates of reported suicide attempts by males who admitted same-sex attraction; however, this particular study found the rate for males who admitted these same-sex relationships was 17.6%, twice the proportional representation of the group in the sample. Although the rates of suicidal ideation and behavior tend to be elevated in the younger homosexual male population, it is uncertain whether this elevation of suicidal risk continues for the older adult male population. The adolescent population may be more at risk because of other factors related to their homosexuality such as depression, stigmatization, and discrimination (Table 29-4). However, it appears that the risk may occur earlier in life and that protective mechanisms lessen the threat of suicide as homosexual men age.[34]

Substance Abuse Disorders

Substance abuse disorders have been shown to be more prevalent in homosexual and bisexual men. Rates of cigarette smoking are very high among homosexual men, sometimes nearly double

heterosexual population rates.[39] Tobacco use as compared in multiple studies among homosexual youth ranges from 38% to 59%, whereas the rate for adult homosexuals is 11–50%. The overall adult smoking rates in these studies was 28%; however, the studies on cigarette smoking by homosexuals were done with convenience samples and with patrons of "gay bars" and other venues commonly associated with alcohol use, which may skew prevalence rates.[40]

Alcohol use has been found to be higher among heterosexual males than homosexual males in more than one study. Even so, it is believed that alcohol use may appear higher in homosexual men because of the frequent survey use of "gay bars" and other venues more likely to be associated with excess alcohol use.[41] The Dutch NEMESIS study of homosexual men and women did not show increased rates of alcoholism in homosexual men compared with heterosexual men.[34] Whether the Dutch findings can be generalized to the US and other national populations is unclear.

Other forms of drug abuse have been established as being higher in the homosexual male population, including the use of marijuana, psychedelic drugs, ecstasy, barbiturates, and stimulants such as amyl or butyl nitrate (i.e., "poppers").[42] A 2003 study co-led by the Chicago Department of Public Health and the CDC discovered an epidemic of methamphetamine use in homosexual men. Up to 10% of homosexual men in the study population had used methamphetamine at least once in the previous year, compared with 0.7% of the general US population. In addition, of homosexual men who admitted using methamphetamine, 20% admitted using it at least once per week.[43] Methamphetamine use has been associated with sexual risk taking and higher incidence of HIV exposure.[44]

Eating disorders are also more prevalent among homosexual males. Anorexia nervosa and bulimia occur in up to 10–15% of all males with approximately 10–42% of the men found to be bulimic or anorexic identifying themselves as homosexual or bisexual.[45] This trend is thought to be caused by an excessive focus on appearance among young homosexual men.[46]

Screening and Counseling

Various national healthcare organizations have developed guidelines for the care of homosexual, bisexual, and other men who have sex with men. Many of the recommendations are for STD surveillance in the general population, not just for homosexual men. Some of these guidelines are evidence based, whereas others are based on expert opinion. Further study and recommendations need to be completed before additional guidelines are developed (Table 29-5).

The CDC has multiple screening guidelines for STDs, several of which are directed toward homosexually active men (strength of recommendation: A). The CDC recommends that clinicians should assess sexual risk in all male patients, which includes routinely inquiring about the sex of patients' sexual partners.[47] Men at risk, including homosexual men, should routinely undergo straightforward, nonjudgmental STD/HIV risk assessment and counseling to reduce the likelihood of acquisition or transmission of HIV and other STDs. At least annually, the following tests should be performed[47]:

- HIV serology, if HIV negative or not previously tested
- Syphilis serology (rapid plasma regain or venereal disease research laboratory)
- Urethral culture or nucleic acid amplification test for gonorrhea
- A urethral or urine test for chlamydia in men with oral-genital exposure
- Pharyngeal culture for gonorrhea in men with oral-genital exposure
- Rectal gonorrhea and chlamydia culture in men who have had receptive anal intercourse

More frequent screening (e.g., at 3–6-month intervals) may be indicated for homosexual men at highest risk, specifically those with multiple anonymous partners, those having sex in conjunction with illicit drug use, and those whose sex partners participate in these activities. If symptoms of STDs are present, physicians should perform diagnostic tests to screen for such diseases.

In addition, the CDC recommends vaccination against hepatitis A and B (strength of recommendation: A) as a means of preventing sexual transmission. Prevaccination serologic testing may be cost-effective in men for whom the presence of hepatitis A and B infection is likely to be high (strength of recommendation: C). The US Preventive Services Task Force (USPSTF)[48] makes recommendations for screening for STDs in the general population with some emphasis on men who have sex with men (strength of recommendation: A). Although the USPSTF concludes the following statements, many recommendations are made on the basis of insufficient evidence. If the patient is a member of a higher-risk population, more complete screening procedures may need to be instituted[48]:

- There is insufficient evidence to recommend for or against routinely screening asymptomatic men for chlamydia infection.
- For gonorrhea, there is insufficient evidence to recommend screening asymptomatic men at increased risk of STDs. (However, recommendations to screen high-risk young men may be made on other grounds.)
- For hepatitis B, routine screening is not recommended unless screening is performed to assess eligibility for hepatitis B vaccination; vaccination with hepatitis B vaccine is recommended at the appropriate times.
- Genital HSV screening is not recommended in asymptomatic persons.
- Routine screening for syphilis is not recommended.
- Periodic screening for HIV is recommended for all persons at increased risk of HIV infection.
- All routine vaccines should be given to homosexual men. In addition, hepatitis A and B immunizations should be given for those at high risk.

Other organizations that have developed screening guidelines for homosexual men include Public Health–Seattle and King County[49] (strength of recommendation: C) and the California STD Controllers Association[50] (strength of recommendation: C). The Seattle and King County guidelines recommend the following:

- The clinician should take a straightforward, nonjudgmental sexual history, especially asking men whether they have had sex with other men in the preceding year.
- All men who have had sex with other men in the preceding year should have the following screening tests at least once a year:
  - HIV serology (if previously HIV negative)
  - Syphilis serology
  - Pharyngeal culture for gonorrhea
- Patients who have had receptive anal intercourse in the preceding year should have the following:
  - Rectal culture for gonorrhea
  - Rectal culture for chlamydia
- More frequent screening with above tests every 3–6 months if any of the following are true:
  - Patient has had anonymous or multiple partners.
  - Patient has used crystal methamphetamine or inhaled nitrites or has had partners who participate in these activities.

Table 29-5. Surveillance for Sexually Transmitted Diseases (STDs) in Healthy Men Who Have Sex with Men of Unknown or Negative HIV Status

Recommendation	CDC STD Guidelines (2002)	US Preventive Services Task Force (1996)	Public Health and Seattle–King County (2001)	AAFP (2005)
Screening recommendation	Routinely inquire of gender of patient's sexual partners; screen at least annually	No recommendation provided	Screen all sexually active men who have sex with men	Counsel patients about risks and preventive strategies
Screening frequency of "high-risk" men	At 3–6-month intervals, screen men who have multiple anonymous sexual partners, who have sex in conjunction with illicit drug use, or who have sexual partners who participate in these activities	No recommendation provided; defines *high-risk patients* as men who have multiple sexual partners	Every 3–6 months, screen men with specific risk behaviors (multiple or anonymous sexual partners, substance abuse)	Counsel patients about risks and preventive strategies
HIV testing	Yes, annually unless high risk	Periodic screening in high-risk individuals	Yes, annually, unless high risk	Yes; if male patient has had sex with men after 1975 (consider periodically unless high risk)
Pharyngeal culture for *Neisseria gonorrhoeae*	Yes, in men with oral-genital exposure (annually, unless high risk)	No recommendation provided	Yes	No recommendation provided
Rectal culture for *N. gonorrhoeae*	Yes, in men who have receptive anal intercourse; include chlamydia culture	No recommendation provided	Yes, in men who have receptive anal intercourse	No recommendation provided
Screen for urethral *N. gonorrhoeae*	Yes, urethral or urine test (culture or nucleic acid amplification)	Insufficient evidence; consider screening high-risk men on other grounds	No	No recommendation provided
Screen for urethral chlamydia	Yes, urethral or urine test (culture or nucleic acid amplification) for men with oral-genital exposure	Insufficient evidence	No	No recommendation provided
Rectal screening for chlamydia	Yes, in men who have receptive anal intercourse	No recommendation provided	If receptive anal intercourse	There is insufficient evidence to recommend for or against routine screening of asymptomatic men for chlamydial infection
Serologic testing for syphilis	Yes	No	Yes	Yes, if multiple sexual partners
Serologic test for herpes simplex type-2 virus	No	Not recommended for asymptomatic persons	Consider	Not recommended for asymptomatic persons

Table continued on following page

Table 29-5. Surveillance for Sexually Transmitted Diseases (STDs) in Healthy Men Who Have Sex with Men of Unknown or Negative HIV Status (Continued)

Recommendation	CDC STD Guidelines (2002)	US Preventive Services Task Force (1996)	Public Health and Seattle–King County (2001)	AAFP (2005)
Immunization for hepatitis A and hepatitis B	Yes; serologic prevaccination testing may be cost-effective in homosexual men with high prevalence of hepatitis A and B in community	Screen high-risk persons to assess eligibility for vaccination; immunize all high-risk persons and young adults not previously immunized	Yes	Yes

HIV, Human immunodeficiency virus; CDC, Centers for Disease Control and Prevention; AAFP, American Academy of Family Physicians. Adapted from: Knight D: Healthcare screening for men who have sex with men, *Am Fam Phys* 69:2149–2156, 2004.

- Screening for urethral infection in asymptomatic men for gonorrhea or chlamydia is not recommended.
- Men who have not been vaccinated against hepatitis A and B should have serologic tests and should be immunized if the test results are negative.
- Some experts recommend HSV serologic testing for homosexually active men.
- If HSV-2 infection is present, men should be informed of a greater risk of acquiring and transmitting HIV.

The California STD Controllers Association guidelines are for HIV-infected men (strength of recommendation: C) and are similar to the Seattle–King County recommendations in that both include a serologic test for syphilis, a pharyngeal culture for gonorrhea, and, if the patient has receptive anal intercourse, a rectal culture for gonorrhea.[50] The California guidelines call for screening for urethral gonorrhea and chlamydia infection, using a nucleic acid amplification test on voided urine. Both the Seattle and California guidelines recommend "consideration" of serologic tests for HSV-2. Both sets of guidelines recommend immunization against hepatitis A and B.[50]

The American Academy of Family Physicians (AAFP) has recommendations for clinical preventive services, some of which apply to homosexual men[51] (strength of recommendation: A). The AAFP Guidelines strongly recommend for immunization against hepatitis A and B in homosexual men and do not recommend routinely screening the asymptomatic population for chronic HBV infection. The AAFP finds insufficient evidence to recommend for or against routine screening for hepatitis C virus in high-risk populations, as it is currently not thought to be an STD. Screening is recommended for HIV in men who have sex with men after 1975 and is strongly recommended for syphilis screening in men who have sex with men and have multiple sexual partners. Insufficient evidence was found regarding screening asymptomatic men for chlamydia or gonorrhea. The AAFP recommends against screening for HSV in asymptomatic adolescents and adults.

Screening guidelines for anal cancer in homosexual men are still lacking. Several studies have tried to estimate the incidence and cost-effectiveness of screening for anal cancer; an Australian study[21] found that it was not cost-effective. However, Goldie and colleagues[20] concluded that, from a financial standpoint, it was reasonable to screen HIV-negative homosexual men every 2–3 years for AIN via anal Pap smear testing (strength of recommendation: C). For HIV-positive men, screening yearly for anal cancer was definitely found to be cost-effective. Further studies are needed to resolve this question of seemingly increased importance.

Recommendations

Bias and negative attitudes prevalent in the American public and among physicians lead patients to limit disclosure of sexual orientation or practice.[7] Failure to determine sexual orientation or practice may lead to a failure to accurately diagnose, treat, or recommend appropriate preventive measures or counseling for a range of conditions. Therefore, physicians must be open to and trained to provide care for the homosexual male (Table 29-6). This population of patients is diverse in income, age, race, national origin, education, and culture; therefore, it is often difficult to determine sexual orientation or sexual behavior of patients. To establish possible homosexual behavior, clinicians should avoid potentially

Table 29-6. Ten Topics Homosexual Men Should Discuss with their Healthcare Providers

Physical
HIV/AIDS, safe sexual practices
STDs
Prostate/testicular/colorectal cancer screening
Hepatitis A and B immunization
HPV, anal papilloma, and screening for anal cancer
Fitness (diet and exercise) and any abnormal eating behaviors
Psychosocial
Tobacco and alcohol use
Substance use
Depression/anxiety
Any suicidal ideation

HIV, Human immunodeficiency virus; AIDS, acquired immunodeficiency syndrome; STDs, sexually transmitted diseases; HPV, human papilloma virus.

Adapted from: The Gay and Lesbian Medical Association Web site. Available at: http://www.glma.org. Accessed January 26, 2006.

stereotypical questions such as "Are you homosexual?" and replace them with questions such as "Do you have sex with men, women, or both?" These questions will more often lead to a correct assessment of a homosexual male's need for specialized healthcare.

Since many men who have sex with men do not consider themselves to be either homosexual or bisexual, they may not perceive themselves to be at risk for various disease conditions and may not respond to labeling with questions regarding homosexual or bisexual activity.[52] Other questions that may be useful include, "Some men, although they are married or have a girlfriend, occasionally have sex with another man. Have you done that?" or "Many men have sex with other men. Have you ever had sex with another man?" To determine specific risks, clinicians should inquire about behaviors with focused questions such as, "Do you engage in anal sex (inserting your penis into a person's rectum or allowing someone to insert his penis into your rectum)?" or "Do you engage in oral sex?" Additional information that is necessary to assess the overall risk of disease transmission includes the number of lifetime and current sexual partners, condom use, and risky sexual practices.

The physician's office and staff should be educated and encouraged to facilitate nondisclosure of homosexuality or homosexual behavior. Intake forms should include appropriate terms

and language such as "relationship status" instead of "marital status" with options such as "partnered." When asking for information, clinicians should use terms such as "partner" or "significant other" along with other terms such as "husband" or "wife."[53] Other helpful suggestions include using gender-neutral terms when discussing sexual partners. Clinicians should ask their male patients to clarify terms with which you may be unfamiliar. It is important to assure patients of confidentiality when discussing private matters and to consider how much information and detail should be documented in the patient's records, according to his wishes.

It is important, especially in adolescents, to question homosexual patients concerning sexual practices and possible psychological problems such as depression, anxiety, suicidal thoughts, and plans. Inquiry about family support and other social supports should be addressed. Many homosexuals may lose traditional social support or be rejected by their "families of origin" after disclosure of their homosexuality.[7]

With homosexual male patients who are highly sexually active with more than one partner, more frequent testing for HIV and other STDs should be suggested. Counseling on effective safer-sex measures and the necessity of condom use during all sexual practices that may carry a risk of disease transmission is imperative. If a homosexual male patient has a history of anal warts or HPV infection, expert opinion states that clinicians should suggest anal Pap smears yearly in HIV-positive patients and every 2–3 years in HIV-negative patients. For patients who show signs and symptoms of STDs, appropriate diagnostic tests and treatment should be facilitated. In male homosexual patients with depression, anxiety disorders, or suicidal ideation or behavior, appropriate medical therapy and referral to appropriate psychological treatment resources should be recommended.

Only a few evidence-based recommendations are available for the care of homosexual males. Due to inherent stigma and prejudice, coupled with the fact that homosexuals represent a minority of the population, lack of funding has limited most research of the homosexual population to small studies with convenience sampling.[7] Large-scale, coordinated, population-based studies and evidence-based guidelines could aid the physician in delivering optimal care for homosexual males. Until this level of evidence is available, clinicians should make use of best practices as advocated by expert panels such as the CDC, the USPSTF, the Healthy People 2010

Companion Document for Lesbian, Gay, Bisexual and Transgendered Health,[54] the AAFP, and the Gay and Lesbian Medical Association (available at: http://www.glma.org).

References

1. Wallick MM, Cabre KM, Townsend MH: How the topic of homosexuality is taught at U.S. medical schools, *Acad Med* 67:601–603, 1992.
2. Boehmer U. Twenty years of public health research: inclusion of lesbian, gay, bisexual and transgender populations, *Am J Public Health* 92:1125–1130, 2002.
3. Lee R. Health care problems of lesbian, gay, bisexual and transgender patients, *West J Med* 172:403–408, 2000.
4. Allen LB, Glicken AD: Adolescent health care experience of gay, lesbian, and bisexual young adults, *J Adolesc Health* 23:212–220, 1998.
5. Skegg KM, Nada-Raja S, Dickson N, et al: Sexual orientation and self-harm in men and women, *Am J Psychiatry* 160:541–546, 2003.
6. The Kinsey Institute: Prevalence of homosexuality: brief summary of US studies compiled June, 1999. Indiana, The Kinsey Institute Web site. Available at: http://www.indiana.edu/~kinsey/resources/bib-homoprev.html. Accessed January 28, 2006.
7. Dean L, Robinson K, Sell R, et al: Lesbian, gay, bisexual, and transgender health: findings and concerns, *J Gay Lesbian Med Assoc* 4:101–151, 2000.
8. Healthy People 2010: Sexually transmitted diseases (infections). Lesbian, gay, bisexual, and transgender health. Available at: http://www.glma.org/policy/hp2010/PDF/HP2010CDLGBTHealth.pdf. Accessed February 9, 2006.
9. Estimated numbers of cases of HIV/AIDS, by year of diagnosis and selected characteristics of persons, 2001–2004. Available at: http://www.cdc.gov/hiv/topics/surveillance/resources/reports/2004report/table1.htm. Accessed February 9, 2006.
10. Barroso PF, Schechter M, Gupta P, et al: Effect of antiretroviral therapy on HIV shedding in semen, *Ann Intern Med* 133:280–284, 2000.
11. Fox K, del Rio C, Holmes KK, et al: Gonorrhea in the HIV era: a reversal in trends among men who have sex with men, *Am J Public Health* 91:959–964, 2001.
12. Centers for Disease Control and Prevention: Increases in unsafe sex and rectal gonorrhea among men who have sex with men–San Francisco, California, 1994–9997, *MMWR Morb Mortal Wkly Rep* 48:45–48, 1999.
13. Sanchez T, Finlayson T, Drake A, et al: Centers for Disease Control and Prevention (CDC): Human immunodeficiency virus (HIV) risk, prevention, and testing behaviors—United States, National HIV Behavioral Surveillance System: men who have sex with men, November 2003–April 2005, *MMWR Morb Mortal Wkly Rep* 55:1–16, 2006.
14. Gonococcal isolate surveillance project (GISP): Percent of urethral *Neisseria gonorrhoeae* isolates obtained from men who have sex with men attending STD clinics, 1988–2004. Available at: http://www.cdc.gov/std/stats/msm.htm. Accessed July 13, 2000.
15. Lafferty WE, Hughes JP, Handsfield HH: Sexually transmitted diseases in men who have sex with men: acquisition of gonorrhea and non-gonococcal urethritis by fellatio and implications for STD/HIV prevention, *Sex Transm Dis* 24:272–278, 1997.
16. Zenilman JM, Weisman CS, Rompal AM, et al: Condom use to prevent incident STDs: the validity of self-reported condom use, *Sex Transm Dis* 22:15–21, 1995.
17. Krone MR, Wald A, Tabet SR, et al: Herpes simplex virus type 2 shedding in human immunodeficiency virus–negative men who have sex with men: frequency, patterns, and risk factors, *Clin Infect Dis* 30:261–267, 2000.
18. Renzi C, Douglas JM, Foster M, et al: Herpes simplex virus type 2 infection as a risk factor for human immunodeficiency virus acquisition in men who have sex with men, *J Infect Dis* 187:19–25, 2003.
19. Primary and secondary syphilis among men who have sex with men—New York City, 2001, *MMWR Morb Mortal Wkly Rep,* 51:853–856, 2002.
20. Goldie SJ, Kuntz KM, Weinstein MC, et al: Cost-effectiveness of screening for anal squamous intraepithelial lesions and anal cancer in human immunodeficiency virus–negative homosexual and bisexual men, *Am J Med* 108:634–641, 2000.
21. Anderson JS, Vajdic C, Grulich AE: Is screening for anal cancer warranted in homosexual men? *Sexual Health* 1137–1144, 2004.
22. Carter PS, De Ruiter A, Whatrup C, et al: Human immunodeficiency virus infection and genital warts as risk factors for anal intraepithelial neoplasia in homosexual men, *Br J Surg* 82:473–474, 1995.
23. Chin-Hong PV, Vittinghoff E, Cranston RD, et al: Age-specific prevalence of anal human papillomavirus infection in HIV-negative sexually active men who have sex with men: the EXPLORE study, *J Infect Dis* 190:2070–2076, 2004.
24. Martin F, Bower M: Anal intraepithelial neoplasia in HIV positive people, *Sex Transm Infect* 77:327–331, 2001.
25. Schlect HP: Why do an anal pap? 2004. In Harvard-wide conference. Available at: http://search.partners.org/highlight/index.html?url=http%3A//www.massgeneral.org/id/intranet/hms/handouts2003 2004/Schlect3_2004.pdf&hltcol=mgh&charset=iso.8859-1&la=en&fterm=hans&fterm=p&fterm=hans+p&search=./Query.html%3Fcharsert%3Diso-8859-1%26style%3Dmgh%26col%3Dmgh%26qt%3Dschlect%252C%2Bhans%2Bp. Accessed January 29, 2006.
26. MacKellar DA, Valleroy LA, Secura GM, et al: Two decades after vaccine license: hepatitis B immunization and infection among young men who have sex with men, *Am J Public Health* 91:965–971, 2001.

27. Kahn J: Preventing hepatitis A and hepatitis B virus infections among men who have sex with men, *Clin Infect Dis* 35:1382–1387, 2002.

28. Jacobs RJ, Meyerhoff AS: Vaccination of sexually active homosexual men against hepatitis A: analysis of costs and benefits, *J Gay Lesbian Med Assoc* 3:51–58, 1999.

29. Fried R, Surawicz C: Proctitis and sexually transmissible diseases of the colon, *Curr Treat Options Gastroenterol* 6:263–270, 2003.

30. Klausner JD, Kohn R, Kent C: Etiology of clinical proctitis among men who have sex with men, *Clin Infect Dis* 38:300–302, 2004.

31. Mays VM, Cochran SD: Mental health correlates of perceived discrimination among lesbian, gay and bisexual adults in the United States, *Am J Public Health* 91:1869–1876, 2001.

32. Gilman SE, Cochran SE, Mays VM, et al: Risk of psychiatric disorders among individuals reporting same-sex sexual partners in the national co-morbidity survey, *Am J Public Health* 91:933–939, 2001.

33. Cochran S, Mays VM: Lifetime prevalence of suicide symptoms and affective disorders among men reporting same-sex sexual partners: results from NHANES III, *Am J Public Health* 90:573–578, 2000.

34. Sandfort TG, de Graaf R, Bijl RV, Schnabel P: Same-sex sexual behavior and psychiatric disorders: findings from the Netherlands mental health survey and incidence study (NEMESIS), *Arch Gen Psychiatry* 58:85–91, 2001.

35. Remafedi G: Suicide and sexual orientation: nearing the end of controversy? *Arch Gen Psychiatry* 56:885–886, 1999.

36. Herrell R, Goldberg J, True WR, et al: Sexual orientation and suicidality: a co-twin control study in adult men, *Arch Gen Psychiatry* 56:867–874, 1999.

37. Remafedi G, French S, Story M, et al: The relationship between suicide risk and sexual orientation: results of a population-based study, *Am J Public Health* 88:57–60, 1998.

38. Russell ST, Joyner K: Adolescent sexual orientation and suicide risk: evidence from a national study, *Am J Public Health* 91:1276–1281, 2001.

39. Stall RD, Greenwood L, Acree M, et al: Cigarette smoking among gay and bisexual men, *Am J Public Health* 89:1875–1878, 1999.

40. Ryan H, Pascale MW, Easton A, et al: Smoking among lesbians, gays and bisexuals: a review of the literature, *Am J Prev Med* 21:142–149, 2001.

41. Drabble L, Midanik LT, Trocki K: Reports of alcohol consumption and alcohol-related problems among homosexual, bisexual and heterosexual respondents: results from the 2000 national alcohol survey, *J Stud Alcohol* 66:111, 2005. Available at: http://infotrac.galegroup.com/itw/infomark/433/301/75361640w1/purl=rc1_HRCA_0_A132050583&dyn=3!xrn_1_0_A132050583?sw_aep=u_amedsci. Accessed March 22, 2006.

42. Dionne S, Odle TG: Gay and lesbian health. *Gale Encyc Med* 2004. Available at: http://infotrac.galegroup.com/itw/infomark/434/301/75361640w1/purl=rc1_HRCA_0_A133987114&dyn=8!xrn_1_0_A 133987114?sw_aep=u_amedsci.Accessed March 22, 2006.

43. Gay and Lesbian Medical Association receives $320,000 grant to study impact of methamphetamine on the gay community 2006. Available at: http://www.glma.org/index.cfm?fuseaction=Feature.showFeature&CategoryID=4&FeatureID=22. Accessed March 22, 2006.

44. Brewer DD, Golden MR, Handsfield HH: Unsafe sexual behavior and correlates of risk in a probability sample of men who have sex with men in the era of highly active antiretroviral therapy, *Sex Transm Dis* 33:250–256, 2006.

45. Russell CJ, Keel PK: Homosexuality as a specific risk factor for eating disorders in men, *Int J Eat Disord* 31:300–306, 2002.

46. Blinder BJ: Anorexia in males. Available at:http://www.ltspeed.com/bjblinder/anmales.htm. Accessed February 23, 2006.

47. Centers for Disease Control and Prevention: Sexually transmitted diseases treatment guidelines 2002, *MMWR Recomm Rep* 51(RR-6):1–78, 2002.

48. Sexually transmitted diseases. In US Preventive Services Task Force: *Guide to Clinical Preventive Services: Report of the U.S. Preventive Services Task Force*, ed 2, Baltimore, MD, 1996, Williams & Wilkins. Available at: http://www.ahrq.gov/clinic/cpsix.htm. Accessed February 9, 2006.

49. Handsfield HH, Wood RW, Celum CL, et al: Sexually transmitted disease and HIV screening guidelines for men who have sex with men, *Sex Transm Dis* 28:457–459, 2001.

50. Gunn RA, Klausner JD, Gandelman A: Guidance for STD clinical preventive services for persons infected with HIV, *Sex Transm Dis* 28:464–467, 2001.

51. AAFP summary of policy recommendations for periodic health examinations Rev 6.0, August 2005, Leawood, KS, 2005, American Academy of Family Physicians. Available at: http://www.aafp.org/exam.xml. Accessed February 6, 2006.

52. Kassler WJ, Wasserheit JN, Cates W: Sexually transmitted diseases. In Woolf S, editor: *Health Promotion and Disease Prevention in Clinical Practice*, Baltimore, MD, 1996, Williams and Wilkins, pp 274–275.

53. Gay and Lesbian Medical Association: Creating a safe clinical environment for men who have sex with men, 2002. Available at: http://ce54.citysoft.com/_data/n_0001/resources/live/GLMA%20guidelines%202006%20FINAL.pdf. Accessed February 23, 2006.

54. Healthy People 2010: Companion document for LGBT health 2001. Available at: http://www.glma.org/_data/n_0001/resources/live/HealthyCompanion Doc3.pdf. Accessed March 4, 2006.

The Transsexual Male

A. Evan Eyler, MD, and Jamie Feldman, MD, PhD

Introduction

This chapter is intended for primary care physicians who wish to provide medical care to transsexual men and female-to-male (FTM) gender-variant persons. The term *gender-variant* refers to persons who experience dissonance between their natal sex and their psychological gender, some of whom will choose hormonal or surgical treatments to resolve this conflict, as well as persons whose *gender presentation* is outside usual male or female norms, and those whose personal *gender identity* is other than fully female or fully male.

Many generalist physicians prescribe androgens to their male-identified transsexual patients, referring only complicated cases for endocrinologic consultation. Some prefer to manage the other aspects of preventive and routine medical care, working closely with an endocrinologist who conducts the hormonal evaluation and prescribes the masculinizing medications. This chapter addresses routine clinical care, preventive care, and some basic principles of hormonal treatment for transgendered male patients.

The Spectrum of Gender Identity and Expression

Western culture has traditionally assumed that anatomic genital sex (male or female) is concordant with gender (i.e., internal, psychological self-perception of maleness or femaleness). In contrast, many non-Western cultures recognize the existence of more than two genders and have different expectations for persons who do not fit either the man's or the woman's role.[1] The *fa' afatama* of traditional Samoan culture are natal females who live in the male social role and are accepted as men.[2] Throughout Western history, some persons have lived "cross-gendered" and have been perceived throughout all or part of adult life as belonging to, or behaving as, the gender not usually associated with their natal, anatomic sex.

Recent years have seen the recognition of persons who do not perceive themselves as being "fully male" or "fully female" and who consider themselves *gender blended*,[3] or differently gendered in some other significant way. Some consider the concept of gender itself as problematic or inapplicable: "Many in the [transgendered] community would see themselves as existing outside of gender, of being oppressed by it but using its icons and signifiers to say who they are."[4]

Like sexual orientation, gender identity can be conceptualized as a continuum.[5] *Cross-dressers* are persons who, at times, dress as the other sex because it is ego-syntonic to do so, but they do not seek medical sex reassignment. Many social scientists consider this a form of gender variance. Bullough and Bullough note:

"The major area in which people depart from societal expectations is in sexual orientation... The second most common area of cross-gender behavior is in the area of the symbolic expression of gender through clothing (including jewelry, tattoos, and other adornments). A smaller group of cross-gendered people seek a complete and permanent identity as a member of the... [other] sex."[6]

Transvestic fetishism is a separate condition, which involves "intense sexually arousing fantasies, sexual urges, or behaviors involving cross-dressing" that cause "clinically significant distress or impairment in social, occupational, or other important areas of functioning."[7] Both cross-dressing and transvestic fetishism occur much more commonly among natal males than natal females.

Transsexual persons are those who seek medical assistance in changing their physical sex to enable their internal self-perception and their physical attributes to become congruent, thus increasing self-comfort and social fit. With regard to terminology concerning gender variance, the World Professional Association for Transgender Health (WPATH) Standards of Care[8] note:

"Between the publication of the Diagnostic and Statistical Manual of Mental Disorders (DSM)-III and DSM-IV, the term *transgender* began to be used in various ways. Some employed it to refer to those with unusual gender identities in a value-free manner—that is, without a connotation of psychopathology. Some people informally used the term to refer to any person with any type of gender identity issues. Transgender is not a formal diagnosis, but many professionals and members of the public found it easier to use informally than GID NOS [Gender Identity Disorder, Not Otherwise Specified], which is a formal diagnosis."[8]

Persons who are FTM transsexual or transgendered are often referred to as *transmen*, or more formally as transsexual (or transgendered) men. *Intersex* is a different medical concept, referring to persons born with ambiguous genitalia or for whom phenotypic and chromosomal sex are discordant (e.g., persons with a 5-alpha reductase deficiency).

Reliable population prevalence estimates for transgendered and transsexual people are difficult to obtain and vary cross-culturally. Data from the Netherlands demonstrate that one in 11,900 natal males and one in 30,400 natal females is transsexual,[8] but persons who identify as transgendered or who cross-dress are likely much more numerous than those who seek sex reassignment surgery.[6,9] Transsexual monozygotic twin pairs have been reported[10]; concordance data appear similar for transsexualism and homosexuality,[11] suggesting that biologic factors strongly influence both gender identity and sexual object choice, but that life experience is also significant. Although biologic influences appear to promote male-to-female (MTF) transsexualism more often than FTM, MTF transition is less common in cultures in which discrimination against women is more pervasive and virulent. In some countries, transgendered persons also experience hate crime victimization, similar to that experienced by gay and lesbian persons.[12] This also restricts the practical ability of persons to gender transition or to be identifiable as transgendered persons.

Transgender Healthcare: General Principles

Primary Care

Transgendered persons often encounter difficulty in obtaining adequate medical services,[13–15] although access may be improving in some respects.[16] Transsexual men who are receiving treatment with androgens but are at a relatively early point in the process of physical transition can present an unusual blend of gender-associated physical characteristics that they can be understandably reluctant to reveal unless the medical environment is supportive.

Some transsexual persons who have completed sex reassignment are indistinguishable from other members of their (new, non-natal) sex and may obtain medical services without routinely revealing their preoperative history. MTF sex-reassignment surgery is currently quite technically advanced, and postoperative MTF persons are often not identifiable as such, even on cursory gynecologic examination. Unfortunately, FTM surgery is currently less sophisticated, and results are more variable. Some postoperative transsexual men are indistinguishable from natal males when nude, but most are not.

Both FTM patients and MTF patients require ongoing hormonal supplementation, which can be managed by generalist physicians who become knowledgeable in this area of practice. In addition, transsexual patients require routine health promotion and preventive services. The general rule is that any intact organ should be cared for (e.g., a woman with a prostate gland may develop disease of this organ). Similarly, FTM reconstructive chest surgery does not remove all of the glandular tissue, as would be the case if a mastectomy were performed for the treatment of breast cancer, so FTM men should, at a minimum, continue self-examination. Older transsexual patients require lower levels of hormone supplementation than their younger peers because the risk of complications rises with age. The healthcare needs of elderly transsexual men are discussed later in this chapter.

Transsexual, transgendered, and cross-dressed patients should be asked how they would like to be addressed. If a legal name change has not been finalized, cross-reference filing of the medical chart under both names may be required.

Multidisciplinary Care and Referrals

Hormonal therapy that modifies the visible sex characteristics and sex-reassignment surgery are life-changing medical interventions that should only be undertaken for patients who have completed an appropriate mental health evaluation and have access to supportive mental health care. In addition, transitioning patients should receive concurrent care from a family physician, an internist, or an endocrinologist who is knowledgeable about hormonal supplementation and general medical care. Professionals in urology, gynecology, plastic surgery, speech therapy, and nursing are consulted when needed, with communication among members of the medical team whenever a treatment change is planned.

All of the care providers should agree to abide by the Standards of Care[8] developed by HBIGDA. Physicians with a strong interest in transsexual medicine or those who wish to provide medical gender transition services are advised to contact HBIGDA (http://www.hbigda.org). Additional information is available at http://www.transcience.org.

Common Clinical Presentations

Physicians who are known in their communities as empathic sources of transgender medical care will find gender-variant patients presenting to their practices for a variety of reasons. Patients will seek initiation of hormonal treatment, prescription medications to replace informally obtained ("street") hormonal preparations, and post-transition medical care. Some persons who are not planning to transition gender, but whose gender presentations or roles are outside societal norms, will also seek care from physicians who are knowledgeable about the spectrum of gender identity and who are known to treat their "non-traditionally gendered" patients with dignity and respect.

The Patient Who Is Seeking Initiation of Hormonal Treatment

A transgendered person who is beginning hormonal treatment may be referred to the physician by a mental health professional or may self-refer. The initial evaluation includes a full health history, a physical examination, and an endocrine assessment. As discussed in the Standards of Care developed by HBIGDA,[8] a mental health evaluation should also be obtained, unless the patient has already been functioning successfully full-time as a member of the psychological gender for a significant period of time (i.e., has already had a substantial real life experience). Communication between the physical and mental health professionals involved in the patient's care is of crucial importance.

The Patient Who Has Been Using Informally Obtained Hormones, and Who Wishes to Begin Taking Prescription Medications

Some people initiate hormone supplementation with testosterone purchased illegally at a fitness center, nonprescription "herbal" preparations, or androgens obtained over the Internet or through veterinary supply. These practices are undertaken for many reasons, including confidentiality concerns, ambivalence about transitioning, the desire to control medication use without "negotiating" with a medical professional, lack of locally available services, and economic need.[16] Regardless of rationale, transgendered persons may eventually wish to begin regular medical care, particularly if a physical problem ensues. Initial evaluation includes the same components (e.g., a full health history, physical examination, and endocrine assessment) as that of patients who are beginning hormone use, as well as a comprehensive history regarding the use of nonprescription preparations. The patient should also be referred to a mental health professional, unless the physician is confident that this is not necessary, as per the Standards of Care.[8]

The Patient Who Is Seeking Surgery

Surgeons who perform FTM genital reconstruction require general medical and mental health referrals regarding their patients before scheduling surgical procedures. In addition, this service is not available in many geographic areas; therefore, patients may have to travel to a surgical center and require some postsurgical care after returning home. Communication between the surgeon and the patient's personal physician will be necessary regarding pre- and post-hospital care.

A comprehensive discussion of FTM surgery is beyond the scope of this chapter. Surgical transition usually includes male chest reconstruction surgery, hysterectomy with bilateral oophorectomy, and the creation of male genitalia through either metaidoioplasty or phalloplasty. The goal of "top surgery" is the creation of an aesthetic-appearing male chest, rather than a postmastectomy flatness. "Bottom surgery" involves either the creation of small but male-appearing genitalia through modification of the tissue around the hormonally enlarged clitoris (metaidoioplasty) or free-flap phalloplasty using tissue from the radial forearm.

The Patient Who Has Completed Medical Transition

Persons who have completed the gender-transition process may change physicians due to geographic relocation, new health insurance plans, and many other reasons. The initial meeting with a new physician can be fraught with anxiety, particularly if the patient's gender history is not known to the new community or employer, or if he has not had genital surgery. Assurances regarding confidentiality of medical records and a calm, welcoming attitude by all members of the office staff can be particularly important under these circumstances.

The Patient Who Is Not Seeking Transition

Some persons who have physical characteristics usually associated with the other gender, or who consider themselves gender blended or having gender identities other than female or male, prefer to obtain medical care from generalist physicians with many transgendered patients in their practices in order to be more readily accepted and understood. As numerous FTM healthcare survey participants noted, having to "educate" one's physician regarding lifestyle and identity issues can be tiresome.[15]

Family Members of Gender-Transitioning Persons

Gender transition requires a substantial and sustained effort in many domains, including medical treatment, social adjustment, and attention to the hundreds of details that accompany living in a gendered world. Transsexual men who are married or partnered are sometimes nevertheless able to continue these relationships during and after transition. In these cases, the couple may become focused on the transition process and neglect other concurrent issues and more routine concerns. It can be helpful to inquire whether the patient's partner is receiving routine medical care and, if not, to invite that person into the clinical practice.

Preventive Care for Transsexual Men

Preventive care is an essential component of healthcare for all persons and is critical to the achievement of many national health objectives.[17]

Primary and secondary prevention of chronic disease has become increasingly important among the transgendered population, due to the aging cohort receiving long-term transgender hormone therapy and a significant number of patients presenting for hormone therapy at older ages with risk factors for chronic disease or comorbid conditions.[13,18] However, transgendered people face significant barriers to receiving adequate preventive services, including a lack of transgender-specific medical knowledge available to generalist physicians. An evidence-based approach to preventive care, and current transgendered male–specific prevention recommendations are discussed below.

Challenges in Providing Preventive Care to the Transgendered Male Population

Delivering high-quality preventive care to patients who are transsexual or transgendered presents several challenges. First, transgender identity and behavior are often socially stigmatized, leading many transsexual men to maintain a traditional female presentation and public role until medical transition is well-established, while keeping their transgender health concerns concealed, and then obliterating evidence of the female past as thoroughly as possible after transition. A Minnesota study of transgender health seminar participants found that 45% had not informed their personal physician of their true gender identity.[19] Lack of healthcare insurance, experience of discrimination in the healthcare setting, lack of access to medical personnel competent in transsexual medicine, and (for some) discomfort with the body can lead transgendered patients to avoid medical care altogether.[14] Thus, transsexual men often lack access to preventive healthcare services and timely treatment of routine health problems.

In addition, most physicians and other healthcare professionals do not receive training in health issues specific to transgendered patients, and they lack ready access to appropriate information or a knowledgeable colleague. Long-term, prospective studies for most transgender-specific health issues are lacking, resulting in variable preventive care recommendations based primarily on expert opinion. However, by using an increasing body of peer-reviewed, scientific research on transgender health, along with relevant data from the general population, one can develop an evidence-based approach to preventive care for male-identified patients who are transgendered or transsexual.

Principles of Evidence-Based Transgender Healthcare

Assembling the Evidence: Methodology

The US Preventive Services Task Force (USPSTF)[20] noted that producing a formal systematic review (consisting of a comprehensive literature search, evaluation of the data, and detailed documentation of methods and findings) is not feasible when addressing many topics in preventive care. Transgender health research consists primarily of many small-sample studies with a variety of methodologies and includes very few randomized trials. Rather than being confined to MEDLINE, the literature on transgender health is spread over many disparate databases.

This chapter follows the USPSTF approach, focusing on a limited number of high-priority topics and reviewing the questions and evidence most critical to making recommendations for medical practice based on the best available evidence. A computerized search of the transgender health literature was performed using the following terms: transsexual*, gender dysphoria, gender identity disorder, sex reassignment, transgender.* Databases across disciplines were searched to facilitate a comprehensive review. The citation databases searched included CINAHL, ERIC (via EBSCO), MEDLINE, PubMed, Science Direct, and Social Sciences Index. The online academic search engines Google Scholar and Scirus were also used to further identify published articles and peer-reviewed presentations. Finally, available abstracts from the HBIGDA symposia from 1999 to 2005 and all articles published in *The International Journal of Transgenderism* were also reviewed. Relevant non-transgender studies were identified through MEDLINE searches, with a focus on meta-analyses, systematic reviews, and large-scale clinical trials.

Peer-reviewed presentations and publications were prioritized over non–peer-reviewed evidence. Wherever possible, evidence showing that preventive services influenced health status per se (e.g., patient-oriented outcomes) was prioritized over evidence that focused on intermediate markers (e.g., disease-oriented outcomes). Lower-level evidence, such as disease-oriented studies or case reports, was not exhaustively reviewed when stronger evidence was available.

An asterisk after a search term means that any extension of that word was also searched; that is, "transsexual" also searched the derivative terms "transsexuals" and "transsexualism."

The evidence was then graded according to the strength of recommendation taxonomy (SORT) classification system.[21]

Incorporating Non-Transgender Evidence into the Transgender-Healthcare Context

Currently, few prospective, large-scale studies exist regarding transgender healthcare, and the health of transsexual men has been less well studied than that of transsexual women. FTM persons represent a numerical minority within the transgendered population, in most cultures. The best available evidence comes from a Dutch retrospective chart review involving 816 MTF and 293 FTM transsexual patients, with duration of hormone use ranging from 2 months to 41 years.[22] Overall mortality and morbidity, including the incidence of venous thromboembolism, cerebrovascular events, coronary events, prostate cancer, breast cancer, hypertension, and liver abnormalities, were compared with age- and gender-specific statistics in the general Dutch population. Because this study did not track a specific cohort over a long period of time, particularly beyond the age of 65 years, the long-term health effects of transgender hormone therapy remain uncertain. According to the SORT criteria, this represents level 2 evidence. The medical literature also contains many smaller-scale transgender-specific studies of particular clinical issues, such as osteoporosis, along with much non–transgender-specific evidence (e.g., studies involving non-transgendered men and women).

Published SORT level 1 transgender-specific evidence is essentially nonexistent. However, level 1 evidence regarding a number of preventive healthcare issues has been gathered for the general population, allowing clinicians to extrapolate evidence-based recommendations for their transgendered patients. When applying knowledge from the general, non-transgendered population, physicians should look for rigorous studies that are highly relevant to the clinical context. For example, a large prospective study involving non-transgendered men using testosterone supplementation for treatment of later life decline in androgen production may be relevant to older transsexual men using similar types of hormone supplements.

Evidence from non-transgender studies can usually be directly applied to similar transgendered patients who have not yet had surgical or hormonal interventions; conclusions from studies involving non-transgendered women are probably applicable to people who are FTM transsexual or transgendered and who have not taken testosterone or had masculinizing surgery. However, subtle physiologic differences between transgendered men and natal women who are not transgendered may exist even before the initiation of hormonal therapy. Bosinski and colleagues[23] compared anthropometric measurements of 15 FTM persons who had not yet initiated treatment with supplemental androgens with 19 non-transsexual female and 21 non-transsexual male control subjects. With regard to 14 sex-dimorphic indices of body build, mean values for the transgendered male participants differed from the non-transsexual females in 7 indices and were indistinguishable from the natal males in 9 indices. In general, the transgendered men presented a more masculine body build relative to the non-transgendered women, particularly with regard to fat distribution and skeletal proportions, even without the use of supplemental testosterone. Although other differences probably exist between transgendered men and non-transgendered women, research conducted with female participants should be considered in the care of transgendered men, particularly before masculinizing treatment and when the conclusions are robust.

In this analysis, non–transgender-specific evidence has been incorporated into the SORT taxonomy by ranking it one level of evidence lower when applied in the transgendered health context. The grade of recommendation for transgender healthcare has not been changed for those areas in which grade A recommendations have been established for non-transgendered patients (based on overwhelming level 1 evidence) and when this would likely be unaffected by hormonal or surgical interventions.

Preventive Care Recommendations for Transsexual and Transgendered Men

Risks and recommendations for screening depend on the patient's hormonal and surgical status. Recommendations specific to each of these patient groups are given below for the following areas: cancer (i.e., breast, cervical, ovarian, and uterine), cardiovascular disease and its risk factors (i.e., hypertension, hyperlipidemia, smoking), diabetes, osteoporosis, blood-borne infections (i.e., human immunodeficiency virus [HIV], hepatitis B and C), and other sexually transmitted infections (STIs). Vaccination recommendations are in keeping with those for non-transgendered

persons, except for hepatitis A and B, as discussed in the HIV/hepatitis section below.

Cancer

Breast Cancer Screening

Patients Who Have Not Yet Had Chest Surgery, With or Without Testosterone Use

- Breast examinations and screening mammography are recommended as for natal females (strength of recommendation: A, based on multiple level 1 studies evaluating mammography for non-transgendered women, as applied to FTM patients not using testosterone; strength of recommendation: B for those with testosterone use).

There is no evidence of increased risk of breast cancer for FTM patients compared with natal females. Conflicting level 3 evidence, including level 2 studies of natal women and disease-oriented evidence, shows either minimally increased or decreased risk for breast cancer among women using exogenous testosterone[24] or with higher levels of endogenous androgens.[25–27]

Patients Who Have Had Chest Surgery, With or Without Testosterone Use

- The risk of breast cancer is reduced with chest surgery but appears higher among FTM men than among natal males (strength of recommendation: B, based on breast reduction studies in non-transgendered women).
- Risk is affected by age at chest surgery and the amount of breast tissue removed (strength of recommendation: C).
- Pre–chest surgery mammography is not recommended unless the patient meets usual natal female recommendations (strength of recommendation: B).
- Yearly chest wall and axillary examinations are recommended, along with education regarding the small but possible risk of breast cancer (strength of recommendation: C).

Transgendered male patients who undergo breast reduction or partial mastectomy (i.e., male chest reconstruction) must retain some degree of underlying breast tissue for good cosmetic results. Multiple studies of non-transgendered women after breast reduction surgery show reduced risk of breast cancer directly related to the amount of tissue removed.[28–30] However, the risk remains higher than in non-transgendered men (level 2). The greatest reduction in risk was seen when patients had the procedure after the age of 40 years. Presurgical mammography does not appear to significantly improve the detection of occult cancers in these patients.[31]

Currently, there are no long-term, prospective studies on the risk of breast cancer among FTM patients. The retrospective study by Van Kesteren and colleagues[22] revealed no breast cancer cases (level 2), but this population may not have been old enough or followed up for long enough to detect any difference. However, the literature contains case series (level 3) of breast cancer among transgendered males who are post–chest surgery and taking testosterone.[32,33]

The incidence of breast cancer among natal males is 1/100th that of natal females. However, the breast cancer risk among men with Klinefelter syndrome is 50 times higher than among non-Klinefelter men.[34] Persons with Klinefelter syndrome have an XXY genotype and have lower testosterone levels, higher estrogen levels, higher gonadotropin levels, and increased gynecomastia relative to XY males. In this regard, transsexual men share some common features with Klinefelter men. This again suggests the possibility of increased risk of breast cancer for FTM persons compared with natal males. A yearly examination for chest masses and axillary adenopathy is a low-cost, low-risk intervention that provides an opportunity for education regarding breast cancer risks.

Cervical Cancer Screening for Transsexual Men

Patients With an Intact Cervix (No Hysterectomy or Subtotal Hysterectomy), With or Without History of Testosterone Use

- Papanicolaou (Pap) smears or other cervical cytology sampling should follow the recommended guidelines for natal females (strength of recommendation: A, based on multiple level 1 studies in non-transgendered women).
- There is no evidence that testosterone increases or reduces the risk of cervical cancer (strength of recommendation: B).
- As testosterone supplementation can result in atrophic changes to the cervical epithelium, mimicking dysplasia, the pathologist should be informed of the patient's hormonal status, that is, that "she" is taking therapeutic testosterone (strength of recommendation: B).
- Total hysterectomy should be considered in the presence of high-grade dysplasia or if the patient is unable to tolerate Pap smears and is at risk for cervical cancer (strength of recommendation: C).

The USPSTF recommends cervical cytology sampling at least every 3 years, until the age of 65 years, for all persons with an intact cervix, and who are at low risk of cervical dysplasia[20] (level 1) with more intensive screening for those at higher risk. Androgen therapy causes significant atrophy in the cervical epithelium, mimicking dysplasia on the Pap smear.[35] However, these changes are not well characterized in the literature, and colposcopy may be indicated for patients at increased cancer risk. For patients otherwise at low risk of cervical cancer, atypical squamous cells of unspecified significance (ASCUS) and low-grade squamous intraepithelial lesion (LSIL). Pap smears are unlikely to represent precancerous lesions, especially in the absence of high-risk strains of human papilloma virus (HPV).[36,37] If the patient has had little sexual activity involving vaginal penetration, speculum examination can be painful or emotionally difficult, and it should be kept to a minimum. As gynecologic examinations may be distressing for transsexual men, hysterectomy should be considered if patients cannot tolerate pelvic examination at reasonable intervals for cancer prevention, particularly if this is desired as part of the transition process.

Patients in need of medical procedures that emphasize conflict between biology and internal self-perception usually benefit from a relaxed, supportive, and neutral approach on the part of their physicians. Helpful messages include the concept that body organs may have little to do with gender identity. Transsexual patients can be reminded that it is important to take care of the body at all stages of the transition process. Some transgender medical practices employ mottos such as "Love your body while you change it," and "Real men get Pap tests.[38] Patients with high levels of discomfort should be scheduled for longer-than-usual appointments to ensure that the visit can proceed in a calm, supportive, and unhurried manner. They can be offered adaptive measures, such as headphones for listening to music during a cervical examination or mild sedation (e.g., 1–2 mg of oral lorazepam) before an endometrial sampling.

Patients Who Have Had Total Hysterectomy (Cervix Completely Removed)

- If there is no prior history of high-grade cervical dysplasia or cervical cancer, no future Pap smears or other cytologic examinations are needed (strength of recommendation: A).
- If there is prior history of high-grade cervical dysplasia or cervical cancer, patients should have periodic Pap smears of the vagina every

1–5 years, as recommended for natal females (strength of recommendation: B).

As noted previously, the USPSTF recommends against screening non-transgendered women after hysterectomy for benign disease[20] (level 1), and the risk of cervical cancer among transgendered male patients after hysterectomy is thus similarly low, even with testosterone therapy. There are no level 1 studies involving FTM patients after hysterectomy with a past history of cervical dysplasia. Level 1 and 2 studies of natal women suggest that patients should continue to undergo periodic screening after hysterectomy[39,40]; however, the optimal frequency of screening has not been determined.

Ovarian and Uterine Cancer Screening for Transsexual Men

Transsexual Men With Intact Ovaries and Uterus (No Hysterectomy), With or Without a History of Testosterone Use

- Screening patients for symptoms and signs of polycystic ovarian syndrome (PCOS) is recommended (strength of recommendation: C).
- Pelvic examinations every 1–3 years are recommended for patients older than 40 years of age or with a family history of ovarian cancer; increase to every year if PCOS is present (strength of recommendation: C).
- Total hysterectomy should be considered if maintenance of fertility is not desired, if the patient is older than 40 years of age, if the patient's health will not be adversely affected by surgery, if the patient is unable to tolerate pelvic examinations (strength of recommendation: C), or if the surgery is desired as part of the transition process.

No recommended screening tests for ovarian cancer exist for any population. Some studies suggest an increased risk of ovarian cancer among FTM patients using testosterone therapy[41,42] and non-transgendered women with PCOS.[43] Several small studies suggest that there may be an increased incidence of PCOS among transsexual men.[23,44,45] PCOS is a hormonal syndrome complex characterized by some or all of the following: infrequent ovulation, absent or infrequent menstrual cycles, multiple cysts on the ovaries (thus the name), hyperandrogenism, hirsutism, acne, hidradenitis suppurativa, acanthosis nigricans, obesity, glucose intolerance, or diabetes. PCOS is associated with infertility as well as with a statistically increased risk of cardiac disease, high blood pressure, and endometrial cancer. The risk of

ovarian cancer increases with age, and pelvic examinations are currently the only screening modality used in any patient population. Because pelvic examinations may be distressing for transsexual men, hysterectomy should be considered if patients wish to stop having them and reduce cancer risk.

As noted above, persons with PCOS have an increased risk of endometrial cancer. The risk of endometrial cancer also increases after the age of 40 years. Although there does not appear to be an increased risk of endometrial carcinoma among patients using masculinizing hormone therapy, dysfunctional uterine bleeding can occur. The endometrium should be evaluated with pelvic ultrasound or endometrial biopsy for unexplained or prolonged vaginal bleeding, especially among patients older than 35 years of age.

Other Cancers

Currently, there is no evidence that transgendered men are at either increased or decreased risk of other cancers, relative to non-transgendered men, independent of other known risk factors. Screening recommendations for other cancers (including colon cancer, lung cancer, and anal cancer) are the same as for non-transgendered male and female patients.

Cardiovascular Disease

All Patients

- Screening for and treatment of modifiable cardiovascular risk is recommended for all transgendered patients, regardless of hormonal status (strength of recommendation: A, based on multiple level 1 studies in numerous non-transgendered populations).
- It is recommend that modifiable cardiovascular risk factors be reasonably controlled before masculinizing endocrine therapy is initiated (strength of recommendation: B).
- Noninvasive cardiac testing (e.g., stress testing) among patients at very high risk for cardiac disease or with any cardiovascular symptoms should be considered before endocrine therapy is initiated (strength of recommendation: C)
- Daily aspirin therapy is recommended for patients at high risk for coronary artery disease (CAD) (strength of recommendation: A, based on multiple level 1 studies in numerous non-transgendered populations).

Assessing and treating cardiovascular risk factors is an essential primary medical care intervention for all patients. There appears to be a high prevalence of cardiovascular risk factors, particularly smoking (see below), among both transsexual men and transsexual women—regardless of hormone status. In the United States, MTF patients tend to present for transgender care at older ages (e.g., early 40s[18]) and with hypertension, diabetes, hyperlipidemia, or other conditions common in middle-aged natal male bodies. FTM patients often present in their teens and 20s—usually before the onset of cardiovascular disease, but they may be at increased risk for hypertension, insulin resistance, and hyperlipidemia due to PCOS, and they will be using masculinizing hormonal treatments for many years. Finally, cardiovascular risk factors are often undiagnosed or undertreated among transgendered patients who do not receive regular medical care. Both masculinizing and feminizing hormonal therapies may further increase cardiovascular risks. Early diagnosis and treatment of cardiovascular risk factors, ideally before the onset of cardiovascular disease, may decrease risks associated with endocrine therapy for these patients.

Coronary Artery Disease, Cerebrovascular Disease, and Masculinizing Therapies

Transsexual Men, Using Testosterone

- Clinical monitoring for cardiac events and symptoms in patients at moderate to high risk for CAD is recommended (strength of recommendation: C).
- Use of testosterone by patients with preexisting CAD may increase the risk of future cardiovascular events (strength of recommendation: C).

The effect of testosterone on cardiovascular events among transgendered male patients is unclear. The retrospective Van Kesteren study from 1997[22] (level 2) found no increase compared with rates in the general population, but the population may not have been old enough or followed long enough to detect any differences. Although hyperandrogen states among non-transgendered women (e.g., PCOS) increase cardiac risk factors such as hyperlipidemia, current evidence of any increase in cardiac morbidity or mortality with PCOS is limited.[46–49] Level 2 studies of testosterone replacement among older hypogonadal men show similar results.[50,51] However, the serum testosterone levels achieved in masculinizing therapy usually exceed those occurring with PCOS and may exceed those achieved in testosterone replacement. Other studies among non-transgendered

men and women (level 3) indicate that low endogenous androgens appear to increase the risk for men, whereas higher endogenous androgens increase the risk for women.[52] However, supraphysiologic levels, including those sometimes achieved by male athletes using androgen supplementation, also increase cardiac risk and sometimes result in premature death.[53] Transsexual men with preexisting CAD who are using testosterone may be at increased risk of future cardiac events. The extent of risk, and of resulting morbidity and mortality, is unclear.

Hypertension

Transsexual Men, Not Currently Using Testosterone

- Screening for and treatment of hypertension should be undertaken as recommended in guidelines for non-transgendered patients (strength of recommendation: A, based on multiple level 1 studies in non-transgendered populations).
- A systolic blood pressure goal of less than 130 mm Hg and a diastolic goal of less than 90 mm Hg should be considered if the patient plans to begin masculinizing endocrine therapy within 1–3 years (strength of recommendation: B).

Transsexual Men, Currently Using Testosterone

- Blood pressure should be monitored at every visit (strength of recommendation: A, based on multiple level 1 non-transgender studies).
- A systolic blood pressure goal of less than 130 mm Hg and a diastolic goal of less than 90 mm Hg should be considered, especially in patients with PCOS (strength of recommendation: B).

The risk of hypertension among transsexual men using testosterone is unclear. The Van Kesteren study from 1997[22] (level 2) reported hypertension in 4.1% of FTM participants, slightly below norms for natal females and well below norms for natal males. However, as noted earlier, this study defined hypertension as being greater than 160/95 mm Hg, which is considerably higher than current North American guidelines.[54] Exogenous testosterone can increase blood pressure,[55,56] and non-transsexual women with PCOS are at increased risk of hypertension.[46] However, a prospective study of healthy FTM participants (n = 28) found no significant change in blood pressure after an average of 18 months of testosterone administration—even among subjects taking twice the usual dose of testosterone.[57] The effect of exogenous testosterone use among patients with known hypertension is not well addressed in the literature. Because hypertension increases the risk of cardiovascular events and strokes, the above recommendations are similar to those from the Joint National Commission for patients with compelling indications for blood pressure control, such as diabetes.[58]

Lipids

Transsexual Men, Not Using Testosterone

- Screening for and treatment of hyperlipidemia according to guidelines for non-transgendered patients is recommended (strength of recommendation: A based on multiple level 1 studies among non-transgendered populations).
- A low-density lipoprotein cholesterol (LDL-C) goal of less than 130 mg/dL should be considered if the patient plans to start masculinizing endocrine therapy within 1–3 years (strength of recommendation: B).

Transsexual Men, Currently Using Testosterone

- A yearly fasting lipid profile is recommended (strength of recommendation: B).
- Supraphysiologic testosterone levels should be avoided, particularly for patients with hyperlipidemia. Daily topical (gel or patch) or weekly intramuscular testosterone regimens are preferable to biweekly or less frequent intramuscular injection programs (strength of recommendation: C).
- Hyperlipidemia should be treated with an LDL-C goal of less than 130 mg/dL for patients at low to moderate risk for CAD and less than 100 mg/dL for high-risk patients (strength of recommendation: B).

Patients receiving masculinizing hormonal regimens experience increases in LDL-C and decreases in high-density lipoprotein cholesterol (HDL-C), putting them at an increased risk of atherosclerotic disease.[59–61] However, no excess cardiovascular morbidity was found in the retrospective Dutch study.[22] Both transsexual men and non-transsexual natal women with PCOS are at increased risk of dyslipidemia, although the effect on the risk of cardiac events is undetermined.[46–49] A meta-analysis concluded that the effects of testosterone enanthate on total, HDL, and LDL cholesterol were small but significant.[62] Also, a 20-week study of supraphysiologic testosterone supplementation in healthy, young, non-transgendered men found no adverse effects on

insulin sensitivity, plasma lipids, or C-reactive protein, except at the highest dose, which produced mean serum testosterone levels of 2370 ng/dL.[63]

To incorporate the effects of masculinizing hormonal therapy into existing evidence-based guidelines, it has been included as an additional cardiac risk factor. Thus, the recommendations above are consistent with the USPSTF guidelines[20] for screening adults older than 20 years with risk factors for CAD. (The USPSTF screening interval is not specified.) Similarly, the recommended goals for the treatment of lipid disorders are consistent with the National Cholesterol Education Program Adult Treatment Panel III (2001) guidelines.[64]

Smoking

- Screening, by history, of all transsexual male patients for past and present tobacco use is recommended (strength of recommendation: A).
- It is recommended to include smoking cessation as part of comprehensive transgender medical care, particularly in association with endocrine therapy (strength of recommendation: C).

Little is known about smoking prevalence or cessation patterns in the transgendered population. Thirty-seven percent of transgendered patients presenting to a Minnesota clinic for hormone therapy were current smokers, compared with 20% for the Minnesota population overall.[65] Many transgendered persons experience multiple commonly identified risk factors for smoking including poverty, stressful living and work environments, and societal marginalization.[66–68]

The risks associated with smoking that are most pertinent to the medical care of transgendered persons include an increased risk of venous thromboembolic events with estrogen therapy, possible increased risk of cardiovascular disease with both feminizing and masculinizing endocrine therapy (especially in persons older than 50 years), and delayed healing after surgery. Smoking also increases the risk of polycythemia with testosterone use, as is discussed below.

Smoking cessation interventions can be effective, particularly if they are incorporated into a comprehensive transgender healthcare program. This approach involves consistent smoking-cessation messages from all members of the clinical staff, frequent supportive follow-up of cessation efforts, and direct communication of the limitations and risks that smoking imposes on hormone therapy.[65] A Minnesota study suggests that initiation of hormone therapy (if desired), combined with a physician-assisted cessation plan, may improve the likelihood of quitting.[65]

Diabetes Mellitus

Transsexual Men, With or Without Testosterone Use

- Screening for and treatment of diabetes mellitus, as for the non-transgendered population, is recommended (strength of recommendation: A).
- Diabetes screening is indicated if PCOS is present (strength of recommendation: B).

As noted above, there is limited evidence of a higher incidence of PCOS, which carries an increased risk of glucose intolerance, among FTM persons. There is no current evidence of an altered risk of type 2 diabetes among transgendered men who are taking testosterone. Testosterone increases visceral fat among FTM patients,[69] and older non-transgendered women with high testosterone levels are at increased risk of developing type 2 diabetes as well.[70] Further research is needed to clarify how these findings affect the risk of diabetes among transsexual men.

Osteoporosis

Transsexual Men, Not Using Testosterone, Without Surgery

- Screening and treatment for osteoporosis, as for natal females, is recommended (strength of recommendation: A).

Transsexual Men, Past or Present Testosterone Use, Without Surgery

- Evidence is mixed with regard to the impact of testosterone on bone density before oophorectomy (strength of recommendation: C).
- Bone density screening should be considered for FTM patients older than 60 years of age with additional risk factors for osteoporosis and who have been taking testosterone therapy for more than 5 years, *or* who had been treated with Depo-Provera (medroxyprogesterone acetate) for more than 5 years (strength of recommendation: C).
- Supplemental calcium (1200 mg daily) and vitamin D (600 units daily) should be considered to maintain bone density (strength of recommendation: C).

Transsexual Men With Current or Previous Testosterone Use, and Post-oophorectomy or Total Hysterectomy

- There is an increased risk of bone density loss after oophorectomy, particularly if testosterone supplementation is reduced or discontinued (strength of recommendation: C).
- Lifelong testosterone therapy is recommended to reduce the risk of bone density loss, if no significant contraindications are present (strength of recommendation: B).
- If there are significant contradictions to testosterone therapy, bisphosphonate therapy (35–70 mg alendronate or 35 mg risedronate weekly, or equivalent) is recommended for osteoporosis prevention (strength of recommendation: B).
- Bone density screening is recommended for persons older than 65 years who are receiving adequate maintenance testosterone supplementation (strength of recommendation: C).
- Bone density screening is recommended at ages 50–60 years for FTM patients with additional risk factors for osteoporosis who have been receiving testosterone therapy for more than 5 years or who have not been continuously receiving adequate maintenance doses of testosterone therapy (strength of recommendation: C).
- Supplemental calcium (1200 mg daily) and vitamin D (600 units daily) is recommended to maintain bone density (strength of recommendation: B).

The USPSTF[20] recommends bone density screening for all women older than 65 years of age, and beginning at the age of 60 years for those women with additional risk factors. The effect of cross-gender hormone treatments on bone density is controversial. Transsexual male patients begin with an average of 10–12% less bone density than natal males, before any hormonal or surgical intervention.[71] Although studies have found that exogenous testosterone use maintains bone density to some degree among FTM patients,[72-76] it may not be sufficient, especially after oophorectomy.[75,77] It is encouraging that one study with longer follow-up (mean, 12.5 years for 24 MTF participants and 7.6 years for 15 FTM participants) found bone densities at or above expected norms, except for five cases of osteoporosis among MTF patients who did not comply with recommended hormonal treatment.[78]

As is the case among non-transsexual middle-aged and elderly persons, hormone deprivation appears to be a primary risk factor for the development of osteoporosis among both FTM and MTF transsexual patients. There is some evidence that luteinizing hormone (LH) suppression may be the best indicator of adequate androgen replacement among FTM men,[73,78] as is the case among natal males receiving treatment for hypergonadotropic hypogonadism.[125]

It is unclear how much testosterone is required to protect against bone loss after gonadal removal. Of note, declining estradiol levels among natal males are more strongly correlated with decreasing bone density than declining testosterone levels.[79–81] Loss of bone density is most likely to occur in patients with other risk factors (e.g., European or Asian ancestry, smoking, family history, high alcohol use, hyperparathyroidism, hyperthyroidism) and those who are not fully adherent to hormone therapy. Of note, some transgendered male patients who are early in the physical process of gender transition use Depo-Provera to produce amenorrhea before hysterectomy. This medication may result in bone density loss with long-term use among non-transgendered women.[82] There are currently no long-term studies examining the degree to which loss of bone density correlates to the risk of clinical fractures among transgendered patients; however, data regarding non-transgendered men and women strongly support this conclusion.[83]

Calcium and vitamin D supplementation and weight-bearing exercise are indicated for all transgendered patients using hormonal therapies who are at risk for osteoporosis. Bone densitometry screening may be indicated for patients at increased risk of osteoporosis, although normative data for transgendered men have not been established. Regardless of hormonal or surgical status, if a transgendered person shows significant bone loss compared with natal sex norms, further intervention is warranted. Bisphosphonates have been demonstrated to increase bone density and decrease fracture risk in non-transgendered men and women[84] and represent a gender-neutral treatment option for transsexual men, who may find the concept of using selective estrogen receptor modulators (SERMs) psychologically unacceptable.

Sexual Health

HIV, Hepatitis B, and Hepatitis C

Because HIV, hepatitis B, and hepatitis C are transmitted by blood exposure as well as through sexual contact (there is limited evidence to support sexual transmission of hepatitis C), HIV and hepatitis prevention and screening are presented separately from STIs, which are discussed below.[85] Transgendered men can be at risk for blood-borne diseases as a result of sharing needles for injection of androgens or illicit drugs.

- Routine screening is recommended, regardless of individual risk, in settings where HIV seroprevalence is at least 1% (strength of recommendation: A, based on evidence-based guidelines for all populations).
- Routine HIV screening is recommended, regardless of individual risk, among populations of FTM men having sex with natal men (strength of recommendation: B).
- Screening is recommended for all patients with current diagnosis of any STI, hepatitis B, or C; past diagnosis of any STI, hepatitis, or tuberculosis; use of shared injection equipment for androgens or illicit drugs; unprotected sex with partner who may be at risk; or unprotected anal or vaginal intercourse with more than one partner (strength of recommendation: A).
- HIV testing should be considered for patients with psychosocial factors that are associated with unsafe sexual practices (e.g., poor self-esteem, lack of safety in a romantic or partnered relationship, substance use, compulsive sex to affirm masculine identity) (strength of recommendation: C).
- HIV testing should be considered for patients with other risks for blood-borne transmission, such as non-professionally performed piercings, tattoos, or other body-modifying procedures (strength of recommendation: C).
- Hepatitis B testing is recommended for all patients who are offered HIV testing and who are not known to be immune (strength of recommendation: A).
- Hepatitis C testing should be considered for all patients who are offered HIV testing, particularly if they are at risk of blood-borne transmission (strength of recommendation: C).
- HIV, hepatitis B, and hepatitis C screening every 6–12 months are recommended to patients with ongoing risk behaviors (strength of recommendation: B). In all other patients, this screening at least once during the lifetime should be considered (strength of recommendation: B).
- All patients with STIs and their partners should be treated according to recommended guidelines for non-transgendered patients to reduce the risk of HIV and

hepatitis B transmission (strength of recommendation: A, based on Centers for Disease Control and Prevention [CDC] guidelines).

- Hepatitis A and B vaccination should be offered to all sexually active patients who are not already immune (strength of recommendation: B).

Evidence-based recommendations from the CDC and USPSTF suggest HIV testing strategies based on prevalence in the clinic setting (e.g., higher in a clinic specializing in STI treatment than in a general medical office) or among the population served (e.g., increased among men who have sex with men).[20] As a whole, the transgendered population appears to have a disproportionately high rate of HIV/AIDS relative to the general population,[86-88] although prevalence varies geographically and by gender identity.

Reported HIV rates from seroprevalence studies in the United States range from 20–35% among MTF transsexual and transgendered women to a 2–3% incidence among FTM men.[89-95] However, a recent study comparing HIV risk behaviors found that FTM persons were less likely than their MTF peers to have used risk-reduction practices with the most recent sexual contact and were also significantly more likely to have engaged in recent high-risk sexual activity.[96] Other studies also have found high levels of sexual risk behavior among transgendered men, and often poor knowledge regarding HIV transmission and its prevention.[97,98] Overall, risks associated with HIV infection (e.g., unprotected sexual activity, multiple sexual partners, sex work, substance use, sexual violence) are more common in transgendered populations.[88,96,99–101] Some transgendered men are also at risk due to sharing injection equipment for androgen use.[102]

Natal males who have sex with men (MSM) are considered a special population in the CDC STI guidelines, which also address HIV testing. As transgendered persons who have sex with men (TSM) shared many of the risk factors for HIV and other STIs with MSM, an argument can be made for extending population health campaigns focused on natal MSM to FTM men who have sex with men and to all transgendered persons of any gender identity who have sex with men (i.e., TSM). This would include CDC recommendations for annual screening for HIV and STIs among sexually active persons and vaccination against hepatitis A and B.

The prevention of HIV involves transgender-specific education and behavioral change.[103–105] HIV testing has been shown to be an effective element in reducing transmission and gaining access to life-extending treatment in all populations. Recent analysis suggests that at least one-time HIV screening for all people, regardless of risk, is a cost-effective public health strategy.[106] A comprehensive discussion of HIV risk and prevention in transgender communities can be found in *Transgender and HIV: Risks, Prevention and Care*.[85,107]

Sexually Transmitted Infections

- Assessment and screening (e.g., gonorrhea, chlamydia, syphilis) is recommended for all transgendered male patients at risk for STIs. These include persons with a current diagnosis of HIV, hepatitis B or C; those with a past diagnosis of STI; persons having unprotected sex with a partner who may be at risk; and persons having unprotected anal or vaginal intercourse with more than one partner (strength of recommendation: A).
- Assessment and screening is recommended for persons with psychosocial factors associated with unsafe sexual practices (e.g., poor self-esteem, lack of safety in a romantic or partnered relationship, substance use, compulsive sexual behavior to affirm masculine identity) (strength of recommendation: B).
- Screening for genital gonorrhea, genital chlamydia, and syphilis every 6–12 months are recommended for all TSMs and other transgendered patients at ongoing risk (strength of recommendation: B). (Because TSM share many of the STI risk factors with MSM, the same screening guidelines are recommended, albeit at a lower grade.)
- All transgendered male patients with STIs and their partners should be treated according to recommended guidelines for non-transgendered patients (strength of recommendation: A).
- It is recommended that transsexual men younger than 25 years of age who have not had genital surgery and are vaginally or anally sexually active, regardless of risk assessment, be screened yearly for gonorrhea and chlamydia to reduce risk of pelvic inflammatory disease (as an extension of recommended guidelines for natal females) (strength of recommendation: A).

The application of evidence-based guidelines for STI screening[20,105] to the transgendered population is somewhat problematic. Sexual orientation and sexual practices among transgendered people show significant variation.[109–112]

Assumptions about sexual activities should be avoided because these can vary depending on the patient's genital anatomy and preferences, as well as that of their partner(s). Although some transgendered men who have not had sex reassignment surgery are genitally decathected, others enjoy genital sexual activity. Transgendered male patients may have participated in receptive (engulfing) or inserting oral, vaginal, or anal intercourse, if the life experience both before and after genital surgery is considered. Some transgendered men form partnerships with gay (natal) males, which may include penovaginal intercourse before FTM sex reassignment surgery. Coleman and colleagues[109] note that this observation "invites us to rethink the genital criterion in the assessment of sexual orientation." Some transgendered men also use silicone sexual aids for vaginal or anal penetration of their partner(s). Although the use of sex toys or hands is considered low risk for HIV transmission, other STIs can be transmitted by unprotected genital touching or the sharing of silicone or other sexual equipment, especially if body fluids are present.

Data regarding the rates of STIs (other than HIV) among transgendered populations are limited. In a 1999 San Francisco study, 31% of FTM participants and 53% of MTF participants reported a prior STI,[113] with 36% reported for both groups in a New York survey.[93] As discussed in the section on HIV, high-risk sexual behaviors reported by transgendered research participants include unprotected sexual activity, sexual participation while intoxicated, and sex with multiple partners or with a single high-risk partner. Cofactors related to unsafe sex, such as depression, suicidal ideation, and physical or sexual abuse, are often also increased among the transgendered population and must be addressed in prevention efforts.* Studies indicate that the need to affirm one's gender identity can lead to participation in high-risk sexual behaviors.[101,103,113] Although the transgendered population as a whole is at increased risk of STIs, individual risks vary greatly. STI screening should be individualized to the patient's anatomy, risk behaviors, and underlying prevalence in the community, if this is known.

The current anatomy of transsexual men affects how screening or diagnostic tests for gonorrhea and chlamydia are performed. A urine-based test of the first 25 mL of non–clean catch urine (e.g., Gen-Probe) can be used regardless of anatomy, making this the ideal testing method for most patients. Alternately, culture can be obtained from the specific site of symptoms or suspected exposure (e.g., pharynx, urethra, cervix, vagina, penis, anus) regardless of the gender identity of the patient, including from the penis of a transsexual man who has had genital surgery or the cervix of a transsexual man who has not.

Prevention education should be focused on the concerns of transgendered persons (e.g., disclosure and discussion with potential partners) and individualized to the patient's anatomic and psychosocial needs. For example, FTM persons who have not had genital surgery and MTF persons who cannot sustain an erection sufficient for intercourse may benefit from discussion of non-penetrative sexual activities and sexual equipment and toys.

Transgender Hormonal Care

Family physicians, general practitioners, and internists often begin transgender medical care by referring their patients to an endocrinologist for hormonal treatment while continuing to provide more routine services. Others prefer to prescribe the hormonal medications themselves, reserving endocrinologic consultation for the more complicated cases. This section offers some basic guidelines for the practice of transgender hormonal treatment in primary care practice.

Initial Consultation

Assessing Initial Expectations and Goals

Personal goals with regard to gender presentation may change with time, particularly with regard to whether FTM surgical sex reassignment is desired. An early, open discussion regarding treatment expectations can foster a more complete understanding of the patient's personal identity and life experience and help to avoid miscommunication or ultimate dissatisfaction with care.

Questions to consider include the following:
- Is the patient seeking full transition, including sex reassignment surgery, or hormone supplementation to facilitate a transgendered presentation on a full- or part-time basis?
- If the goal is to transition, has the patient formed a mental "timeline," and is it realistic?
- Has he discussed the decision to begin hormone treatment with the significant others in his life, or more broadly?

---

*References 88, 91, 101, 114, 115.

- Is the patient aware that hormonal transition may sometimes be initiated before full disclosure (i.e., "coming out"), but that progress will then be limited by the need to conceal the physical changes from public notice, such as in the work environment?

Defining Realistic Expectations of Hormone Use at the Beginning of the Treatment Process

Androgen supplementation fosters the development of the male secondary sexual characteristics, but does not "undo" the female sexual development that has already taken place. Androgen use will cause male pattern hair growth (and sometimes male pattern baldness) and deepening of the voice, but breast atrophy will be minimal. Both androgens and estrogens will cause some degree of body habitus change, but individual results vary greatly, and basic skeletal structure will not be affected more than slightly. (Some transgendered men experience growth in the hands and feet with testosterone use.) Common effects of treatment with androgens, after natural female puberty, are summarized in Table 30-1.

Sexual changes may or may not occur, as the response to hormonal therapy is quite individual in this regard. Most transgendered men taking testosterone experience increased libido and a shift to more "genitally focused" and less "total body" orgasms, consistent with usual beliefs about male sexual release.[116] These changes are likely both physiologic and social in etiology. (Interestingly, some transgendered women also experience an increase in libido, despite nearly complete suppression of testosterone production, due to the erotically powerful psychological experience of [at last!] finding the physical body coming into harmony with the internal gender self-perception.)

Similarly, emotional changes demonstrate significant individual variation. Emotional experience is generally a result of a mix of factors, including personality structure; previous life experience; medical health and illness, including hormonal status; environmental cues and prompts, such as the personal enjoyment that can accompany taking on the appearance of the preferred gender; and the response of other persons to self-presentation. Patients beginning treatment with hormones should be informed that, although their basic personality and personhood will not change, the combination of the new social presentation and hormone use can facilitate some shifting of emotional experience.

Table 30-1. Common Effects of Androgen Supplementation After Cessation of Natural Puberty

Usual Effects
Masculinization of body habitus
Increase in upper body strength, mass
Male pattern body hair growth (and sometimes male pattern baldness)
Beard growth
Deepening of vocal pitch (though the larynx will not enlarge)
Clitoral enlargement
Subjective well-being and increased libido
Increased erythrocytosis
Acne
Weight gain
Conditions Requiring Clinical Caution
Cardiac, vascular, or renal disease, or hypertension, due to the retention of sodium and fluids
Breast cancer
Hyperlipidemias
Polycythemia
Sleep apnea
Migraine
Androgen sensitive epilepsy
Hepatic impairment
Bleeding disorders (use gel or transdermal patch formulations, not injections)
Smoking

Note: Testosterone undergoes some peripheral conversion to estradiol, so bioavailable estrogen may increase with androgen supplementation.
Adapted from: Conway AJ, Handelsman DJ, Lording DW, et al: Use, misuse and abuse of androgens: the Endocrine Society of Australia consensus guidelines for androgen prescribing, *Med J Aust* 172:220–224, 2000.

Some persons experience a broadening of emotional range even before the initiation of treatment with hormones, or very early in the treatment process. For example, some transsexual men who have newly begun treatment with testosterone feel free to act out sexually or aggressively, even before androgen levels have exceeded female norms. Similarly, some natal males who are not seeking full transition feel more free to laugh, cry, and express affection in feminine ways when dressed *en femme*, even before beginning estrogen supplementation. Patients should be cautioned that androgen use (like estrogen use) is never an excuse for socially inappropriate behavior.

A frank discussion regarding shared goals and medical concerns should be undertaken before treatment with hormones is begun. The message is one of strong support for the patient's personal identity and the process of transition, *and* a commitment to safe and effective medical treatment. Attempting to hasten the transition process by using very high doses of hormone preparations will not improve the end result but will increase the risk of medical complications, which can interfere with the individual's ultimate physical goals. For example, a transgendered man who develops polycythemia while using a very high testosterone dose may be unable to continue hormonal treatment until this condition has been evaluated and resolved.

Hormonal medications are readily available without prescription in many countries and can be obtained via the Internet and other means. Caring for patients without full knowledge of the prescription and nonprescription medications they are using can be both challenging and dangerous. A reasonable condition for treatment is the commitment to taking only prescribed medications and taking them as directed. This should be discussed openly at the first medical visit, before hormone prescription. Evidence that the patient has not openly disclosed the use of hormones received through alternate sources should be confronted in the same manner as would a breach of the clinical relationship in the treatment of any other medical condition, such as chronic pain.

Baseline Endocrine Laboratory Evaluation

It is useful to know the baseline hormonal status of the patient before treatment with supplemental hormones is initiated. If serum testosterone and estradiol levels differ significantly from expected norms, based on natal sex and age, additional investigation is usually indicated to determine whether an endocrinopathy is present or whether the patient has already been using hormones obtained informally or through other medical sources. Other age-appropriate laboratory evaluations, such as screening for hyperlipidemia and glucose intolerance, can be performed concurrently if these have not already been obtained.

Smoking Cessation Counseling Before the Initiation of Androgen Supplementation

The medical risks associated with androgen use are significantly increased by smoking, particularly the risks of polycythemia and polycythemic

stroke.[117] A candid discussion regarding the risks of smoking should take place before the first testosterone prescription.

The time between the initial presentation for gender transition medical services and the first prescription of androgens can be a particularly auspicious opportunity for smoking cessation. The patient is likely to be more involved in the healthcare process (engaging in medical and mental health evaluations and establishing treatment plans) than he has been previously and is often feeling more optimistic about the future than has been the case in the past. The combination of a strengthened sense of self-efficacy (demonstrated by making the decision to physically confirm his authentic psychological gender) and new, *personalized* information about the risks of smoking can provide fertile ground for motivational assessment and behavior change.[118,119]

Patients who stop smoking should be given full support in accordance with current practice, such as brief cognitive-behaviorally based education and pharmacotherapy with nicotine replacement, bupropion, or other agents.[20] Counseling is aimed at identifying cues to smoking, breaking the link between triggers and smoking behavior, and management of cravings. A brief, evidence-based guideline for smoking cessation has been produced by the US Public Health Service.[120] This can be easily adapted to the situation of the transitioning person and used by family physicians and nurses in the course of routine clinical care.

Androgen Supplementation

Simple, "Steady-State" Testosterone Supplementation Programs Are Preferred

Androgen supplementation has traditionally been administered by injection of testosterone cypionate or testosterone enanthate every 1–3 weeks. These treatment programs produce an initial peak in serum testosterone, sometimes at a supraphysiologic level, followed by a gradual diminution over the time preceding the next injection. This pattern is quite different than the usual minor diurnal variations experienced by natal males. Many physicians are now prescribing testosterone patches or gel for their transgendered male patients. These preparations provide less variability in serum testosterone levels, and the patches somewhat mimic the usual diurnal variation of natal males.[121] Testosterone 1% gel is easy to use, aesthetic, and generally well accepted by transgendered male patients,[122] although some develop skin irritation. In addition, patches and gel can be administered by the patient without the need for training in injection technique.

Serum Hormone Levels Should Guide Hormone Dosage

Great individual variation exists in pharmacokinetic processing of hormonal medications.[123] Two persons of the same age and natal sex can require substantially different doses of the same estrogen or androgen preparation to achieve the same serum level. It is important to measure serum testosterone levels periodically to guard against under- or overdosing. Patient symptom report is not sufficient as a sole criterion to guide dosage adjustment. However, a report of new adverse symptoms, whether physical (e.g., headaches) or emotional (e.g., emotional lability, aggressive irritability) should prompt a reassessment of serum testosterone level.

Gender Transition Health Care, Including Hormonal Supplementation, Should Be Reassessed Across the Life Span

During the gender-transition process, the focus of the patient and his helping professionals often narrows to the immediate medical and social exigencies of the transition itself. (Is adequate physical transition being safely achieved? Is it time to inform the patient's employer of the change in identity, and is the patient emotionally prepared to do this?) However, once body modification has been accomplished, the focus of both medical care and social development must shift to a more long-term perspective.

Patients should be advised early in treatment that health maintenance is a lifelong process. Transsexual men have the same need for preventive care as their non-transsexual peers. In addition, decisions regarding use of hormones will need to be periodically revisited during mid life and older age. Testosterone production declines by approximately 50% between the ages of 30 and 80 years among natal males,[124] and the appropriateness of routine androgen supplementation for older men is currently a matter of debate.[117,124] Gradually reducing testosterone dosage as the transsexual man ages has intuitive appeal, but evidence regarding best practices in this regard is currently lacking. Physicians and their transsexual male patients will need to reassess the practical aspects of hormonal care in the years ahead, as the current cohort of transsexual men ages and as better evidence-based practices are defined.

Care of Elderly Transgendered Male Patients

It is not currently possible to offer truly evidence-based guidelines for the care of elderly transgendered male patients because applicable data are so limited. Nonetheless, as the US and world geriatric populations continue to expand, it is worthwhile to consider the hormonal treatment of older transgendered men in light of available information, although recommendations will be largely extrapolated from the experience of non-transgendered older men *and* based on expert opinion rather than robust data.

Androgen supplementation among non-transsexual elderly men is currently controversial,[117,124] and data regarding testosterone use by elderly transsexual men are few. Testosterone production in natal males declines slowly from mid life through old age, eventually by nearly 50%. Average serum testosterone levels among 30-year-old men are approximately 600 ng/dL, or 20.8 nmol/liter; mean values for 80-year-old men are approximately 400 ng/dL, or 13.9 nmol/L. This "andropause" results in a decrease in muscle strength and mass, bone strength (though it is primarily the androgen-derived estrogen that maintains bone density), erythrocytosis, and subjective well-being. Frailty often increases over time.

Androgen replacement has been suggested as a means of maintaining vigor and robustness among elderly men. However, because of the associated risks, androgen supplementation is not recommended by most professional bodies, including the Institute of Medicine, for routine use. Supplemental testosterone is used primarily in deficiency states accompanied by clinical evidence of resultant problems,[125] particularly if the morning serum testosterone level falls below 300 ng/dL.[126] Some authors recommend 200 ng/dL as the value below which men should be considered hypogonadal, regardless of age and other factors.[127]

Estrogens also exert significant effects on male physiology, including maintenance of the bone mass.[128] In natal males, estrogens are derived from the conversion of endogenous testosterone, from supplemental androgens, from phytoestrogens, and from medications and substances with estrogenic effects.[128] The effects of oophorectomy and androgen supplementation on the physiology and health of elderly transsexual men are currently unknown.

Elderly transsexual men require ongoing testosterone supplementation, particularly if oophorectomy has been performed. At present, few data are available regarding optimal androgen dosing and monitoring in this population. Initiation of androgen use in the elder years, for the purpose of gender transition, is even less common than continuation of treatment begun earlier in the life course. Clinical considerations are therefore based on experience with testosterone use by non-transsexual men.

Risks Associated with Supplemental Testosterone Use

Research among non-transsexual men using supplemental testosterone has identified the following adverse effects and health risks: acne and oily skin; breast enlargement and tenderness, especially early in treatment; fluid retention and peripheral edema; sleep apnea; worsening of prostate disease (fortunately not a consideration for transsexual men); the development of polycythemia; and possibly negative effects on androgen-sensitive epilepsy and some conditions consistent with migraine headaches.[125–127]

Some authors consider a personal history of breast (or prostate) cancer to be an absolute contraindication to use of supplemental testosterone,[125] although clinicians often make this decision on a case-by-case basis. Relative contraindications include chronic obstructive pulmonary disease (particularly among patients who are overweight or who smoke tobacco[127]) and renal or cardiac conditions (e.g., congestive heart failure, uncontrolled hypertension) that may be worsened by temporary fluid expansion. The presence of sleep apnea, migraine, and epileptic syndromes should be taken into account in clinical decision making.[125]

Although cardiac effects, in the absence of significant existing disease, have generally been neutral overall,[129] the long-term impact of testosterone on cardiovascular disease remains unknown[127,130] and may be subtly different in natal males, natal females, and possibly FTM transsexual persons, as discussed earlier in this chapter. Testosterone increases thrombogenicity and platelet aggregation, although the American Association of Clinical Endocrinologists Hypogonadism Task Force[131] has noted that resultant clinical problems have not been observed among natal males receiving replacement doses of testosterone. Whether this is equally true among transgendered men is unknown.

Supratherapeutic androgen administration, such as is sometimes used by male bodybuilders, is associated with cardiac disease and other serious complications[54] and is thoroughly contraindicated for both transsexual men and natal males. An excellent discussion of the risks of supraphysiologic testosterone use is found in the recent *Sports Illustrated* series about illicit steroid use among major league baseball players.[132] Patients may find this more understandable and personally relevant than medical explanations offered during clinical care.

Polycythemia

Testosterone supplementation results in increased erythrocyte production in both natal females and natal males. Although this may provide therapeutic benefit to elderly persons experiencing decreased erythropoiesis, occasionally hemoglobin and hematocrit elevate to pathologic levels, particularly if the serum testosterone is above the usual male range. Arterial and venous thromboembolic events may ensue, particularly if other cardiac risk factors (especially smoking) are present.[133] Elderly patients are at higher risk due to the vascular changes that accompany the aging process. Wald and colleagues[127] note, "The main risk factor for polycythemia with testosterone administration appears to be age, and the incidence...was reported to be higher with intramuscular rather than transdermal preparations."

Older FTM patients should be advised about the possible consequences of polycythemia and should have hemoglobin and hematocrit levels monitored periodically. An annual evaluation may suffice when the testosterone dosage and hematocrit have stabilized over time; more frequent monitoring should be obtained earlier in the treatment process. The American Society of Andrology recommends physical examination and hematocrit determination before the initiation of treatment; at 3, 6, and 12 months; and then annually thereafter for non-transgendered male patients receiving androgen supplementation.[126] Hematocrit monitoring every 6 months for at least the first 18 months has also been recommended.[127]

There is currently no evidence suggesting that FTM transsexual patients who develop polycythemia should be treated differently than non-transsexual men who develop this condition while using androgen supplementation for treatment of hypogonadism. Reduction in testosterone dosage or a moratorium on supplementation is usually required when hemoglobin and hematocrit levels elevate to or above the upper limit of the normal male range (hematocrit 52%). When hematocrit elevates above 54%, phlebotomy should be undertaken to reduce it below

45% to prevent vascular occlusive complications.[134] Actual polycythemia vera may be insufficiently responsive to phlebotomy alone and may require treatment with chemotherapy.

Choice of Testosterone Preparation

Testosterone can be administered by a variety of routes, including transdermally, intramuscularly, orally, and buccally. Hepatic dysfunction and malignancies have previously been observed among men using oral testosterone preparations,[135] although a newer preparation of testosterone undecenoate dissolved in castor oil appears to be acceptably safe[136] and is used in Canada and parts of Europe.

Although intramuscular testosterone preparations have long been the mainstay of FTM hormonal treatment, other routes of administration, particularly the transdermal patches and gels, offer some advantages in the treatment of elderly patients. Elderly persons generally exhibit less muscle mass than their younger peers and may experience more difficulties with injection pain and other sequelae. Transdermal administration also provides less variability in average testosterone levels than most injection programs. Among natal males, transdermal patches, applied nightly, produce a mean total testosterone profile that mimics the male circadian pattern.[137] Some patients cannot tolerate the dermal irritation that the patch can produce; this may be a greater problem among older patients because of age-associated dermal changes. Topical testosterone gel does not produce the circadian pattern associated with patch use[137] but is easy to use and is generally well accepted by FTM patients.[122] Buccal testosterone administration also appears to be safe and effective[138] although its role in the treatment of older patients, who are more likely than their younger peers to experience problems maintaining oral health, remains to be determined.

Although additional clinical research regarding use of hormonal treatments by elderly transsexual men is clearly needed, current information suggests the following recommendations:

- Treatment with androgens during mid life and the later years is associated with significant benefits and medical risks. Patients should be advised of the risks, benefits, and possible adverse effects associated with androgen use and should be assisted in making an informed decision about its use (strength of recommendation: B).
- Transsexual men who begin hormonal treatment in mid life or at later ages should be evaluated for indications of cardiovascular disease, chronic obstructive pulmonary disease, polycythemia, and other chronic conditions that may be worsened by the use of testosterone (strength of recommendation: C).
- Androgens should be used with extreme caution, or not at all, by older transsexual men with uncontrolled concurrent health risks—particularly polycythemia, conditions susceptible to worsening from fluid overload due to sodium and fluid retention (e.g., cardiac or renal disease, uncontrolled hypertension), or a history of breast cancer. Informed consent is extremely important in such cases (strength of recommendation: C).
- Elderly transsexual men wishing to begin treatment with testosterone should be advised of the fact that optimum use of androgen supplementation is not yet well understood, but that doses resulting in modest serum levels (i.e., not above the norms for natal males of similar age) should be used (strength of recommendation: C).
- Hemoglobin levels should be monitored periodically (at least annually when therapy is well established) among both transsexual and non-transsexual men who use supplemental androgens (strength of recommendation: C).
- When possible, transdermal preparations (i.e., gel or patches) should be used (strength of recommendation: C).
- Transsexual men who use androgens should not smoke. This is particularly important later in life. Physicians should assist their older patients in smoking cessation (strength of recommendation: A).

Surgery

Research regarding the surgical experience of elderly transsexual patients is scant. Many outcome studies have included small numbers of elderly participants, but none have specifically evaluated the experience of this population. Anecdotal information suggests that the results of genital surgery for elderly transsexual patients are often not as good as those achieved by younger persons due to the relative lack of tissue distensibility, the age-related genital shrinkage that may have occurred before initiation of hormonal supplementation, and the loss of tissue tone.[139,140] Nonetheless, transsexual elders may experience the same emotional relief of gender dysphoria and sense of completion as their younger peers. For many older persons, the joy of personal fulfillment is tempered by regret that opportunity for gender transition, including gender confirmation surgery, did not arise until so late in the life course.

Decisions regarding candidacy for the surgical procedures associated with gender transition are made on the basis of the health status of the patient, rather than on the basis of chronologic age, per se. Some older patients who are in good health may be reasonable candidates for genital surgery, though a thorough preoperative evaluation should be performed. Medical and surgical history, current cardiovascular health status, and complexity of the planned procedure, including estimated anesthesia time, cardiovascular stress, and physiologic fluid shifting should be weighed by the patient's personal physician and anesthesiologist.[141] Genital surgeries are usually scheduled far in advance of the surgery date, allowing ample opportunity for cardiopulmonary evaluation to be conducted on an outpatient basis during the months before the planned procedure.

Postsurgical recovery times generally lengthen with aging. Older persons undergoing surgery usually need more in-home support during the weeks after surgery than their younger peers. Assessing the degree of family support and other resources available is a crucial aspect of the surgical planning process, particularly in the United States, where hospitalizations are often relatively brief and much postsurgical recovery and care occurs in the home setting. The recovery process may be further complicated if empathic, nonjudgmental personal care assistants are not available during the postoperative period.

Conclusion

Gender is a fundamental aspect of human experience. Like sexual orientation, it can be conceptualized as a continuum and is at least somewhat culturally defined. Caring for gender-variant persons, including transsexual male patients, can be an intellectually stimulating and emotionally rewarding experience for physicians and other clinical professionals.

Meeting the transsexual patient before physical transition has begun and making this clinical journey with him or her can be a life-changing experience for the treating physician. Many clinicians report that working with gender-transitioning persons has profoundly affected their personal beliefs regarding the nature of masculinity and femininity and, indeed, the concept of gender itself.

The medical care of transsexual and transgendered men is currently largely based on extrapolation from data from other clinical populations (e.g., non-transgendered women and men) and on small, population-specific studies and case reports. Until more robust and relevant data are available, physicians must use the available evidence, tempered with clinical judgment and consideration of each patient's individual medical presentation, to assist their transsexual male patients in achieving medically safe gender transition and long-term good health.

References

1. Ramet SP, editor: *Gender Reversals and Gender Cultures: Anthropological and Historical Perspectives,* New York, 1996, Routledge.
2. Connolly PH: The Fa'afafine in contemporary Samoa: new psychobiosocial challenges, *Sex Disabil* 22(1):88–89, 2004.
3. Devor H: *Gender Blending: Confronting the Limits of Duality,* Bloomington IN, 1989, University of Indiana Press.
4. Whittle S: Gender fucking or fucking gender? current cultural contributions to theories of gender blending. In Ekins R, King D, editors: *Blending Genders: Social Aspects of Cross-Dressing and Sex-Changing,* New York, 1996, Routledge.
5. Eyler AE, Wright, K: Gender identification and sexual orientation among genetic females with gender-blended self-perception in childhood and adolescence, *Int J Transgenderism* 1:1 1997. Available at: http://www.symposion.com/ijt/ijtc0101.htm.
6. Bullough V, Bullough B: *Cross Dressing, Sex and Gender,* Philadelphia, 1993, University of Pennsylvania Press.
7. American Psychiatric Association: *Diagnostic and Statistical Manual of Mental Disorders,* ed 4, Washington, DC, 1994, American Psychiatric Association Press.
8. Meyer W 3rd, Bockting WO, Cohen-Kettenis P, et al: The standards of care for the care of gender identity disorders, ed 6, *Int J Transgenderism* 5:1, 2001. Available at: http://www.symposion.com/ijt/soc_2001/index.htm.
9. Janus SS, Janus CL: *The Janus Report on Sexual Behavior,* New York, 1993, John Wiley and Sons, pp 110–111, 120–121.
10. Green R: Family co-occurrence of "gender dysphoria": ten sibling or parent-child pairs, *Arch Sex Behav* 29(5):499–507, 2000.
11. Diamond M: Transsexualism and intersexuality: different views of sexual development [abstract], XVIII Biennial Symposium of the Harry Benjamin International Gender Dysphoria Association, 2003.
12. Witten TM, Eyler AE: Hate crimes against the transgendered: an invisible problem, *Peace Rev* 11 (3):461–468, 1999.

13. Witten TM: Transgender aging: an emerging problem and an emerging need, *Revue Sexologies* 12 (4):15–20, 2003.
14. Kammerer N, Mason T, Connors M: Transgender health and social service needs in the context of HIV risk, IJT 3,1+2, 1999. Available at: http://www.symposion.com/ijt/hiv_risk/kammerer.htm.
15. Eyler AE, Witten TM, Cole SS: Assessing the health-care needs of the transgender community: preliminary survey results [abstract], XV Harry Benjamin International Gender Dysphoria Association Symposium: the state of our art and the state of our science. Vancouver, BC, Canada, September 12, 1997.
16. Nemoto T, Opertario D, Keatley J: Health and social services for male-to-female transgender persons of color in San Francisco, *Int J Transgenderism* 8(2/3):5–19, 2005.
17. US Department of Health and Human Services: *Healthy People 2010: Understanding and Improving Health*, ed 2, Washington, DC, 2000, US Government Printing Office.
18. Blanchard R: A structural equation model for age at clinical presentation in nonhomosexual male gender dysphorics, *Arch Sex Behav* 23(3):311–320, 1994.
19. Bockting WO, Rosser B, Simon R, Coleman E: Transgender HIV prevention: a model education workshop, *JGLMA*, 2000, pp 175–183.
20. US Preventive Services Task Force: *The Guide to Clinical Preventive Services*, AHRQ Pub. No. 05-0570, Washington DC, 2005, Agency for Health Care Research and Quality.
21. Ebell MH, Siwek J, Weiss BD, et al: Strength of recommendation taxonomy (SORT): a patient-centered approach to grading evidence in the medical literature, *Am Fam Phys* 69(3):548–556, 2004.
22. van Kesteren PJ, Asscheman H, Megens JA, Gooren LJ: Mortality and morbidity in transsexual subjects treated with cross-sex hormones, *Clin Endocrinol* 47(3):337–342, 1997.
23. Bosinski HA, Peter M, Bonatz G, et al: A higher rate of hyperandrogenic disorders in female-to-male transsexuals, *Psychoneuroendocrinology* 22(5):361–380, 1997.
24. Dimitrakakis C, Jones RA, Liu A, Bondy CA: Breast cancer incidence in postmenopausal women using testosterone in addition to usual hormone therapy, *Menopause* 11(5):531–535, 2004.
25. Manjer J, Johansson R, Berglund G, et al: Postmenopausal breast cancer risk in relation to sex steroid hormones, prolactin and SHBG (Sweden), *Cancer Causes Control* 14(7):599–607, 2003.
26. Missmer SA, Eliassen AH, Barbieri RL, Hankinson SE: Endogenous estrogen, androgen, and progesterone concentrations and breast cancer risk among postmenopausal women, *J Natl Cancer Inst* 96(24):1856–1865, 2004.
27. Liao DJ, Dickson RB: Roles of androgens in the development, growth, and carcinogenesis of the mammary gland, *J Steroid Biochem Mol Biol* 80(2):175–189, 2002.
28. Boice JD Jr, Friis S, McLaughlin JK, et al: Cancer following breast reduction surgery in Denmark, *Cancer Causes Control* 8(2):253–258, 1997.
29. Boice JD Jr, Persson I, Brinton LA, et al: Breast cancer following breast reduction surgery in Sweden, *Plast Reconstr Surg* 106(4):755–762, 2000.
30. Brinton LA, Persson I, Boice JD Jr, et al: Breast cancer risk in relation to amount of tissue removed during breast reduction operations in Sweden, *Cancer* 91(3):478–483, 2001.
31. Hage JJ, Karim RB: Risk of breast cancer among reduction mammoplasty patients and the strategies used by plastic surgeons to detect such cancer, *Plast Reconstr Surg* 117(3):727–735, 2006.
32. Eyler AE, Whittle ST: FTM breast cancer: community awareness and illustrative cases, XVII Harry Benjamin International Gender Dysphoria Association Symposium. Galveston, TX, November 2, 2001, The San Luis Resort and Conference Center.
33. Burcombe RJ, Makris A, Pittam M, Finer N: Breast cancer after bilateral subcutaneous mastectomy in a female-to-male trans-sexual, *Breast* 12(4):290–293, 2003.
34. Hultborn R, Hanson C, Kopf I, et al: Prevalence of Klinefelter's syndrome in male breast cancer patients, *Anticancer Res* 17(6D):4293–4297, 1997.
35. Miller N, Bedard YC, Cooter NB, et al: Histological changes in the genital tract in transsexual women following androgen therapy, *Histopathology* 10(7):661–669, 1986.
36. Melnikow J, Nuovo J, Willan AR, et al: Natural history of cervical squamous intraepithelial lesions: a meta-analysis, *Obstet Gynecol* 92(4 Pt 2):727–735, 1998.
37. Sherman ME, Lorincz AT, Scott DR, et al: Baseline cytology, human papillomavirus testing, and risk for cervical neoplasia: a 10-year cohort analysis, *J Natl Cancer Inst* 95(1):46–52, 2003.
38. Weigel Stanley CF, Eyler AE: Personal communication from the University of Michigan Comprehensive Gender Services Program, Ann Arbor, MI, March, 2000.
39. Kalogirou D, Antoniou G, Karakitsos P, et al: Vaginal intraepithelial neoplasia (VAIN) following hysterectomy in patients treated for carcinoma in situ of the cervix, *Eur J Gynaecol Oncol* 18(3):188–191, 1997.
40. Mouithys P, Papadopoulos C, Allier G, et al: Is it necessary to make screening pap smears after hysterectomy? *Gynecol Obstet Fertil* 31(7–8):620–623, 2003.
41. Hage JJ, Dekker JJ, Karim RB, et al: Ovarian cancer in female-to-male transsexuals: report of two cases, *Gynecol Oncol* 76(3):413–415, 2000.
42. Pache TD, Chadha S, Gooren LJ, et al: Ovarian morphology in long-term androgen-treated female to male transsexuals: a human model for the study of polycystic ovarian syndrome? *Histopathology* 19(5):445–452, 1991.
43. Schildkraut JM, Schwingl PJ, Bastos E, et al: Epithelial ovarian cancer risk among women with polycystic ovary syndrome, *Obstet Gynecol* 88(4 Pt 1):554–559, 1996.

44. Futterweit W: Endocrine therapy of transsexualism and potential complications of long-term treatment, *Arch Sex Behav* 27(2):209–226, 1998.

45. Balen AH, Schachter ME, Montgomery D, et al: Polycystic ovaries are a common finding in untreated female to male transsexuals, *Clin Endocrinol (Oxf)* 38(3):325–329, 1993.

46. Cibula D, Cifkova R, Fanta M, et al: Increased risk of non–insulin dependent diabetes mellitus, arterial hypertension and coronary artery disease in perimenopausal women with a history of the polycystic ovary syndrome, *Hum Reprod* 15(4):785–789, 2000.

47. Loverro G: Polycystic ovary syndrome and cardiovascular disease, *Minerva Endocrinol* 29(3):129–138, 2004.

48. Pierpoint T, McKeique PM, Isaacs AJ, et al: Mortality of women with polycystic ovary syndrome at long-term follow-up, *J Clin Epidemiol* 51(7):581–586, 1998.

49. Legro RS: Polycystic ovary syndrome and cardiovascular disease: a premature association? *Endocr Rev* 24(3):302–312, 2003.

50. Hajjar RR, Kaiser FE, Morley JE: Outcomes of long-term testosterone replacement in older hypogonadal males: a retrospective analysis, *J Clin Endocrinol Metab* 82(11):3793–3796, 1997.

51. Tan RS, Culberson JW: An integrative review on current evidence of testosterone replacement therapy for the andropause, *Maturitas* 45(1):15–27, 2003.

52. Hak JW, Elisabeth A, et al: Low levels of endogenous androgens increase the risk of atherosclerosis in elderly men: the Rotterdam study, *J Clin Endocrinol Metab* 87(8):3632–3639, 2002.

53. Pärssinen M, Seppälä T: Steroid use and long-term health risks in former athletes, *Sports Med* 32(2):83–94, 2002.

54. National High Blood Pressure Education Program: the Seventh Report of the Joint National Committee on Prevention, Detection, Evaluation, and Treatment of High Blood Pressure (JNC 7). Available at: http://www.nhlbi.nih.gov/guidelines/hypertension.

55. Steinbeck A: Hormonal medication for transsexuals, *Venereology* 10(3):175–177, 1997.

56. Rhoden EL, Morgentaler A: Risks of testosterone-replacement therapy and recommendations for monitoring, *N Engl J Med* 350(5):482–492, 2004.

57. Meyer WJ III, Webb A, Stuart CA, et al: Physical and hormonal evaluation of transsexual patients: a longitudinal study, *Arch Sex Behav* 15(2): 121–138, 1986.

58. Chobanian AV, Bakris GL, Black HR, et al: Seventh report of the Joint National Committee on Prevention, Detection, Evaluation, and Treatment of High Blood Pressure, *Hypertension* 42(6):1206–1252, 2003.

59. Goh HH, Loke DF, Ratnam SS: The impact of long-term testosterone replacement therapy on lipid and lipoprotein profiles in women, *Maturitas* 21(1):65–70, 1995.

60. McCredie RJ, McCrohon JA, Turner L, et al: Vascular reactivity is impaired in genetic females taking high-dose androgens, *J Am Coll Cardiol* 32(5): 1331–1335, 1998.

61. Asscheman H, Gooren LJ, Megens JA, et al: Serum testosterone level is the major determinant of the male-female differences in serum levels of high-density lipoprotein (HDL) cholesterol and HDL2 cholesterol, *Metabolism* 43(8):935–939, 1994.

62. Whitsel EA, Boyko EJ, Matsumoto AM, et al: Intramuscular testosterone esters and plasma lipids in hypogonadal men: a meta-analysis, *Am J Med* 111 (4):261–269, 2001.

63. Singh AB, Hsia S, Alaupovic P, et al: The effects of varying doses of T on insulin sensitivity, plasma lipids, apolipoproteins, and C-reactive protein in healthy young men, *J Clin Endocrinol Metab* 87 (1):136–143, 2002.

64. Executive Summary of The Third Report of The National Cholesterol Education Program (NCEP) Expert Panel on Detection Evaluation, and Treatment of High Blood Cholesterol In Adults (Adult-TreatmentPanel III), *JAMA*, 285(19):2486–2497, 2001.

65. Feldman J, Bockting W: Transgender health, *Minn Med* 86(7):25–32, 2003.

66. Gruskin EP, Hart S, Gordon N, Ackerson L: Women enrolled in a large health maintenance organization, *Am J Public Health* 91(6):976–979, 2001.

67. Tang H, Greenwood GL, Cowling DW, et al: Cigarette smoking among lesbians, gays, and bisexuals: how serious a problem? (United States), *Cancer Causes Control* 15(8):797–803, 2004.

68. Gilman SE, Abrams DB, Buka SL: Socioeconomic status over the life course and stages of cigarette use: initiation, regular use, and cessation, *J Epidemiol Community Health* 57(10):802–808, 2003.

69. Elbers JM, Asscheman H, Seidell JC, Gooren LJ: Effects of sex steroid hormones on regional fat depots as assessed by magnetic resonance imaging in transsexuals, *Am J Physiol* 276(2 Pt 1):E317–E325, 1999.

70. Oh JY, Barrett-Connor E, Wedick NM, et al: Endogenous sex hormones and the development of type 2 diabetes in older men and women: the Rancho Bernardo study, *Diabetes Care* 25(1):55–60, 2002.

71. Campion JM, Maricic MJ: Osteoporosis in men, *Am Fam Phys* 67(7):1521–1526, 2003.

72. Schlatterer K, Yassouridis A, von Werder K, et al: A follow-up study for estimating the effectiveness of a cross-gender hormone substitution therapy on transsexual patients, [review], *Arch Sex Behav* 27(5):475–492, 1998.

73. van Kesteren P, Lips P, Gooren LJ, et al: Long-term follow-up of bone mineral density and bone metabolism in transsexuals treated with cross-sex hormones, *Clin Endocrinol (Oxf)* 48(3):347–354, 1998.

74. Turner A, Chen TC, Barber TW, et al: Testosterone increases bone mineral density in female-to-male transsexuals: a case series of 15 subjects, *Clin Endocrinol (Oxf)* 61(5):560–566, 2004.

75. Goh HH, Ratnam SS: Effects of hormone deficiency, androgen therapy and calcium supplementation on bone mineral density in female transsexuals, *Maturitas* 26(1):45–52, 1997.

76. Lips J, van Kesteren PJ, Asscheman H, Gooren LJ: The effect of androgen treatment on bone metabolism in female-to-male transsexuals, *Bone Miner Res* 11(11):1769–1773, 1996.

77. Tangpricha V, Turner A, Malabanan A: Effects of testosterone therapy on bone mineral density in the FTM patient, *Int J Transgenderism* 5.4 (2001).

78. Ruetsche AG, Kneubuehl R, Birkhaeuser MH: Cortical and trabecular bone mineral density in transsexuals after long-term cross-sex hormonal treatment: a cross-sectional study, *Osteoporosis Int* 16(7):791–798, 2005.

79. Amin S, Zhang Y, Sawin CT, et al: Association of hypogonadism and estradiol levels with bone mineral density in elderly men from the Framingham study, *Ann Intern Med* 133(12):951–963, 2000.

80. Riggs BL, Khosla S, Melton LJ III: A unitary model for involutional osteoporosis: estrogen deficiency causes both type I and type II osteoporosis in postmenopausal women and contributes to bone loss in aging men, *J Bone Miner Res* 13(5):763–773, 1998.

81. Greendale GA, Edelstein S, Barrett-Connor E: Endogenous sex steroids and bone mineral density in older women and men: the Rancho Bernardo Study, *J Bone Miner Res* 12(11):1833–1843, 1997.

82. Scholes D, LaCroix AZ, Ichikawa LE, et al: Change in bone mineral density among adolescent women using and discontinuing depot medroxyprogesterone acetate contraception, *Arch Pediatr Adolesc Med* 159(2):139–144, 2005.

83. De Laet CE, van Hout BA, Burger H, et al: Bone density and risk of hip fracture in men and women: cross sectional analysis, *BMJ* 315(7102): 221–225, 1997.

84. Watts NB: Treatment of osteoporosis with bisphosphonates, *Rheum Dis Clin North Am* 27(1): 197–214, 2001.

85. Centers for Disease Control and Prevention: Sexually transmitted diseases treatment guidelines 2002, *MMWR Recomm Rep* 51(RR-6):1–78, 2002.

86. Asscheman H, Gooren LJ, Eklund PL: Mortality and morbidity in transsexual patients with cross-gender hormone treatment, *Metabolism* 38(9): 869–873, 1989.

87. Boles J, Elifson KW: The social organization of transvestite prostitution and AIDS, *Soc Sci Med* 39(1):85–93, 1994.

88. Clements-Nolle K, Marx R, Guzman R, Katz M: HIV prevalence, risk behaviors, health care use, and mental health status of transgender persons: implications for public health intervention, *Am J Public Health* 91(6):915–921, 2001.

89. Kellogg TA, Clements-Nolle K, Dilley J, et al: Incidence of human immunodeficiency virus among male-to-female transgendered persons in San Francisco, *J Acquir Immune Defic Syndr* 28(4): 380–384, 2001.

90. Xavier J: *The Washington, DC Transgender Needs Assessment Survey: Final Report for Phase Two,* Washington, DC, 2000, Gender Education and Advocacy.

91. Kenagy GP: HIV among transgendered people, *AIDS Care* 14(1):127–134, 2002.

92. Kenagy G, Bostwick W: Health and social service needs of transgender people in Chicago. 1–26, 2001, unpublished.

93. Simon PA, Reback CJ, Bemis CC: HIV prevalence and incidence among male-to-female transsexuals receiving HIV prevention services in Los Angeles County, *AIDS* 14(18):2953–2955, 2000.

94. McGowan CK: *Transgender Needs Assessment,* New York, 1999, New York City Department of Health.

95. Risser J, Shelton A: *Behavioral Assessment of the Transgender Population, Houston, Texas,* Galveston, TX, 2002, University of Texas School of Public Health.

96. Kenagy GP, Hsieh CM: The risk less known: female-to-male transgender persons' vulnerability to HIV infection, *AIDS Care* 17(2):195–207, 2005.

97. Namaste V: HIV/AIDS and female-to-male transsexuals and transvestites: results from a needs assessment in Quebec. In Bockting W, Kirk S, editors: *Transgender and HIV: Risks, Prevention and Care,* New York, 2001, Haworth Press, pp 91–99.

98. Hein D, Kirk M: Education and soul-searching: the Enterprise HIV Prevention Group. *Int J Transgenderism* 1999. Available at: http://www.symposion.com/ijt/hiv_risk/hein.htm.

99. Avery EN, Cole CM, Meyer WJ: Transsexuals and HIV/AIDS risk behaviors (poster presentation). XIV International Symposium of the Harry Benjamin International Gender Dysphoria Association, University of Ulm, Kloster Irsee, Germany, September 9, 1995.

100. Gross J, Davis M: *Female to Male Transgenders and HIV Risk Behaviors in Los Angeles,* Los Angeles, 2004, International AIDS Society.

101. Nemoto T, Operario D, Keatley J, Villegas D: Social context of HIV risk behaviours among male-to-female transgenders of colour, *AIDS Care* 16(6):724–735, 2004.

102. Nemoto T, Luke D, Mamo L, et al: HIV risk behaviours among male-to-female transgenders in comparison with homosexual or bisexual males and heterosexual females, *AIDS Care* 11(3):297–312, 1999.

103. Bockting WO, Robinson BE, Rosser BRS: Transgender HIV prevention: a qualitative needs assessment, *AIDS Care* 10(4):505–526, 1998.

104. Nemoto T, Keatley J, Operario D, et al: Implementing HIV prevention, drug abuse treatment, and mental health services in the transgender community in San Francisco (poster presentation). XVI International AIDS Conference, Barcelona, Spain, July, 2002.

105. Sausa LA: The HIV prevention and educational needs of trans youth: A qualitative study (UMI No. 3087465), *Dis Abstr Internat* 64(4):1186, 2003.

106. Sanders GD, Bayoumi AM, Sundaram V, et al: Cost-effectiveness of screening for HIV in the era of highly active antiretroviral therapy, *N Engl J Med* 352(6):570–585, 2005.

107. Bockting W, Kirk S, editors: *Transgender and HIV: Risks, Prevention, and Care,* Binghampton, NY, 2001, Haworth Press.

108. Bockting W, Avery E, editors: *Transgender Health and HIV Prevention Needs Assessment Studies from Transgender Communities across the United States,* Binghamton, NY, 2005, Haworth Press.

109. Coleman E, Bockting WO, Gooren L: Homosexual and bisexual identity in sex-reassigned female-to-male transsexuals, *Arch Sex Behav* 22(1):37–50, 1993.

110. Devor H: Sexual orientation identities, attractions and practices of female to male transsexuals, *J Sex Res* 30(4):303–315, 1993.

111. Lawrence AA: Sexuality before and after male-to-female sex reassignment surgery, *Arch Sex Behav* 34(2):147–166, 2005.

112. Bockting WO, Robinson BE, Forberg J, Scheltema K: Evaluation of a sexual health approach to reducing HIV/STD risk in the transgender community, *AIDS Care* 17(3):289–303, 2005.

113. Clements-Nolle K, Marx R, Guzman R, Katz M: HIV prevalence, risk behaviors, health care use, and mental status of transgender persons: Implications for public health intervention, *Am J Public Health* 91(6):915–921, 2001.

114. Keatley J, Nemoto T, Operario D, Soma T: The impact of transphobia on HIV risk behaviors among male to female transgenders in San Francisco, Poster presented at XVI International AIDS Conference, Barcelona, Spain, 2002.

115. Mathy R: Transgender identity and suicidality in a nonclinical sample: sexual orientation, psychiatric history, and compulsive behaviors, *J Psychol Human Sexuality* 13(1):31–54, 2002.

116. Lawrence AA: Factors associated with satisfaction or regret following male-to-female sex reassignment surgery, *Arch Sex Behav* 32(4):299–315, 2003.

117. Darby E, Anawalt BD: Male hypogonadism: an update on diagnosis and treatment, *Treat Endocrinol* 4(5):293–309, 2005.

118. DiClemente CC: Motivational interviewing and the stages of change. In: Miller WR, Rollnick S: *Motivational Interviewing: Preparing People for Change*, ed 2, New York, 2002, The Guilford Press.

119. Bandura A: *Self-efficacy: The Exercise of Control*, New York, 1997, Worth Publishers.

120. US Public Health Service: Treating tobacco use and dependence. 2000. Available at: http://www.surgeongeneral.gov/tobacco.

121. Mazur N, Belld N, Wu J, et al: Comparison of the steady-state pharmacokinetics, metabolism, and variability of a transdermal testosterone patch versus a transdermal testosterone gel in hypogonadal men, *J Sex Med* 2(2):213–226, 2005.

122. Feldman J: Masculinizing hormone therapy with testosterone 1% topical gel. XIX Biennial Syposium, Harry Benjamin International Gender Dysphoria Association, Universita Degli Studi di Bologna, Bologna, Italy, April 8, 2005.

123. Speroff L, Fritz MA: *Clinical Gynecologic Endocrinology and Infertility*, ed 7, Philadelphia, 2005, Lippincott, Williams & Wilkins, p 867.

124. Snyder PJ: Hypogonadism in elderly men—what to do until the evidence comes, *N Engl J Med* 350(5):440–442, 2004.

125. Conway AJ, Handelsman DJ, Lording DW, et al: Use, misuse and abuse of androgens: the Endocrine Society of Australia consensus guidelines for androgen prescribing, *Med J Aust* 172:220–224, 2000.

126. American Society of Andrology: Testosterone replacement therapy for male aging: ASA position statement, *J Androl* 27(2):133–134, 2006.

127. Wald M, Meacham RB, Ross LS, et al: Testosterone replacement therapy for older men, *J Androl* 27(2):126–132, 2006.

128. Gooren LJ, Toorians AW: Significance of oestrogens in male (patho)physiology, *Ann Endocrinol (Paris)* 64(2):126–135, 2003.

129. Tan RS, Salazar JA: Risks of testosterone replacement therapy in ageing men, *Expert Opin Drug Saf* 3(6):599–606, 2004.

130. Tenover JL: Testosterone replacement therapy in older adult men, *Int J Androl* 22(5):300–306, 1999.

131. American Association of Clinical Endocrinologists Hypogonadism Task Force: American Association of Clinical Endocrinologists medical guidelines for clinical practice for the evaluation and treatment of hypogonadism in adult male patients—2002 update, *Endocr Pract* 8:439–456, 2002.

132. Fainaru-Wada M, Williams L: : The truth about Barry Bonds and steroids, *Sports Illustrated* March 13, 2006; excerpted from their book, Fainaru-Wada M, Williams L, editors: *Game of Shadows*, New York, 2006, Gotham Books.

133. Hachulla E, Rose C, Trillot N, et al: What vascular events suggest a myeloproliferative disorder? *J Mal Vasc* 25(5):382–387, 2000.

134. Pearson TC, Messinezy M: Idiopathic erythrocytosis, diagnosis and clinical management, *Pathol Biol (Paris)* 49(2):170–177, 2001.

135. Nieschalg E, E, Behre HM, HM, editors: *Testosterone: Action, Deficiency, Substitution*, ed 2, New York, 1998, Springer.

136. Gooren LJ, Bunck MC: Androgen replacement therapy: present and future, *Drugs* 64:1861–1891, 2004.

137. Mazer N, Bell D, Wu J, et al: Comparison of the steady-state pharmacokinetics, metabolism, and variability of a transdermal testosterone patch versus a transdermal testosterone gel in hypogonadal men, *J Sex Med* 2(2):213–226, 2005.

138. Dobs AS, Matsumoto AM, Wang C, et al: Short-term pharmacokinetic comparison of a novel testosterone buccal system and a testosterone gel in testosterone deficient men, *Curr Med Res Opin* 20(5):729–738, 2004.

139. Kuzon W: Personal communication from the Director of Surgical Services, Ann Arbor, 2000, University of Michigan Comprehensive Gender Services Program.

140. Wilson N: Personal communication, from the Chief of the Division of Plastic Surgery, Hutzel Hospital, Detroit, Michigan, 2006.

141. King MS: Preoperative evaluation, *Am Fam Phys* 62:387–396, 2000.

Portions of this chapter previously appeared in Principles of Transgender Medicine and Surgery, Chapter 2 ("Primary Medical Care of the Gender–Variant Patients"), Chapter 3 ("Preventive Care of the Transgendered Patient: An Evidence–based Approach") and Chapter 14 ("Transgender Aging and the Care of the Elderly Transgendered Patient") (Binghamton, NY: The Haworth Press, Inc., 2007). Chapter copies available from The Haworth Document Delivery Service: 1–800–HAWORTH. E-mail address: docdelivery@haworth-press.com.

Index

Note: Page references followed by "*f*" indicate figures and by "*t*" indicate tables.